## Free personal online access for 12 months

The copy of the *Oxford Textbook of Transplant Anaesthesia and Critical Care* you have purchased entitles you to free personal online access to the supporting website for 12 months.

Customers outside North and South America, please visit: **https://subscriberservices.sams.oup.com/token** to set up access.

Customers in North and South America, please visit: **https://ams.oup.com/order/OTANATPSCRIP** to set up access.

To register, enter the code at the top of this card.
Please keep this card for future reference as, in the event of a query, you may be asked to return it. Please note that as part of the registration process you will be informed of our terms and conditions, and will be asked to accept these to confirm your online access.

| unique code: | JY15554625684492 |
| --- | --- |

The online access provided free with this book is for individuals who have purchased a personal copy only, and this will be verified as part of the access process. Users of library copies should ask their librarian about access in their institution.

### Customer support

Customers outside North & South America
**Tel:** +44 (0) 1865 353705
**Email:** accesstokens@oup.com

Customers in North & South America
**Tel:** 1-800-334-4249 ext. 6484
**Email:** oxfordonline@oup.com

of
ant
esia and
Care

# Oxford Textbooks in Anaesthesia

**Oxford Textbook of Anaesthesia for the Elderly Patient**
Edited by Chris Dodds, Chandra M. Kumar, and Bernadette Th. Veering

**Oxford Textbook of Anaesthesia for Oral and Maxillofacial Surgery**
Edited by Ian Shaw, Chandra M. Kumar, and Chris Dodds

**Principles and Practice of Regional Anaesthesia, Fourth Edition**
Edited by Graeme McLeod, Colin McCartney, and Tony Wildsmith

**Oxford Textbook of Cardiothoracic Anaesthesia**
Edited by R. Peter Alston, Paul S. Myles, and Marco Ranucci

**Oxford Textbook of Transplant Anaesthesia and Critical Care**
Edited by Ernesto A. Pretto, Jr., Gianni Biancofiore, Andre De Wolf, John R. Klinck, Claus Niemann, Andrew Watts, and Peter D. Slinger

# Free personal online access for 12 months

Individual purchasers of this book are also entitled to free personal access to the online edition for 12 months on *Oxford Medicine Online* (<www.oxfordmedicine.com>). Please refer to the access token card for instructions on token redemption and access.

Online ancillary materials, where available, are noted at the end of the respective chapters in this book. Additionally, *Oxford Medicine Online* allows you to print, save, cite, email, and share content; download high-resolution figures as Microsoft PowerPoint slides; save often-used books, chapters, or searches; annotate; and quickly jump to other chapters or related material on a mobile-optimized platform.

We encourage you to take advantage of these features. If you are interested in ongoing access after the 12-month gift period, please consider an individual subscription or consult with your librarian.

# Oxford Textbook of

# Transplant Anaesthesia and Critical Care

Editor-in-Chief

**Ernesto A. Pretto, Jr.**

Editors

**Gianni Biancofiore**

**Andre De Wolf**

**John R. Klinck**

**Claus Niemann**

**Andrew Watts**

Contributing Editor

**Peter D. Slinger**

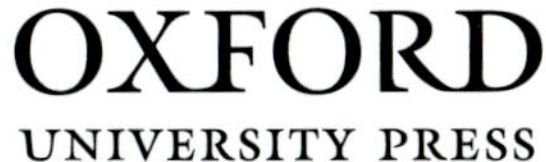

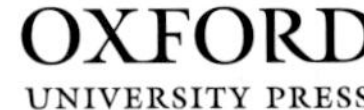

Great Clarendon Street, Oxford, OX2 6DP,
United Kingdom

Oxford University Press is a department of the University of Oxford. It furthers the University's objective of excellence in research, scholarship, and education by publishing worldwide. Oxford is a registered trade mark of Oxford University Press in the UK and in certain other countries



First Edition Published in 2015

Impression: 1



Published in the United States of America by Oxford University Press
198 Madison Avenue, New York, NY 10016, United States of America

British Library Cataloguing in Publication Data
Data available

Library of Congress Control Number: 2014948994

ISBN 978–0–19–965142–9

Printed in China by
Asia Pacific Offset Ltd.

# Foreword

Organ transplantation began with kidney transplantation in the early 1950s and expanded to heart, lung, liver, pancreas, multiviscera, and xenograft transplantation. Its evolution over the past 50 years or so has been dramatic. The experimental stage of organ transplantation (1960–1980) evolved into the developmental stage (1980–1990) and refinement stage (1991–present) with excellent clinical outcomes. This evolution has been made possible by better understanding of the scientific basis of transplantation, which includes immunology and pathophysiology and continuously improving surgical technique and perioperative care. It is noteworthy that the role of anaesthesiologists and intensivists has been vital in its progression, because organ transplantation is a medical field that requires a multidisciplinary approach by dedicated physicians and scientists of all medical fields.

I am extremely pleased to witness the publication of the *Oxford Textbook of Transplant Anaesthesia and Critical Care* edited by Drs Biancofiore, De Wolf, Klinck, Niemann, Pretto, Slinger, and Watts, who are my respected colleagues and experts in the transplantation field. The major strength of this textbook can be found in its comprehensiveness and the inclusion of scientific bases. It begins with the history of organ transplantation and includes ethics, organ donation, and perioperative management of all transplanted organs. The molecular basis of organ transplantation should encourage further exploration in organ preservation, prevention of ischaemic injury, and modulation of rejection phenomena. The book presents many ideas and concepts to guide the future direction of transplant anaesthesiology, critical care and research, a vital issue for further development of organ transplantation.

Organ transplantation, particularly the field of anaesthesiology and critical care medicine, was once believed to be a 'black hole'—an amorphous unknown object with a huge mass absorbing all resources without a trace. We now have a much better understanding of that black hole, and I believe that we are better equipped to explore the unknown universe with the guidance of this textbook. As a long-time anaesthesiologist in the transplantation field, I sincerely appreciate all editors and contributors for their life-time dedication to organ transplantation.

Yoogoo Kang, MD
Professor, Anesthesiology
Director, Hepatic Transplantation Anesthesiology
Thomas Jefferson University

# Preface

So the LORD GOD caused a deep sleep to fall upon the man, and he slept; then He took one of his ribs and closed up the flesh at that place

—*Genesis 2:21*

Organ transplantation is a relatively new medical science that has made it possible for patients with an irreversibly damaged organ, and little hope of long-term survival, to receive a replacement organ from another human-being, living or deceased. This ancient idea, once also the purview of science-fiction novels, has become reality, and it is revolutionizing medical care by bringing renewed hope for healing to thousands of patients worldwide, every day. The only limitation to a much wider application of this life-saving technology is the scarcity of suitable organs.

The successful and steady evolution of the field of clinical organ transplantation over the past 100 years or so is directly attributable to the multidisciplinary nature and scientific basis of transplant care. In fact, only since 1995 during which time medical technology has made great strides forward have we seen marked improvements in long-term survival, including among recipients of the most complex transplant procedures. In particular, advances in perioperative and critical care management of the transplant recipient have accounted to a great extent for these recent improvements in outcomes.

One of those seminal achievements was the initiation by a group of anaesthesiologists and intensive care physicians at the University of Pittsburgh of a multidisciplinary approach to liver transplantation. The first gathering of this group in 1982 was called 'Anesthesia and Perioperative Care in Liver Transplantation', which later became the International Liver Transplantation Society (ILTS). In a letter dated 5 August 1993 by Dr Thomas Starzl, a renowned American liver transplant pioneer, to Dr Peter Safar, a critical care medicine pioneer and founding Chairman of the Department of Anesthesiology and Critical Care Medicine at the University of Pittsburgh, who was then director of what is now known as the Safar Center for Resuscitation Research, Starzl wrote:

> *. . . I have always taken pains to point out how what we do would be utterly impossible without the marvelous collaboration of our unselfish colleagues who work in the operating room and slave over these terribly sick patients afterwards. In a much more professionally meaningful but less public way, we have promoted the interests of the anesthesia and ICU physicians by passing the leadership baton onto Kang et al., for the organization of the International Liver Transplantation Society that will be meeting for the second time this year in Canada. Dr. Kang's efforts and those of his intensive care colleagues were responsible for the birth of this very important organization. . . .*

In the same vein, the American Society of Anesthesiologists (ASA) described the nature of anaesthesia practice for organ transplantation, and those anaesthesiologists and intensivists engaged in its delivery, in the following manner:

> *The complexity of transplant surgeries requires the expertise and specialty of a transplant anesthesiologist who is an integral part of the transplant team. Transplant anesthesiologists have an extensive background in critical care medicine, cardiac anesthesiology and/or pediatric anesthesiology. This type of anesthesiologist also provides consultation in both the preoperative and intraoperative stages of care.*

This statement was a first step in the direction of defining the knowledge base, required training and experience, and scope of practice of the 'transplant anaesthesiologist'.

Likewise, a recent 'landmark' decision by the Organ Procurement and Transplantation Network (OPTN)/United Network for Organ Sharing (UNOS) (the principal government-mandated agency overseeing organ procurement and sharing in the US), in partnership with the ASA Committee on Transplantation, has promulgated guidelines for the qualifications and clinical responsibilities of the director of liver transplant anaesthesia programmes, as follows:

*The director of liver transplant anesthesia should have one of the following:*

1. *Fellowship training in Critical Care Medicine, Cardiac Anesthesiology, or a Liver Transplant Fellowship, that includes the peri-operative care of at least 10 liver transplant recipients.*
2. *Experience in the peri-operative care of at least 20 liver transplant recipients in the operating room, within the last 5 years. Experience acquired during postgraduate residency training does not count for this purpose.*

*The director of liver transplant anesthesia has clinical responsibilities that include but are not limited to the following:*

- *Pre-operative assessment of transplant candidates*
- *Participation in candidate selection*
- *Intra-operative management*
- *Post-operative visits*
- *Participation on the Selection Committee*
- *Consultation pre-operatively with subspecialists as needed*
- *Participation in morbidity and mortality (M&M) conferences (UNOS Bylaws)*

These guidelines provide official recognition that expertly trained anaesthesiologists are critical to optimizing transplant care. The UNOS bylaws endorse transplant anaesthesiologists' active participation in medical decision-making in all facets of transplant care.

We believe these guidelines should not be limited to the care of liver transplant recipients alone but that the benefits of multidisciplinary care and specialized training in transplant anaesthesia will inevitably lead to improved care for all types of organ transplant recipients, as well as organ donors. Other than pain management and critical care medicine, perhaps there is no other subspecialty of anaesthesiology where our involvement has been as important to improved outcomes and as valued by our professional counterparts.

Therefore the impetus for a book on '*Transplant Anaesthesia and Critical Care*' derives from the same spirit of collaboration and collegiality that seeks to affirm the current trend towards greater specialization in transplant anaesthesia and critical care. Specifically, this book attempts to define the normative body of scientific and clinical knowledge, skill, and training that is essential to the expertise of the anaesthesiologist involved in the care of the organ donor as well as the organ transplant recipient.

On behalf of the editors, the expectation is that the appearance of this book is timely, relevant, and true to the present state-of-the-art and that it will bolster the continued development of the burgeoning field of transplant anaesthesia and critical care. As you will see on initial perusal of the table of contents we have taken a holistic approach to the scope of practice of transplant anaesthesia. In so doing we cover in depth many aspects of transplantation of the major organ systems. Moreover, we have assembled a cadre of multidisciplinary transplant experts from several continents that present updated evidence-based information on various topics related to transplantation, including data on organ transplant practices in leading countries, as well as some of the ethical challenges facing the field of organ transplantation today.

We hope this book will be well received by the medical and scientific communities and that it will serve as the authoritative reference work in the field, thereby forming the basis for the design of curricula for teaching and training of medical students, anaesthesia residents, transplant anaesthesia fellows, nurse anaesthetists, and attending anaesthesiologists in transplant care.

Finally, we believe that the future of transplant anaesthesia relies heavily on discovery. As such we hope this book will provide the reader with key insights into cellular mechanisms of ischaemia–reperfusion injury that will inspire transplant anaesthesiologists to engage in basic and clinical research, and in so doing contribute to the collective advancement of the science of transplantation.

Ernesto A. Pretto, Jr., MD, MPH
Miami Transplant Institute

# Contents

# Abbreviations

| | |
|---|---|
| 2,3DPG | 2,3-diphosphoglycerate |
| 31P-NMR | phosphorus-31 nuclear magnetic resonance |
| 6-MWT | 6-minute walk test |
| 7DS | seventh day syndrome |
| 99TcMAA | technetium-99-radiolabelled macro-aggregated albumin |
| A/C | assist-control |
| A2ALL | Adult to Adult Living Donor Liver Transplantation Cohort Study |
| A–a | alveolar–arterial |
| AAA | aromatic amino acid |
| AAMR | acute antibody-mediated rejection |
| AASLD | American Association for the Study of Liver Diseases |
| AAT | α1-antitrypsin |
| ABG | arterial blood gas |
| ABOi | ABO-incompatible |
| ACC | American College of Cardiology |
| ACDA | acid citrate dextrose solution A |
| ACE | angiotensin-converting enzyme |
| ACLF | acute-on-chronic liver failure |
| ACO | approved combined organs |
| ACS | American College of Surgeons |
| ACTH | adrenocorticotropic hormone |
| ADA | American Diabetes Association |
| ADH | antidiuretic hormone |
| ADP | adenosine diphosphate |
| AE | adverse event |
| AF | atrial fibrillation |
| AFP | alpha-fetoprotein |
| AHA | American Heart Association |
| aHUS | atypical haemolytic–uraemic syndrome |
| AICD | automatic implantable cardioverter-defibrillator |
| AIDS | acquired immunodeficiency syndrome |
| AKBR | arterial ketone body ratio |
| AKI | acute kidney injury |
| ALF | acute liver failure |
| ALG | antilymphocyte globulin |
| ALI | acute lung injury |
| ALS | amyotrophic lateral sclerosis |
| ALT | alanine transaminase |
| AMP | adenosine monophosphate |
| AMR | antibody-mediated rejection |
| ANT | adenosine nucleotide translocator |
| AOPO | Association of Organ Procurement Organizations |
| APC | antigen-presenting cells |
| APRV | airway pressure release ventilation |
| aPTT | activated partial thromboplastin time |
| AR | acute rejection |
| ARB | angiotensin-receptor |
| ARDS | acute respiratory distress syndrome |
| ARDSNET | Acute Respiratory Distress Syndrome Network |
| ARF | acute respiratory failure |
| ASN | American Society of Nephrology |
| ASPEN | American Society of Parenteral and Enteral Nutrition |
| AST | American Society of Transplantation |
| AST | aspartate aminotransferase |
| ASTS | American Society of Transplant Surgeons |
| ATG | antithymocyte globulin |
| ATN | acute tubular necrosis |
| ATP | adenosine triphosphate |
| AUC | area under the curve |
| AV | arteriovenous |
| BAL | bronchoalveolar lavage |
| BCAA | branched-chain amino acid |
| BH | Berlin Heart EXCOR® |
| BiPAP | bilevel positive airway pressure |
| BIS | bispectral index |
| BiVAD | biventricular assist device |
| BM | bone marrow |
| BMI | body mass index |
| BNP | brain natriuretic peptide |
| BOB | bronchiolitis obliterans |
| BODE | body mass, airflow obstruction, dyspnoea, and exercise capacity |
| BSA | body surface area |
| BSLTx | bilateral sequential lung transplantation/transplant |
| BUN | blood urea nitrogen |
| CABG | coronary artery bypass grafting |
| CAD | coronary artery disease |
| CAHPS | Consumer Assessment of Healthcare Providers and Systems |
| CARS | compensatory anti-inflammatory response syndrome |

| | |
|---|---|
| CAV | cardiac allograft vasculopathy |
| CAVH | continuous arteriovenous haemofiltration |
| CAVHD | continuous arteriovenous haemodialysis |
| CAVHDF | continuous arteriovenous haemodiafiltration |
| CBC | complete blood count |
| CBIG | catastrophic brain injury guideline |
| CCO | continuous cardiac output |
| CDC | Centers for Disease Control and Prevention |
| CESAR | conventional ventilatory support versus extracorporeal membrane oxygenation for severe adult respiratory failure trial |
| CF | cystic fibrosis |
| CFTR | cystic fibrosis transmembrane conductance regulator gene |
| cGMP | cyclic guanosine monophosphate |
| CHD | congenital heart disease |
| CHF | congestive heart failure |
| CI | cardiac index |
| CIT | cold ischaemia time |
| CKD | chronic kidney disease |
| CM-AR | cell-mediated acute rejection |
| CMP | cardiomyopathy |
| $CMRO_2$ | cerebral metabolic rate for oxygen |
| CMS | Centers for Medicare and Medicaid Services |
| CMV | cytomegalovirus |
| CNI | calcineurin inhibitor |
| CNS | central nervous system |
| CNT | National Council of Transplantation |
| CO | cardiac output |
| COOLDonor | Cooling to Optimize Organ Live in Donor Study |
| COPD | chronic obstructive pulmonary disease |
| CPAP | continuous positive airway pressure |
| CPB | cardiopulmonary bypass |
| CPM | central pontine myelinolysis |
| CPP | cerebral perfusion pressure |
| CPX | cardiopulmonary exercise |
| CR | chronic rejection |
| Cr | creatinine |
| CRBSI | catheter-related bloodstream infection |
| CRRT | continuous renal replacement therapy |
| CSF | cerebrospinal fluid |
| CT | computed tomography |
| CTA | computed tomography angiography/angiogram |
| CTLA4-Ig | cytotoxic T-lymphocyte antigen-4 immunoglobulin |
| CTP | Child–Turcotte–Pugh |
| CUSUM | cumulative summation |
| CV | cardiovascular |
| CVA | cerebrovascular accident |
| CVC | central venous catheter |
| CVD | cardiovascular disease |
| CVP | central venous pressure |
| CVVH | continuous venovenous haemofiltration |
| CVVHDF | continuous venovenous haemodialysis and filtration |
| CYP3A | cytochrome P-450 IIIA |
| DAD | diffuse alveolar damage |
| DBD | deceased brain donors |
| DCCT | Diabetes Control and Complications Trial |
| DCD | donation after circulatory death |
| DCDD | donation after circulatory determination of death |
| DCM | dilated cardiomyopathy |
| DDAVP | 1-desamino-8-D-arginine vasopressin |
| DGF | delayed graft function |
| DI | diabetes insipidus |
| DIC | disseminated intravascular coagulation |
| DIOS | distal intestinal obstruction syndrome |
| DLA | donor-specific antibodies |
| DLCO | diffusing capacity of the lungs for carbon monoxide |
| DLTx | double-lung transplantation/transplant |
| DMADV | define, measure, analyse, design, verify |
| DMAIC | define, measure, analyse, improve, control |
| DMG | donor management goal |
| DNDD | donation/donors after neurological determination of death |
| DNR | do not resuscitate |
| DOB | delta over baseline |
| DPA | dorsal pancreatic artery |
| DR | donor–recipient |
| DRESS | drug-related eosinophilic syndrome |
| DRI | donor risk index |
| DSA | donor-specific antibodies |
| DSE | dobutamine stress echocardiography |
| DXR | delayed xenograft rejection |
| EASD | European Association for the Study of Diabetes |
| EASL | European Association for the Study of the Liver |
| EBMT | European Group for Blood and Marrow Transplantation |
| EBS | European Board of Surgery |
| EBV | Epstein–Barr virus |
| EC | endothelial cell |
| ECD | expanded criteria donor |
| ECG | electrocardiography |
| ECHO | echocardiography |
| ECHOT4 | Evaluation of the Efficacy and Safety of Levothyroxine in Brain Death Organ Donors: a Randomized Controlled Trial |
| ECMO | extracorporeal membrane oxygenation |
| EC-MPA | enteric-coated mycophenolic acid |
| EEG | electroencephalography |
| EF | ejection fraction |
| EGDT | early goal-directed therapy |
| EHR | electronic health record |
| EJ | external jugular |
| ELITA | European Liver and Intestinal Transplant Association |
| ELTR | European Liver Transplant Registry |
| EMB | endomyocardial biopsy |
| EPTS | estimated post-transplant survival |
| ERCP | endoscopic retrograde cholangiopancreatography |
| ESA | European Society of Anaesthesiologists |
| ESDP | Eurotransplant Senior DR-compatible Program |
| ESLD | end-stage liver disease |
| ESOT | European Society of Organ Transplantation |
| ESP | Eurotransplant Senior Program |
| ESPEN | European Society for Clinical Nutrition and Metabolism |

| | |
|---|---|
| ESRD | end-stage renal disease |
| EU | European Union |
| EVLP | ex-vivo lung perfusion |
| EVLWi | extravascular lung water index |
| FDA | Federal Drug Administration |
| FEV | forced expiratory volume |
| FFP | fresh frozen plasma |
| FGF-1 | fibroblast growth factor-1 |
| FIH | factor-inhibiting hypoxia-inducible factor |
| FiO2 | fraction of inspired oxygen |
| FKBP | FK506 binding protein |
| FMS | Fluid Management System |
| FPG | fasting plasma glucose |
| FRC | functional residual capacity |
| FRETEP | Renal Graft Function After Treatment with Erythropoetin |
| FSGS | focal segmental glomerulosclerosis |
| FSH | follicle-stimulating hormone |
| FTc | corrected flow time |
| FVC | forced vital capacity |
| GABA | gamma-aminobutyric acid |
| GAD | glutamic acid decarboxylase |
| Gal | galactose |
| GalT | galactosyltransferase |
| G-CSF | granulocyte-colony stimulating factor |
| GEDV | global end-diastolic volume |
| GFR | glomerular filtration rate |
| GI | gastrointestinal |
| GJ | gastrojejunostomy |
| GORD | gastro-oesophageal reflux disease |
| GVH | graft versus host |
| GVHD | graft versus host disease |
| H1N1 | influenza A virus type H1N1 |
| H-2 | histocompatibility 2 |
| HAART | highly active antiviral therapy |
| HAR | hyperacute rejection |
| HAT | hepatic artery thrombosis |
| HAV | hepatitis A virus |
| Hb | haemoglobin |
| HBsAg | hepatitis B surface antigen |
| HBV | hepatitis B virus |
| HCAHPS | Hospital Consumer Assessment of Healthcare Providers and Systems |
| HCC | hepatocellular carcinoma |
| HCM | hypertrophic cardiomyopathy |
| HCV | hepatitis C virus |
| HD | haemodialysis |
| hDAF | human decay accelerating factor |
| HDL | high-density lipoprotein |
| HE | hepatic encephalopathy |
| HELPP | haemolysis, elevated liver enzymes, and low platelets |
| HES | hydroxyethyl starch |
| HHS | Health and Human Services |
| HIF | hypoxia-inducible factor |
| HIV | human immunodeficiency virus |
| HLA | human leucocyte antigen |
| HLHS | hypoplastic left heart syndrome |
| hMCP | human membrane cofactor protein |
| HOPE | HIV Organ Policy Equity |
| HPS | hepatopulmonary syndrome |
| HRCT | high-resolution computed tomography |
| HRQOL | Health-Related Quality of Life |
| HRS | hepatorenal syndrome |
| HRSA | Health Resources and Services Administration |
| HTK | histidine–tryptophan–ketoglutarate |
| HTN | hypertension |
| HTx | heart transplantation/transplant |
| HU | high urgency |
| HVG | host versus graft |
| HX | hypoxanthine |
| I/R | ischaemia–reperfusion |
| IA-1 | zinc finger protein IA-1 |
| IABP | intra-aortic balloon pump |
| IAK | islet after kidney |
| IAP | intra-abdominal pressure |
| ICAM-1 | intercellular adhesion molecule 1 |
| ICG | indocyanine green |
| ICP | intracranial pressure |
| ICS | intraoperative red blood cell salvage |
| ICT | intracardiac thrombosis |
| ICU | Intensive Care Unit |
| IDF | International Diabetes Federation |
| IEq | islet equivalents |
| IFG | impaired fasting glycaemia |
| IFN-$\gamma^3$ | interferon-gamma |
| Ig | immunoglobulin |
| IGT | impaired glucose tolerance |
| IHD | ischaemic heart disease |
| IJ | internal jugular |
| IL | interleukin |
| IL-2R | interleukin-2 receptor |
| ILTS | International Liver Transplantation Society |
| IM | intramuscular |
| IMA | inferior mesenteric artery |
| IMPDH | inosine monophosphate dehydrogenase |
| IMPDH1 | inosine 5-monophosphate dehydrogenase 1 |
| IMV | inferior mesenteric vein |
| INCORT | National Institute of Transplant Coordination |
| INH | isoniazid |
| iNO | inhaled nitric oxide |
| INOP | Iranian Network for Organ Procurement |
| INR | International Normalized Ratio |
| IoC | index of covariance |
| IPC | ischaemic preconditioning |
| IPF | initial poor function |
| IPF | idiopathic pulmonary fibrosis |
| IS | immunosuppressive regimens |
| ISCT | International Society for Cellular Therapy |
| ISHLT | International Society for Heart and Lung Transplantation |
| ISO | International Organization for Standardization |
| ITA | islet transplant alone |
| ITBV | intrathoracic blood volume |
| ITBVi | intrathoracic blood volume index |
| ITCO | intermittent thermodilution cardiac output |
| ITx | intestinal transplantation/transplant |
| IV | intravenous |

| | |
|---|---|
| IVC | inferior vena cava |
| IVIG | intravenous immunoglobulin |
| IVS | interventricular septum |
| JCV | John Cunningham virus |
| JDRFI | Juvenile Diabetes Research Foundation International |
| J–E | jaundice–encephalopathy |
| JKTNW | Japan Kidney Transplant Network |
| JNK | c-Jun N-terminal kinase |
| JOTNW | Japan Organ Transplant Network |
| KCC | King's College Criteria |
| KO | knockout |
| KTx | kidney transplantation |
| LA | left atrial |
| LAS | lung allocation score |
| LD | live donor |
| LDF | leucocyte depletion filter |
| LDL | low-density lipoprotein |
| LDLT | living donor liver transplantation |
| LFA-1 | leucocyte function antigen |
| LFT | liver function test |
| LH | luteinizing hormone |
| LICAGE | Liver Intensive Care Group of Europe |
| LiMax | maximal enzymatic liver function capacity |
| LPD | low potassium dextran |
| LRD | living related donor |
| LTx | lung transplantation/transplant |
| LV | left ventricle |
| LVAD | left ventricular assist device |
| LVEDA | left ventricular end-diastolic area |
| LVEF | left ventricular ejection fraction |
| MA | maximum amplitude |
| MAC | minimum alveolar concentration |
| MACE | major adverse cardiac events |
| MAGE | mean amplitude of glycaemic excursions |
| MAP | mean systemic arterial pressure |
| MAPK | mitogen-activated protein kinase |
| MARS® | Molecular Adsorbent Recirculating System |
| Mb | megabase |
| MCA | middle cerebral artery |
| MCF | maximum clot firmness |
| MCP | membrane cofactor protein |
| MCT | medium chain triglycerides |
| MDRD | modification of diet in renal disease |
| MELD | Model for End-stage Liver Disease |
| MET | mean exercise tolerance |
| MGH | Massachusetts General Hospital |
| mHag | minor histocompatibility antigen |
| MHC | major histocompatibility complex |
| MI | myocardial infarction |
| MMF | mycophenolate mofetil |
| MMR | measles, mumps, and rubella |
| MMRC | Modified Medical Research Council |
| MMVTx | modified multivisceral transplantation/transplant |
| MOF | multi-organ failure |
| MPA | mycophenolic acid |
| mPAP | mean pulmonary artery pressure |
| MPSC | Membership and Professional Standards Committee |
| MPT | mitochondrial permeability transition |
| MPTP | mitochondrial permeability transition pore |
| MRA | magnetic resonance angiography/angiogram |
| MRI | magnetic resonance imaging |
| MRSA | methicillin-resistant Staphylococcus aureus |
| mTOR | mammalian target of rapamycin |
| MVTx | multivisceral transplantation/transplant |
| Nabs | natural antibodies |
| NAC | N-acetyl-cysteine |
| NADPH | nicotinamide adenine dinucleotide phosphate |
| NAFLD | non-alcoholic fatty liver disease |
| NASH | non-alcoholic steatohepatitis |
| NATCO | North American Transplant Coordinators Organization |
| NF-κB | nuclear factor kappa-light-chain-enhancer of activated B cells |
| NGSP | National Glycohemoglobin Standardization Program |
| NHANES | National Health and Nutrition Examination Survey |
| NHBD | non-heart-beating donor |
| NHL | non-Hodgkin lymphoma |
| NHS | National Health Service |
| NICE | National Institute for Health and Clinical Excellence |
| NIH | National Institutes of Health |
| NIRS | near-infrared spectroscopy |
| NIV | non-invasive ventilation |
| NK | natural killer |
| NKT | natural killer T |
| NMDA | N-methyl-D-aspartate |
| n-NOS | nitric oxide synthetase |
| $NO^-$ | nitric oxide |
| NOTA | National Organ Transplant Act |
| NPO | nil per os |
| NQF | National Quality Forum |
| NSQIP | National Surgical Quality Improvement Program |
| NTPR | National Transplantation Pregnancy Registry |
| NVASRS | National Veterans Administration Surgical Risk Study |
| NYHA | New York Heart Association |
| O:E | observed to expected |
| OGD | oesophagogastroduodenoscopy |
| OGTT | oral glucose tolerance test |
| $OH^-$ | hydroxyl radical |
| OKT3 | muromonab-CD3 |
| OLT | orthotropic liver transplantation |
| OLV | one-lung ventilation |
| ONT | Spanish National Transplant Organization |
| $OONO^-$ | peroxynitrite |
| OPO | organ procurement organization |
| OPTN | Organ Procurement and Transplantation Network |
| OR | operating room |
| OTPD | organs transplanted per donor |
| P:F | $PaO_2$:$FiO_2$ ratio |
| PA | pulmonary artery |
| PAC | pulmonary artery catheter |
| PACU | post-anaesthesia care unit |
| PAD | pulmonary artery diastolic pressure |

PAFC pulmonary artery flotation catheter
PAH pulmonary artery hypertension
PAK pancreas after kidney
PAKTx pancreas after kidney transplantation/transplant
$PaO_2$ arterial partial pressure of oxygen in arterial blood
PAOP pulmonary arterial occlusion pressure
PAP pulmonary artery pressure
$PaCO_2$ partial pressure of carbon dioxide
PAT pancreas alone transplant
PAWP pulmonary artery wedge pressure
PBC primary biliary cirrhosis
PBPC peripheral blood progenitor cells
PCA patient-controlled analgesia
PCI percutaneous coronary intervention
PCMR Pediatric Cardiomyopathy Registry
PCP pneumocystis pneumonia
PCR polymerase chain reaction
PCWP pulmonary capillary wedge pressure
PD peritoneal dialysis
PDF primary liver dysfunction
PDGF platelet-derived growth factor
PDK pyruvate dehydrogenase kinase
PDSA plan, do, study, act
PE pulmonary embolus
PedsQL4.0 Pediatric Quality of Life Inventory 4.0
PEEP positive end-expiratory pressure
PELD paediatric end-stage liver disease
PERV porcine endogenous retrovirus
PET positron emission tomography
PFO patent foramen oval
PG prostaglandin
PGD primary graft dysfunction
PGNF Primary Graft Non-Function
PHD prolyl hydroxylase
PHT pulmonary hypertension
PHTS Pediatric Heart Transplant Study
PICC percutaneous intravenous catheter
PICU paediatric intensive care unit
Pinsp inspiratory pressure
PIP peak inspiratory pressure
PLE protein-losing enteropathy
PML progressive multifocal leucoencephalopathy
PN parenteral nutrition
PNF primary non-function
PNH paroxysmal nocturnal haemoglobinuria
po per os
POC point of care
POCD postoperative cognitive dysfunction
PP pancreatic polypeptide
P-PASS preprocurement pancreas allocation suitability score
PPH primary pulmonary hypertension
PPHTN portopulmonary hypertension
ppm parts per million
PPV pulse pressure variation
PRA panel reactive antibody
PRBC packed red blood cell
PRN pro re nata
PRS postreperfusion syndrome
PSE portosystemic encephalopathy
PSR Program-Specific Report
PT prothrombin time
PTFE polytetrafluoroethylene
PTH parathyroid hormone
PTLD post-transplant lymphoproliferative disorder
PTT partial thromboplastin time
PTxA pancreas transplant alone
PV pulmonary vein/venous
PVR pulmonary vascular resistance
QALY quality-adjusted life expectancy
qds four times a day
QOL quality of life
QOLI quality of life index
RA right atrium
RAAS renin–angiotensin–aldosterone system
RAP right atrial pressure
RBC red blood cell
RCM restrictive cardiomyopathy
RCPCH Royal College of Paediatrics and Child Health
RCT randomized clinical trial
RE response entropy
RFLP restriction fragment length polymorphism
RIPCOD Remote Ischemic Preconditioning in Neurological Death Organ Donors
RIPCOT Remote Ischemic Preconditioning in Abdominal Organ Transplantation
RIS rapid infusion system
ROS reactive oxygen species
ROTEM® rotational thromboelastometry
RRT renal replacement therapy
RV right ventricle/ventricular
RVAD right ventricular assist device
RVSP right ventricular systolic pressure
SA sinoatrial
SA splenic artery
SAC standard acquisition charge
SAM systolic anterior motion
SATA Society for the Advancement of Transplant Anesthesia
SBP spontaneous bacterial peritonitis
SBS short bowel syndrome
SCD standard criteria donor
SCM sternocleidomastoid
SCUF slow continuous ultrafiltration
$ScvO_2$ central venous oxygen saturation
SE state entropy
SEOPF Southeast Organ Procurement Foundation
SEROPP Southeastern Regional Organ Procurement Program
SFSS small-for-size syndrome
SIK simultaneous islet–kidney
SIMV synchronized intermittent mandatory ventilation
SIRS systemic inflammatory response syndrome
$SjO_2$ jugular bulb oxygen saturation
$SjvO_2$ jugular venous oxygen saturation
SKPT simultaneous kidney–pancreas transplant
SLA swine leucocyte antigen
SLTx single-lung transplantation/transplant

| | |
|---|---|
| SMA | superior mesenteric artery |
| SMV | superior mesenteric vein |
| SPAD® | Single Pass Albumin Dialysis |
| SPECT | single photon emission computed tomography |
| SPKTx | simultaneous pancreas–kidney transplantation/ transplant |
| $SpO_2$ | peripheral capillary oxygen saturation |
| SPRT | sequential probability ratio test |
| SREBP | sterol regulatory element binding protein |
| SRTR | Scientific Registry of Transplant Recipients |
| SVC | superior vena cava |
| $SvO_2$ | mixed venous oxygen saturation |
| SVR | systemic vascular resistance |
| SVV | stroke volume variation |
| T1DR | type 1 diabetes recurrence |
| T3 | tri-iodothyronine |
| T4 | thyroxin |
| TACO | transfusion-associated circulatory overload |
| TA-GVHD | transfusion-associated graft versus host disease |
| TAP | transversus abdominis plane |
| TB | tuberculosis |
| TCD | transcranial Doppler |
| TCR | Transplant Candidate Registration Form |
| TEA | thoracic epidural anaesthesia |
| TEB | transthoracic electrical bioimpedance |
| TED | thromboembolic deterrent |
| TEG | thromboelastography/gram |
| TEM-A | ThromboElastoMeter-Automated |
| TGF-β | transforming growth factor β |
| TGH | Toronto General Hospital |
| THAM | tris(hydroxymethyl)aminomethane |
| THAM | tromethamine |
| TIA | transient ischaemic attack |
| TIPS | transjugular intrahepatic portosystemic shunt |
| TIVA | total intravenous anaesthesia |
| TMA | thrombotic microangiopathy |
| TNF | tumour necrosis factor |
| TOE | transoesophageal echocardiography |
| TOF/PA | tetralogy of Fallot with pulmonary atresia |
| TOR | target of rapamycin |
| TPE | therapeutic plasma exchange |
| TPG | transpulmonary gradient |
| TPM | Transplant Procurement Management |
| TPN | total parenteral nutrition |
| TRALI | transfusion-related acute lung injury |
| TRF | Transplant Recipient Follow-up Form |
| TRICC | Transfusion Requirements in Critical Care |
| TRIM | transfusion-related immunomodulation |
| TRR | Transplant Recipient Registration Form |
| TSH | thyroid-stimulating hormone |
| TTE | transthoracic echocardiogram |
| TTS | the Transplantation Society |
| UAGA | Uniform Anatomical Gift Act |
| UCLA | University of California, Los Angeles |
| UEMS | Union Européenne des Médecins Spécialistes |
| UFR | ultrafiltration rate |
| UIP | usual interstitial pneumonia |
| UKELD | United Kingdom Model for End-Stage Liver Disease |
| UNOS | United Network for Organ Sharing |
| USRDS | US Renal Data System |
| UTI | urinary tract infection |
| UW | University of Wisconsin |
| VA | Veterans Administration |
| VAD | ventricular assist device |
| VA-ECMO | venoarterial extracorporeal membrane oxygenation |
| vCJD | variant Creutzfeldt–Jakob disease |
| VDAC | voltage-dependent anion channels |
| VEGF | vascular endothelial growth factor |
| VHA | viscoelastic haemostatic assay |
| VO2 | peak oxygen consumption |
| VRE | vancomycin-resistant Enterococcus |
| VSD | ventricular septal defect |
| VT | ventricular tachycardia |
| VTE | venous thromboembolic |
| VVB | venovenous bypass |
| vWF | von Willebrand factor |
| WBC | white blood cell |
| WHO | World Health Organization |
| WIT | warm ischaemia time |
| WU | Woods Units |
| XD | xanthine dehydrogenase |
| XO | xanthine oxidase |
| ZnT8 | zinc transporter 8 |
| α1AT | alpha-1-antitrypsin |
| αFP | alpha-fetoprotein |
| γGT | serum glutamyl transferase |

# Editors

## Editor-in-Chief

**Ernesto A. Pretto, Jr., MD, MPH**
Professor and Chief
Division of Transplant and Vascular Anesthesia
Department of Anesthesiology, Perioperative Medicine and Pain Management
Miami Transplant Institute
University of Miami
Leonard M. Miller School of Medicine/Jackson Memorial Hospital
Miami
Florida
USA

## Editors

**Gianni Biancofiore, MD**
Head Anestesia e Rianimazione SSN
Azienda Ospedaliera Pisana
Ospedale di Cisanello
Pisa
Italy

**Andre De Wolf, MD**
Professor of Anesthesiology
Director, Transplant Anesthesiology Service
Department of Anesthesiology
Feinberg School of Medicine
Northwestern University
Chicago
Illinois
USA

**John R. Klinck, MD, FRCPC, FRCA**
Consultant in Anaesthesia
Division of Perioperative Care
Cambridge University Hospitals
Cambridge
UK

**Claus Niemann, MD**
Professor of Anesthesia & Surgery
Department of Anesthesia and Perioperative Care
Department of Surgery, Division of Transplantation
University of California
San Francisco
California
USA

**Andrew Watts, MD, FANZCA**
Consultant in Anaesthesia
Head of Transplant Anaesthesia
Royal Prince Alfred Hospital
Sydney
Australia

## Contributing Editor

**Peter D. Slinger, MD, FRCPC**
Associate Professor and Staff Anesthesiologist
Toronto General Hospital
University of Toronto
Toronto
Canada

# Contributors

**Luz Aguina**
Fellow
Solid Organ Transplant and Vascular Anesthesia
University of Miami
Leonard M. Miller School of Medicine
Miami
Florida
USA

**Gabriella Amorese**
Division of General and Transplant Surgery and Division of Anesthesia and Intensive Care
Cisanello University Hospital
Pisa
Italy

**Faisal Anis**
Transplant Anesthesia Fellow
Division of Solid Organ Transplant and Vascular Anesthesia
Department of Anesthesiology, Perioperative Medicine and Pain Management
University of Miami
Leonard M. Miller School of Medicine/Jackson Memorial Hospital
Miami
Florida
USA

**Alan Ashworth**
Consultant in Anaesthesia & ICU
University Hospital of South Manchester
Manchester
UK

**Oliver Bagshaw**
Consultant in Anaesthesia and Intensive Care
Birmingham Children's Hospital
Birmingham
UK

**Kumar Belani**
Professor of Anesthesiology
University of Minnesota
Minneapolis
Minnesota
USA

**James Bennett**
Consultant Anaesthetist
Birmingham Children's Hospital
Birmingham
UK

**Gabriela A. Berlakovich**
Medical University Vienna
Department of Surgery
Inerim. Head Division of Transplantation
Vienna
Austria

**Gianni Biancofiore**
Head Anestesia e Rianimazione SSN
Azienda Ospedaliera Pisana
Ospedale di Cisanello
Pisa
Italy

**Martin Birch**
Assistant Professor of Anesthesiology
University of Minnesota
Minneapolis
Minnesota
USA

**Matthew B. Bloom**
Trauma Surgery and Surgical Critical Care
Cedars-Sinai Medical Center
Los Angeles
California
USA

**Ugo Boggi**
Professor of Surgery
Director of Kidney and Pancreas Transplantation Program
University School of Medicine
Pisa
Italy

**Peter Bromley**
Consultant Anaesthetist
Birmingham Children's Hospital
Birmingham
UK

**Daniel M. Bruggebrew**
Donor Network
West California
USA

**George Burke**
Professor of Surgery, Chief
Division of Kidney and Kidney–Pancreas
University of Miami
Leonard M. Miller School of Medicine
Miami
Florida
USA

**Richard Charlewood**
Transfusion Medicine Specialist
New Zealand Blood Service
Auckland
New Zealand

**Linda Chen**
Assistant Professor
DeWitt Daughtry Department of Surgery
Surgical Director, Liver Kidney Live Donor Program
Miami Transplant Institute
University of Miami
Leonard M. Miller School of Medicine/Jackson Memorial Hospital
Miami
Florida
USA

**Gaetano Ciancio**
Professor of Surgery
Division of Kidney and Kidney–Pancreas
University of Miami
Leonard M. Miller School of Medicine
Miami
Florida
USA

**Maria Gabriella Costa**
Associate Professor of Anesthesiology and Critical Care Medicine
Department of Anesthesia and Critical Care Medicine
University School of Medicine
Udine
Italy

**Marcelo Cypel**
Assistant Professor of Surgery
University of Toronto and Toronto General Hospital
Toronto
Canada

**Andrea De Gasperi**
Director of Abdominal Transplant Anesthesia and Critical Care Service 2, Ospedale Niguarda Ca' Granda
Milan
Italy

**Kerry Gunn**
Specialist Anaesthetist
Department of Anaesthesia and Perioperative Medicine
Auckland City Hospital
Auckland
New Zealand

**Giorgio Della Rocca**
Professor of Anesthesiology and Critical Care Medicine
Department of Anesthesia and Critical Care Medicine
University School of Medicine
Udine
Italy

**M. Francesca Egidi**
Professor of Nephrology Head, Department of Nephrology
University School of Medicine
Pisa
Italy

**Obi Ekwenna**
Assistant Professor of Urology and Transplantation
Department of Urology
University of Toledo Medical Center
Ohio
USA

**Mazen Faden**
Assistant Professor
Department of Anesthesia and Critical Care
King Abdulaziz
University Jeddah
Saudi Arabia

**James Y. Findlay**
Associate Professor of Anesthesiology and Consultant
Department of Anesthesiology and Critical Care Medicine
Mayo Clinic
Rochester
Minnesota
USA

**Robin N. Fiore**
Institute for Bioethics and Health Policy
University of Miami
Leonard M. Miller School of Medicine
Miami
Florida
USA

**Haran Fisher**
Assistant Professor
Division of Solid Organ Transplant and Vascular Anesthesia
Department of Anesthesiology, Perioperative Medicine and Pain Management
University of Miami
Leonard M. Miller School of Medicine/Jackson Memorial Hospital
Miami
Florida
USA
and
Department of Anaesthesia
Schneider Children's Hospital
Tel Aviv
Israel

**Kyota Fukazawa**
Assistant Professor of Clinical Anesthesiology
Department of Anesthesiology
University of Miami
Leonard M. Miller School of Medicine
Miami
Florida
USA

**Mark Hayman**
Department of Anaesthesia
Royal Prince Alfred Hospital
Sydney
Australia

**Benjamin E. Hippen**
Metrolina Associates PA
Charlotte
North Carolina
USA

**Ryutaro Hirose**
Professor in Clinical Surgery
Department of Surgery
Division of Transplantation
Associate Director
Surgical Residency Program
University of California
San Francisco
California
USA

**Katherine G. Hoctor**
Voluntary Assistant Professor of Anesthesiology
University of Miami
Leonard M. Miller School of Medicine
Jackson Memorial Hospital
Miami
Florida
USA

**Gyu-Sam Hwang**
Department of Anesthesiology and Pain Medicine
Asan Medical Centre
University of Ulsan
Seoul
Korea

**Anurag Johri**
Department of Anesthesiology, Perioperative Medicine and Pain Management
University of Miami
Leonard M. Miller School of Medicine/Jackson Memorial Hospital
Miami
Florida
USA

**Lydia M. Jorge**
Assistant Professor of Pediatric Anesthesia
Department of Anesthesiology
University of Miami
Miami
Florida
USA

**John R. Klinck**
Consultant in Anaesthesia
Division of Perioperative Care
Cambridge University Hospitals
Cambridge
UK

**Michael C. Lewis**
Professor and Chairman
Department of Anesthesiology
University of Florida College of Medicine
Jacksonville
Florida
USA

**Darren J. Malinoski**
Assistant Chief of Surgery
Portland VA Medical Center
Associate Professor of Surgery
Oregon Health & Science University
Portland
Oregon
USA

**Piero Marchetti**
Associate Professor of Endocrinology and Metabolic Diseases
Director
Unit of Endocrinology and Cellular and Solid Organ Transplantation Metabolism
University School of Medicine
Pisa
Italy

**Paul Martin**
Professor of Medicine and Director Division of Hepatology
University of Miami
Leonard M. Miller School of Medicine
Miami
Florida
USA

**Stuart Andrew McCluskey**
Department of Anesthesia and Pain Management
Toronto General Hospital
University of Toronto
Toronto
Canada

**Kirstin Naguit**
Department of Anaesthesia
Concord Repatriation General Hospital
Sydney
Australia

**Richard Neal**
Consultant in Intensive Care
Birmingham Children's Hospital
Birmingham
UK

**Nikole Neidlinger**
Medical Director
Donor Network West
California
USA

**Jamie Lindemann Nelson**
Professor of Philosophy
Associate Faculty
Center for Ethics and Humanities in the Life Science
Michigan State University
Michigan
USA

**Claus Niemann**
Professor of Anesthesia & Surgery
Department of Anesthesia and Perioperative Care
Department of Surgery, Division of Transplantation
University of California
San Francisco
California
USA

**Seigo Nishida**
Professor of Clinical Surgery
DeWitt Daughtry Department of Surgery
Miami Transplant Institute
University of Miami
Leonard M. Miller School of Medicine/Jackson Memorial Hospital
Miami
Florida
USA

**Margherita Occhipinti**
Department of Clinical and Experimental Medicine
Cisanello University Hospital
Pisa
Italy

**John O'Grady**
Professor of Hepatology
Institute of Liver Sciences
King's College Hospital
London
UK

**Andrea Olmos**
Department of Anesthesia and Perioperative Care
University of California
San Francisco
California
USA

**Justin Parekh**
Assistant Professor of Transplant Surgery
University of Texas
Southwestern Dallas
Texas
USA

**Vishal C. Patel**
Research Fellow
Institute of Liver Sciences
King's College Hospital
London
UK

**William Peruzzi**
Professor of Anesthesiology, Perioperative Medicine & Pain Management
Chief Medical Officer, Alameda Health System
California
USA

**Antonello Pileggi**
Professor of Surgery, Microbiology and Immunology, and Biomedical Engineering
Cell Transplant Center, Diabetes Research Institute
University of Miami
Leonard M. Miller School of Medicine
Miami
Florida
USA

**Livia Pompei**
Associate Professor of Anesthesiology
Department of Anesthesia and Critical Care Medicine
University School of Medicine
Udine
Italy

**Ernesto A. Pretto, Jr.**
Professor and Chief
Division of Transplant and Vascular Anesthesia
Department of Anesthesiology, Perioperative Medicine and Pain Management
Miami Transplant Institute
University of Miami
Leonard M. Miller School of Medicine/Jackson Memorial Hospital
Miami
Florida
USA

**J. Sudharma Ranasinghe**
Professor of Clinical Anesthesiology
University of Miami
Leonard M. Miller School of Medicine
Director of Obstetric Anesthesia
Jackson Memorial Hospital
Miami
Florida
USA

**Karina Rando**
Assistant Professor in Anesthesiology
Consultant Anesthesiologist in the Liver Transplant Unit National Center of Liver and Pancreas Surgery (UDA)
Central Hospital of the Army (H.C.FF.AA)
Montevideo
Uruguay

**Shariq S. Raza**
Department of Surgery
Section of Trauma and Surgical Critical Care
Temple University Hospital
Philadelphia
Pennsylvania
USA

**Camillo Ricordi**
Professor of Surgery and Scientific Director
Diabetes Research Institute
University of Miami
Leonard M. Miller of Medicine
Miami
Florida
USA

**Andrew Roscoe**
Toronto General Hospital
Toronto
Canada

**Derek Rosen**
University of Toronto and Toronto General Hospital
Toronto
Canada

**Phillip Ruiz**
Professor of Surgery and Pathology
Director Immunopathology
Department of Pathology
University of Miami
Leonard M. Miller School of Medicine
Miami
Florida
USA

**Junichiro Sageshima**
Department of Surgery
University of California
Davis
California
USA

**Mauricio Sainz-Barriga**
Abdominal Transplant
Surgery Department
University Hospitals
Leuven
Belgium

**Ali Salim**
Professor of Surgery
Harvard Medical School
Chief, Division of Trauma, Burns, and Surgical Critical Care
Brigham and Women's Hospital
Boston
Massachusetts
USA

**Joseph Scalea**
Transplantation Biology Research Center
Massachusetts General Hospital
Harvard Medical School
Boston
Massachusetts
USA

**Giuseppe Segoloni**
Professor of Nephrology
Head Department of Nephrology
University School of Torino
Torino
Italy

**Anand Sharma**
Senior Consultant (Anesthesia)
Medanta Institute of Critical Care and Anesthesia
Gurgaon
Haryana
India
University of Toronto and
University of Ulsan
Korea

**Robby Sikka**
Department of Anesthesiology
University of Minnesota Medical Center
Minneapolis
Minnesota
USA

**Peter D. Slinger**
Associate Professor and Staff Anesthesiologist
Toronto General Hospital
University of Toronto
Toronto
Canada

**Thomas Soliman**
Division of Transplantation
Department of Surgery
Medical University of Vienna
Vienna
Austria

**Fouad G. Souki**
Assistant Professor, Clinical Anesthesiology
Division of Solid Organ Transplant and Vascular Anesthesia
University of Miami
Miami
Florida
USA

**Andrew C. Steel**
Toronto General Hospital
Toronto
Canada

**Elod Szabo**
Assistant Professor
Department of Anesthesia
The Hospital for Sick Children
University of Toronto
Toronto
Canada

**Hui-Hui Tan**
Department of Gastroenterology and Hepatology
Singapore General Hospital
Singapore

**Masayuki Tasaki**
Transplantation Biology Research Center
Massachusetts General Hospital
Harvard Medical School
Boston
Massachusetts
USA

**Sean Van Slyck**
Vice President Organ Program
Donor Network West
California
USA

**Samantha Vizzini**
Department of Anesthesiology, Perioperative Medicine and Pain Management
University of Miami
Leonard M. Miller School of Medicine/Jackson Memorial Hospital
Miami
Florida
USA

**Gebhard Wagener**
Department of Anesthesiology
Columbia University
New York
USA

**Marcin Wąsowicz**
Department of Anesthesia and Pain Management
Cardiovascular Intensive Care Unit
Toronto Genaral Hospital
University Health Network
University of Toronto
Toronto
Canada

**Andrew Watts**
Consultant in Anaesthesia
Head of Transplant Anaesthesia
Royal Prince Alfred Hospital
Sydney
Australia

**Andre De Wolf**
Professor of Anesthesiology
Director, Transplant Anesthesiology Service
Department of Anesthesiology
Feinberg School of Medicine
Northwestern University
Chicago
Illinois
USA

**Kazuhiko Yamada**
Professor of Surgery
Columbia University Medical Center
Department of Medicine Immunology
Irving Cancer Center
New York
USA

SECTION 1

# Introduction

# CHAPTER 1

# History of organ transplantation

John R. Klinck and Ernesto A. Pretto, Jr.

## Introduction

The scientific and technical foundations of organ transplantation were established in the first two decades of the twentieth century, with the advent of techniques of vascular anastomosis, auto-transplant experiments in animals, and efforts to define and manipulate the immune response (see Figure 1.1). Human kidney transplants were attempted, as early as in the 1930s, and in the 1940s the pioneers of immunology began to characterize rejection and tolerance. This knowledge led to successful human kidney transplantation, first carried out in identical twins in the 1950s, demonstrating that with immune tolerance a single kidney could sustain life for many years. Corticosteroids, dialysis machines, heart–lung bypass, and organ cooling were also introduced in the 1950s, furthering the quest for wider application of transplantation. The 1960s saw the introduction of azathioprine and the evolution of microsurgical techniques, fostering intensive small-animal experimentation. Important advances were made in organ preservation, as the techniques of both ex-vivo perfusion and cold storage were refined, while tissue typing and the development of antilymphocyte sera supported the belief that the lethal obstacle of rejection might soon be overcome. The first human liver, lung, and heart transplants were performed in 1963 and 1968, although rejection frustrated these premature efforts. The 1960s also witnessed the widespread introduction of artificial ventilation, from which the concept of brain death emerged. This would soon open the door to heart-beating cadaveric donation.

The pivotal breakthrough, however, came in the late 1970s with the discovery of cyclosporine. This humble fungal derivative offered effective immunosuppression without life-threatening side effects. It transformed long-term outcomes and propelled clinical transplantation into the mainstream. These benefits were consolidated in the 1980s, when rapid expansion of transplant services, in particular the development of committed multidisciplinary teams and organ procurement organizations (OPOs), heralded transplantation as the treatment of choice for most forms of organ failure. Funding for clinical transplantation and pharmaceutical research increased enormously in the 1980s and 1990s, leading to further advances in immunosuppression and in most aspects of clinical care. This chapter highlights some of these developments, emphasizing the roles of basic science and clinical liver transplantation in the development of transplant perioperative care.

## Early development

The modern era of clinical organ transplantation began in the 1950s, but depended on key advances in vascular surgery, immunology, and experimental transplantation dating from the earliest years of the twentieth century. Jaboulay and Carrel pioneered the techniques of vascular anastomosis in France, and Carrel described their use in kidney and heart transplantation in animals in his famous paper of 1902. Awarded the Nobel Prize in 1912, Carrel continued this work with Guthrie in Chicago and first described the use of cold storage for tissue preservation. The same pre-war decade saw important advances in the understanding of host responses to foreign tissue, including recognition of the lymphocyte, many aspects of its behaviour, and its suppression by both chemicals and radiation. These developments and the aims of future research in organ transplantation were presciently summarized by Carrel at a landmark international meeting of the International Society of Surgery in New York in 1914, but he did not pursue these himself, and much of the new knowledge, published in German and French, fell into obscurity with the outbreak of World War I. In the post-war years, leadership in medical research passed to a more affluent, English-speaking North America, and this early scientific momentum was lost. No further international conference addressing the challenges of transplantation would take place until 1948. Historians refer to this early period of promising but unsustained progress as the 'lost era' of organ transplantation (Hamilton, 2012).

In the 1930s Carrel resumed work in the field, collaborating with the famous aviator and inventor Charles Lindbergh to develop an ex-vivo perfusion apparatus that anticipated later organ preservation techniques. In the period 1933–1949, the Soviet surgeon Yuri Voronoy performed the first human kidney allografts (Hamilton and Reid, 1984; Matevossian et al., 2009), using Carrel's techniques to graft kidneys from cadaveric donors to the femoral vessels of recipients under local anaesthetic. He hoped to achieve life-saving temporary function in the setting of mercury ingestion. This was a common form of suicide associated with splenic and lymph node atrophy, and he believed that rejection might be attenuated. However, since he accepted the contemporary dogma that prolonged warm ischaemia was desirable and that mismatching of blood groups was not important, the grafts invariably failed. Further progress in clinical transplantation awaited the advances in laboratory immunology and chemical immunosuppression of the 'modern' era, beginning in the 1950s.

## The concept of immune rejection and the first immunosuppressive agents

For decades, rejection was thought to be a non-specific inflammatory process directed against foreign tissue, until Peter Medawar's groundbreaking work with skin grafts in the 1940s revealed that it was an acquired, donor-specific response. Medawar and

| | |
|---|---|
| **1900–1920** | |
| Paul Ehrlich, Elie Metchnikoff, Georg Schone | "Lost Era" of transplant immunology: discovery of humoral and cellular immune responses, chemical and radiation-induced immunosuppression |
| Alexis Carrel, Charles Guthrie | Techniques of vascular anastomosis; observations on tissue cooling; Carrell's "road map" to organ transplantation 1914 |
| **1920s** | |
| James Murphy, Leo Loeb | Genetic control of cellular immune response: non-specific inflammatory mechanism of rejection disproved |
| **1930s** | |
| Yu Yu Voronoy | Extracorporeal human kidney allografting confirms short term viability |
| Alexis Carrell | Extracorporeal organ perfusion |
| Key supporting advance: | Laboratory tests of kidney function |
| **1940s** | |
| George Snell, Peter Medawar, Peter Gorer | Modern era of transplant immunology: lymphocyte role in graft rejection shown to be acquired and donor-specific; HLA system and genetics of rejection elucidated. |
| Key supporting advance: | Invention of dialysis machine |
| **1950s** | |
| Key supporting advances: | Discovery and synthesis of corticosteroids; dialysis used successfully in Korean War, development of organ cooling and heart-lung bypass |
| Joseph Murray, David Hume | Kidney transplant between identical twins confirms graft longevity |
| **1960s** | |
| | Technical success with deceased donor organs: |
| Murray & Hume | Kidney transplant |
| James Hardy | Lung transplant |
| Richard Lillehei, William Kelly | Pancreas/kidney transplant |
| Thomas Starzl, Roy Caine | Liver transplant |
| Christiaan Barnard, Norman Shumway | Heart transplant |
| Folkert Belzer, Geoffrey Collins | Ex-vivo machine preservation, Static cold preservation |
| Paul Terasaki | Tissue typing |
| Henry Beecher | Harvard Ad Hoc Committee: concept of brain death enables cadaveric heart-beating donation |
| Key supporting advances: | Azathioprine, steroid-azathioprine combination; growth of mechanical ventilation and ICUs; microsurgical techniques and intensive animal experimentation; anti-lymphocyte sera; cardiac catheterization; Uniform Anatomical Gift Act |
| **1970s** | |
| Key supporting advances: | Legislative recognition of brain death |
| | Kidney transplantation officially funded |
| Jean Borel, David White | Discovery and experimental study of cyclosporin |
| **1980s** | |
| Roy Caine, Thomas Starzl | Successful clinical use of cyclosporin propels kidney and liver transplant to mainstream |
| Bruce Reitz, Michael DeBakey, Joel Cooper | Heart, lung, and heart-lung transplants re-established |
| Key supporting advances: | Wide public acceptance and rapid expansion of transplant services; multidisciplinary teams; organ procurement organizations; tacrolimus, monoclonals |
| **1990s** | |
| | Pancreas, intestinal, multi-visceral transplants established; living donation of kidney, liver and lung |
| **2000-present** | |
| | Globalization of organ transplant and growth of living donation in kidney and liver transplant; focus on increasing supply of deceased donor organs; tissue transplants: hand and face |

**Fig. 1.1** A chronology of organ transplantation.

others also confirmed that immune rejection was predominantly lymphocyte-mediated, as 'lost era' investigators had suggested. This led to experiments in the 1950s with whole-body radiation and donor bone marrow infusion, known to induce tolerance in animals. Corticosteroids, isolated in the 1930s and synthesized at huge expense in the late 1940s after rumours that Luftwaffe pilots in World War II had used them, were also discovered to have immunosuppressive effects and were used in human kidney transplants. Although dramatic results obtained in inflammatory and autoimmune diseases were not replicated in transplantation, steroids continued to be used when radiation was found to be too dangerous, and they soon found a place in combination with another important agent.

The suppressive effects of nitrogen mustard ('mustard gas') on the bone marrow and immunity were known from tragic experience in both World Wars, and analogues were synthesized for treatment of lymphoid cancers in the mid-1940s. In the 1950s, the capacity of purine analogues to suppress immunity was recognized, and Roy Calne demonstrated that 6-mercaptopurine yielded much better results than radiation in animals. He speculated correctly that a dominant effect on cell-mediated as opposed to humoral immunity might account for this. This countered the contemporary belief that all immunosuppression affected T- and B-cell function equally, thereby inevitably exposing the recipient to lethal infection. Working with Joseph Murray in Boston, Calne showed even better experimental results with another purine analogue, azathioprine. However, clinical outcomes with this agent, as with radiation and with combinations of the two, remained poor.

The next major advance in immunosuppression awaited an empiric discovery in the early 1960s, by Willard Goodwin and

Thomas Starzl, that high-dose steroid treatment reversed acute rejection in kidney recipients receiving azathioprine. Starzl extended this important observation, suggesting that combining prophylactic low-dose steroids and azathioprine might be beneficial. This proved to be the case and rapidly became the standard immunosuppressive regime. Aided by advances in human leucocyte antigen (HLA) tissue matching and wider availability of dialysis, kidney transplantation units proliferated. Small-animal models of kidney, heart, and liver transplants, designed to study immunosuppression, were by then well established and the pace of experimental work in the field quickened (Bradley and Hamilton, 2001). The scientific basis of immune rejection and immunosuppression in organ transplantation is presented in Chapter 11.

## Evolution of organ preservation techniques and solutions

The development of organ preservation techniques has been vital to progress in solid organ transplantation. The earliest attempts evolved from an interest in evaluating physiological function. Le Gallois (1813) predicted that organ function could be restored by perfusion with arterial blood, and Von Cyon, Ringer, and Langendorff later studied the effects of ex-vivo normothermia, mostly with isolated mammalian hearts (Toledo-Pereyra, 1984; Miller, 2004). Carrel described the benefits of cold storage of explanted vessels and, with Lindbergh, developed a pumped perfusion apparatus able to maintain organs for 20–40 days with normothermic serum. This laid the groundwork for later improvements in organ preservation by continuous perfusion (Malinin, 1996).

The value of cooling the perfusate was explored in the 1950s. In 1956 a canine kidney autograft functioned after 24 hours of hypothermic perfusion preservation (Murray et al., 1956), and the preservation of kidneys with cold perfusate was widely adopted by the early 1960s. Belzer et al. (1967) extended experimental preservation times, obtaining consistent function after 72 hours through the use of continuous pulsatile perfusion at 10°C with a cryoprecipitate plasma preparation. Toledo-Pereyra et al. (1976) added silica gel to plasma protein fraction, obtaining even better results.

However, early perfusion preservation required the use of complex, non-portable devices, hampering its widespread application. This difficulty was compounded by the emergence of HLA matching for clinical kidney transplants in the late 1960s, which increased distances between matched donor–recipient pairs. The impracticality of moving donors or perfusion apparatus and the need for longer preservation times stimulated further research into simple cold storage. Although well described in the 1950s and widely adopted in experimental liver and heart transplantation in the 1960s, simple cold storage with solutions then available could not sustain viability long enough for clinical kidney transplants. A breakthrough came in 1969 when Collins and Terasaki introduced a novel preservation solution effective enough to replace hypothermic perfusion. This was a crystalloid constituted to resemble intracellular fluid, thereby reducing sodium influx and osmotic cell swelling, and allowing unperfused cold storage of the kidney for up to 30 hours. Although machine perfusion remained in use in some centres and portable pumps were soon developed, Collins' solution and its simpler derivative, Euro Collins, rapidly became the mainstay of solid organ preservation worldwide.

The next significant advance in organ preservation was reported in 1992 by Belzer at the University of Wisconsin (UW) with the introduction of UW solution (Belzer et al., 1992). This solution contained impermeants, shown to further reduce cell swelling, as well as antioxidants and other agents thought to preserve adenosine triphosphate (ATP) production and attenuate ischaemia–reperfusion injury. It was shown to be very effective in the preservation of kidney and liver grafts, though less effective in pancreas and heart preservation. In the 1990s Bretschneider introduced histidine–tryptophan–ketoglutarate (HTK) solution (Gubernatis et al., 1990). UW and HTK solutions have safely extended kidney preservation times to 24 hours or longer, thereby facilitating organ sharing across large geographic regions. The scientific foundations of organ preservation, including a review of the basic biochemistry and molecular pathways of cell injury and death, are presented in Chapter 10.

## Brain death and heart-beating donation

Advances in clinical transplantation in the 1960s focused attention on legal issues related to organ donation. In many countries no legal framework existed and removal of organs from cadavers depended only on approval by authorities in local hospitals. Where laws existed, they addressed donation for anatomical teaching and corneal grafting, not rapid removal for transplant. As results in renal and experimental transplantation improved, most developed countries moved to allow individuals to register consent to tissue donation on death, or for relatives to consent in the absence of known wishes.

In the same decade, advances in anaesthesia had an important impact on the progress of organ transplantation. Muscle relaxants and mechanical ventilators, introduced during the 1950s, improved patients' tolerance for lengthy operations, allowed them to be ventilated postoperatively, and could prevent immediate death of those patients with severe head injuries. Biochemical and blood gas measurements facilitated this, and specialist respiratory care wards were created. Peter Safar, a pioneer of cardiopulmonary resuscitation, set up such a unit at Baltimore City Hospital in 1958, coining the term 'Intensive Care'. This was soon replicated in Boston, where admissions increased six-fold between 1961 and 1966.

As management became more skillful, it was recognized that some patients who were admitted to the Intensive Care Unit (ICU) were kept alive without hope of neurological recovery, causing distress to staff and families. Robert Schwab, a neurologist at Massachusetts General Hospital, addressed this in an analysis of prognostic signs associated with consistent postmortem findings of extensive, irreversible brain injury. His confidence in these signs led to determination of 'brain death' and consensual termination of artificial ventilation in an increasing number of patients in the mid-1960s. The definition of death was debated in medical, religious, and legal circles but not resolved. At a meeting of leading transplant surgeons in London in 1966, the removal of organs from a 'brain-dead' donor was reported but essentially rejected by Calne, Starzl, and others. Their views were echoed by Norman Shumway at the University of California, Los Angeles (UCLA) the following year. He acknowledged the great advantage this would offer, particularly in cardiac transplantation, but agreed that attitudes in both the medical profession and society would need to change before this would be possible. Nonetheless, transplant surgeons began to consider the possibility of heart-beating donation and to seek the opinions of colleagues in critical care and neurology.

Henry Beecher, Professor of Anesthesia Research at Harvard, pursued this matter as chair of the medical faculty's Standing Committee on Human Studies. Motivated by what he regarded as the indignity of prolonged, futile artificial ventilation, he established a subcommittee, the Harvard Ad Hoc Committee on Brain Death. The committee's groundbreaking report was published in the *Journal of the American Medical Association* in August 1968, amid growing public disquiet at poor results of human heart transplants around the world. An association was inevitably inferred between the redefinition of death to prevent fruitless prolongation of intensive care and the needs of organ transplantation, undermining trust in the medical profession and deterring legislators from changing the law. Although critical care physicians readily adopted the Harvard Committee's recommendations from the outset, this was without legal support. As a result, brain death was not legally recognized in the US or UK until the early 1980s.

## Kidney transplantation

Several surgical teams in France and the US undertook experimental kidney transplantation in humans in the early 1950s, including one mother-to-son living donation. These were now blood group compatible and some recipients were treated with a costly new immunosuppressant, hydrocortisone. In Boston, a newly developed haemodialysis machine, pioneered by Willem Kolff in the Netherlands during World War II, supported recipients. Senior physicians in New England met this device with scepticism, but innovative US Army doctors at a specialist renal failure treatment facility proved its use during the Korean War. Dialysis could optimize recipients' pretransplant status and allowed time for ischaemic grafts to recover post transplant. However, the problem of rejection consistently frustrated these efforts. Joseph Murray in Boston achieved success in 1954 by transplanting kidneys between identical twins. This was done without the use of immunosuppressive agents and confirmed immunologists' predictions that immune reactivity in this setting would be minimal. Success in twins was replicated in other centres and proved beyond doubt that technical problems had been mastered and that a transplanted kidney could sustain good health for decades. Murray became a leading figure in the experimental and clinical development of renal transplantation and was awarded the Nobel Prize in 1990.

## Heart transplantation

Carrel and Guthrie reported a canine heterotopic heart transplant in 1905 and continued work on the extracorporeal perfusion of explanted organs into the 1930s. Frank Mann also experimented with heterotopic heart transplantation in 1933, commenting on the histology and lethal significance of rejection. Downie, Demikhov, and others continued animal experimentation based on Mann's technique in the 1950s, and knowledge of cardiac physiology was greatly advanced by Richards and Cournand, whose pioneering work on cardiac catheterization was rewarded with the Nobel Prize in 1956.

In-situ (orthotopic) replacement, however, awaited the development of methods of preserving the donor heart and of keeping the recipient alive during implantation. Hypothermia was found to address both these issues, allowing up to 30 minutes of circulatory arrest, as described in a 1953 report of canine en-bloc heart–lung transplants. The development of the heart–lung machine, pioneered by Gibbon in the early 1950s, was another vital technical advance. Both these techniques were adopted and refined by Shumway and Lower in their classic series of experimental orthotopic heart transplants dating from the late 1950s. They also introduced important improvements in surgical technique, including the use of a left atrial cuff to reduce the number of venous anastomoses. Since Reemtsma had demonstrated in 1958 that immunosuppressive agents could delay rejection and improve survival of the transplanted heart, Shumway and colleagues became convinced that immunologic rejection was the only remaining obstacle to successful clinical heart transplantation.

Reports of better immunosuppression with azathioprine and steroids in the mid-1960s, however, appeared to make clinical heart transplantation feasible. Although Shumway's group, after systematic and painstaking experimentation, was poised to begin clinical heart transplantation, Christian Barnard, a South African surgeon who had worked with the Shumway group at Stanford, performed the first human heart transplant in December 1967. Although the patient survived for only 18 days, many other centres around the world followed suit. However, results beyond the early postoperative period were poor, and the number of heart transplants worldwide dropped from 100 in 1968 to just 18 in 1970. The surgical hubris behind this 'Year of the Heart', while capturing the public imagination at its outset, ultimately undermined public confidence in transplantation and led to a decade-long moratorium in heart transplantation while a solution to the problem of graft rejection was sought. However, the intense media interest surrounding these events stimulated important changes in the legal definition of death in most western countries and focused public attention on organ transplantation as never before.

## Lung and heart–lung transplantation

Carrel and Guthrie reported experimental lung transplantation in 1905, and Demikhov described both isolated lung and heart–lung replacement in dogs in the late 1940s. Further attempts were made in the 1950s in several units in the US, but technical success was uniformly followed by rejection. Hardy, Lillehei, and others performed human lung transplants in the 1960s. They identified the problems of bronchial anastomotic leaks, necrosis, and stenosis before the inevitable onset of rejection, sepsis, and/or multi-organ failure. No further attempts were made until the cyclosporine era. Long-term success in lung grafting was first achieved in a series of patients from Toronto, beginning in 1983 (Cooper et al., 1987). Bilateral en-bloc lung transplant was described by Patterson in 1988 but was associated with a high incidence of tracheal necrosis. This was rapidly superseded by a sequential bilateral technique, often without cardiopulmonary bypass, still standard today (Pasque et al., 1990).

Successful clinical en-bloc heart–lung transplantation was first reported by Reitz in 1981 after extensive experimental work in primates. Many transplant programmes performed this procedure during the 1980s, mainly for cystic fibrosis and primary pulmonary hypertension. However, the indications for this procedure have declined progressively since the 1990s as a result of the success of lung transplantation, the high demand for isolated hearts, and the added risk of cardiac rejection and other complications.

## Pancreas, kidney–pancreas, intestinal, and multivisceral transplantation

Kelly and Lillehei performed a series of seven pancreas and kidney–pancreas transplants in the 1960s, but only one patient survived to a year. Technical problems, especially with enzyme leaks, proved as disastrous as rejection, and further interest in the procedure was limited to a few surgical programmes, notably in Minneapolis, Munich, Lyon, and Stockholm, until the appearance of cyclosporine. These programmes addressed the formidable problems of exocrine drainage with varying success. The alternative techniques of bladder versus enteric exocrine drainage were developed, along with systemic versus portal venous drainage. Immunosuppression also proved a far greater challenge than seen in other solid organs, and the advent of tacrolimus and antilymphocyte monoclonal antibodies led to progressive improvement in results through the 1990s. Isolated pancreas and combined kidney–pancreas transplants became widely accepted treatments by the year 2000.

Intestinal transplantation was performed experimentally by Lillehei and others starting in the late 1950s but was thwarted by graft-versus-host disease in non-immunosuppressed animals and rejection in those on azathioprine and steroids. Although clinical demand was reduced by the introduction of total parenteral nutrition from the late 1960s, rejection continued to frustrate occasional attempts in humans well into the 1980s, despite the introduction of cyclosporine. Grant first reported success in 1990 in a series of combined liver and small bowel transplants, suggesting that simultaneous grafting of the liver conferred an immunological advantage. This was later debated, but the introduction of tacrolimus in 1988 was an undisputed turning point. It provided the superior immunosuppression required, as demonstrated by the excellent results obtained in Starzl's series of multivisceral transplants reported in 1989 (Starzl et al. 1989). Tacrolimus also transformed results in isolated small bowel transplantation, and both small bowel and multivisceral transplants (now typically including pancreas and stomach) became established therapies in the late 1990s.

## Liver transplantation

Welch performed the first experimental liver transplant in a canine model in 1955 by placing a liver graft in the abdomen heterotopically (without removal of the native organ) (Welch, 1955). The liver was found to be less vulnerable to rejection than the kidney, but without portal inflow it rapidly atrophied and was thus unsuitable for studies of immunosuppression. This problem, combined with a belief at the time that the liver mediated rejection and that the grafted organ might be tolerated if the native liver was removed, soon prompted the development of the orthotopic procedure. Rejection was not prevented, but the orthotopic technique created an enduring model for experimental immunosuppression and a method of implantation that remains the standard today. With confidence in the surgical technique and useful experimental data on azathioprine and steroid-based immunosuppression, Starzl performed the first human liver transplant in Denver, Colorado, in 1963 on a 3-year-old child with biliary atresia (Starzl and Demetris, 1990). Four more liver transplants were attempted soon afterward, but all patients died within 23 days, most from primary ischaemic injury to the graft, but one intraoperative death was from haemorrhage. A self-imposed moratorium followed while Starzl considered technical refinements.

Calne moved from a pig model to clinical liver transplantation in Cambridge in 1967 (Calne, 1983). Starzl resumed clinical transplants in Denver and both continued experimental work on surgical technique, preservation, and immunosuppression. Despite a public and academic climate unfavourable to clinical transplantation following the disastrous 'Year of the Heart', they persevered with human liver transplants during the late 1960s and throughout the 1970s, making incremental progress. However, survival at 1 year remained less than 25%, and it was not until the discovery of cyclosporine and its introduction into clinical practice in the late 1970s that rejection could be controlled. This provided the breakthrough needed to move liver transplantation and the entire field of organ replacement into mainstream medical care.

The National Institutes of Health (NIH) Consensus Conference on Liver Transplantation in 1983 signalled recognition of the operation as worthy of broader introduction. At that time, four pioneering liver transplant centres (Denver, Cambridge, Hanover, and Groningen) presented results of 540 orthotopic liver transplant procedures, and demonstrated much better outcomes compared with matched controls with end-stage liver disease (ESLD) who were given conventional treatment. In cyclosporine-treated recipients, 1-year survival was 60%, versus 25–35% in the pre-cyclosporine era. Organ donation legislation, using the Harvard Criteria to define brain death, and other important advances in liver procurement and preservation facilitated the use of liver grafts from brain-dead donors, contributing to this success.

From 1983 continuing into the 1990s, a positive cycle was created that produced rapid growth in liver transplant procedures with long-term survival. Better results brought more referrals, and more experience yielded even better results. Specialists in a range of supporting disciplines were attracted to the challenges presented by transplant patients and brought wider expertise to liver transplant teams, further enhancing care. Today, according to the World Health Organization (WHO), more than 20,000 patients receive liver transplants each year. One-year survival is > 85–90%, while 5- and 10-year survival and quality of life for the majority of recipients are excellent. Advances in liver transplantation have also facilitated the development of intestinal and multivisceral transplantation.

### Evolution of surgical technique in liver transplantation (caval replacement versus piggyback and the introduction of venovenous bypass)

Although both main techniques of whole-liver grafting, namely caval replacement (classical) and caval preservation (piggyback), date from the first clinical descriptions in the 1960s, the relative simplicity and greater laboratory experience with caval replacement led to its rapid adoption as the standard method. Also, while in animal models full caval and portal clamping caused fatal splanchnic stasis and hypotension unless an extracorporeal portosystemic shunt was used, it was tolerated in humans without shunting, further reducing the incentive to apply the more demanding piggyback technique.

However, most of the early liver transplant recipients were children or relatively fit adults with tumours, and with more experience it became clear that some recipients tolerated caval clamping poorly. Moreover, the deteriorating state of the patient during the anhepatic phase meant that implantation needed to be performed quickly, by a very experienced surgeon, which made teaching difficult. Passive shunts were tried, but some clotted or caused fatal thromboembolism. In Cambridge, Calne developed a technique of venoarterial (femoral vein to femoral artery) pumped perfusion with heparinization and an oxygenator, which was implemented in five patients intolerant of a trial clamping of the inferior vena cava (IVC). This was reported to restore arterial blood pressure, clearly by increasing and redistributing arterial blood volume rather than supporting venous return. All survived the transplant but 4/5 died within a few weeks of surgery. An intraoperative death in Pittsburgh in 1982 partly attributed to severe splanchnic stasis led to development of a roller-pump-driven portofemoral to axillary (venovenous) bypass circuit with systemic heparinization (Denmark et al., 1983). Although this device was successful in several patients, deaths from uncontrolled bleeding soon followed. Late in 1982 a newly developed centrifugal pump, causing less turbulence than conventional roller pumps and already in use without heparin in patients on membrane oxygenators, was successfully used in animal transplant models. This was introduced in human liver recipients in 1983 and, with the later addition of heparin-bonded tubing, became standard care in adult liver transplants in Pittsburgh for the next 20 years (Shaw et al., 1984).

The adoption of venovenous bypass was widespread thereafter, given the pre-eminence of Pittsburgh in the development of liver transplantation and as the sole liver transplant surgical training centre in the US at the time. A percutaneous technique for outflow and return was developed independently in several centres in the mid-1980s, reducing the incidence of wound infection and lymphocele associated with venous cut-downs. These modifications continue to be used.

However, the routine use of venovenous bypass has declined progressively since 2000 for several reasons. First, many long-established programmes have used it only occasionally, including Cambridge (UK), London, Ontario, the University of Minnesota, and University of California, San Francisco, and it has never been used routinely in children. A number of fatalities have been associated with its use, mainly due to perforation of central veins when large-bore percutaneous access is used, and observational studies have not shown any clear benefit. Probably most significant is that the piggyback technique has become more widely practised, providing better haemodynamic stability by preserving some caval flow during the implantation phase.

## Evolution of anaesthesia and perioperative care in liver transplantation

Early descriptions of anaesthesia for clinical liver transplantation come from Denver (Aldrete, 1969), Cambridge (Calne, 1983; Carmichael et al., 1985), and Pittsburgh (Kang et al., 1985). J. Antonio Aldrete provided perioperative care for Starzl's first 180 liver transplants at the University of Colorado, Denver. In 1981, Starzl moved to the University of Pittsburgh, where Yoogoo Kang, John Sassano, Jose Marquez, Douglas Martin, and Ake Grenvik further defined the principles of liver transplant anaesthesia and critical care. John Farman and Michael Lindop successfully addressed the same challenges in Cambridge, working with Roy Calne. One author of this chapter (J.K.) trained as a resident in this unit from 1980.

During the early 1980s, the classic perioperative problems were identified, including profound haemodynamic instability after reperfusion (postreperfusion syndrome (PRS)), massive haemorrhage, hypocalcaemia, hypothermia, and acidosis. Changes in cardiac output and alterations in systemic vascular resistance were identified and noted in Pittsburgh (Martin et al., 1981) and Cambridge (Carmichael et al., 1985), the two leading liver transplant centres at that time. Cardiovascular depression due to citrate-induced hypocalcaemia was also recognized around the same time (Marquez et al., 1986). Transient but occasionally severe reperfusion hyperkalaemia was described, which remains an occasional cause of intraoperative cardiac arrest and death to this day. Use of the pulmonary artery (PA) catheter was routine in the early years both in the operating room and critical care setting but declined sharply after a randomized trial in sepsis published in 2005 demonstrated little benefit to its use. However, the oximetric PA catheter is still widely employed in cardiac surgery and liver transplantation, where the diagnosis and management of pulmonary hypertension and frequent measurement of cardiac index and mixed venous oxygen saturation ($SvO_2$) still provide compelling reasons for its use. Today, many centres are routinely using transoesophageal echocardiography (TOE) in liver transplantation, although often in combination with a PA catheter. Rapid point-of-care measurement of blood gases, available only from the late 1970s, was gradually extended to include sodium, potassium, ionized calcium, haemoglobin, and lactate over the next 20 years and has been a standard of care for many years.

General anaesthetic agents used in the earliest descriptions of liver transplantation included fluoroxene, trichloroethylene, and nitrous oxide. Halothane was widely used in the 1970s but avoided in liver surgery because of rare but severe hepatotoxicity. Enflurane (from 1975), isoflurane (from 1982 and still widely used), and later desflurane became the agents of choice, influenced by the work of Gelman and others on the effects of anaesthetic agents on splanchnic blood flow (Gelman et al., 1987). High-dose fentanyl (50–100 μg/kg) as a sole anaesthetic agent, then popular in cardiac surgery but associated with reports of awareness, was used in some centres in the 1980s but was largely replaced by the ultra-short-acting opiate remifentanil plus isoflurane or desflurane from the late 1990s.

Changes in coagulation and the use of coagulation tests including factor assays and serial thromboelastograms (TEG) were well described in early reports. Groth (1969) reported hyperfibrinolysis, unexpected venous thrombosis, treatment with epsilon-aminocaproic acid, and indications for fibrinogen, heparin, and protamine. He also observed that a functioning graft was critical to normalization of clotting. The use of fresh whole blood was described by Aldrete and also advocated by Farman (Carmichael et al., 1985). Kang et al. (1985) provided the first detailed report on the intraoperative use of TEG and on the diagnosis and management of hyperfibrinolysis in liver recipients, establishing TEG as a valuable point-of-care modality. It is now widely used and refinements continue to be developed (see Chapter 37).

The use of targeted antifibrinolytic therapy as demonstrated by Kang was extended to prophylactic use in many liver transplant units following the publication of a randomized trial of aprotinin in cardiac surgery. Significant reduction in blood loss during liver transplants was later demonstrated in double-blind randomized trials of tranexamic acid and aprotinin. However, aprotinin was removed from the market in 2008 when studies in cardiac surgery suggested an increased risk of multi-organ failure and death. Selective use of tranexamic acid for prophylaxis or treatment of established fibrinolysis continues in many units.

Further early improvements in perioperative care included adequate fluid warming, warm-water mattresses, and forced-air warming from the mid-1980s. Commercial cell salvage systems were developed in the early 1980s, coinciding with the rapid growth of cardiac and major vascular surgery and liver transplantation. Concerns about the safety of donated blood, given the epidemic of human immunodeficiency virus (HIV) at that time, and the rising costs of transfusion were major stimuli to the introduction of this technology. The first commercially available rapid infusion system (Haemonetics RIS, Braintree, Massachusetts) was developed in Pittsburgh by anaesthesiologist John Sassano in 1982. It used a fluid reservoir, mechanical roller pump, and countercurrent fluid warming and air detectors to deliver up to 1.5 L of blood per minute. This device became commercially available in the mid-1980s and was widely used in liver transplant and trauma centres until recently. More compact venous infusion systems such as the Fluid Management System (FMS) manufactured by Belmont Corporation (Braintree, Massachusetts) are now used in most liver transplant and trauma units and for combat casualty care (Chapter 37). Rapid infusion systems have proved indispensable in solid organ transplantation, especially multivisceral procedures.

### Fast-tracking and early postoperative care

Early reports of clinical liver transplantation describe elective postoperative ventilation for up to 24 hours (Calne, 1983; Carmichael et al., 1985). The rapid growth in surgical and anaesthetic experience through the 1980s and 1990s, introduction of shorter-acting anaesthetic agents, muscle relaxants, and analgesics, and better prevention of hypothermia and bleeding led to efforts to wean patients from mechanical ventilation earlier. Improved patient selection, shorter operative times, cost considerations, and limited availability of critical care beds also contributed. Several units reported safe extubation of selected patients in the operating room from the mid-1990s, and a multicentre trial demonstrated cost-effectiveness (Mandell et al., 2007). 'Fast-tracking', or extubation in the operating room with subsequent admission to a high-dependency area, is now well established, although in most units a policy of ICU admission and extubation within a few hours is usual. Safe early extubation after liver transplant depends on several key criteria, including good graft function, minimal comorbidity, and low operative blood loss.

### Trends in liver disease, donation, and organ allocation

Since 1990 the success of liver transplantation has led to a huge increase in referrals for treatment. Epidemics of hepatitis C, alcohol-related disease, non-alcoholic fatty liver disease, and hepatocellular carcinoma in aging populations have compounded this effect. However, the supply of heart-beating, donation after brain death (DBD) donors has been level or declining since the early 1990s, a result of demographic changes and improvements in traffic safety and emergency and critical care. Waiting-list mortality has increased, stimulating the development of alternative sources of organs for transplant. Technical innovations such as split-liver donation to two recipients have helped, but few donor livers are suitable for this. Livers from marginal donors are increasingly used, and research allowing better prediction of graft function in older and otherwise suboptimal donors continues.

Living donor liver transplantation (LDLT) has also developed to meet this need and to allow treatment of patients in countries where the use of heart-beating donors is outside cultural norms. LDLT programmes have grown rapidly since the first successful adult-to-child living donor procedure by Strong and Lynch in Brisbane in 1989 (Garcea et al., 2009). Although living donation peaked in the US in 2001 at over 500 transplants, it has since fallen in the US and Europe after donor deaths. Nonetheless, it is the main source of organs in Japan, Korea, Hong Kong, Taiwan, Turkey, India, and the Middle East. Recipient survival is now as good as that obtained in cadaveric donation, but significant donor morbidity and mortality remain a striking negative feature.

Donation after circulatory death (DCD) has been a source of donor organs for many years in some centres, particularly in Spain, but has recently gained wider acceptance in the US and in other European countries. This has the potential to make a significant difference to donation rates, although outcomes, especially in terms of biliary complications, remain poorer than those seen in DBD. Research into improved preservation techniques in this setting, including normothermic extracorporeal membrane oxygenation (ECMO), continues (Magliocca et al., 2005).

The management of waiting lists and organ allocation has evolved significantly since 1985. The choice of recipient from among size- and blood group-matched peers was typically carried out by transplant centre physicians, based on geography, subjective judgements of need or benefit based on poorly validated prognostic scoring, or even length of time on the waiting list. A move to a 'sickest first' model based on the Model for End-stage Liver Disease (MELD) was implemented in the US in 2002 and has now been adopted in varying forms in most other countries. The MELD score is derived from three simple laboratory assays—International Normalized Ratio of the prothrombin time (INR), creatinine, and bilirubin—and was developed at the Mayo Clinic, Rochester, Minnesota, to predict survival in ESLD patients after transjugular intrahepatic portosystemic shunting (Malinchoc et al., 2000). It has been shown to predict transplant waiting-list mortality and to improve overall survival when used to prioritize listed patients, although exception rules are needed in conditions such as hepatocellular carcinoma. This allocation system has been criticised, however, since it does not maximize 'transplant benefit' or life-years gained after transplantation.

## Worldwide growth, regulation, and academic organizations

The number of organ transplant programmes in the US and Europe increased rapidly after the introduction of cyclosporine in 1979–80 and following NIH endorsement of liver transplantation in 1983, slowing only in the mid-1990s when the donor supply reached a plateau. From about 2000, economic development initiated a second phase of rapid expansion, mainly in China, Eurasia, the Middle East, India, and South America. Living donation has accounted for much of this growth. Established in Japan, Korea, and China since the mid-1990s, living donor programmes have grown rapidly in Turkey, Egypt, and India since 2005, and continued expansion is likely. There are now more than 500 liver transplant centres in 81 countries across the world (Wahlia and Schumann, 2008; Busuttil, 2010) and many more kidney transplant programmes. The number of intestinal and multivisceral transplant programmes has also increased steadily since the turn of the century.

Organizations to promote and coordinate organ procurement and distribution and to monitor and maintain standards in organ transplantation have been created in all countries in which national legislation addressing transplantation has been passed. The best known is the United Network for Organ Sharing (UNOS), which funds the Scientific Registry of Transplant Recipients (SRTR) in the US. There are comparable bodies in European, Australasian, Asian, and South American countries, although data quality, transparency of outcomes, and overall effectiveness are reported to vary between organizations.

National and international academic societies contribute enormously to progress in the field by supporting education, mentorship, and research and by advising on standards. These include the following:

- International Liver Transplantation Society (ILTS)
- The Transplantation Society (TTS)
- American Association for the Study of Liver Diseases (AASLD)
- European Association for the Study of the Liver (EASL)
- American Society of Transplantation (AST)
- European Society of Organ Transplantation (ESOT)
- American Society of Transplant Surgeons (ASTS)
- Liver Intensive Care Group of Europe (LICAGE)
- European Liver and Intestinal Transplant Association (ELITA)
- Society for the Advancement of Transplant Anesthesia (SATA)

Many smaller national societies are also very active in the field.

## Conclusion

Despite the remarkable progress in organ transplantation achieved thus far, important challenges remain, many of which could be effectively addressed by anaesthesiologists and intensivists in the perioperative period. Key goals include increasing the supply of donor organs, improving the preservation of organs from non-heart-beating and extended criteria donors, optimizing the long-term function and survival of transplanted grafts, and preserving function in other organs. All of these could be pursued in interventional studies led by perioperative and critical care physicians. Well-designed observational studies relating to the care of organ donors and recipients in the perioperative period would also greatly enhance progress in this field. Initiatives to collect standardized data on comorbidity, perioperative techniques, and outcomes should be supported. Efforts in this direction are underway, supported by many of the authors in this book.

## References


Aldrete JA (1969) Anesthesia and intraoperative care. In: Starzl TE, Putnam CW (eds) *Experience in Hepatic Transplantation*, pp. 83–111. WB Saunders, Philadelphia.

Belzer FO, Sterry Ashby B, Englebert Dunphy J (1967) 24-Hour and 72-hour preservation of canine kidneys. *Lancet*, **290**(7515):536–539.

Belzer FO, D'Alessandro AM, Hoffmann RM, et al. (1992) The use of UW solution in clinical transplantation: a 4-year experience. *Ann Surg*, **215**(6):579–585.

Bradley JA, Hamilton DN (2001) Organ transplantation: an historical perspective. In: Hakim NS, Danovitch GM (eds) *Transplantation Surgery*. Springer, London.

Busuttil RW (2010) International Liver Transplantation Society 2009 presidential address: the internationalization of liver transplantation. *Liver Transpl*, **16**:558–566.

Calne RY (ed) (1983) *Liver Transplantation: The Cambridge-King's College Hospital Experience*. Grune and Stratton, London.

Carmichael FJ, Lindop MJ, Farman JV (1985) Anaesthesia for hepatic transplantation: cardiovascular and metabolic alterations and their management. *Anesth Analg*, **64**:108–116.

Collins GM, Bravo-Shugarman M, Terasaki PI (1969) Kidney preservation for transportation. Initial perfusion and 30 hours' ice storage. *Lancet*, **2**(7632):1219–1222.

Cooper JD, Pearson FG, Patterson GA, et al. (1987) Technique of successful lung transplantation in humans. *J Thorac Cardiovasc Surg*, **93**:173–181.

Denmark SW, Shaw BW Jr, Starzl TE, Griffith BP (1983) Veno-venous bypass without systemic anticoagulation in canine and human liver transplantation. *Surg Forum* **34**:380–382.

Garcea G, Nabi H, Maddern GJ (2009) Russell Strong and the history of reduced-size liver transplantation. *World J Surg*, **33**(8): 1575–1580.

Gelman S, Dillard E, Bradley EL Jr (1987) Hepatic circulation during surgical stress and anesthesia with halothane, isoflurane, or fentanyl. *Anesth Analg*, **66**(10):936–943.

Groth CG (1969) Changes in coagulation. In: Starzl TE, Putnam CW (eds) *Experience in Hepatic Transplantation*, pp. 159–175. WB Saunders, Philadelphia.

Gubernatis G, Pichlmayr R, Lamesch P, et al. (1990) HTK-solution (Bretschneider) for human liver transplantation. *Langenbecks Arch Chir*, **375**(2):66–70.

Hamilton D (2012) *A History of Organ Transplantation*. University of Pittsburgh Press, Pittsburgh.

Hamilton DN, Reid WA (1984) Yuri Voronoy and the first human kidney allograft. *Surg Gynecol Obstet*, **159**(3):289–294.

Kang YG, Martin DJ, Marquez J, et al. (1985) Intraoperative changes in blood coagulation and thrombelastographic monitoring in liver transplantation. *Anesth Analg*, **64**(9):888–896.

Le Gallois M (Julien Jean Cesar) (1813) *Expériences sur le principe de la vie*. Translated by NC and JG Nancrede. Experiments on the principle of life, and particularly on the principle of the motions of the heart, and on the seat of this principle: including the report made to the first class of the institute, upon the experiments relative to the motions of the heart. M. Thomas, Philadelphia. Microform in English, 1813.

Magliocca JJF, Magee JC, Rowe SA, et al. (2005) Extracorporeal support for organ donation after cardiac death effectively expands the donor pool. *J Trauma*, **58**(6):1095–1102.

Malinchoc M, Kamath PS, Gordon FD, Peine CJ, Rank J, ter Borg PC (2000) A model to predict poor survival in patients undergoing transjugular intrahepatic porto-systemic shunts. *Hepatology*, **31**(4):864–871.

Malinin TI (1996) Remembering Alexis Carrel and Charles Lindbergh. *Heart Inst J*, **23**(1):28–35.

Mandell MS, Stoner TJ, Barnett R, et al. (2007) A multicenter evaluation of safety of early extubation in liver transplant recipients. *Liver Transpl*, **13**(11):1557–1563.

Marquez JM Jr, Martin D (1986) Anesthesia for liver transplantation. In: Winter PW, Kang YD (eds) *Hepatic Transplantation*, pp. 44–57. Praeger, New York.

Marquez J, Martin D, Virji MA, et al. (1986) Cardiovascular depression secondary to ionic hypocalcemia during hepatic transplantation in humans. *Anesthesiology*, **65**(5):457–461.

Martin DJ, Marquez JM, Kant JG, Shaw BW, Pinsky MR (1981) Liver transplantation: hemodynamic and electrolyte changes seen immediately following revascularization. *Anesth Analg*, **63**:246A.

Matevossian E, Kern H, Hüser N, et al. (2009) Surgeon Yurii Voronoy (1895–1961)—a pioneer in the history of clinical transplantation: in memoriam at the 75th anniversary of the first human kidney transplantation. *Transpl Int*, **22**(12):1132–1139.

Miller DJ (2004) Sydney Ringer; physiological saline, calcium and the contraction of the heart. *J Physiol*, **555**(Pt 3):585–587.

Murray JE, Lang S, Miller BJ, et al. (1956) Prolonged functional survival of renal autografts in the dog. *Surg Gynecol Obstet*, **103**:15.

National Institutes of Health (1984) National Institutes of Health Consensus Development Conference Statement: Liver Transplantation, 20–23 June. *Hepatology*, **4**:107S–110S.

Pasque MK, Cooper JD, Kaiser LR, et al. (1990) Improved technique for bilateral lung transplantation: rationale and initial clinical experience. *Ann Thorac Surg*, **49**:785–791.

Shaw BW Jr, Martin DJ, Marquez JM, et al. (1984) Venous bypass in clinical liver transplantation. *Ann Surg*, **200**(4):524–534.

Starzl TE, Demetris AJ (1990) *Liver Transplantation: A 31-Year Perspective*. Year Book Medical Publishers, Chicago.

Starzl TE, Demetris, AJ, Van Thiel D (1989) Liver transplantation. *N Engl J Med*, **321**:1014–1022.

Toledo-Pereyra LH (1984) A study of the historical origins of cardioplegia. Dissertation/thesis in English.

Toledo-Pereyra LH, Simmons RL, Najarian JS, Condie RM (1976) Effective use of silica gel fraction for kidney preservation after 2-yr room storage. *Surg Forum*, **27**(62):311–312.

Wahlia A, Schumann R (2008) The evolution of liver transplant practices. *Curr Opin Organ Transpl*, **13**(3):275–283.

Welch CS (1955) A note on transplantation of the whole liver in dogs. *Transpl Bull*, **2**:54–55.

# CHAPTER 2

# The development of organ donation systems and regulatory bodies in the United States

Nikole Neidlinger, Sean Van Slyck, and Daniel M. Bruggebrew

## The Uniform Anatomical Gift Act

The original Uniform Anatomical Gift Act (UAGA) was promulgated in 1968. Accepted in every jurisdiction, the UAGA formally created the power to donate organs to any potential recipient that might need an organ to survive. In 1987, the National Conference of Commissioners on Uniform State Laws revised the UAGA to address changes in circumstances and in practice. Only 26 US states enacted the 1987 UAGA, resulting in non-uniformity. The 2006 UAGA was an effort to resolve inconsistencies and produce more effective nationwide organ sharing.

The 2006 Act further simplifies the document of gift and accommodates driver's licence 'donor dots' and similar registrations. Importantly, this version of the UAGA strengthens the language that bars others from overriding the potential donor's decision to make an anatomical gift. The practice of organ procurement organizations (OPOs) seeking affirmation even when the donor has clearly made a gift has occasionally resulted in a reversal of the donor's wishes. If an individual does not prepare a document of gift, organs may still be donated by the legal next-of-kin or designee. Further, the 2006 UAGA encourages and establishes standards for donor registries and better enables OPOs to gain access to these registries (Uniform Law Commission, 2006).

## The development of interhospital and regional sharing

Until the mid-1960s transplant surgeons matched donors and recipients mainly by blood type, with recipients waiting for a matching donor in the same hospital where they were being treated. At Leiden University in the Netherlands, Dr Jon J. van Rood experimentally determined that, beyond blood type alone, the HLA-type of donors and recipients influenced the outcome of kidney transplantation (Jansen, 2007). However, the probability of finding a donor with a matching tissue type within a limited geographic region was low. To make the best possible matches, van Rood needed a central database of all patients waiting for a donor kidney.

So, van Rood founded Eurotransplant in 1967. Twelve transplant centres in three countries volunteered to share their transplant candidates' information. At the end of 1970 Eurotransplant was active at 68 centres in six countries: Austria, Belgium, Luxembourg, West Germany, the Netherlands, and Switzerland. Eventually Switzerland withdrew from Eurotransplant, but in 1999 Slovenia joined, followed by Croatia in 2007.

In 1969 three hospitals in London described the requirements and organization for improving the matching of random cadaveric kidneys by prospective tissue typing and exchanging of kidneys between centres. They utilized computer analysis of the frequency of 13 HLA specificities in a population of 180 renal patients and healthy volunteers in the London region to show that a pool size of greater than 120 is required to enable close matching (one or less difference between donor and recipient) of all kidneys that become available (Festenstein et al., 1969).

In similar American studies in the late 1960s it was found that 'matched' kidney transplantation had superior outcomes, both for graft and recipient survival, over 'mismatched' (Lee et al., 1967). With this understanding, and with the recent development of preservation solutions to maintain kidneys outside of the human body for limited times by hypothermic maintenance, regional sharing soon became a reality in the US as well (Tanaka et al., 1971). The Southeastern Regional Organ Procurement Program (SEROPP) was founded in 1968 and was composed of eight institutions including Johns Hopkins University and Georgetown University. By 1971, at the University of California, Los Angeles, 864 waiting recipients from 61 transplant centres in the US and Canada were on a computerized waiting list, maintained by the National Transplant Communications Network, which facilitated interhospital cooperation and sharing of kidneys (Terasaki et al., 1971).

SEROPP became the Southeast Organ Procurement Foundation (SEOPF) in 1975, and by 1982 there were active members throughout the US. SEOPF implemented the first computer-based organ matching system, the 'United Network for Organ Sharing' (UNOS), in 1977. Five years later SEOPF established the Kidney Center for round-the-clock assistance in placing donated organs. Further, in 1984, UNOS separated from SEOPF and was incorporated as an independent non-profit organization.

## The National Organ Transplant Act

The National Organ Transplant Act (NOTA), passed by the US Congress in 1984, provides authority to the Secretary of Health and Human Services (HHS) to make grants for the planning, establishment, reimbursement, and certification of OPOs (US Congress, 1984). The US was divided into geographical regions and assigned to local OPOs to ensure effectiveness in the procurement and distribution of organs. NOTA stipulates that OPOs shall:

- Identify and acquire all usable organs from potential organ donors
- Arrange for the acquisition and preservation of donated organs
- Arrange for tissue typing and disease testing

## The Organ Procurement and Transplantation Network

NOTA calls for the Organ Procurement and Transplantation Network (OPTN) to be operated by a private, non-profit organization under federal contract. Responsibilities of the OPTN include:

- Developing and operating a secure internet-based computer system to maintain the nation's organ transplant waiting list and recipient/donor organ characteristics
- Facilitating the organ matching and placement process through the use of a computer system and a fully staffed Organ Center operating twenty-four hours a day
- Developing consensus-based policies and procedures for organ recovery, allocation, and transportation
- Collecting and managing scientific data about organ donation and transplantation
- Providing data to the government, the public, students, researchers, and the Scientific Registry of Transplant Recipients, for use in the field of solid organ allocation and transplantation
- Providing professional and public education about donation and transplantation, the activities of the OPTN, and the critical need for donation

Under US federal law, all transplant centres and OPOs must be members of the OPTN to receive funds through Medicare. Other members of the OPTN include independent histocompatibility laboratories involved in organ transplantation; relevant medical, scientific, and professional organizations; relevant voluntary health and patient advocacy organizations; and members of the general public with a particular interest in donation and/or transplantation.

## The United Network for Organ Sharing

On 1 October 1986, after being awarded a federal contract by the Health Resources and Services Administration (HRSA), UNOS officially began administering the OPTN (Pierce, 1996). Between 1983 and 1986 the OPTN/UNOS wait-list system grew from 5,120 to 9,681 renal candidates and from 97 to 892 extrarenal candidates awaiting donation. Due to the rapid growth of the wait-list it was realized that a universal organ allocation policy was necessary for fair and equitable distribution (Williams et al., 2004).

The first national guidelines were established using former SEOPF policies and algorithms that had been developed at the University of Pittsburgh (Starzl et al., 1987). This method continues to operate today by use of an interconnected system for donor–recipient matching:

- Potential transplant recipients are listed in the wait-list system by organ type
- Donors are registered through the DonorNet® system
- At the time of organ allocation, donor-specific 'match runs' are generated, taking into account UNOS policies, that place all potential transplant recipients in real-time rank order by organ type

Today UNOS maintains a centralized computer network, UNet℠, which links all OPOs and transplant centres. UNet℠ maintains listings for 123,203 potential transplant candidates as of 26 February 2015, and that number continues to rise.

## The Final Rule

Effective 16 March 2000, the HHS implemented a Final Rule establishing a regulatory framework for the structure and operations of the OPTN. Under the terms of the Final Rule, policies intended to be binding upon OPTN members are developed through the OPTN committees and Board of Directors and then submitted to the Secretary for final approval. The Final Rule requires that the OPTN shall admit and retain the following as members: all OPOs, transplant hospitals participating in the Medicare or Medicaid programmes, and other organizations, institutions, and individuals that have an interest in the fields of organ donation or transplantation (Department of Health and Human Services, 1998).

## The governing body of OPTN/UNOS

OPTN/UNOS policies are developed by its members through a committee system using a data-driven, democratic, process. The success of this system is dependent on thousands of hours of volunteer time by both professional and lay members (Williams et al., 2004). The Board of Directors—which consists of 41 elected members representing transplant coordinators; OPOs; histocompatibility experts; transplant candidates, recipients, donors, and donor family members; transplant hospitals, physicians, and surgeons; professionals in transplant-related fields such as medical examiners, hospital administration, and emergency personnel; and the general public—is the governing body that oversees and participates in developing policies for operating the OPTN (Department of Health and Human Services, 1998).

OPTN/UNOS committees develop and review proposed policies and provide assessments to the Board of Directors, taking into account historical, legal, and operational considerations, as well as public comments. The President, with approval of the Board of Directors, appoints the chairs and members of committees for 2-year terms (two exceptions are the Patient Affairs and Ethics Committees members who serve 3-year terms). There are currently 22 committees, including Kidney Transplantation, Minority Affairs, and Paediatric Transplantation Committees, with approximately 400 members.

## HIV-positive donors and PHS increased risk guidelines

Developed in 1994 by the Centers for Disease Control and Prevention (CDC), the Public Health Service guidelines designate organ donors as 'increased risk' if they meet any of the criteria for increased-risk behaviours that present an increased chance of HIV transmission (Rogers et al., 1994). This designation is intended to alert and protect transplant candidates from the risks of infection, because even negative antibody testing of potential donors does not entirely eliminate the possibility of disease transmission due to the window period between infection and seroconversion (Kucirka et al., 2009). In 2013, the CDC updated these guidelines in a document meant to provide guidance to organ procurement and transplantation personnel with regard to reducing the risk of HIV, hepatitis B virus, and hepatitis C virus transmission through organ donation (Seem et al., 2013).

In 1988, an amendment to the NOTA explicitly stated that potential organs from individuals known to be infected with HIV shall not be procured for transplantation. However, HIV is no longer a medical contraindication to transplantation, and since 1990 has become a manageable chronic disease. For HIV-infected candidates on the organ waiting list, HIV-infected deceased donors could attenuate the organ shortage and wait-list mortality. Deceased HIV-infected patients represent a potential of approximately 500–600 donors per year. In the current era of HIV management, a legal ban on the use of these organs may be unwarranted (Boyarsky et al., 2011). In November 2013, US President Barack Obama signed the HIV Organ Policy Equity Act, also known as the HOPE Act, which ended the ban on use of HIV-positive organs (Rhodan, 2013). Though organs from HIV-positive donors have not yet been utilized, the HOPE Act paved the way for critical research to identify best practices for organ transplants between HIV-positive donors and recipients.

## The structure of organ procurement organizations

### Geographic boundaries of organ allocation in the US

Prior to NOTA, many OPOs were operating independently in regions around the US. For instance, the New England Organ Bank was established as the nation's first OPO in 1968, with its mission being to serve Massachusetts and the surrounding states (Ojo et al., 2005). Today there are 58 federally designated OPOs, with each transplant centre being a member of a single OPO. Because of the historical boundaries prior to NOTA, there is wide variation among OPOs in terms of geographical size (multiple states versus a single metropolitan area), population served (1.2–17.4 million people), and number of eligible deaths for organ donation (6–14% of all hospital deaths) (Ojo et al., 2005). Additionally, there is wide variety in quality performance metrics among OPOs, including rates of referral of eligible donors from local hospitals and rates of authorization from next-of-kin (Nathan et al., 2003).

With some exceptions, organs procured from deceased donors within the boundaries of an OPO are preferentially allocated to waiting recipients listed at local transplant centres that are members of that OPO, then to potential recipients in the OPO's region (one of eleven), and finally to those waiting in the nation. There are 11 regions in the US designated by UNOS for administrative purposes; each region contains several OPOs (UNOS, 2013a). The reason organs are allocated in this manner is historically based on the premise of 'local primacy'. Local primacy assumed when creating the allocation scheme that donation would be better supported and received by the public, as well as by hospital and OPO employees, if donated local organs would benefit local waiting patients (Roberts, 2001).

The end result is that the geographical boundaries for distributing organs historically was not be aligned with the geographical need or acuity of illness in waiting recipients in the same area. For many years, the organ being allocated was not offered to patients outside the OPO, regardless of their priority, until it has been refused for all of the patients within the OPO. Advocates of this system cite the benefit of minimizing cold ischaemia and travel time by preferentially allocating organs locally. Opponents of this system cite geographic inequities in waiting time and acuity of illness among wait-listed patients as a reason to consider different allocation schemes or different geographic borders in allocation versus the current system that uses boundaries of the OPO (Roberts, 2001).

Additionally, opponents of this system cited that the Final Rule expects 'equitable allocation of organs from most to least medically urgent... distributing organs over as broad a geographic area as feasable.' On 18 June 2013, a new UNOS policy (UNOS, 2013b) mandated that liver allografts from deceased donors be offered to candidates within the donor's UNOS region with a MELD score >35, regardless of whether these candidates are in the donor's local service area. The net effect was that regional allocation increased significantly (over local allocation), with expected increases in transport distance and time. Additionally, cold ischaemia time was largely unaffected and organ discard rates decreased (Feng et al., 2015). Following this broader sharing of liver allografts, a new kidney allocation system emerged on 4 December 2014, which encouraged broader national and regional sharing of kidneys to patients who are difficult to match, as well as patients with longest time on haemodialysis. The net effect of these changes has also been an increase in geographical sharing of organs (Hampton, 2015).

### Governing structure of the OPO

NOTA defined the composition of each OPO's governing Board of Directors as follows: a transplant surgeon from each transplant centre in the OPO, a physician with expertise in the field of neurology or neurosurgery, an individual with expertise in histocompatibility laboratory practices, members of the lay public, hospital administrators, intensive care or emergency department personnel, members of voluntary health organizations, and tissue-bank representatives. In addition, OPOs must employ an executive director to provide administrative guidance and a physician for medical consultation (Johnson and Broznick, 1996).

### Funding and financing of OPOs

Transplantation is often the only available therapy for end-stage organ failure. Today 80% of potential recipients are waiting for a kidney transplant. As a part of the End Stage Renal Disease (ESRD) Program, the federal government pays for medical treatment for nearly all Americans affected by kidney failure. While most ESRD patients are treated with dialysis, about 10% of patients are treated by kidney transplant. In 1972 a Social Security Amendment guaranteed access to kidney transplant for potential recipients regardless of ability to pay. As a result, Medicare Part A reimburses the costs of renal transplant (Holloway and Hauff, 2006). A subsequent law in 1974 established an 'organ acquisition cost center' to define the acceptable costs associated with acquiring a deceased donor kidney for transplantation. The costs included fees associated with identifying, managing, and recovering a deceased donor kidney, and included donor hospital fees, tissue typing, surgeons' fees, preservation materials, operating room cost, and administrative and overhead costs. These collective costs are referred to as the standard acquisition charge (SAC) (Festenstein et al., 1969, 1971). Since ESRD patients represent 80% of the US transplant waiting list, Medicare is the main source of financing for OPOs through the kidney SAC (Prottas, 1989).

There is tremendous variability in SAC for renal and extrarenal organs across the US, mainly due to the variation in demographics, size, performance, and geography of the OPO. For instance, some OPOs service a geographical area of several hundred thousand kilometres, and acquire the increased cost associated with travel throughout such a large area in order to provide a service. Regulatory aspects of procurement have also had an impact on cost. Even well-meaning legislative policies such as a 1997 Medicare ruling that all deaths be reported to the OPO have raised operating cost for OPOs, given the additional expense required to establish high-volume call centres to respond to the vast number of referrals (Holloway and Hauff, 2006). Despite the wide variance in costs and SAC, the key to efficient OPO operation lies in the ability to identify and convert at least 75% of eligible organ donors into actual donors, and to maximize the number of recovered and billable organs per deceased donor.

## Measuring OPO performance

As the federal government and the Centers for Medicare and Medicaid Services (CMS) oversee, and are a primary source of, OPO reimbursement, standard performance expectations and metrics have been developed to estimate the potential organ donor pool and to measure OPO performance (Ojo et al., 2005).

### The 'Collaborative'

As OPOs began public reporting of donation metrics in 2002, wide variation was identified in performance. The ability to identify and convert an eligible donor into an organ donor varied widely from 0 to 100%. Furthermore, data reporting identified that the vast majority of potential organ donors were found in a small number of acute care hospitals. This prompted a focus on 'best practices' by evaluating the highest-performing OPOs and acute care hospitals, referred to as the Collaborative.

The Collaborative was launched with the goal of creating a system that ensured timely referral of potential organ donors, effective screening and consent practices, optimal donor management, and efficient organ recovery systems. It was designed to swiftly identify best practices and distribute ideas, to promote quality improvement, and to achieve measurable and reproducible results. Some of the best practices identified included early referral of potential donors by hospitals, multidisciplinary team communication 'huddles' in the donation process, aggressive pursuit of every potential organ donor, and focus on donor family support and care. The Collaborative also implemented specific nationwide goals of a 75% donation rate, zero medical examiner denials, 100% of potential donor families approached by a trained requestor, and 100% timely referral rate.

The Collaborative created industry-specific standards and definitions based on best practices, and improved donation rates nationwide within 1 year by 10.8%. Among hospitals that participated in the Collaborative donation increased by 16%, versus only 9% in all other hospitals. The strategies identified through the Collaborative are continually analysed and improved upon to promote efficiency of OPOs (Shafer et al., 2006).

### Potential organ donors per million population

One method of establishing expectations for the potential organ donor pool has been statistical evaluation of populations based on the number and characteristics of deaths in a geographic region (Sheehy and Brigham, 2003). However, there are wide geographic disparities in causes, mechanisms, and locations of death across the US. Moreover, variation in end-of-life care and de-escalation of life-support practices may contribute to variation in potential organ donors (Ojo et al., 2005). These geographical differences are not amenable to intervention by the OPO or hospital; as such, additional means of defining potential donors have evolved.

### Eligible death

HRSA defines eligible deaths as heart-beating individuals aged 70 or below meeting the criteria for neurological death and having no exclusionary criteria for donation. The exclusionary criteria are defined by HRSA based on classification of disease codes and are listed in Box 2.1. Individuals who have been classified as having 'eligible deaths' more accurately represent the potential

**Box 2.1** Inclusionary criteria for eligible organ donors

Individuals aged 70 years or younger who have been declared dead by neurological criteria with no evidence of:

- Tuberculosis
- HIV
- Creutzfeldt–Jacob disease
- Herpetic septicaemia
- Rabies
- Reactive hepatitis B surface antigen
- Any retroviral infection
- Active malignant neoplasm other than primary central nervous system (CNS) or skin tumour
- History of lymphoma, leukaemia, or multiple myeloma
- History of aplastic anaemia
- Agranulocytosis
- Fungal or viral meningitis or encephalitis
- Gangrene of the bowel
- Extreme immaturity
- Miscellaneous carcinomas

donor pool and allow for more meaningful comparison of OPO potential. However, eligible deaths are discovered through a labour-intensive process of thorough review of hospital death records and rely on self-reporting by both hospitals and OPOs and are, therefore, subject to bias and variability (Ojo et al., 2005).

As the definition of eligible deaths encompasses those individuals who have met the criteria for neurological death, those patients with imminent neurological death or loss of brainstem reflexes that have not been formally declared brain dead by a physician will be omitted from the pool, as will individuals with donor potential who are older than 70 and heart-beating individuals who are candidates for donation after circulatory death. Though the eligible death rate is more accurate than population analysis, HRSA, OPTN, and OPOs are evaluating more accurate and meaningful methods of determining true donor potential.

### Conversion rate

The conversion rate is a measure of an OPO's donation rate. It is a calculation of the percentage of eligible deaths that became organ donors and is a surrogate for OPO performance. At the commencement of the 2003 Collaboratives, the mean conversion rate in the US was 51.5%; in 2014 it was 77.9% and above the national goal of 75%, though disparities remain among acute care hospitals and OPOs (Shafer et al., 2006; AOPO, 2014).

### Organs transplanted per donor

Once a deceased donor is identified and authorization for donation has been granted, evaluation and management of the potential donor becomes critical. A thorough medical, social, and behavioural history is obtained from the legal next-of-kin and serologic testing is performed. Neurological death is associated with a complex set of physiological disturbances, including haemodynamic instability, coagulopathy, metabolic and electrolyte imbalances, diabetes insipidus, endocrine insufficiency, and hypoxaemia. Prompt identification and management of these clinical derangements is paramount to effective care of the donor and preservation of organs for transplantation (Powner, 2006). The goal of all donation opportunities is to maximize the number of organs transplanted per donor (OTPD). OTPD, however, is complex and depends on many donor factors including age, comorbidity, and appropriate clinical management. In 2011, the mean number of OTPD across US donor service areas was 3.1 and varied widely depending on the classification of the donor (AOPO, 2011).

Individuals are classified as DCD if death is declared by circulatory rather than neurological criteria. These DCD donors have lower potential OTPD based on lower thoracic organ potential, as well as more stringent criteria for minimal time between extubation and declaration of death (warm ischaemia time). DCD donors represented 13% of the US donor pool in 2011 with an average OTPD of 2.

Expanded criteria donors (ECD) are donors who are older than 60 years or those who are older than 50 with two of the three following comorbidities: death by stroke, history of hypertension, or terminal creatinine of ≥ 1.5 mg/dL. ECD donors represented 22% of all deceased donors in the US in 2011 with an average OTPD of 1.85 (AOPO, 2011). Standard criteria donors (SCD) do not meet the criteria for ECD or DCD and represent younger, lower risk, healthier donors with higher potential number of organs for transplantation. The national goal for OTPD defined by the Collaborative is 3.75, and this represents a performance gap in the current procurement system. However, it is important to consider that donor shortages coupled with increased waiting time and demand continue to drive aggressive pursuit of individuals once considered to be unsuitable donors (Ojo et al., 2005). Each year the percentage of the donor pool represented by ECD and DCD increases.

## Responsibilities of OPOs

OPOs serve as intermediaries between community donor hospitals and transplant centres in their efforts to maximize every donation opportunity. Table 2.1 shows the interaction between the three estates during a typical donation process.

### Community and professional education

Predisposition of individuals toward the value of organ donation is one task of the OPO that is handled by the Community Development department. Through community outreach and education about organ donation, OPOs attempt to increase the number of people who are willing to donate. Public education includes focused attention on specialized groups such as high schools, local primary care clinics, faith-based societies, and minority and ethnic communities (AOPO, 2011).

Many OPOs also focus efforts on first-person authorization, primarily through drivers' licence bureaus. Approximately 42% of the US population has signed up on their state registry, and in 2011 the milestone of 100 million organ donors nationwide was achieved. At that time, Alaska and Montana boasted that 78% of licenced drivers had designated their intent to donate (Donate Life America, 2011). Signing up on the registry has earned the same authority as a legal advanced directive in many states and is referred to as 'first person authorization'. Signing up on the donor registry has been identified as one of the most important factors for families and legal next-of-kin when considering end-of-life options, as many families who do not authorize donation cite being unsure of the wishes of the deceased at the time they are approached (Siminoff, 2006).

### Hospital development

Organ recovery starts with identification of a potential donor referral from a donor hospital affiliated with the OPO. Of all the aspects of recovery, obtaining timely hospital referrals has been one of the most challenging, as the referrals most often come from physicians or nurses with no direct benefit in the organ donation process and whose attentions and responsibilities are directed elsewhere. The hospital development of an OPO focuses on persuading the medical staff at donor hospitals that involvement in organ donation is worth their personal and professional time, despite the lack of incentive other than to promote altruism. The Collaborative identified that 75% of potential organ donors are found in only 483 of the more than 6,000 acute care hospitals in the US (Shafer et al., 2006). These hospitals are, in general, larger trauma centres with specialized resources including neurologists and neurosurgeons.

This focus on fewer hospitals allows for targeted education and marketing of information on organ donation to affiliated hospitals and represents one of the most important areas of OPO outreach. In fact, most OPOs spend more time attempting to create collaborations and relationships with donor hospitals than they do in actual organ recovery. This is because donor hospitals represent

**Table 2.1** The three estates of organ donation and transplantation in the US (<http://optn.transplant.hrsa.gov/contentdocuments/optn_policies.pdf>)

| Donor hospital | OPO | Transplant centre |
|---|---|---|
| Refer potential donor to the OPO<br>◆ Ventilated patients with imminent death (GCS 3–5) | Receive and triage initial referral | *Independent of the donor process*<br>New patient referral |
| Optimize patient end-organ function<br>◆ Normalize electrolytes<br>◆ Treat diabetes insipidus<br>◆ Optimize pulmonary function | Onsite response to evaluate referral for suitability<br>◆ Absolute contraindications: HIV, metastatic cancer | Evaluate patient for listing |
| Brain death evaluation and declaration(s) | Provide family with grief support and authorization discussion<br>◆ Secure first person authorization or obtain written authorization | Patient wait-listed with UNOS |
| **Donor work-up**<br>Collaborate with OPO during donor work-up<br>◆ Physician consultations and procedures (echo, bronchoscopy, pathology, pharmacy, etc.) | ◆ Infectious disease testing (HIV, HCV, HBV, EBV, CMV), other optional tests (West Nile Virus, Chagas, Toxoplasmosis)<br>◆ Optimize end-organ function (steroid administration, normalize electrolytes, hormone replacement, etc.)<br>◆ Organ-specific evaluation (echo, cath, bronchoscopy, prerecovery liver biopsy) | Maintain patient on UNOS wait-list |
| **Organ allocation** | Commence organ allocation<br>◆ Execute UNOS organ-specific match runs<br>◆ Allocate via the DonorNet® electronic allocation system | Surgeon receives patient-specific organ offer<br>◆ Evaluate donor specifics<br>◆ Evaluate patient status (health and insurance status)<br>◆ Accept/decline the organ offer |
| **Organ recovery**<br>◆ Provide: operating room, anaesthesia support (for brain-dead donors), scrub tech, and circulator | ◆ Coordinate arrival of all recovery teams at donor hospital (flight vs ground transportation considerations)<br>◆ Organ perfusion: provide organ flush and storage supplies (Viaspan®, HTK, cardioplegia, pulmoplege, etc.)<br>◆ Ensure appropriate packaging and labelling<br>◆ Provide donor documentation<br>◆ Coordinate distribution of recovered organs to appropriate transplant centres | ◆ Identify appropriately qualified recovery surgeon(s)<br>◆ Send team to donor hospital to procure organ(s)<br>◆ Return to transplant centre with transplantable organ(s) |
| Donor placed in morgue (until mortuary recovers the body) | Postrecovery family notifications | Transplant surgery |
| Post-case follow-up with OPO<br>◆ Outcome data, process improvement, etc. | Family follow-up<br>◆ Immediate and long-term donor family correspondence<br>Opportunity for donor family and recipient contact | Post-transplant patient monitoring<br>◆ Immediate and long term |

GCS, Glasgow Coma Scale; HIV, human immunodeficiency virus; HCV, hepatitis C virus; HBV, hepatitis B virus; EBV, Epstein–Barr virus; echo, echocardiogram; CMV, cytomegalovirus; WNV, ; Chagas, ; Toxo, ; cath, cardiac catheterization; scrub tech, a technician who assists the surgeon during surgery; HTK, histidine–tryptophan–ketoglutarate.

the organ supply, in which there is a critical shortage, whereas organ distribution to transplant centres and surgeons is far less of a problem, given demand (Prottas, 1989).

## Donor family support and the organ donor authorization process

In order to succeed in converting potential eligible donors to actual donors, OPOs must obtain authorization for organ donation. Effective communication with the hospital staff and grieving family is paramount for success and has been extensively studied by the transplantation and donation community. Communication research has identified that the method of approach is pivotal in encouraging authorization. For instance, messages that dispel myths are more persuasive, as are statistical messages that include specific factual information about the donation process (Siminoff, 2006). Families report having questions about a potential increase in hospital bills, funeral arrangements, possible mutilation, ability to selectively decide which organs are donated, and other myths and misconceptions about access to transplantation. Addressing these issues as part of the discussion, even if the family has not raised them, has been shown to improve the donation authorization rate (Siminoff et al., 2001).

The environment in which the authorization process takes place also has an impact on the outcome. Appropriate timing and ability for the family to comprehend brain death contributed to an increase in authorization, whereas families who felt pressured or hurried were more likely to decline. Additionally, families who perceived the requestor as sensitive and empathetic to their needs were more likely to donate (Siminoff et al., 2001).

OPOs have developed specific training programmes in effective requesting, and the OPO family coordinator is specially trained to be the designated requestor for organ donation. Other aspects of successful requesting are creation of a supportive and private environment for the donation discussion, time spent gaining rapport with the family, passionate advocacy for organ donation, including positive messages and endorsement, and the ability to explain brain death in simple, unequivocal terms (Siminoff, 2006).

In addition to supporting donor families during the acute grieving process, OPOs have specially trained staff that assist families with bereavement literature, grief counselling and referrals, follow-up letters regarding case outcomes, donor family gatherings and support groups, and events to honour and remember organ donors. The OPO family department also coordinates correspondence between recipients and donor families and continues the support process for months to years following the death of a loved one.

### Clinical donor management

After the diagnosis of neurological death, focus shifts from that of saving a life to maintaining viable organs for transplantation. Brain death is accompanied by a myriad of clinical findings that can jeopardize end-organ function. The goal of the OPO's clinical services department is to maintain optimal organ function after death in order to ensure functional organs after transplantation.

Some of the changes associated with brain death include haemodynamic collapse, coagulopathy, loss of temperature regulation, electrolyte imbalance, pulmonary dysfunction, myocardial stunning, and endocrine abnormalities (Arbour, 2005). Although the specifics of donor management are beyond the scope of this chapter, OPO clinical services are aimed at maximizing the organ donation gift, and clinical pathways have been designed to guide the care of organ donors (Holmquist et al., 1999).

### Organ allocation

As evidenced in the earlier review of regulatory requirements (see section 'The United Network for Organ Sharing'), the common theme represented across all agencies is the need to ensure a system for the fair and equitable distribution of organs to those patients awaiting transplant (US Congress, 1984; Department of Health and Human Services, 1998). The organ allocation process commences when the potential organ donor is registered with DonorNet® and the OPO coordinator executes organ-specific match runs. These match runs serve as the list of potential transplant recipients, who are ranked according to such criteria as medical urgency, blood type, size matching, and wait-time. The OPO coordinator's role is to relay the relevant donor information to surgeons, or their representative, for each potential transplant recipient. The Final Rule stipulates that 'an "organ offer" is made when all information necessary to determine whether to transplant the organ into the potential recipient has been given to the transplant hospital' (Department of Health and Human Services, 1998). The organ offer process has evolved over time from one in which the OPO coordinator primarily utilized a verbal report of information over the phone to one in which the OPO coordinator now utilizes DonorNet® as the primary source of data transfer from the OPO to the surgeon (US Congress, 1984; Department of Health and Human Services, 1998).

OPOs utilize a variety of staffing models for their organ allocation efforts, ranging from off-site organ placement staff, usually in a call centre, to on-site organ procurement coordinators (those clinically managing the donor), or a combination of both. Additionally, UNOS staffs the 24-hour Organ Center with organ placement specialists who are meant to assist OPOs with organ allocation efforts.

### Surgical recovery

Once all organs are allocated, the OPO focuses on the next phase of the donor process: surgical recovery of the donated organs. The OPO is responsible for coordination of the surgical recovery teams, appropriate packaging and labelling of the recovered organs, ensuring appropriate transportation of the organ to the transplant programme, and postmortem donor care (Department of Health and Human Services, 1998).

Coordinating the arrival of multiple recovery teams (both local and non-local) in concert as required by UNOS policy, a common task of all OPOs, requires significant logistical efforts. With the continued focus on limiting geographic disparities in access to organs and the resultant changes to OPTN allocation policies, non-local recovery teams are travelling to distant locations with greater frequency to recover transplantable organs (Donate Life America, 2011).

During the intraoperative surgical recovery phase of the donation process, the host OPO often utilizes a specialized recovery staff member, in addition to the organ procurement coordinator, who is responsible for oversight of the surgical process. The recovery coordinator's role will vary depending on the OPO but often entails providing perfusion and packaging supplies for the recovery, assisting organ recovery staff with the room setup, assisting the surgical team with perfusion of the organs, documenting surgical findings in the donor record, and ensuring each organ is packaged and labelled in accordance with OPTN policy. Upon completion of the surgical recovery, the OPO recovery coordinator is responsible for transport of the donated organs to the respective transplant centres (US Congress, 1984). Once the surgical process is complete, the incision has been closed, and the surgical teams have departed, the OPO coordinator will assist hospital staff with postmortem care. .

## Notable organ sharing systems abroad

### Spain

The Spanish Transplantation Law was first enacted in 1979 and contained the basic elements of any transplantation law (Matesanz, 1998). In 1989 the Spanish National Transplant Organization

(ONT) was created, conceived as a technical agency of the Ministry of Health in charge of overseeing donation and transplantation activities in the country (Matesanz et al., 2011). The ONT arranges processes between donors and recipients based on criteria established by healthcare professionals, edits consensus documents, and promotes policies aimed at benefitting transplantation through a national forum (Manyalich et al., 2011). Any national decision is agreed upon by the Transplantation Commission of the Health Interterritorial Council, which is comprised of the ONT as chair and 17 regional coordinators (Matesanz et al., 2011).

The first transplant coordination team in Spain was created in 1985 at the Hospital Clinic of the University of Barcelona (Beltran et al., 1985). It was found that by incorporating transplant coordinators into medical institutions the activity of transplant programmes increased (Manvalich et al., 1997). The Transplant Procurement Management (TPM) project was launched in 1991, under the auspices of the University of Barcelona and with technical and financial support from the ONT, as a specialist professional training programme for transplant coordinators who are responsible for coordinating all aspects that make organ transplantation possible (Manyalich et al., 2011). These coordinators are in-house professionals and members of staff (the majority of whom are critical care physicians) at the 170 participating procurement hospitals (Matesanz et al., 2011).

### Japan

The Japan Kidney Transplant Network (JKTNW) was founded in April 1995 under the guidance of the Ministry of Health and Welfare, using UNOS as a model. Prior to its establishment, transplants were conducted mainly through kidney banks located in each prefecture, with recipients in the same facility as the donor usually given priority. Delayed enactment of necessary laws regarding organ transplants from brain-dead donors forced the JKTNW to limit its function to cadaveric kidney transplantation and to exclude the other solid organs from consideration. JKTNW set up a UNet$^{SM}$-like system whereby donors and recipients would be matched at the national level.

In 1997 the Organ Transplant Law took effect, reorganizing JKTNW into the Japan Organ Transplant Network (JOTNW), which expanded to heart and liver transplants in addition to kidneys. This law permitted donations of organs by a brain-dead donor only if '. . . the donor expressed in writing prior to death his/her intent to agree to donate his/her organs, and his/her family members did not object to the donation'. In 2009, in response to the Declaration of Istanbul, the issue was discussed in the Diet of Japan, and a bill to revise the Organ Transplant Act was promulgated. Rules regarding organ donation after brain death have been eased and even if an individual's intention is unclear, donation of his/her organs has become possible with family consent. As a result, donation of organs after brain death by children under the age of 15 has also become possible (Japan Organ Transplant Network, 2012).

### Iran

In Iran the Iranian Network for Organ Procurement (INOP) conducts organ allocation. The INOP is part of the Management Centre for Transplantation and Special Diseases, affiliated with the Ministry of Health and Medical Education. It maintains a national waiting list, and organ sharing follows a geographic distribution order (locally, then regionally, then nationally). Independent procurement units operate out of each medical science university, and these units interact with the INOP to facilitate organ exchange between centres (Kazemeyni et al., 2004).

## Worldwide authorization practices

The gap between the supply and demand of organs continues to be the rate-limiting step in achieving transplantation for all waiting recipients. The most common reason that potential organ donors are not converted to actual donors is the inability to obtain authorization (Hartwell, 1999). Organizations and task forces that have addressed barriers to authorization and donation have focused on authorization policies and how they impact organ donation. Internationally there are a wide variety of approaches to authorization, as well as a wide variability in the number of organ donors per million population, which ranges from 0.6 per million in Malaysia to 34 per million in Spain (Chow, 2011).

Historically, most countries used the policy of voluntary 'opting in' for donation in the early years of transplantation. However, in the 1980s, with unrest over the organ shortage and improving outcomes in transplantation, some nations abandoned this in favour of an 'opt-out' policy (Hartwell, 1999).

### Opt-in systems

The US, UK, Ireland, Denmark, Netherlands, and most countries in Latin America utilize the opt-in system. This system requires the explicit consent of the donor by signing up on the local donor registry or authorization of the donor's next-of-kin or authorizing party for those that have not indicated their intent via the registry. Opt-in systems allow individuals the autonomy to choose donation in the context of their own values and cultural and spiritual beliefs (Kazemeyni et al., 2004).

### Opt-out systems

The opt-out system was first utilized by Singapore, and several European nations have followed suit. Opt-out systems maintain the humanitarian idea that organ donation is the 'right thing to do' and that, unless they have specifically chosen not to donate, all individuals would desire to donate organs upon their death (also referred to as 'presumed consent'). Advocates of this system cite that this approach results in a higher rate of donation and life-saving transplants and is ethically justified in that it benefits society. Opponents cite that proceeding without discussing the process with a willing next-of-kin could result in missing critical past medical history (NHS Blood and Transplant, 2012). Additionally, opponents note that an individual's failure to 'opt out' may not necessarily be related to a desire to donate, but could instead indicate one's inability to understand the system, and that individual autonomy is lost.

Nations utilizing an opt-out policy include Austria, Spain, Belgium, Finland, Sweden, Portugal, the Czech Republic, Slovakia, Hungary, and Poland (Kazemeyni et al., 2004; Rithalia et al., 2009). However, these nations vary in actual practice. In some nations such as Austria, donation moves forward with little or no discussion with the next-of-kin, referred to as 'hard presumed consent'. In nations with this type of practice, families are told about organ donation in order to explain the time lapse between death declaration and the time when the remains will be available for burial (Hartwell, 1999). On the other hand, nations such as Spain practise 'soft' presumed consent. In Spain physicians involved with transplant coordination still ask the families about organ donation and ensure that the family does not object. Advocates of the Spanish system cite presumed consent as one reason for the high number of organ donors per million, but others cite different factors such as early identification and referral as the key to Spain's success.

The impact of presumed consent was the focus of a 2009 systematic review that attempted to identify the impact of this type of system on donation rates and attitudes toward donation (Rithalia et al., 2009). The review included five 'before-and-after' studies in nations with new legislation introducing presumed consent, as well as eight studies comparing nations with opt-in versus opt-out donation policies. Additionally, 13 surveys regarding attitudes toward donation were included. The study found that presumed consent appeared to increase organ donation rates after the legislation was introduced but that the studies did little to address possible confounding factors or biases that may have impacted the results. Presumed consent was associated with increases of 21–30% and with 2.7–6.1 more donors per million population; however, other important factors were identified that impacted donation rate and were not associated with presumed consent. Attitude surveys showed support for presumed consent in recent studies in the UK, though results were variable (Rithalia et al., 2009).

### Professional societies

Along with the growth of transplantation and the development of OPOs came a multitude of professional societies dedicated to supporting the evolving field of donation and transplantation. While certainly not an exhaustive list, here are a few notable professional societies:

- The Association of Organ Procurement Organizations (AOPO) is the professional organization representing the 58 OPOs in existence today that is 'dedicated to the special concerns of OPOs, providing education, information sharing, research and technical assistance and collaboration with other healthcare organizations and federal agencies'. AOPO began as the Association of Independent Organ Procurement Agencies in 1984 and adopted its current name in 1988 when its standards were adopted by the Health Care Financing Administration and subsequently applied to the entire OPO community. AOPO offers a voluntary peer-review accreditation process, based upon its ethical and organizational standards, which occurs every 3 years.
- The North American Transplant Coordinators Organization (NATCO) is a volunteer association, which was formed in 1976 in an effort to address transplant coordinators' educational needs. NATCO continues to thrive today, with focused efforts on legislative and regulatory advocacy, education, collaboration, and communication and social media.
- The American Society of Transplant Surgeons (ASTS) was founded in 1974 in an attempt to unite transplant surgeons in the up and coming field of transplant. ASTS is committed to 'fostering and advancing the practice and science of transplantation for the benefit of patients and society' and its membership is over 2,000 surgeons, scientists, physicians, and allied health professionals.
- The International Society for Heart and Lung Transplantation (ISHLT) is a 'professional organization dedicated to improving the care of patients with advanced heart or lung disease through transplantation, mechanical support and innovative therapies via research, education and advocacy'. ISHLT began in 1981 and now has over 2,500 members from all over the world who are responsible for the treatment and management of end-stage heart and lung disease.

## Conclusion

The field of organ transplantation is rooted in legislation that defines the circumstances and conditions of death, the process of organ donation, the organizational framework for the procurement and sharing of donated organs, and guidelines for the protection of the rights and dignity of organ donors and their families, as well as prohibitions on the commercialization of organs. The critical elements in this process were identified immediately after the first transplantation of cadaveric organs and have remained essentially unaltered in the intervening years. The main theme represented across all organ procurement and recovery agencies worldwide is the need to ensure a system for the fair and equitable distribution of donated organs of the highest quality possible for the benefit of patients awaiting transplantation. Internationally there are a wide variety of approaches to organ procurement and allocation. These agencies will continue to evolve to ensure that every available donated organ serves the purpose of prolonging the quality of life of those patients who receive them.

## References


AOPO (2011) *Data on Donation and Transplantation.* <http://www.aopo.org/related-links-data-on-donation-and-transplantation/>.

Arbour R (2005) Clinical management of the organ donor. *AACN Clin Issues*, **16**:551–580; quiz 600–601.

Beltran JJ, Fornaguera JM, Manalich M, Sentis J, Planella VL, Nalda MA (1985) Removal of organs from patients attended in an emergency resuscitation unit. *Rev Esp Anestesiol Reanim*, **32**:234–235.

Boyarsky BJ, Hall EC, Singer AL, Montgomery RA, Gebo KA, Segev DL (2011) Estimating the potential pool of HIV-infected deceased organ donors in the United States. *Am J Transplant*, **11**:1209–1217.

Chow TS (2011) WHO: rate of donation in Malaysia among lowest in the world. *George Town Star*, 6 June. <http://thestar.com.my/news/story.asp?file=/2011/6/6/nation/8844674&sec=nation>.

Department of Health and Human Services (1998) *The 'Final Rule'. Department of Health and Human Services 42 CFR Part 121 Organ Procurement and Transplantation Network; Final Rule (63 Federal Register 16295, at 16332, April 2, 1998).* <http://www.nap.edu/openbook.php?record_id=9628&page=199>.

Donate Life America (2011) *Donate Life America announces 100 millionth organ, eye, and tissue donor registered in the U.S.* <http://donatelife.net/donate-life-america-announces-100-millionth-organ-eye-and-tissue-donor-registered-in-the-u-s/>.

Feng S, O'Grady J (2015) Share 34: a liver in time saves lives? *Am J Transplant*, **15**:581–582.

Festenstein H, Oliver RT, Hyams A, et al. (1969) A collaborative scheme for tissue typing and matching in renal transplantation. *Lancet*, **2**:389–391.

Festenstein H, Oliver RT, Sachs JA, et al. (1971) Multicentre collaboration in 162 tissue-typed renal transplants. The London and Regional Transplant Group, March, 1969, to December, 1970. *Lancet*, **2**:225–228.

Hampton T (2015) New kidney allocation system. *JAMA*, **313**(4):346.

Hartwell L (1999) Global organ donation policies around the world. *Contemp Dialysis Nephrol*, December.

Holloway GK, Hauff HM (2006) The economics of organ donation and transplantation. In: Lapointe Rudow D, Ohler L, Shafer T (eds) *A Clinician's Guide to Donation and Transplantation*. NATCO, Lenexa, Kansas.

Holmquist M, Chabalewski F, Blount T, Edwards C, McBride V, Pietroski R (1999) A critical pathway: guiding care for organ donors. *Crit Care Nurse*, **19**:84–98; quiz 99–100.

Jansen J (2007) Jon van Rood: pioneer at the crossroad of human leukocyte antigens and transplantation. *Transfus Med Rev*, **21**:159–163.

Japan Organ Transplant Network (2012) *Organ Transplanting in Japan*. <http://www.jotnw.or.jp/english/>.

Johnson HK, Broznick BA (1996) Organ procurement organizations. In: Phillips MG (ed) *UNOS Organ Procurement, Preservation and Distribution in Transplantation*, 2nd edn. UNOS, Richmond, Virginia.

Kazemeyni SM, Bagheri Chime AR, Heidary AR (2004) Worldwide cadaveric organ donation systems (transplant organ procurement). *Urol J*, **1**:157–164.

Kucirka LM, Namuyinga R, Hanrahan C, Montgomery RA, Segev DL (2009) Formal policies and special informed consent are associated with higher provider utilization of CDC high-risk donor organs. *Am J Transplant*, **9**:629–635.

Lee HM, Hume DM, Vredevoe DL, Mickey MR, Terasaki PI (1967) Serotyping for homotransplantation. IX. Evaluation of leukocyte antigen matching with the clinical course and rejection types. *Transplantation*, **5**(Suppl):1040–1045.

Manyalich M, Cabrer C,Sanchez-Ibanez J, et al. (1997) The Spanish model: keys to procurement: transplant procurement management. In: Phillips G, Strong DM, von Versen R, Nather A (eds) *Advances in Tissue Banking*. World Scientific, Hackensack, New Jersey.

Manyalich M, Mestres CA, Balleste C, Paez G, Valero R, Gomez MP (2011) Organ procurement: Spanish transplant procurement management. *Asian Cardiovasc Thorac Ann*, **19**:268–278.

Matesanz R (1998) Cadaveric organ donation: comparison of legislation in various countries of Europe. *Nephrol Dial Transpl*, **13**:1632–1635.

Matesanz R, Dominguez-Gil B, Coll E, de la Rosa G, Marazuela R (2011) Spanish experience as a leading country: what kind of measures were taken? *Transpl Int*, **24**:333–343.

Nathan HC, Held P, McCullough K, Pietroski RS, Ojo A (2003) Organ donation in the United States. *Am J Transpl*, **3**:29–40.

NHS Blood and TransplantUnited Kingdom Transplant (2012) *Opt In or Opt Out*. <http://www.uktransplant.org.uk/ukt/newsroom/statements_and_stances/statements/opt_in_or_out.jsp>.

Ojo A, O'Connor K, McGowan J, Dickinson D (2005) Quantifying organ donation rates by donation service area. *Am J Transpl*, **5**:958–966.

Pierce GE (1996) UNOS history. In: Phillips MG (ed) *Organ Procurement, Preservation, and Distribution in Transplantation*. UNOS, Richmond, Virginia.

Powner DJ (2006) Adult clinical donor care. In: Shafer T, Zampiello F, Chessare J, Wagner D, Perdue J (eds) *A Clinician's Guide to Donation and Transplantation*. NATCO, Lenexa, Kansas.

Prottas JM (1989) The organization of organ procurement. *J Health Politic Pol Law*, **14**:41–55.

Rhodan, M. (2013) President signs HOPE Act, clearing the way for HIV-positive organ donation. *Time*, 22 November 2013.

Rithalia A, McDaid C, Suekarran S, Myers L, Sowden A (2009) Impact of presumed consent for organ donation on donation rates: a systematic review. *BMJ*, **338**:a3162.

Roberts JP (2001) *Prioritization and Distribution of Organs for Liver Transplantation*. CenterSpan, <http://www.centerspan.org/pubs/liver/roberts1.htm>.

Rogers MF, Simonds RJ, Lawton KE, Moseley RR, Jones WK (1994) Guidelines for preventing transmission of human immunodeficiency virus through transplantation of human tissue and organs. Centers for Disease Control and Prevention. *MMWR Recomm Rep*, **43**:1–17.

Seem DL, Lee I, Umscheid CA, Kuehnert MJ (2013) PHS guideline for reducing human immunodeficiency virus, hepatitis B virus, and hepatitis C virus transmission through organ transplantation. *Public Health Reports*, **128**:247.

Shafer T, McBride V, Zampiello F, Chessare J, Wagner D, Perdue J (2006) The organ donation breakthrough collaborative. In: Lapointe Rudow D, Shafer T (eds) *A Clinican's Guide to Donation and Transplantation*. NATCO, Lenexa, Kansas.

Sheehy E, Brigham LE (2003) Estimating the number of potential organ donors in the United States. *New Engl J Med*, **349**:667–674.

Siminoff L (2006) Requesting organ donation: effective communication. In: Shafer T, Zampiello F, Chessare J, Wagner D, Perdue J (eds) *A Clinician's Guide to Organ Donation and Transplantation*. NATCO, Lenexa, Kansas.

Siminoff LA, Hewlett J, Arnold RM (2001) Factors influencing families; consent for donation of solid organs for transplantation. *JAMA*, **286**:71–77.

Starzl TE, Hakala TR, Tzakis A, et al. (1987) A multifactorial system for equitable selection of cadaver kidney recipients. *JAMA*, **257**:3073–3075.

Tanaka N, Stevens LE, Terasaki PI (1971) Storage and transport of 83 human kidneys by simple hypothermia. *Transplantation*, **12**:348–352.

Terasaki PI, Wilkinson G, McClelland J (1971) National transplant communications network. *JAMA*, **218**:1674–1678.

Uniform Law Commission (2006) *Anatomical Gift Act (2006)*. <http://www.nccusl.org/actsummary.aspx?title=anatomical gift act>.

UNOS (2013a) *UNOS Facts and Figures*. <http://www.unos.org/docs/unos_factsfigures.pdf>.

UNOS (2013b) *Code of Federal Regulations, Title 42, Part 121.8*. UNOS, Richmond, Virginia.

US Congress (1984) The National Organ Transplant Act. In: *Public Law 98-507, 98 stat 2339*. Weekly compilation of presidential documents.

Williams MC, Creger JH, Belton AM, et al. (2004) The Organ Center of the United Network for Organ Sharing and twenty years of organ sharing in the United States. *Transplantation*, **77**:641–646.


## Further reading


AOPO: <http://aopo.server280.com/public-education-a45>.

ASTS: <http://www.asts.org>.

Eurotransplant International Foundation: <http://www.eurotransplant.org/cms/index.php?page=history>.

ISHLT: <http://www.ishlt.org/>.

JOTNW: <http://www.jotnw.or.jp/english/03.html>.

NATCO: <http://www.natco1.org/>.

NHS Blood and Transplant: <http://www.uktransplant.org.uk/ukt/newsroom/statements_and_stances/statements/opt_in_or_out.jsp>.

OPTN: <http://optn.transplant.hrsa.gov/policiesandbylaws/policies.asp>; <http://optn.transplant.hrsa.gov/members/bodqa.asp>; <http://optn.transplant.hrsa.gov/publiccomment/pubcommentpropsub_238.pdf>.

Transplant Living: <http://www.unos.org/donation/index.php?topic=organ_allocation>.

UNOS: <http://www.unos.org>; <http://www.unos.org/donation/index.php?topic=history>; <http://www.unos.org/donation/index.php?topic=organ_allocation>; <http://www.unos.org/donation/index.php?topic=fact_sheet_1>.

# CHAPTER 3

# Organ donor allocation and transplant logistics: the European perspective

Gabriela A. Berlakovich and Thomas Soliman

## Donor selection

The demographics of the donor population have changed since 1995. This is due in part to the fact that mortality after motor vehicle crashes has decreased; however, this has also meant a progressive decline in the availability of grafts from optimal and standard donors (i.e. < 40 years old). Therefore if criteria for organ donation had remained unaltered, donation activity would have dramatically decreased. To overcome this gap, donor criteria had to be extended. For example, donor age increased significantly in all solid organ transplants, but the most impressive increase was seen among liver donors. Actually the median age of a liver donor is the same as for a kidney donor (Figure 3.1).

DBD remains the main source of transplantable organs, particularly by expanding the donor pool through the greater acceptance and use of ECD. This trend has applied to all solid organs since around 1995. Compared to donor demographics in the US, the European donor population employs a higher proportion of ECD, especially with regard to age and cause of death (Braat et al., 2012).

A distinct alternative source of donor organs has been DCD. Europe has had a leading role in the development of the concept of 'non-heart-beating' donation (Booster et al., 1993; Wijnen, 1995). There are two principal types of DCD donor. Donor protocols differentiate between 'controlled' and 'uncontrolled' DCD donors, and these have been subclassified into four subtypes (Kootstra et al., 1995). DCD categories I (dead on arrival) and II (resuscitation attempted without success) are classified as uncontrolled DCD, and because of the severe haemodynamic instability and a long warm ischaemic time mostly only kidneys are procured from these donors. In contrast, in DCD categories III (awaiting cardiac arrest at the ICU) and IV (cardiac arrest while brain-dead diagnostic) cardiac death occurs under controlled conditions. The recent increase in DCD in some European countries has contributed to an increase in the number of transplants. But still, not all European countries have specific legislation mandating the use of DCD donors for organ transplantation. However, in those countries that adhere to the legal framework for DCD, the use of these organs has not necessarily resulted in an increase in the total number of organs transplanted. The biggest concern about DCD is that these donors are not considered a reliable source of viable grafts. As data from the Netherlands (Roels and Rahmel, 2011) and the UK (Monbaliu et al., 2012) indicate, the use of DCD organs has merely caused a shift from potential DBD (heart-beating donors) to DCD (Figures 3.2 and 3.3).

Furthermore, there is evidence that intensive care professionals are encouraging DCD to avoid prolonging the ICU management until brain death occurs. However, this trend may have been reversed in the last few years (Dominguez-Gil et al., 2011). A second specific problem with DCD is that the procedure results in an extended period of warm ischaemia from circulatory arrest and is followed by cold ischaemia, which causes a more pronounced reperfusion injury with an elevated incidence of primary non-function and delayed graft function. However, at least in kidney transplantation, long-term patient and graft survival are almost identical to DBD (Barlow, 2009). In the future, extracorporeal machine perfusion immediately following circulatory arrest may mitigate ischaemia–reperfusion injury of these grafts. Various techniques to mitigate ischaemic injury of these grafts have been investigated in animal studies and clinical investigations (Moers et al, 2009; Luer et al, 2010; Cobert et al., 2011; Fondevila et al, 2011; Gallinat et al, 2012). Preliminary data indicate that extracorporeal perfusion immediately following cardiac death may have the ability to 'recondition' the damaged organ that has undergone warm ischaemic injury during DCD procurement. Considering organ shortage and death on the waiting list, DCD grafts remain a small but valuable source of organs, with potential to play a more important role in organ donation in the future.

Besides expanding the deceased donor pool, another way of overcoming the organ shortage is the widespread promotion of living donation. The patients who may benefit the most are those suffering from ESRD, with the advantage of potentially pre-emptive living donor kidney transplantation (Meier-Kriesche and Kaplan, 2002). Huge disparities exist among European countries in terms of rates of living donor kidney transplantation, ranging from < 10% to > 50% of all kidney transplants performed. The reason

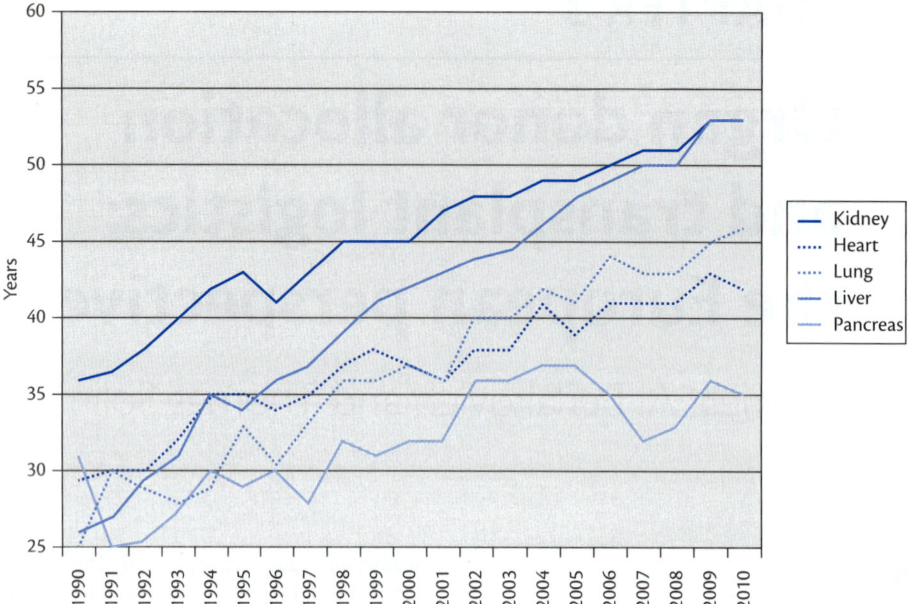


**Fig. 3.1** Median age of deceased donors used for a transplant in Eurotransplant. (Reproduced from Eurotransplant International Foundation (2013) <http://www.eurotransplant.org>. Retrieved March 2013.)

might be differences in the availability of deceased organs, as well as major cultural differences.

## Legislation

National donor legislation is quite different among European countries. These differences mainly concern two types of consent for donation from deceased donors. With 'presumed consent', organ donation is automatically considered in deceased persons, unless prior to dying they had previously specifically registered their wish not to donate. Several countries with presumed consent law have developed a non-donor registry in order to collect persons' objections during life. However, the registration rate in these registries is rather low. Another option for documentation of presumed consent is keeping a written statement in the form of an official document (e.g. a driver's licence or national identification card). In these cases, no formal request of the potential donor family is required before proceeding with organ procurement. In practice, in most countries with presumed consent the families are informed about organ procurement for transplantation, although there exists no requirement by law to do so. Mostly this is an attempt to determine whether the deceased person ever objected to organ donation during his or her lifetime.

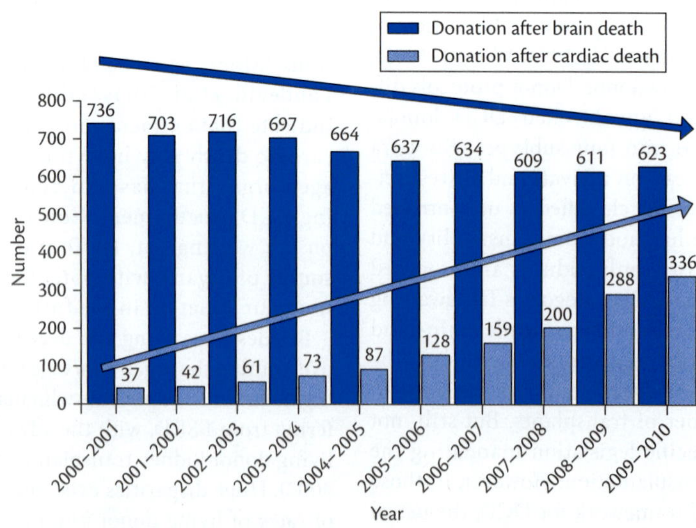


**Fig. 3.2** In the UK, an increase in the number of DCD donors is accompanied by a decrease in the number of DBD (Monbaliu et al., 2012). (This figure was published in *Journal of Hepatology*, 56, Monbaliu et al, 'Liver transplantation using Donation after Cardiac Death donors', pp. 474–485, Copyright © 2012 Elsevier and the European Association for the Study of the Liver (EASL).)

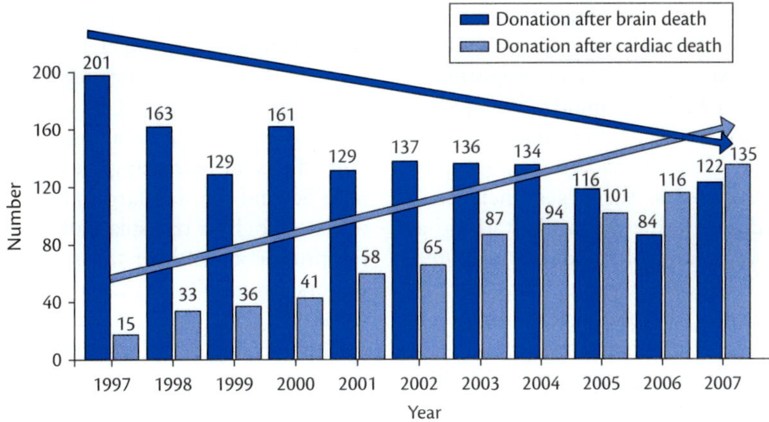


**Fig. 3.3** In the Netherlands, an increase in the number of DCD donors is accompanied by a decrease in the number of DBD (Roels and Rahmel, 2011). (Reproduced with permission from Roels L, and Rahmel A, 'The European Experience', *Transplant International*, 24, pp. 350–367, Wiley. © 2011 Roels, L. & Rahmel. Transplant International © 2011 European Society for Organ Transplantation.)

The other principle that governs organ donation is informed consent, i.e. that deceased persons have to have given explicit consent for organ donation during their lifetime. In the absence of such informed consent, most laws require the deceased's next-of-kin to consent to postmortem removal.

Similar to non-donor registries, the registration rate for organ donation is quite low. Since the early 1990s several educational programmes based on the Spanish model have been established in Europe. Transplant coordinators, nurses, and physicians are trained in communication, especially in delivering bad news to the family in an appropriate and compassionate manner, and can present families with the option of organ donation at the same time (Blok, 1999; Roels et al., 2002).

## Transplant logistics

As a general rule, OPOs try to achieve optimal use of available donor organs and to provide society with a transparent and objective allocation system. Furthermore, they assess risk factors for waiting-list mortality and study transplant outcomes. Last but not least, OPOs promote, support, and coordinate organ donation and transplantation. In Europe OPOs are organized at the national level, such as in Spain, France, and Italy, or regionally (multinational level), such as in Scandinavian countries. However, even within a multinational OPO framework, national legislation takes precedence over the international interests of the organization, i.e. presumed or informed consent for organ donation.

Scandiatransplant is the regional organ exchange organization of the Nordic countries and covers a population of 24.5 million inhabitants in five countries (Denmark, Finland, Iceland, Norway, and Sweden). NHS Blood and Transplant covers the UK and Republic of Ireland, with a total population of 65.4 million. Eurotransplant International Foundation is the largest European OPO and covers Central Europe, with a population of 124.7 million inhabitants in seven countries (Austria, Belgium, Croatia, Germany, Luxemburg, the Netherlands, and Slovenia).

Organ-specific rules for allocation are comparable among the different OPOs in Europe. Usually deceased organs are allocated to blood-group-identical patients on the waiting list for reasons of justice and equity. In living donation, compatible blood groups are accepted, as there is no immunological disadvantage. Moreover, in recent years protocols for ABO-incompatible living donation kidney transplantation have been standardized (Wilde et al., 2009). Patient and graft survival as well as kidney function among ABO-incompatible living donor kidney transplants have been comparable to those of ABO-compatible living donor kidney transplants, with an incidence of antibody-mediated rejection reported to be 0% (Genberg, 2010).

For paediatric transplantation there are special regulations with a priority status in all European countries and paediatric donor organs are allocated preferentially to paediatric recipients.

### Kidney

Protocols for allocation of kidneys follow an algorithm that takes into account donor and recipient immunological matching (cross-match, percentage panel reactive antibodies, HLA-A, HLA-B, HLA-donor–recipient (DR) matching), waiting time, and donor region. The latter is considered in order to avoid long-distance shipping of organs, thereby keeping cold ischaemic times short and maintaining an even balance of donated organs and kidney transplants within a country/region. Despite this effort, immunological matching and waiting time take precedence over other considerations, resulting in kidneys having the highest exchange rates across OPOs, with the exception of Scandiatransplant. In the Nordic countries the overall exchange rate of deceased kidneys has stabilized at around 12% in recent years, with one-third of kidney transplants performed from living donors (Grunnet, 2010). As mentioned in the section 'Donor selection', in kidney transplantation there is clear-cut evidence for a significant advantage in post-transplant survival after living donation (Meier-Kriesche and Kaplan, 2002). Despite immunological mismatch, the rate of delayed graft function is significantly lower than in DBD kidneys because of the extremely short cold ischaemic time and perfect organ quality.

In contrast to other solid organ transplants, kidneys from DCD donors have had a major impact on overall numbers of donors, with DCD representing a proportion of up to 30–40% of total deceased donors (Roels and Rahmel, 2011) in some countries. The incidence of delayed graft function is about two-fold higher than in DBD kidneys, but the management of the perioperative period with renal replacement therapy is not challenging and long-term graft survival is comparable to DBD kidney transplantation (Barlow, 2009).

In kidney allocation there exist more special programmes than in any other organs, e.g. for highly immunized recipients, long-waiting recipients (> 5 years), and very old recipients.

Since the 1990s there have been significant demographic changes in both donors and recipients. The largest increase in patients awaiting deceased donor kidney transplantation has been in the group aged 65 years and older (de Fijter, 2009). Consequently, an 'old for old' allocation strategy was devised in many European programmes whereby aged kidneys are preferentially allocated to aged recipients irrespective of HLA mismatch. In the Eurotransplant Senior Program (ESP), kidneys from donors over 65 years are assigned with priority to registered ESP recipients. In order to keep cold ischaemic time as short as possible these kidneys are preferentially allocated to local recipients with panel reactive antibodies < 5% without prospective HLA matching (Frei, 2008). A new initiative is the Eurotransplant Senior DR-compatible Program (ESDP), which considers full HLA-DR compatibility, defined as zero HLA-DR mismatches, while maintaining the ESP principle (de Fijter, 2009).

## Liver

Protocols for liver allocation are similar in all European OPOs and consist of a two-tiered candidate system, defined by medical urgency. In this scheme allocation is prioritized for high urgency (HU) requests. HU liver candidates are defined as recipients with acute liver failure without pre-existing liver disease (e.g. fulminant hepatitis B, intoxication, Wilson's disease) or acute retransplantation because of primary non-function or graft thrombosis early after transplantation. All other candidates enter a second-tier priority allocation, which is based on the MELD score. HU requests that do not fit standard criteria are audited.

In HU requests the next-available appropriate organ within an OPO is offered to the requisitioning transplant centre. Liver exchange thereafter follows a payback system, which means that the recipient centre has to offer the next-available donor liver of the same blood group to the previously donating centre. Second priority goes to approved combined organ (ACO) transplantation, third priority to local allocation within the donor region, and fourth priority to allocation within the OPO. In non-HU requests allocation is performed more or less according to the MELD score (Wiesner, 2001), which predicts the waiting-list survival at 3 months. Since the severity of some underlying liver diseases is not reflected in the laboratory MELD score, standard exceptions (match MELD) were defined. Countries are divided into those pursuing a patient-based allocation system according to match MELD and those following a centre-oriented allocation system, where medical urgency is usually defined by MELD but waiting time still plays a role.

According to an initiative within NHS Blood and Transplant, donor livers are not allocated to patients but are centre-specific, as per the 'Donor Organ Sharing Scheme' prepared by the Liver Advisory Group. Following these general principles, DR matching should be provided, especially for livers derived from donors with extended criteria. Remarkably, within Scandiatransplant the liver is the most frequently exchanged organ among centres, followed by the heart.

Since the 1990s the limited supply of suitable liver grafts has been insufficient to meet the still-rising demand for organs. Against this background, regardless of the various organ allocation policies adopted by different transplant programmes, waiting-list mortality remains a major concern. The most important efforts for increasing the liver donor pool are extending criteria beyond the standard in brain-death donors (ECD) and the initiation of liver transplantation from DCD donors. An increasing proportion of liver transplants are now derived from DCD donors (Monbaliu et al., 2012), especially in the Netherlands (21%), Belgium (18%), and the UK (12%). However, the biliary epithelium is particularly vulnerable to ischaemia–reperfusion injury and a high incidence of biliary strictures and/or bile cast syndrome (de Vera, 2009; Detry, 2010) has become a concern. Ischaemic cholangiopathy has been reported in 9–50% of DCD recipients, leading often to graft loss and retransplantation. Furthermore, as in all DCD transplants, the rate of primary non-function and delayed graft function is significantly higher in DCD livers compared to DBD livers. In all other organ transplants artificial devices to support failing organs are available as a bridge to transplantation, such as renal replacement therapy in patients with end-stage kidney disease or ventricular assist devices and extracorporeal membrane oxygenation for patients with end-stage heart disease. Unfortunately the only treatment modality for ESLD is transplantation. Patient and graft survival rates similar to those of DBD liver transplantation can be achieved by using controlled DCD grafts but only after very restrictive criteria are employed, despite a higher risk of biliary stricture (Dubbeld, 2010).

LDLT is predominantly performed in paediatric recipients; adult-to-adult has no significant impact on overall numbers. The reasons might be that the willingness for donation as well as the number of suitable donors is quite low and the outcome is inferior compared to deceased whole liver transplantation. Recipients have a higher risk of primary non-function or dysfunction due to small-for-size and a significantly higher risk of technical failures, especially biliary and vascular complications. Additionally, the mortality risk of 0.2% and morbidity risk of 11–28% for donors represent non-negligible limitations for the use of LDLT grafts. Actually, LDLT accounts for less than 5% of liver transplants in Europe (according to the European Liver Transplant Registry (ELTR) and OPTN).

## Pancreas

The procedure for pancreas allocation is rather simple and comparable among the European OPOs. Allocation for vascularized pancreas transplantation is primarily patient-oriented. The main issue is active waiting time, and national recipients are prioritized over international patients in order to minimize cold ischaemic time.

Patients listed for pancreas only and combined kidney–pancreas transplantation have equal access to donor organs. Special requests are reserved for acute retransplantation due to graft thrombosis.

Pancreas transplant activity among European countries and even among different centres within a country is likely to be multifactorial. Various proportions of pancreas utilization from deceased donors are observed and the rate of organs accepted for transplantation and finally transplanted differs from 20% to 80% (according to Eurotransplant) and may reflect the increasing number of aged deceased donors. The numbers of deceased donors and other solid organ transplantation increased in most countries, but pancreas transplant activity showed variability regardless of these evolutions (González-Posada et al., 2010).

Despite the trend in other solid organ transplants, donor criteria are implemented very slowly and carefully, as can be seen in the acceptance of donor age since the 1990s. Only a slight increase in donor age can be observed in pancreas donors, and the median age still shows younger than in all other organ donors (Figure 3.1). The preprocurement pancreas allocation suitability score (P-PASS) developed from the Eurotransplant database (Vinkers, 2008a) considers donor age, body mass index, length of stay in the ICU, pre-existing cardiac arrest, serum sodium level, serum amylase or lipase level, and use of vasopressive agents. Unfortunately, P-PASS did not reach broad implementation in practice due to conflicting results (Vinkers, 2008b; Schenker, 2010).

On the other hand, the pancreas transplant waiting list has increased significantly since 2005, especially by accepting older recipients, while the number of donor organs has been stable or even decreased (according to Eurotransplant; González-Posada et al., 2010). A recent analysis from a European center demonstrated that graft survival and the risk of death from cardiovascular complications was not significantly different between recipients with an age younger than 50 years and 50 years plus. The group 50 plus had selective cardiovascular work-up during evaluation, in 94% coronary angiography was performed, and as long as coronary lesions were correctable by stenting or bypass, the candidate was accepted for pancreas transplantation (Schenker, 2011).

Considering an incidence of about 30% reoperation following pancreas transplantation, with consequently negative impact on patient and graft survival (Perez-Saez, 2011), DCD and living donation actually have not had an impact on the number of pancreas transplantations, but promising results have been published by single centers (Fernandez, 2005; Sutherland, 2012).

## Thoracic organs

The ranking of potential recipients in Europe is mainly based on medical urgency status and waiting time. In multinational OPOs the country balance is also considered for allocation. Requests for an HU status are regulated by audits. Transplantation of ACO is subject to audits, with prioritization following the urgent status.

In practice the allocation algorithm is rather complicated, at least in Eurotransplant, as there are two HU statuses, the HU national status and the HU international status, respectively. Furthermore, there exist several diverging national and international regulations.

Expanding the donor pool in heart transplantation is nearly exclusively limited to ECD, primarily older donors, vasopressor requirement, and donor hearts with some degree of abnormalities by echocardiography (Wittwer and Wahlers, 2008; Smits, 2012). Donor hearts with one- or two-vessel coronary artery disease requiring back-table coronary bypass grafting before transplantation are not accepted anymore because of poor outcome (Marelli, 2003). Heart transplantation in the setting of domino transplantation has no significant impact on overall numbers. Since 2008 only one living donor heart transplant has been performed within the Eurotransplant area.

Lung donor shortages have resulted in the critical appraisal of deceased donor criteria and relaxation of strict guidelines in DBD (Aigner, 2005; Smits, 2011; Schiavon, 2012). Ex-vivo perfusion for reconditioning of initially rejected donor lungs (Aigner, 2012; Sanchez, 2012) appears to be a promising development but is actually only performed in especially experienced centers. Moreover, successful techniques such as segmental resection and lobe transplantation have been developed (Aigner et al., 2004). Therefore transplantations of lungs from DCD (de Antonio and de Ugarte, 2008; De Vleeschauwer, 2009; Zych, 2012) as well as from living donors have increased over the past few years.

A very recent initiative within some regions in Eurotransplant is the lung allocation score (LAS) that was implemented in the US in 2005. Recipient-derived and outcome-oriented variables are considered within the LAS but donor-derived variables are not integrated. The score is constructed using estimated mortality on the waiting list and the probability of success following lung transplantation. According to this allocation policy, the patient with the highest medical urgency and the greatest expected benefit is the first to receive the lung.

# Conclusion

Looking at a map, you may find in some typical European way a great number of different systems for donor allocation and transplant logistics. Side by side there are pure national as well as binational and multinational organizations to coordinate local clinical transplantation activities. Moreover, different countries even in the same organization often have different legislation about organ donation regardless of whether based on informed or presumed consent, which might have consequences for DBD, DCD, and living donation.

However, despite this great organizational disparity, allocation itself and donor selection are very similar within these organizations, following the same evidence-based guidelines that are used in almost all established transplant centers throughout the world. Finally, all organizations are common in facing the problem of organ shortage. Their first general strategy to overcome this problem was to expand the donor criteria mainly by accepting older donors and implementing age-matched programs like the ESP; the second sustained attempt was to initiate DCD in order to widen the potential number of organ donors; and, last but not least, they increased the number of eligible grafts from these donors.

So, in coming years, organ shortage will continue to be the main focus of the work of all European organizations for donor allocation and transplant logistics, leading to a closer, particularly scientific, cooperation between these organizations.

# Acknowledgements

We thank Andreas Zuckermann, MD (Division of Cardiac Surgery), for providing us with information on the allocation and transplantation of thoracic organs.

# References

Aigner C, Mazhar S, Jaksch P, Seebacher G, Taghari S, Marta G (2004) Lobar transplantation, split lung transplantation and peripheral segmental resection—reliable procedures for downsizing donor lungs. *Eur J Cardio-Thorac Surg*, **25**:179–183.

Aigner C, et al. (2005) Extended donor criteria for lung transplantation—a clinical reality. *Eur J Cardio-Thorac Surg*, **27**:757–761.

Aigner C, et al. (2012) Clinical ex vivo lung perfusion—pushing the limits. *Am J Transplant*, **12**:1839–1847.

Barlow, AD, Metcalfe MS, Johari Y, Elwell R, Veitch PS, Nicholson ML (2009) Case-matched comparison of long-term results of non-heart beating and heart-beating donor renal transplants. *Br J Surg*, **96**:685–691.

Blok, GA, Van Dalen J, Jager KJ, et al (1999) The European Donor Hospital Education Programme (EDHEP): addressing the training needs of doctors and nurses who break bad news, care for the bereaved, and request donation. *Transpl Int*, **12**:161–167.

Booster MH, Wijnen RM, Ming Y, Vroeman JP, Kootstra G. (1993) In situ perfusion of kidneys from non-heart-beating donors: the Maastricht protocol. *Transplant Proc*, **25**:1503–1504.

Braat AE, Blok JJ, Putter H (2012) The Eurotransplant donor risk index in liver transplantation: ET-DRI. *Am J Transplant*, **12**:2789–2796.

Cobert ML, Merritt ME, West LM, Jessen ME, Peltz M (2011) Differences in regional myocardial perfusion, metabolism, MVO2, and edema after coronary sinus machine perfusion preservation of canine hearts. *ASAIO J*, **57**:481–486.

de Antonio DG, de Ugarte AV (2008) Present state of nonheart-beating lung donation. *Curr Opin Organ Transpl*, **13**:659–663.

de Fijter JW (2009) An old virtue to improve senior programs. *Transpl Int*, **22**:259–268.

Detry O, Donckier V, Lucidi V, et al. (2010) Liver transplantation from donation after cardiac death donors: initial Belgian experience 2003–2007. *Transpl Int*, **23**:611–618.

de Vera ME, Lopez-Solis R, Dvorchik I, et al. (2009) Liver transplantation using donation after cardiac death donors: long-term follow-up from a single center. *Am J Transplant*, **9**:773–781.

De Vleeschauwer S, Van Raemdonck D, Vanaudenaerde B, et al. (2009) Early outcome after lung transplantation from non-heart-beating donors is comparable to heart-beating donors. *J Heart Lung Transplant*, **28**:380–387.

Dominguez-Gil B, Haase-Kromwijk B, Van Leiden H (2011) Current situation of donation after circulatory death in European countries. *Transpl Int*, **24**:676–686.

Dubbeld J, Hoekstra H, Farid W, et al. (2010) Similar liver transplantation survival with selected cardiac death donors and brain death donors. *Br J Surg*, **97**:744–753.

Fernandez LA, Di Carlo A, Odorico JS, et al.(2005) Simultaneous pancreas–kidney transplantation from donation after cardiac death: successful long-term outcomes. *Ann Surg*, **242**:716–723.

Fondevila C, Hessheimer AJ, Maathuis MH, et al. (2011) Superior preservation of DCD livers with continuous normothermic perfusion. *Ann Surg*, **254**:1000–1007.

Frei U, et al (2008) Prospective age-matching in elderly kidney transplant recipients—a 5-year analysis of the Eurotransplant Senior Program. *Am J Transplant*, **8**:50–57.

Gallinat A, et al (2012) Hypothermic reconditioning of porcine kidney grafts by short-term preimplantation machine perfusion. *Transplantation*, **94**:809–813.

Genberg H, et al (2010) Isoagglutinin adsorption in ABO-incompatible transplantation. *Transfus Apher Sci*, **43**:231–235.

Grunnet N, Bödvarsson M, Jakobsen A, Kyllönen L, Pfeffer P, Sørensen SS (2010) Scandiatransplant report 2009. *Transplant Proc*, **42**:4429–4431.

Kootstra G, Daemen JH, Oomen AP (1995) Categories of non-heart-beating donors. *Transplant Proc*, **27**:2893–2894.

Luer B, Koetting M, Efferz P, Minor T (2010) Role of oxygen during hypothermic machine perfusion preservation of the liver. *Transpl Int*, **23**:944–950.

González-Posada JM, Marrero D, Hernández D, et al. (2010) Pancreas transplantation: differences in activity between Europe and the United States. *Nephrol Dial Transplant*, **25**:952–959.

Marelli D, et al (2003) Results after transplantation using donor hearts with preexisting coronary artery disease. *J Thorac Cardiovasc Surg*, **126**:821–825.

Meier-Kriesche HU, Kaplan B (2002) Waiting time on dialysis as the strongest modifiable risk factor for renal transplant outcomes: a paired donor kidney analysis. *Transplantation*, **74**:1377–1381.

Moers C, Smits JM, Maathuis MH, et al. (2009) Machine perfusion or cold storage in deceased-donor kidney transplantation. *N Engl J Med*, **360**:7–19.

Monbaliu D, Pirenne J, Talbot D (2012) Liver transplantation using donation after cardiac death donors. *J Hepatol*, **56**:474–485.

Perez-Saez MJ, Toledo K, Navarro MD, et al. (2011) Long-term survival of simultaneous pancreas–kidney transplantation: influence of early posttransplantation complications. *Transplant Proc*, **43**:2160–2164.

Roels L, Rahmel A (2011) The European experience. *Transpl Int*, **24**:350–367.

Roels L, Cohen B, Gachet C, Miranda BS (2002) Joining efforts in tackling the organ shortage: the Donor Action experience. *Clin Transpl*, 2002: 111–120.

Sanchez PG, Bittle GJ, Burdorf L, Pierson RN 3rd, Griffith BP (2012) State of art: clinical ex vivo lung perfusion: rationale, current status, and future directions. *J Heart Lung Transplant*, **31**:339–348.

Schenker P, Vonend O, Ertas N, Wunsch A, Traska T, Viebahn R (2010) Preprocurement pancreas allocation suitability score does not correlate with long-term pancreas graft survival. *Transplant Proc*, **42**:178–180.

Schenker P, Vonend O, Kruger B, et al. (2011) Long-term results of pancreas transplantation in patients older than 50 years. *Transpl Int*, **24**:136–142.

Schiavon M, Falcoz PE, Santelmo N, Masard G (2012) Does the use of extended criteria donors influence early and long-term results of lung transplantation? *Interact Cardiovasc Thorac Surg*, **14**:183–187.

Smits JM, van der Bij W, Van Raemdonck D, et al. (2011) Defining an extended criteria donor lung: an empirical approach based on the Eurotransplant experience. *Transpl Int*, **24**:393–400.

Smits JM, De Pauw M, de Vries E, et al. (2012) Donor scoring system for heart transplantation and the impact on patient survival. *J Heart Lung Transplant*, **31**:387–397.

Sutherland DE, Radosevich D, Gruessner R, Gruessner A, Kandaswamy R (2012) Pushing the envelope: living donor pancreas transplantation. *Curr Opin Organ Transpl*, **17**:106–115.

Vinkers MT, Rahmel AO, Slot MC, Smits JM, Schareck WD (2008a) How to recognize a suitable pancreas donor: a Eurotransplant study of preprocurement factors. *Transplant Proc*, **40**:1275–1278.

Vinkers MT, Rahmel AO, Slot MC, Smits JM, Schareck WD (2008b) Influence of a donor quality score on pancreas transplant survival in the Eurotransplant area. *Transplant Proc*, **40**:3606–3608.

Wiesner RH, McDiarmid SV, Kamath PS, et al. (2001) MELD and PELD: application of survival models to liver allocation. *Liver Transpl*, 7:567–580.

Wijnen RM, Booster MH, Stubenitzky BM, et al (1995) Outcome of transplantation of non-heart-beating donor kidneys. *Lancet*, **345**:1067–1070.

Wilde B, Pietruck F, Kribben A, Witzke O (2009) Isoagglutinin titre adsorption: breaking the barrier in major ABO-incompatible organ transplantation. *Transfus Apher Sci*, **41**:45–48.

Wittwer T, Wahlers T (2008) Marginal donor grafts in heart transplantation: lessons learned from 25 years of experience. *Transpl Int*, **21**:113–125.

Zych B, Popov AF, Amrani M, et al. (2012) Lungs from donation after circulatory death donors: an alternative source to brain-dead donors? Midterm results at a single institution. *Eur J Cardio-Thorac Surg*, **42**:542–549.

## Further reading

European Liver Transplant Registry: <http://www.eltr.org>.

Eurotransplant International Foundation: <http://www.eurotransplant.org>.

NHS Blood and Transplant: <http://www.organdonation.nhs.uk>.

Organ Procurement and Transplantation Network: <http://optn.transplant.hrsa.gov>.

Scandiatransplant: <http://www.scandiatransplant.org>.

SECTION 2

# Introduction to transplant ethics

# CHAPTER 4

# Acquiring organs ethically: problems and prospects

Jamie Lindemann Nelson

## Introduction

Transplanted human organs can sustain lives that would otherwise end soon, and they can enhance lives that would otherwise be significantly impaired. Thousands of people benefit in these crucial ways every year. Thousands more who could benefit, don't.

While the size of the gap between the available supply of organs and the potential benefit of their transplantation is more complicated than it is sometimes painted, it is plain that organ transplantation as a medical practice falls tragically short of doing as much good as it might. In some countries—the US is a conspicuous example—one reason for this shortfall is the general problem of limited access to healthcare (Axelrood et al., 2010). But the access problem with organ transplantation is not solely fiscal; fundamentally, the organs themselves are not supplied in sufficient quantities to meet the need. Human decisions and social arrangements, not natural necessities or technological limitations, account for a good deal of the lost years and diminished health.

Transplantation involving living providers might seem more straightforward. Most of the moral heavy lifting would seem to be done by the familiar device of fully informed, fully voluntary consent—but this appearance is at least partially deceiving. Informed consent as such is not a simple idea, even in contexts where the aim of an intervention is fully therapeutic. When the intervention inflicts surgical morbidity and removes vital body parts, sometimes without a clear sense of long-term consequences, the issue becomes even more complex. Are there any moral limitations we face in taking organs from those who are still alive, apart from getting valid consent? If valid consent can authorize some degree of harm to the provider (for example, harm caused to renal donors), why can't it authorize others (harm that would be caused to, say, cardiac donors)? Who can consent—or refuse—on my behalf, under what conditions, with what limits?

Further, whether we're worried about the quick or the dead, we have to struggle with questions concerning the nature of organs themselves. Are organs part of what constitutes a human person, intimate parts of that which has 'not . . . a price, but . . . dignity' (Kant, 1998), and therefore transferable to others only in the ways that any intimate transaction can be authorized, via a person's express consent to bestow a gift? Or are they best seen as the property of the person within whose body they are located? Then why may not organs—or future interests in them—be bought and sold on the market?

Still further, organ acquisition raises questions about the nature of our moral and political ties to one another. On our deaths our organs become useless to us. They may remain, however, of enormous potential value to some among the living. Why, then, is it not flatly wrong to withhold them? Why may not they be considered public goods, to be taken by the state and allocated according to social need?

These tough and disparate questions about the ethical dimensions of organ procurement draw this discussion in a number of directions. Yet there is an overarching theme: thinking to any serious purpose about the ethics of obtaining organs cannot be detached from some of the most profound questions humans know how to ask: quandaries about death, about consent and the will, about harm and benefit, and about what we owe to others, and what we are free to do ourselves. Positions on such perennial problems will strongly colour how we think about the questions addressed here—'brain death' and donation after circulatory death, 'presumed consent' and markets in organs and organ futures, about family consent and family vetoes—as well as many others—e.g. about 'directed donation' and organ procurement 'chains'—which space precludes addressing. The aim here is not to offer resolutions to any of these questions, but to make it plain that organ procurement ethics requires struggling toward the best answers we can provide. If decisions about practice and policy are to be as sound as we can make them, our understandings of the fundamental issues should be explicit and defensible.

## Maximizing organ acquisition: practical means, moral challenges, and maintaining trust

Given the life-and-death stakes involved, though, it is powerfully tempting to think that the primary question is straightforward to pose, if not easy to answer: how can the number of available organs be maximized? Moral objections to procurement schemes that hold out reasonable promise of added efficiency should, it seems, face a very high bar. Apart from a more-or-less refined idea that money is dirty and commercial motivations ignoble, why should laws forbid markets in organs? Are not markets famously efficient solutions to problems of scarcity? Do they not reinforce individual liberty and honour choice? Apart from more or less refined squeamishness, why should governments not take useable organs on a person's death? Governments have powers of taxation and conscription, and in taking money or turning civilians into soldiers they take items—our money, our time, even our lives—which presumably have considerable worth for us. They can already mandate cutting into our corpses for important social reasons—autopsies. Why should it not take items precious to others that can no longer do us any significant good at all? Why should not the choice between such alternatives be completely pragmatic: find out which approach will spare the most lives and the most suffering, and choose that one?

The 'high bar' point is serious; those who object to commodifying or conscripting organs, who support families who block donations, or who think it clearly on the side of the angels to block racists from donating only to 'their own', need to be very clear on the cost of their positions. If they prevail, many may die soon who would otherwise live longer. Yet reflection indicates that unwillingness to cut through these knots in quite such a Gordian fashion may not be merely callous. After all, many social policy changes might well have life-saving, extending, and enhancing effects. High degrees of economic stratification in a society have been correlated with bad health outcomes; there is, for example, reason to think that even the wealthiest are less healthy when income differentials are large than they are where the distribution of wealth is more tightly compacted (Daniels et al., 2011). More progressive taxation might make everyone healthier and longer-lived. Stricter environmental regulations might well cost fewer deaths connected to environmental degradation. What we eat and how we exercise can have significant health impacts, but there are not serious government-provided incentives or penalties for such lifestyle choices. Gun violence takes many lives; so do car crashes. Yet, in the US at least, gun ownership is at least as sacred as freedom of worship, and safety is one consideration among others in automotive design, not a trumping value.

Saving lives and improving health are, plainly, not the only outcomes we care about: whether this schedule of values is reasonable is another matter, but it is clear that we are willing to forego aggregate health benefits for personal autonomy, for economic opportunity, and for other values as well. Maybe the 'high bar' point needs to be stood on its head: why should we want to do anything to improve organ procurement efficiency if it would cost us more or threaten our other values? Why is dying from a specific medical cause—end-stage organ disease—so *particularly* worth averting?

## Practical means

It is not hard to forward possible explanations drawing on how our psychologies work, rather than justifications drawing on a rationally defensible understanding of relevant moral values. We can, perhaps, identify more with people with end-stage organ failure than with those who would likely have much longer and healthier lives if tax policy, or gun policy, or automotive policy, or healthcare policy changed; psychologically, the difference between people one can give a name to and merely statistical lives is very salient. But the question is really how important saving, lengthening, and substantially improving human lives should be to us, individually and jointly. For almost everyone, reducing premature death and serious illness count as good things; if increasing the supply of transplantable organs helps achieve those ends, it would seem a good thing too. Yet the lesson in the way our values are reflected in our practices seems to be that saving lives doesn't run roughshod over everything else that matters to us. Other things that are significant to us—e.g. respect for a person's sovereignty over her body, concerns about market norms driving out other understandings of what matters most to us, the special roles that families play in many people's lives—are all still in play.

## Moral challenges

If more ambitious strategies for organ procurement are to survive their political and philosophical contests with such values, reminding people that more lives would be saved and served if more organs were available is only part of the argument. People involved in this discussion should consider that there may be benefits ensuing from, or values honoured by, various forms of organ provision and transplantation that go beyond simply lengthened life and enhanced quality for individuals as such. If even carefully regulated markets in organs chip away at values that should be protected from commercialization, they might also make providers or their survivors as well as recipients substantially better off; if opt-out systems don't convey a fully robust appreciation of individual autonomy, they may at the same time provide the basis for a richer awareness of social solidarity, reinforcing values associated with the thought that 'we are all in this together' (Nelson, 2010, 2011).

Further, if commodifying organs or simply conscripting them seem morally dangerous, or if shifting from 'opt-in' to 'opt-out' systems, or providing donor families with incentives (such as defraying funeral expenses) seem ethically troubling, there is nothing so safe about simply sticking with an inefficient status quo. Pointing out that human societies are sensitive to other values than saving life doesn't mean that any appeal to such countervailing values ought to succeed in a given instance. To make this point more vividly, it might help to consider a concrete case—the organ procurement system in Spain, for example. There the organ donation rate—about 34 per million population—comes close to doubling the average in European Union (EU) countries, and exceeds what is yielded by the US system as well—typically reported at roughly 26 per million population (Directorate-General for Health & Consumers, undated). Although the precise reasons for Spain's success are controversial, these results emerge from a system that combines a legal presumption that if the recently dead had had objections to providing organs, they would have expressed them—an opt-out system—coupled with highly dedicated and skilled procurement teams. The result: proportionally less people die waiting for a transplant in Spain than in the US or elsewhere in the world.

The Spanish organ procurement system suggests that it is possible to generate considerably more organs for transplant in ways that seem broadly acceptable to a democratic polity. There may be solid cultural reasons why Spanish-like policies wouldn't transfer to other countries, of course, but if someone thinks that what is distinctive about the Spanish system is fundamentally immoral, then it would be important to make that case. While taking steps that would yield more efficient procurement of organs may turn out to be morally discretionary—something a society may choose or not choose to do, in the context of its entire range of policies and procedures—that's a case that needs making too. It is dubious that simply citing conflicting values would be a sufficient justification for retaining systems that could be reformed to yield more medical benefit.

Even in commodification-banning, opt-in systems of the sort prevalent in much of the world (e.g. the US, the UK, the

Netherlands, New Zealand, Canada) there are mechanisms in place that would, in principle, allow us to do much more good than is now being done. What stands in the way is not an absolute shortage of fiscal resources, or even of organs. What seems scant is will, and perhaps moral imagination. Many individuals won't register as organ donors; many families won't donate on the deaths of their loved ones; recent studies done in the UK, the US, and Australia indicate that requests for organ donation are refused by families between 40% and 50% of the time (Wilkinson, 2007).

As matters stand, families have the right to withhold donation when the decedent has left no indication of her choice and, in effect, they have the power to block organ retrieval even when the decedent has. But such actions may offend, and perhaps even outrage, values of compassion, solidarity, or beneficence. Indeed, they may serve as paradigm examples of how exercising a prerogative may be legitimate, insofar as it validly protects a person from interference from coercive power of the state, but leaves her fair game for moral critique.

The prevailing donation rhetoric of 'gift' and 'altruism' may have distracted people from other ways of speaking of organ provision—the language of 'obligation' and 'responsibility', for example. From the perspective of the prospective donor, so to speak, failing to authorize the transplantation of organs will in many cases be akin to foregoing an opportunity of easy rescue. Walking by the child drowning in a pond when you could save her with very little trouble and the loss of nothing of value to you will strike many as a shockingly horrible thing to do. Why should not potential donors, or at least those for whom donation would not violate core religious tenets or devastate their families—that is, those for whom the rescue would genuinely not be easy—see their own disinclination to authorize donation on their death in the same manner?

We face, then, serious moral reasons to increase organ availability—in the US alone, the waiting list at the end of 2014 stood at more than 123,000 and climbing (according to the OPTN)—but we also have both moral and solely practical reasons to be cautious about whether we properly understand and properly respect the moral principles, intuitions, or even 'gut feelings' that stand against proposals that could increase the supply. Organ procurement, in particular, and the entire transplant system, in general, rest on a foundation of social trust. When such trust in lacking, the whole system is damaged. Some indication of the impact of a lack of trust emerges in the attitudes and actions of socially marginalized people.

For example, in the UK, families of people of non-white heritage refuse to donate relatives' organs at a higher rate than the population average (Bird and Harris, 2010). Even for people whose background does not include any systematic evidence that the healthcare system is untrustworthy, or untrustworthy for people in their demographic, concerns about the ethical reliability of the system seem to persist. For example, consider the fairly widely read transplantation-driven dystopic fantasies played out in novels such as Kazuo Ishiguro's Booker-Prize finalist *Never Let Me Go* (Ishiguro, 2005) and Ninni Holmqvist's *The Unit* (Holmqvist, 2008). In Ishiguro's novel, people have been cloned to serve as a repository of organs for their genetic doubles. In Holmqvist's novel, those who are single, childless, aging, and not employed in 'progressive' industries are mandatory organ providers. These literary novels were not bestsellers, but neither did they fall dead born from the press; Ishiguro's book was the basis for the 2010 movie directed by Mark Romanek and starring Kiera Knightley. This would seem to provide some reason for thinking that something about organ transplantation, and procurement in particular, continues to prompt some level of social anxiety. Even proposals for increasing supply that are impeccable from the point of view of sound moral reflection may fail to be acceptable if they erode trust.

## Maintaining trust

As trust is the social good that fundamentally enables the transplant enterprise, then shifts in policy or practice ought to proceed on the basis of public, transparent, defensible deliberation. It's not always clear that transplant-enabling policies have been enacted in such ways in the past—there is some basis for thinking that shifts in what is technically feasible push medical professionals, bioethicists, and others to alter critical moral and philosophical understandings in a more accommodating direction. Consider the increasing use of living organ providers, one of the chief responses to the persistent shortfall of cadaver organs. In the US the number of living donors rivals that of postmortem donors; they provide kidneys and, more controversially, extrarenal organs or organ parts—lung, liver lobes, pancreas, intestines—for transplantation (OPTN, 2010).

Living donation is assumed to require thoroughly informed and voluntary consent—or, perhaps more accurately, substantial efforts to make such consent possible. There are, of course, serious questions about what constitutes such consent. How much information need be provided? How much uptake is necessary? What makes an act of consent fully voluntary? A mother, on learning that her child requires a liver transplant, immediately wants to provide a lobe of her own; indeed, she cannot imagine the possibility of any contrary desire. Nothing she is subsequently told about death rates or long-term consequences has any impact on her eagerness. Is she operating as an autonomous, informed agent? Or is she acting as a loving parent, whose power to authorize the use of her organs comes from sources other than an impartial or even altruistic calculation of interests?

The big question that arises concerning shifts in moral understandings, however, is whether fully informed and voluntary consent can even be a *sufficient*, not merely *necessary*, condition for removing organs. Seeing consent as sufficient to authorize interventions runs against the longstanding medical ethical norm that healthcare providers 'do no harm' to their patients or, more realistically interpreted, do nothing that isn't justified by a reasonable expectation of a positive balance of potential benefits versus harm and risk of harm. Cutting into healthy people and taking their organs looks a good deal like a clear harm that is uncompensated by the prospect of benefit—surely not *medical* benefit—for the surgical patient.

The Ethics Committee of the Transplant Society provides a clear statement of what is generally taken as the justification for the risks of transplantation to living donors:

> In principle, the Ethics Committee of TTS recommends that live lung, liver, pancreas, and intestine donation should only be performed when the aggregate benefits to the donor–recipient pair (survival, quality of life, psychological, and social well-being) outweigh the risks to the donor–recipient pair (death, medical, psychological and social morbidities) (Pruett et al., 2006).

This view assumes, perhaps too blithely, that the harms, risks, and potential benefits to each party in the transplant relationship can be meaningfully aggregated. Can surgical morbidity, the chances of complications, and the possibility of death for a liver lobe donor be measured against the chances of 5 years of extra life on an antirejection regimen minus the odds of earlier graft failure leading to further morbidity and death for the recipient? Even if a good positive answer can be found, what justifies such an aggregative way of thinking about the provider and recipient in the first place, particularly given medicine's traditional fidelity to the interests of individual patients? The leading possibility would seem to be the donor's consent—she provides the treatment team with permission to aggregate her interests with those of the recipient, and, along with the recipient, provides the only authoritative answer about the harm, risk, and potential benefits tradeoff—not that her authority necessarily stems from any clear sense about how those factors stack up even in her own case.

Yet if the provider's consent is fully authoritative about her own contribution to the aggregate assessment, the aggregate move may be beside the point. Presumably, aggregative assessment of harms and benefits was to be a reasonable successor to a principle of 'do no (overall) harm' to patients, conceived as a moral norm independent of consent—an additional constraint that expresses the traditional value of fidelity to the medical best interest of the individual under one's care. If aggregate risk:benefit ratio is to be credited with that kind of normative independence, there must be some non-arbitrary basis for healthcare professionals to judge that the threats to the potential provider either do or do not outweigh the potential gains to the recipient.

Nor is this the only reason to worry that the drive to maximize the potential of transplantation medicine may incline professionals to forge new norms rather than follow old, less accommodating values. 'Brain death', that conceptual innovation so crucial to post-mortem organ retrieval, has been largely accepted among theoreticians, practitioners, politicians, and the public for many years and incorporated into public life. Recently, however, that consensus has shown signs of theoretical erosion.

In *Death, Dying and Organ Transplantation*, Frank Miller and Robert Truog (2011) have argued that it is not plausible to regard human beings who are 'brain dead' as simply and straightforwardly dead. As they argue, there is simply too much brain-dead individuals, properly supported, can do—for example, grow, heal, even gestate—for people in that condition to be seen as dead in the traditional sense. The removal of vital organs from the 'brain dead' is, in sober fact, the real cause of their deaths: in their view, transplant surgeons kill such organ providers in the course of trying to save organ recipients.

Not that there is anything wrong with that. While organ provision may kill the persons whose organs are removed, Miller and Truog do not see this as morally very important. If those persons have previously expressed willingness to donate and have suffered the kind of massive and irremediable brain damage that counts as 'brain death', then causing them to die via the removal of organs will neither wrong nor harm them; they are being killed with their permission and their death does not set back their interests. Miller and Truog press an analogy with the removal of life support for those patients who have decided that, under certain conditions, further technological support does not provide them with a net benefit.

If this analysis is on track, then another moral constraint on defensible organ procurement independent of consent—the 'doctors must not kill' principle—has been effectively vitiated. Moreover, even if one is not persuaded by these antibrain death considerations, it is hard to deny that the fundamental tension between removing organs while they are still usable and not killing providers in the process has been handled by a willingness to refigure the criteria of the death concept, tweaking them a bit to allow timely removal of vital organs. In 'donation after circulatory death' protocols now in place in many transplantation centres, organs are harvested from those who have not undergone brain death. In a carefully controlled setting, circulatory support is withdrawn, a short waiting period begins after the heart stops, and then organs are quickly removed for use elsewhere. The worry here is that the procedure essentially sidesteps a core feature of the common understanding of death—death is irreversible. But as is powerfully suggested by successful cardiac transplantation from circulatory death donors, irreversibility is not the point: the operative understanding is that a donor is dead when the heart stops and a properly authorized decision not to attempt resuscitation has been made. Again, everything seems to hinge on consent, whether provided by someone who expects to walk away from providing organs or on behalf of someone who cannot have any expectations about anything.

Miller and Truog's view about how to justify organ procurement-killings involves a substantive position on a highly controversial issue: the moral equivalence of killing and letting die. If the appeal to refusal of life-extending therapy is going to have the authority with which they invest it, the differences between such cases and organ procurement have to be morally superficial; the fact that what professionals do in withholding life support is describable as 'letting die' while taking out a person's heart is more aptly described as 'killing' can make no significant moral difference (for further discussion see Nelson, 2012).

Another crucial question for procurement ethics is whether their view constrains the kind of acceptable consent to organ provision. If Miller and Truog are right, a person's consent for 'post-mortem' organ removal is not consent to organ provision after her death but consent to be killed via organ provision—would it be reasonable to 'presume' such consent? What about the range of familial authority over provisions—can families authorize organ procurement if doing so involves killing their relative? It might be replied that families authorize treatment withdrawal all the time—if the 'killing/letting die' equation is accepted (a reasonably large 'if'), family authority would seem to be left just where it is now. Yet, as the justification of organ provision is to provide for others' needs, causing people to die to give others organs might seem more problematic than it is in end-of-life scenarios, where the justification is typically that medical treatment no longer promotes the patient's interests.

## Opt-out organ provision and the moral status of dead people

Perhaps, however, the insistence on the sufficiency of valid consent that seems now to drive actually existing procurement procedures—even opt-out regimes typically draw on the idea of 'presumed consent'—is sufficient to maintain public trust. Surprisingly, perhaps, the *necessity* of consent has its challengers too. The Oxford political philosopher Cecile Fabré, for example, has argued that, in principle, conscripting organs from all those whose chances of a decent life would not be substantially set back by their provision to those whose life chances would be substantially advanced by reception is a requirement of justice (Fabré, 2006). Restricting attention to dead donors, David Hershenov and James Delaney (2009) have argued that the reasons that justify state-mandated autopsies could also in principle justify mandatory organ provision. Jamie L. Nelson (2009) has argued that a minimal understanding of the duty of beneficence—generating an 'easy rescue' obligation—provides the living with a presumptive duty to do nothing to block the retrieval of usable organs on their death; while people could refuse to be providers ('opt-out'), that refusal would be seen as a conscientious dissent, not a mere assertion of will.

All these authors believe that the considerations they advance support procurement systems that default toward organ retrieval, although how powerful the presumption is differs. It is worth underscoring, however, that none of them is based on the assumption of 'presumed consent'. The moral consideration authorizing removal is not consent, presumed or performed, but rather justice in Fabré's case, beneficence in Nelson's, and what might be described as consistency with significant settled social practice in Delaney and Hershenov's. Fabré's proposal would not exclude recognizing conscientious objection, but the bar would be set very high; it isn't clear precisely what is Hershenov and Delaney's view on allowing exemptions from postmortem organ provision, as their view is driven by the analogy to mandatory autopsy, from which exemption in many jurisdictions is rare (NHS Choices, 2013). Nelson's view, however, would make dissent effective simply on registering an objection—the presence of an objection being seen as 'good enough' evidence that any potential 'rescue' effected by a person's organs after her death would not be, for that individual, 'easy'.

Procurement systems generally, but 'opt-out' proposals especially, are haunted by the possibility that the dead can be wronged. If in a routine retrieval system organs were taken from a dead person who had or would have objected, does that action wrong the organ provider? If so, the confident assumption that retrieving organs from the recently dead could not harm or otherwise offend the provider in any way—supporting in particular proposals based, like Nelson's, on the presumption of 'easy rescue'—would need further attention.

Intuitions run both ways on this matter. It might seem most straightforward to assert that, at least given a naturalistic understanding of death, there is no one to serve as the subject of any putative harm or wrong to the dead person. This doesn't preclude the possibility that prior to death someone might find the prospect of having her organs removed after death deeply troubling, nor that those specially bound to a dead organ provider might not justifiably complain; such scenarios support making 'opt-out' readily available. However, it surely seems likely to affect the set of acceptable possibilities for reforming procurement practices if the dead provider herself could be harmed or offended by what is done to her body.

There are social practices and moral understandings concerning the dead that suggest that they are thought to continue to have some kind of direct moral standing: we think it important to honour wills, for example, and that it would be wrong to spread vicious lies about a dead person. If a person's life work fails immediately after her death, or if her children are harmed or turn out badly, there is a tendency to think that things have gone less well *for her* than they otherwise would have done.

There are, of course, ways to accommodate our sense that something goes wrong if such lies are told or wills are dishonoured that don't seem to make any essential reference to those who are dead. Yet many think that people can be wronged or harmed by events about which they never learn and which have no impact on their experience at all. Many think that people who are under the illusion that their spouse truly loves them, when in fact their spouse despises and betrays them, have, in that respect, a life of less quality than they would have had if their belief were true; our interest is not only in thinking that we are loved by those who matter most to us, but in its being in fact the case that we are so loved. If we can be harmed or wronged even by acts that have no impact on our thoughts or feelings, why can't we wrong a person in a persistent vegetative state, for instance? And if we can wrong such a person—completely insentient and never capable of any further awareness—why not a person who is dead? It is tempting to say, 'Well, with the living, no matter how badly off they are, there is someone there, someone you can point at. After death there simply is no such person.' Yet the dead do not altogether vanish; we can still *refer* to the dead and predicate properties of them—there is someone in particular we mean when we speak of Shakespeare and claim that he wrote *Titus Andronicus*.

Drawing on work by the moral philosophers George Pitcher and Joel Feinberg, Timothy M. Wilkinson (2011) has argued that we offend against the sovereignty people have over their own body if we, for example, remove organs against their previously stated wishes. The object of the wrong is the 'antemortem self'—that is, the living person, but as she figures into our thought and talk after she is dead. But how can an event that happens after my death—in the future—make me worse off now? Pitcher points out that not all harms are made up of events that first occur and then cause their victim to be worse off: when a child dies it is at the moment of the death that parents are harmed, even if they don't find out about it for days afterwards. This view does not require that causation be instantaneous. The relationship between the harm and its subject is more like the relationship between a person's being the antepenultimate president of a club, to use an example suggested by Wilkinson. If the club goes out of existence unexpectedly, two presidents down the line, that person is, at this moment, the antepenultimate president, despite the fact that the event that gives her that status occurs only in the future.

It is possible, then, if this line of thought is correct, that removing organs from those who would object (or, possibly, *not* removing organs from people who had desired, or even elected, to donate, as might happen if family vetoes are honoured) can harm or otherwise wrong the dead—which is to say, they offend the living, but considered from an antemortem perspective. They are harmed because their interest in, say, being buried intact was set back by the actions of others; they were wronged because their desires to help others were not honoured by others.

One still might try to rescue opt-out procurement on traditional 'presumed consent' grounds, arguing that those who object to organ removal after death could easily and effectively make their wishes known, as they would do, one assumes, if they cared about the matter. This approach seems unavailable to Nelson, as an 'easy rescue' view is not based on consent, presumed or otherwise. Neither the Fabré nor the Hershenov–Delaney views are based on a presumption of consent either. Yet they do not seem as vulnerable to postmortem harm objections: Fabré, of course, as she is in principle willing to remove non-vital organs from the living, takes considerations of justice presumptively to trump any harms that might be involved in organ conscription, and Hershenov and Delaney might reply that whatever harms or wrongs that post-mortem organ procurement involves are presumably at stake in mandatory autopsy as well; *if* such autopsies are licit, presumably mandatory organ provision is too.

What the entire postmortem harm mechanism tends to neglect, however, is the possibility of postmortem wrongs not done to the dead but done by the dead. The doing involved in the wrong doing, of course, needs to occur during the lifetime of the antemortem person. Yet if the possibility of postmortem harm is credited, that might not be a fatal objection. Imagine a procurement system that defaults to removal and a person who finds the idea of her heart ever beating in someone else's chest to be distasteful. However, the same person might regard it equally distasteful to wade into murky water to pull out a drowning child; it is hard to imagine that mere distaste could insulate such a person against the charge that they had behaved horribly were they to let the child drown on such a plea—the rescue remains, in the relevant sense, easy. If the analogy holds, neither could mere squeamishness excuse a person of her presumptive duty to make her organs available after her death. Just as harming and wronging are functions of values and interests held by the living but which can be thwarted or dishonoured by events occurring after their deaths, so too do people have duties based in values they endorse while alive whose occasion for performance (or failure) occurs after they are dead.

Therefore the claim that the living have a presumptive duty to provide useful organs after their deaths is not clearly refuted even if we can be wronged after death, since similar considerations support the claim that we can also do wrong after death, and there seems reason to believe that not every kind of reluctance to provide organs would successfully rebut the 'easy rescue' presumption. Yet differences between shallow ponds and hospitals abound; some are even imaginable between autopsies and transplants. The question remains as to whether those differences constitute moral dis-analogies or not. If the weight of the argument suggests there are morally inconsequential differences, we then face the practical problems: what accounts for the resistance of some countries to accept opt-out provision? Is it likely that efforts to reform procurement systems in the direction of opt-out will succeed—as they conspicuously did not, recently, in the UK—and make more organs available to those who so gravely need them (Bird and Harris, 2010)? Or might they rather have an opposite effect, eroding the fabric of trust that makes organ transplant possible at all.

## Organ vendors: three kinds of critique

Innovative opt-out or conscription strategies tend to be rather muted on the subject of whether human organs as such have a special moral status: they are assumed to be like actions, which can in some cases be the subject of a moral demand. Or they are assumed to be like goods, which can be redistributed according to the demands of justice. Or they assume that it makes no difference whether organs are to be put inside of someone else or not: if they can be removed to, say, further a criminal investigation, they can be removed to implant into a different person for medical reasons.

But the status quo, whether opt-in as, for example, in the US, the UK, New Zealand, and Canada (and many other countries), or opt-out, as in Spain, France, Belgium, and Austria (and many other countries), assumes that organs are the kind of entity whose transfer to others needs to be specially authorized, in ways that are somewhat reminiscent of how societies license the provision of other expressions of intimacy—as gifts. Those who believe that a market in human organs could substantially relieve the supply problem challenge the notion that organs are somehow morally special in that sense.

The case for marketing organs seems straightforward. It draws on a reasonable expectation that a market would increase the availability of organs, thus extending and improving many human lives, and on a facially plausible view that organs are the property of those whose bodies they help make up during life, and of the decedent's heirs after death—whose body is it, after all? As suggested by the continuing resistance to even regulated organ markets, however, there is a case—indeed, several cases—for the other side. A purely consequentialist antimarket case stands or falls on the claim that, contrary to the assumptions of organ market proponents, allowing people to either sell or buy organs would not improve the availability of organs overall—what some might be motivated to give as a priceless gift of life, they would not be motivated to sell for $3,000—or, more commonly, a market would cause harms to organ vendors substantial enough to overbalance whatever gains would be achieved overall—that is, taking both vendors and purchasers into account.

A more mixed view, drawing on consequences and 'in-principle' considerations, would not need to maintain that, overall, the harms connected with markets outweigh their benefits. It could hold, rather, that the harms would be unjustly distributed, too much falling on those who are worst off, say, to warrant a market in organs even if the overall benefits were substantial; this concern is clearly close to the worry that vendors would typically be poorly off overall and would expose themselves to risks of substantial harm for fleeting economic benefits. The poor economic situation of providers undermines consent and renders them vulnerable to exploitation as a respect offence, as well as to the harms and risks of organ provision.

Presumably, various forms of regulation could reduce or possibly even avoid these problems. Restricting the market in organs to postmortem provision would obviously substantially lessen risks and harms to vendors. A person's heirs might benefit financially or, possibly, the organ provider herself could vend a 'future interest' in her organs, agreeing to allow retrieval should she die in propitious circumstances, for a price (which, presumably, would be rather modest, as most don't die in circumstances that lend themselves to organ retrieval). Of course, these restrictions might also substantially decrease the potential yield from vended organs. Other forms of restriction that would allow some people to vend some organs might strike an acceptable balance—restricting sellers to those who face a small risk of bad long-term consequences by insisting on a standard of health, on the reliable availability to the vendor of quality healthcare, and only allowing transplant of organs for which there is a reasonably robust history supporting projections of long-term acceptable consequences to sellers. Medical professionals might have moral reason to insist on such restrictions, even if vendors do not. Even given the persistence of economic disparities between purchasers and vendors, such regulations might reduce the worry that sellers were being exploited. Further, if the only allowable purchaser of organs were in effect the government, opening up organ sales might not at the same time skew considered moral judgements concerning who should receive organs—a central buyer and distributer could ensure that organs did not go to the highest bidder (who might be someone whose interest in human organs were not transplant at all) but to those who were neediest, or whose need was most urgent, or whose chance of benefiting was the best, or employing whatever criteria were regarded as most defensible as a matter of a just social policy.

More decidedly, 'in principle' or deontic arguments are not so easy to accommodate with market restrictions, but neither are they as straightforward to make. The customary start is probably with Kantian-style objections to commodifying persons that revolve around the insistence that people have 'dignity, not price'. If a proper understanding of the most central and defensible of our moral values flatly forbids the selling of persons to other persons, there might be an argument that, as people are significantly composed of organized, animate matter, treating non-renewable parts of ourselves (at least) as though they could be properly bought and sold dishonours the same values that most clearly support the non-commodifiability of people as such. A related thought is based on the recognition that the values expressed in market transactions are not appropriate for all goods, and that we have reason to resist the tendencies in contemporary culture that operate as if this were not so: we should regard certain things—human lives, or certain relationships such as friendship or intimacy, or certain actions, such as voting—in ways that recognize the non-economic valuation variously appropriate to them. Otherwise we risk eroding the ability to mark certain features of our life as playing special roles, with respect to which we can effectively express a rich range of affective and evaluative attitudes: respect, love, awe, equity, and so forth (Anderson, 1995).

Another related notion is that seeing organs as something that we can alienate for a price suggests that they are property. This may seem an altogether natural assumption—how can we understand a person's special relationship with her own organs apart from the idea that they are her property, and hence, the thought continues, items that she has a right to sell if she likes and can find a willing buyer? There may be consequences of unregulated transactions that justify some constraints on the exercise of that right, but the presumption is that people may alienate their own, as they like.

The answer, of course, is that there are indeed other ways of understanding the relationship between a person and her organs: children, for example, belong to their parents, but not in the sense of being their property. Property, the argument has it, is not a natural relationship: we do not 'own' anything, including our organs, outside of a system of social practices and understandings that includes a certain conception of property and within which ownership rights are assigned. One of the 'blocked transactions' in ongoing schemes of social cooperation is sale of one's self; a person may not legally sell herself into slavery, for example. As our organs are integral parts of what constitutes us when alive, it might seem reasonable to extend this prohibition to them. Or, of course, organs might be better understood as analogous to aspects of our lives that are saleable: many forms of human labour, and many of the items that labour produces, including aesthetic and intellectual productions that seem to be deeply connected with the fundamental character of the person who produces them. The chief point here is not that reflection on the conventional character of property forbids commodification of organs. Rather, it makes it easier to appreciate the possibility that other ways of regarding organs as property might express conventions that, all things considered, make more sense. If among the reasons to recognize a human organ as a commodity is increasing the availability of organs, there might be even more efficient ways of achieving that goal. It might, for example, be a better convention to regard any organs after death that remain viable as items that no one is free to sell, as they are already owned by those whose lives will go very badly without them.

Of course, mixed solutions are possible here: a procurement system could be envisaged in which useful organs are presumptively retrieved at a person's death, but in which they—or some of them—can also be sold during a person's life. Incentives prompting organ donation that fall short of paying what a market would bear—defraying funeral expenses, for example—might be understood as 'nudges' in the direction of donation that do not trigger moral reservations about more complete forms of commodification.

## Organ procurement and families

In many organ procurement regimens, whether officially 'opt-in' or 'opt-out', families can effectively veto the removal of organs from dead providers; in opt-in systems they can opt-in on behalf of a dead relative. That is a fair amount of power for families to wield—is so much deference to their decisions defensible?

Families' diverse and dynamic character makes it hard to get an accurate picture of the nature and limits of their authority to license, decline, or overrule donation decisions, but that diversity and dynamism needs to be accommodated by any adequate understanding of procurement ethics. Indeed, as procurement practice often allows families authority not recognized by relevant laws, transplantation medicine itself might be seen to have expressed an openness to the view that the nature of families cannot be pinned down by explicit legislation. Of course, an open attitude toward who counts as families presumably won't lessen interfamilial conflicts about organ retrieval. That, however, is a problem that has to be faced whatever understandings of what constitutes a family achieve recognition. It is also possible that different grounds for claiming family standing may be perfectly valid but draw on different factors—and perhaps factors of different strengths—to support claims to control over the disposition of relatives' bodies. However, in the hope of getting a decent glimpse of the basic structure of issues concerning families and organ procurement, the ever-developing range of familial connections will be acknowledged but not explored.

## Familial authorization

In T.M. Wilkinson's nicely nuanced view, families can properly convey the *willingness* of a deceased relative to donate, even if the relative never officially or explicitly *consented* to provide post-mortem organs. Wilkinson regards this as completely consistent with the appropriate respect for a person's sovereignty over her body, even after death. Reasonable beliefs concerning the willingness of the decedent to donate are sufficient; therefore on the basis of a person's willingness to provide organs upon death, a family may—and likely ought to—consent on behalf of the decedent (Wilkinson, 2011).

Perhaps Wilkinson can be gone one better: just as willingness to provide can be distinguished from consent to provide, a 'latent' willingness might be distinguishable from express willingness; a family member might say to a close relative, 'I knew you'd like that' and be quite right, even if the relative hadn't previously given the matter any thought. Might some families reliably infer what their loved one would have wanted and validly authorize consent (or refusal) on such grounds?

One reason for a positive answer lies in thinking of family members—or, to put the matter more carefully, of *some* members of *some* families—as standing in a relationship that can amount to a kind of *shared agency*, based on long and reliable histories of making joint decisions on the basis of common values, common reasons for honouring those values, and common conceptions of the physical and social world (Rovane, 1997). People whose relation to the decedent is as close as that might have grounds to not only convey any actual past decisions or explicitly expressed willingness concerning procurement choices, but also actively extend the decedent's agency, authorizing donation on the grounds that coming to a current situation of choice in the vivid and urgent way that occurs in real-time cases *would have lead* the potential provider to change her mind, given her underlying values (Nelson, 2003).

Families who could validly extend—as opposed to hijack—agency in this way might of course be rare and hard to identify reliably. In any event, the supporting considerations might seem arcane at best. Yet the reason such possibilities need to be considered at all might also be seen as based on arcane considerations—that is, on the view that death does not end a person's sovereignty over her body and that the dead remain vulnerable to certain kinds of wrongs. Without that assumption, familial authority to donate seems even clearer: at least without revising standing conventions concerning property, the decedent's body can as reasonably be regarded as belonging to the family as to anyone else, and at least if there is consensus within the family (and possibly even if there is not), procurement would seem something that the family could clearly authorize, if their relative died without any indication of willingness to donate, whether expressed or constructed.

## Familial veto

Probing the intricacies of familial permission to provide organs raises some significant theoretical problems, but, in practice, it is seldom challenged. What is a matter of considerable controversy is the notion that families have the authority to veto organ removal, not just when the decedent's attitude to provide organs is unknown (and not confidently reconstructable), but even when a decedent is known to have consented to donate. In the UK, the US, and Australia, for example, studies indicate that requests for provision are effectively refused between 40% and 50% of the time, and that explicit decisions to donate are overridden in nearly 10% of cases, even though in most jurisdictions the legal basis for familial refusal is unclear or non-existent (Kirby, 2009).

Similar issues emerge over refusals as over authorizations. If death does not void personal sovereignty, then it seems as though refusing to honour the decedent's decisions about the disposition of her body—indeed, refusing to honour the decedent's express desire to achieve what she herself may have thought of as 'easy rescue'—could well represent a serious respect offence. Yet, as so often, there are countervailing considerations, even assuming that death does not undermine the reasons we have to respect a person's special authority over her body. It is family members who will continue to live and to feel and who may find organ removal an unmanageable extra source of pain at a time that may seem to them to be already intolerable. Further, any desire that the decedent may have had on the subject of organ provision was presumably not the only thing she desired; the family's pain at the notion of organs being removed from their lost loved-one could also be considerations that might have moved the decedent had she vividly anticipated them.

These considerations speak most eloquently to cases in which a recently dead person had left no explicit instructions and whose family is dealing not with consent to donate but with willingness to do so. There seems reason to believe that in such cases families are not acting indefensibly if they factor in their own distress to the whole range of things about which their relative had attitudes. It seems likelier that families are in a weaker position, morally, to expect that their contrary wishes should control the matter if their relative left an express consent; the fact that families do sometimes effectively veto such acts of consent might appear a concession to fear of lawsuits, or of reluctance to distressing further a bereaved and very present family, at the cost of the pain that the bereaved, remote family of the person who dies for the want of a timely transplant will feel. Arguments have been made in the literature that medical professionals who do not contest the family's refusal are at fault (Shaw, 2012).

But the cupboard of response on behalf of the family isn't bare, even here. If costless or nearly costless rescue remains an ethical obligation—and even one whose discharge may be facilitated by state action—it isn't clearly covered by cases where families are deeply distressed by the prospect of organ retrieval, organ transplant, or both. It is true that failure to remove the organs will very likely allow considerably more disutility—otherwise deferrable deaths, and all their accompanying pain and loss—to exist in the world than would be caused by removing them. Yet this observation recalls the earlier discussion of the height of the bar that objections to more efficient procurement have to clear. If the life-saving card trumps every other one, then disallowing familial vetoes of explicit postmortem consent on the part of the decedent seems the least of its implications. We ought then, it seems, look with much more friendly eyes on the whole idea of routine postmortem retrieval of organs. If we aren't ready to take that step, perhaps the family's distress needs to be respected in theory as in practice.

It is true that other kinds of familial distress, even if extreme, do not as a matter of course derail other expressions of a deceased relative's judgement, as in the case of ordinary wills. Still, there may be room for an argument that a loved-one's body has a different relationship to her survivors than does her property (in part because it is not an object useful to relatives, as property may be; the body's value would seem wholly expressive, residing in how it figures into the meaningfulness of specific forms of response to death).

## Conclusion

The technologies and human skills that make organ transplantation a great success from a technical point of view are still to be fully matched by the kind of refiguring of moral and social attitudes that would allow transplantation to have its optimal impact on human health and longevity. It may be the case that those attitudes will never, in fact, 'catch up', if that is the correct way to put the matter; technical progress may allow xenograft or perhaps stem-celled-based therapies to provide people facing end-stage organ failure with outcomes that are as good as or better than those transplant organs can now provide. All things considered, this would probably count as a great advance. Still, there may be something to regret in that, whether as individuals or societies and whatever the appropriate understanding of personal sovereignty, familial authority, or personal obligation might be, the enterprise of organ provision and transplantation has not been able to strike more of us as a morally attractive outcome. The growth in living donation is surely inspiring. It is also, however, typically an expression of a kind of powerful bond between people already close to each other. Organ provision to strangers after death represents a way to affirm a fundamental solidarity among us all, and it is something of a shame that we have not been better able to embrace it.

Research for this essay (and the supporting publications Nelson 2009, 2010, and 2011) was conducted with the support of a sabbatical leave provided by Michigan State University, and a generous internal grant as well.

## References

Anderson E (1995) *Values in Ethics and Economics*. Harvard University Press, Cambridge, Massachusetts.

Axelrod DA, Millman DM, Abecassis MM (2010) U.S. health care reform and transplantation, part one: overview and impact on access and reimbursement in the private sector. *Am J Transplant*, **10**(10):2197–2202.

Bird SM, Harris J (2010) Time to move to presumed consent for organ donation. *BMJ*, **340**(c2188):1010–1013.

Daniels N Kennedy B, Kawachi I (2011) *Is Inequality Bad for our Health?* Beacon Press, Boston.

Directorate-General for Health & Consumers (undated) Key facts and figures on EU organ donation and transplantation. <http://ec.europa.eu/health/ph_threats/human_substance/oc_organs/docs/fact_figures.pdf>.

Fabré C (2006) *Whose Body Is it, Anyway?* Oxford University Press, Oxford.

Hershenov DB, Delaney J (2009) Mandatory autopsy and organ conscription. *Kennedy Inst of Ethics J*, **19**(4):367–391.

Holmqvist N (2008) *The Unit*. Translated by Marlaine Delargy. Other Press, New York.

Ishiguro I (2005) *Never Let Me Go*. Vintage, New York.

Kant I (1998) Groundwork of the metaphysics of morals (trans. Mary Gregory), p. 42. Cambridge University Press, Cambridge.

Kirby JC (2009) Organ donation: who *should* decide?—A Canadian perspective. *J Bioeth Inq*, **6**(1):123–128.

Miller F, Truog R (2011) *Death, Dying, and Organ Transplantation*. Oxford University Press, Oxford.

Nelson J (2003) *Hippocrates' Maze*. Rowman and Littlefield, Totowa, Maryland.

Nelson JL (2009) Dealing death and retrieving organs. *J Bioeth Inq*, **6**(3):285–291.

Nelson JL (2010) Donation by default. *Int J Feminist Approach Bioeth*, **3**(1):23–42.

Nelson JL (2011) Internal organs, integral selves, and good communities. *Theoretical Med Bioethics*, **32**(5):289–300.

Nelson JL (2012) Doctors kill a lot of people. Get over it. *Hastings Center Rep*, **42**(3):46–47.

NHS Choices (2013) *Post-mortem*. <http://www.nhs.uk/conditions/post-mortem/pages/introduction.aspx>.

OPTN (2010) *2010 SRTR and OPTN Annual Report*. UNOS, Richmond, Virginia.

Pruett TL, Tibell A, Alabdulkareem A, et al. (2006) The ethics statement of the Vancouver Forum on the live lung, liver, pancreas, and intestine donor. *Transplantation*, **81**(10):1386–1387.

Rovane C (1997) *The Bounds of Agency*. Princeton University Press, Princeton, New Jersey.

Shaw D (2012) We should not let families stop organ donation from dead relatives. *BMJ*, **345**:e5275.

Wilkinson TM (2007) Individual and family decisions about organ donation. *J Appl Philos*, **24**(1):26–40.

Wilkinson TM (2011) *Ethics and the Acquisition of Organs*. Oxford University Press, Oxford.

## Further reading

United Network for Organ Sharing: <http://www.unos.org/>.

# CHAPTER 5

# Organ allocation: a guide for the perplexed

Benjamin E. Hippen

## Introduction

Over six decades of organ procurement and transplantation, controversies over the proper structure and justification of how organs are allocated have never fully receded from public discussion and debate. Medical innovation, far from being an ameliorating force, has merely made it possible to plausibly consider candidates for transplantation who were previously thought to be too high risk, and innovation has allowed more and more patients who might have previously succumbed to their disease to survive long enough to join the ranks of those in demand for a solid organ transplant. The hope that regenerative medicine might stave off the need for an organ transplant, or provide an endless supply of transplantable organs, has not been realized and is unlikely to be realized in the near future. Around the world there are far more individuals who might benefit from transplantation compared to the number of organs available for transplant. Unfortunately, creative efforts to significantly increase the supply of organs from deceased donors have not proven to be very successful.

Readers familiar with the terrain of organ allocation debates will find that this chapter follows an unusual path. Rather than focus on the tension between competing moral values, which emerge in discussions of allocating a scarce resource, the author has chosen to linger over a number of premises that are typically taken for granted in discussions of organ allocation. It may come as a surprise to some that not all agree that there is a shortage of organs or that the sense of crisis which follows should be cause for suspicion rather than a search for solutions. Discussions of organ allocation presume that there is a disparity between demand and supply, and so this presumption should not be merely taken for granted. Furthermore, organ allocation does not occur in a social vacuum. It involves the deliberate expenditure of large amounts of (limited) resources, resources that might be spent elsewhere. The opportunity costs of organ transplantation, as well as the particulars of an organ allocation system, have different stakes for individuals, societies, and healthcare delivery systems in different parts of the world, and these opportunity costs are worthy of awareness.

Next, organ allocation systems are integrated into the practical necessities of how organs are procured, transported, and transplanted and the extant political economy of transplantation, which is the regulatory and financial frameworks that structure incentives and disincentives for how transplant centres behave in approaching the evaluation and acceptance of patients for transplantation. Well before any discussion of how to distribute X number of organs to X + n number of recipients and why, there is a great deal of 'allocation' which occurs beforehand, in the form of practices that impact access to transplant evaluation, access to the waiting list, removal from the waiting list, organ acceptance practices, etc. Who gets which kidney and why is not unimportant but is far from the whole story and may not be the most important vantage for thinking about the moral dimensions of organ allocation.

## Shortage or sham?

Most discussions of organ allocation begin with a nod toward the dimensions of the shortage of organs and proceed into a discussion of philosophical concepts, which have been applied, to address how and why a scarce resource ought to be dispensed. It is not especially controversial to note that there is substantive disagreement about how resources should be allocated under conditions of scarcity, but it should be noted at the outset that the conditions of scarcity that are at the heart of allocation debates are not universally accepted as simple facts of the matter. For critics such as the anthropologist Nancy Scheper-Hughes, the alleged 'fact' of scarcity is in fact a social construct created by self-interested transplant professionals to create a social urgency to increase organ procurement (Scheper-Hughes, 1995), wrongly recasting the discussion of organ procurement as a matter of 'lifeboat ethics' (Scheper-Hughes, 2007) and creating a state of affairs that serendipitously yields additional professional and financial benefits to these very same transplant physicians and surgeons (Scheper-Hughes, 1995). Were society to start looking askance at efforts by the medical establishment to, as Scheper-Hughes charges, avoid death at all costs and reject what she construes as the fetishization of a false promise of immortality, then the disparity between demand and supply would not appear as a disparity at all. To be sure, this is a jaundiced view of the transplant enterprise which has been not only soundly rejected by transplant professionals (whose protests might be dismissed as merely defensive self-interest) but also belied by verifiable facts regarding the relative benefits in terms of survival and quality of life of transplantation for a broad range of patients with renal failure.

The purpose of highlighting Scheper-Hughes' criticism at the outset of this chapter is not to highlight its veracity but rather to point out the temptation to avoid discussions of allocation, a discussion that deliberately divides needy individuals into groups that will be conspicuously better or worse off as a result of a deliberate and conscious decision. Ethically (and emotionally) speaking, it is far preferable to face a condition of scarcity with a solution that manages to circumvent the tradeoffs in thinking about scarcity. Even if it is an overstatement to argue that the demand for organ transplantation is an ideologically freighted illusion, it might be more plausibly argued that the apparent demand for organs is overstated compared to the 'real' demand, and by extension the conditions of scarcity too are equally overstated. For those more sympathetic to the transplant enterprise, the opportunity to show that conditions of scarcity are overstated has the same obvious benefit of not being complicit in a system of tradeoffs which deliberately leave some better off and some worse off.

In 2008 the *Washington Post* published a story which reported that as many as a third of patients currently listed for a kidney transplant in the US were not actually eligible to receive a transplant (Stein, 2008). This was met with suitable outrage from members of the transplant community. A community member of the board of directors of UNOS commented, 'The list is what [the transplant community] use for propaganda. It's the marketing tool. It's always: the waiting list, the waiting list, the growing waiting list. It's what they use to argue that we need more organs. It's dishonest.' Bioethicist and University of Pennsylvania professor Arthur Caplan opined, 'You can't have one-third of the list out there that doesn't really belong... you can't inflate the numbers' (Stein, 2008). In fact, the patients referred to in the story were listed as Status 7, a designation that allows candidates to accrue time on the waiting list without being offered an organ. In an allocation system that privileges waiting time, there are a great many reasons why a candidate would be listed under this designation, temporarily or even for long periods of time.[1] In actuality, the ultimate disposition of patients who are initially listed as Status 7, who are initially listed for transplant and subsequently transition to Status 7 and back, is not well understood. What is better understood is that perhaps one-third of these patients are ultimately taken off the transplant list, which is to say that perhaps 10% of all listed patients are ultimately removed from the list for various reasons, including death. But this is far from establishing the premise that patients who are listed to accrue waiting time but are not currently appropriate for an organ offer were never appropriate for an organ offer and/or will never be appropriate for an organ offer. It is easier to worry less about scarcity if there are readily available premises which assure that no such scarcity exists.

However, organ transplantation does operate under conditions of actual scarcity. Scarcity in transplantation exists along multiple dimensions and only some of these dimensions are conspicuous. The most conspicuous form of scarcity is the disparity between the demand for and supply of available organs for transplantation. The fact that there is a scarcity of organs depends on the premise that there is a given cohort of patients for whom an organ transplant would confer measurable benefit, in terms of additional quantity and/or quality of life, compared to not receiving a transplant. But this is only one dimension of scarcity. The austere and much-invoked principles of 'efficiency' and 'equity' belie the true costs, in blood and treasure, of what is at stake in debates over organ allocation.

Consider the ESRD programme in the US by way of example. In 2009, the US Federal Government spent nearly $29 billion on dialysis and transplantation, amounting to 6.5% of the Medicare budget on 0.6% of all Medicare beneficiaries. (Private insurers spend another $12 billion on top of that.) Of that $29 billion, some $1.8 billion was spent on kidney transplantation, despite the fact that a kidney from a deceased donor extends the life of a recipient 100% over 5 years, compared to the same candidate who remains on dialysis (median 5-year patient survival of 75% with transplant compared to a 5-year survival of 35% with haemodialysis (HD)/peritoneal dialysis (PD)) (USRDS, 2012). On average, the cost of a kidney transplant reaches a break-even point of the cost of maintenance dialysis in the US after 18 months, beyond which a transplant is cost-effective compared to dialysis (Matas, 2003). So, discussions regarding organ allocation have a direct impact on the political economy of renal replacement therapy, a therapy that involves an allocation of finite resources (namely the public's money) and the opportunity costs involved in spending resources on some therapies rather than others, or continuing a rate of spending that is simply unsustainable.

Similarly, in many developing countries, the cost of chronic dialysis is within the reach of only the wealthiest citizens of these countries, which means that transplantation is the only plausible, practical option for patients with kidney failure. In Pakistan the financial burden of dialysis means that it is available only as a limited 'bridge' therapy to transplantation, rather than the destination therapy it is in many countries in the developed world, such that allocation discussions revolve around which patients shall continue to receive chronic dialysis and which patients shall be withdrawn for lack of an available, willing, and able living donor (Moazam, 2006). The rise and growth of kidney transplantation in Iran, a country in which the State provides healthcare to its citizens, was fuelled by the rise in identified cases of kidney disease and kidney failure and the concomitant financial burden of chronic dialysis on the State's coffers. The lack of a legal framework (until the 2000s) that recognized death by whole-brain criteria as death and a relatively moribund biologically related living donor programme in the 1980s prompted the Iranian government to institute a patchwork of local-charity-run regional systems to provide financial incentives to unrelated living donors, a process that led to a rapid growth in the volume of kidney transplants in Iran which persists to this day (Hippen, 2008; Mahdavi-Mazdeh, 2012).

The point is that while discussions of organ allocation usually focus on the benefits (and less commonly the harms) conferred on individual candidates, actual systems of organ allocation also have non-trivial economic implications, which will manifest in different ways for different communities and different healthcare delivery systems. From the vantage of a patient with ESRD, the therapeutic options are death, dialysis, or transplantation. But, from the vantage of a healthcare delivery system, a debate over

[1] A non-exhaustive list of examples include: patients on the waiting list who develop reversible problems (e.g. an infection, a major surgery, a slow-healing diabetic foot ulcer) which require resolution before transplantation; patients whose kidney function is sufficient to accrue waiting time but whose kidney disease has an indolent rate of progression and who may not be appropriate for an immediate organ offer; patients listed at a centre with very long waiting times and in which the centre defers medical testing until the candidate has accrued enough waiting time to make it closer to the top of the list, so as to avoid repeated/redundant testing; patients who may have living donors but for whom there is uncertainty if their living donors will be accepted as donor candidates; and patients who have various forms of cancer which can recur after transplant and who require a waiting period between the time of cure and the time of transplant.

one or another system of organ allocation might reasonably take into account and weigh relative opportunity costs. So one way of allocating kidneys from deceased donors would be to ensure that the youngest, healthiest candidates receive the 'best' quality organs. Since dialysis is more expensive than transplantation after the first 18 months and since young, healthy donors tend to live longer both on dialysis and after transplantation, preferentially allocating the best organs to the youngest, healthiest candidates is the most cost-effective organ allocation system. If financial resources are fungible, the less money that needs to be spent on ESRD, the more money there is available for spending on other goods (or simply spending less in general). However, allocating an organ to a candidate who might otherwise be at high rate of graft failure and return to dialysis would be a cost-ineffective approach to organ allocation, since the cost of an early graft failure and return to dialysis far exceeds the cost of simply remaining on dialysis, unless the patient dies relatively soon after the graft fails. Dwelling on these apparently cold-blooded concerns should not be mistaken as arguing that these concerns ought to have priority in debates over organ allocation. Rather, the point is to show that the scarcity of organs is not the only, or even the most important, dimension of scarcity at work when thinking about organ allocation.

Discussions of just organ allocation must also take into account evolving trends in organ procurement. Alarmingly, despite the steady growth in the number of candidates added to the waiting list for a kidney, the growth in the total number of organs from deceased donors and from living donors has not kept pace (according to the SRTR). In deceased donation, the total number of organs from SCD has fallen, and the total number of organs from deceased donors has barely kept pace by a concomitant increase in the number of kidneys for ECD and DCD, organs that have been observed to have a higher rate of complications and failures compared to kidneys from SCD. Additionally, for reasons that are not clear, the total number of organs from living donors has also fallen, and precipitously so, from biologically related donors (according to the SRTR). As might be expected, since 2005 there has been a steady increase in the number of candidates on the waiting list who die waiting for a kidney (now exceeding 8% annually), as well as other candidates who are removed from the list due to physiological deterioration.

It has long been observed that the average age of patients on the waiting list is increasing. While the median survival of a new-incident ESRD patient initiating dialysis has not improved since 2000, the median age of a new-incident ESRD patient initiating dialysis has increased by a decade, from 55 to 66, over the same time frame. The age distribution of the waiting list reflects this trend: the vast majority of those currently on the waiting list for a kidney transplant is made up of candidates over the age of 50, and nearly a third are 65 and older. Older candidates tend to die sooner on dialysis and tend to be removed from the waiting list due to deterioration or death more frequently than younger candidates. Thus the stakes of the debate over kidney allocation are considerably higher for older candidates, since older candidates are generally more physiologically vulnerable and tend to suffer a much higher rate of complications (including higher rates of death and graft failure) after receiving a kidney from an ECD compared to receiving a kidney from a younger, healthier donor. In this sense, older transplant candidates face a panoply of vulnerabilities, not only from their physiological state but also more saliently from allocation decisions which serve to demote the claims of older candidates in favour of the claims of younger candidates.

Next, the current composition of the waiting list may not represent the true demand for organs. One study of the US ESRD population showed that there are between 80,000 and 130,000 additional dialysis-dependent patients that (based on demographics) would theoretically benefit from receiving a transplant compared to remaining on dialysis but are never referred for transplantation (Schold et al., 2007). If even a fraction of this 'invisible' demand were to be realized, the disparity between demand and supply would be further exacerbated, and the current median waiting time for an organ would in many instances exceed the median survival for all but the youngest and most physiologically robust of candidates.

A related and underappreciated fact relevant to the practice of organ allocation is the increased emphasis on publicly reported outcomes measurement for transplant centres and the impact of these metrics on candidate selection. Transplant centres in the US publicly report outcomes for patient and graft survival, and centres are held to account for their reported outcomes by government regulatory agencies and private insurance companies (Howard, 2007). Failures to achieve a sufficient outcome threshold for patient and graft survival can and have had significant implications for transplant centres, including but not limited to a loss of insurance contracts, regulatory sanctions, and even the involuntary closure of transplant centres. This regulatory milieu encourages centres that are at risk of falling below expected outcomes (for a sense of what the bar is here, the national average for 1-year patient and graft survival in the US is 99% and 95%, respectively) to be conservative in their organ acceptance practices, as well as in candidate selection and listing. While expected outcomes for individual centres are 'risk adjusted' based on a number of reported donor and candidate demographics, candidate comorbidities which pose an increased risk for patient death or graft failure but are not included as variables in the risk-adjustment model which sets the bar for 'expected' outcomes result in the transplant centre 'taking on' unadjusted risk in accepting such a candidate for listing and transplantation. Too much realized unadjusted risk puts transplant centres at regulatory and financial risk, which means that centres are powerfully incentivized to avoid accepting such candidates for listing.

Since all transplant centres operate under the same regulatory framework and therefore under the same structure of incentives and disincentives, it reasonably follows that a conservative approach to risk tolerance which systematically excludes whole categories of candidates (specifically, candidates believed to have risk of death or graft failure after transplant which are not captured by the risk-adjusted model) might proliferate and become the practice norm. A robust operational precautionary principle is itself a kind of allocation decision, albeit one that involves controlling (limiting) access to transplantation rather than a comparative judgement regarding who ought to have more or less priority for an organ. Of course, if a centre's risk tolerance is too conservative, that is, if a centre ends up 'cherry picking' very low risk candidates and donor organs, the risk-adjusted expected patient and graft survival ends up being very high. If the centre fails to meet that very high standard (which might occur with only a few patient deaths or graft losses after transplant), the same regulatory penalties would apply. Adhering to these regulatory realities, in turn, will substantially alter the actual composition of patients on the waiting list well before any discussion of how to allocate organs comes into play. But deliberate practices, or the unintended consequences of regulatory policies, which alter access to the supply of organs are themselves a robust form of allocation. It is easy to overlook this fact if the focus of discussion is on how to allocate X organs to X + n candidates. It is commonly overlooked that allocation decisions involve decisions about not only the distribution of a limited supply but also the size and composition of those who are actually permitted by a centre to participate in the pool of demand in the first place.

In sum, a discussion of the normative dimensions of organ allocation is usefully supplemented by an exploration of the political economy of organ transplantation specifically and healthcare delivery generally in different societies. Detaching discussions of allocation from these contexts might leave the reader with the mistaken impression that the gladiatorial contest of competing moral principles is conducted on a metaphysical plane detached from a host of important, if sometimes mundane, social realities.

## Principles of allocation: efficiency and equity, and the spectre of uncertainty

### Sidebar—property and authority

Any system of organ allocation rests on a theory of property rights in organs, since an organ allocation system must have organs to allocate and must have the authority to disposition the property right in the organs. In most countries, and with very limited exceptions, the property rights in organs from deceased donors are held by the State. While consent for organ donation after death must be obtained from surrogates of the deceased (or, in rare instances, the decedent him-/herself before death), once organs are procured, the right to dispose of the property rights in the organ rests with the State and its designees (organ procurement organizations and transplant centres). That disposition includes either allocating the organ to an individual or discarding the organ altogether. In unusual instances, some locales permit the families of a decedent to exert a property right usually reserved for the State, by requesting a directed donation to an individual. But the infrequency with which this occurs underscores the rule: organs procured from deceased donors become the property of the State, up and until the State relinquishes the property right by allocating the organ to an individual transplant recipient.

It is worth lingering over how unusual this widely, tacitly accepted arrangement is. In western societies many recognized property rights of individuals are conferred to the individual's estate after death, to be subsequently dispositioned according to estate law. An individual's property is not simply forfeit to the State upon the individual's death. Premortem individuals can create legal instruments to dictate how their assets and possessions are to be managed after their death, including their wishes regarding burial, cremation, or (within limits) other plans for the ultimate disposition of their corpse, but they have no such right over the disposition of their organs, except for the sole decision as to whether or not to be an organ donor after death. One reason supporting the view that organs donated after death should be the sole property of the State is that property rights in an organ are tied to an individual's interest in keeping his/her organs while alive and that the State has a societal interest in procuring and allocating organs from decedents. Once the individual dies, so too does the interest in keeping one's organs, and absent this interest, the property rights in one's organs are forfeit to the State.

This is an argument that has been offered in defence of organ conscription after death by the State: if an individual's interest in keeping his organs vanishes after he dies because his property rights in his own organs rest solely on his interest in keeping them while alive, then deceased individuals have no property rights in their organs. Furthermore, the decedent's surrogates have no property rights preventing the procurement of organs after the decedent's death, since all that follows upon an individual's death is that the individual's property rights in his/her organs expire with the individual, not that these property rights are conferred by default either to surrogates or to the State (Spital, 2003). The State, in asserting a property right over organs from the deceased, must rely on the additional claim that there is a positive societal benefit in procuring organs from the deceased, and this positive societal benefit successfully competes against other claims of benefits and harms which might be the basis for conflicting claims for property rights in organs from the deceased.

But if property rights are based on an individual's interest in maintaining those rights while alive and those interests expire after death, then it raises the question of the moral justification for allocation of any property rights to an individual's 'estate' after death. Why then should money, real estate, and other assets remain the private property of a decedent's estate? If, on the other hand, a coherent argument can be made that there are some interests that individuals cultivate which persist after the individual's death, it raises the question of whether or not property rights in one's organs might be included in that list of surviving interests. It isn't hard to imagine that individuals (if asked) might have detailed, considered preferences regarding the preferential allocation of their organs to fellow members of an individual's moral community, and that just as individuals might have interests in how their assets are distributed after death, they might have directly analogous interests in how and to whom their organs are allocated, interests that are almost uniformly ignored by most organ allocation systems. My point here is not to stake out a particular position on with whom or with what entity property rights in organs from the deceased should ultimately lie. But the very possibility of an organ allocation system rests on some theory of property rights in organs which confers these rights on the entity doing the allocating, and the widespread assumption that organs become the property of the State after procurement is an unusual exception to how most property rights of individuals are dispositioned after death, and the justification for this exception for organs from the deceased, an exception that dispenses with the need to account for the postmortem interests of individuals, is not obvious. Insofar as the basis for those property rights changes or is undermined, the right of an entity to allocate organs might change or be undermined.

Even if we grant that the State ought to always have the right to dispose of organs from deceased donors in a manner it sees fit so as to achieve a positive social benefit, the authority whereby allocation is undertaken on behalf of the State's (stipulated, for now) property rights in deceased donor organs remains a separate concern. The philosopher Robert Veatch has convincingly argued that decisions regarding how organs ought to be allocated should not be left to the medical profession. Veatch (2008) argues that while transplant physicians can surely be understood as possessing clinical expertise, the issues at stake in organ allocation are fundamentally ethical and not clinical concerns. It does not follow that by virtue of being an authority on clinical matters that clinicians should be in authority regarding how properly to allocate organs. Clinical expertise can and should inform ethical reflection, but clinical expertise alone does not provide answers to ethical questions. Given that the State's property rights in organs are predicated on the positive benefits for society of more organs for transplantation, presumably the authority to render ethical judgements regarding how best to allocate organs rests with society.

So, what is 'society' and how does it speak on its own behalf? Veatch argues that '. . . it is the general lay public that creates the money pool to support dialysis and creates the pool of cadaver organs to be allocated. They should be the ones making the moral choices relating to medical and nonmedical goods and relating the pursuit of maximum benefit to maximum justice or fairness in allocation' (Veatch, 2008, p. 284). Even if we stipulate that Veatch is right about this, there is no such thing as a 'general lay public', available and waiting to substantively opine on such matters. Instead there is a broad array of professional societies, patient rights organizations, as well as many species of public intellectual gadfly with particular interests in how organs ought to be allocated. These are the actual voices heard and the arguments aired when it comes to actually rendering policy decisions about organ allocation, which are not obviously the only voices and the only arguments worthy of consideration. Any system of allocation will result in benefits to some and harms to other members of 'society', and it is not at all obvious that society speaks with one voice on how organs ought to be allocated or that substantive disagreements within society regarding how organs ought to be allocated are soluble. The sum total of these active participants make up a minuscule fraction of taxpayers, donor families, and transplant candidates, and the majority of institutions and individuals who do participate in and substantively influence these policy discussions have little claim to being representative of the considered views of taxpayers, donor families, and/or transplant candidates, assuming large swaths of these fellow citizens have considered views on organ allocation strategies to begin with.

In short, the familiar discussion of organ allocation as a conflict of competing ethical principles rests on a number of contentious premises regarding property rights in organs from deceased donors, as well as the assumption that the moral authority of a small, interested coterie of commentators can speak in broad terms and without distortion on these matters on behalf of the various values and commitment of stakeholders in diverse and morally pluralistic societies and so arrive at 'consensus'; this should be understood to be as dubious as it sounds. To be sure, if organ transplantation is a social good which ought to be promoted and paid for, if there is a shortage of organs relative to the population who might benefit from them, if organs have to be allocated somehow, then having a system of organ allocation is inevitable. These sceptical reflections regarding where the property rights in organs from the deceased are located and why and how one should think about the relationship between the moral authority of theoretical 'society' to pronounce on the ethical questions raised by organ allocation and the actual, self-identified participants who shape and determine the direction and substance of organ allocation policy should be cause for approaching the familiar discussion with a large helping of humility.

## Efficiency—a multivalent concept

In the US literature on kidney allocation, the terms 'efficacy' and 'equity' are frequently invoked as concepts that need to be 'balanced' by any just system of organ allocation. Unfortunately, several ideas are packed into the term 'efficiency', and it is useful to unpack and examine these ideas separately.

In any organ allocation system, 'ought implies can'. In other words, an organ allocation system must respect certain clinical realities regarding the successful procurement, placement, and function of different solid organs. Call this requirement Ef1. A system that did not respect these realities, and by extension regularly resulted in poor outcomes, would be per se unjustifiable. In this usage one narrow definition of the concept of efficiency is the timely allocation and transplant of a procured and allocated organ, such that a system which respects efficiency is one that accedes to the clinical realities that solid organ transplantation from deceased donors operates under time constraints, constraints that can only be negotiated at the margins at the direct cost of the performance of the organ after transplantation. So-called cold ischaemic time limits are different for different organs. Hearts, lungs, and livers tolerate much shorter cold ischaemic times compared to kidneys, which in turn means that there is a higher priority to procure and disposition those organs compared to the kidneys from any given donor. Also, technological advances can sometimes change the clinical realities in ways that may or may not have implications for allocation, but which are worth keeping in mind if the structure of an allocation system is ethically disputed. The way to think about this is that evolutions in what is clinically possible circumscribe the normative limits on a system of allocation: when what 'can' happen changes, it may in turn affect what 'ought' to happen.

So, for example, the introduction and widespread use of cold-perfusion pumping systems for kidneys has allowed them to be successfully transplanted with much longer cold ischaemic times (that is, well beyond 24 hours) than was previously possible. This in turn permits the transfer of kidneys not simply across locales but across continents without additional risk to the function of the organ after transplant, save the various things that can go wrong in the course of packaging and transport of an organ. If organs can be preserved for longer periods of time ex vivo, this theoretically expands the geographic boundaries of where an organ can be shipped without the cost of worse graft function after transplant, which in turn makes allocation systems which emphasize eliminating geographic disparities in access to transplantation clinically possible. If it is true for the purposes of discussing organ allocation that 'ought implies can', it is useful and necessary to understand what can be accomplished before a discussion of how organs ought to be allocated.

Another sense of efficiency (Ef2) has to do with assuring the rapid, reliable, reproducible, transparent, and ultimately flexible disposition of an organ to a rank-ordered list of candidates. When an organ offer is made, the rank-ordered list of candidates who have a claim to that organ must be able to be generated quickly and according to criteria that is both publicly available and clear. Potential candidates must be contacted to determine if they are sufficiently healthy to proceed with transplant, and they must be clinically evaluated in person in the hospital setting in order to be cleared to proceed to transplant, a process that takes time and effort. Such a system must be sufficiently flexible to respond to situations in which a candidate who is offered an organ and is found to be unsuitable for proceeding to transplant after an in-person evaluation can be quickly passed over and candidates next in lexical priority can be similarly mobilized for evaluation. A system in which candidates are identified and screened ad hoc is inefficient in the Ef2 sense and sets the stage for both clinical errors and the ethical criticism of arbitrariness.

Efficiency is often discussed in a third sense (Ef3), which tacitly assumes an account of Ef1 and Ef2 but largely overlaps where it is not completely indistinguishable from 'utility', though compared to the vast literature in moral philosophy on utilitarianism and its implications, the notion of utility invoked here is quite parochial. In the first place, representative views of Ef3 as utility skip over crucial questions and controversies well explored (if not often solved) within utilitarian thought.

## The measurement of utility

In contemporary organ allocation discussions, utility is measured in the coin of years of survival after transplantation (UNOS proposal). Identifying utility with 'life years' has the prima facie virtue of being reliably and reproducibly measurable and easily comprehended. The rationale for any solid organ transplant procedure is that a successful transplant will confer a benefit (however defined) to a patient and that the benefit conferred is superior (however defined) to not pursuing a transplant. Survival is a common measure of benefit but is not the only possible measure of benefit, nor is it obviously the most morally important measure of benefit; additional years of life lived may not be especially attractive if those additional years are of very low quality from the standpoint of the individual living them. But survival measurements have the virtue of being comparable across individuals; a year of survival for A is quantitatively equal to a year of survival for B, C, and D.

The use of a common metric is also important in addressing the problem of interpersonal comparisons of utility (see the section 'Sidebar—interpersonal comparisons of utility'), because if it is morally important for a system of allocation to distribute quantifiable utility between discrete persons, one has to have a way of assuring the potential that utility can, indeed, be distributed to the persons in question. This may seem a pedestrian point, but if the utility in question to be distributed is 'happiness', it is clear that the process and verification of 'distributing' happiness becomes rather more complicated, because of substantive disagreements between individuals over what constitutes happiness and whether it is meaningful to say that happiness is a thing that can be reliably and reproducibly distributed in more or fewer quantities by some mechanism like an allocation system. (In such a system, perhaps the chronically dysthymic need not apply.) For simplicity's sake, efficiency in the Ef3 sense has come to mean more utility in the sense of increasing the number of years of survival after transplantation using one allocation scheme instead of different, competing approaches to allocation. But, as elsewhere, it should suffice for now to conclude here that 'keeping it simple' for the purposes of measuring utility requires skipping over a number of pertinent questions.

## Sidebar—*interpersonal comparisons of utility*

While the metric of 'life years after transplant' has obvious methodological advantages in thinking through distributive approaches, it has proven to be unsatisfactory, as the exercise of substituting 'happiness' for 'years of survival' shows. Individuals can and verifiably do value certain aspects of their lives quite differently; individuals value different things at different junctures in life, to say nothing of the fact that what individuals actually say they value does not necessarily correspond to observed behaviours. The recognition that each of us has substantively different views of the good life, and that robust generalizations about what constitutes the good life for all are demonstrably false, is a part of the justification in the West for negative liberty rights, the right (within limits) to be left alone to pursue our designs of the life well lived without outside interference, and the requirement for informed consent from individuals before their bodies are violated by the medical profession, even if ostensibly for the individual's 'benefit'. Quite understandably, grappling with the diversity of attitudes toward the good life and what constitutes life's quality is mostly passed over in silence in allocation debates, since taking that challenge seriously would make a hash of how these entities would be measured between persons and whether it is metaphysically possible to parse and distribute discrete 'quality' units.

The 'fair innings' argument can be understood as a limited response to the charge that 'survival years' as a measure of utility is shallow. There are several versions of the 'fair innings' argument, but Alan Williams (1997, p. 119) offers a useful and broadly accepted version: '[The fair innings argument] reflects the feeling that everyone is entitled to some "normal" span of health (usually expressed in terms of life years, e.g. 'three score and ten'). The implication is that anyone failing to achieve this has in some sense been cheated, whilst anyone getting more than this is "living on borrowed time"'. Fair innings introduces the claim that not all years of survival are equal, that some years of survival while young are more valuable than years of survival when older, and that there is an injustice which should be ameliorated when an expectation of a normal lifespan is not achieved. Since organ allocation is zero sum, that is, an organ allocated to one individual is an organ not allocated to another, organs should be preferentially allocated to younger candidates at the explicit expense of older candidates. As framed by Williams, not only does fair innings confer on society a duty to individuals to help them lead a normal lifespan, but also society itself has an interest in fulfilling this end. Williams himself favourably quotes a paper commissioned by the World Bank to the effect that 'Most societies attach more importance to a year of life lived by a young or middle-aged adult than to a year of life lived by a child or an elderly person' and '. . . people of different ages have a different (social) value (which in turn reflects their likely life stage)', as graphically illustrated in Figure 5.1 (Williams, 1997, pp. 126–127).

There is much to commend a 'fair innings' approach, even as one might dispute where the lines are drawn regarding relative quality measurements from the vantage of individuals or society. Fair innings approaches frankly acknowledge the zero-sum nature of organ allocation decisions under conditions of scarcity, and by extension that benefits for some come at the expense of losses for

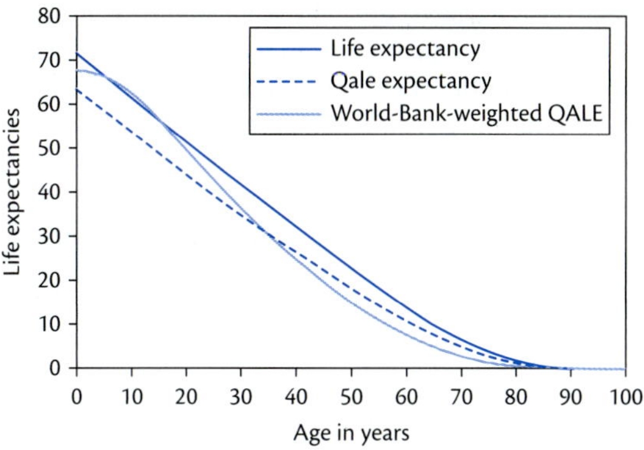


**Fig. 5.1** Williams' approach to fair innings takes this 'societal worth' graph and uses it to modify individual claims against society for the opportunity to live a normal lifespan, as illustrated by the comparison between life expectancy (solid line) and societal worth (shaded line, as estimated by the World Bank graph). This combination both respects the individual's claim to have a right to a normal lifespan and is slightly weighted for the different quantified social worth over an individual's lifespan. QALY, Quality-adjusted life expectancy. (Reproduced with permission from Williams A, 'Intergenerational equity: An exploration of the 'fair innings' argument', *Health Economics*, 6, pp. 117–132. © 1992 John Wiley and Sons.)

others. It is a useful and illustrative attempt to balance the claims of individuals with the interests of society. Accordingly, the flaws in the fair innings approach are representative of the flaws in any system of allocation that relies on broad generalizations about interpersonal comparisons of utility and confident assertions about the worth of individuals to society across the lifespan.

To take the last point first, any assertions about calculating and employing the 'social worth' of individuals for the purposes of organ allocation would have to contend with the sordid history of how 'social worth' arguments have been ruthlessly employed against all manner of disadvantaged and disenfranchised persons. Examples of this, just in organized medicine in the first half of the twentieth century alone, are sufficient to fill several volumes, and to even pick out a few from the list of horribles would be to risk failing to do justice to many others. Insofar as the requisite reticence and care that would be required to address this extensive litany of wrongs is even possible, it is highly unlikely that the resulting conclusions from such an intellectual exertion would yield anything more than the most qualified and tentative of conclusions, such that they would be of little use to contemporary discussions of organ allocation.

Setting that elephantine challenge aside, Williams acutely characterizes the claims of individuals against society for providing the opportunity for a normal lifespan as a 'feeling', but it is not at all clear that this claim is anything more than the articulation of a feeling. Why should matters of biological misfortune uncontroversially become matters to be corrected in the name of social justice, rather than just an unfortunate state of affairs to be noted and perhaps regretted (whereas disability activists sharply dispute that biological misfortune should be cast as 'misfortune' and that the choice of terminology is revealing of deeper prejudices)? Why should the quality of one's lived life as a whole be understood as synonymous with longevity? Is it obvious that individuals tend to value their young adult years more than their later years? Why is the opportunity of some to be young inexorably more valuable than the opportunity of others to grow old? The central problem with the fair innings argument is that it can only grant the claim of individuals to have a right to achieve a normal lifespan, but must (arbitrarily) cut off or sharply limit further ruminations on the difficulties posed by assessing the value of individual lives and comparing valued lives with one another without substantially truncating what it is that is being 'valued' for the purposes of comparison. Just as with the identification of what counts as utility, fair innings is only convincing if one is prepared to set aside a whole set of troubling normative questions.

From measurement to prediction: a prospectively implemented organ allocation system designed to maximize utility (efficiency in the Ef3 sense) must be able to not only define utility as a measurable, distributable unit but also predict the utility conferred by an organ allocation decision. An organ allocation system in which conferred utility could only be assessed retrospectively, with no means of predicting conferred utility prospectively, would be useless. This does not necessarily mean that the formula used to predict utility must reliably and reproducibly predict utility gained in individual cases of organ allocation, but the formula must at least predict the total utility conferred by applying the formula to a group of allocation decisions. Still, whether a utility prediction formula performs more or less well at predicting conferred utility in individual cases, for specific groups of donor–candidate pairings, or for the entire system is morally relevant. If, for some reason, a prediction model frequently yields the wrong answer, then the moral case for applying a formula designed to maximize utility must be tempered by the unfortunate fact that the prediction model employed will frequently not achieve that end. The options then are to either (1) find a different prediction model less hobbled by error, (2) think through the moral implications of using a prediction model that will be wrong a certain percentage of the time, or (3) abandon the use of a prediction model altogether. Option (3) would entail abandoning the goal of using an allocation system to maximize utility, since if there is no means of predicting utility conferred by an allocation system, there is no way to design an allocation system to maximize utility, except perhaps by accident.

In debates over kidney allocation in the US, the utility prediction formula, which has been under discussion for several years, is a mathematical formula generated from a retrospective examination of many years of data collected on patient outcomes after transplantation in the US. The estimated post-transplant survival (EPTS) formula, which measures candidate age, length of time on dialysis, whether the candidate had a prior transplant, and whether the patient had diabetes, generates a numerical score that ostensibly correlates with survival after transplantation. Higher EPTS scores entail lower rates of survival after transplantation (OPTN, 2012). The formula is as follows:

> EPTS score = (0.047 × (Age – 25, 0)) + (–0.015 × Diabetes × (Age – 25, 0)) + (0.398 × Prior organ transplant) + (–0.237 × Diabetes × Prior organ transplant) + (0.315 × log (Years on dialysis + 1)) + (–0.099 × Diabetes × log (Years on dialysis + 1)) + (0.130 × (Years on dialysis = 0)) + (–0.348 × Diabetes × (Years on dialysis = 0)) + (1.262 × Diabetes)

One need not require a degree in statistics to notice that this derived mathematical formula makes little clinical sense. 'Diabetes' as a cause of ESRD is well appreciated to result in worse outcomes for patients on dialysis as well as after transplantation compared to similar patients without diabetes as the cause of their ESRD. Also length of time on dialysis has been associated with lower patient survival after transplantation. (In both instances this is almost certainly related to the acceleration of cardiovascular disease.) However, in the EPTS formula, diabetes as a variable both increases and decreases the overall EPTS score, as does the number of years on dialysis. There is no measurement of cardiovascular disease burden in this prediction model, nor in any other prediction model currently under discussion. The reason is because the existing patient databases mined for transplant outcomes do not measure cardiovascular disease burden because it is difficult to categorically measure between patients, and even if agreement might be reached on how to do so, data would need to be collected for years before a formula similar to EPTS could be generated. Furthermore, 'diabetes' as a cause of ESRD is a different clinical entity than 'diabetes' as a comorbid condition but not as a cause of ESRD. In other words, a 60-year-old patient with 30 years of diabetes and ESRD from diabetes is probably clinically different than a 60-year-old patient with ESRD from IgA nephropathy and 3 years of diabetes with no established end-organ damage. But, for the purpose of EPTS calculations, both patients 'have diabetes' (Hippen, 2009).

It shouldn't be a surprise, then, that the inability of EPTS to distinguish between vastly different clinical entities means that the ability of the EPTS to reliably predict survival after transplantation is poor. One way to gauge this quantitatively is to measure the index of covariance (IoC) of a predictive model. A predictive model with an IoC of 0.5 is correct 50% of the time, and a predictive model with an IoC of 1.0 is correct 100% of the time. A predictive model with an IoC of 0.5 is as accurate as a coin flip. An allocation model in which organ allocation was determined by the flip of a coin as defined by years of survival after transplant could seamlessly replace a predictive model with an IoC of 0.5, ostensibly designed to maximize utility. Thus it is morally relevant to know that the EPTS prediction model has an IoC of 0.693, which is to say that the EPTS has a 69% chance of being correct (and therefore a 31% chance of being wrong) in predicting patient survival after transplantation (UNOS, 2012, p. 15). Furthermore, there are no prediction models in circulation (including EPTS) that have been prospectively validated in actual clinical settings, which only adds further caveats to the predictive power attributed to the EPTS score.

In the interests of creating some sort of allocation system, a reasonable response might be to grant the limited predictive power of the EPTS with the plea that this is 'the best we can do with what we have'. But if 'the best we have' is wrong 30% of the time, using the EPTS scoring system to make decisions about organ allocation will mis-triage, and thereby harm, 30% of candidates. Utilitarian calculations include not only a measurement of the additional benefits conferred by an allocation system but also a rigorous attempt to define, measure, and minimize disutility, or harm.

Let us stipulate a system in which patients predicted to have better post-transplant survival receive allocation priority for the best quality organs, and stipulate that A has a better predicted post-transplant survival compared to B, C, and D. In a zero-sum system, an organ allocated to patient A is an organ not allocated to patient B, C, or D. Whatever benefits A accrues, it comes at the expense of B, C, or D. If B subsequently dies on the waiting list and B would not have died on the list if he had received the organ instead of A, then B has suffered a harm, a harm that must be weighed against the benefit of allocating the organ to A. Suppose now that A is predicted to have a superior post-transplant survival to B, C, and D but the prediction is wrong: B actually has the longer survival. In that instance the allocation priority enjoyed by A is wrongly conferred, which is a harm to B (since B has been mis-triaged through no fault of his own), but C and D are also harmed, since A's accidental benefit undermines C's and D's ostensibly equal claims to the organ allocated to A, once maximization of utility is no longer a consideration. This is not to say that A has harmed B, C, and D, but that the breakdown in the moral premise which justifies the allocation system which allocated the kidney to A has resulted in B, C, and D being harmed by the allocation system, although B is harmed in a different way compared to C and D. All candidates, including A, are harmed by the sheer capriciousness of the system, which turns out to be a kind of fraud, unlike the use of a coin flip or a lottery system for distributing organs, where the probabilities of getting an organ are roughly equally distributed among the candidates and all of the candidates are in a position to understand this. But an error rate of 30% for EPTS means that though candidates may think they understand the rationale for their own place in the rank-ordered list of candidates to receive a transplant, that rationale is undermined 1/3 of the time, such that some candidates who should receive priority do not and some candidates who should not receive priority get priority.

If these prediction models for utility are 'the best we have' right now, then the transplant community, policy-makers, and regulators should simply acknowledge that even if the considerable difficulties in defining, measuring, and comparing utility can be successfully surmounted, on its own terms, current utility prediction models are just not suitable for use in organ allocation. If ought implies can, and utility prediction models cannot reliably and reproducibly predict utility, then utility prediction models ought not to be used for organ allocation. That this conclusion might be widely demoralizing does not make it less sound.

## Equity: of what, for who, and why

Whether or not it ought to be so, it is widely the case that property rights in deceased donor organs are held and dispositioned by the State. If it is the case that individuals who require an organ transplant have a prima facie equal claim to an organ from the State, it is then left to an organ allocation system to further distinguish and prioritize the claims of individuals. Competing individual claims to an organ are in the first instance distinguished by efficiency claims in the Ef1 and Ef2 sense described in the section 'Efficiency—a multivalent concept'. So an individual's claim to a particular donated organ may be invalidated if it is clinically inadvisable to allocate that organ (or any organ) to that candidate or if it is technically unfeasible to transport and transplant that organ to that recipient.

Time on the waiting list is another means distinguishing competing individual claims to an organ. Waiting time has the virtue of being easy to quantify and measure and is easy to compare between individuals: a year for A is numerically identical to a year for B. So if A and B have prima facie equal claims to an organ, one way to treat A's and B's claim equally is to allocate an organ to whomever has accumulated more waiting time.[2] A central complaint of those who would supplement a waiting time-based allocation system with utility calculations is that waiting time is

[2] When an individual's waiting time should begin is open to debate. In the US it has been proposed that waiting time should begin when a candidate's glomerular filtration rate is documented at <= 20 cc/min or the date of onset of ESRD, rather than the current practice of starting waiting time at the time the candidate is registered on a list at a transplant centre. In principle, as long as the clock starts for the same time for all individuals, when an individual's waiting time begins is of secondary concern.

not efficient in the Ef3 sense: young candidates may receive organs that do not last as long or have more complications, and older candidates may receive kidneys from younger donors and die well before the organ itself fails.

And so, the critics argue, the current system that privileges waiting time must be supplemented with utility considerations. But, as we have reviewed at some length, utility considerations are beset by problems and controversy at every step, from what counts as utility, to what sort of utility can actually be measured, compared between individuals, predicted, and distributed. The virtue of waiting time as a means of distinguishing otherwise equal claims is simple: waiting time does not require the enormous exercise in question-begging, controversy aversion, and predictive uncertainties one must labour through to bring forth a useable account of utility to the discussion of organ allocation.

To be sure, all candidates do not endure waiting time equally. Young, healthier candidates are typically much more likely to survive on the waiting list compared to older and sicker candidates. Herein lies a biological inequality, which is not ameliorated by waiting time as a metric. But waiting time does not imply that 'fair innings' considerations should apply either to the young (so that they might receive a better quality organ and enjoy the opportunity to live a more 'normal' lifespan) or to the old.[3] That an individual is in need of a kidney at an older age rather than a younger age (and vice versa) just *is* the case, and it is perhaps unfortunate, but it is not obviously unjust. The priority of waiting time is compatible with the resoundingly sceptical approach toward utility measurements I have argued for here. Unless and until utility's proponents improve upon their assertions, metrics, interpersonal comparisons, and predictive tools, there is little reason to doubt the ethical superiority of an organ allocation system predicated on waiting time.

## Conclusion

Moral pluralism, fundamental disagreements about the right and the good, is a hallmark of modern western societies (Engelhardt, 1996). In defending our parochial views of morality, we reference our reason, our views of happiness and how to get it (or more of it), our community, our sense of self-worth, our god (or his absence), and quite often some pastiche of these. It should therefore not be overly surprising that problems such as organ allocation should generate controversies that are not obviously or easily resolved by reference to normative icons that not all of us respect, or at least respect in the same ways. Recognition of this state of affairs need not lead to nihilism, relativism, or quietist despair. Rather, it offers the opportunity to approach the thorny moral problems of organ allocation with a spirit of humility, one generated by taking a sceptical approach toward robust, substantive generalizations about what constitutes the good life, how to measure it, how to predict it, and how to dole it out in the right way. Understanding why it is difficult to generate comprehensive, convincing, enduring answers to thorny moral questions can set the stage for trying again. But until then, it is more ethically reliable to base a system of organ allocation on premises that can actually be articulated, examined, and defended.

[3] An idiosyncratic but no less defensible version of fair innings is one that takes account of the additional vulnerability of older candidates on the waiting list and is designed to minimize death on the waiting list rather than maximize the lifespan of the youngest and healthiest. Since the youngest and healthiest can wait longer on the list, they are less likely to die than older candidates. Here one faces yet another utility comparison: the harm of death for the old compared to the further extension of life for the young. It is of interest that organ allocation systems for livers, hearts, and lungs, in taking a 'sickest first' approach, prioritize the avoidance of death and the minimization of harm rather than the maximization of survival. Unlike ESRD, where chronic dialysis is widely available (and with the modest exception of the destination left ventricular assist device (LVAD)), allocation choice for these organs is one of life or death.

## References

Engelhardt HT (1996) *The Foundations of Bioethics*, 2nd edn. Oxford University Press, Oxford.

Hippen BE (2008) Organ sales and moral travails: lessons from the living kidney vendor program in Iran. *Cato Policy Analysis*, No. 614, 20 March 20. <http://www.cato.org/publications/policy-analysis/organ-sales-moral-travails-lessons-living-kidney-vendor-program-iran>.

Hippen BE (2009) The kidney allocation score: methodological concerns, moral objections and unintended consequences. *Am J Transpl*, **9**:1507–1512.

Howard R (2007) The challenging triangle: balancing outcomes, transplant numbers and costs. *Am J Transpl*, **7**:2443–2445.

Mahdavi-Mazdeh M (2012) The Iranian model of living renal transplantation. *Kidney Int*, **82**:627–634.

Matas A, Schnitzler M (2003) Payment for living donor (vendor) kidneys: a cost-effectiveness analysis. *Am J Transpl*, **4**:216–221.

Moazam F (2006) *Bioethics and Organ Transplantation in a Muslim Society: A Study in Culture, Ethnography and Religion*. Indiana University Press, Bloomington.

OPTN (2012) *Proposal to substantially revise the kidney allocation system*. <http://optn.transplant.hrsa.gov/publiccomment/pubcommentpropsub_311.pdf>.

Scheper-Hughes N (1995) The primacy of the ethical: propositions for a militant anthropology. *Curr Anthropol*, **36**:409–440.

Scheper-Hughes N (2007) The tyranny of the gift: sacrificial violence in living donor transplantation. *Am J Transpl*, **3**:507–511.

Schold J, Srinivas TR, Kayler LK, Meier-Kriesche HU (2007) The overlapping risk profile between dialysis patients listed and not listed for renal transplantation. *Am J Transpl*, **8**:58–68.

Spital A (2003) Conscription of cadaveric organs for transplantation: neglected again. *Kennedy Inst Ethics J*, **13**,169–174.

Stein R (2008) A third of patients on transplant list are not eligible. *Washington Post*, 22 March. <http://www.washingtonpost.com/wp-dyn/content/article/2008/03/21/ar2008032102981.html>.

US Renal Data System, USRDS (2012) *Annual Data Report: Atlas of Chronic Kidney Disease and End-Stage Renal Disease in the United States*. National Institutes of Health, National Institute of Diabetes and Digestive and Kidney Diseases, Bethesda, Maryland.

Veatch R (2000) *Transplantation Ethics*. Georgetown University Press, Washington, DC.

Williams A (1997) Intergenerational equity: an exploration of the 'fair innings' argument. *Health Econ*, **6**:117–132.

# CHAPTER 6

# Ethical issues in transplant tourism and organ commercialism

Robin N. Fiore

## Global context of kidney disease and renal replacement therapies[1]

Chronic kidney disease is a worldwide public health problem and consumes a significant percentage of health resources in both developed and developing countries. Worldwide, nearly 2 million people are being kept alive by renal replacement therapies—dialysis and transplant (Couser et al., 2011). These figures are expected to increase significantly in the next decade due to population aging, urbanization, and increased access to care. Approximately 80% of those receiving renal replacement therapy live in Japan, the US, Brazil, and Europe; fewer than 10% of patients in India and Pakistan who need renal replacement therapy receive it and there is little or no access to renal replacement therapies in Africa (White et al., 2008; and according to the United States Renal Data System). Nearly 1 million people die from renal failure or complications of end-stage renal disease (ESRD) each year in low-income countries where renal replacement therapy is unavailable or unaffordable (Barsoum, 2006; White et al., 2008).

For ESRD patients, transplantation offers the only prospect of restoring a healthy, productive life. Compared with dialysis, transplantation improves both survival and quality of life. According to a recent systematic review of 110 studies including almost 2 million participants, compared with dialysis, kidney transplantation not only is associated with reduced risk of mortality and cardiovascular events but also imposes far fewer constraints on day-to-day activities (Tonelli et al., 2011). In the US transplant recipients aged 20–39 years will live almost 17 years longer than dialysis patients (Wolfe et al., 1999). Transplantation is also the most cost-effective renal replacement therapy in terms of cost per life-year gained. In high-income countries the ongoing annual cost of maintaining a functioning transplant is approximately one-third to one-quarter that of dialysis (White et al., 2008). In the UK, for instance, the cost of transplant to the National Health Service (NHS) in year 1 is greater than the cost of dialysis, but by year 2 the cumulative costs of dialysis outweigh transplant costs; by year 5 the cumulative costs of dialysis are approximately 1.5 times the cost of transplant (Kerr, 2012).

[1] Although commercialism applies to human cells and tissues as well as several types of human organs, the focus of this chapter will be commercial activities in connection with kidney transplantation, the most commonly needed and most transplanted organ.

Tragically, the benefits of kidney transplantation remain unrealized to a large degree because kidney donation has not kept pace with the number of patients in need of organs. The annual rate of kidney donation from deceased donors has remained relatively flat in the last decade. Living donor transplants, especially from unrelated donors, have increased as a result of technical advances, including, among others: surgical techniques that reduce donor discomfort and recovery time, directed donation, desensitization protocols that permit transplantation from a wider donor pool, and unconventional organ donation variations such as kidney swaps ('paired donation' and 'non-simultaneous extended altruistic donor chains'). However, the number waiting for transplantation far outweighs the number of suitable organs available, despite efforts to increase donation rates.

The most common argument justifying transplant commercialism is that it will spur donations and thereby lead to fewer deaths of transplant candidates who are waiting for an organ. A brief look at data on wait times is instructive: according to the OPTN, 93,860 patients were registered on the kidney transplant waiting list in the US as of 1 October 2012; although the median wait time was 2.6 years, the wait exceeded 4 years for some regions. More than 8% die per year while waiting for transplant; and more than 40% of candidates listed in a given year will die while waiting, according to estimates (Matas, 2006). As of 31 December 2013, according to Eurotransplant, there were 10,757 people waiting for a kidney transplant in the EU (Eurotransplant International Foundation, 2013); and there were 6,348 people registered on the kidney transplant waiting list in the UK (excluding multi-organ transplants involving kidneys) (NHS Blood and Transplant, 2014a). The median waiting time to transplant in the UK for adult patients registered on the kidney-only transplant list is 1,082 days–slightly less than 3 years–and as high as 1,768—slightly less than 5 years—in some regions (NHS Blood and Transplant, 2014b).

The bleak outcomes associated with dialysis, projected increases in chronic kidney disease and renal failure, and severe shortage of suitable organs make it imperative to increase rates of both deceased and living kidney donation. The challenge has been acknowledged by individual governments, transplant consortia, and collaborating non-governmental organizations, but growth in the number of candidates exceeds growth in organ donations. Meanwhile, markets are one way to fill the gap, at least for those who have means.

Before addressing particular practices of concern, it is useful to briefly describe the regulatory background against which debates about commercialism play out.

## Legislating altruism

The first successful kidney transplants were followed by the formation of transplant physician societies, the development of organ procurement mechanisms, and the passage of enabling legislation with respect to anatomical gifts, determination of death, and insurance coverage for ESRD. Policy-makers in the West lined up on the side of altruistic donation despite the otherwise for-profit nature of medicine and healthcare.

In the US, NOTA, passed in 1984, criminalized buying and selling human organs, punishable by fines and prison:

> It shall be unlawful for any person to knowingly acquire, receive, or otherwise transfer any human organ for valuable consideration for use in human transplantation if the transfer affects interstate commerce. (NOTA, 1984)

Note that the unfortunate wording of the law has the unintended consequence of disallowing almost all incentives to donate, including charitable tax deductions.

The WHO and most European countries issued similar bans. The WHO *Guiding Principles on Human Cell, Tissue and Organ Transplantation* (1987) states:

> Cells, tissues and organs should be donated freely, without any monetary payment or other reward of monetary value. Purchasing, or offering to purchase, cells, issues or organs for transplantation, or their sale by living persons or by next of kin for deceased person, should be banned (Guiding Principle 5). (World Health Organization, 2015)

The accompanying Commentary to Guiding Principle 5 makes clear that one of the aims of this guidance is 'to affirm the special merit of *donating* [emphasis mine] human materials to save and enhance life' (World Health Organization, 2015).

Without irony, the Ethics Committee of the Transplantation Society, a non-governmental organization associated with the WHO, issued the following policy on the involvement of transplant professionals in transplant commercialism:

> No transplant surgeon/team shall be involved directly or indirectly in the buying or selling of organs/tissues or in any transplant activity aimed at commercial gain to himself/herself or an associated hospital or institute. (Council of the Transplantation Society, 1985)

The prohibition on selling human organs reflects western views about the vulgarity of markets and the moral superiority of certain kinds of motivation. According to this view, donation-without-benefit-to-self contributes to social solidarity and reinforces the virtues of charity and compassion. The distinction between gift and sale echoes the traditional separation between private and public spheres of human activity, each with its different constitutive values. It reflects also a view about human dignity and the sanctity of the human body that is offended by commodification and attributing instrumental valuation to humans and human body parts (John Paul II, 1995). These attitudes are reiterated in historical policy debates about the abolition of slavery, the decriminalization of prostitution, surrogate gestation contracts, and compensation for research participation.

More recently, the EU adopted the now familiar principles of voluntary, unpaid donation and non-profit procurement, but added the further ban on advertising the need for, or availability of, organs with a view to offering or seeking financial gain (Article 13) (European Union, 2012a). Although the primary stated aim of this EU Directive is the safety and quality of organs, Article 7 states that it 'explicitly contributes indirectly to combating organ trafficking through the establishment of competent authorities, the authorization of transplantation centers, the establishment of conditions of procurement and systems of traceability' (European Union, 2012b). The anti-trafficking objective relies on standards of traceability and non-profiteering applied to organ exchanges between EU members states and between EU members and third countries.

In sum, the consensus among public policy-makers, ethicists, and medical professionals has long been and continues to be that organ donors should not be financially compensated or advantaged, say, by receiving a priority organ allocation. With few exceptions—in some cases reimbursement for certain limited expenses—a donor should be motivated purely by altruism. In this view, even well-regulated or intrastate markets in organs are ruled out.

A number of bioethicists and transplant professionals have challenged 'the great consensus' by refocusing moral concern on the human lives lost from prohibiting commercial organ activities. In addition they argue that the actual consequences of commercialization depend crucially on the particular institutional arrangements through which organ sales are implemented (Cherry, 2005; Friedman and Friedman, 2006).

## Scarcity and commercialism

The main impediment to providing transplantation at (or near) the level of need is a severe shortage of organ donors, a dearth that shows no sign of abating under the established regimes. In the US, an opt-in or affirmative consent country, both deceased and living kidney donation rates have remained flat in terms of absolute numbers since 2005 despite public information campaigns and programmes aimed at increasing cadaveric donation. Presumed consent or so-called opt-out approaches dominate in European countries but remain controversial in the US, where autonomy considerations typically trump social welfare. The US at 26.3 deceased donors per million population ranked behind Spain and Portugal, both presumed-consent nations, at 34.1 per million and 26.7 per million, respectively. A recent systematic review concludes that presumed consent alone is unlikely to explain the variation in organ donation rates between opt-in and opt-out systems because the custom of obtaining family agreement makes presumption moot (Rithalia et. al., 2009). Other possible reasons for the differences include culture, social solidarity, and attitudes toward medical professionals.

Strict presumed consent could increase the supply of organs from deceased donors, though it may also engender mistrust and end up discouraging living donors. Wait-lists for organs grow year by year, with appalling consequences, while cadaveric donation alone is manifestly insufficient. As need exceeds legitimate supply by a factor greater than ten, patients must choose between transplant tourism and death. In the US alone, no fewer than 373 patients from 34 states are known to have received foreign transplants in 35 countries between 1987 and 2006 (Merion et al., 2008).

Absolute legal prohibitions expose potential kidney purchasers to 'uncontrolled free enterprise'. Indeed, 'there is much more scope for exploitation and abuse when a supply of desperately wanted goods is made illegal' (Radcliffe-Richards et al., 1998). As with other recognized demand-driven activities—gambling, prostitution, alcohol and substance use, etc.—prohibition does not reduce demand so much as it drives it underground, or, in the case of kidneys, across borders.

## Transplant tourism and organ trafficking

Travel across borders for locally unavailable medical care has been commonplace: national health patients avoiding health system limits, women travelling for reproductive services, candidates for sexual reassignment seeking non-judgemental surgeons, and so forth. Entrepreneurial medical professionals and third-party payers have packaged travel and discount medical care at distant network 'centres for excellence' and renowned medical centres have arranged visas and transportation for wealthy foreign patients. Increased patient mobility and globalization significantly increase the chances that patients will travel to satisfy medical needs. Nevertheless, cross-border travel for organ transplants is not merely medical tourism for transplant purposes.

Before continuing, it will be useful to distinguish between transplant commercialism, transplant tourism, and organ trafficking. Transplant commercialism, broadly understood, refers to a policy or practice in which an organ is treated as a commodity, including its being bought or sold or used primarily to produce profit. Transplant tourism involves the movement of organs, donors, recipients, or transplant professionals across jurisdictional borders for the purpose of transplantation.

At its most benign, transplant tourism might involve expatriates returning to their country of origin to participate, as a donor or recipient, in a living related donor (LRD) transplant where there is a genetic or familial relationship. However, more often it is a commercial transaction, involving an unrelated organ seller or 'vendor' who is either induced to provide an organ for financial considerations or, worse, coerced for the financial benefit to a third party.

Transplant tourism is widely condemned and prohibited by law in most countries. It should be noted, however, that such laws typically apply to the purchase of organs within one's own jurisdiction and not extraterritorially. Transplant tourists are, in principle, subject to the laws of the jurisdiction in which they are travelling, but, in practice, laws are loosely enforced in common organ-selling destinations. Moreover, upon returning to one's home country there are rarely legal consequences. In other words, while 'the purchase of organs is illegal, the purchase of organs will not (always) be *punishable*' (Ambagtsheer and Weimar, 2012).

Transplant tourism destinations often lack comprehensive patient registries and auditing functions, so reliable data for transplant tourism are not available. The WHO estimates that as much as 10% of organs transplanted worldwide are the result of commercial transplant activity, with most of it taking place in India, Pakistan, the Philippines, and China, identified by WHO as the primary 'organ-exporting' countries (Shimazono, 2007). Each of these countries represents a different 'version' of transplant tourism. India, for instance, long known as 'the great organ bazaar', had a legal organ market before passing legislation in 1994 banning kidney sales. Since then, illegal schemes have been uncovered regularly, including 'kidney tours' in which vendors (paid donors) were transported to other countries for the removal and subsequent transplant of their kidneys. Since the 1980s, prisoners sentenced to death constituted China's chief source of organs, as much as 90%. Human rights groups have long criticized China for creating an incentive for prisons to execute prisoners in order to profit from selling their organs. In 2012 China announced plans to end the practice of transplanting organs from executed prisoners within 3–5 years. In the Philippines the sale of human organs has been officially illegal since 2003, but the Filipino government failed to provide an enforcement mechanism until 2012 (Official Gazette, 2012) .

In 2008 Israel passed a law banning the sale and brokerage of organs and ended health insurance system funding for foreign transplants. Prior to this, Israel's health system did not restrict payment for transplantation services, with the result that 'its citizens purchase, proportionally, the largest number of organs in the global market' (Scheper-Hughes, 2002). Israel's wait-list for kidney transplants dropped from 705 days to 509 days during 2001–2005. However, a side effect of the policy was the transfer of one's duty (life saving) to others, as seen in the single-digit rates of living donations, including LRD during the same period. Similarly, LRD dropped off precipitously in Pakistan, Korea, and Hong Kong with the availability of purchased kidneys (Ambagtsheer and Wimar, 2012). Before the British transferred sovereignty to mainland China, living donors accounted for nearly half of all kidney transplants in Hong Kong. Since then, with transplant candidates able to travel to China to purchase kidneys, the number of living donor transplants in Hong Kong has fallen to only 15–20% of all kidney transplants performed there (Danovitch and Leichtman, 2006).

A common type of policy argument is that organ sales should not be prohibited because doing so allows both the person who objects to selling and the person who does not object each to exercise their moral preference without impediment. That is, the objector is able to refrain while the non-objector is able to participate. The experiences of Israel and Hong Kong function as 'natural experiments', revealing the insidious effect of compensation on altruism and the manner in which 'the moral commitment to do one's duty can be weakened by financial compensation and monetary reward' (Danovitch and Leichtman, 2006).

The ethical objection to transplant commercialism, then, is that a profit motive changes the moral nature of the transaction from one of rescue, charity, and self-sacrifice, and thereby brings about perverse consequences for vendor, recipient, the community, and the health system. First, organ sellers or vendors are unable to enforce contracts or bring actions for non-payment, fraud, negligence, etc. and are therefore at the mercy of often unscrupulous brokers and entrepreneurs. Second, transplant tourism activities lack oversight and quality control, with the result that travellers/recipients may receive poor quality organs or organs that come with undetected bacterial, viral, or fungal infections. Third, the exporting of local kidneys to global recipients diminishes the health, vigour, and resiliency of the community. Fourth, health resources are overwhelmed with foreign patients and are unavailable to the local population, precipitating poorer health and quality of life overall.

The lack of institutional infrastructure and data in organ markets means that evidence is lacking for most such claims. However, the handful of extant studies consistently reports a lack of individual economic improvement following the sale of kidneys in India and Pakistan (Goyal et al., 2002; Moazam et al., 2009). For example, a widely cited study of 305 individuals in Chennai, India, who had sold a kidney an average of 6 years before the survey found that nearly all had sold kidneys to pay off debts, but most were still in debt at the time of the survey (Goyal et al., 2002). Moreover, seller health status deteriorated and seller income declined following nephrectomy and most said they would not recommend selling a kidney to others. It remains to be determined whether these outcomes are necessarily related to commercial organ provision per se or to a lack of regulation.

The example of Iran may support the latter. Rather than ban compensation for kidney donation, Iran banned foreign transplant tourism, creating a regulated intrastate system closed to non-Iranians. The government acts as broker, paying all expenses in connection with a kidney transplant and providing health insurance and monetary awards to living donors. Non-Iranians are not permitted to donate or to receive kidneys from Iranian living donors. According to official reports, by 1999 the renal wait-list in Iran had been eliminated under this programme (Akoh, 2012). It should be noted that the experiences reported by vendors was less encouraging. Those vendors for whom donating was purely financial were dissatisfied, in large part because promised inducements to donate were reneged upon. Three-quarters of the respondents agreed with the statement that kidney sales should be banned and responded that, were they to make such a decision again, they would prefer begging or loans with crippling interest rates to becoming a paid kidney donor (Zargooshi, 2001a, 2001b).

## Exploiting kidney vendors

Kidney vendors are usually poor, uneducated, lacking healthcare, unemployed, and more likely to be female (Khajehdehi, 1999). Although buyers, too, are desperate, they are at the same time privileged: typically from high-income countries, male, white or Asian, with health insurance and some college education. The danger of commodification is that 'organs are being thought of as "just organs", rather than as living parts of a person' by buyers and brokers (Fox and Swazey, 1992).

A central ethical objection to permitting organ sales rests on several different types of worries about the exploitation of the poor, as Radcliffe-Richards and colleagues (1998) astutely argue. In the first type, potential kidney vendors need to be protected because they are, arguably, incapable of giving valid informed consent because they are, variously, uneducated or cannot conceive of the risks but only the benefits, or because their reasoning is compromised by the anxieties of their economic situation. In response, Radcliffe-Richards and colleagues. point out that there are accepted methods for enhancing capacity and obtaining informed consent, ranging from education and counselling to appointing an authorized decision-maker or independent advocate.

The second type of worry is that the range of choices available to the poor is too constricted and therefore their choice to sell a kidney is one in which they lack alternatives. Radcliffe-Richards and colleagues argue that the worse we think the selling of a kidney, the worse should seem the position of the vendors when that option is removed. In other words, their choice to sell a kidney was the best of their options, and all the options that remain to them, if we remove the option of selling, must be, by their estimation, worse than selling a kidney. Thus we do not improve matters for the poor by removing the best option when all their other choices are worse. If we care about exploiting the poor, we must take actions that make organ vending a less preferred option, by either reducing poverty or expanding their opportunities. Of course, as a practical matter, we cannot wait to establish a market for kidneys until all of the poor have been made better off. We could, however, institute a level of guaranteed payments that would be sufficient to improve their lives, all things considered. Such guarantees would require institutionalizing kidney commerce so that black markets were disestablished and traffickers had no way to sell coerced kidneys.

The third type of concern has to do with the asymmetrical risks that living donors and poor vendors undertake. The poor enter the transaction less healthy and with greater health deficits; selling a kidney can exacerbate ill health and needs for resources in ways that are not the case for healthy donors. These objections can, of course, be met with some guarantee of access to healthcare resources, whether by insurance or contract. The risks of underpayment or fraud are better met with a regulated system than a black market.

In sum, the argument for protecting poor would-be organ vendors from exploitation fails to justify prohibiting organ sales. Moreover, the insistence that altruism opposes kidney selling also fails; the kidney vendor may be selling a kidney for altruistic reasons, to improve the life of his or her family, or, even more directly, to pay for needed healthcare. It is reasonable to conclude with Radcliffe-Richards et al. (1998): 'The weakness of the familiar arguments suggests that they are attempts to justify the deep feelings of repugnance which are the real driving force of prohibition, and feelings of repugnance among the rich and healthy, no matter how strongly felt, cannot justify removing the only hope of the destitute and dying.'

## The relation between transplant tourism and trafficking

The WHO justified its complete ban of organ trade, in part, on the grounds that it would lead to trafficking in human beings. The Commentary to Guiding Principle 5 states:

> Payment for [. . .] organs is likely to take unfair advantage of the poorest and most vulnerable groups, undermines altruistic donation, and leads to profiteering and human trafficking. Such payment conveys the idea that some persons lack dignity, that they are mere objects to be used by others. (World Health Organization, 2015)

By 2000, the *Protocol to Prevent, Suppress and Punish Trafficking in Persons, Especially Women and Children* avoided causal claims but redefined trafficking to include 'payment in order to obtain consent for organ removal'. Article 3 of the Protocol states:

> (a) 'Trafficking *in persons*' shall mean the recruitment, transportation, transfer, harboring or receipt of persons, by means of the threat or use of force or other forms of coercion, of abduction, of fraud, of deception, of the abuse of power or of a position of vulnerability or of the giving or receiving of payments or benefits to achieve the consent of a person having control over another person, for the purpose of exploitation. Exploitation shall include, at a minimum, the

exploitation of the prostitution of others or other forms of sexual exploitation, forced labor or services, slavery or practices similar to slavery, servitude or *the removal of organs* [emphasis mine]; (b) The consent of a victim of trafficking in persons to the intended exploitation . . . shall be irrelevant where any of the means set forth in subparagraph (a) have been used. . . . (UNHCR, 2000)

The influential *Declaration of Istanbul* (2008), signed by 150 representatives from 78 countries, includes brokering by third parties in the definition of trafficking and maintains that they are equally problematic crimes:

*Organ trafficking* is the recruitment, transport, transfer, harboring or receipt of living or deceased persons or their organs by means of the threat or use of force or other forms of coercion, of abduction, of fraud, of deception, of the abuse of power or of a position of vulnerability, or of the giving to, or the receiving by, a third party of payments or benefits to achieve the transfer of control over the potential donor, for the purpose of exploitation by the removal of organs for transplantation. (Steering Committee of the Istanbul Summit, 2008)

It has become common to blur the line between transplant tourism and trafficking and to condemn all organ commercialism, thus avoiding considering potentially useful though ethically imperfect alternatives that achieve the goals of rescue without exploiting others. Banning organ sales on account of worries about trafficking leads to more trafficking. The reduced risks to vendors in a legal market and the increased payments from elimination of brokers will bring an end to black markets. In addition, supply and demand will come in line, avoiding untold suffering and death.

## Conclusion

Demand for transplantable organs continues to outpace availability, despite intensive efforts to increase supply, efficiency, and utility. In the face of organ scarcity—both natural and structural—various forms of transplant commercialism have arisen. Many oppose every form of commercialism relating to human bodies and body parts as intrinsically immoral. Transplant tourism and organ trafficking are two forms of commercialism that raise substantial ethical concerns. However, given the suffering and unnecessary loss of life associated with diseases most commonly treated with solid organ transplant, moral arguments for limited and strategic commercial approaches rather than outright prohibition must be considered.

## References


Akoh JA (2012) Key issues in transplant tourism. *World J Transplant*, **2**(1):9–18.

Ambagtsheer F, Weimar W (2012) A criminological perspective: why prohibition of organ trade is not effective and how the Declaration of Istanbul can move forward. *Am J Transplant*, **12**(3):171–175.

Barsoum RS (2006) Chronic kidney disease in the developing world. *N Engl J Med*, **354**:997–999.

Cherry MJ (2005) *Kidney for Sale by Owner: Human Organs, Transplantation and the Market.* Georgetown University Press, Washington, DC.

Council of the Transplantation Society (1985) Commercialization in transplantation, the problems and some guidelines for practice. *Lancet*, **2**:715.

Couser WG, Remuzzi G, Mendis S, Tonelli M (2011) The contribution of chronic kidney disease to the global burden of major noncommunicable diseases. *Kidney Int*, **80**(12):1258–1270.

Danovitch GM, Leichtman AB (2006) Kidney vending, the 'Trojan Horse' of organ transplantation. *Clin J Am Soc Nephrol*, **1**:1122–1145.

European Union (2012a) Article 13, European Union, The European Parliament and the Council *Directive 2010/53/EU* on standards of quality and safety of human organs intended for transplantation. <http://eur-lex.europa.eu/lexuriserv/lexuriserv.do?uri=celex,32010l0053,en,not>.

European Union (2012b) Article 17, European Union, The European Parliament and the Council *Directive 2010/53/EU* on standards of quality and safety of human organs intended for transplantation. <http://eur-lex.europa.eu/lexuriserv/lexuriserv.do?uri=celex,32010l0053,en,not>.

Eurotransplant International Foundation (2013) *Annual Report 20 13. Table 4.5(i) Active Eurotransplant waiting lists at year end, from 2009 to 2013*, p. 50. <https://www.eurotransplant.org/cms/mediaobject.php?file=AR20135.pdf>.

Fox R, Swazey P (1992) *Spare Parts: Organ Replacement in American Society.* Oxford University Press, New York.

Friedman EA, Friedman AL (2006) Payment for donor kidneys: pros and cons. *Kidney Int*, **69**(6):960–962.

Goyal M, Mehta RL, Schneiderman LJ, Sehgal AR (2002) Economic and health consequences of selling a kidney in India. *JAMA*, **288**(13):1589–1593.

John Paul II (1995) *Evangelium Vitae.* Encyclical letter on the value and inviolability of human life. 25 March 25. <http://www.vatican.va/holy_father/john_paul_ii/encyclicals/documents/hf_jp-ii_enc_25031995_evangelium-vitae_en.html>.

Kerr M (2012) Quality and productivity in kidney care services. <www.kidneycare.nhs.uk>.

Khajehdehi P (1999) Living non-related versus related renal transplantation—its relationship to the social status, age and gender of recipients and donors. *Nephrol Dialysis Transplant*, **14**(11):2621–2624.

Matas A (2006) Why we should develop a regulated system of kidney sales: a call for action! *Clin J Am Soc Nephrol*, **1**(6):1129–1132.

Merion RM, Barnes AD, Lin M, et al. (2008) Transplants in foreign countries among patients removed from the US transplant waiting list. *Am J Transplant*, **8**(4 Pt 2):988–996.

Moazam F, Zaman RM, Jafarey AM (2009) Conversations with kidney vendors in Pakistan, an ethnographic study. *Hastings Center Report*, **39**(3):29–44.

NHS Blood and Transplant (2014a) *Annual Report on Kidney Transplantation: Report for 2013/2014. Patients on the Kidney Transplant List 2005*, pp. 9–10. <http://www.odt.nhs.uk/pdf/organ_specific_report_kidney_2014.pdf>.

NHS Blood and Transplant (2014b) *Annual Report on Kidney Transplantation: Report for 2013/2014. Median Waiting Time to Kidney Only Transplant in the UK*, pp. 14–15. <http://www.odt.nhs.uk/pdf/organ_specific_report_kidney_2014.pdf>.

NOTA (1984) *National Organ Transplant Act.* Public Law 98-507-Oct. 19, 1984. <http://history.nih.gov/research/downloads/pl98-507.pdf>.

Official Gazette (2012) Republic Act No. 10364. *Expanded Anti-Trafficking in Persons Act of 2012.* <http://www.gov.ph/2013/02/06/republic-act-no-10364/>.

Radcliffe-Richards J, Daar AS, Guttmann RD, et al. (1998) The case for allowing kidney sales. *Lancet*, **351**(9120):1950–1952.

Rithalia A, McDaid C, Suekarrran S, Norman G, Myers L, Sowden A (2009) A systematic review of presumed consent systems for deceased organ donation. *Health Technol Assess*, **26**:1–95.

Scheper-Hughes N (2002) The ends of the body: commodity fetishism and the global traffic in organs. *SAIS Review*, **XXII**(1):72.

Shimazono Y (2007) The state of international organ trade, a provisional picture. *Bull World Health Organ*, **85**:955–962.

Steering Committee of the Istanbul Summit (2008) The Declaration of Istanbul on Organ Trafficking and Transplant Tourism. Participants in the International Summit on Transplant Tourism and Organ

Trafficking Convened by the Transplantation Society and International Society of Nephrology, 30 April–2 May, Istanbul. *Transplantation*, **86**(8):1013–1018.

Tonelli M, Wiebe N, Knoll G, et al. (2011) Systematic review, kidney transplantation compared with dialysis in clinically relevant outcomes. *Am J Transplant*, **11**:2093–2109.

UNHCR (2000) *Protocol to Prevent, Suppress and Punish Trafficking in Persons, Especially Women and Children*, supplementing the *UN Convention Against Transnational Organized Crime*. <http://www2.ohchr.org/english/law/protocoltraffic.htm>.

White SL, Chadban SJ, Jan S, Chapman JR, Cass A (2008) How can we achieve global equity in provision of renal replacement therapy? *Bull World Health Organ*, **86**:229–237.

Wolfe RA, Ashby VB, Milford EL, et al. (1999) Comparison of mortality in all patients on dialysis, patients on dialysis awaiting transplantation, and recipients of a first cadaveric transplant. *N Engl J Med*, **341**:1725–1730.

World Health Organization (2015) *Guiding Principles on Human Cell, Tissue and Organ Transplantation*, WHA 63.22/2010. <http://www.who.int/transplantation/en/>.

Zargooshi J (2001a) Quality of life of Iranian kidney 'donors'. *J Urol*, **166**(5):1790–1799.

Zargooshi J (2001b) Iranian kidney donors, motivations and relations with recipients. *J Urol*, **165**(2):386–392.

## Further reading

Global Registry on Transplantation and Donation: <http://www.transplant-observatory.org/pages/home.aspx>.

Organ Procurement and Transplant Network: <http://optn.transplant.hrsa.gov/latestdata/rptdata.asp>.

United States Renal Data System, National Institutes of Health, National Institute of Diabetes and Digestive and Kidney Diseases: <http://www.usrds.org/>.

SECTION 3

# The organ donor

# CHAPTER 7

# Neurological determination of death and organ donation

Shariq S. Raza, Ali Salim, and Darren J. Malinoski

## Introduction

As of March 2015, there were over 123,000 patients on the OPTN/UNOS waiting list. In 2012, however, only 28,052 organ transplantations were performed from 14,013 donors, while over 6,000 patients died while waiting for an available organ (according to OPTN data). This disparity between need and supply of transplantable organs is growing steadily in the US, with the waiting list far surpassing the number of available donors and organs. In addition to the obvious benefits that transplant recipients gain from the act of organ donation, the psychological and social benefits of organ donation for patients with catastrophic brain injuries and their families are being increasingly recognized (Merchant et al., 2008). When one considers that over 75% of families consent to organ donation when approached by an appropriate requestor (OPTN data January 2008–June 2010) and that more than 50% of the adult population in the US is currently registered to be an organ donor on a state registry (according to the Donate Life America National Donor Designation Report Card), it is evident that the desire to donate organs is prevalent in both our patients and their families.

In order to respect and carry out these wishes, the Revised Uniform Anatomical Gift Act requires OPOs and donor hospitals to have the necessary policies and procedures in place to preserve the option of donation for every patient and their family (Uniform Law Commission, 2008). This includes avoiding a deceleration in the critical care provided to patients with catastrophic brain injuries until the desire to donate has been elucidated in an appropriate manner (Uniform Law Commission, 2008).

The majority of transplanted organs come from donors after neurological determination of death (DNDD, previously termed 'brain death'). Being that all of these donors enter the ICU at some point during their treatment, intensivists of all types are often involved in the diagnosis, referral, and initial stabilization of patients with severe brain injuries. When these injuries would not benefit from neurosurgical or neurological intervention and are deemed to be non-survivable, they are deemed 'catastrophic brain injuries'. The intensivist's goals shift from optimizing cerebral perfusion pressure to maintaining haemodynamic stability and diagnosing neurological death, should it occur; preparing the family for devastating news; allowing them to begin the grieving process and consider their end-of-life options; preserving the option of organ donation for every patient and their family; and honouring donor registry first-person authorizations for organ donation. Intensivists are often intimately involved in discussions of end-of-life care as well as the critical care management of patients with catastrophic brain injuries, resulting in a potentially significant impact on organ donation processes and transplantation outcomes.

In efforts to maximize organ donation outcomes, the American College of Surgeons (ACS) qualitatively evaluates each hospital's organ donation practices during the trauma centre verification process (American College of Surgeons, 2006). Specifically, the ACS requires verified trauma centres to: (1) establish a relationship with an OPO, (2) develop policies for notification of the OPO when there is a patient with the potential for neurological death, (3) review organ donation rates, and (4) implement protocols for the determination of death by neurological criteria (American College of Surgeons, 2006). In addition, the creation of a multidisciplinary organ donor council with support from a trauma programme as well as the hospital administration has been associated with improved organ donation outcomes (Kong et al., 2010). Recent data have shown that having specific catastrophic brain injury guidelines (CBIGs) and the presence of a trauma surgeon on an organ donor council were associated with significantly higher rates of organ donors amongst trauma admissions (Malinoski et al., 2012b).

This chapter focuses on the diagnosis and pathophysiology of neurological death and critical care management strategies for patients with catastrophic brain injuries; it also provides an overview of the organ donation process and discusses the benefits of organ donation to the families of patients in the ICU.

## Determination of death by neurological criteria

The concept of 'brain death' has caused great controversy in medicine and politics. It is debated by ethicists, law professors, government agencies, and healthcare workers (Capron, 2001; Sheehy et al., 2003; Hanto, 2007; Shemie et al., 2007). First introduced by Mollaret and Goulon in 1959, 'brain death' was originally described as a persistent vegetative state or permanent coma (Wijdicks, 2001). After 1959 the definition evolved, until 1968 when the Harvard Medical School Ad Hoc Committee created the current definition, which was later affirmed by the Uniform Determination of Death Act in 1981 (Wijdicks, 2001; Todd et al., 2007). Due to some difficulties in understanding both the similarities and the distinctions between 'brain death' and 'cardiac death', it has been proposed that new terminology be utilized in order to more easily equate the permanence and legality of these two terms: 'neurological determination of death' and 'circulatory determination of death'. In this new schema, death can be declared by two different methods, but there is only one kind of 'death'.

In general, neurological death is the irreversible loss of all brain function. Ultimately, the brainstem controls brain function and is responsible for regulating breathing, heart rate, and reflexes such as gagging or coughing when the airway is obstructed, withdrawal from pain, and pupillary function. Without a functioning brainstem, life cannot exist. Therefore, diagnosing brain death requires the absence of brainstem function.

To establish a diagnosis of neurological death the clinician must first identify the underlying causes and determine that they are irreversible (Wijdicks, 2001). Trauma, stroke, cerebral hypoxia, intracranial haemorrhage, tumours, meningitis, and encephalitis are all well-known causes (Karcioglu et al., 2003). All confounding factors must be eliminated, such as hypothermia (<35°C), hypoxia, intoxication by legal or illegal drugs, shock/hypotension, and severe electrolyte disturbances (Wijdicks, 2001). Figure 7.1 shows an example of a neurological death declaration note.

The clinical brain death assessment is usually made in the ICU. This evaluation involves three steps: verifying unconsciousness, documenting absent brainstem reflexes, and the apnoea test. To verify unconsciousness, a score of 3 on the Glasgow Coma Scale is required. The five brainstem reflexes that should be assessed in adults are shown in Figure 7.2 (Wijdicks, 2001). If all brainstem reflexes are absent, an apnoea test is performed. Before embarking on the apnoea test, the patient should have a partial pressure of arterial carbon dioxide ($PaCO_2$) within the normal range and be preoxygenated with 100% fraction of inspired oxygen ($FiO_2$). The apnoea test ensures the patient has lost the drive to breathe, and confirms the diagnosis of neurological death.

An overview of the procedure and an example of a neurological death declaration protocol are shown in Table 7.1 and Figure 7.1, respectively. Criteria for a positive apnoea test are: no attempt to breathe while disconnected from the ventilator (as oxygen is still delivered to the airway), a $PaCO_2 \geq 60$ mmHg or a rise $\geq 20$ mmHg above baseline, and an arterial pH $\leq 7.3$. It usually takes 5–10 minutes of apnoea for the $PaCO_2$ to meet criteria and we recommend drawing blood gasses every 3 minutes until either brain death is confirmed or the patient becomes haemodynamically unstable, at which point the patient should be reconnected to the ventilator. Some institutions recommend that the clinical examination, including the apnoea test, be performed twice, 6 hours apart for adults and as much as 48 hours apart for neonates, but the need for a second assessment remains controversial (Wijdicks, 2001; Shemie et al., 2007).

If the patient is haemodynamically unstable and would not tolerate even a few minutes off the ventilator for fear of causing cardiopulmonary arrest, other confirmatory tests may be used. These are detailed in Table 7.2. Historically, the most common in the US is cerebral angiography. If the carotid arteries' flow cuts off at the base of the skull and there is no blood flow within the calvarium, the patient is declared brain dead. Recently, clinicians have used magnetic resonance angiograms (MRA) or computed tomography angiograms (CTA) in lieu of more invasive traditional angiography (Young et al., 2006).

| | **BRAIN DEATH DECLARATION FORM** | |
|---|---|---|
| | **RESULTS** | |
| **Initial Evaluation** | **Check Box** | **Comments** |
| Mechanism consistent with brain death | ☐ Yes ☐ No | |
| Other causes of death excluded, for example: | ☐ Yes ☐ No | |
| Toxins I drugs (no contributory abnormalities) Metabolic parameters (no contributory abnormalities) | | |
| **Vital Signs** | | |
| Temperature (> 35°C) (record:) | ☐ Yes ☐ No | |
| Blood pressure normal for age (record) | ☐ Yes ☐ No | |
| Oxygen saturation 1> 90%) (record:) | ☐ Yes ☐ No | |
| **Neurological Examination** | | |
| Response to verbal stimuli absent | ☐ Yes ☐ No | |
| Pupils fixed and dilated | ☐ Yes ☐ No | |
| Corneal reflex absent | ☐ Yes ☐ No | |
| Oculocephalic Telex absent {pt not in C-spine precautions) | ☐ Yes ☐ No | |
| Oculovestibular reflex absent (pt in C-spine precautions) | ☐ Yes ☐ No | |
| Motor respome .lo noxious stimulation absent | ☐ Yes ☐ No | |
| **For infants Only** | | |
| Sucking/rooting reflexes absent (for infants) | ☐ Yes ☐ No | |
| **Apnea Test (no respiratory effort in the setting of):** | | |
| pH ≤ 7.30 AND EITHER | ☐ Yes ☐ No | |
| pCO2 ≥ 60 mmHg OR ≥ 20 mm Hg over baseline | ☐ Yes ☐ No | |
| **Other Confirmatory Tests (as needed)** | | |
| 4-vessel cerebral angiography | ☐ Yes ☐ No | |
| Radionuclide cerebral blood flow study | ☐ Yes ☐ No | |
| EEG | ☐ Yes ☐ No | |
| Doppler/Ultrasound | ☐ Yes ☐ No | |

*AFTER ALL CLINICAL CRITERIA ARE MET, EITHER AN APNEA OTR OTHER CONFIRMATORY TEST IS REQUIRED TO COMPLETE THE FIRST EXAM. THE SECOND EXAM CAN REFER TO THE APNEA OR OTHER CONFIRMATORY TEST OF THE FIRST EXAM.

I certify that the above tests have been performed and That according to hospital policy this patient is brain dead.

California Licensed Physician's Signature ______ License Number ______ Date Time ______

Indicate if examination is first or second examination: ______

If second exam, indicate: Identity of the first examiner: ______

Date and time of the first exam: ______

**Fig. 7.1** Neurological (brain) death declaration form. (Reproduced with permission from Dixon TD and Malinoski DJ, 'Devastating Brain Injuries: Assessment and Management. Part I: Overview of Brain Death', *Western Journal of Emergency Medicine*, 10 pp. 11–17, Copyright 2009 the Authors.)

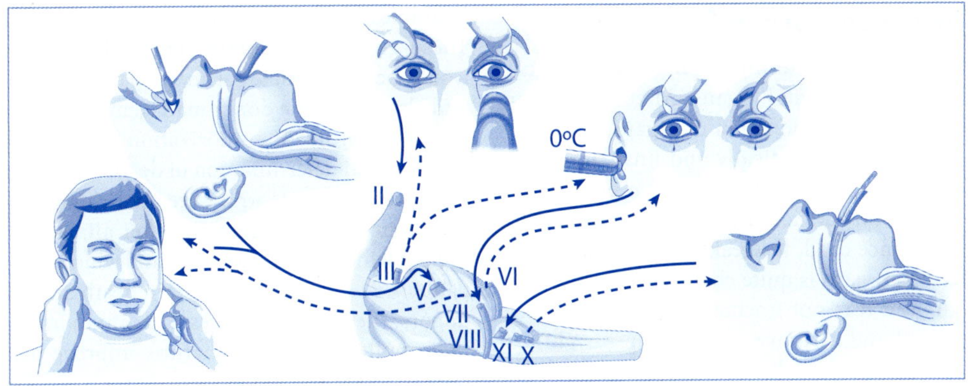


**Fig. 7.2** Steps in a clinical examination to assess brainstem reflexes. Tested cranial nerves are indicated by Roman numerals; solid arrows represent afferent limbs and broken arrows efferent limbs. Depicted are absence of grimacing or eye opening with deep pressure on both condyles at the level of the temporomandibular joint (afferent nerve V and efferent nerve VII), absent corneal reflex elicited by touching the edge of the cornea (V and VII), absent light reflex (II and III), absent oculovestibular response toward the side of the cold stimulus provided by ice water (pen marks at the level of the pupils can be used as reference) (VIII and III and VI), and absent cough reflex elicited through introduction of a suction catheter deep in the trachea (IX and X). (Adapted from Wijdicks EFM, 'Brain death', *New England Journal of Medicine*, 2001, 344, pp. 1215–1221, Lippincott Williams & Wilkins, Massachusetts Medical Society. Used with permission of Mayo Foundation for Medical Education and Research. All rights reserved.)

Electroencephalography (EEG) is a well-validated modality and is frequently utilized to confirm brain death with absence of electrical activity. The disadvantage of EEG is that devices in the ICU may cause artifacts, leading to spurious results (Wijdicks, 2001). Other tests include transcranial Doppler ultrasound to assess cerebral blood flow and nuclear imaging to assess uptake of tracer in the brain. This last method is preferred for secondary confirmation in many institutions. However, none of these confirmatory tests replaces the clinical exam. Due to variations in practice around the country, a standard practice has been advocated by the American Academy of Neurology (Wijdicks et al., 2010).

Since children are more resilient than adults, a longer time between assessments has been advocated (Wijdicks, 2001). Additionally, many institutions require other confirmatory tests, in addition to the apnoea test, in children less than 1 year of age. Deciding who is qualified to determine death by neurological criteria is another difference. Some centres advocate that at least two clinicians concur on the diagnosis and that at least one of those clinicians is a neurologist or neurosurgeon. Similar to adults, consensus guidelines have also recently been updated for paediatric patients (Nakagawa et al., 2011).

**Table 7.1** Apnoea test sequence

1. Preoxygenate the patient with 100% $FiO_2$
2. Ensure the patient is not hypo-/hypercarbic via ABG (goal baseline $PaCO_2$ 45–55 mmHg)
3. Disconnect the ventilator but supply 'blow-by' oxygen via the endotracheal tube
4. Monitor the patient for any signs of respiration or haemodynamic instability
5. Obtain ABGs at selected intervals (q3–4 min)
6. Stop the test and return to mechanical ventilation if:
   a: haemodynamic instability occurs, or
   b: the patient exhibits attempts to breathe, or
   c: the $PaCO_2$ is ≥ 60 mmHg or rises ≥ 20 mmHg above baseline in the setting of an arterial pH ≤ 7.3

$FiO_2$, Fraction of inspired oxygen; ABG, arterial blood gas; $PaCO_2$, partial pressure of arterial carbon dioxide.

Once declared dead by neurological criteria, the patient may become an organ donor with family authorization and/or an advanced directive. This may be verified by living wills or other applicable legal documents, e.g. registration when obtaining a driver's licence in the US (United Network for Organ Sharing, 2007). Neurological death can be a challenging concept to grasp for a patient's family, and it is important to equate 'brain death' with the layperson's understanding of bodily death, which usually means that the heart has stopped. The essential connection between brain function and conscious thought may not be obvious to laypersons and should be stated explicitly.

It is imperative to separate end-of-life discussions surrounding neurological death and the withdrawal of medical support from conversations about organ donation to avoid any perceived conflict of interest. It is highly recommended that healthcare providers not approach family members about organ donation without first consulting with their local OPO. In general, representatives from the OPO who are formally trained to talk with families about organ donation make the first, formal approach after end-of-life discussions have taken place and the family understands the concept of neurological death. Healthcare providers with a close relationship to the family may be involved in the process as well.

**Table 7.2** Additional confirmatory testing for the determination of brain death

- Cerebral angiography
- Electoencephalography (EEG)
- Transcranial Doppler ultrasonography
- Cerebral scintigraphy (technetium Tc 99m hexametazime)
- Computed tomography angiography (CTA)
- Magnetic resonance angiography (MRA)

## Neurological death and organ function

The goal prior to and after the determination of neurological death is to maintain perfusion of vital organs. After a family or advanced directive authorizes the donation of organs, the OPO assumes care of the donor, both medically and financially, but physician involvement is still important to perform procedures and provide expert critical care advice. The brain is so central to bodily homeostasis that, once dead, it wreaks havoc on all other organ systems. Preserving organs is quite challenging in the face of neurological death, and it is not uncommon to lose donors to the spiral of hormonal and cardiovascular collapse. While a detailed discussion of the pathophysiological effects of brain death is undertaken in Chapter 8, it is worth mentioning that the critical care provided to patients with catastrophic brain injuries can be challenging and, when done correctly, can positively impact the organ donation process.

Many hospitals have adopted CBIGs to assist in the management of patients with neurological injuries and a very poor prognosis. Examples of such protocols can be found in Figures 7.3 and 7.4. These guidelines contain standard critical care practices that would be appropriate for many patients with survivable injuries and also reflect the donor management protocols that many OPO personnel utilize if authorization for donation is obtained after neurological determination of death. With the use of these guidelines, some patients who were once thought to have fatal injuries may neurologically improve; after all, we are not always able to predict which injuries are fatal and which are salvageable. Even for patients who do regress to brain death and subsequently become donors, these ICU practices that aim to improve perfusion of the brain will also, by their nature, improve perfusion of the other organs. In the end, good patient care is good organ donor care.

While it has been found that there are more organs transplanted per donor when more critical care endpoints are met by the OPO prior to organ recovery (Merchant et al., 2008; Hagan et al., 2009; Malinoski et al., 2011), ongoing work in UNOS Region 5 (Southwestern US) has also recently demonstrated that having these critical care endpoints achieved in the donor hospital ICU

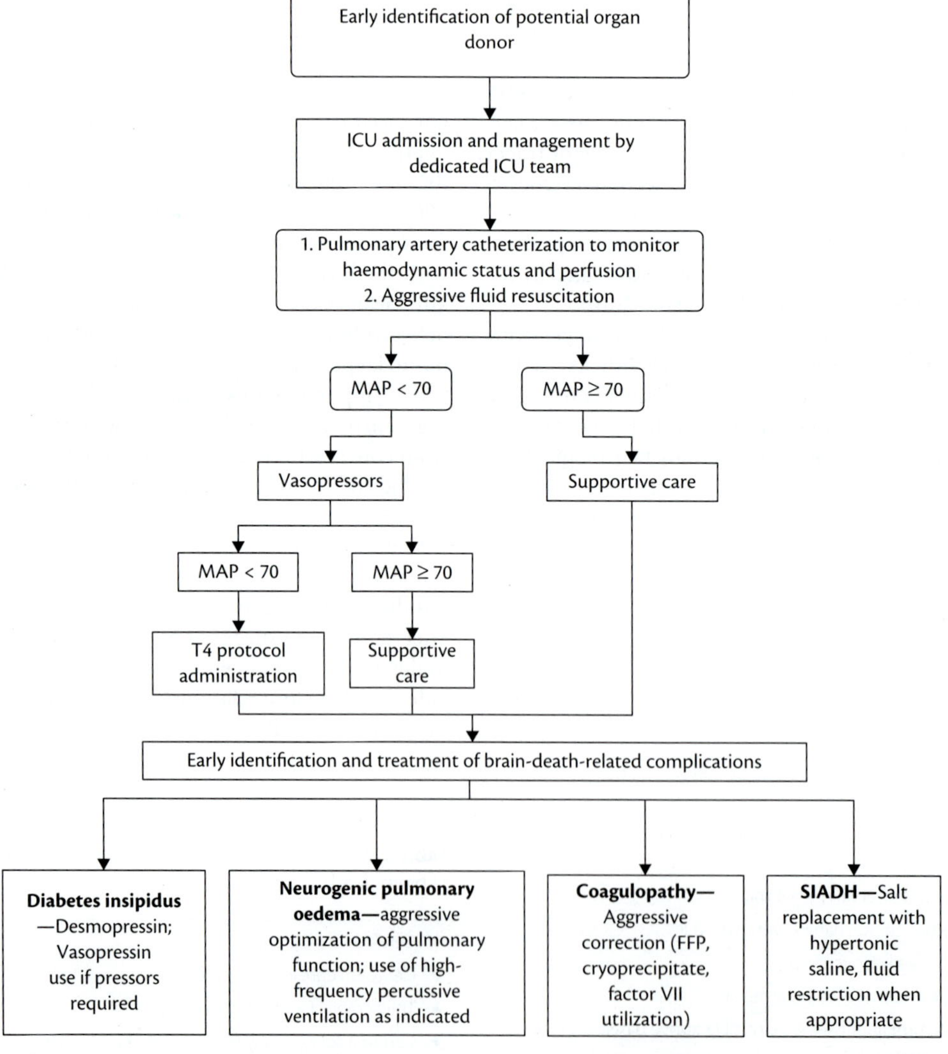


**Fig. 7.3** Protocol for aggressive management of patients with catastrophic brain injuries and imminent neurological death. FFP, Fresh frozen plasma; MAP, mean arterial pressure; ICU, intensive care unit; SIADH, syndrome of inappropriate antidiuretic hormone secretion. (Joseph DuBose and Ali Salim, *Journal of Intensive Care Medicine*, 'Aggressive Organ Donor Management Protocol', 23, 6, pp. 367–375, copyright © 2008 by Sage Publications. Reprinted by Permission of SAGE Publications.)

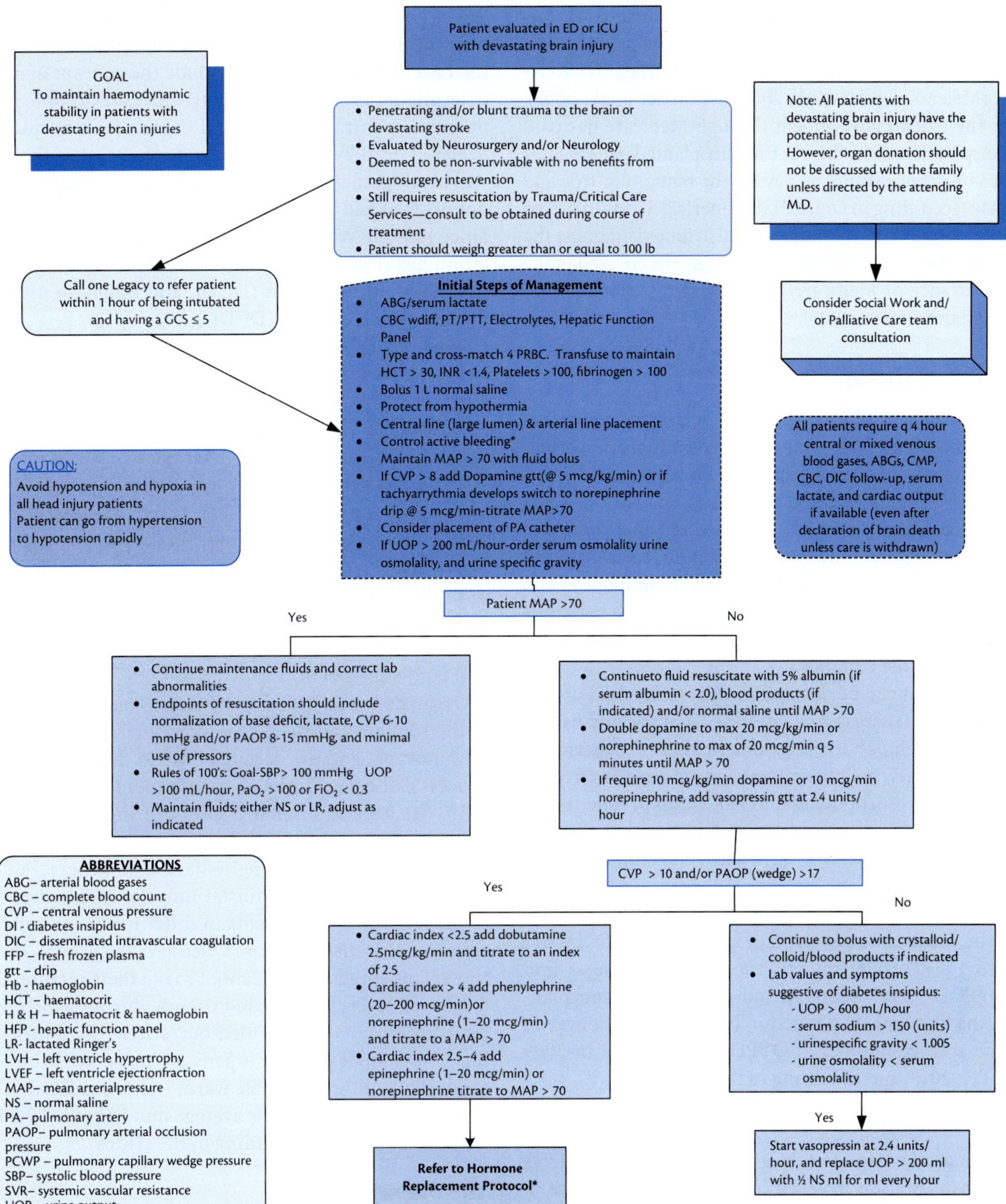


**Fig. 7.4** Detailed protocol for aggressive management of patients with catastrophic brain injuries and imminent neurological death. (Reproduced with permission from Dixon TD and Malinoski DJ, 'Devastating Brain Injuries: Assessment and Management. Part I: Overview of Brain Death', *Western Journal of Emergency Medicine*, 2009, 10 pp. 11–17. Copyright 2009 the Authors)

* The Hormone Replacement Protocol consists of intravenous boluses of 1 amp D50, 2 g methylprednisolone, 20 units of regular insulin, and 20 mcg of levothyroxine (not given unless serum $K^+ > 3.5$ mmol/L). This is followed by a thyroxine infusion (200 mcg in 500 mL 0.9% NaCl) beginning at 10 mcg/hour, titrated to blood pressure and cardiac index. Vasopressin infusions can also be used for hypotension in the setting of diabetes insipidus.

prior to authorization for donation is associated with both more organs transplanted per donor and less delayed graft function in the recipients of kidneys from these patients (Malinoski et al., 2012a, 2013). Therefore, optimizing the care of patients with devastating neurological injuries has the potential to benefit these patients as well as the recipients of their organs for those who go on to donate.

The intensive care of the DNDD does increase overall cost of care, but there is no cost to the donor's estate or family (according to Donate Life America). The cost-effectiveness of transplantation has been well established and has been most extensively reviewed for kidney transplantation (Suthanthiran and Strom, 1994; Evans and Kitzmann, 1998; Oostenbrink et al., 2005; Kim, 2006; Hagan et al.,

2009; Nakagawa et al., 2011). Furthermore, it is imperative to remember that the care of the donor potentially benefits eight patients with end-stage organ failure, and many more who will benefit from tissue donation (Meier-Kriesche et al., 2005; Schnitzler et al., 2005). Traditionally, the federal government through Medicare has paid for 75% of transplantations in the US; the transplanted patient and/or the patient's insurance company pay for the remaining 16% and 9%, respectively (according to Donate Life America). Costs incurred while caring for the DNDD are ultimately distributed amongst the patients receiving the donated organs and are usually covered in the US through insurance or Medicare/Medicaid (US Department of Health and Human Services, 2008).

## Types of organ donor

In a patient with a catastrophic brain injury, once a determination has been made that there is no chance of a meaningful recovery, a declaration of death by neurological criteria is the next logical step. Under ideal circumstances, a referral to an OPO is made before such a declaration in order to ensure optimal preservation of the option to donate and timely action once a decision to donate has occurred. Once the patient is legally declared dead and the process of organ donation has been authorized, the patient is deemed an organ donor and his or her organs are evaluated for their suitability for transplantation.

The solid organs that can be donated include abdominal organs such as kidneys, liver, pancreas, and intestine. Thoracic organs that can be transplanted include both lungs and the heart. Furthermore, the liver could potentially be split and transplanted into two recipients. There is thus the great potential to benefit up to nine recipients with solid organs from a single donor. Additional tissues that can be donated include the cornea, skin, bone, and tendons.

### Standard criteria donors

The SCD is the most common type of organ donor. SCDs are declared dead by neurological criteria and are younger and healthier than ECDs; their organs are more suitable for transplantation due to the fact that they function better and last longer in recipients. The average number of OTPD from an SCD in 2009 was 3.67 (OPTN, 2010; and according to the HRSA).

### Expanded criteria donor

The severe shortage of organs and the growing number of patients waiting for transplantation have led to more widespread use of organs from donors not commonly used in the past. ECDs are also declared dead by neurological criteria but are older and have more medical comorbidities. There is typically an increased risk of early and late graft failure and delayed graft function inherent with the use of organs from ECDs.

The criteria for an ECD have been defined by UNOS as the following: any donor aged over 60, or over 50 years with at least two of the following conditions: hypertension, serum creatinine > 1.5 mg/dL, or cause of death from cerebrovascular accident (OPTN, 2014). The average number of OTPD per ECD in 2009 was 1.81 (OPTN, 2010; and according to the HRSA).

### Donation after circulatory determination of death

Historically, early transplantation operations were performed with organs from donors who had recently died of cardiopulmonary arrest, for the 'Dead Donor Rule' stipulates that the removal of organs for transplantation cannot be the cause of one's death. As the idea of death evolved to include the concept of a neurological determination of death, patients with catastrophic brain injuries became a substantial source of organs for transplantation once declared dead by neurological criteria. Because their hearts were still beating, their organs were better preserved than the previous donors who had been declared dead by cardiopulmonary criteria. Since 1995, however, the scarcity of organs available for transplantation has renewed interest in 'non-heart-beating donors', donation after cardiac death (DCD), and donation after circulatory determination of death (DCDD).

Potential DCDD donors are patients who either do not have a neurological injury or otherwise do not meet the criteria for brain death yet have no meaningful chance of survival due to their injuries/illness and are likely to suffer a cardiac arrest if life support is withdrawn. Examples of such patients include ventilator-dependent amyotrophic lateral sclerosis (ALS) patients, high spinal cord injuries, and severe traumatic brain injury/stroke/anoxic brain injury patients who do not regress to neurological death. It is critical to recognize that the decision to withdraw life-sustaining measures must precede any conversation about organ donation in order to remove any real or perceived conflicts of interest among healthcare providers, OPO personnel, and family members.

Organ donation in such patients may occur after the withdrawal of life support and the declaration of circulatory death, which is how most patients are declared dead in the hospital. This planned process can occur in the operating room, the pre-op area, or the ICU. The general unpredictability of the time period until the donor's expected death following removal of mechanical support can also be a challenging factor. In general, a DCDD must experience asystole within 60 minutes of planned withdrawal of life-sustaining treatments in order for his or her organs to be suitable for transplantation. Once asystole occurs, the recovering transplant surgery team cannot make their incision until a 3- to 5-minute observation period occurs, during which the potential for autoresuscitation is ruled out. After this waiting period, an incision is made and the organs are preserved with ice and cold fluids. Due to the inevitable warm ischaemia that occurs prior to the recovery of organs, the average number of OTPD in 2009 was 2 (OPTN, 2010; and according to the HRSA).

### The live organ donor

As surgical and anaesthetic techniques have advanced and our understanding of organ function has evolved, the options to donate an organ while one is alive and healthy have also become viable. Donation in such a manner is referred to as living donation, and this category now represents 44% of all donors (OPTN, 2014). This usually encompasses transplants amongst close relatives, although non-related living donations are becoming increasingly common.

## Conclusion

The active participation of all healthcare providers involved in the care of patients with severe neurological insults preserves the option of organ donation for patients and their families. This care usually occurs in the ICU and operating room and can be greatly influenced by intensivists and anaesthesiologists. While the benefits of organ donation for transplant recipients are widely recognized, it is also important to realize that the families of patients who suffer catastrophic brain injuries and regress to neurological death can experience an improved bereavement process if their loved one goes on to donate organs (Merchant et al., 2008). As intensivists who care for critically ill patients, it is important that we preserve this option as a part of quality end-of-life care. The use of CBIGs can assist in these efforts and is associated with improved organ donation outcomes. First and foremost, achieving the critical care endpoints that are targeted by these management protocols has the potential to benefit our patients by turning a devastating neurological injury into a survivable one. When that doesn't happen, it preserves the option of donation for those patients and families who choose to donate organs and tissues.

## Acknowledgements

The data and analyses reported in the 2010 Annual Data Report of the US Organ Procurement and Transplantation Network and the Scientific Registry of Transplant Recipients have been supplied by UNOS and the Minneapolis Medical Research Foundation under contract with HHS/HRSA. The authors alone are responsible for reporting and interpreting these data; the views expressed herein are those of the authors and not necessarily those of the US Government.

## References

American College of Surgeons (2006) *Resources for Optimal Care of the Injured Patient*. ACS, Chicago.

Capron AM (2001) Brain death—well settled yet still unresolved. *N Engl J Med*, **344**(16):1244–12446.

Evans RW, Kitzmann DJ (1998) An economic analysis of kidney transplantation. *Surg Clin N Am*, **78**(1):149–174.

Hagan ME, McClean D, Falcone CA, et al. (2009) Attaining specific donor management goals increases number of organs transplanted per donor: a quality improvement project. *Prog Transplant*, **19**(3):227–231.

Hanto DW (2007) Ethical challenges posed by the solicitation of deceased and living organ donors. *N Engl J Med*, **356**(10):1062–1066.

Karcioglu O, Ayrik C, Erbil B (2003) The brain-dead patient or a flower in the vase: the emergency department approach to the preservation of the organ donor. *Eur J Emerg Med*, **10**:52–57.

Kim SJ, Gordon EJ, Powe NR (2006) The economics and ethics of kidney transplantation: perspectives in 2006. *Curr Opin Nephrol Hypertens*, **15**:593–598.

Kong AP, Barrios C, Salim A, et al. (2010) A multidisciplinary organ donor council and performance improvement initiative can improve donation outcomes. *Am Surg*, **76**(10):1059–1062.

Malinoski DJ, Daly MC, Patel MS, et al. (2011) Achieving donor management goals before deceased donor procurement is associated with more organs transplanted per donor. *J Trauma*, **71**(4):990–995; discussion 996.

Malinoski DJ, Patel MS, Daly MC, et al. (2012a) The impact of meeting donor management goals on the number of organs transplanted per donor: results from the United Network for Organ Sharing Region 5 prospective donor management goals study. *Crit Care Med*, **40**:2773–2780.

Malinoski DJ, Patel MS, Lush S, et al. (2012b) Impact of compliance with the American College of Surgeons trauma center verification requirements on organ donation-related outcomes. *J Am Coll Surg*, **215**(8):186–192.

Malinoski DJ, Patel MS, Ahmed O, et al. (2013) The impact of meeting donor management goals on the development of delayed graft function in kidney transplant recipients. *Am J Transplant*, **13**(4):993–1000.

Meier-Kriesche H, Schold JD, Gaston RS, et al. (2005) Kidneys from deceased donors: maximizing the value of a scarce resource. *Am J Transpl*, **5**:1725–1730.

Merchant SJ, Yoshida EM, Lee TK, et al. (2008) Exploring the psychological effects of deceased organ donation on the families of the organ donors. *Clin Transplant*, **22**(3):341–347.

Nakagawa TA, Ashwai S, Mathur M, et al. (2011) Guidelines for the determination of brain death in infants and children: an update of the 1987 Task Force Recommendations. *Crit Care Med*, **39**(9):2139–2156.

Oostenbrink JB, Kok ET, Verheul RM (2005) A comparative study of resource use and costs of renal, liver and heart transplantation. *Transpl Int*, **18**:437–443.

OPTN (2010) *2010 SRTR and OPTN Annual Data Report*. UNOS, Richmond, Virginia.

OPTN (2014) *Policy 3.5: Organ Distribution—Allocation of Deceased Kidneys, 3.5-1*. <http://optn.transplant.hrsa.gov/policiesandbylaws2/policies/pdfs/policy_7.pdf>.

Schnitzler MA, Whiting JF, Brennan DC, et al. (2005) The life-years saved by a deceased organ donor. *Am J Transplant*, **5**:2289–2296.

Sheehy E, Conrad SL, Brigham LE, et al. (2003) Estimating the number of potential organ donors in the United States. *N Engl J Med*, **349**(7):667–674.

Shemie SD, Pollack MM, Morioka M, et al. (2007) Forum. *Lancet Neurol*, **6**:87–92.

Suthanthiran M, Strom TB (1994). Renal transplantation. *N Engl J Med*, **331**(6):365–376.

Todd PM, Jerome RN, Jarquin-Valdivia AA (2007) Organ preservation in a brain dead patient: information support for neurocritical care protocol development. *J Med Libr Assoc*, **95**(3):238–245.

Uniform Law Commission (2008) Revised Uniform Anatomical Gift Act. <http://uniformlaws.org/shared/docs/finals_nc/uaga_final_nc.doc>.

Wijdicks EFM (2001) The diagnosis of brain death. *N Engl J Med*, **344**(16):1215–1221.

Wijdicks EF, Varelas PN, Gronseth GS, et al. (2010) Evidence-based guideline update: determining brain death in adults: report of the Quality Standards Subcommittee of the American Academy of Neurology. *Neurology*, **74**(23):1911–1918.

Young GB, Shemie SD, Doig CJ, et al. (2006) Brief review: the role of ancillary tests in the neurological determination of death. *Can J Anesth*, **53**:533–539.

## Further reading

Donate Life America: <http://www.donatelife.net>.
OPTN: <http://optn.transplant.hrsa.gov>.
United Network for Organ Sharing: <http://www.unos.org>.
US Department of Health and Human Services: <http://www.hrsa.gov>.

# CHAPTER 8

# Critical care of the organ donor

Matthew B. Bloom, Ali Salim, and Darren J. Malinoski

## Introduction

Optimal and aggressive critical care of the potential donor begins long before the declaration of a neurological determination of death (brain death). In order to maximize the gift of transplantation, however, it must continue through the entire process of referral, consent, and organ recovery.

CBIGs have been put in place in many ICUs to optimize the management of patients with severe neurological injuries. With the use of these guidelines, patients who were once thought to have neurologically devastating injuries may improve. For the subset of patients who regress to neurological death and subsequently become donors, these same practices improve perfusion and function of the remaining organs as well. Ultimately, optimizing the care of patients with severe brain injuries has the potential to benefit both these patients as well as the recipients of their organs, for those who go on to donate.

There is, however, one important distinction to be made. Dramatic and severe physiological changes accompany the transition to neurological death and require specialized knowledge on the part of the treating physician. Care is no longer aimed at maximizing neurological recovery but shifts to the maintenance of the remaining organ systems. Often the optimal treatment for one system is in conflict with the best treatment for another. The use of a checklist of standardized critical care endpoints, or DMGs, serves as a set of targets to ensure a course steered towards a middle ground and optimizes the number of organs suitable for transplant from DNDD.

Unfortunately, patients who are declared dead by neurological criteria are often not managed aggressively by their responsible teams. At times, such patients are 'written off', and the level of response to their fluctuating haemodynamics may be far from optimal. Because the time from declaration of neurological death to the time of organ recovery may be prolonged due to social, medical, or administrative reasons, many potentially transplantable organs are lost before reaching the operating room. In addition, the physiology of neurological death exists before pronouncement occurs and the haemodynamic instability that often accompanies neurological death can even delay the ability to perform confirmatory tests. In such cases, maintaining standard critical care practices aimed at normalizing physiological parameters as much as possible serves to obtain a diagnosis for patients and their families, while simultaneously preserving the option of donation.

## Pathophysiology of neurological death

Neurological death is caused by the herniation of cerebral contents due to supranormal intracranial pressures. Early pontine ischaemia results in a catecholamine surge with hypertension, known commonly as the first stage of the Cushing reflex. As ischaemia progresses caudally to the vagal nucleus in the medulla oblongata, the loss of baroreflector reflexes and unopposed sympathetic activity results in a profound hyperdynamic state—or the 'sympathetic storm' (Tuttle-Newhall et al., 2003). Systemically, sympathetic vasoconstriction causes compromise of end-organ perfusion.

As the brain continues to herniate, a sudden cardiovascular collapse can develop, in part due to direct catecholamine-induced myocardial injury and subsequent cardiac dysfunction, as well as destruction of pontine and medullary vasomotor centres (Bittner et al., 1995; Ryan et al., 2003). The effects of this haemodynamic instability can cause marked damage to potentially donatable end organs. Profound hypotension develops due to loss of sympathetic tone, amplified by the development of DI due to the infarcted posterior pituitary.

Major swings in hormone levels are seen. Cortisol, vasopressin, thyroxine, and insulin are a few of the important and powerful hormones whose end effects often amplify one another and cause dramatic physiological swings. The treating intensivist must understand the role that each of these mediators plays in order to properly supplement and maintain haemodynamic stability and organ perfusion.

The physiological changes that manifest as different portions of the brain become injured during the herniation process present a multifaceted challenge to the treating intensivist. These physiological alterations result in diffuse vascular regulatory disturbances and widespread cellular injury (Novitzky et al., 1989). Severe alterations also occur in metabolism (Novitzky et al., 1988), immunology (Kusaka et al., 2000), and coagulopathy (Salim et al., 2006). In sum, these disturbances frequently lead to the development of multi-organ system failure and cardiovascular collapse.

### The cardiovascular system

Two distinct, and in many ways opposite, profiles of haemodynamic activity are seen during the process of neurological death. Brainstem ischaemia causes a catecholamine surge, in particular of epinephrine and norepinephrine, as the medulla endeavours to maintain cerebral perfusion pressure and improve local tissue oxygenation. This response manifests as increases in heart rate, blood pressure, cardiac output, and systemic vascular resistance. This surge of catecholamines can challenge the balance between myocardial supply and demand. Several autopsy studies have demonstrated left ventricular subendocardial necrosis (Kolin and Norris, 1984; Cooper et al., 1989). Electrocardiography (ECG) changes and cardiac arrhythmias are common and are thought to be due to both metabolic and electrolyte abnormalities as well as infarction of the conduction system. The use of standard anti-arrhythmic therapy is appropriate. An important caveat to remember is that vagus nucleus disruption in the brainstem may result in a bradyarrhythmia which is resistant to the effects of atropine, and a beta-adrenergic agonist such as isoproterenol or epinephrine may be required (Wood et al., 2004). Untreated arrhythmias may become completely refractory to management if not treated early and aggressively.

The second phase of cardiovascular activity, characterized by haemodynamic collapse, coincides with brainstem herniation and results in the loss of sympathetic activity causing profound vasodilatation, myocardial depression, and low levels of serum catecholamines. The haemodynamic effects can be amplified by hypovolaemia due to DI, which is often present concurrently. Additional myocardial depression may be due to a concurrent reduction in tri-iodothyronine (T3) production as well as direct mitochondrial inhibition.

At a minimum, all DNDDs should have a central venous pressure (CVP) monitor to guide resuscitation and support. Pulmonary artery catheter-directed resuscitation is aimed at optimizing cardiac output and maintaining normal preload and afterload. After the achievement of adequate fluid resuscitation, vasopressin is the currently recommended first-choice haemodynamic therapy, due to its catecholamine sparing effects and ability to counteract vasodilatation. Vasopressin also acts to inhibit the diuresis of DI that is often present. Low to absent levels of vasopressin occur in up to 90% of organ donors (Howlett et al., 1989). Vasopressin is usually seen to be deficient in donors who require catecholamine support (Chen et al., 1999). After vasopressin, additional agents such as dopamine, phenylephrine, or norepinephrine are titrated as needed to maximize end-organ perfusion.

ECG is routinely used to assess the left ventricular function of a potential donor heart. Cardiac catheterization may be more selectively employed for donors > 55 years of age and younger patients with a history of cocaine use, or those with three or more risk factors for coronary artery disease, such as hypertension, diabetes, dyslipidaemia, prolonged smoking history, or family history of premature coronary artery disease (Zaroff et al., 2002). In the setting of left ventricular dysfunction, pulmonary artery catheter-directed management can maximize donor recovery. Knowledge of the patient's cardiac output and left ventricular filling pressures allows for optimal management of vasopressors and fluids. It has been shown that properly managed younger hearts with left ventricular dysfunction can markedly recover function after transplantation (Milano et al., 1993). The role of adjunctive hormone therapy to improve cardiac function is discussed in the section 'The role of thyroxine'.

## The pulmonary system

The systemic inflammatory response syndrome (SIRS) seen in neurological death takes its toll upon the pulmonary system of potential donors, resulting in utilization rates of potential lungs of only around 20%. Increased systemic pressures and left atrial pressures during the catecholamine surge can result in elevated pulmonary artery pressures and subsequent endothelial damage, leading to direct pulmonary damage due to capillary leak. During cardiovascular collapse, intravenous fluid administration needed to maintain systemic blood pressure can cause further pulmonary damage due to volume overload, pulmonary capillary leak, and resultant development of pulmonary oedema.

The 'ideal' environment for the lungs of mildly fluid-positive euvolaemia is in contrast with a more aggressive fluid regiment to optimize renal function. Increased pulmonary capillary permeability as well as decreased pulmonary resistance makes the lungs particularly sensitive to increases in volume loading. A marked difference in Alveolar–arterial (A–a) gradients has been demonstrated between a CVP of 8–10 mmHg and 4–6 mmHg (Rosengard et al., 2002; Kutsogiannis et al., 2006). Pulmonary-artery-driven resuscitation directed by donor management guidelines serves to optimize the greatest number of organs, unless it is known that a particular organ is not suitable for transplantation, and the direction of management can be skewed in favour of residual organ optimization. Targets of CVP 6–8 mmHg or pulmonary capillary wedge pressure (PCWP) 8–12 mmHg are moderate.

Lung-protective strategies commonly used in the ICU should continue to be performed in the potential organ donor. In the brain-injured patient, hyperventilatory strategies are often employed aimed at promoting hypocapnia and lower intracranial pressures through cerebral vasoconstriction. These same alkinalizing strategies can exasperate bronchospasm, airway oedema, and pulmonary microvascular permeability (Laffey et al., 2000). High-minute ventilation strategies should be reversed after the declaration of neurological death. Strategies to minimize atelectasis and promote alveolar recruitment should be employed. Protective modes of ventilation should be used to achieve a target $PaO_2$ (arterial partial pressure of oxygen in arterial blood):$FiO_2$ (P:F) ratio of >300. The protective strategies of the Acute Respiratory Distress Syndrome Network (ARDSNET) goals of low tidal volumes (6–8 mL/kg) and low plateau pressures (< 30 cm $H_2O$) (Brower et al., 2000) serve to minimize alveolar shear injury, volutrauma, and barotrauma. Appropriate pressure control modes or other newer modes such as airway pressure release ventilation (APRV) can minimize lung injury and improve P:F ratios (Hanna et al., 2011). Adjustments of the respiratory rate to achieve a $PaCO_2$ of 40–45 mmHg and of $FiO_2$ to obtain $PaO_2$ of 90 mmHg or greater are often employed (Mascia et al., 2010).

Pulmonary toilet manoeuvres such as chest percussion, postural drainage, recruitment manoeuvres, and serial bronchoscopy can also improve lung function. Protocols with built-in lung recruitment manoeuvres of brief periods of increased positive end-expiratory pressure (PEEP) to 30 cm $H_2O$ have been shown to improve gas exchange and increase the number of suitable lungs for transplantation (Noiseux et al., 2009). Bronchoscopy allows for evaluation of individual lungs, as one may be suitable for transplant and the other injured from a process such as contusion or aspiration pneumonitis. Bronchoscopy and lavage for microbiology is a routine part of the donation work-up. Bronchial colonization or infection with bacteria or yeast is seen in up to 80% of organ donors and correlates with lung recipient survival (Avlonitis et al., 2003). High endotracheal cuff pressures can minimize aspiration into the lungs, an important risk in this patient population with likely earlier neurological injury and loss of cough reflex (Hanna et al., 2011).

The use of steroids has been shown to improve pulmonary function and lead to the use of lungs that may have been previously deemed unacceptable for transplantation (Follette et al., 1998).

The larger role of steroids is discussed in the section 'The role of steroids'.

## The renal system

Sympathetic storm and subsequent cardiovascular collapse have a deleterious effect upon the renal system. Hypoperfusion of the juxtaglomerular cells of the kidney activates the renin–angiotensin–aldosterone axis, causing salt and water retention as well as vasoconstriction, which in turn can lead to compromised renal blood flow, glomerular and tubular injury, and ultimately renal insufficiency. This directly compromises kidney viability and post-transplantation function and underscores the need for active haemodynamic management in donors.

While dopamine administration is no longer recommended as a first-line vasopressor in the management of the DNDD because of its tachycardic and pro- arrhythmic effects, transplanted kidneys that come from donors treated with low-dose dopamine have been shown to have better graft function post transplantation. Specifically, recipients have been shown to require a shorter duration of haemodialysis after transplantation (Schnuelle et al., 1999). It is thought that preconditioning of the transplanted organs with dopamine may make them better able to withstand ischaemic damage during cold preservation (Gottmann et al., 2006).

Hyperglycaemia is well known to impact renal function. Multiple causes have been suspected, including the impairment of autoregulation of glomerular capillary pressure (Hostetter et al., 1981), upregulation of glucose transporter 1 and 2 expression (Chen et al., 1999; Gnudi et al., 2007), and increased production of multiple inflammatory molecules, as well as transforming growth factor beta 1 (Mehta, 2007) and nitric oxide (De Vriese et al., 2001). Poor glucose control in potential donors has been shown to be directly associated with declining renal function prior to organ recovery (Blasi-Ibanez et al., 2009).

The maintenance of urine output to a minimum of 0.5 cc/kg/hour while avoiding the massive diuresis of DI is the goal of renoprotective resuscitation.

## The hepatic system

While the overall inflammatory process of brain death can take its toll on the liver as well, hypernatraemia has been associated with increased rates of transplanted liver allograft loss. Donor plasma sodium >155 mmol has been suggested as the cause in several studies (Gonzalez et al., 1994; Totsuka et al., 1999), although more recent studies have refuted this finding (Mangus et al., 2010). It is theorized that hypernatraemia promotes the influx of osmotic molecules into hepatocytes, which then promote water influx and cell lysis when transplanted into a eunatraemic recipient.

While cellular dysfunction is clearly observed (Okamoto et al., 1998; Sato et al., 1998; van Der Hoeven et al., 2000), perhaps because of its tremendous metabolic reserve, the organ as a whole appears more tolerant to the dramatic changes that occur around the time of neurological death than other solid organs (Compagnon et al., 2002).

## The endocrine and metabolic systems

### Hormonal deficiencies

Multiple endocrine derangements occur in the setting of neurological death. Ischaemia of the hypothalamic–pituitary axis can lead to diminished circulating levels of adrenocorticotropic hormone (ACTH), thyroid-stimulating hormone (TSH), and vasopressin, resulting in important endocrine derangements with marked systemic effects. The stress response to DNDD causes the activation of leucocytes and a pronounced inflammatory response.

### The role of vasopressin

Once intravascular volume has been repleted with crystalloid or colloid, the treatment of hypotension with vasopressors is appropriate. Dopamine was previously used as the initial therapy to treat hypotension in these patients, but consensus has led to the use of vasopressin as first-line treatment. Severe intracranial swelling leads to disruption of the function of the posterior pituitary and causes decreased levels of vasopressin and development of neurogenic DI. Up to 90% of DNDDs are noted to have a severe deficiency in vasopressin, which contributes to the cardiovascular collapse and resultant hypotension (Pennefather et al., 1995; Chen et al., 1999). Neurogenic DI is present in nearly half of all DNDDs (Salim et al., 2006). When uncontrolled, this results in a massive hypo-osmolar diuresis and electrolyte abnormalities. This loss of intravascular volume contributes to a profound hypotension. The correction of DI, as well as of fluid status, is of paramount importance to preserve perfusion.

Vasopressin (or antidiuretic hormone, ADH) acts upon its V1 subtype receptors, found in vascular smooth muscle which are responsible for its vasopressor activity, as well as the V2 subtype, found in renal collecting duct epithelia which increases water permeability and is responsible for vasopressin's antidiuretic activity. 1-Desamino-8-D-arginine vasopressin (DDAVP) is highly selective for the V2 subtype alone and may be used as an adjunctive treatment for DI.

### The role of thyroxine

Diminished circulating levels of thyroxine have been implicated as a reason for haemodynamic instability in DNDDs. Resulting decreased energy stores lead to diminished production of adenosine triphosphate, causing myocardial dysfunction and resultant circulatory collapse.

It is known from animal studies that this cardiovascular deterioration is associated with impaired oxygen use, a shift from aerobic to anaerobic metabolism, a depletion of glycogen and myocardial high-energy stores, and the accumulation of lactate (Novitzky et al., 1988; Cooper et al., 1989; Salter et al., 1992). This irregular metabolism has been associated with low levels of T3, thyroxin (T4), and to a lesser extent cortisol and insulin (Novitzky et al., 1986, 1987, 1988; Wicomb et al., 1986). Therapeutic replacement with T3 has been associated with complete reversal of anaerobic metabolism and subsequent stabilization of cardiac function when applied to DNDDs (Novitzky et al., 1986; Gonzalez et al., 1994). In addition, the use of T3 has been associated with significant improvements in cardiovascular status, reductions in inotropic support, and decreases in donors lost from cardiac instability (Cooper et al., 1989; Novitzky et al., 1990, 1996; Zuppa et al., 2004). It has been demonstrated that haemodynamically unstable organ donors require a significant decrease in, or complete lack of, vasopressor support after T4 administration (Salim et al., 2001). In another study in DNDDs, T4 administration was associated with significantly more organs procured per donor group (3.9 ± 1.7 vs 3.2 ± 1.7, $P = 0.048$) (Salim et al., 2007). The aetiology of this functional 'hypothyroid state' is poorly understood but may be a result of lower than normal TSH levels caused by the irreversible damage to the hypothalamus and pituitary from ischaemia. Another explanation is a decrease in the peripheral conversion of T4 to its more potent analogue T3, similar to the euthyroid sick syndrome (Masson et al., 1990; DuBose and Salim, 2008).

### The role of insulin

Severe glucose abnormalities may be also present in prerecovery donors. After the development of neurological death, insulin levels have been measured to decrease to 50% of baseline at 3 hours, and even further to 20% at 13 hours (Wicomb et al., 1986). The resulting pronounced hyperglycaemia has many potentially harmful effects and leads to increased risk of allograft dysfunction.

Protein glycosylation from uncontrolled glucose levels promotes tissue damage, especially of the renal system. Osmotic diuresis resulting from glucose spillage may overtax renal medullary function and contribute to the diuresis seen in brain death. It is thought that maintaining tight control with glucose levels under 150 mg/dL using parenteral insulin yields renal allografts with lower creatinine levels (Blasi-Ibanez et al., 2009). Several studies have demonstrated concern for exceeding tight glucose control leading to hypoglycaemic episodes, but in the setting of neurological death the concern for brain injury or stroke resulting from hypoglycaemia no longer applies. Hence, strict glucose control to attain levels between 80 and 110 mg/dL may lead to improved renal allograft function. A risk of bloodstream infections related to hyperglycaemia in ICU patients still exists and may confound the transplantation process.

### The role of steroids

Another systemic response experienced by the body following brain death is a massive inflammatory response characterized by elevations in plasma levels of inflammatory mediators such as interleukin-6 and tumour necrosis factor. Rapid expression of these cytokines, along with cellular adhesion molecules and major histocompatibility complex class II antigens, occurs in DNDDs (Pratschke et al., 2000). This cytokine surge can be detrimental to the function and survival of grafts from these potential organ donors (Deng et al., 1995). A study in 2008 demonstrated a correlation between increased plasma levels of interleukin-6 and decreased graft survival (Murugan et al., 2008). Animal studies have demonstrated the effect of neurological death upon intercellular adhesion molecule 1 (ICAM-1) expression and leucocyte infiltration into peripheral organs, as well as a time-dependent progression of immune-mediated organ dysfunction (van Der Hoeven et al., 2000). Steroids have well-known anti-inflammatory effects by decreasing levels of serum cytokines (Kuecuek et al., 2005). Such decreases in serum cytokines can lead to improved post-transplant organ viability (Kotsch et al., 2008). Steroids also act to overcome a relative adrenal insufficiency as a result of the stress of traumatic brain injury (Howlett et al., 1989).

## Disorders of coagulation and thermoregulation

Disorders of coagulation are a direct consequence of the release of thromboplastin, cerebral gangliosides, and plasminogen-rich substrate from traumatized brain tissue (Miner et al., 1982). Hypothermia and acidosis, along with the dilution of clotting factors, fibrinogen, and platelets, can contribute to a state of disseminated intravascular coagulation and uncontrollable bleeding (Hefty et al., 1993). Massive transfusion protocols including the use of fresh frozen plasma (FFP), platelets, and cryoprecipitate are often required. Recent consensus has recommended transfusion of packed red blood cells to a hematocrit > 30% for organ donors to maximize end-organ oxygen delivery (Zaroff et al., 2002).

Hypothermia rapidly develops due to the loss of hypothalamic thermoregulation and promotes further haemodynamic instability, coagulopathy, and myocardial depression and arrhythmias. It should be proactively addressed with patient warming devices, including heated intravenous fluids and ventilated gases.

## Treatment strategies

### The use of defined donor management goals

The majority of organ donation candidates present after a neurological determination of death and may have been earlier managed with the goal of optimizing brain tissue outcome. After the declaration of neurological death, however, the treating intensivist may now ignore haemodynamic effects upon the brain such as intracranial pressure (ICP) and focus on maximizing the well-being of as many other end organs as possible. Often, the physiological milieu which might best benefit a particular organ might be contrary to the best interests of another. For example, elevated capillary wedge pressure and its beneficial effects on the renal perfusion can cause deleterious effects on the pulmonary system. Unless the intensivist knows a priori that a particular organ will not be suitable for transplantation, one is faced with a delicate balancing act between the competing needs of several different organ systems. The development of DMG has created specific physiological targets for the OPO and intensivist to achieve, aimed at maximizing the total number of transplantable organs.

It has been shown that adoption of specific standardized donor management techniques led to resuscitation of 92% of organs that initially did not meet transplant criteria. Further, the optimization of cardiac function in DNDDs improves the viability of other transplantable organs (Wheeldon et al., 1995). In order to stabilize the haemodynamic derangements that occur secondary to pituitary dysfunction and subsequent DI in the majority of DNDDs, aggressive fluid resuscitation is recommended to maintain a CVP of 8–12 mmHg and a systolic arterial pressure of between 90 and 140 mmHg (Hunt et al., 1996). However, in lung donors it has been shown that maintenance of a CVP between 8 and 10 mmHg may result in an increased alveolar arterial oxygen gradient when compared with potential donors maintained between 4 and 6 mmHg (Pennefather et al., 1993). Meeting DMGs prior to organ recovery is an independent predictor for achieving ≥ 4 OTPD. The early and persistent attainment of DMGs is critical for maximizing the number of OTPD (Malinoski et al., 2011, 2012).

A sample checklist of DMGs utilized by the procurement officers in UNOS Region 5 (Southwestern US) is shown in Table 8.1. Not only has it been found that there are more organs transplanted per donor when these goals are met by the OPO prior to organ recovery (Hagan et al., 2009; Franklin et al., 2010; Malinoski et al., 2011), but also recent work in Region 5 has demonstrated that having these critical care endpoints achieved in the donor hospital ICU prior to authorization for donation is associated with both more OTPD and less delayed graft function in the recipients of kidneys from these patients (Malinoski et al., 2012, 2013).

**Table 8.1** UNOS Region 5 donor management goals (Reproduced from Malinoski DJ, 'The Impact of Meeting Donor Management Goals on the Development of Delayed Graft Function in Kidney Transplant Recipients', American Journal of Transplantation, 13, 4, pp. 993–1000, copyright 2013, with permission from The American Society of Transplantation and the American Society of Transplant Surgeons)

| Donor management goals | Parameters |
|---|---|
| Mean arterial pressure | 60–110 mm Hg |
| Central venous pressure | 4–12 mm Hg |
| Ejection fraction | ≥ 50% |
| Vasopressors | ≤ 1 and low dose[a] |
| Arterial blood gas pH | 7.3–7.5 |
| P:F | ≥ 300 |
| Serum sodium | ≤ 155 mEq/L |
| Blood glucose | ≤ 180 mg/dL |
| Urine output | ≥ 0.5 cc/kg/hour over 4 hours |

[a] Low dose of vasopressors is defined as: dopamine ≤ 10 mcg/kg/min, phenylephrine ≤ 60 mcg/min, or norepinephrine ≤ 10 mcg/min.

### Hormone replacement strategies

Management of brain-dead organ donors begins with fluid resuscitation and vasomotor support. However, given the derangements described in the section 'The endocrine and metabolic systems' , many of these patients require hormonal support as well. It has been shown that the use of multidrug hormone replacement therapy results in an approximate 25% increase in mean number of organs procured per patient compared with donors not receiving such therapy (Rosendale et al., 2003). This illustrates the importance of hormone replacement therapy on organ donation. One example of such a protocol (see Figure 8.1) consists of 1 amp 50% dextrose, 2 g solumedrol, 20 units of regular insulin, and 20 μg of thyroid hormone (T4), followed by a continuous infusion of 10 μg/hour. The use of such a comprehensive protocol can ensure that the major hormonal derangements which occur during the process of neurological death and organ donation are anticipated and optimally treated.

## Additional considerations during organ recovery

Once an organ donor has been successfully managed in the ICU and organs have been allocated for recovery and transplantation, care shifts to the anaesthesiologist in the operating room. The goals of management continue to be the maintenance of haemodynamic stability and other physiological parameters/DMGs, but there are a few unique practices during the surgical recovery process that are worthy of note.

Chemical neuromuscular paralysis is commonly administered in order to block muscle twitching caused by spinal reflexes to painful stimuli. Positive haemodynamic responses to stimuli are also still present in the DNDD and may include spinal reflexes and reflex arc-mediated adrenal medullary stimulation (Wetzel et al., 1985; Gelb and Robertson, 1990).

Prostaglandins may be administered for their lung-protective effects. These agents in particular can cause a profound hypotension, for which the anaesthesiologist must be prepared. Around

**Harmone Replacement Proloccl (to be initiated only after Primary Attending approval)**

**Goal: To maintain hemodynamic stability in patients with devastating brain injuries**

**Pretreatment**

1. Continue resuscitation to minimum CVP of 7 mmHg
2. Transfuse to achieve an Hct > 30
3. Maintain K +, CA++, Mg ++
   and Phosphorous within normal limits

**Prerequisite:**

Patient is requiring a combined vasopressor need greater that 15 mcg (all VP added as mcg/kg/min or mcg/min) to maintain a systolic pressure of 100 after pre-treatment is completed.

**Harmone Replacement Protocol**

1. Administer IV boluses of the following in rapid succession:
   1 amp of 5% Dextrose
   2 g of Methlyprednisoione
   2 units Regular insulin
   Insulin drip to maintain glucose between
   8–15 mg/dl, minimum rate 1 unit/hr
   20 mcg Levothyroxine (Thyroid Harmone)
   (do not given unless serum K+ >3.5)
2. Start a drip of 200 mcg thyroxine in 500 ml NS (0.4 mcg/ml). Administer at 25 ml (1 mcg) per hour initialily.
   Reduce levels of other pressors as much as possible and then adjust thyroxine as necessary to maintain desired pressuer per M.D. order
3. Monitor K+ levels carefully. The only perceived complication of the Harmone replacement protocol identified to this point is an unusually high K+ requirement (hypokalemia) in some cases.
4. Maintain CVP at desired level by replacing urine output if over 200ml/hour.

**Note: thyroxine may lead to tachycardia and hyperthermia within 30 min of initiation

**Common Problems and Special Considerations**

- DIC: If a patient has clinical signs of DIC, transfuse immediately 4-6 units of FFP. Delaying transfusion while waiting for lab results with uncontrolled hemorrhage is not indicated. Maintain Hct >3 with pRBC.
- DI: If patient is normotensive, serum sodium >150 and UOP >600 ml/hr, give 1-2 micrograms of DDAVP IVP (q 6 hours as needed) and replace UOP ml for ml with ½ NS q hour for UOP > 200 (example : for UOP of 1000 ml replace with 800 ml of ½ NS). If patient is hypotensive, then use vasopressin gtt as described in above protocol. Common error. Assuming high UOP is from DI, but is really from ED lasix and/or mannitol. Replace diuretic fluid loss with NS or LR. (Another marker of DI: urine specific gravity <1.005)
- **Tachycardia and hypertension**: This commonly occurs prior to complete hemiation and should only be treated with short acting medication (esmolol) as patients can quickly change to a hypotensive state
- **Neurogenic pulmonary edemia**: This may occur and decrease the PO2; increase ventilator support as needed. With severe problems of oxygenation, use the oscillating ventilator.
- **Hyperglycemia or hypokalemia**: Use insulin gtt and replace as needed.
- **Cardiac arrest**: Follow ACLS code guidelines. Epinephrine boluses and gtt are often needed

**Fig. 8.1** Example of a hormone replacement protocol as devised by Darren Malinoski for use at UC Irvine Medical School

the time of aortic cross-clamping, mannitol and lasix are often administered to protect renal function, and the resulting diuresis may promote hypotension as well.

The role of the anaesthesiologist is generally limited to the time of aortic cross-clamping. The exception is in the case of lung recovery, which will require the anaesthesiologist to manually ventilate the lungs until their removal.

Lastly, the operating room can become the site of many procurement professionals working simultaneously and expeditiously in tight quarters. Effective communication between all providers and the establishment of an overall leader directing the process as a whole make the procurement proceed optimally.

## Conclusion

Donation and transplantation critical care requires specialized knowledge. Multiple complex systemic effects occur in the setting of neurological death and can require treatment strategies outside of the routine practice of critical care. The effects of pronounced changes in hormone levels and systemic inflammation can turn organs from potential life-saving gifts to unusable tissue if not properly managed.

DMGs serve as a treatment outline to optimize the critical care of the DNDD population. Their goals represent haemodynamic and physiological targets for the intensivist to achieve. They take into account the needs of competing organ systems and optimize the health of the maximum number of potential organs. Repeatedly, the attainment of DMGs has been shown to increase the number of organs per donor that are suitable for transplantation. The ready use of multidrug hormone replacement therapy is an important adjunct to the care of DNDDs. Treatment with multidrug hormone replacement therapy can significantly increase the chances of a DNDD reaching the stage of organ transplantation and can improve the viability of the organs recovered.

Understanding the process of neurological death and its unique effects upon end organs improves both the quality and quantity of available grafts and maximizes the gift of donation.

## Acknowledgements

The authors wish to thank Dr Nancy Knudson and Dr Steven Colquhoun for their help in preparing this manuscript.

## References

Avlonitis VS, Krause A, Luzzi L, et al. (2003) Bacterial colonization of the donor lower airways is a predictor of poor outcome in lung transplantation. *Eur J Cardio-Thorac Surg*, **24**:601–607.

Bittner HB, Kendall SW, Chen EP, Craig D, Van Trigt P (1995) The effects of brain death on cardiopulmonary hemodynamics and pulmonary blood flow characteristics. *Chest*, **108**:1358–1363.

Blasi-Ibanez A, Hirose R, Feiner J, et al. (2009) Predictors associated with terminal renal function in deceased organ donors in the intensive care unit. *Anesthesiology*, **110**:333–341.

Brower RG, Matthay MA, Morris A, et al. (2000) Ventilation with lower tidal volumes as compared with traditional tidal volumes for acute lung injury and the acute respiratory distress syndrome. *N Engl J Med*, **342**:1301–1308.

Chen JM, Cullinane S, Spanier TB, et al. (1999) Vasopressin deficiency and pressor hypersensitivity in hemodynamically unstable organ donors. *Circulation*, **100**:II244–II246.

Compagnon P, Wang H, Lindell SL, et al. (2002) Brain death does not affect hepatic allograft function and survival after orthotopic transplantation in a canine model. *Transplantation*, **73**:1218–1227.

Cooper DK, Novitzky D, Wicomb WN (1989) The pathophysiological effects of brain death on potential donor organs, with particular reference to the heart. *Ann Roy Coll Surg Engl*, **71**:261–266.

De Vriese AS, Stoenoiu MS, Elger M, et al. (2001) Diabetes-induced microvascular dysfunction in the hydronephrotic kidney: role of nitric oxide. *Kidney Int*, **60**:202–210.

Deng MC, Erren M, Kammerling L, et al. (1995) The relation of interleukin-6, tumor necrosis factor-alpha, IL-2, and IL-2 receptor levels to cellular rejection, allograft dysfunction, and clinical events early after cardiac transplantation. *Transplantation*, **60**:1118–1124.

Dubose J, Salim A (2008) Aggressive organ donor management protocol. *J Int Care Med*, **23**:367–375.

Follette DM, Rudich SM, Babcock WD (1998) Improved oxygenation and increased lung donor recovery with high-dose steroid administration after brain death. *J Heart Lung Transplant*, **17**:423–429.

Franklin GA, Santos AP, Smith JW, Galbraith S, Harbrecht BG, Garrison RN (2010) Optimization of donor management goals yields increased organ use. *Am Surg*, **76**:587–594.

Gelb AW, Robertson KM (1990) Anaesthetic management of the brain dead for organ donation. *Can J Anaesth*, **37**:806–812.

Gnudi L, Thomas SM, Viberti G (2007) Mechanical forces in diabetic kidney disease: a trigger for impaired glucose metabolism. *J Am Soc Nephrol*, **18**:2226–2232.

Gonzalez FX, Rimola A, Grande L, et al. (1994) Predictive factors of early postoperative graft function in human liver transplantation. *Hepatology*, **20**:565–573.

Gottmann U, Brinkkoetter PT, Bechtler M, et al. (2006) Effect of pre-treatment with catecholamines on cold preservation and ischemia/reperfusion-injury in rats. *Kidney Int*, **70**:321–328.

Hagan ME, McClean D, Falcone CA, Arrington J, Matthews D, Summe C (2009) Attaining specific donor management goals increases number of organs transplanted per donor: a quality improvement project. *Progr Transpl*, **19**:227–231.

Hanna K, Seder CW, Weinberger JB, Sills PA, Hagan M, Janczyk RJ (2011) Airway pressure release ventilation and successful lung donation. *Arch Surg*, **146**:325–328.

Hefty TR, Cotterell LW, Fraser SC, Goodnight SH, Hatch TR (1993) Disseminated intravascular coagulation in cadaveric organ donors. Incidence and effect on renal transplantation. *Transplantation*, **55**:442–443.

Hostetter TH, Troy JL, Brenner BM (1981) Glomerular hemodynamics in experimental diabetes mellitus. *Kidney Int*, **19**:410–415.

Howlett TA, Keogh AM, Perry L, Touzel R, Rees LH (1989) Anterior and posterior pituitary function in brain-stem-dead donors. A possible role for hormonal replacement therapy. *Transplantation*, **47**:828–834.

Hunt SA, Baldwin J, Baumgartner W, et al. (1996) Cardiovascular management of a potential heart donor: a statement from the Transplantation Committee of the American College of Cardiology. *Crit Care Med*, **24**:1599–1601.

Kolin A, Norris JW (1984) Myocardial damage from acute cerebral lesions. *Stroke J Cereb Circ*, **15**:990–993.

Kotsch K, Ulrich F, Reutzel-Selke A, et al. (2008) Methylprednisolone therapy in deceased donors reduces inflammation in the donor liver and improves outcome after liver transplantation: a prospective randomized controlled trial. *Ann Surg*, **248**:1042–1050.

Kuecuek O, Mantouvalou L, Klemz R, et al. (2005) Significant reduction of proinflammatory cytokines by treatment of the brain-dead donor. *Transplant Proc*, **37**:387–388.

Kusaka M, Pratschke J, Wilhelm MJ, et al. (2000) Activation of inflammatory mediators in rat renal isografts by donor brain death. *Transplantation*, **69**:405–410.

Kutsogiannis DJ, Pagliarello G, Doig C, Ross H, Shemie SD (2006) Medical management to optimize donor organ potential: review of the literature. *Can J Anaesth*, **53**:820–830.

Laffey JG, Engelberts D, Kavanagh BP (2000) Buffering hypercapnic acidosis worsens acute lung injury. *Am J Resp Crit Care Med*, **161**:141–146.

Malinoski DJ, Daly MC, Patel MS, Oley-Graybill C, Foster CE 3rd, Salim A (2011) Achieving donor management goals before deceased donor procurement is associated with more organs transplanted per donor. *J Trauma*, **71**:990–995; discussion 996.

Malinoski DJ, Patel MS, Daly MC, Oley-Graybill C, Salim A (2012) The impact of meeting donor management goals on the number of organs transplanted per donor: results from the United Network for Organ Sharing Region 5 prospective donor management goals study. *Crit Care Med*, **40**:2773–2780.

Malinoski DJ, Patel MS, Ahmed O, et al. (2013). The impact of meeting donor management goals on the development of delayed graft function in kidney transplant recipients. *Am J Transplant*, **13**(4):993–1000.

Mangus RS, Fridell JA, Vianna RM, et al. (2010) Severe hypernatremia in deceased liver donors does not impact early transplant outcome. *Transplantation*, **90**:438–443.

Mascia L, Pasero D, Slutsky AS, et al. (2010) Effect of a lung protective strategy for organ donors on eligibility and availability of lungs for transplantation: a randomized controlled trial. *JAMA*, **304**:2620–2627.

Masson F, Thicoipe M, Latapie MJ, Maurette P (1990) Thyroid function in brain-dead donors. *Transpl Int*, **3**:226–233.

Mehta RL (2007) Glycemic control and critical illness: is the kidney involved? *J Am Soc Nephrol*, **18**:2623–2627.

Milano A, Livi U, Casula R, et al. (1993) Influence of marginal donors on early results after heart transplantation. *Transplant Proc*, **25**:3158–3159.

Miner ME, Kaufman HH, Graham SH, Haar FH, Gildenberg PL (1982) Disseminated intravascular coagulation fibrinolytic syndrome following head injury in children: frequency and prognostic implications. *J Pediatr*, **100**:687–691.

Murugan R, Venkataraman R, Wahed AS, et al. (2008) Increased plasma interleukin-6 in donors is associated with lower recipient hospital-free survival after cadaveric organ transplantation. *Crit Care Med*, **36**:1810–1816.

Noiseux N, Nguyen BK, Marsolais P, et al. (2009) Pulmonary recruitment protocol for organ donors: a new strategy to improve the rate of lung utilization. *Transplant Proc*, **41**:3284–3289.

Novitzky D (1996) Novel actions of thyroid hormone: the role of triiodothyronine in cardiac transplantation. *Thyroid*, **6**:531–536.

Novitzky D, Cooper DK, Reichart B (1986) Value of triiodothyronine (T3) therapy to brain-dead potential organ donors. *J Heart Transplant*, **5**:486–487.

Novitzky D, Cooper DK, Reichart B (1987) Hemodynamic and metabolic responses to hormonal therapy in brain-dead potential organ donors. *Transplantation*, **43**:852–854.

Novitzky D, Cooper DK, Morrell D, Isaacs S (1988) Change from aerobic to anaerobic metabolism after brain death, and reversal following triiodothyronine therapy. *Transplantation*, **45**:32–36.

Novitzky D, Horak A, Cooper DK, Rose AG (1989) Electrocardiographic and histopathologic changes developing during experimental brain death in the baboon. *Transplant Proc*, **21**:2567–2569.

Novitzky D, Cooper DK, Chaffin JS, Greer AE, Debault LE, Zuhdi N (1990) Improved cardiac allograft function following triiodothyronine therapy to both donor and recipient. *Transplantation*, **49**:311–316.

Okamoto S, Corso CO, Nolte D, et al. (1998) Impact of brain death on hormonal homeostasis and hepatic microcirculation of transplant organ donors. *Transplant Int*, **11**(Suppl 1):S404–407.

Pennefather SH, Bullock RE, Dark JH (1993) The effect of fluid therapy on alveolar arterial oxygen gradient in brain-dead organ donors. *Transplantation*, **56**:1418–1422.

Pennefather SH, Bullock RE, Mantle D, Dark JH (1995) Use of low dose arginine vasopressin to support brain-dead organ donors. *Transplantation*, **59**:58–62.

Pratschke J, Wilhelm MJ, Kusaka M, et al. (2000) Accelerated rejection of renal allografts from brain-dead donors. *Ann Surg*, **232**:263–271.

Rosendale JD, Kauffman HM, McBride MA, et al. (2003) Aggressive pharmacologic donor management results in more transplanted organs. *Transplantation*, **75**:482–487.

Rosengard BR, Feng S, Alfrey EJ, et al. (2002) Report of the Crystal City meeting to maximize the use of organs recovered from the cadaver donor. *Am J Transplant*, **2**:701–711.

Ryan JB, Hicks M, Cropper JR, et al. (2003) Functional evidence of reversible ischemic injury immediately after the sympathetic storm associated with experimental brain death. *J Heart Lung Transplant*, **22**:922–928.

Salim A, Vassiliu P, Velmahos GC, et al. (2001) The role of thyroid hormone administration in potential organ donors. *Arch Surg*, **136**:1377–1380.

Salim A, Martin M, Brown C, Belzberg H, Rhee P, Demetriades D (2006) Complications of brain death: frequency and impact on organ retrieval. *Am Surg*, **72**:377–381.

Salim A, Martin M, Brown C, et al. (2007) Using thyroid hormone in brain-dead donors to maximize the number of organs available for transplantation. *Clin Transplant*, **21**:405–409.

Salter DR, Dyke CM, Wechsler AS (1992) Triiodothyronine (T3) and cardiovascular therapeutics: a review. *J Cardiac Surg*, **7**:363–374.

Sato T, Asanuma Y, Yasui O, Kurokawa T, Shibata S, Koyama K (1998) Impaired hepatic mitochondrial function reserve in brain-dead pigs. *Transplant Proc*, **30**:4351–4355.

Schnuelle P, Lorenz D, Mueller A, Trede M, Van Der Woude FJ (1999) Donor catecholamine use reduces acute allograft rejection and improves graft survival after cadaveric renal transplantation. *Kidney Int*, **56**:738–746.

Totsuka E, Dodson F, Urakami A, et al. (1999) Influence of high donor serum sodium levels on early postoperative graft function in human liver transplantation: effect of correction of donor hypernatremia. *Liver Transplant Surg*, **5**:421–428.

Tuttle-Newhall JE, Collins BH, Kuo PC, Schoeder R (2003) Organ donation and treatment of the multi-organ donor. *Curr Problems Surg*, **40**:266–310.

Van Der Hoeven JA, Ter Horst GJ, Molema G, et al. (2000) Effects of brain death and hemodynamic status on function and immunologic activation of the potential donor liver in the rat. *Ann Surg*, **232**:804–813.

Wetzel RC, Setzer N, Stiff JL, Rogers MC (1985) Hemodynamic responses in brain dead organ donor patients. *Anesth Analg*, **64**:125–128.

Wheeldon DR, Potter CD, Oduro A, Wallwork J, Large SR (1995) Transforming the 'unacceptable' donor: outcomes from the adoption of a standardized donor management technique. *J Heart Lung Transplant*, **14**:734–742.

Wicomb WN, Cooper DK, Novitzky D (1986) Impairment of renal slice function following brain death, with reversibility of injury by hormonal therapy. *Transplantation*, **41**:29–33.

Wood KE, Becker BN, Mccartney JG, D'Alessandro AM, Coursin DB (2004) Care of the potential organ donor. *N Engl J Med*, **351**:2730–2739.

Zaroff JG, Rosengard BR, Armstrong WF, et al. (2002) Consensus conference report: maximizing use of organs recovered from the cadaver donor: cardiac recommendations, 28–29 March, Crystal City, Vancouver. *Circulation*, **106**:836–841.

Zuppa AF, Nadkarni V, Davis L, et al. (2004) The effect of a thyroid hormone infusion on vasopressor support in critically ill children with cessation of neurological function. *Crit Care Med*, **32**:2318–2322.

# CHAPTER 9

# Research in organ donors: future directions

Claus Niemann and Andrea Olmos

## Introduction

The shortage of organs available for transplantation continues to be a national crisis. According to figures from the OTPN, as of March 2012 there were over 113,000 candidates awaiting organ donation, while only 28,535 solid organ transplants were performed in 2011. The disparity between the demand for donor organs and the supply of organs available for transplantation will likely continue to grow as organ transplantation remains the treatment of choice for qualifying patients with organ failure and as post-transplantation outcomes continue to improve. In an effort to bridge this gap between organ supply and demand, the transplant community has found ways to increase the organ supply, such as expanding the use of living organ donation and utilizing more suboptimal donors, including ECD and DCD donors (Chang et al., 2003; Nathan et al., 2003; Saidi et al., 2007; Sung et al., 2008). Furthermore, beginning in 2003 the US Department of Health and Human Services launched the Organ Donation Breakthrough Collaboratives, setting ambitious goals for organ procurement and transplantation and encouraging the adoption of best practices for identifying potential donors and obtaining consent for deceased organ donation (Howard et al., 2007).

Given that deceased donors currently contribute the majority of organs for transplantation, maximizing the number of transplantable organs from this donor pool remains the best method for increasing the number of organs available for transplantation (Salim et al., 2007).

An important strategy to improve organ utilization from this donor pool involves the use of novel donor management therapies designed to protect organs from the physiological disturbances associated with brain death (Salim et al., 2006). Brain death results in profound haemodynamic, endocrine, and metabolic dysfunction that is frequently associated with major complications in the potential donor. If not treated appropriately, such complications can progress to cardiovascular collapse and, ultimately, the loss of potentially transplantable organs (Mackersie et al., 1991; DuBose and Salim, 2008). In order to optimize organ viability and function in deceased donors, aggressive donor management protocols to restore and stabilize physiological functions have been advocated. A limited number of these standardized donor management protocols have been shown to increase the number and quality of transplantable organs and to reduce the number of donors lost due to medical failures (Wheeldon et al., 1995; Follette et al., 1998; Rosendale et al., 2002, 2003a; Straznicka et al., 2002; Salim et al., 2005; Angel et al., 2006; Venkateswaran et al., 2008). However, most evidence for aggressive donor management protocols is retrospective and there are conflicting results regarding which management practices significantly impact organ yield (Hagan et al., 2009; Franklin et al., 2010; Malinoski et al., 2011). This lack of quality data on optimal donor management strategies is an obstacle to uniform, evidenced-based donor management practices (Shemie et al., 2006). As a result, donor management practices remain inconsistent across different donation service areas in the US and there remains a persistent shortage of organs for transplantation.

Despite the acute need for donor management techniques that can increase the number and quality of organs available for transplantation, deceased donor management is one of the most neglected areas in transplantation medicine and research (Shah, 2008). Efforts to identify interventions that protect organs during the donation process remain very limited, and rigorous evidence to support the various proposed management protocols is lacking (Feng, 2010). Furthermore, there are a number of unique challenges posed by research in the deceased organ donor. These obstacles include a long list of stakeholders, the logistics and ethics of individual and institutional informed consent for the donor and organ recipients, and the lack of a sound research infrastructure to facilitate collaborative prospective interventional trials (Feng, 2010). Still, innovation in donor management offers the most realistic hope to improve both the quality and size of the current organ supply. Rigorous research in deceased donors is necessary to advance the field of donor management and optimize organ utilization. More specifically, the science of clinical trial design needs to be applied to the implementation of donor management studies.

## The current state of donor research

There is a wealth of basic science research examining the complex processes of brain death that affect deceased donors. Furthermore, a wide range of mechanisms for possible therapeutic interventions to protect donor organs from the profound physiological disturbances caused by brain death has emerged from experimental animal models (Takada et al., 1998; Kotsch et al., 2006; Bouma et al., 2009; Oto et al., 2009; Ollinger and Pratschke, 2010; Danobeitia et al., 2011). However, most of these mechanisms have not been tested in organ donors. The clinical science investigating deceased donor management is quite sparse and has been largely limited to retrospective cohort studies.

Multiple publications have reported that aggressive donor management protocols improve organ quality and increase the number of organs transplanted per donor. For example, several observational studies have found that aggressive lung donor management protocols are associated with an increased number of lungs available for transplantation (Follette et al., 1998; Straznicka et al., 2002; Angel et al., 2006). In 2006, Angel et al. demonstrated that implementation of the San Antonio Lung Transplant protocol for managing potential lung donors within the Texas Organ Sharing Alliance was associated with an increased rate of lung donation (including procurement from donors initially rated as unacceptable) and lung transplantation without adversely affecting the clinical outcomes of lung transplant recipients (Angel et al., 2006). Another large retrospective study by Rosendale et al. demonstrated that the use of three-drug hormonal resuscitation in deceased donors is associated with significant increases in organs transplanted per donor (Rosendale et al., 2003b).

Results from such studies and recognition of the inconsistencies in donor care have led to a national push to implement a standardized checklist of critical care endpoints as DMGs. These goals are aimed at restoring and stabilizing the physiological functions of deceased donors and include measurement of haemodynamic, pulmonary, acid-base, renal, electrolyte, and endocrine functions. Recently, the HRSA recommended that OPOs adopt DMGs to increase organ yield (Malinoski et al., 2011). In a retrospective cohort study, Malinoski et al. demonstrated that meeting at least eight of these ten DMGs in deceased donors prior to organ procurement was significantly associated with more organs transplanted per donor. Furthermore, certain DMGs were found to be independent predictors of OTPD (Malinoski et al., 2011). However, these results conflict with other similarly designed studies regarding which specific DMGs significantly impact organ yield (Hagan et al., 2009; Franklin et al., 2010). Large prospective randomized controlled studies are necessary to verify DMGs and other aggressive donor management protocols and, more importantly, to quantify the extent to which specific donor interventions might enhance organ recovery and outcomes among transplant recipients.

## Donor management intervention trials, past and present

In the current literature only a handful of published donor intervention trials are aimed at optimizing donor organ quality and quantity and improving graft function in recipients. In 2008 Kotsch et al. published a prospective randomized trial of methylprednisolone treatment in deceased donors to improve liver graft function in recipients (Kotsch et al., 2008). In this small single-centre study 100 donors were randomized to receive treatment with methylprednisolone (250 mg intravenous bolus followed by continuous infusion at 100 mg/hour) from the point at which consent for donation is obtained until organ recovery or no treatment. Methylprednisolone treatment reduced intragraft and serum cytokine expression in donors and ameliorated ischaemia–reperfusion injury in liver recipients. Lower rates of acute rejection following liver transplantation were also observed.

A second published donor intervention trial examined the use of dopamine in deceased donors to improve kidney transplant outcomes (Schnuelle et al., 2009). The study was a randomized multicentre parallel group trial of 264 haemodynamically stable brain-dead donors with preserved renal function and 487 subsequent renal transplants. Donors were randomized to receive or not receive a continuous dopamine infusion at a standard dose of 4 μg/kg/min after confirmation of brain death and until cross-clamping. Dopamine decreased the need for multiple dialysis treatments in recipients following renal transplantation. Multiple-dialysis treatments were strongly correlated with 3-year allograft failure. A follow-up retrospective multicentre retrospective cohort study nested in the database of the dopamine trial by Schnuelle et al. (2009) investigated the association between donor exposure to desmopressin before organ retrieval and renal transplant outcomes (Benck et al., 2011). Desmopressin was associated with improved 2-year kidney graft survival. Furthermore, dopamine pretreatment in the donors enhanced the graft survival benefit of desmopressin, while assignment of the donor to the non-dopamine group abolished the graft survival benefit.

In a more recently published study, Mascia et al. tested whether use of a lung-protective strategy in deceased donors increased the number of lungs available for transplantation (Mascia et al., 2010). The study was stopped early due to termination of funding. This was a multicentre randomized controlled trial of potential lung donors conducted at 12 European ICUs. One hundred and eighteen donors were randomized to either the conventional or protective-lung ventilatory strategy, which was applied during the 6-hour observation period required for declaration of brain death and maintained until donors arrived in the operating room for organ recovery. Significantly more donors in the protective strategy group met lung donor eligibility criteria after the 6-hour observation period and had their lungs recovered. Table 9.1 contains a list of published donor intervention trials aimed at increasing the quantity of transplantable organs and/or optimizing transplanted organ function.

A small number of donor intervention trials are currently listed on the <http://www.clinicaltrials.gov> website. A list of the trials can be found in Table 9.2. Several of these trials address the use of ischaemic preconditioning in deceased donors to improve post-transplantation outcomes. One of the more novel ongoing studies is designed to examine the effect of intravenous beta-epoietin administered to deceased donors 1 hour before organ recovery on kidney function in recipients of renal graft transplants (NCT01450878). Two other studies compare the use of therapeutic hypothermia in deceased donors with the standard maintenance of normothermia (NCT01544530 and NCT01680744).

While the presence of recently published and ongoing donor intervention trials is encouraging, many of these studies are single-centre with relatively small enrollments. Furthermore, most of these studies extend pre-existing concepts rather than exploring the multitude of novel mechanistic approaches that have emerged from basic science research and animal models (Feng, 2010). Examples of promising strategies for protecting donor organs that have been investigated in animal models but have yet to be tested in organ donors include modulation of the inflammatory response to brain death (a key pathway of organ injury during the donation process) as well as upregulation of cytoprotective proteins, such as heme-oxygenase-1 to reduce

**Table 9.1** Published prospective donor intervention trials

| Author | Study design | Enrolment (number) | Study intervention | Study results |
|---|---|---|---|---|
| Kotsch et al. 2008 | Prospective randomized controlled | 100 | Methylprednisolone 250 mg IV bolus at time of organ donation consent, followed by 100 mg/hour continuous infusion | Methylprednisolone resulted in reduced intragraft and serum cytokine expression in donors, lower rates of acute rejection following liver transplantation |
| Schnuelle et al. 2009 | Prospective randomized controlled, open-label | 264 | Low-dose dopamine infusion, 4 μg/kg/min | Dialysis requirement reduced in recipients of kidney grafts from donors in dopamine group |
| Mascia et al. 2010 | Prospective randomized controlled | 118 | Lung-protective strategy (tidal volumes 6–8 mL/kg, PEEP 8–10 cm water, apnoea test performed using CPAP, closed circuit for airway suction) | More lungs recovered from donors in lung-protective strategy group (trial terminated early) |
| Kellum et al. 2008 | Prospective randomized, open-label, feasibility study | 8 | Cytokine removal with haemoadsorption device | Cytokine removal across haemoadsorption device ranged from 4% to 30%, with overall removal greatest for IL-6, TNF |
| Koneru et al. 2005 | Prospective randomized controlled | 62 | 5 minutes of liver IPC by hilar clamping in deceased donors | IPC did not cause haemodynamic instability in donors and did not decrease graft injury in liver recipients |
| Amatscheck et al. 2012 | Prospective randomized placebo-controlled, blinded | 90 | Methylprednisolone 1,000 mg 6 hours prior to organ recovery | Recipients of livers from donors in the treatment and placebo groups had similar early graft function, 3-year survival rates, and acute rejection rates |
| Kainz et al. 2010 | Prospective randomized placebo-controlled | 269 | Methylprednisolone 1,000 mg at least 3 hours prior to organ recovery | Incidence of acute renal failure (more than one dialysis incidence in first week after renal transplantation) in recipients of kidneys from donors in treatment and placebo groups did not differ |

PEEP, Positive end-expiratory pressure; CPAP, continuous positive airway pressure; IPC, ischaemic preconditioning; IL, interleukin; TNF, tumour necrosis factor.

dysfunctional inflammation (Takada et al., 1998; Kotsch et al., 2006; Bouma et al., 2009; Oto et al., 2009; Ollinger and Pratschke, 2010; Danobeitia et al., 2011). In the meantime, the current recommendations on donor treatment are based on physiological rationale, experiential reasoning, and only sparse evidence from observational studies, while controlled clinical data using reasonable endpoints for the assessment of transplantation outcomes remain limited (Kirschbaum and Hudson, 2010).

## Challenges of conducting research in deceased organ donors

Many components contribute to the lack of randomized prospective trials in donor management; however, a major factor is the unique challenges posed by research in deceased organ donors. A number of substantial barriers specific to the field of organ transplantation impede progress in this important investigative area. One of the major obstacles to innovation in donor management is the large list of different stakeholders to consider when undertaking trials involving deceased donors. The first stakeholder is the principal investigator of the donor intervention trial. The principal investigator must first approach the OPO staff and medical board, who then pass the intervention proposal along to transplant physicians across the community for scientific and clinical consideration. If the aforementioned parties support the proposal, then it is presented to the physicians, nurses, and administration and institutional review boards of the various donor hospitals within the donation service area(s). Furthermore, the intervention proposal must be presented to donor families (Feng, 2010). Ultimately, a proposed donor intervention must be approved by a large group of parties scattered throughout a community, each party with its own concerns and interests. Reaching consensus across such a diverse collection of interests and backgrounds can be extremely challenging and presents a significant barrier to innovation in donor management (Feng, 2010).

## Individual and institutional informed consent for deceased organ donor research

Other substantial barriers to conducting donor research are the logistics and complex ethical considerations of individual and institutional informed consent for both the deceased donor and the potential organ recipients. Donor management intervention trials present unique ethical and regulatory challenges for which there are no consensus guidelines available nationally or internationally (Pentz et al., 2005). Brain-dead potential organ donors have been declared dead and therefore are not considered human subjects under existing federal policy (Rey et al.,

**Table 9.2** Donor intervention studies listed in ClinicalTrials.gov

| ClinicalTrails.gov number | Start date | End date (projected) | Study title | Study status | Enrolment (projected number) | Study design |
|---|---|---|---|---|---|---|
| NCT00245830 | 10/03 | 3/07 | Ischemic Preconditioning of Liver in Cadaver Donors | Completed | 100 | Treatment, randomized, single blind, parallel assignment, efficacy study |
| NCT00238030 | 12/04 | 10/10 | Thyroxine Replacement in Organ Donors | Competed | 34 | Treatment, randomized, double blind, single group assignment, efficacy study |
| NCT00998972 | 9/06 | 6/11 | N-acetyl-cysteine (NAC) and Kidney Graft Function | Completed | 236 | Treatment, randomized, single blind, parallel assignment, efficacy study |
| NCT00310401 | 4/07 | 6/11 | The Effect of Nebulized Albuterol on Donor Oxygenation | Completed | 507 | Treatment, randomized, double blind, parallel assignment, efficacy study |
| NCT00718575 | 8/08 | 14/10 | The Effects of Glucose/Ischemic Preconditioning on Reperfusion Injury in Deceased-Donor Liver Transplantation | Suspended | 100 | Treatment, randomized, single blind, parallel assignment, safety/efficacy study |
| NCT01140035 | 1/09 | 9/11 | Intensive Insulin Therapy in Deceased Donors | Completed | (200) | Treatment, randomized, single blind, parallel assignment, efficacy study |
| NCT00975702 | 4/09 | (12/12) | Remote Ischemic Preconditioning in Abdominal Organ Transplantation (RIPCOT) | Enrolling by invitation | (580) | Treatment, randomized, double blind, parallel assignment, safety/efficacy study |
| NCT00987714 | 8/09 | (8/11) | Monitoring Organ Donors to Increase Transplantation Results | Recruiting | (960) | Supportive care, randomized, open-label, parallel assignment |
| NCT01939171 | 6/10 | 2/12 | Thymoglobulin in Cadaver Donor | Completed | 20 | Prevention, randomized, open-label, parallel assignment, safety/efficacy study |
| NCT01515072 | 7/11 | (8/14) | Remote Ischemic Preconditioning in Neurological Death Organ Donors (RIPNOD) | Recruiting | (320) | Treatment, randomized, open-label, parallel assignment, efficacy study |
| NCT01450878 | 12/11 | (11/14) | Renal Graft Function After Treatment with Erythropoetin (FRETEP) | Recruiting | (166) | Treatment, randomized, double blind, parallel assignment, efficacy study |
| NCT01544530 | 3/12 | (3/14) | Cooling to Optimize Organ Live in Donor Study (COOLDonor) | Recruiting | (60) | Treatment, randomized, open-label, parallel assignment, safety/efficacy study |
| NCT01680744 | 5/12 | 11/14 | The Effect of Therapeutic Hypothermia on Deceased Donor Renal Graft Outcomes—a Randomized Controlled Trial From the Region 5 Donor Management Goals Workgroup | Completed | 370 | Prevention, randomized, single blind, single group assignment, efficacy study |
| NCT01860716 | 5/13 | (12/13) | Impact of Melatonin in the Pretreatment of Organ Donor and the Influence in the Evolution of Liver Transplant | Not yet open for participant recruitment | (60) | Prevention, randomized, double blind, parallel assignment, safety/efficacy study |
| NCT02211053 | 7/14 | (7/16) | Evaluation of the Efficacy and Safety of Levothyroxine in Brain Death Organ Donors: a Randomized Controlled Trial (ECHOT4) | Recruiting | (60) | Supportive care, randomized, double blind, parallel assignment, efficacy study |

2011). As a result, the US federal requirement that all human research undergo review by an institutional review board does not extend to research with deceased donors (Wicclair and DeVita, 2004; Pentz et al., 2005). Despite the lack of a federal mandate, oversight of deceased donor research by an institutional review board has been the prevailing practice in the US. While the Office for Human Protection does not require that deceased research subjects be protected via the institutional review board process, an institution can mandate such oversight on its own accord. For example, the Committee for the Oversight of Research Involving the Dead at the University of Pittsburg School of Medicine and Medical Center requires the following for studies involving the dead: (1) a review process to ensure scientific merit of studies; (2) informed consent from the patient or surrogate; (3) institutional oversight to determine whether studies are within ethical and societal norms and whether information derived from studies may impact the deceased's family; and (4) procedures limiting time from consent to releasing the body to the family (Committee for the Oversight of Research Involving the Dead, 2003).

Similarly, because deceased donors are legally dead and not considered human subjects, it is unclear whether consent is or should be required under the current regulatory framework and, if so, whom it should be obtained from. There is a lack of uniform practices and, as a result, consent practices have varied across different donor management intervention trials (Koneru et al., 2005; Kotsch et al., 2008; Schnuelle et al., 2009; Feng, 2010; Rey et al., 2011). The purpose of informed consent in human subject research is to promote individuals' autonomy, respect their values and interests, and protect them from exposure to risks or harm without their knowledge (Emanuel et al., 2000). It is unclear that consent for deceased organ donors could serve the purpose that it is intended to serve in living human subjects. For example, the deceased are not capable of making decisions; therefore it might seem counterintuitive to protect their autonomy with consent. However, society regularly respects the autonomy and values of the deceased. For example, we require consent for organ donation from either the donor or a surrogate (Rey et al., 2011). One of the key functions of informed consent is to make individuals aware of the potential risks of participating in a study. In the case of deceased organ donors, the potential research participant is not capable of understanding the risks and benefits of a study and of making an informed decision to participate in or abstain from a study. Furthermore, the potential for harm after death seems minor, bringing into question the purpose of informed consent for research from deceased donors (Rey et al., 2011).

Despite the fact that deceased donors are not considered human subjects and despite the uncertainty surrounding the function of consent for research from the deceased, informed consent from the donor family is now expected and standard. Obtaining consent for research from the donor family allows the transplant community to respect and protect the deceased donor, minimize the family's distress, and maintain public trust in the medical profession (Feng, 2010). Although the tragic circumstances of deceased organ donation make it difficult to obtain consent from the donor's family, securing consent is crucial for the continuing growth and the future success of donor research.

## Recipient-informed consent for deceased organ donor research

Standards and uniform practices are also lacking regarding consent from the recipients or potential recipients of organs procured from donors enrolled in research studies. More often than not, published donor management interventional trials do not explicitly address recipient consent. There are currently no regulatory mechanisms to accommodate the ethical arguments for and against requiring recipient consent for donor management studies. However, when considering whether to require recipient consent in donor management research, two factors must be evaluated: (1) whether recipients are considered research subjects; and (2) whether reasons exist to waive general requirements for subjects' consent (Rey et al., 2011). Most donor management trials are designed to assess and collect data on both donor and recipient outcomes; therefore recipients involved in such studies would be classified as human subjects and require informed consent. However, arguments could be made for waiving recipient consent using the emergency research consent waiver or the minimal risk research waiver. For example, the study in which a recipient will participate is often not known until the organ becomes available. This does not allow enough time to obtain truly informed recipient consent before the organ is placed; therefore the emergency research consent waiver could be invoked (Halpern et al., 2008). Also, most donor interventions, such as tight glucose control and therapeutic hypothermia, will rarely pose unique risks to recipients and will therefore meet criteria for minimal risk (Morris and Nelson, 2007). However, interventions exposing donors to new compounds could potentially put recipients at risk for harm and thus would not meet minimal risk criteria.

Beyond these regulatory concerns, requiring recipient consent for donor intervention studies raises both logistic and ethical concerns. Many organs are placed late in the donation process and often even after organ procurement. This means that most recipients are unknown until well into the donor management period or even after organ recovery when the donor study intervention has already been initiated or completed. Requiring institutional review board approval and individual recipient consent would pose a substantial barrier to donor intervention trials and would not make the research feasible (Feng, 2010). Mandating consent from potential recipients of organs from donors involved in management studies also poses ethical dilemmas. Part of the problem stems from the time-sensitive nature of the organ donation and transplantation process. Prolonging organ placement in order to secure consent for research participation from the potential recipients of those organs would cause delay that could be detrimental to the outcomes of transplantation. Even if recipient consent precedes donor treatment, coercion is a significant concern given the stress of the transplant process. Furthermore, the recipient may feel pressured to consent for a study in order to qualify for that specific transplantation opportunity (Feng, 2010). The recipient may feel that he/she does not actually have a choice to abstain from participation in the research if doing so means that he/she becomes ineligible for transplantation. In this case, consent is not serving the function of promoting an individual's autonomy as intended. The potential recipient's consent could be sought before enrolling the identified donor in the study, such that the recipient could decline to participate in the study but still receive the transplant. However, giving recipients authority over donor management is ethically problematic and would introduce biases into the research (Freedman, 1987; Rey et al., 2011).

## Transplant research infrastructure

The lack of an established research infrastructure amongst transplant centres or OPOs in the US is also a significant obstacle to conducting robust clinical trials. Most of the observational studies and clinical trials have been limited to single institutions or single donation services areas and vary widely in data quality and data collection methods. UNOS Region 5 was the first to conduct a collaborative, prospective DMG study, in which all eight OPOs in the region agreed to evaluate and then implement the same ten critical care endpoints (DMGs) as goals at the beside of every deceased donor. This study by Malinoski et al. (2011) found that meeting at least eight of ten DMGs in deceased donors prior to organ procurement was significantly associated with more OTPD.

While this collaboration produced encouraging results, inconsistent and inefficient data quality and collection methods have made it difficult to establish uniform, evidence-based, donor management practices. An appropriate research infrastructure is absolutely necessary to address these shortcomings and conduct prospective interventional studies on a large enough scale to draw meaningful conclusions and impact the donation and transplantation community as a whole. A successful and sound research infrastructure will need to include multiple donation services areas to enable collaborative prospective randomized interventional trials. It will also need an integrated researchable database for evaluating the impact of interventions on donor and recipient outcomes and facilitating meaningful review of DMG data. A current study investigating the impact of therapeutic hypothermia on renal protection during the donation process is attempting to achieve this goal.

One way to develop such an infrastructure is to gradually expand an existing and successful research framework to additional donation services areas. For example, the California Transplant Donor Network and the University of California San Francisco successfully completed a randomized prospective trial across 40 hospitals in Northern California and Nevada examining the effects of intensive insulin therapy in deceased organ donors on renal function at the time of organ recovery and on early graft function in kidney recipients (NCT01140035). The investigators of this trial have expanded this research infrastructure to a second donation services area (Southern California, OneLegacy) in order to conduct a large-scale prospective randomized interventional trial of therapeutic hypothermia in deceased donors, which will have access to approximately 10% of all the deceased donors in the US. They have also created a web portal for real-time donor management data entry, including donor demographic information, data on achievement of DMGs from the time of referral to the OPO through the time of organ recovery, as well as specific variables for the proposed hypothermia trial. The database will also be used to track subsequent organ utilization and graft function data in the recipient. Applying existing knowledge and lessons learned from establishing the infrastructure and logistics of the previous intensive insulin therapy trial will help to overcome obstacles in the second donation services area.

This strategy of gradually expanding a research infrastructure to a limited number of donation services areas, rather than to an entire region or even larger area, makes a successful execution more likely. Another advantage of progressively developing and expanding an existing and successful research infrastructure is that it allows investigators to ensure better trial protocol compliance and data quality. It also limits the number of stakeholders, which can facilitate communication, problem-solving, and face-to-face meetings between participating investigators. By leveraging an existing research infrastructure and expanding it, investigators could potentially demonstrate the feasibility of a donor intervention across different donation services areas, validate findings in different practice environments, and make substantial progress towards establishing uniform, evidence-based donor management practices that can increase the quantity and quality of transplantable organs.

## Additional barriers to donor interventional studies

However, even with the appropriate research infrastructure in place, trial design poses another barrier to donor interventional studies with regard to safety, efficacy, and scientific validity. For donor trials in which a systemic intervention is administered to improve the function of a particular organ, the intervention may have an impact on other organs, including potentially transplantable organs, and ultimately on the recipients of these organs. Such an intervention may improve the function of the organ of interest but compromise the function or quality of another potentially transplantable organ (Feng, 2010). Many donor intervention trials are intended to improve early graft function in corresponding recipients. However, there is currently a lack of validated endpoints for early graft function.

This makes it challenging to select meaningful endpoints for donor intervention trials. The commonly used outcomes of graft survival and recipient survival lack granularity. For the kidney, occurrence of delayed graft function (DGF), defined as the need for dialysis within 1 week of transplantation, is a frequently used endpoint for donor intervention trials and is somewhat more discriminating than graft or recipient survival (Feng, 2010). DGF has the benefit of being correlated with both graft and patient survival and, therefore, can be used as a surrogate for these outcomes. DGF is also consistently documented in the UNOS database, which makes it an accessible endpoint. However, there is no general agreement among nephrologists about the criteria for dialysis requirement postkidney transplantation. The decision to dialyze a patient following kidney transplantation and the timing of dialysis is quite subjective, yet DGF is used as an objective assessment of early kidney graft function.

Finally, assessing the effects that a donor management intervention has on the recipients of the corresponding organs is very challenging. When the predictor variable is being measured in one population (the donors) and the outcome of interest is being measured in a separate heterogeneous population (the recipients) with its own set of interacting variables, it becomes very difficult to control for all interactions. Using DGF as an example, multiple risk prediction models have identified several recipient factors, including male gender, African-American race, higher body mass index, and diabetic ESRD, which are significantly associated with DGF (Irish et al., 2003, 2010). Other studies have also found recipient race, gender, duration of pretransplant dialysis, and panel reactive antibody status to be correlated to the incidence of DGF (Ojo et al., 1997; McLaren et al., 1999; Halloran and Hunsicker, 2001; Patel et al., 2008). Although donors in an intervention trial are randomized, recipient factors may obscure correlations between the donor intervention and recipient outcomes.

## Conclusion

The number of transplant candidates awaiting organ donation far outnumbers the supply of organs available for transplantation. This disparity will likely continue to grow as organ transplantation remains the treatment of choice for qualifying patients with organ failure and as post-transplantation outcomes improve. Deceased donor management interventions may serve to bridge this gap between organ supply and demand by increasing the quantity and quality of organs available for transplantation. In particular, large prospective randomized controlled studies are necessary to quantify the extent to which specific donor interventions might enhance organ recovery and outcomes among transplant recipients. However, there are currently substantial logistical, ethical, and scientific obstacles unique to the transplantation setting that hinder innovation in deceased donor management through clinical trials. Furthermore, there is no precedent for how to appropriately conduct donor intervention studies and no governing body or regulatory mechanism to provide structure or oversight to this unique and relatively young research field.

Thus far, donor research oversight has occurred on an institutional basis and has varied widely. However, the issues that confront donor management research extend beyond the reach of individual investigators or even individual institutions. A larger body will be necessary to clearly define these issues and then approach them (Feng, 2010). This will require agreement among the stakeholders in the organ transplantation process, including investigators, transplant centres, OPOs, the OPTN, Regional Review Boards, and community members. New regulatory structures will need to be established outside of the existing Institutional Review Board and, instead, at the level of OPOs, the OPTN, and Regional Review Boards. These structures will help optimize the efficiency of study proposal reviews and the consistency of oversight (Rey et al., 2011). Furthermore, these structures may create a more favourable environment for collaborative donor intervention studies across multiple donation services areas and potentially across multiple donor regions. Such a system would offer protection to research participants while helping to promote collaborative, large-scale research efforts in this vital field of investigation.

## References


Amatschek S, et al. (2012) The effect of steroid pretreatment of deceased organ donors on liver allograft function: a blinded randomized placebo-controlled trial. *J Hepatol* 2012;**56**:1305–9.

Angel LF, Levine DJ, Restrepo MI, et al. (2006) Impact of a lung transplantation donor-management protocol on lung donation and recipient outcomes. *Am J Respir Crit Care Med*, **174**(6):710–716.

Benck U, Gottmann U, Hoeger S, et al. (2011) Donor desmopressin is associated with superior graft survival after kidney transplantation. *Transplantation*, **92**(11):1252–1258.

Bouma HR, Ploeg RJ, Schuurs TA (2009) Signal transduction pathways involved in brain death-induced renal injury. *Am J Transplant*, **9**(5):989–997.

Chang GJ, Mahanty HD, Ascher NL, Roberts JP (2003) Expanding the donor pool: can the Spanish model work in the United States? *Am J Transplant*, **3**(10):1259–1263.

Committee for the Oversight of Research Involving the Dead (2003) Policy for research involving the dead. *Crit Care Med*, **31**(5 Suppl):S391–393.

Danobeitia JS, Sperger JM, Hanson MS, et al. (2011) Early activation of the inflammatory response in the liver of brain-dead non-human primates. *J Surg Res*, **176**(2):639–648.

DuBose J, Salim A (2008) Aggressive organ donor management protocol. *J Intensive Care Med*, **23**(6):367–375.

Emanuel EJ, Wendler D, Grady C (2000) What makes clinical research ethical? *JAMA*, **283**(20):2701–2711.

Feng S (2010) Donor intervention and organ preservation: where is the science and what are the obstacles? *Am J Transplant*, **10**(5):1155–1162.

Follette DM, Rudich SM, Babcock WD (1998) Improved oxygenation and increased lung donor recovery with high-dose steroid administration after brain death. *J Heart Lung Transplant*, **17**(4):423–429.

Franklin GA, Santos AP, Smith JW, Galbraith S, Harbrecht BG, Garrison RN (2010) Optimization of donor management goals yields increased organ use. *Am Surg*, **76**(6):587–594.

Freedman B (1987) Scientific value and validity as ethical requirements for research: a proposed explication. *IRB*, **9**(6):7–10.

Hagan ME, McClean D, Falcone CA, et al. (2009) Attaining specific donor management goals increases number of organs transplanted per donor: a quality improvement project. *Prog Transplant*, **19**(3):227–231.

Halloran PF, Hunsicker LG (2001) Delayed graft function: state of the art. Summit Meeting, 10–11 November, Scottsdale, Arizona. *Am J Transplant*, **1**(2):115–120.

Halpern SD, Shaked A, Hasz RD, Caplan AL (2008) Informing candidates for solid-organ transplantation about donor risk factors. *N Engl J Med*, **358**(26):2832–2837.

Howard DH, Siminoff LA, McBride V, Lin M (2007) Does quality improvement work? Evaluation of the organ donation breakthrough collaborative. *Health Serv Res*, **42**(6 Pt 1):2160–2173; discussion 2294–2323.

Irish WD, McCollum DA, Tesi RJ, et al. (2003) Nomogram for predicting the likelihood of delayed graft function in adult cadaveric renal transplant recipients. *J Am Soc Nephrol*, **14**(11):2967–2974.

Irish WD, Ilsley JN, Schnitzler MA, Feng S, Brennan DC (2010) A risk prediction model for delayed graft function in the current era of deceased donor renal transplantation. *Am J Transplant*, **10**(10):2279–2286.

Kainz A, et al. (2010) Steroid pretreatment of organ donors to prevent postischemic renal allograft failure: a randomized, controlled trial. *Ann Intern Med* 2010;153:222–30.

Kellum et al. (2008) Effects of hemoadsorption on cytokine removal and short-term survival in septic rats. *Crit Care Med*. 2008 May; 36(5): 1573–1577.<http://www.ncbi.nlm.nih.gov/entrez/eutils/elink.fcgi?dbfrom=pubmed&retmode=ref&cmd=prlinks&id=18434884>7

Kirschbaum CE, Hudson S (2010) Increasing organ yield through a lung management protocol. *Prog Transplant*, **20**(1):28–32.

Koneru B, Fisher A, He Y, et al. (2005) Ischemic preconditioning in deceased donor liver transplantation: a prospective randomized clinical trial of safety and efficacy. *Liver Transpl*, **11**(2):196–202.

Kotsch K, Francuski M, Pascher A, et al. (2006) Improved long-term graft survival after HO-1 induction in brain-dead donors. *Am J Transplant*, **6**(3):477–486.

Kotsch K, Ulrich F, Reutzel-Selke A, et al. (2008) Methylprednisolone therapy in deceased donors reduces inflammation in the donor liver and improves outcome after liver transplantation: a prospective randomized controlled trial. *Ann Surg*, **248**(6):1042–1050.

Mackersie RC, Bronsther OL, Shackford SR (1991) Organ procurement in patients with fatal head injuries. The fate of the potential donor. *Ann Surg*, **213**(2):143–150.

Malinoski DJ, Daly MC, Patel MS, Oley-Graybill C, Foster CE 3rd, Salim A (2011) Achieving donor management goals before deceased donor procurement is associated with more organs transplanted per donor. *J Trauma*, **71**(4):990–995; discussion 996.

Mascia L, Pasero D, Slutsky AS, et al. (2010) Effect of a lung protective strategy for organ donors on eligibility and availability of lungs for transplantation: a randomized controlled trial. *JAMA*, **304**(23):2620–2627.

McLaren AJ, Jassem W, Gray DW, Fuggle SV, Welsh KI, Morris PJ (1999) Delayed graft function: risk factors and the relative effects of early function and acute rejection on long-term survival in cadaveric renal transplantation. *Clin Transplant*, **13**(3):266–272.

Morris MC, Nelson RM (2007) Randomized, controlled trials as minimal risk: an ethical analysis. *Crit Care Med*, **35**(3):940–944.

Nathan HM, Conrad SL, Held PJ, et al. (2003) Organ donation in the United States. *Am J Transplant*, **3**(Suppl 4):29–40.

Ojo AO, Wolfe RA, Held PJ, Port FK, Schmouder RL (1997) Delayed graft function: risk factors and implications for renal allograft survival. *Transplantation*, **63**(7):968–974.

Ollinger R, Pratschke J (2010) Role of heme oxygenase-1 in transplantation. *Transpl Int*, **23**(11):1071–1081.

Oto T, Calderone A, Li Z, Rosenfeldt FL, Pepe S (2009) p38 mitogen-activated protein kinase inhibition reduces inflammatory cytokines in a brain-dead transplant donor animal model. *Heart Lung Circ*, **18**(6):393–400.

Patel SJ, Duhart BT, Jr, Krauss AG, et al. (2008) Risk factors and consequences of delayed graft function in deceased donor renal transplant patients receiving antithymocyte globulin induction. *Transplantation*, **86**(2):313–320.

Pentz RD, Cohen CB, Wicclair M, et al. (2005) Ethics guidelines for research with the recently dead. *Nat Med*, **11**(11):1145–1149.

Rey MM, Ware LB, Matthay MA, et al. (2011) Informed consent in research to improve the number and quality of deceased donor organs. *Crit Care Med*, **39**(2):280–283.

Rosendale JD, Chabalewski FL, McBride MA, et al. (2002) Increased transplanted organs from the use of a standardized donor management protocol. *Am J Transplant*, **2**(8):761–768.

Rosendale JD, Kauffman HM, McBride MA, et al. (2003a) Aggressive pharmacologic donor management results in more transplanted organs. *Transplantation*, **75**(4):482–487.

Rosendale JD, Kauffman HM, McBride MA, et al. (2003b) Hormonal resuscitation yields more transplanted hearts, with improved early function. *Transplantation*, **75**(8):1336–1341.

Saidi RF, Elias N, Kawai T, et al. (2007) Outcome of kidney transplantation using expanded criteria donors and donation after cardiac death kidneys: realities and costs. *Am J Transplant*, **7**(12):2769–2774.

Salim A, Velmahos GC, Brown C, Belzberg H, Demetriades D (2005) Aggressive organ donor management significantly increases the number of organs available for transplantation. *J Trauma*, **58**(5):991–994.

Salim A, Martin M, Brown C, Rhee P, Demetriades D, Belzberg H (2006) The effect of a protocol of aggressive donor management: implications for the national organ donor shortage. *J Trauma*, **61**(2):429–433; discussion 433–435.

Salim A, Martin M, Brown C, et al. (2007) Using thyroid hormone in brain-dead donors to maximize the number of organs available for transplantation. *Clin Transplant*, **21**(3):405–409.

Schnuelle P, Gottmann U, Hoeger S, et al. (2009) Effects of donor pretreatment with dopamine on graft function after kidney transplantation: a randomized controlled trial. *JAMA*, **302**(10):1067–1075.

Shah VR (2008) Aggressive management of multiorgan donor. *Transplant Proc*, **40**(4):1087–1090.

Shemie SD, Ross H, Pagliarello J, et al. (2006) Organ donor management in Canada: recommendations of the forum on medical management to optimize donor organ potential. *CMAJ*, **174**(6):S13–32.

Straznicka M, Follette DM, Eisner MD, Roberts PF, Menza RL, Babcock WD (2002) Aggressive management of lung donors classified as unacceptable: excellent recipient survival one year after transplantation. *J Thorac Cardiovasc Surg*, **124**(2):250–258.

Sung RS, Galloway J, Tuttle-Newhall JE, et al. (2008) Organ donation and utilization in the United States, 1997–2006. *Am J Transplant*, **8**(4 Pt 2):922–934.

Takada M, Nadeau KC, Hancock WW, et al. (1998) Effects of explosive brain death on cytokine activation of peripheral organs in the rat. *Transplantation*, **65**(12):1533–1542.

Venkateswaran RV, Patchell VB, Wilson IC, et al. (2008) Early donor management increases the retrieval rate of lungs for transplantation. *Ann Thorac Surg*, **85**(1):278–286; discussion 286.

Wheeldon DR, Potter CD, Oduro A, Wallwork J, Large SR (1995) Transforming the "unacceptable" donor: outcomes from the adoption of a standardized donor management technique. *J Heart Lung Transplant*, **14**(4):734–742.

Wicclair MR, DeVita M (2004) Oversight of research involving the dead. *Kennedy Inst Ethics J*, **14**(2):143–164.

SECTION 4

# The scientific basis of organ transplantation

# CHAPTER 10

# Organ resuscitation

Ernesto A. Pretto, Jr., Kyota Fukazawa, and Antonello Pileggi

## Introduction

In terms of pathophysiology, organ transplantation consists of three main phases and five stages (see Figure 10.1). The period of time preceding and immediately following catastrophic brain injury of the organ donor is the 'pre-ischaemic' phase. During the 'ischaemic' phase the organ is removed from the body of the donor and preserved but sustains cold ischaemic injury during storage or perfusion preservation and warm ischaemic injury before revascularization. In the 'post-ischaemic' phase there is restoration of blood flow to the graft in the recipient. These events result in ischaemia–reperfusion and inflammatory insult to the graft, increasing the likelihood of organ damage and failure. Aggressive intensive care management of the donor is critical to preventing deterioration of organ function. However, there is preliminary evidence to indicate there may be improved graft function when therapy to protect or precondition the graft is initiated in the donor, prior to organ recovery (see Chapter 9). This chapter provides a detailed review of the underlying cellular mechanisms that lead to impaired graft function. It also highlights proposed key molecular targets that are essential for the future development of novel resuscitative therapies/interventions.

## The 'organ transplant continuum'

In order to more clearly conceptualize the pathophysiological and molecular stresses organs are subjected to during transplantation, a detailed phased risk analysis of the transplant process may be helpful. Therefore we will describe known cellular and molecular mechanisms associated with organ transplantation, from the moment of brain death certification in the donor to reperfusion of the graft in the recipient. We will focus on mechanisms common to most cell and tissue types. To clinically contextualize these biochemical and molecular events we have characterized injury mechanisms according to when (timing) and why (risks) they occur, during procurement, preservation, and transplantation (see Table 10.1).

### Phase I: pre-ischaemia–anoxia

Attempts to protect, also called preconditioning of, organs for transplantation ideally must be instituted immediately after brain death certification. At this time, organ donor management consists simply of meticulous critical care and intraoperative management (see Chapter 7). Pathophysiological and metabolic changes resulting from massive brain injury contribute to extracerebral organ dysfunction. For example, massive brain ischaemia triggers the release of catecholamines, proinflammatory cytokines, and chemokines (TNF-α, IL-1β, IL-8, CCL2/MCP-1, amongst others). This results in profound haemodynamic, hormonal, and metabolic derangements. Additionally, these mediators lead to 'immune'-activation of the graft (i.e. increased major histocompatibility complex (MHC) class I and II antigens as well as costimulation of antigens and selectins) that increase immunogenicity in the postreperfusion period, triggering innate immunity and increasing the incidence of acute and chronic rejection phenomena that can shorten graft lifespan (Takada et al., 1998; Endo et al., 2000; Weiss et al., 2007; Ogliari et al., 2008; Hoeger et al., 2009; Ilmakunnas et al., 2010). Indeed, higher rates of preserved graft function and lower episodes of rejection are observed after transplantation of organs obtained from living donors.

#### Stage 1: pre-ischaemia: the transition to and moment of brain death certification

Risk factors for organ injury or damage include pre-existing comorbidities, such as age, race, diabetes, hypertension, lifetime alcohol intake or drug abuse, exposure to hepatitis virus, fatty liver, fibrosis, and other irreducible causes of organ damage associated with aging (senescence) and chronic disease.

Additionally, life-support interventions aimed at reversing terminal illness, albeit futile, may or may not compromise systemic organ function. Episodes of cardiac arrest with successful resuscitation during the process of terminal illness in the yet-to-become donor, as well as the warm ischaemic phase in the deceased cardiovascular donor, will invariably result in a major adverse impact on short- and long-term graft function in the recipient. The extent to which these interventions will compromise graft function is impossible to predict at this time.

### Phase II: ischaemia–anoxia

#### Stage 2: pre-preservation: the process of cerebral death

The risks of organ injury after brain death (donor risk factors) are: cerebral injury (traumatic vs cerebrovascular brain injury); haemodynamic derangements leading to compromised systemic blood supply and oxygen delivery, with reduced organ perfusion pressure resulting in aggravated tissue ischaemia and anoxia (i.e. cardiac arrest); electrolyte disturbances (hypernatraemia); and hormonal imbalances. Prolongation of this period is associated with high risk of graft failure (donor risk index > 1.7) (see Chapter 7).

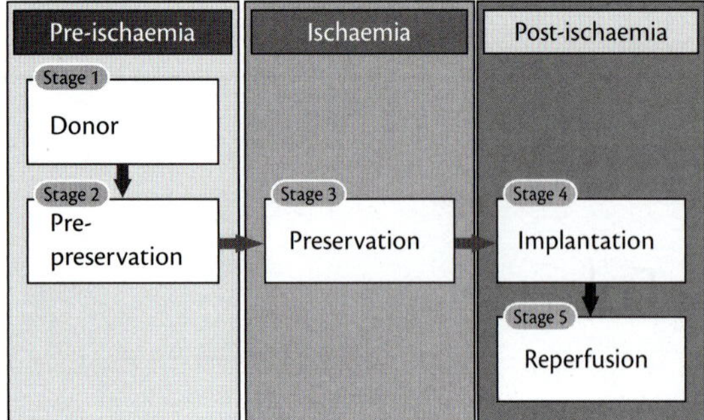


**Fig. 10.1** Pathophysiological phases and stages during organ transplantation

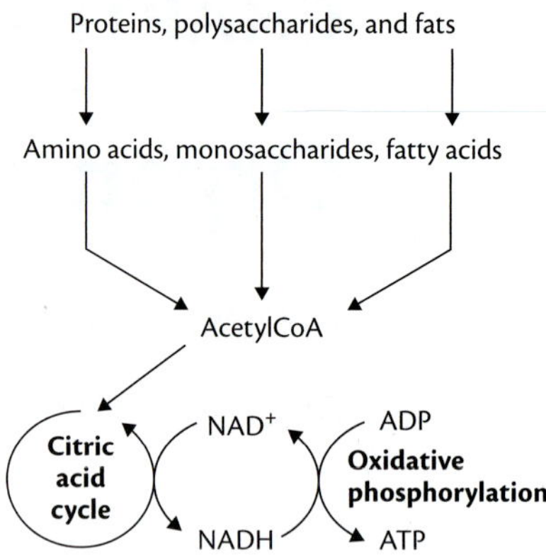


**Fig. 10.2** Abbreviated scheme of cellular oxygen and energy metabolism (the mitochondrion)

### *Biochemical events in ischaemia and anoxia*

Ischaemia is defined as a decrease in the blood supply to a body organ, tissue, or part caused by constriction or obstruction of the blood vessels. Anoxia is a condition characterized by an absence of oxygen supply to an organ or a tissue. Both conditions occur simultaneously in organ transplantation, hence the term ischaemia–anoxic injury. Cellular energy is produced in general terms at two intracellular locations: in the cytosol, through a process called glycolysis, when glucose or glycogen is the fuel, and in the mitochondria, where oxidative phosphorylation occurs through the citric acid cycle and the electron transport chain (see Figure 10.2).

However, during ischaemia–anoxia the citric acid cycle may exhibit opposing directionalities (Chinopoulos, 2013) (see Figure 10.3).

**Table 10.1** The organ transplant continuum: phases, stages, and major events

| | |
|---|---|
| **Phase I** | **Pre-ischaemia** |
| *Stage 1* | The moment of brain death certification (donor) |
| **Phase II** | **Ischaemia–anoxia** |
| *Stage 2* | Prepreservation: the time interval and events during terminal illness and brain death prior to organ recovery: |
| | 2a. Period of terminal illness |
| | 2b. Brain death derangements |
| *Stage 3* | Cold preservation: the time interval and events from the moment of aortic cross-clamp (cellular events triggered by global ischaemia–anoxia during cold storage or perfusion) |
| *Stage 4* | Rewarming ischaemia–anoxia (implantation): the time interval and events after removal of the organ from cold storage or perfusion preservation and before revascularization |
| **Phase III** | **Post-ischaemia–anoxia** |
| *Stage 5* | Reperfusion: the time interval and events following revascularization and reperfusion of the graft in the recipient |

The end product of metabolism is the production of ATP, which is an unstable molecule with high energy content (ATP has two high-energy phosphate bonds), and this is utilized as the principal source of energy in all cells to maintain vital cellular function. Intracellular ATP levels are maintained by a two-step metabolism of glucose, which is: (1) glucose to pyruvate ('glycolysis', producing two molecules of ATP from one molecule of glucose); and (2) pyruvate to water and carbon dioxide ('Krebs cycle' and 'electron transport chain', producing 36 molecules of ATP from one molecule of glucose). The second step utilizes oxygen as a cofactor for oxidative reaction. Cessation of oxygen supply during recovery of organs impairs Krebs cycle and electron transport chain reactions. Glycolysis is increased to maintain ATP production, resulting in excess pyruvate, which is metabolized to lactic acid by lactic dehydrogenase.

The process of metabolizing pyruvate whether to lactic acid or acetyl-CoA by pyruvate dehydrogenase is actively managed by the hypoxia-inducible factor (HIF)-1, depending on available oxygen. HIF-1 activates the expression of lactate dehydrogenase-A and pyruvate dehydrogenase kinase 1 (PDK1), thus tipping the balance from oxidative to glycolytic metabolism. This is considered an innate protection mechanism against hypoxia and promotes cell survival during ischaemia. To increase survival of cells during transplantation the aims of current organ preservation techniques/solutions include: energy conservation and maintenance of ATP production (glucose), reduction of oedema via extracellular oncotic pressure (lactobionate, raffinose, mannitol, sorbitol, hespan, etc.), patency of the microcirculation (perfusion preservation), in addition to decreased metabolic demand (cooling), and provision of antioxidants (glutathione).

When glucose or glycogen is the primary substrate, the rate of the initial reaction sequence, the glycolytic pathway, is regulated by the enzyme phosphofructokinase (PFK), which is activated by adenosine diphosphate (ADP), adenosine monophosphate (AMP), and inorganic phosphate. This enzyme is inhibited by moderate levels of ATP and by citrate. Hence, when the citric acid cycle and the electron transport chain are actively generating citrate and ATP, glycolysis is retarded. The overall efficiency is exceedingly low, producing about 3–7% of normal ATP. Nevertheless, this constitutes the only means of ATP production in the absence of oxygen. Fatty acids and ketone bodies are also oxidized aerobically in the citric acid cycle with an overall efficiency similar to

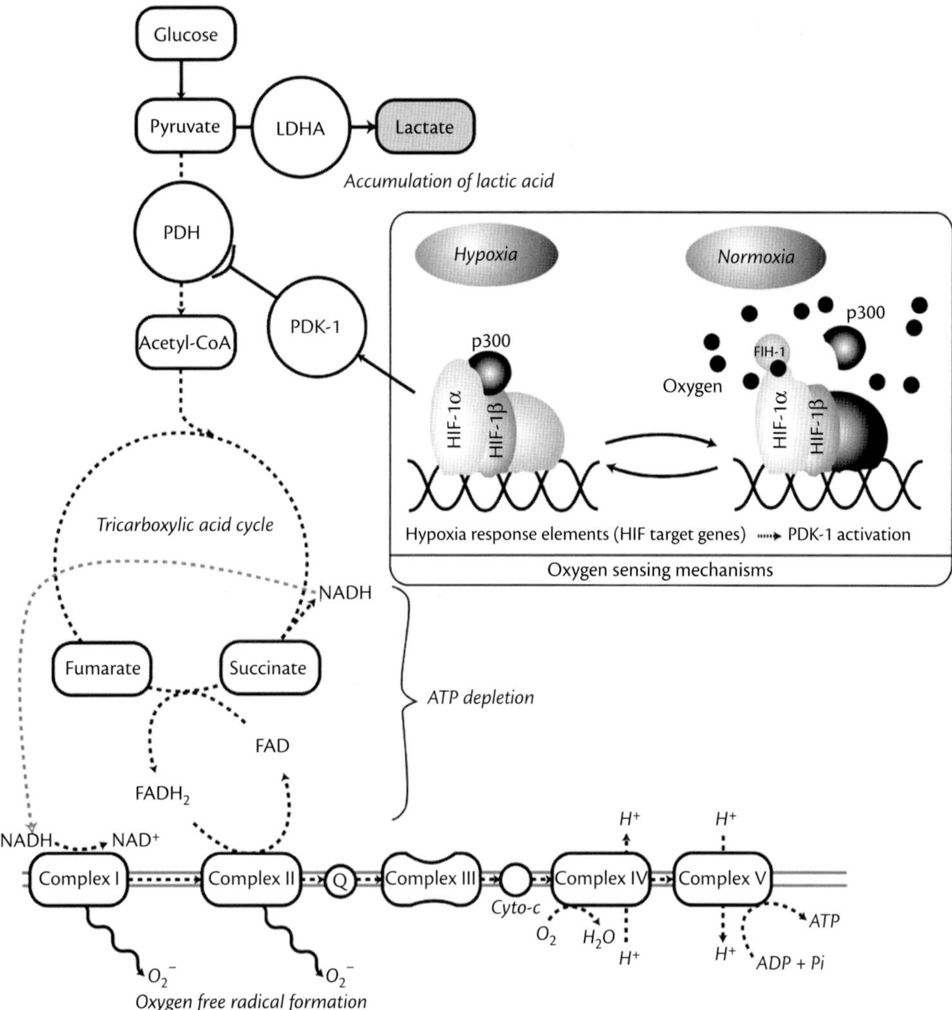


**Fig. 10.3** Intracellular ATP production and its regulation under anaerobic conditions. Under hypoxia, binding of p-300 to HIF-α activates expression of lactate dehydrogenase-A and pyruvate dehydrogenase kinase 1 (PDK1), thus tipping the balance from oxidative to glycolytic metabolism. ATP, Adenosine-5'-triphosphate; Cyto-c, cytochrome-c; FAD, flavin adenine dinucleotide; FIH, factor-inhibiting HIF; HIF, hypoxia-inducible factor; LDHA, lactate dehydrogenase A; NADH, nicotinamide adenine dinucleotide; PDH, pyruvate dehydrogenase; PDK-1, pyruvate dehydrogenase lipoamide kinase isozyme 1; Q, coenzyme Q

that of carbon dioxide, namely 40–50%. Whether produced by anaerobic glycolysis or aerobic means, trapped energy is stored as the high-energy compounds ATP and ADP, and their concentration as determined through various laboratory assays and imaging techniques, such as phosphorus-31 nuclear magnetic resonance (31P-NMR), provides a convenient index of the energy status of cells and tissues (Slade et al., 2006).

Other cellular functions that are energy dependent and essential for survival include the regulation of ions and water across cell membranes between cells and their environment, regulation of intracellular calcium homeostasis, and the translation and synthesis of proteins. Cells generate energy through cellular processes that are common to all. The mechanism by which cells expend energy in the form of ATP, however, differs from tissue to tissue depending on the degree of cell specialization. This characteristic of individual cells and tissues is what defines specialization of organ function. For example, in the kidney, energy is expended predominantly via sodium reabsorption in the proximal tubules. In the heart, energy is expended mostly during myofibrillar contraction and relaxation. Calcium ($Ca^{2+}$) uptake across the sarcolemmal membrane and its subsequent release from the sarcoplasmic reticulum in the intracellular compartment is essential to myocardial function. In the liver most of the energy expended goes toward protein synthesis and drug metabolism, and so forth. Therefore temporary suspension or a pharmacologic 'downregulation' of the metabolic rate prior to an ischaemic–anoxic insult can lead to energy conservation that contributes to cell protection, thereby enhancing viability post insult (Boutilier, 2001). Since these processes are mediated via enzymatic reactions, a down-regulation of energy utilization can also be achieved through induced hypothermia. Cooling reduces the metabolic rate or oxygen consumption, promoting energy conservation (Boutilier, 2001). Therefore suspension of cellular functions for the purposes of inducing a state of energy conservation or 'hibernation' prior to ischaemic–anoxic insult forms one of the cornerstones of cellular protection–preservation strategy in organ transplantation.

Within a few seconds of the institution of ischaemia–anoxia (i.e. aortic cross-clamping), even after cooling, the tissue demand for oxygen exceeds the supply available, and thus intracellular ATP concentration and oxygen tension decrease rapidly. Simultaneous with the onset of ischaemia, energy metabolism switches directions, from mitochondrial oxidative metabolism to anaerobic glycolysis (see Figure 10.4). Cellular functions continue, even in the presence of reduced energy, resulting in the eventual depletion of high-energy phosphates.

The quantities of ATP generated by anaerobic glycolysis stored in the form of creatine phosphate become inadequate and ATP is broken down to hypoxanthine (HX), which accumulates in the cytosol (Figure 10.4).

Also, the lack of ATP and accumulation of lactic acid due to anaerobic metabolism leads to a decrease of cytosolic pH (acidosis) and to the release of calcium from intracellular stores, resulting in a marked increase in cytosolic calcium. This in turn activates proteases that, among other ATP-utilizing reactions, trigger the conversion of intracellular xanthine dehydrogenase (XD) to xanthine oxidase (XO), especially in endothelial tissue of the liver and intestines, which contain larger concentrations of XD. During ischaemia both XO and its substrate HX continue to accumulate in the intracellular compartment, which sets the stage for oxidative radical formation at reperfusion. After sustained and severe ischaemia, glycogen stores and antioxidants such as glutathione are also depleted.

In the heart, ATP depletion leads to loss of sarcolemmal membrane integrity with extracellular uptake of $Ca^{2+}$, loss of intracellular regulation of $Ca^{2+}$ with release of $Ca^{2+}$ ions from intracellular stores, and increased cytosolic $Ca^{2+}$ concentration. Mitochondrial buffering of excess cytosolic $Ca^{2+}$ leads to mitochondrial failure, opening of the mitochondrial transition pore, and subsequently impaired contractile function and delayed myofibrillar relaxation during diastole (Pilcher et al., 2012).

The ischaemic period is characterized by changes in transcriptional control of gene expression (transcriptional reprogramming). The lack of oxygen during ischaemia–anoxia causes impairment in the activity of oxygen-sensing prolyl hydroxylase (PHD) enzymes. This triggers the post-translational activation of hypoxia and inflammatory signalling cascades, which in turn control the transcription factors, HIF, and nuclear factor kappa-light-chain-enhancer of activated B cells (NF-κB), respectively (Eltzschig and Carmeliet, 2011).

### Stage 3: cold preservation

During this stage, injury risk is associated with several factors: global anoxia (absence of oxygen) and cooling, the rate of cooling, and the lowest graft temperature achieved during cold storage, as well as the duration of cold preservation. Because cooling is uncontrolled during cold storage preservation, the risk of differential cooling, with cell crystallization and 'thermal shock' of tissue, exists. In the liver, graft sinusoidal endothelial cell (EC) injury exposes the hepatocyte microvilli where polymorphs attach, releasing multiple mediators that accumulate later, thus amplifying the inflammatory process when released in the recipient. In all transplanted organs, platelets and leucocytes adhere to and 'plug' the microcirculation during absence of flow in cold storage

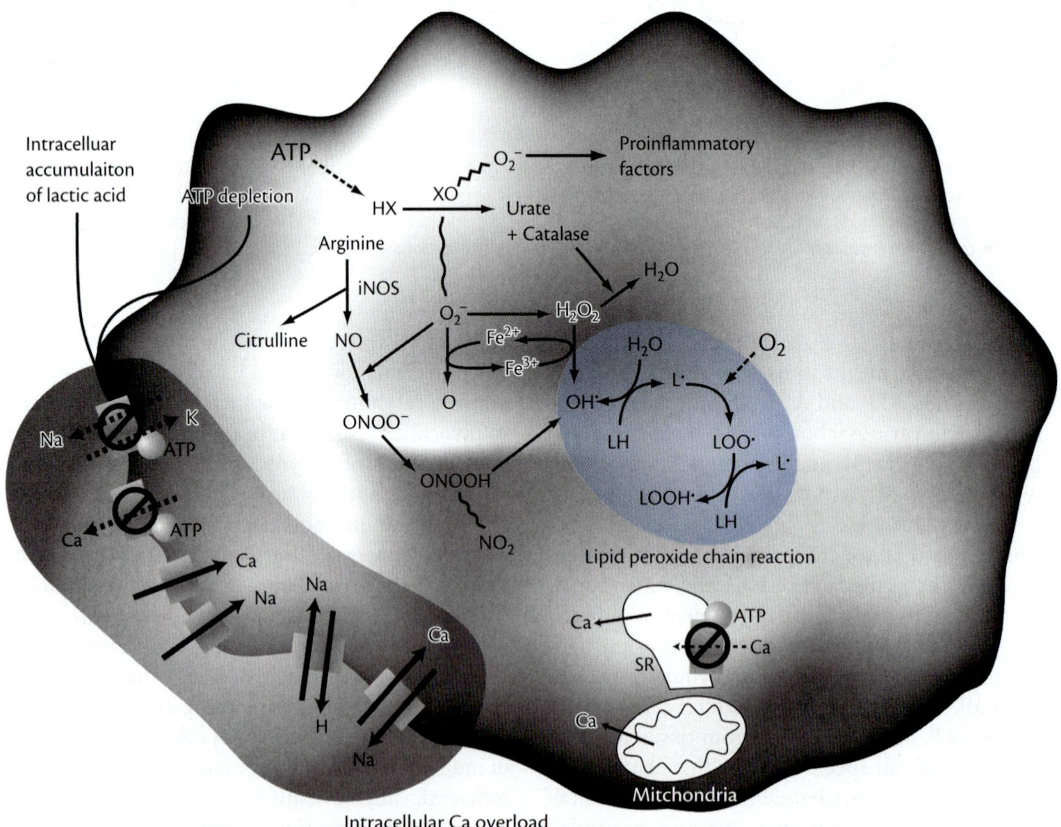


**Fig. 10.4** Generation of reactive oxygen species following ischaemia-anoxia. Severe depletion of ATP causes intracellular accumulation of its degenerative product, hypoxanthine (HX). ATP, Adenosine-5'-triphosphate; HX, hypoxanthine; NO, nitric oxide; XO, xanthine oxidase

preservation, and almost immediately upon reperfusion aggravate the degree of ischaemic injury by procoagulant and mechanical mechanisms, leading to the no-reflow phenomenon with areas of persistent ischaemia, despite restoration of blood flow.

### *Cold preservation injury*

Cooling, which, on the one hand, is beneficial to the organ by reducing oxygen demand and slowing down ATP utilization, may have detrimental effects on some cellular biological processes. For example, despite a continuing, albeit rapidly diminishing, supply of cellular ATP during preservation, at very low temperatures the cell is increasingly incapable of utilizing ATP. Therefore at temperatures commonly used for preservation there is essentially no $Na^+$-$K^+$-ATPase activity in most, if not all, cells. This inhibition of membronal ion pump mechanisms promotes cell swelling. Cell swelling, in turn, contributes to microvascular failure and worsening of the no-reflow phenomenon after reperfusion. Cold storage injury is further aggravated by a non-uniform rate of organ cooling, which is dependent on multiple external factors such as temperature inside the box, size of the graft organ, ambient temperature, and duration of transport.

Perfusion preservation affords better control over temperature and preserves the integrity of the microcirculation better than cold storage. Preservation injury occurs during cold storage and affects mainly non-parenchymal ECs (Caldwell-Kenkel et al., 1989). In contrast, warm ischaemia primarily affects parenchymal cells (Ikeda et al., 1992). Cold anoxia is associated with diffuse EC damage, which does not manifest itself until 30–60 minutes following reperfusion. The degree of EC damage correlates well with functional impairment of the graft following transplantation.

### *Stage 4: rewarming ischaemia–anoxia (implantation)*

Risk of warm ischaemic injury starts with the removal of the graft from cold storage or interruption of perfusion preservation and placement of the organ on the warm operative field. This damage is variable and depends on the duration of the implantation period and aforementioned environmental factors. Immediately prior to implantation, organs preserved in cold storage are 'rinsed' by gravity flow with crystalloid solution, albumin, or blood to flush out preservation solution and to clear clogged venous channels of cellular debris (leucocytes, platelets, etc.). However, because this process occurs by gravity and without sustaining an adequate perfusion pressure, it does not guarantee that the microcirculation is washed out completely. Depending on the duration of cold and warm ischaemia–anoxia, energy stores (glycogen, ATP) are further depleted. An antioxidant-containing solution for rinsing grafts called the Carolina rinse solution has been developed, with demonstrated clinical benefits over conventional rinse solutions (Gao et al., 1991; Currin et al., 1996; Bachmann et al., 1997; Yin et al., 2002).

## Phase III: post-ischaemia–anoxia

Attempts to modulate cell injury and death of the graft following extended periods of ischaemia–anoxia constitute organ 'postconditioning'. The combination of treatments for organ protection/preconditioning, coupled with perfusion preservation allowing better control over rate and duration of cooling, and the use of treatments intended to target reperfusion injury of the graft in the recipient may afford the best opportunity to ensure maximum viability of the organ. The sum total of these sequential interventions is what in this chapter we term 'organ resuscitation'. However, this research is still in its infancy, limited by the lack of multicentre prospective randomized clinical trials.

### Stage 5: reperfusion

The primary risk for cell injury during this stage is 'reperfusion injury', which is the sentinel event leading to graft injury and failure after preservation. Reperfusion of the graft in the recipient flushes out residual preservation solution and releases accumulated byproducts of anaerobic cellular metabolism but also triggers the production of oxygen-derived free radicals or reactive oxygen species (ROS), which in turn signals cellular production of pro-inflammatory mediators, further altering EC function, both within the graft and occasionally beyond (Figure 10.4).

### *Reperfusion injury*

Does cell injury cease with the re-establishment of blood flow at the time of revascularization of the graft in the recipient? In recent years experimental evidence has been accumulating to suggest that ischaemia constitutes but one component of organ damage and that reperfusion or the re-introduction of oxygen may be the primary component.

Reperfusion injury is two-fold, comprising the following:

(1) The no-reflow phenomenon or disseminated microvascular failure: defined as poorly reperfused and persistently ischaemic areas of the graft that can be identified by macroscopic inhomogeneity in the distribution of oxygenated blood leading to localized microscopic or macroscopic infarcts. As described above, this phenomenon is most likely due to organ oedema and plugging of the microcirculation (Yellon and Hausenloy, 2007). This process can be appreciated macroscopically in the solid organ graft by the mottled appearance of the graft surface immediately following reperfusion (i.e. unclamping). Persistent surface inhomogeneity (> 5 minutes) indicates worse no-reflow phenomenon. Furthermore, reperfusion is associated with increased vascular permeability, tissue inflammation, an imbalance between mediators of vasodilation and vasoconstriction, as well as an activation of coagulation and the complement system. Microvascular failure postgraft reperfusion can lead to dysfunction of distant organs such as the lung, leading to increased EC permeability, disruption of the alveolar-capillary membrane, and pulmonary oedema and hypoxaemia (Klausner et al., 1989).

(2) Reoxygenation injury: the magnitude of the release of ROS (primarily singlet oxygen and superoxide) and subsequently the enzymatic generation and release of peroxide and hydroxyl radicals may be a function of the duration of ischaemia that immediately precedes reperfusion (Zar et al., 1998). The release of ROS is attenuated by hypothermia (Zar et al., 1999). Since intracellular calcium binding is an active process, the lack of ATP leads to the release of calcium from storage sites, ending in cytosolic calcium overload, which in turn triggers the activation of proteases that catalyze the conversion of XD to XO, primarily in or on the EC surface. Subsequently, $Ca^{2+}$, XO, and its substrate HX accumulate in the cytosol during ischaemia–anoxia. The longer the duration of ischaemia–anoxia, the greater the accumulation of the aforementioned metabolic end products. Reperfusion of ischaemic

tissues of the brain-injured terminally ill patient or of the graft in the recipient results in ROS production from the conversion of accumulated HX to urate and $H_2O$ in the presence of $O_2$, which is catalyzed by the enzyme XO. Excess ROS production in turn triggers an inflammatory response. Glycogen stores and antioxidants such as glutathione, catalase, and superoxide dismutase scavenge excess ROS but are rapidly depleted. In the liver, Kupffer cells are primed for activation. Superoxide in the presence of free iron and copper and $H_2O_2$ react to trigger the formation of hydroxyl radical ($OH^-$) by the Fenton reaction. Subsequently, the ROS chain reaction with the excessive production of $HO^-$ may trigger breakdown of lipids to free fatty acids by lipid peroxidation. Iron catalyzes the lipid peroxidation chain reaction sustained by lipid alkyl and peroxyl radicals. Superoxide also reacts with nitric oxide ($NO^-$) to form peroxynitrite ($OONO^-$). $OONO^-$ causes nitrosylation of tyrosyl residues in proteins and also decomposes to hydroxyl radical-like species. Superoxide liberation activates the intracellular signalling mechanism, promoting the induction of NF-κB, which ultimately induces the expression of a host of pro-inflammatory mediators: complement factors, leucocyte adhesion molecules, cytokines, and growth factors.

It is theorized that the catalyst–substrate combination of XO-HX, when liberated into the interstitial space and bloodstream in the presence of oxygen, may constitute a continuing source of ROS generation, in turn signalling the activation, production, and diapedesis of neutrophils, and causing microvascular inflammatory damage in the liver and extrahepatic organs such as the heart (Parks and Granger, 1988).

Therefore we theorize that the release of XO-HX during reperfusion may contribute to SIRS and to adverse organ interaction or 'cross-talk' (i.e. hepatorenal syndrome). Other mechanisms of oxidative radical production involve the calcium-triggered activation of phospholipase A2 which causes breakdown of membrane lipid into its constituents following two primary pathways, lipo-oxygenase and cyclo-oxygenase metabolism of arachidonate. In addition, leucotriene activation of polymorphonuclear-neutrophil-stimulated nicotinamide adenine dinucleotide phosphate (NADPH) oxidase results in further ROS formation (Ernster, 1988; Hernandez and Granger, 1988; Parks and Granger, 1988; McCord and Omar, 1993; Nishino et al., 1997; Jaeschke, 2002; Braunersreuther and Jaquet, 2012).

Finally, these molecular pathways, if left unabated, will lead to cell death by one of two mechanisms: necrosis (cell dissolution) or apoptosis (induction of death genes), or a combination of both (necro-apoptosis). In addition, they contribute to increasing the immunogenicity of the graft in the early post-transplant period, which, in turn, results in worse clinical outcomes, with heightened incidence of rejection episodes that shorten graft survival. In this final phase during the transplant continuum, novel therapies must be developed to target suppression of the initial burst (spark) of ROS formation to interrupt signalling, therefore avoiding the induction of the cascade of biochemical events leading to cell injury and, subsequently, SIRS.

Ischaemia–reperfusion causes cell death via necrosis or activates the cascade of biochemical events that lead to programmed cell death, which is also known as apoptosis. On the other hand, 'autophagy' is a highly regulated, catabolic, intracellular phenomenon associated with synthesis, degradation, and recycling of cellular components through the lysosomal system to preserve cell survival in conditions of starvation or stress, and hence may be less relevant to ischaemic damage sustained during organ transplantation. The process through which necrosis or apoptosis result in death is determined by a phenomenon called the mitochondrial permeability transition (MPT). We will briefly review these processes.

*Necrosis* is a passive mechanism of cell death due to overwhelming injury, characterized by early cell and organelle swelling, ion deregulation, ATP depletion, and activation of degradative enzymes. These processes culminate in the rupture of the cell membrane and extrusion or release of intracellular proteins, metabolites, and ions—potent stimuli for immune response or inflammatory processes that characterize necrosis. Necrotic cells signal the immune system, leading to inflammatory cell infiltration and cytokine production (see Figure 10.5).

*Apoptosis* is a tightly regulated mechanism of programmed cell death, by which normal cells die during development or in the maintenance of cell number in tissues with rapid turnover. It is a systematic enzymatic (caspase-signalling) cascade or self-contained programme of cell death, with shrinkage of the cell and its nucleus. In contrast to necrosis, the integrity of the plasma membrane remains largely intact until later in the process of cell death. For this reason it is believed to be less immune-stimulatory. However, recent studies have detected ATP release via membronal channels (pannexin hemichannels) that can attract phagocytes. In fact, ATP appears to be involved in the inflammation process and innate immune responses in injured tissues, which may contribute to the amplification of adaptive immune responses associated with allograft rejection. Experimental models have demonstrated improved allograft survival and tolerance induction upon modulation of ATP binding with its purinergic receptors using ATP-agonists on T lymphocytes (Vergani et al., 2013a, 2013b). Pharmacological inhibition of apoptosis may have potential as an effective therapeutic strategy against ischaemia–reperfusion injury. Pilot clinical trials using pan-caspase inhibitors yielded promising results in improving hepatic cold ischaemia–reperfusion injury (Baskin-Bey et al., 2007).

Massive apoptosis only occurs pathologically and is divided into three stages. In the first phase, the 'initiation phase', there is initial activation of tightly regulated molecular machinery involving various proteases. In the second phase, the 'effector phase', the molecular machinery becomes fully activated, as shown by the ability of the cytosolic extracts of committed cells to induce apoptotic changes in the nuclei. Only after this phase do the hallmarks of apoptosis become evident. These include morphologic changes that include DNA fragmentation and the formation of apoptotic bodies. Both forms of cell death coexist (necro-apoptosis) in ischaemia–reperfusion–preservation injury, and there is now evidence that halting the activation and the effector phases of apoptosis is associated with increased survival after reperfusion (see Figure 10.6).

*Autophagy* ('self eating') is defined as a process of cell degradation through the lysosomal machinery, involving the sequestration of cytoplasmic components into double-membrane autophagosomes that fuse with lysosomes, where their content undergoes degradation and recycling. This process is regulated by a series of autophagy proteins. Normally, autophagy is a survival

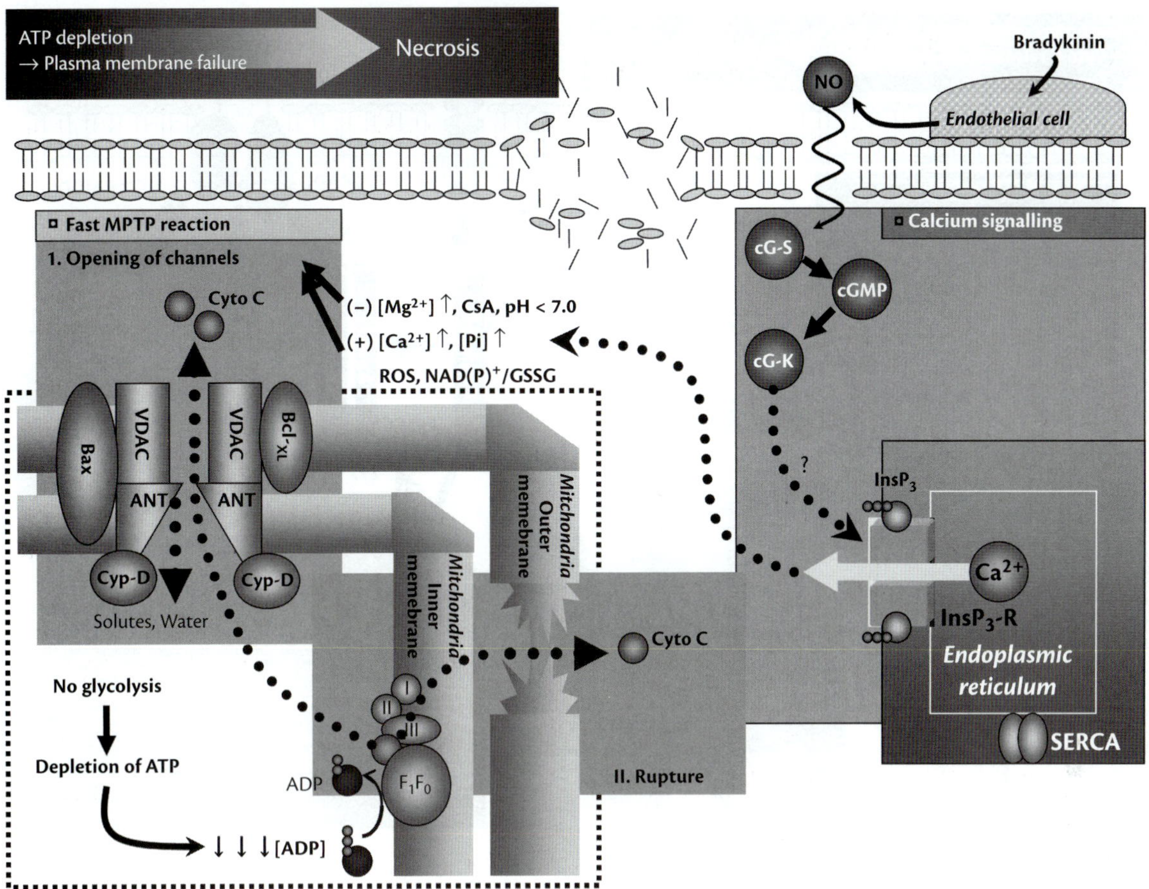


**Fig. 10.5** Pathways of cell necrosis. Bradykinin stimulates release of NO from endothelial cells. Diffusion of NO into hepatocytes stimulates c-GMP generation and subsequent cGMP-dependent pathway toward $InsP_3$ receptor activation. A rapid rise in intracellular pH during reperfusion, along with translocation of Bax to the mitochondrial surface, increased calcium, and generation of ROS open a very conductive permeability transition pore (MPTP), which is composed of cyclosphilin D, adenosine nucleotide translocator (ANT), and voltage-dependent anion channels (VDAC). Mitochondrial membrane become very permeable to solute, leading to mitochondrial swelling and uncoupling of oxidative phosphorylation. Subsequently $F_1F_0$ adenosine triphosphatase (ATPase), which hydrolyse ATP to ADP, are activated, leading to ATP depletion. ATP depletion causes plasma membrane bleb formation and cell volume expansion, which is the hallmark of cell lysis. ADP, Adenosine diphosphate; ANT, adenine nucleotide translocator; ATP, adenosine-5′-triphosphate; Bax, Bcl-2–associated X protein; Bcl-XL, B-cell lymphoma extra large; s-GC, soluble guanylate cyclase; cGK, cGMP protein kinase; cGMP, cyclic guanosine monophosphate; CsA, cyclosporine A; Cyp-D, cyclophilin D; Cyto c, cytochrome-c; $F_1F_0$, F-type ATPase ($F_0$ and $F_1$ domain); GSSG, glutathione disulphide; $InsP_3$-R, inositol trisphosphate receptor; NAD(P), nicotinamide adenine dinucleotide (phosphate); NO, nitric oxide; ROS, reactive oxygen species; SERCA, sarco-/endoplasmic reticulum $Ca^{2+}$-ATPase; VDAC, voltage-dependent anion channels

mechanism under stress conditions by clearing cellular debris and contributing to cell homeostasis (Mizumura et al., 2012; Ryter and Choi, 2012; Choi et al., 2013).

## The mitochondrial permeability transition in cell injury and death

The MPT is defined as an increase in the permeability of inner and outer mitochondrial membranes or pores to molecules of less than 1,500 Daltons. It results from the opening of a mitochondrial permeability transition pore (MPTP). The MPTP is a protein pore in the inner membrane of the mitochondria resulting from ischaemic–anoxic and ischaemic–reperfusion conditions, evident during oxygen deprivation of ex-vivo cells, tissues, and organs. Increased mitochondrial permeability leads to mitochondrial swelling and cell death via either necrosis or apoptosis.

Various factors trigger MPTP opening. High levels of $Ca^{2+}$ within mitochondria can cause the MPT pore to open. This is possibly because $Ca^{2+}$ binds to and activates $Ca^{2+}$ binding sites on the matrix side of the MPTP. MPT induction is also due to the changes in the transmembrane potential. The presence of ROS during reperfusion injury is another result of excessive cytosolic $Ca^{2+}$ and can also cause opening of the MPT pore. Other factors include the presence of certain fatty acids, inorganic phosphate, and rapid correction of low intracellular pH. However, these factors cannot open the pore without $Ca^{2+}$, though at high enough concentrations $Ca^{2+}$ alone can induce MPT. Stress in the endoplasmic reticulum can be a factor in triggering MPT.

Conditions that cause the pore to close or remain closed include acidic conditions (low pH) and high concentrations of ADP, ATP, and NADH. $Mg^{2+}$ can also inhibit MPT, because it can compete with $Ca^{2+}$ for the $Ca^{2+}$ binding sites on the matrix and/or cytoplasmic side of the MPTP.

The induction of MPT, which increases mitochondrial membrane permeability, causes mitochondria to become further

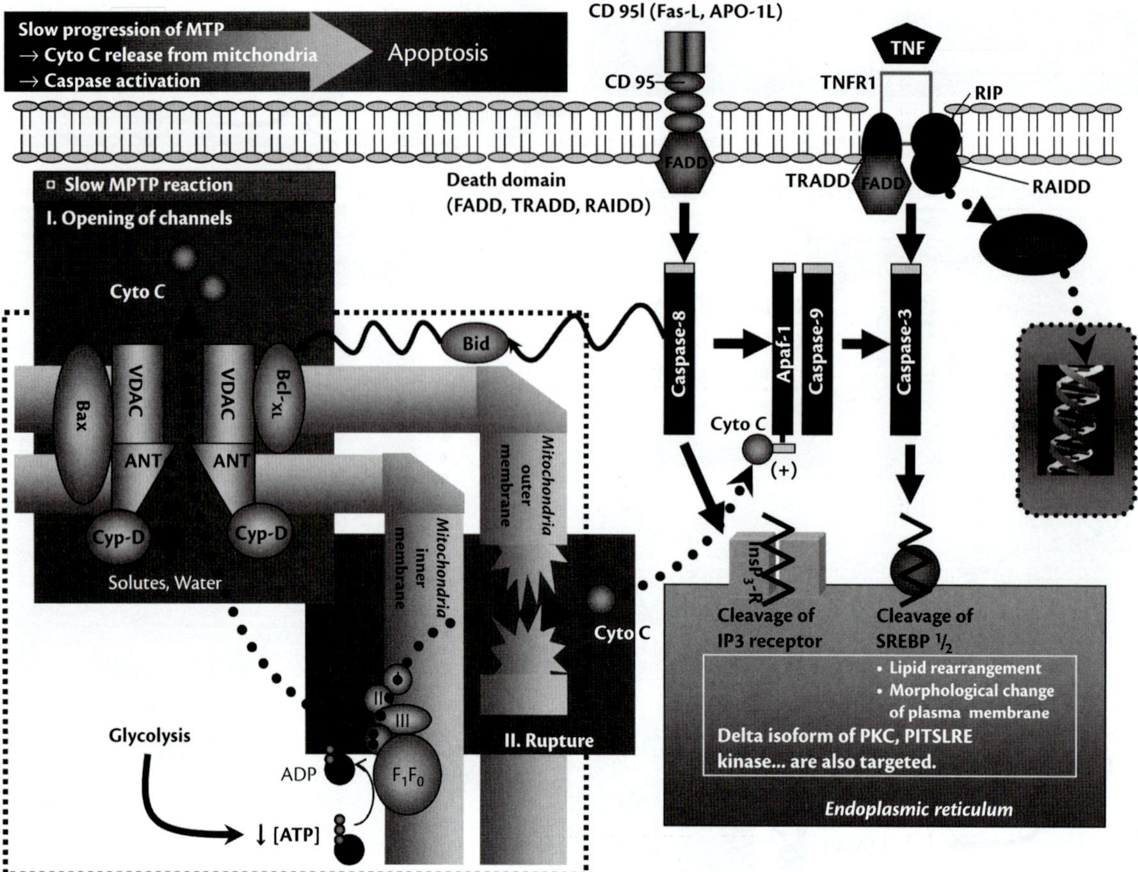


**Fig. 10.6** Pathways of cell apoptosis: binding of Fas ligand/Fas receptor and TNF-α/TNF-α receptor initiate the apoptosis process. The apoptosis process includes: (1) sterol regulatory element binding proteins (SREBP)-1/2 are cleaved by caspase 3, (2) the delta isoform of protein kinase C is targeted by caspases during TNF-α or CD-95-mediated apoptosis; and (3) PISTLRE kinase is targeted by caspases in CD-95-mediated apoptosis. ADP, Adenosine diphosphate; ANT, adenine nucleotide translocator; Apaf-1, apoptotic protease activating factor 1; APO-1L, apoptosis antigen-1 ligand; ATP, adenosine-5'-triphosphate; Bax, Bcl-2-associated X protein; Bcl-XL, B-cell lymphoma extra large; Bid, BH3-interacting domain death agonist; CD95, cluster of differentiation 95; Cyp-D, cyclophilin D; Cyto c, cytochrome-c; FADD, Fas-associated protein with death domain; Fas-L, Fas ligand; $F_1F_0$, F-type ATPase ($F_0$ and $F_1$ domain); $InsP_3$-R, inositol trisphosphate receptor; PITSLRE, serine/threonine-protein kinase; PKC, protein kinase C; SREBP, sterol regulatory element-binding proteins; TNF, tumour necrosis factor; TNFR1, tumour necrosis factor-1 receptor; TRADD, tumour necrosis factor receptor type 1-associated death domain protein; RAIDD, RIP-associated Ich-1/CED homologous protein with death domain; RIP, receptor-interacting protein; VDAC, voltage-dependent anion channels

depolarized, meaning that the membrane potential is abolished. When this is lost, hydrogen ions and some molecules are able to flow across the outer mitochondrial membrane uninhibited. Loss of membrane potential interferes with the production of ATP, the cell's main source of energy, because mitochondria must have an electrochemical gradient to provide the driving force for ATP production. MPT also allows $Ca^{2+}$ to leave the mitochondrion, which can place further stress on nearby mitochondria, which in turn can activate harmful calcium-dependent proteases.

ROS are also produced as a result of MPT pore opening. MPT can allow glutathione, an antioxidant, to exit mitochondria, reducing the organelles' ability to neutralize free radicals. In addition, the electron transport chain may produce more free radicals due to loss of its components, such as cytochrome c, through the MPTP, with escape of electrons from the chain, which can then reduce molecules and form free radicals. Much research has found that the fate of the cell after an insult depends on the extent of MPT.

In summary, if MPT occurs to only a slight extent, the cell may recover, whereas if it occurs more, it may undergo apoptosis. If it occurs to an even larger degree, the cell is likely to undergo necrosis.

## The concept of 'organ resuscitation'

Previous research on organ preservation has focused primarily on the development of solutions to 'cool' and 'pickle' organs during storage and transportation (cold storage). The aims of cold storage are to reduce cellular metabolism by cooling, reduce cellular oedema with the use of large non-permeable molecules, maintain intracellular electrolyte milieu with a high extracellular osmolar environment to prevent intracellular loss of electrolytes, and replenish antioxidants such as glutathione, purportedly consumed during preservation due to oxidative stress. However, organ resuscitation envisions a paradigm shift towards the development of pharmacological regimens to induce protection or preconditioning in the donor, enhanced preservation by substituting cold storage

**Table 10.2** The transplant continuum viewed from the perspective of organ resuscitation

| Phases | Interventions |
|---|---|
| Phase I | Preconditioning (cytoprotection) |
| Phase II | Preservation (hypothermic and normothermic perfusion preservation) |
| Phase III | Postconditioning (prevention of reperfusion injury of the graft) |

with perfusion preservation with nutrients, anti-apoptotic agents and antioxidants, and instituting postconditioning regimens in the recipient (see Table 10.2).

## Donor preconditioning

Ischaemic preconditioning refers to inflow occlusion of the vascular supply of an organ to generate transient (minutes) warm ischaemia followed by reperfusion. Another form is 'remote' ischaemic preconditioning, whereby transient warm ischaemia–reperfusion of other body parts (i.e. limbs) is induced, followed by reperfusion. The putative mechanisms by which ischaemic preconditioning confers protection to organs seem to rely on the induction of natural intracellular response to ischaemia (i.e. via the upregulation of HIF-1α, cytoprotective molecules such as heat shock proteins, anti-apoptotic genes, and reduction of oxygen-derived free radicals, amongst other molecular mechanisms), which renders the tissues more resilient to subsequent ischaemic insult (Adam et al., 1998; Clavien et al., 2000; Franchello et al., 2009; Beck-Schimmer et al., 2012; Chouker et al., 2012; Della-Morte et al., 2012; Hogan et al., 2012; Pilcher et al., 2012; Albrecht et al., 2013).

## Pharmacological preconditioning

The use of pharmacological means of preconditioning organs while still in the body of the donor is appealing and may help to maximize organ utilization and clinical outcomes after transplantation. Experimental studies have shown the salutary effects on organ function of selectively targeting signal transduction pathways involved in tissue damage upon hypoxia, such as inhibitors of c-Jun N-terminal kinases (JNKs) (Uehara et al., 2004; Noguchi et al., 2009; Kanellis et al., 2010) and mitogen-activated protein kinase (MAPK) p38 (Yoshinari et al., 2001; Hashimoto et al., 2002; Koike et al., 2004; Ito et al., 2008; Oto et al., 2009) (see Figure 10.7). There is evidence that inhalational agents (isoflurane and sevoflurane) can also induce pre- and postconditioning in the donor when administered prior to recovery of organs (see Chapter 9).

## Perfusion preservation

Recent research in kidney preservation has shown that perfusion preservation is superior to cold storage preservation. This has triggered a shift in research and development away from cold storage methods and towards the development of novel artificial circulatory devices for continuous organ perfusion preservation. This

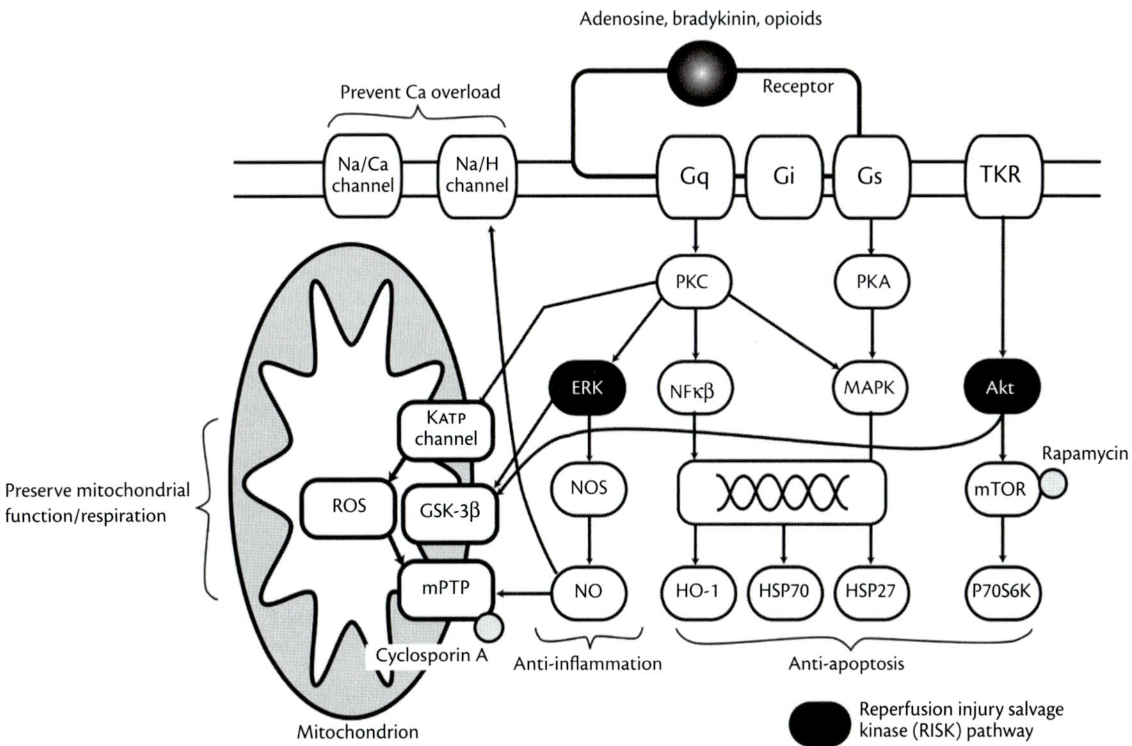


**Fig. 10.7** Molecular targets for organ resuscitation. ERK, Extracellular signal-regulated kinases; Gs, Gi, Gq (G protein subunits: Gs, stimulatory; Gi, inhibitory; Gq, regulate phospholipase C (PLC) pathway); GSK-3β, glycogen synthase kinase 3; HO-1, haemeoxygenase 1; HSP, heat shock protein; mTOP, mammalian target of rapamycin; MAPK, mitogen-activated protein kinases; mPTP, mitochondrial permeability transition pore; NF-κB, nuclear factor kappa-light-chain-enhancer of activated B cells; NO, nitric oxide; NOS, nitric oxide synthases; PKA, protein kinase A; PKC, protein kinase C; p70S6K, p70S6 kinases; ROS, reactive oxygen species; TKR, tyrosine kinase receptor

modality has many advantages and facilitates ex-vivo assessment of organ function as well as the prevention of microvascular perfusion failure (Van Raemdonck et al., 2013). Perfusion preservation of kidneys has been shown to prevent clinically significant deterioration in organ function, especially of the organ that is recovered from a donor of marginal quality or ECD.

### Recipient postconditioning (modulation of cell death)

Recipient postconditioning is an attempt to modulate cell death and entails the interruption of molecular pathways that lead to irreversible cell damage and ultimately graft dysfunction or primary non-function in the recipient. In order to further explore and develop potential postconditioning therapeutic strategies it is important to understand the key molecular pathways and when they are activated during the transplant continuum.

## Conclusion

In summary, in order to ensure maximum organ viability in the recipient it will be necessary in the future to explore in multicentre randomized prospective clinical trials promising interventions that inhibit reoxygenation injury, necrosis, apoptosis and the inflammatory process that results from ischaemia–reperfusion injury. In particular, therapeutic trials must focus on the prevention of post-ischaemic calcium overload, maintenance of mitochondrial integrity through the prevention of the MPT, and anti-inflammatory regimens. The new paradigm will most likely result in a multifactorial approach by simultaneously targeting key molecular pathways, including genomic and proteomic mechanisms that may favourably modulate or prevent cell injury and death. This approach must aim to enhance cell viability via inhibition of various injury pathways (i.e. antinecrosis, anti-apoptosis, and antinecro-apoptosis treatments). In order to achieve the number of cases needed for statistical power in prospective trials in organ transplantation it will be necessary to develop research partnerships across various institutions and across organ systems and for both donor and recipient research. Moreover, since these cellular mechanisms are common to most if not all organ systems, it would not be unscientific to include all patients undergoing solid or thoracic organ transplantation in clinical trials of promising therapies. We await the creation of national and international research consortia dedicated to organ transplant research. Anaesthesiologists are well suited to engage in these endeavours at all levels and may be facilitated through non-profit institutions, such as the Society for the Advancement of Transplant Anesthesia (<http://www.transplantanesthesia.org>).

## References


Adam R, Arnault I, Bao YM, Salvucci M, Sebagh M, Bismuth H (1998) Effect of ischemic preconditioning on hepatic tolerance to cold ischemia in the rat. *Transpl Int*, **11**(Suppl 1):S168–170.

Albrecht M, Zitta K, Bein B, et al.(2013) Remote ischemic preconditioning regulates HIF-1 alpha levels, apoptosis and inflammation in heart tissue of cardiosurgical patients: a pilot experimental study. *Basic Res Cardiol*, **108**(1):314.

Bachmann S, Bechstein WO, Keck H, et al. (1997) Pilot study: Carolina rinse solution improves graft function after orthotopic liver transplantation in humans. *Transplant Proc*, **29**(1–2):390–392.

Baskin-Bey ES, Washburn K, Feng S, et al. (2007) Clinical trial of the pan-caspase inhibitor, IDN-6556, in human liver preservation injury. *Am J Transplant*, **7**(1):218–225.

Beck-Schimmer B, Breitenstein S, Bonvini JM, et al. (2012) Protection of pharmacological postconditioning in liver surgery: results of a prospective randomized controlled trial. *Ann Surg*, **256**(5):837–844; discussion 844–845.

Boutilier RG (2001) Mechanisms of cell survival in hypoxia and hypothermia. *J Exp Biol*, **204**(Pt 18):3171–3181.

Braunersreuther V, Jaquet V (2012) Reactive oxygen species in myocardial reperfusion injury: from physiopathology to therapeutic approaches. *Curr Pharm Biotechnol*, **13**(1):97–114.

Caldwell-Kenkel JC, Currin RT, Tanaka Y, Thurman RG, Lemasters JJ (1989) Reperfusion injury to endothelial cells following cold ischemic storage of rat livers. *Hepatology*, **10**(3):292–299.

Chinopoulos C (2013) Which way does the citric acid cycle turn during hypoxia? The critical role of alpha-ketoglutarate dehydrogenase complex. *J Neurosci Res*, **91**(8):1030–1043.

Choi AM, Ryter SW, Levine B (2013) Autophagy in human health and disease. *N Engl J Med*, **368**(7):651–662.

Chouker A, Ohta A, Martignoni A, Lukashev D, Zacharia LC, Jackson EK, Schnermann J, Ward JM, et al. (2012) In vivo hypoxic preconditioning protects from warm liver ischemia-reperfusion injury through the adenosine A2B receptor. *Transplantation*, **94**(9):894–902.

Clavien PA, Yadav S, Sindram D, Bentley RC (2000) Protective effects of ischemic preconditioning for liver resection performed under inflow occlusion in humans. *Ann Surg*, **232**(2):155–162.

Currin RT, Caldwell-Kenkel JC, Lichtman SN, et al. (1996) Protection by Carolina rinse solution, acidotic pH, and glycine against lethal reperfusion injury to sinusoidal endothelial cells of rat livers stored for transplantation. *Transplantation*, **62**(11):1549–1558.

Della-Morte D, Guadagni F, Palmirotta R, et al. (2012) Genetics and genomics of ischemic tolerance: focus on cardiac and cerebral ischemic preconditioning. *Pharmacogenomics*, **13**(15):1741–1757.

Eltzschig HK, Carmeliet P (2011) Hypoxia and inflammation. *N Engl J Med*, **364**(7):656–665.

Endo A, Yagi T, Nakao A, et al. (2000) Cytokine-mediated, deteriorative effects of brain death on porcine liver transplantation: intervention of sympathoadrenal pathway in cerebrohepatic organ interaction. *Transplant Proc*, **32**(7):1637–1642.

Ernster L (1988) Biochemistry of reoxygenation injury. *Crit Care Med*, **16**(10):947–953.

Franchello A, Gilbo N, David E, et al. (2009) Ischemic preconditioning (IP) of the liver as a safe and protective technique against ischemia/reperfusion injury (IRI). *Am J Transplant*, **9**(7):1629–1639.

Gao WS, Takei Y, Marzi I, et al. (1991) Carolina rinse solution—a new strategy to increase survival time after orthotopic liver transplantation in the rat. *Transplantation*, **52**(3):417–424.

Hashimoto N, Takeyoshi I, Yoshinari D, et al. (2002) Effects of a p38 mitogen-activated protein kinase inhibitor as an additive to Euro-Collins solution on reperfusion injury in canine lung transplantation. *Transplantation*, **74**(3):320–326.

Hernandez LA, Granger N (1988) Role of antioxidants in organ preservation and transplantation. *Crit Care Med*, **16**(5):543–549.

Hoeger S, Petrov K, Reisenbuechler A, et al. (2009) The additional detrimental effects of cold preservation on transplantation-associated injury in kidneys from living and brain-dead donor rats. *Transplantation*, **87**(1):52–58.

Hogan AR, Doni M, Molano RD, et al. (2012) Beneficial effects of ischemic preconditioning on pancreas cold preservation. *Cell Transplant*, **21**(7):1349–1360.

Ikeda T, Yanaga K, Kishikawa K, Kakizoe S, Shimada M, Sugimachi K (1992) Ischemic injury in liver transplantation: difference in injury sites between warm and cold ischemia in rats. *Hepatology*, **16**(2):454–461.

Ilmakunnas M, Hockerstedt K, Makisalo H, Siitonen S, Repo H, Pesonen EJ (2010) Hepatic IL-8 release during graft procurement is associated with impaired graft function after human liver transplantation. *Clin Transplant*, **24**(1):29–35.

Ito T, Omori K, Rawson J, et al. (2008) Improvement of canine islet yield by donor pancreas infusion with a p38MAPK inhibitor. *Transplantation*, **86**(2):321–329.

Jaeschke H (2002) Xanthine oxidase-induced oxidant stress during hepatic ischemia-reperfusion: are we coming full circle after 20 years? *Hepatology*, **36**(3):761–763.

Kanellis J, Ma FY, Kandane-Rathnayake R, et al. (2010) JNK signalling in human and experimental renal ischaemia/reperfusion injury. *Nephrol Dial Transplant*, **25**(9):2898–2908.

Klausner JM, Paterson IS, Mannick JA, Valeri R, Shepro D, Hechtman HB (1989) Reperfusion pulmonary edema. *JAMA*, **261**(7):1030–1035.

Koike N, Takeyoshi I, Ohki S, Tokumine M, Matsumoto K, Morishita Y (2004) Effects of adding P38 mitogen-activated protein-kinase inhibitor to celsior solution in canine heart transplantation from non-heart-beating donors. *Transplantation*, **77**(2):286–292.

McCord JM, Omar BA (1993) Sources of free radicals. *Toxicol Ind Health*, **9**(1–2):23–37.

Mizumura K, Cloonan SM, Haspel JA, Choi AM (2012) The emerging importance of autophagy in pulmonary diseases. *Chest*, **142**(5):1289–1299.

Nishino T, Nakanishi S, Okamoto K, et al. (1997) Conversion of xanthine dehydrogenase into oxidase and its role in reperfusion injury. *Biochem Soc Trans*, **25**(3):783–786.

Noguchi H, Matsumoto S, Onaca N, et al. (2009) Ductal injection of JNK inhibitors before pancreas preservation prevents islet apoptosis and improves islet graft function. *Hum Gene Ther*, **20**(1):73–85.

Ogliari AC, Caldara R, Socci C, et al. (2008) High levels of donor CCL2/MCP-1 predict graft-related complications and poor graft survival after kidney-pancreas transplantation. *Am J Transplant*, **8**(6):1303–1311.

Oto T, Calderone A, Li L, Rosenfeldt FL, Pepe S (2009) p38 Mitogen-activated protein kinase inhibition reduces inflammatory cytokines in a brain-dead transplant donor animal model. *Heart Lung Circ*, **18**(6):393–400.

Parks DA, Granger DN (1988) Ischemia-reperfusion injury: a radical view. *Hepatology*, **8**(3):680–682.

Pilcher JM, Young P, Weatherall M, Rahman I, Bonser RS, Beasley RW (2012) A systematic review and meta-analysis of the cardioprotective effects of remote ischaemic preconditioning in open cardiac surgery. *J R Soc Med*, **105**(10):436–445.

Ryter SW, Choi AM (2012) Regulation of autophagy in oxygen-dependent cellular stress. *Curr Pharm Des*, **19**(15):2747–2756.

Slade JM, Towse TF, Delano MC, Wiseman RW, Meyer RA (2006) A gated 31P NMR method for the estimation of phosphocreatine recovery time and contractile ATP cost in human muscle. *NMR Biomed*, **19**(5):573–580.

Takada M., Nadeau KC, Hancock WW, et al. (1998) Effects of explosive brain death on cytokine activation of peripheral organs in the rat. *Transplantation*, **65**(12):1533–1542.

Uehara T, Xi Peng X, Bennett B, et al. (2004) c-Jun N-terminal kinase mediates hepatic injury after rat liver transplantation. *Transplantation*, **78**(3):324–332.

Van Raemdonck D, Neyrinck A, Rega F, Devos T, Pirenne J (2013) Machine perfusion in organ transplantation: a tool for ex-vivo graft conditioning with mesenchymal stem cells? *Curr Opin Organ Transplant*, **18**(1):24–33.

Vergani A, Fotino C, D'Addio F, et al. (2013a) Effect of the purinergic inhibitor oxidized-ATP in a model of islet allograft rejection. *Diabetes*, **62**(5):1665–1675.

Vergani A, Tezza S, D'Addio F, et al. (2013b) Long-term heart transplant survival by targeting the ionotropic purinergic receptor P2X7. *Circulation*, **127**(4):463–475.

Weiss S, Kotsch K, Francuski M, et al. (2007) Brain death activates donor organs and is associated with a worse I/R injury after liver transplantation. *Am J Transplant*, **7**(6):1584–1593.

Yellon DM, Hausenloy DJ (2007) Myocardial reperfusion injury. *N Engl J Med*, **357**(11):1121–1135.

Yin M, Currin RT, Peng XX, Mekeel HE, Schoonhoven R, Lemasters JJ (2002) Carolina rinse solution minimizes kidney injury and improves graft function and survival after prolonged cold ischemia. *Transplantation*, **73**(9):1410–1420.

Yoshinari D, Takeyoshi I, Kobayashi M, et al. (2001) Effects of a p38 mitogen-activated protein kinase inhibitor as an additive to University of Wisconsin solution on reperfusion injury in liver transplantation. *Transplantation*, **72**(1):22–27.

Zar HA, Tanigawa K, Kim YM, Lancaster JR Jr (1998) Rat liver postischemic lipid peroxidation and vasoconstriction depend on ischemia time. *Free Radic Biol Med*, **25**(3):255–264.

Zar HA, Tanigawa K, Kim YM, Lancaster JR Jr (1999) Mild therapeutic hypothermia for postischemic vasoconstriction in the perfused rat liver. *Anesthesiology*, **90**(4):1103–1111.

## CHAPTER 11

# Transplant immunology

Phillip Ruiz, Junichiro Sageshima, George Burke, Linda Chen, and Gaetano Ciancio

## The immunobiology of tissue rejection

The introduction of a solid organ allograft into a recipient presents a potential scenario whereby the host immune system can initiate and promulgate a vigorous and sustained response towards the graft that can culminate in decreased function and ultimately the demise of the transplant. This phenomenon was delineated by the studies of Billingham et al. (1953) who were among the first to recognize in animals that allogeneic skin grafts, but not autologous grafts, were rejected and that the failure of organ transplantation was secondary to immunological reactions. As a result of animal experimentations, several tenets of organ transplantation became apparent, including that (1) solid organ grafts may be recognized as antigenic and the graft may also be a source of immune cells, (2) this immune response between recipient and donor obliges a need for immunosuppression for the survival of the graft and the host, and (3) the definitive objective should be the induction and maintenance of immunological tolerance.

Based on these studies and others, a concept evolved that the grafts genetically bore an inherent level of immunogenicity when presented to hosts within the same species (i.e. alloimmunity). George Snell and Peter A. Gorer, via their development of inbred mice, observed that normal and tumour grafts were accepted between certain inbred animals but not between animals of different strains. They termed the principal gene locus responsible for the graft rejection histocompatibility 2 (H-2) (Snell, 1957). Additional investigation revealed the locus to be genetically complex, and the concept of the major histocompatibility complex (MHC) was born, providing the foundation for transplantation immunology and immunogenetics (Gorer and Boyse, 1959). In humans the MHC was outlined based on the discovery of agglutinating antibodies between different persons that had been transfused; the antigens that were being recognized were termed HLA and were found to be analogous with H-2 in the mouse (Dausset et al., 1965). Ultimately it was discovered that MHC gene region (a 4-megabase (Mb) region on chromosome 6) products are vital in the regulation of immune responses since they present peptide antigens to T-cell receptors in a restricted fashion only with identical and corresponding molecules (Doherty and Zinkernagel, 1975). Aside from their antigen-presenting capability, the MHC molecules themselves are among the most antigenic molecules when presented into another host (i.e. transplantation) and serve as allograft antigens. As such, identification of MHC molecules became the most significant gauge of biological incompatibility when considering potential recipient and donor combinations. These genes play a crucial role in host immune responses and possible susceptibility to several autoimmune diseases.

This degree of genetic disparity between recipient and donor at the MHC is one of the principal factors that influence the robustness of an immunologically based antidonor response. The MHC of humans encodes two major classes of proteins that are extremely polymorphic: HLA class I (HLA-A, HLA-B, and HLA-C) and HLA class II (HLA-DP, HLA-DQ, and HLA-DR) (Marsh et al., 2005; Marsh, 2012). The distribution of class I molecules is on the plasma membranes of practically all nucleated cells, whereas class II molecules are expressed chiefly by B lymphocytes, macrophages, and dendritic cells. However, the expression of class I and II molecules varies in density between cells and it is not static, since molecules such as interferon-gamma (IFN-$^{3}$) can upregulate their expression. Since the basic function of class I and II molecules is antigen presentation (Hennecke and Wiley, 2001), this variation in their expression greatly influences levels of local and systemic immune responses.

The intraspecies polymorphism of the MHC enables the group to have a superior shared immunity against continuously mutating pathogens. However, as mentioned before, this polymorphism serves as a formidable antigenic barrier when tissues are transplanted among genetically dissimilar members of that species and the MHC molecules themselves effectively induce an alloimmune response.

In addition to MHC glycoproteins, other immunogenic families of molecules operate as 'transplantation' antigens. So-called minor histocompatibility antigens (mHags) were discovered when HLA-identical transplants showed rejection, in some cases directed to Y chromosome encoded molecules (Goulmy, 1996 , 2006). The mHags are presented as peptides on the cell surface primarily by MHC class I and occasionally by class II molecules (Robertson et al., 2007). Other molecules including MICA/MICB (Boukouaci et al., 2009) and KIR (Kwakkel-van Erp et al., 2008) not only serve as immunogenic molecules but also provide indicators to the function of certain cells of the immune response and their participation in processes such as graft versus host disease (GVHD). Finally, there are another group of antigens expressed on allografts that are restricted to various tissues and are termed tissue-specific antigens. These molecules are also relatively polymorphic but not well understood at this point. Cellular and humoral immune responses can be generated to these antigens and clearly they serve as a potential source of graft dysfunction when immunologically targeted (Mathew et al., 1991; Joyce et al., 1992).

The proliferation and maturation of the effector cells and molecules as part of the adaptive immunity directed to the graft represents the injurious phase of the antigraft response and this is what is targeted by immunosuppressive therapy. Although there are several forms and means by which allografts are injured aside from the adaptive immune response, including ischaemia, innate immune activation, protracted non-specific inflammation with secretion of soluble factors, infections, and recurrent/de-novo immune diseases, we will focus on the adaptive alloimmune response in this chapter.

## Host versus graft response

The antigenic variances between the donor and recipient result in a variety of immune cellular and humoral networks that become activated and participate in alloreactive effector responses as well as regulatory responses. If the immune effector response predominates and is not pharmacologically inhibited, this is clinically manifested as host versus graft (HVG) or as graft versus host (GVH) responses. Sustained responses of this type result in the loss of the graft or GVHD and can culminate in the death of the patient. Regulatory cell-rich responses may by comparison lead to graft acceptance and true immunological tolerance. The donor-derived cellular and humoral immune responses to transplantation antigens are often classified in several forms of graft rejection, including hyperacute, acute, subacute, and chronic (Suthanthiran and Strom, 1994). Hyperacute responses occur within minutes, are antibody-mediated, and tend to be irreversible. Acute and subacute responses largely are cell-mediated and/or antibody-mediated, ensue in a span of days to months, and can be tempered with a variety of immunosuppressive reagents. Chronic rejection (CR) occurs in the span of months to years, is archetypally not responsive to current therapy, and has emerged as the foremost problem facing transplant survival.

The presentation of donor alloantigens to the recipient immune system can be via either the direct or indirect antigen presentation pathways. In the direct pathway, complete donor class I and II MHC or other transplantation antigen molecules on donor APC are directly recognized by recipient CD8+ and CD4+ T-cells, respectively, whereas in the indirect pathway, donor allopeptides are processed and presented in the context of MHC molecules on self or recipient APC to self CD8+ and CD4+ T-cells (Krensky, 1997; Jiang et al., 2004). The proportion of the T-cell repertoire responding in the direct pathway tends to be high, while a lower frequency of alloreactive T-cells is seen with the indirect pathway. Direct allorecognition is the predominant response for early rejection episodes, while indirect allorecognition is the prevalent response in late rejection events.

Acute rejection (AR) of allografts may be primarily antibody-driven, cell-mediated, or a combination of both processes. Acute antibody-mediated rejection (AAMR) occurs in response to any antigens but chiefly to ones expressed on endothelium of allografts (Akalin and Watschinger, 2007; Truong et al., 2007). AAMR may occur due to preformed anti-HLA antibody regularly present in persons sensitized by preceding antigen exposure, which can be due to prior transplantation, pregnancy, or transfusions. In addition, natural antibodies to the ABO blood group antigens can participate in AAMR.

Antibodies directed against HLA molecules tend to be IgG class, while anti-ABO antibodies are of IgM class; however, anti-HLA antibodies can be found in all classes of immunoglobulins. The early acute phase of AAMR is associated with deposition of these antibodies along the endothelium (Baldwin et al., 1999; Shimizu and Colvin, 2005), initiation of the complement cascade, and thereafter a series of events that injure the vessel, with possible thrombus formation and ischaemic injury due to vascular occlusion. Complement split products, such as C3d and C4d, are often present and their detection has allowed them to often be reliable tissue markers of AAMR. For example, immunostaining of kidney graft peritubular capillaries for C4d in biopsy specimens has been a useful marker for AAMR (Feucht et al., 1991, 1993). However, C4d immunostaining may also appear and disappear within days on serial biopsies and may be variable over time (Banasik et al., 2007). Interestingly, positive immunostaining for C4d correlates with poor graft survival (Truong et al., 2007), and this marker has been incorporated into grading criteria for kidney and cardiac allograft rejection as one of the defining features of AAMR (Akalin and Watschinger, 2007; Nickeleit and Andreoni, 2007; Solez et al., 2007).

T-cell-mediated AR, also known as cell-mediated acute rejection (CM-AR), originates from T-cells recognizing direct alloantigens or alloantigens indirectly presented (described above) and is characterized by infiltration of cells into interstitial areas of organ grafts. The activated and proliferating T-cells directly and indirectly injure the tissue via numerous interactions propagated through adhesion and ligand molecules as well as homing receptors (e.g. CD40/CD40L, CD103) that enhance infiltration through basement membranes of various parenchymal cell structures.

The kinetics of T-cell infiltration into allografts in CM-AR varies according to time post-transplant, the degree of disparity, and the numbers of memory cells (e.g. CD45RO phenotype) (Azzawi et al., 1998; Erren et al., 1999; Wang et al., 1999). Established AR in several organ allografts has a predominance of memory cells and the formation of tertiary germinal centres. Some markers of CM-AR include perforin and granzyme B in the allograft (D'Errico et al., 2003; Wagrowska-Danilewicz and Danilewicz, 2003; Mengel et al., 2004), which are lytic enzymes expressed by cytotoxic T-cells.

Aside from the predominant T-cells, B-cells, natural killer (NK), natural killer T (NKT) cells, and monocytes/macrophages (Ashokkumar et al., 2012) are also present during CM-AR. These non-T-cells may play a pivotal role in CM-AR as they are capable of antigen presentation (Chantranuwat et al., 2004; Hammond et al., 2005) and may serve some effector functions. Upon activation they can produce tissue injury by releasing free radicals and other toxic mediators and can activate the coagulation cascade.

Protracted inflammation secondary to AR or other causes ultimately results in fibrosis in allografts that is a central component of CR. The entity identified as 'chronic rejection' tends to be variable in its phenotype and is influenced by numerous immune and non-immune variables (Takeda et al., 2011). Cellular infiltrates of T lymphocytes and monocytes/macrophages have been identified as central components in fibrosis induction within allografts (Allan et al., 2002; Ozdemir et al., 2002) due to their initiation of fibrosis, via production of fibrogenic factors and matrix proteins. CD4+ and CD8+ T-cells are present in graft infiltrates in experimental and clinical CR (Racusen, 2003), with these T-cells (and macrophages) often being in aggregates and perivascular distribution.

Ongoing antibody-mediated immune injury likely plays a prominent role in the pathogenesis of CR (O'Leary et al., 2011) and this is pathologically supported by the presence of C4d staining in biopsies from a subgroup of patients with CR (Mauiyyedi et al., 2001). Increased expression of adhesion molecules may also be present in chronic allograft vasculopathy (Suzuki et al., 1997; Zembala et al., 1997). Localized expression of factors, such as transforming growth factor β (TGF-β) (Csencsits et al., 2006; Rintala et al., 2006), angiotensin II (Barocci et al., 1999), and plasminogen activator inhibitor (Ikegami et al., 1995), has been implicated in the pathogenesis of CR. Fibroblast growth factor-1 (FGF-1) and receptor are upregulated with CR (Kerby et al., 1997), and platelet-derived growth factor (PDGF) A and B have been detected in smooth muscle cells and macrophages present in vessels with allograft vasculopathy (Lemstrom et al., 2004).

Chemokines (e.g. RANTES/CCL5) also play a role in CR and inflammation in allografts (Hancock et al., 2003) such that antagonism of chemokine receptors tempers chronic vasculopathy development by reducing mononuclear cell recruitment to the transplanted hearts (Yun et al., 2004).

Interstitial fibrosis progression is a central lesion of CR enhanced by fibroblasts differentiating into myofibroblasts in the grafted organs (Pedagogos et al., 1997). Proliferating myofibroblasts have also been seen in glomerular mesangium (Pilmore et al., 2002) and in the intima of vessels with allograft vasculopathy (Subramanian et al., 2002). Matrix component accumulation also contributes to CR fibrosis, with collagen type III progressively increasing with time in allografts (Waller et al., 2004), as well as increased expression of laminin β2 and collagen 4α3 (Paczek et al., 1996; Bakker et al., 2003), tenascin, and fibronectin (Paczek et al., 1996).

In addition to ongoing AAMR and CM-AR, infectious complications occurring in transplants such as viral infections can lead to fibrosis in allografts. Viral infections have been implicated in the pathogenesis of chronic allograft vasculopathy in a number of solid organ allografts (Streblow et al., 2008).

## Clinical immunology of tissue typing and organ matching

Since the HLA complex encodes the most immunogenic molecules on a transplanted organ to a genetically disparate host, they serve as the primary targets of allograft rejection, making the MHC molecules the most important barriers in allotransplantation within any species and in xenotransplantation. Specialized *histocompatibility clinical laboratories* are critical and central in their support of a transplant programme, since they identify the class I and II HLA molecules present on the cadaveric or living-related donor and potential recipient. The histocompatibility labs are also responsible for monitoring of recipient immune sensitization to specific donor histocompatibility antigens, whether in the form of antibodies (humoral sensitization) (Platt and Cascalho, 2011) or as immune effector cells (cellular sensitization). As such, a variety of standard histocompatibility and molecular-based tests are utilized after the transplant in the monitoring and clinical maintenance that is required for successful long-term transplantation.

These HLA proteins can be expressed at different levels and/or restricted to select cellular types, so that a transplanted organ (e.g. liver) may not be as immunogenic as another (e.g. kidney) for a particular donor–recipient pair. Regardless, a high level of HLA antigen compatibility or matching between the donor and recipient tends to augment the chances for a successful transplant acceptance by the recipient due to a lower level of immune response to the donor (Cecka, 2010), whereas the chance of graft rejection is heightened with a significant level of histo-incompatibility or mismatching. The incredible diversity in the number of HLA alleles or polymorphisms provides populations with heterogeneity and immune vigour but also makes matching HLA alleles very challenging; the majority of human transplantation combinations for donors and recipients will have some degree of MHC incompatibility between each other. In general, collective mismatches at HLA-A, HLA-B, HLA-C, HLA-DR, and HLA-DQ are associated with poorer graft survival. Thus, it is incumbent for a transplant programme to be able to identify these major and in many cases minor mismatched differences and try to arrive at the best acceptable combination possible for the potential transplant recipient.

The methodologies used to determine HLA compatibility have evolved significantly since first attempted in the early 1960s. HLA typing is still performed by serological assays in some centres, although the majority of techniques currently used are molecular-based assays (Eng and Leffell, 2011). These molecular techniques include southern blotting, polymerase chain reaction (PCR), restriction fragment length polymorphism (RFLP) analysis of PCR products (PCR-RFLP), and sequence-based typing (Dunn, 2011).

Two sources can be used for class I and II HLA typing: DNA or the expression of these antigens on leucocyte cell surfaces. The most common class I antigens that are identified or typed are HLA-A, HLA-B, and HLA-C, while in class II it is HLA-DR, HLA-DRB1, HLA-DP, and HLA-DQ. Molecular HLA typing is accomplished at several levels of discrimination between alleles, with the categories being low, medium, and high resolution. Low resolution characterizes broad families of alleles that may have many members. High-resolution typing is an attempt to definitively identify the allele residing at a given locus for the recipient. Medium resolution lies between high and low, narrowing the choices to fewer subtypes than by low-resolution typing. In general, solid organ transplant combinations can generally operate well with low-resolution typing, while bone marrow programmes need the support of high-resolution typing to promote long-term graft survival and minimize GVHD.

## Pharmacological modulation of the immune response

Although immunological tolerance—donor-specific unresponsiveness without maintenance immunosuppressive medication while preserving intact immune function against infection or malignancy—may be the ultimate goal of transplant immunology, this condition has been established only sporadically in a limited number of patients, and the majority of transplant recipients require life-long immunosuppressive medication. Pharmacological modulation of the host immune response often starts in an operating room before the graft reperfusion, and it is essential for a transplant anaesthesiologist to understand the basic immunological and pharmacological properties of these medications. This section briefly summarizes immunosuppressive agents in current clinical use; however, the reader should refer to the package insert of each product before actual use because this section is not intended to cover dosing and administration guidelines entirely and includes 'off-label' use of medication.

## Corticosteroids

Corticosteroids, originally supplemented azathioprine (Imuran) in the 1960s, have played a central role in pharmacological modulation of the recipient's immune system (Murray et al., 1963; Starzl et al., 1963). Although newer immunosuppressive medications and their combinations (i.e. protocols) may allow significant dose reduction or withdrawal of corticosteroids shortly after the transplantation, high-dose corticosteroids are often infused during transplant surgery. In addition to their immunological properties to suppress alloimmune responses on lymphocytes and macrophages, their broad actions affect the innate immune system and suppress non-specific inflammatory responses in ischaemia–reperfusion injury of transplanted organs (Feola et al., 1976). Owing to their strong inhibition of numerous cytokine expressions, they are also used as premedication for biological immunosuppressive agents (i.e. monoclonal and polyclonal antibodies, as described in the next sections) to minimize cytokine-release syndrome. Methylprednisolone (Solu-Medrol) and hydrocortisone (Solu-Cortef) are the commonly used preparations. Among their well-known side effects, hypertension, hyperglycaemia, and leucocytosis are often seen perioperatively. Steroids psychosis may be observed in patients, especially the elderly in an ICU setting after transplant surgery.

## Antithymocyte globulin

The polyclonal antibody preparations antithymocyte globulin (ATG) and antilymphocyte globulin (ALG) have been used in clinical and experimental transplantation since the 1960s (Starzl et al., 1967; Lance and Batchelor, 1968; Russell, 1968). Activated human thymocytes or lymphocytes are injected into a rabbit (or horse) and immune globulin is purified and pasteurized from the sera of the animals. This immunosuppressive product contains cytotoxic antibodies directed against antigens expressed on human lymphocytes, including CD2, CD3, CD4, CD8, CD11a, CD25, CD44, CD45, CD80, CD86, and HLA class I and II (Mohty, 2007). These polyclonal antibodies as well as some monoclonal antibodies such as alemtuzumab (Campath 1H, anti-CD52 monoclonal antibody) and now obsolete muromonab-CD3 (Orthoclone OKT3, first-generation anti-CD3 antibody) are sometimes called 'depleting antibodies' due to their T-cell-depleting capacities, whereas anti-CD25 monoclonal antibodies are non-depleting. Rabbit ATG (Thymoglobulin, Genzyme) has largely replaced equine ATG (Atgam, Pfizer) for solid organ transplantation in the US market (Brennan et al., 1999; Hardinger et al., 2004) and rabbit ATG (ATG-Fresenius S, Fresenius) is marketed outside of the US. The standard dose of Thymoglobulin (1–1.5 mg/kg/day × 4–10 days, total dose 6–15 mg) exerts profound T-cell depletion—especially CD4+ T-cells—and its (at least partial) effect along with standard maintenance immunosuppression can last for years after administration (Sageshima et al., 2011).

While the only Federal Drug Administration (FDA)-approved indication is the treatment of renal transplant AR (Webster et al., 2006), Thymoglobulin has often been used for induction therapy—to prevent rejection (Nashan, 2005; Gaber et al., 2010) and to decrease ischaemia–reperfusion injury (Goggins et al., 2003; Bogetti et al., 2005)—and also in non-renal organ transplantation (Burke et al., 2004; Bogetti et al., 2005; Soliman et al., 2007; Goland et al., 2008; Vianna et al., 2008; Farney et al., 2009). Because rapid infusion can cause infusion-associated reactions (e.g. cytokine release syndrome), it should be infused over 4–6 hours into a high-flow vein. If there is no central venous or arteriovenous fistula access, addition of hydrocortisone (Solu-Cortef) 20 mg and heparin 1,000 units to a high-volume (> 500 mL saline) carrier solution may decrease the risk of thrombophlebitis. To prevent infusion-associated reactions, premedication with diphenhydramine (Benadryl), acetaminophen (Tylenol), and corticosteroids is often used. Although serum sickness is rare when used with high-dose steroids, cytokine release syndrome, including pulmonary oedema in patients with fluid overload, needs to be monitored carefully. Leucopaenia and/or thrombocytopaenia are common. The Thymoglobulin dose should be reduced by one-half if the white blood cell (WBC) count is below 3,000/mm$^3$ or if the platelet count is below 75,000/mm$^3$, and stopping Thymoglobulin treatment should be considered if they are below 2,000 or 50,000/mm$^3$, respectively. Profound lymphocyte depletion may possibly lead to serious infection including cytomegalovirus (CMV) infection (Akalin et al., 2004) and malignancies including post-transplant lymphoproliferative disorder (PTLD) (Marks et al., 2011).

## Alemtuzumab (anti-CD52 monoclonal antibody)

Alemtuzumab (Campath-1H, Genzyme), a recombinant humanized CD52-specific complement-fixing (cytotoxic-lympho-depleting) IgG1 monoclonal antibody, was first introduced to kidney transplantation by Calne in the late 1990s with low-dose cyclosporine A monotherapy (Calne et al., 1998), with the hope of establishing 'prope' or near tolerance. However, subsequent studies have demonstrated that alemtuzumab alone or in combination with low-dose maintenance immunosuppression (e.g. sirolimus) can result in a higher incidence of AR and it does not induce tolerance (Kirk et al., 2003, 2005; Knechtle et al., 2003). Some studies have also shown a higher incidence of antibody-mediated rejection (AMR) (Bloom et al., 2009; Willicombe et al., 2011) and the concept of alemtuzumab as a tolerogenic agent has been abandoned (Ciancio and Burke, 2008).

Nonetheless, with a wide distribution of CD52 glycoprotein on various peripheral blood mononuclear cells and high affinity of alemtuzumab to the CD52 antigen, single-dose alemtuzumab infusion can induce profound and prolonged depletion of peripheral lymphocytes (Sageshima et al., 2011). While its use for solid organ transplantation (i.e. induction therapy or treatment of rejection) is not approved by the FDA, its relatively low cost and ease of use have made alemtuzumab an attractive alternative lymphocyte-depleting agent (Ciancio and Burke, 2008; Morgan et al., 2012), and its application extends to non-renal organ transplantation (Tzakis et al., 2003; Farney et al., 2009; Teuteberg et al., 2010; Shyu et al., 2011). Typically, one vial (= 30 mg) or 0.3 mg/kg of alemtuzumab is infused over 2–4 hours intraoperatively. Diphenhydramine (Benadryl) and acetaminophen (Tylenol) along with corticosteroids are recommended to use as premedication 30 minutes prior to the first infusion in order to prevent infusion-associated reactions. When the second dose is administered, dose modification is required based on neutropaenia or thrombocytopaenia. In some protocols, subcutaneous administration of alemtuzumab has also been used (Clatworthy et al.,

2007; Vo et al., 2008b). The risks of viral infection and PTLD might be similar to other depleting antibodies, requiring appropriate CMV prophylaxis (Ciancio et al., 2005; Walker et al., 2007).

### Basiliximab and daclizumab (anti-CD25 (interleukin-2 receptor) monoclonal antibodies)

Since interleukin-2 (IL-2) plays a critical role in T-cell activation and proliferation, antibodies against [α] subunit (CD25) of the IL-2 receptor were introduced to experimental and clinical transplantation in the late 1980s (Tighe et al., 1988; Kirkman et al., 1991). Although initial murine monoclonal antibodies had limited efficacy due to high immunogenicity and short half-life, chimeric Basiliximab (Simulect, Novartis) and humanized Daclizumab (Zenapax, Roche) have prolonged half-lives and demonstrate stable CD25 saturation for 1–3 months (Kahan et al., 1999b; Onrust and Wiseman, 1999).

In contrast to antithymocyte globulin and alemtuzumab, these antibodies cause T-cell dysfunction but are non-depleting (Onrust and Wiseman, 1999). They aim to decrease AR rates early after transplantation when the incidence of rejection is high (i.e. they act as induction agents to prevent rejection but not to treat rejection), while maintaining the pre-existing immune responses of other cells (Vincenti et al., 1997, 1998; Beniaminovitz et al., 2000; Ciancio et al., 2002; Neuhaus et al., 2002). Although their efficacy in immunologically high-risk patients (e.g. repeat transplant, highly sensitized, young African-American) may be limited, various protocols have demonstrated the lower incidence of AR episodes in low-to-standard immunological risk patients with remarkably high safety profiles (Nashan, 2005; Sageshima et al., 2009; Webster et al., 2010). Fixed doses of Basiliximab (Simulect, 20 mg per dose for adult and paediatric patients weighing ≥ 35 kg, and 10 mg per dose for paediatric patients weighing < 35 kg) are usually given on day 0 and day 4 post-transplant. In contrast, while discontinued in the US market, Daclizumab (Zenapax) is used as weight-adjusted dosing. In an original study, 1 mg/kg doses are given every 2 weeks for a total of 5 doses, while many subsequent protocols include limited dosage (mainly 2 doses) of 1–2 mg/kg infusion (ter Meulen et al., 2001). Hypersensitivity might occur, but infusion-associated reactions are rare for both agents and premedication is not mandatory. The risks of infection (including CMV), malignancy, and other transplant-related adverse effects of patients receiving these agents seem to be similar to patients not receiving an induction therapy (Sageshima et al., 2009; Webster et al., 2010).

### Rituximab (anti-CD20 monoclonal antibody)

Rituximab (Rituxan, Genentech-Biogen/Roche), approved by the FDA for B-cell non-Hodgkin's lymphoma in 1997, is a genetically engineered, chimeric murine/human monoclonal antibody directed against the CD20 antigen found on the surface of B-lymphocytes (Leget and Czuczman, 1998; Pescovitz, 2006). As the role of B-cell is recognized to a greater extent in transplant immunology, its use for transplant patients is expanding. In addition to the indication to treat B-cell lymphoma or PTLD in transplant recipients (Faye et al., 1998), more attention has been paid to its property to control humoral immunity (Bohmig et al., 2011; Clatworthy, 2011; Jordan et al., 2011a). Rituximab has largely replaced pretransplant splenectomy for ABO-incompatible transplantation with similar long-term results (Tanabe et al., 2009, 2010; Crew and Ratner, 2010), leaving splenectomy as a post-transplant rescue therapy only for refractory AMR caused by anti-A and/or anti-B antibodies.

Often in combination with other modalities to control humoral immunity (i.e. plasmapheresis or intravenous immunoglobulin (IVIG)), rituximab has been used to decrease preformed antibody levels in patients waiting for deceased-donor transplantation and patients who have antibodies specific to their potential living donors (Stegall et al., 2006; Vo et al., 2008a; Bohmig et al., 2011). Rituximab, along with other antibody-targeted immunotherapies, has also successfully been used in the treatment of AMR (Jordan et al., 2010). A unique application of this agent is the treatment or prevention of recurrent focal segmental glomerulosclerosis (FSGS) and other nephrotic glomerulopathy after kidney transplantation (Ponticelli and Glassock, 2010; Fornoni et al., 2011).

Rituximab seems to have a direct effect on podocytes in stabilizing and decreasing urine protein excretion. Single or multiple doses of rituximab (375 mg/m$^2$ body surface area (BSA)) are often used, but a reduced dosage may be equally effective as a standard dose regimen in selected indications (Toki et al., 2009). To minimize the risk of infusion-associated reactions (e.g. hypotension, arrhythmia, and respiratory distress) especially after the first infusion, a slow escalating infusion rate with appropriate premedication is used. While progressive multifocal leucoencephalopathy (PML) has been reported after rituximab therapy, overall incidences of infection and malignancy seem to be acceptable when compared with other immunotherapies (Gea-Banacloche, 2010).

### Belatacept (cytotoxic T-lymphocyte antigen-4 immunoglobulin (CTLA-4 Ig))

The full activation of T-cells requires costimulatory signals (signal 2). Belatacept (Nulojix, Bristol-Myers Squibb), a fusion protein of the Fc fragment of human IgG1 immunoglobulin and the extracellular domain of CTLA-4, binds to CD80 (B7-1) and CD86 (B7-2) on antigen-presenting cells and blocks costimulatory signals to CD28 (B7 receptor) on T-cells (Sayegh and Turka, 1998; Vincenti et al., 2005). It is designed to prevent kidney allograft rejection without nephrotoxic calcineurin inhibitors (CNIs, cyclosporin and tacrolimus) (Durrbach et al., 2010; Vincenti et al., 2010). Starting the day of transplant, 6 doses of Belatacept (10 mg/kg) are infused during a 3-month initial phase. Afterwards, the maintenance dose (5 mg/kg) is given every 4 weeks. It is to be infused over 30 minutes and no premedication is required. Because of a higher incidence of PTLD predominantly involving the central nervous system, Belatacept can be used only in patients who are Epstein–Barr virus (EBV) seropositive. John Cunningham virus (JCV)-associated PML and other serious infections were also reported, but there seems to be no significant increase in overall incidence of infection or malignancy.

### Bortezomib (proteasome inhibitor)

Bortezomib (Velcade, Millennium) is a proteasome inhibitor which is approved in the US for treating relapsed multiple myeloma and mantle cell lymphoma (Adams, 2002). From its apoptotic effects on plasma cells and suppression of T-cell functions, Bortezomib—alone or in combination with other modalities—has been used for pretransplant desensitization and prevention and treatment of acute and chronic AMR in transplantation (Jordan et al., 2010; Woodle et al., 2011). Peripheral neuropathy is a relatively common side effect and neutropaenia and thrombocytopaenia from myelosuppression can also occur.

### Eculizumab (anti-C5 monoclonal antibody)

Eculizumab (Soliris, Alexion) is a recombinant humanized monoclonal antibody targeting complement protein C5, preventing the formation of the terminal complement complex C5b-9. It has been approved by the FDA for paroxysmal nocturnal haemoglobinuria (PNH) and atypical haemolytic–uraemic syndrome (aHUS). In transplantation, Eculizumab has been used to prevent and treat post-transplant aHUS or thrombotic microangiopathy (Chatelet et al., 2009; Zimmerhackl et al., 2010); it has also been used for prevention and treatment of AMR (Locke et al., 2009). Although intravenous infusion of Eculizumab is well tolerated, it can increase the risk of infections by encapsulated organisms such as meningococcus (McKeage, 2011).

### Intravenous immune globulins

IVIGs are pooled gammaglobulin preparations from human donor plasma. Their mechanism of action is complex, including effects on T-cells, B-cells, antibodies, and cytokines; it is rather immunomodulatory than immunosuppressive (Jordan et al., 2011b). High-dose IVIG has been used to decrease levels of sensitization in patients awaiting transplantation (Stegall et al., 2006); IVIGs have also been used to treat or prevent AMR (Jordan et al., 2010). The standard dose of high-dose IVIG is 2 g/kg, but the dose may be split specifically for volume-sensitive patients. Diphenhydramine (Benadryl), acetaminophen (Tylenol), and corticosteroids are used before slow infusion (over 4–8 hours) of IVIG. In addition to minor infusion-associated reactions, acute renal failure can occur, often osmotic nephrosis with sucrose-containing products, and they should be used with caution for patients with base-line renal impairment (Dickenmann et al., 2008). Low-dose IVIG (100–150 mg/kg) is frequently combined with plasmapheresis (Stegall et al., 2006; Montgomery et al., 2011); CMV high-titre immune globulin (Cytogam, CSL Behring) may be selected for this dose.

### Cyclosporine and tacrolimus (calcineurin inhibitors)

Since the original introduction of cyclosporine in the 1980s, CNIs have played a major role in transplant immunosuppression (Calne et al., 1978; Morris et al., 1983, Starzl et al., 1989; European FK506 Multicentre Liver Study Group, 1994; US Multicenter FK506 Liver Study Group, 1994; Mayer et al., 1997; Pirsch et al., 1997; Mentzer et al., 1998; OPTN 2012;). Both cyclosporine and tacrolimus bind to cytoplasmic receptor proteins, i.e. cyclophilin- and tacrolimus-binding protein (FK506 binding protein (FKBP)), respectively, and inhibit the function of calcineurin, limiting certain cytokine production and lymphocyte proliferation (Thomson and Starzl, 1993). Their mechanism of action is more selective than their predecessors (e.g. azathioprine and steroids), and their introduction significantly decreased AR rates and increased graft and patient survival rates with fewer infectious complications. Although both agents have intravenous formulae, an enteral route by mouth or via a gastric tube is often preferred. Because of significant inter- and intrapatient variability of absorption and metabolism, therapeutic drug monitoring is mandatory for these agents (Kelly and Kahan, 2002).

While the original formulation of cyclosporine (Sandimmune, Novartis) depends on bile for absorption, the microemulsion formulation of cyclosporine (Neoral, Novartis) and tacrolimus (Prograf, Astellas) does not depend on bile. The trough concentration (the level immediately before next dose) and occasionally C2 (the level 2 hours after dose, only for Neoral) correlates well with the area under the curve (AUC) and is usually used for clinical therapeutic drug monitoring (Kelly and Kahan, 2002; Knight and Morris, 2007). CNIs are metabolized by the cytochrome P-450 IIIA (CYP3A) in the liver and the gastrointestinal tract, and are known to have significant drug interactions with co-administered medication that can modify CYP3A activity (Kelly and Kahan, 2002). Cyclosporine and tacrolimus share the majority of their side-effect profiles including nephrotoxicity, but cyclosporine commonly causes more hypertension and dyslipidaemia, whereas tacrolimus causes more hyperglycaemia and neurotoxicity (Webster et al., 2005).

### Mycophenolate mofetil and mycophenolic acid (inosine monophosphate dehydrogenase (IMPDH) inhibitors)

Mycophenolate mofetil (MMF) (CellCept, Roche) and enteric-coated mycophenolic acid (EC-MPA) (Myfortic, Novartis), both as MPA, inhibit IMPDH and de-novo purine synthesis, blocking T-cell and B-cell proliferation and antibody production (Thomson and Starzl, 1993). Since their introduction to clinical transplantation in 1995 (CellCept) (European Mycophenolate Mofetil Cooperative Study Group, 1995; Sollinger, 1995) and 2004 (Myfortic) (Budde et al., 2004; Salvadori et al., 2004), they largely replaced azathioprine (OPTN, 2012), which is the same class but a less selective antimetabolite. While some studies suggest certain benefits of AUC measurement of MPA (Bennett, 2003), clinical therapeutic drug monitoring is not routinely employed. Oral liquid and intravenous formulae are also available for MMF. Gastrointestinal side effects (e.g. diarrhoea and nausea) are common for both agents, and bone marrow suppression (especially neutropaenia) often necessitates dose reduction of MMF or EC-MPA, which can increase incidence of AR episodes (Budde et al., 2004; Salvadori et al., 2004; Ciancio et al., 2008a).

### Sirolimus and everolimus (mammalian target of rapamycin (mTOR) inhibitors)

While sirolimus (or rapamycin, Rapamune, Pfizer) (Groth et al., 1999; Kahan et al., 1999a; Kahan, 2000; MacDonald, 2001; Flechner et al., 2002; Larson et al., 2006) and everolimus (Zortress (US) and Certican (Europe), Novartis) (Vitko et al., 2004; Lorber et al., 2005) bind to the same cytoplasmic receptor proteins as tacrolimus (FKBP), their complex inhibits mTOR instead of calcineurin, leading to inhibition of lymphocyte activation and proliferation (Kahan, 2001). They are metabolized by CYP3A and p-glycoprotein; concomitant administration of mTOR inhibitors and CNIs significantly modifies drug exposure of mTOR inhibitors (Zimmerman et al., 2003). A trough concentration reflects AUC and is usually used for therapeutic drug monitoring. As compared with CNIs, mTOR inhibitors were initially thought to be less nephrotoxic, but they can still delay recovery from acute tubular necrosis following renal transplantation (McTaggart et al., 2003), and concomitant administration of mTOR inhibitors and standard-dose CNIs potentiates nephrotoxicity (Lorber et al., 2005; Ciancio et al., 2006). Proteinuria is common either de novo or as exaggeration of pre-existing proteinuria, and close monitoring is required for any proteinuric patients (Lorber et al., 2005; Buchler et al., 2007). Thrombocytopaenia and dyslipidaemia are common especially when combined with other immunosuppressive medication causing such side effects (i.e. mycophenolate and cyclosporine, respectively) (Groth et al., 1999). Fluid retention, pneumonia, and delayed wound healing are occasionally observed. Because of their antitumour properties—in fact, higher-dose everolimus (Afinitor) is marketed for certain neoplastic diseases—mTOR inhibitors may be of particular value in transplant patients with or at high risk for post-transplant neoplasms (e.g. skin cancer) (Stallone et al., 2005; Campistol et al., 2006).

### Azathioprine

Azathioproine (Imuran, Prometheus) is the oldest immunosuppressive medication that has been used for transplantation (Murray et al., 1963; Starzl et al., 1963); however, newer agents (described in the section 'Mycophenolate mofetil and mycophenolic acid (inosine monophosphate dehydrogenase (IMPDH) inhibitors), sirolimus, and everolimus (mammalian target of rapamycin (mTOR) inhibitors) have replaced its role in most clinical transplant settings. It can still be used for patients who cannot tolerate other medications or for long-term low-cost immunosuppressive protocols (Farney et al., 2010). It is a derivative of 6-mercaptopurine and inhibits purine nucleotide synthesis. Bone marrow suppression is a well-known side effect and hepatotoxicity is also common.

### Immunosuppressive protocols

Because each immunosuppressive agent described above has a different mechanism of action and a side-effect profile, a wide variety of their combinations has been tested to maximize their immunosuppressive effects and to minimize side effects (OPTN, 2012). The goal of these combinations (i.e. protocols) is to obtain the least rejection rate, and consequently to avoid long-term immunological graft loss, and at the same time to achieve the minimal mortality and morbidity rates, especially from infectious, neoplastic, and cardiovascular complications. Because each patient population has different immunological risks and susceptibility to side effects of immunosuppressive medication there is no single immunosuppressive protocol that fits all transplant patients and organs.

#### Induction therapy

To prevent AR episodes early after transplantation while the risk of rejection is highest, intense immunosuppression—often using depleting antibodies—is employed in immunologically high-risk patients who receive immunogenic organs (Ciancio et al., 2008b; Goland et al., 2008; Vianna et al., 2008; Farney et al., 2009; Gaber et al., 2010; Aliabadi et al., 2011). In contrast, initial intense immunosuppression may increase the risk of infectious complications, specifically in patients with pre-existing infectious (e.g. viral hepatitis, HIV) or immunocompromised (e.g. malnutrition, chronic steroid use) conditions (Burroughs, 2002). Relatively mild induction therapies using non-depleting antibody or no induction were generally preferred for patients with a low immunological risk (Nashan, 2005; Sageshima et al., 2009; Campara et al., 2010; Webster et al., 2010); recently, however, more protocols tend to include intense induction therapies even for these low-risk populations, aiming for less maintenance immunosuppression (i.e. steroid- or CNI-sparing protocols) to avoid long-term side effects (Buchler et al., 2007; Pascual et al., 2009; Woodle et al., 2010; Ciancio et al., 2011).

#### Maintenance therapy

Corticosteroids and CNIs have been the mainstream of maintenance immunosuppressive therapy. They are used as dual or triple therapy often with an IMPDH inhibitor or an mTOR inhibitor. Although these combinations have decreased AR rates and improved short-term graft survival, side effects of immunosuppressive medication are still troublesome, and long-term survival, as well as quality of life, has yet to be enhanced (OPTN, 2012). Because poor graft and patient survival is in part associated with long-term steroid and CNI use, dose reduction or discontinuation of these agents have been evaluated using many different protocols.

To avoid short- and long-term side effects of corticosteroids, transplant centres have reported steroid-sparing (i.e. avoidance or withdrawal) protocols in renal (Pascual et al., 2009; Knight and Morris, 2010; Woodle et al., 2010; Lightner et al., 2011) and non-renal (Lerut et al., 2009; Mineo et al., 2009; Knight and Morris, 2011) transplantation. The majority of them have shown equivalent, if not superior, outcomes, but yet long-term follow-up is required to determine the risk:benefit ratio of each protocol. In contrast, most of the CNI-sparing protocols have demonstrated a higher incidence of rejection as compared with conventional immunosuppressive protocols, leaving CNIs a key component of post-transplant immunosuppression (Mulay et al., 2005; Guerra et al., 2007; Danger et al., 2008; Farkas et al., 2009; Zuckermann and Aliabadi, 2009; Penninga et al., 2012). Nonetheless, a recent protocol using Belatacept, MMF, and corticosteroids (but no CNIs) has demonstrated a promising outcome—a similar rejection rate as cyclosporin-treated patients with superior kidney graft function—in primarily low-risk renal transplant recipients (Durrbach et al., 2010; Larsen et al., 2010; Vincenti et al., 2010; Vanrenterghem et al., 2011). Its application to other patient populations and long-term results are of most interest in CNI-sparing protocols.

## Conclusion

The exponential growth in our knowledge of basic immunological processes has fostered the tremendous gains made in our comprehension of alloimmune reactions occurring in human hosts of allogeneic solid organ transplants. We now have clear delineation of many of the molecular pathways and initiating events that drive the recipient's adaptive and innate immune pathways to identify and injure the targets seen as 'foreign' on the transplanted organ. Our understanding of these processes is now being translated into more precise clinical laboratory methodologies that greatly facilitate the identification of the most suitable donor–recipient pairs and which provide more accurate assessment of possible immunological complications such as AR and CR reactions. Our enhanced knowledge base of the processes involved in the immune interactions between host and transplant has also led to an amazing progress in new pharmaceutical and biological agents that disrupt and inhibit arms of the immune system in increasingly precise fashion. As our general knowledge base, immunodiagnostics, and transplant immunosuppressive regimens improve, so will in similar fashion the survival and success of all forms of solid organ transplantation.

## References


Adams J (2002) Proteasome inhibition: a novel approach to cancer therapy. *Trends Molec Med*, **8**:S49–S54.

Akalin E, Watschinger B (2007) Antibody-mediated rejection. *Semin Nephrol*, **27**:393–407.

Akalin E, Bromberg JS, Sehgal V, Ames S, Murphy B (2004) Decreased incidence of cytomegalovirus infection in thymoglobulin-treated transplant patients with 6 months of valganciclovir prophylaxis. *Am J Transplant*, **4**:148–149.

Aliabadi A, Grommer M, Zuckermann A (2011) Is induction therapy still needed in heart transplantation? *Curr Opin Organ Transplant*, **16**:536–542.

Allan JS, Madsen JC, Allan JS, Madsen JC (2002) Recent advances in the immunology of chronic rejection. *Curr Opin NephrolHypertens*, **11**:315–321.

Ashokkumar C, Gabriellan A, Ningappa M, Mazariegos G, Sun Q, Sindhi R (2012) Increased monocyte expression of sialoadhesin during acute cellular rejection and other enteritides after intestine transplantation in children. *Transplantation*, **93**:561–564.

Azzawi M, Hasleton PS, Geraghty PJ, et al. (1998) RANTES chemokine expression is related to acute cardiac cellular rejection and infiltration by CD45RO T-lymphocytes and macrophages. *J Heart Lung Transplant*, **17**:881–887.

Bakker RC, Koop K, Sijpkens YW, et al. (2003) Early interstitial accumulation of collagen type I discriminates chronic rejection from chronic cyclosporine nephrotoxicity. *J Am Soc Nephrol*, **14**:2142–2149.

Baldwin WM 3rd, Samaniego-Picota M, Kasper EK, et al.(1999) Complement deposition in early cardiac transplant biopsies is associated with ischemic injury and subsequent rejection episodes. *Transplantation*, **68**:894–900.

Banasik M, Boratynska M, Nowakowska B, et al. (2007) C4D deposition and positive posttransplant crossmatch are not necessarily markers of antibody-mediated rejection in renal allograft recipients. *Transplant Proc*, **39**:2718–2720.

Barocci S, Ginevri F, Valente U, Torre F, Gusmano R, Nocera A (1999) Correlation between angiotensin-converting enzyme gene insertion/ deletion polymorphism and kidney graft long-term outcome in pediatric recipients: a single-center analysis. *Transplantation*, **67**:534–538.

Beniaminovitz A, Itescu S, Lietz K, et al. (2000) Prevention of rejection in cardiac transplantation by blockade of the interleukin-2 receptor with a monoclonal antibody. *N Engl J Med*, **342**:613–619.

Bennett WM (2003) Immunosuppression with mycophenolic acid: one size does not fit all. *J Am Soc Nephrol*, **14**:2414–2416.

Billingham RE, Brent L, Medawar PB (1953) Actively acquired tolerance of foreign cells. *Nature*, **172**:603–606.

Bloom D, Chang Z, Pauly K, et al. (2009) BAFF is increased in renal transplant patients following treatment with alemtuzumab. *Am J Transplant*, **9**:1835–1845.

Bogetti, D., Sankary, H. N., Jarzembowski, T. M., et al. (2005). Thymoglobulin induction protects liver allografts from ischemia/ reperfusion injury. *Clin Transplant*, **19**:507–511.

Bohmig GA, Wahrmann M, Bartel G (2011) Transplantation of the broadly sensitized patient: what are the options? *Curr Opin Organ Transplant*, **16**:588–593.

Boukouaci W, Busson M, Peffault de Latour R, et al. (2009) MICA-129 genotype, soluble MICA, and anti-MICA antibodies as biomarkers of chronic graft-versus-host disease. *Blood*, **114**:5216–5224.

Brennan DC, Flavin K, Lowell JA, et al. (1999) A randomized, double-blinded comparison of Thymoglobulin versus Atgam for induction immunosuppressive therapy in adult renal transplant recipients. *Transplantation*, **67**:1011–1018.

Buchler M, Caillard S, Barbier S, et al. (2007) Sirolimus versus cyclosporine in kidney recipients receiving thymoglobulin, mycophenolate mofetil and a 6-month course of steroids. *Am J Transplant*, **7**:2522–2531.

Budde K, Curtis J, Knoll G, et al. (2004) Enteric-coated mycophenolate sodium can be safely administered in maintenance renal transplant patients: results of a 1-year study. *Am J Transplant*, **4**:237–243.

Burke GW, 3rd, Kaufman DB, Millis JM, et al. (2004) Prospective, randomized trial of the effect of antibody induction in simultaneous pancreas and kidney transplantation: three-year results. *Transplantation*, **77**:1269–1275.

Burroughs AK (2002) Induction immunosuppression for patients who underwent transplantation for cirrhosis caused by hepatitis C? The answer is no! *Liver Transplant*, **8**:S47–S49.

Calne RY, White DJ, Thiru S, et al. (1978) Cyclosporin A in patients receiving renal allografts from cadaver donors. *Lancet*, **2**:1323–1327.

Calne R, Friend P, Moffatt S, et al. (1998) Prope tolerance, perioperative campath 1H, and low-dose cyclosporin monotherapy in renal allograft recipients. *Lancet*, **351**:1701–1702.

Campara M, Tzvetanov IG, Oberholzer J (2010). Interleukin-2 receptor blockade with humanized monoclonal antibody for solid organ transplantation. *Expert Opin Biol Ther*, **10**:959–969.

Campistol JM, Eris J, Oberbauer R, et al. (2006) Sirolimus therapy after early cyclosporine withdrawal reduces the risk for cancer in adult renal transplantation. *J Am Soc Nephrol*, **17**:581–589.

Cecka JM (2010) HLA matching for organ transplantation . . . why not? *Int J Immunogenet*, **37**:323–327.

Chantranuwat C, Qiao JH, Kobashigawa J, Hong L, Shintaku P, Fishbein M C (2004) Immunoperoxidase staining for C4d on paraffin-embedded tissue in cardiac allograft endomyocardial biopsies: comparison to frozen tissue immunofluorescence. *Appl Immunohistochem Mol Morphol*, **12**:166–171.

Chatelet V, Fremeaux-Bacchi V, Lobbedez T, Ficheux M, Hurault de Ligny B (2009) Safety and long-term efficacy of eculizumab in a renal transplant patient with recurrent atypical hemolytic-uremic syndrome. *Am J Transplant*, **9**:2644–2645.

Ciancio G, Burke GW 3rd (2008) Alemtuzumab (Campath-1H) in kidney transplantation. *Am J Transplant*, **8**:15–20.

Ciancio G, Burke GW, Suzart K, et al. (2002) Daclizumab induction, tacrolimus, mycophenolate mofetil and steroids as an immunosuppression regimen for primary kidney transplant recipients. *Transplantation*, **73**:1100–1106.

Ciancio G, Burke GW, Gaynor JJ, et al. (2005) A randomized trial of three renal transplant induction antibodies: early comparison of tacrolimus, mycophenolate mofetil, and steroid dosing, and newer immune-monitoring. *Transplantation*, **80**:457–465.

Ciancio G, Burke GW, Gaynor JJ, et al. (2006) A randomized long-term trial of tacrolimus/sirolimus versus tacrolimums/mycophenolate versus cyclosporine/sirolimus in renal transplantation: three-year analysis. *Transplantation*, **81**:845–852.

Ciancio G, Burke GW, Gaynor JJ, et al. (2008a) Randomized trial of mycophenolate mofetil versus enteric-coated mycophenolate sodium in primary renal transplant recipients given tacrolimus and daclizumab/thymoglobulin: one year follow-up. *Transplantation*, **86**:67–74.

Ciancio G, Burke GW, Gaynor JJ, et al. (2008b) Campath-1H induction therapy in African American and Hispanic first renal transplant recipients: 3-year actuarial follow-up. *Transplantation*, **85**:507–516.

Ciancio G, Gaynor JJ, Sageshima J, et al. (2011) Randomized trial of dual antibody induction therapy with steroid avoidance in renal transplantation. *Transplantation*, **92**:1348–1357.

Clatworthy MR (2011) Targeting B cells and antibody in transplantation. *Am J Transplant*, **11**:1359–1367.

Clatworthy MR, Sivaprakasam R, Butler AJ, Watson CJ (2007) Subcutaneous administration of alemtuzumab in simultaneous pancreas-kidney transplantation. *Transplantation*, **84**:1563–1567.

Crew RJ, Ratner LE (2010) ABO-incompatible kidney transplantation: current practice and the decade ahead. *Curr Opin Organ Transplant*, **15**:526–530.

Csencsits K, Wood SC, Lu G, et al. (2006) Transforming growth factor beta-induced connective tissue growth factor and chronic allograft rejection. *Am J Transplant*, **6**:959–966.

D'Errico A, Corti B, Pinna AD, et al. (2003) Granzyme B and perforin as predictive markers for acute rejection in human intestinal transplantation. *Transplant Proc*, **35**:3061–3065.

Danger R, Giral M, Soulillou JP, Brouard S (2008) Rationale and criteria of eligibility for calcineurin inhibitor interruption following kidney transplantation. *Curr Opin Organ Transplant*, **13**:609–613.

Dausset J, Rapaport FT, Colombani J, Feingold N (1965) A leucocyte group and its relationship to tissue histocompatibility in man. *Transplantation*, **3**:701–705.

Dickenmann M, Oettl T, Mihatsch MJ (2008) Osmotic nephrosis: acute kidney injury with accumulation of proximal tubular lysosomes due to administration of exogenous solutes. *Am J Kidney Dis*, **51**:491–503.

Doherty PC, Zinkernagel RM (1975) A biological role for the major histocompatibility antigens. *Lancet*, **1**:1406–1409.

Dunn PPJ (2011) Human leucocyte antigen typing: techniques and technology, a critical appraisal. *Int J Immunogenet*, **38**:463–473.

Durrbach A, Pestana JM, Pearson T, et al. (2010) A phase III study of belatacept versus cyclosporine in kidney transplants from extended criteria donors (BENEFIT-EXT study). *Am J Transplant*, **10**:547–557.

Eng HS, Leffell MS (2011) Histocompatibility testing after fifty years of transplantation. *J Immunolog Meth*, **369**:1–21.

Erren M, Arlt M, Willeke P, et al. (1999) Predictive value of the CD45RO positive T-helper lymphocyte subset for acute cellular rejection during the early phase after kidney transplantation. *Transplant Proc*, **31**:319–321.

European FK506 Multicentre Liver Study Group (1994) Randomised trial comparing tacrolimus (FK506) and cyclosporin in prevention of liver allograft rejection. *Lancet*, **344**:423–428.

European Mycophenolate Mofetil Cooperative Study Group (1995) Placebo-controlled study of mycophenolate mofetil combined with cyclosporin and corticosteroids for prevention of acute rejection. *Lancet*, **345**:1321–1325.

Farkas SA, Schnitzbauer AA, Kirchner G, Obed A, Banas B, Schlitt HJ (2009) Calcineurin inhibitor minimization protocols in liver transplantation. *Transplant Int*, **22**:49–60.

Farney AC, Doares W, Rogers J, et al. (2009) A randomized trial of alemtuzumab versus antithymocyte globulin induction in renal and pancreas transplantation. *Transplantation*, **88**:810–819.

Farney AC, Doares W, Kaczmorski S, Rogers J, Stratta RJ (2010) Cost-effective immunosuppressive options for solid organ transplantation: a guide to lower cost for the renal transplant recipient in the USA. *Immunotherapy*, **2**:879–888.

Faye A, van den Abeele T, Peuchmaur M, Mathieu-Boue A, Vilmer E (1998) Anti-CD20 monoclonal antibody for post-transplant lymphoproliferative disorders. *Lancet*, **352**:1285.

Feola M, Rovetto M, Soriano R, Cho SY, Wiener L (1976) Glucocorticoid protection of the myocardial cell membrane and the reduction of edema in experimental acute myocardial ischemia. *J Thorac Cardiovasc Surg*, **72**:631–643.

Feucht HE, Felber E, Gokel MJ, et al. (1991) Vascular deposition of complement-split products in kidney allografts with cell-mediated rejection. *Clin Exp Immunol*, **86**:464–470.

Feucht HE, Schneeberger H, Hillebrand G, et al. (1993) Capillary deposition of C4d complement fragment and early renal graft loss. *Kidney Int*, **43**:1333–1338.

Flechner SM, Goldfarb D, Modlin C, et al. (2002) Kidney transplantation without calcineurin inhibitor drugs: a prospective, randomized trial of sirolimus versus cyclosporine. *Transplantation*, **74**:1070–1076.

Fornoni, A., Sageshima, J., Wei, C., et al. (2011) Rituximab targets podocytes in recurrent focal segmental glomerulosclerosis. *Sci Translation Med*, **3**:85ra46.

Gaber AO, Knight RJ, Patel S, Gaber LW (2010) A review of the evidence for use of thymoglobulin induction in renal transplantation. *Transplant Proc*, **42**:1395–1400.

Gea-Banacloche JC (2010) Rituximab-associated infections. *Sem Hematol*, **47**:187–198.

Goggins WC, Pascual MA, Powelson JA, et al. (2003) A prospective, randomized, clinical trial of intraoperative versus postoperative Thymoglobulin in adult cadaveric renal transplant recipients. *Transplantation*, **76**:798–802.

Goland S, Czer LS, Coleman B, et al. (2008) Induction therapy with thymoglobulin after heart transplantation: impact of therapy duration on lymphocyte depletion and recovery, rejection, and cytomegalovirus infection rates. *J Heart Lung Transplant*, **27**:1115–1121.

Gorer PA, Boyse EA (1959) Pathological changes in F1 hybrid mice following transplantation of spleen cells from donors of the parental strains. *Immunology*, **2**:182–193.

Goulmy E (1996) Human minor histocompatibility antigens. *Curr Opin Immunol*, **8**:75–81.

Goulmy E (2006) Minor histocompatibility antigens: from transplantation problems to therapy of cancer. *Hum Immunol*, **67**:433–438.

Groth CG, Backman L, Morales JM, et al. (1999) Sirolimus (rapamycin)-based therapy in human renal transplantation: similar efficacy and different toxicity compared with cyclosporine. Sirolimus European Renal Transplant Study Group. *Transplantation*, **67**:1036–1042.

Guerra G, Srinivas TR, Meier-Kriesche HU (2007) Calcineurin inhibitor-free immunosuppression in kidney transplantation. *Transplant Int*, **20**:813–827.

Hammond ME, Stehlik J, Snow G, et al. (2005) Utility of histologic parameters in screening for antibody-mediated rejection of the cardiac allograft: a study of 3,170 biopsies. *J Heart Lung Transplant*, **24**:2015–2021.

Hancock WW, Wang L, Ye Q, Han R, Lee I (2003) Chemokines and their receptors as markers of allograft rejection and targets for immunosuppression. *Curr Opin Immunol*, **15**:479–486.

Hardinger KL, Schnitzler MA, Miller B, et al. (2004) Five-year follow up of thymoglobulin versus ATGAM induction in adult renal transplantation. *Transplantation*, **78**:136–141.

Hennecke J, Wiley DC (2001) T cell receptor-MHC interactions up close. *Cell*, **104**:1–4.

Ikegami M, Nagano T, Hara Y, et al. (1995) Tissue type plasminogen activator (t-PA) and plasminogen activator inhibitor (PAI) in transplanted kidneys. *Nippon Hinyokika Gakkai Zasshi*, **86**:991–995.

Jiang S, Herrera O, Lechler RI (2004) New spectrum of allorecognition pathways: implications for graft rejection and transplantation tolerance. *Curr Opin Immunol*, **16**:550–557.

Jordan SC, Reinsmoen N, Peng A, et al. (2010) Advances in diagnosing and managing antibody-mediated rejection. *Pediatr Nephrol*, **25**:2035–2048.

Jordan SC, Kahwaji J, Toyoda M, Vo A (2011a) B-cell immunotherapeutics: emerging roles in solid organ transplantation. *Curr Opin Organ Transplant*, **16**:416–424.

Jordan SC, Toyoda M, Kahwaji J, Vo AA (2011b) Clinical aspects of intravenous immunoglobulin use in solid organ transplant recipients. *Am J Transplant*, **11**:196–202.

Joyce S, Mathew JM, Flye MW, Mohanakumar T (1992) A polymorphic human kidney-specific non-MHC alloantigen. Its possible role in tissue-specific allograft immunity. *Transplantation*, **53**:1119–1127.

Kahan BD (2000) Efficacy of sirolimus compared with azathioprine for reduction of acute renal allograft rejection: a randomised multicentre study. The Rapamune US Study Group. *Lancet*, **356**:194–202.

Kahan BD (2001) Sirolimus: a comprehensive review. *Expert Opin Pharmacother*, **2**:1903–1917.

Kahan BD, Julian BA, Pescovitz, MD, Vanrenterghem Y, Neylan J (1999a) Sirolimus reduces the incidence of acute rejection episodes despite lower cyclosporine doses in caucasian recipients of mismatched primary renal allografts: a phase II trial. Rapamune Study Group. *Transplantation*, **68**:1526–1532.

Kahan BD, Rajagopalan PR, Hall M (1999b) Reduction of the occurrence of acute cellular rejection among renal allograft recipients treated with basiliximab, a chimeric anti-interleukin-2-receptor monoclonal antibody. United States Simulect Renal Study Group. *Transplantation*, **67**:276–284.

Kelly P, Kahan BD (2002) Review: metabolism of immunosuppressant drugs. *Curr Drug metab*, **3**:275–287.

Kerby JD, Luo KL, Ding Q, et al. (1997) Immunolocalization of acidic fibroblast growth factor and receptors in the tubulointerstitial compartment of chronically rejected human renal allografts. *Transplantation*, **63**:988–995.

Kirk AD, Hale DA, Mannon RB, et al. (2003) Results from a human renal allograft tolerance trial evaluating the humanized CD52-specific monoclonal antibody alemtuzumab (CAMPATH-1H). *Transplantation*, **76**:120–129.

Kirk AD, Mannon RB, Kleiner DE, et al. (2005) Results from a human renal allograft tolerance trial evaluating T-cell depletion with alemtuzumab combined with deoxyspergualin. *Transplantation*, **80**:1051–1059.

Kirkman RL, Shapiro ME, Carpenter CB, et al.(1991) A randomized prospective trial of anti-Tac monoclonal antibody in human renal transplantation. *Transplantation*, **51**:107–113.

Knechtle SJ, Pirsch JD, Fechner HJ Jr, et al. (2003) Campath-1H induction plus rapamycin monotherapy for renal transplantation: results of a pilot study. *Am J Transplant*, **3**:722–730.

Knight SR, Morris PJ (2007) The clinical benefits of cyclosporine C2-level monitoring: a systematic review. *Transplantation*, **83**:1525–1535.

Knight SR, Morris PJ (2010) Steroid avoidance or withdrawal after renal transplantation increases the risk of acute rejection but decreases cardiovascular risk. A meta-analysis. *Transplantation*, **89**:1–14.

Knight SR, Morris PJ (2011) Steroid sparing protocols following nonrenal transplants; the evidence is not there. A systematic review and meta-analysis. *Transplant Int*, **24**:1198–1207.

Krensky AM (1997) The HLA system, antigen processing and presentation. *Kidney Int*, **58**:S2–7.

Kwakkel-van Erp JM, van de Graaf EA, Paantjens AWM, et al. (2008) The killer immunoglobulin-like receptor (KIR) group A haplotype is associated with bronchiolitis obliterans syndrome after lung transplantation. *J Heart Lung Transplant*, **27**:995–1001.

Lance EM, Batchelor JR (1968) Selective suppression of cellular immunity by antilymphocyte serum. *Transplantation*, **6**:490–491.

Larsen CP, Grinyo J, Medina-Pestana J, et al. (2010) Belatacept-based regimens versus a cyclosporine A-based regimen in kidney transplant recipients: 2-year results from the BENEFIT and BENEFIT-EXT studies. *Transplantation*, **90**:1528–1535.

Larson TS, Dean PG, Stegall et al. (2006) Complete avoidance of calcineurin inhibitors in renal transplantation: a randomized trial comparing sirolimus and tacrolimus. *Am J Transplant*, **6**:514–522.

Leget GA, Czuczman MS (1998) Use of rituximab, the new FDA-approved antibody. *Curr Opin Oncol*, **10**:548–551.

Lemstrom KB, Nykanen AI, Tikkanen JM, et al. (2004). Role of angiogenic growth factors in transplant coronary artery disease. *Annal Med*, **36**:184–193.

Lerut J, Bonaccorsi-Riani E, Finet P, Gianello P (2009) Minimization of steroids in liver transplantation. *Transplant Int*, **22**:2–19.

Lightner A, Concepcion W, Grimm P (2011) Steroid avoidance in renal transplantation. *Curr Opin Organ Transplant*, **16**:477–482.

Locke JE, Magro CM, Singer AL, et al. (2009) The use of antibody to complement protein C5 for salvage treatment of severe antibody-mediated rejection. *Am J Transplant*, **9**:231–235.

Lorber MI, Mulgaonkar S, Butt KM, et al. (2005) Everolimus versus mycophenolate mofetil in the prevention of rejection in de novo renal transplant recipients: a 3-year randomized, multicenter, phase III study. *Transplantation*, **80**:244–252.

Macdonald AS (2001) A worldwide, phase III, randomized, controlled, safety and efficacy study of a sirolimus/cyclosporine regimen for prevention of acute rejection in recipients of primary mismatched renal allografts. *Transplantation*, **71**:271–280.

Marks WH, Ilsley JN, Dharnidharka VR (2011) Posttransplantation lymphoproliferative disorder in kidney and heart transplant recipients receiving thymoglobulin: a systematic review. *Transplant Proc*, **43**:1395–1404.

Marsh SG (2012) Nomenclature for factors of the HLA system, update January 2012. *Tissue Antigen*, **79**:393–397.

Marsh SGE, Albert ED, Bodmer WF, et al. (2005) Nomenclature for factors of the HLA system, 2004. *Tissue Antigen*, **65**:301–369.

Mathew JM, Joyce S, Lawrence W, Mohanakumar T (1991) Evidence that antibodies eluted from rejected kidneys of HLA-identical transplants define a non-MHC alloantigen expressed on human kidneys. *Transplantation*, **52**:559–562.

Mauiyyedi S, Pelle PD, Saidman S, et al. (2001) Chronic humoral rejection: identification of antibody-mediated chronic renal allograft rejection by C4d deposits in peritubular capillaries. *J Am Soc Nephrol*, **12**:574–582.

Mayer AD, Dmitrewski J, Squifflet JP, et al. (1997) Multicenter randomized trial comparing tacrolimus (FK506) and cyclosporine in the prevention of renal allograft rejection: a report of the European Tacrolimus Multicenter Renal Study Group. *Transplantation*, **64**:436–443.

McKeage K (2011) Eculizumab: a review of its use in paroxysmal nocturnal haemoglobinuria. *Drugs*, **71**:2327–2345.

McTaggart RA, Gottlieb D, Brooks J, et al. (2003) Sirolimus prolongs recovery from delayed graft function after cadaveric renal transplantation. *Am J Transplant*, **3**:416–423.

Mengel M, Mueller I, Behrend M, et al. (2004) Prognostic value of cytotoxic T-lymphocytes and CD40 in biopsies with early renal allograft rejection. *Transplant Int*, **17**:293–300.

Mentzer RM Jr., Jahania MS, Lasley RD (1998) Tacrolimus as a rescue immunosuppressant after heart and lung transplantation. The U.S. Multicenter FK506 Study Group. *Transplantation*, **65**:109–113.

Mineo D, Sageshima J, Burke GW, Ricordi C (2009) Minimization and withdrawal of steroids in pancreas and islet transplantation. *Transplant Int*, **22**:20–37.

Mohty M (2007) Mechanisms of action of antithymocyte globulin: T-cell depletion and beyond. *Leukemia*, **21**:1387–1394.

Montgomery RA, Lonze BE, King KE, et al. (2011) Desensitization in HLA-incompatible kidney recipients and survival. *N Engl J Med*, **365**:318–326.

Morgan RD, O'Callaghan JM, Knight SR, Morris PJ (2012) Alemtuzumab induction therapy in kidney transplantation: a systematic review and meta-analysis. *Transplantation*, **93**(12):1179–1188.

Morris PJ, French ME, Dunnill MS, et al. (1983) A controlled trial of cyclosporine in renal transplantation with conversion to azathioprine and prednisolone after three months. *Transplantation*, **36**:273–277.

Mulay AV, Hussain N, Fergusson D, Knoll GA (2005) Calcineurin inhibitor withdrawal from sirolimus-based therapy in kidney transplantation: a systematic review of randomized trials. *Am J Transplant*, **5**:1748–1756.

Murray JE, Merrill JP, Harrison JH, Wilson RE, Dammin GJ (1963) Prolonged survival of human-kidney homografts by immunosuppressive drug therapy. *N Engl J Med*, **268**:1315–1323.

Nashan B (2005) Antibody induction therapy in renal transplant patients receiving calcineurin-inhibitor immunosuppressive regimens: a comparative review. *BioDrugs*, **19**:39–46.

Neuhaus P, Clavien PA, Kittur D, et al. (2002) Improved treatment response with basiliximab immunoprophylaxis after liver transplantation: results from a double-blind randomized placebo-controlled trial. *Liver Transplant*, **8**:132–142.

Nickeleit V, Andreoni K (2007) The classification and treatment of antibody-mediated renal allograft injury: where do we stand? (Comment.) *Kidney Int*, **71**:7–11.

O'Leary JG, Kaneku H, Susskind BM, et al. (2011) High mean fluorescence intensity donor-specific anti-HLA antibodies associated with chronic rejection postliver transplant. *Am J Transplant*, **11**:1868–1876.

Onrust SV, Wiseman LR (1999) Basiliximab. *Drugs*, **57**:207–213; discussion 214.

OPTN (2012) Organ Procurement and Transplantation Network and Scientific Registry of Transplant Recipients 2010 data report. *Am J Transplant*, **12**(Suppl 1):1–156.

Ozdemir BH, Ozdemir FN, Gungen Y, Haberal M (2002) Role of macrophages and lymphocytes in the induction of neovascularization in renal allograft rejection. *Am J Kidney Dis*, **39**:347–353.

Paczek L, Bartlomiejczyk I, Gradowska L, et al. (1996) Intraglomerular fibronectin and laminin turn-over in chronically rejected kidney allografts in humans. *Annal Transplant*, **1**:41–43.

Pascual J, Zamora J, Galeano C, Royuela A, Quereda C (2009) Steroid avoidance or withdrawal for kidney transplant recipients. *Cochrane Database Syst Rev*, 15(9):CD005632.

Pedagogos E, Hewitson TD, Walker RG, Nicholis KM, Becker GJ (1997) Myofibroblast involvement in chronic transplant rejection. *Transplantation*, **64**:1192–1197.

Penninga L, Wettergren A, Chan AW, Steinbruchel DA, Gluud C (2012) Calcineurin inhibitor minimisation versus continuation of calcineurin inhibitor treatment for liver transplant recipients. *Cochrane Database Systc Rev*, **3**:CD008852.

Pescovitz MD (2006) Rituximab, an anti-cd20 monoclonal antibody: history and mechanism of action. *Am J Transplant*, **6**:859–866.

Pilmore HL, Yan Y, Eris JM, Hennessy A, McCaughan GW, Bishop GA (2002) Time course of upregulation of fibrogenic growth factors and cellular infiltration in a rodent model of chronic renal allograft rejection. *Transplant Immunol*, **10**:245–254.

Pirsch JD, Miller J, Deierhoi MH, Vincenti F, Filo RS (1997) A comparison of tacrolimus (FK506) and cyclosporine for immunosuppression after cadaveric renal transplantation. FK506 Kidney Transplant Study Group. *Transplantation*, **63**:977–983.

Platt JL, Cascalho M (2011). Donor specific antibodies after transplantation. *Pediatr Transplant*, **15**:686–690.

Ponticelli C, Glassock RJ (2010) Posttransplant recurrence of primary glomerulonephritis. *Clin J Am Soc Nephrol*, **5**:2363–2372.

Racusen LC (2003) Immunopathology of organ transplantation. *Springer Seminar Immunopathol*, **25**:141–165.

Rintala JM, Savikko J, Rintala SE, von Willebrand E (2006) The effect of leflunomide analogue FK778 on development of chronic rat renal allograft rejection and transforming growth factor-BETA expression. *Transplant Proc*, **38**:3239–3240.

Robertson NJ, Chai JG, Millrain M, et al. (2007) Natural regulation of immunity to minor histocompatibility antigens. *J Immunol*, **178**:3558–3565.

Russell PS (1968) Antilymphocyte serum as an immunosuppressive agent. *Annal Intern Med*, **68**:483–486.

Sageshima J, Ciancio G, Chen L, Burke GW 3rd (2009) Anti-interleukin-2 receptor antibodies-basiliximab and daclizumab-for the prevention of acute rejection in renal transplantation. *Biologics*, **3**:319–336.

Sageshima J, Ciancio G, Guerra G, et al. (2011) Prolonged lymphocyte depletion by single-dose rabbit anti-thymocyte globulin and alemtuzumab in kidney transplantation. *Transplant Immunol*, **25**:104–111.

Salvadori M, Holzer H, de Mattos A, et al. (2004) Enteric-coated mycophenolate sodium is therapeutically equivalent to mycophenolate mofetil in de novo renal transplant patients. *Am J Transplant*, **4**:231–236.

Sayegh MH, Turka LA (1998) The role of T-cell costimulatory activation pathways in transplant rejection. *N Engl J Med*, **338**:1813–1821.

Shimizu A, Colvin RB (2005) Pathological features of antibody-mediated rejection. *Curr Drug Targets*, **5**:199–214.

Shyu S, Dew MA, Pilewski JM, et al. (2011) Five-year outcomes with alemtuzumab induction after lung transplantation. *J Heart Lung Transplant*, **30**:743–754.

Snell GD (1957) The genetics of transplantation. *Annal N Y Acad Sci*, **69**:555–560.

Solez K, Colvin RB, Racusen LC, et al. (2007) Banff '05 Meeting Report: differential diagnosis of chronic allograft injury and elimination of chronic allograft nephropathy ('CAN'). *Am J Transplant*, **7**:518–526.

Soliman T, Hetz H, Burghuber C, et al. (2007) Short-term induction therapy with anti-thymocyte globulin and delayed use of calcineurin inhibitors in orthotopic liver transplantation. *Liver Transplant*, **13**:1039–1044.

Sollinger HW (1995) Mycophenolate mofetil for the prevention of acute rejection in primary cadaveric renal allograft recipients. U.S. Renal Transplant Mycophenolate Mofetil Study Group. *Transplantation*, **60**:225–232.

Stallone G, Schena A, Infante B, et al. (2005) Sirolimus for Kaposi's sarcoma in renal-transplant recipients. *N Engl J Med*, **352**:1317–1323.

Starzl TE, Marchioro TL, Waddell WR (1963) The reversal of rejection in human renal homografts with subsequent development of homograft tolerance. *Surg Gynecol Obstetr*, **117**:385–395.

Starzl TE, Marchioro TL, Hutchinson DE, Porter KA, Cerilli GJ, Brettschneider L (1967) The clinical use of antilymphocyte globulin in renal homotransplantation. *Transplantation*, **5**(Suppl):1100–1105.

Starzl TE, Todo S, Fung J, Demetris AJ, Venkataramman R, Jain A (1989) FK 506 for liver, kidney, and pancreas transplantation. *Lancet*, **2**:1000–1004.

Stegall MD, Gloor J, Winters JL, Moore SB, Degoey S (2006) A comparison of plasmapheresis versus high-dose IVIG desensitization in renal allograft recipients with high levels of donor specific alloantibody. *Am J Transplant*, **6**:346–351.

Streblow DN, Dumortier J, Moses AV, Orloff SL, Nelson JA (2008) Mechanisms of cytomegalovirus-accelerated vascular disease: induction of paracrine factors that promote angiogenesis and wound healing. *Curr Topic Microbiol Immunol*, **325**:397–415.

Subramanian SV, Kelm RJ, Polikandriotis JA, Orosz CG, Strauch AR (2002) Reprogramming of vascular smooth muscle alpha-actin gene expression as an early indicator of dysfunctional remodeling following heart transplant. *Cardiovasc Res*, **54**:539–548.

Suthanthiran M, Strom TB (1994) Renal transplantation. *N Engl J Med*, **331**:365–376.

Suzuki J, Isobe M, Yamazaki S, Horie S, Okubo Y, Sekiguchi M (1997) Inhibition of accelerated coronary atherosclerosis with short-term blockade of intercellular adhesion molecule-1 and lymphocyte function-associated antigen-1 in a heterotopic murine model of heart transplantation. *J Heart Lung Transplant*, **16**:1141–1148.

Takeda A, Horike K, Ohtsuka Y, et al. (2011) Current problems of chronic active antibody-mediated rejection. *Clin Transplant*, **25**(Suppl 23):2–5.

Tanabe K, Ishida H, Shimizu T, Omoto K, Shirakawa H, Tokumoto T (2009) Evaluation of two different preconditioning regimens for ABO-incompatible living kidney donor transplantation. A comparison of splenectomy vs. rituximab-treated non-splenectomy preconditioning regimens. *Contrib Nephrol*, **162**:61–74.

Tanabe M, Kawachi S, Obara H, et al. (2010) Current progress in ABO-incompatible liver transplantation. *Eur J Clin Invest*, **40**:943–949.

Ter Meulen CG, Baan CC, Hene RJ, Hilbrands LB, Hoitsma AJ (2001) Two doses of daclizumab are sufficient for prolonged interleukin-2Ralpha chain blockade. *Transplantation*, **72**:1709–1710.

Teuteberg JJ, Shullo MA, Zomak R, et al. (2010) Alemtuzumab induction prior to cardiac transplantation with lower intensity maintenance immunosuppression: one-year outcomes. *Am J Transplant*, **10**:382–388.

Thomson AW, Starzl TE (1993) New immunosuppressive drugs: mechanistic insights and potential therapeutic advances. *Immunol Reviews*, **136**:71–98.

Tighe H, Friend PJ, Collier SJ, et al. (1988) Delayed allograft rejection in primates treated with anti-IL-2 receptor monoclonal antibody Campath-6. *Transplantation*, **45**:226–228.

Toki D, Ishida H, Horita S, Setoguchi K, Yamaguchi Y, Tanabe K (2009) Impact of low-dose rituximab on splenic B cells in ABO-incompatible renal transplant recipients. *Transplant Int*, **22**:447–454.

Truong LD, Barrios R, Adrogue HE, Gaber LW (2007) Acute antibody-mediated rejection of renal transplant: pathogenetic and diagnostic considerations. *Arch Pathol Lab Med*, **131**:1200–1208.

Tzakis AG, Kato T, Nishida S, et al. (2003) Preliminary experience with campath 1H (C1H) in intestinal and liver transplantation. *Transplantation*, **75**:1227–1231.

US Multicenter FK506 Liver Study Group (1994) A comparison of tacrolimus (FK 506) and cyclosporine for immunosuppression in liver transplantation. *N Engl J Med*, **331**:1110–1115.

Vanrenterghem Y, Bresnahan B, Campistol J, et al. (2011) Belatacept-based regimens are associated with improved cardiovascular and metabolic risk factors compared with cyclosporine in kidney transplant recipients (BENEFIT and BENEFIT-EXT studies). *Transplantation*, **91**:976–983.

Vianna RM, Mangus RS, Fridell JA, Weigman S, Kazimi M, Tector J (2008) Induction immunosuppression with thymoglobulin and rituximab in intestinal and multivisceral transplantation. *Transplantation*, **85**:1290–1293.

Vincenti F, Lantz M, Birnbaum J, et al. (1997) A phase I trial of humanized anti-interleukin 2 receptor antibody in renal transplantation. *Transplantation*, **63**:33–38.

Vincenti F, Kirkman R, Light S, et al. (1998) Interleukin-2-receptor blockade with daclizumab to prevent acute rejection in renal transplantation. Daclizumab Triple Therapy Study Group. *N Engl J Med*, **338**:161–165.

Vincenti F, Larsen C, Durrbach A, et al. (2005) Costimulation blockade with belatacept in renal transplantation. *N Engl J Med*, **353**:770–781.

Vincenti F, Charpentier B, Vanrenterghem Y, et al. (2010) A phase III study of belatacept-based immunosuppression regimens versus cyclosporine in renal transplant recipients (BENEFIT study). *Am J Transplant*, **10**:535–546.

Vitko S, Margreiter R, Weimar W, et al. (2004) Everolimus (Certican) 12-month safety and efficacy versus mycophenolate mofetil in de novo renal transplant recipients. *Transplantation*, **78**:1532–1540.

Vo AA, Lukovsky M, Toyoda M, et al. (2008a) Rituximab and intravenous immune globulin for desensitization during renal transplantation. *N Engl J Med*, **359**:242–251.

Vo AA, Wechsler EA, Wang J, et al. (2008b) Analysis of subcutaneous (SQ) alemtuzumab induction therapy in highly sensitized patients desensitized with IVIG and rituximab. *Am J Transplant*, **8**:144–149.

Wagrowska-Danilewicz M, Danilewicz M (2003) Immunoexpression of perforin and granzyme B on infiltrating lymphocytes in human renal acute allograft rejection. *Nefrologia*, **23**:538–544.

Walker JK, Scholz LM, Scheetz MH, et al. (2007) Leukopenia complicates cytomegalovirus prevention after renal transplantation with alemtuzumab induction. *Transplantation*, **83**:874–882.

Waller JR, Brook NR, Bicknell GR, Nicholson ML (2004) Differential effects of modern immunosuppressive agents on the development of intimal hyperplasia. *Transplant Int*, **17**:9–14.

Wang P, Zhu L, Liu T, Zhang X, Qiu Y (1999) Intragraft CD45 RO gene expression is an early marker to detect small bowel allograft rejection in rats. *Microsurgery*, **19**:348–350.

Webster A, Woodroffe RC, Taylor RS, Chapman JR, Craig JC (2005) Tacrolimus versus cyclosporin as primary immunosuppression for kidney transplant recipients. *Cochrane Database Syst Rev*, **19**(4):CD003961.

Webster A, Pankhurst T, Rinaldi F, Chapman JR, Craig JC (2006) Polyclonal and monoclonal antibodies for treating acute rejection episodes in kidney transplant recipients. *Cochrane Database Syst Rev*, **19**(2):CD004756.

Webster AC, Ruster LP, Mcgee R, et al. (2010) Interleukin 2 receptor antagonists for kidney transplant recipients. *Cochrane Database Syst Rev*, **20**(1):CD003897.

Willicombe M, Roufosse C, Brookes P, et al. (2011) Antibody-mediated rejection after alemtuzumab induction: incidence, risk factors, and predictors of poor outcome. *Transplantation*, **92**:176–182.

Woodle ES, Peddi VR, Tomlanovich S, Mulgaonkar S, Kuo PC (2010) A prospective, randomized, multicenter study evaluating early corticosteroid withdrawal with Thymoglobulin in living-donor kidney transplantation. *Clin Transplant*, **24**:73–83.

Woodle ES, Walsh RC, Alloway RR, Girnita A, Brailey P (2011) Proteasome inhibitor therapy for antibody-mediated rejection. *Pediatr Transplant*, **15**:548–556.

Yun JJ, Whiting D, Fischbein MP, et al. (2004) Combined blockade of the chemokine receptors CCR1 and CCR5 attenuates chronic rejection. *Circulation*, **109**:932–937.

Zembala M, Wojnicz R, Zakliczynski M, et al. (1997) Cellular adhesion molecules changes in myocardium during first year post heart transplant. *Annal Transplant*, **2**:16–19.

Zimmerhackl LB, Hofer J, Cortina G, et al. (2010) Prophylactic eculizumab after renal transplantation in atypical hemolytic-uremic syndrome. *N Engl J Med*, **362**:1746–1748.

Zimmerman JJ, Harper D, Getsy J, Jusko WJ (2003) Pharmacokinetic interactions between sirolimus and microemulsion cyclosporine when orally administered jointly and 4 hours apart in healthy volunteers. *J Clin Pharmacol*, **43**:1168–1176.

Zuckermann AO, Aliabadi AZ (2009) Calcineurin-inhibitor minimization protocols in heart transplantation. *Transplant Int*, **22**:78–89.

# CHAPTER 12

# Xenotransplantation

Kazuhiko Yamada, Joseph Scalea, and Masayuki Tasaki

## Introduction

Transplantation is the only cure end-stage liver, kidney, heart, and lung disease. Although improvements in operative technique and immunosuppression have paved the way for increases in the organ donor pool through living donor kidney donation, there remains a vast disparity between the number of organs available for transplantation and the demand for these organs. Indeed, progress has been made in the fields of regenerative medicine and stem cell technologies (Takahashi and Yamanaka 2006; Takahashi et al., 2007; Ott et al., 2008; Kobayashi et al., 2010; Green et al., 2011 ); yet, at the present time, de-novo and regenerated tissues are not capable of sustaining life in animal models. However, these are not the only options for organ replacement. Xenotransplantation, or the transplantation of organs across species, would provide an inexhaustible supply of donor organs. This necessity has led to a resurgence of interest in the clinical potential of xenotransplants since 2005.

The first xenotransplants were carried out long before allogeneic transplantation. However, until recently, these attempts resulted in failure, partly due to a lack of understanding of the immunological significance of interspecies antigenicity. Recently, enormous progress has been made in the quest for successful xenotransplantation, but the field remains one of preclinical research, not of clinically available therapy. Because the field of xenotransplantation is heavily dependent on large animal models and because the technical aspects are surgically complex, in this chapter we will attempt to explain with clarity the nuances of clinical xenotransplantation as they relate to the surgeon and to the anaesthesiologist.

## A brief history of solid organ xenotransplantation

Although the anecdotal history of xenotransplantation dates back to ancient times, it was not until the 1960s, with the advent of immunosuppressive drugs, that serious attempts at clinical xenotransplantation began. In 1963 Reemtsma transplanted a kidney from a rhesus monkey into a 43-year-old male across a concordant xenogeneic barrier, using an immunosuppressive approach to prevent rejection (Reemtsma et al., 1964). The patient died 63 days post-transplantation. The following year he transplanted a chimpanzee kidney into a patient, who survived for 9 months; this remains the longest known surviving xenotransplanted organ (Reemtsma et al., 1964). Also in 1964, Hardy conducted the first cardiac xenotransplantation, replacing a human heart with that of a chimpanzee (Hardy et al., 1964), but the patient died 90 minutes after the transplant. Soon thereafter, Hitchcock and Starzl transplanted baboon kidneys into six human patients, with variable survival ranging from 19 to 98 days (Starzl et al., 1964). In 1969 Bertoye and Marion reported two liver transplants, from baboon to human, with one patient surviving 4 months and the other 39 hours (Bertoye et al., 1969). In the early 1970s Starzl reported liver xenotransplantation from chimpanzee to human, with survivals up to 15 days (Giles et al., 1970; Starzl et al., 1974). Clearly, the early results with xenotransplantation were not encouraging.

Based largely on these results, clinical xenotransplantation almost vanished, as interest and understanding of allogeneic transplantation intensified. However, as allogeneic transplantation became increasingly successful, the inability of supply to meet demand became quickly apparent and there was again interest in xenotransplantation. In 1984 Bailey transplanted an ABO-incompatible baboon heart into a 12-day-old baby girl named Baby Fae (Bailey et al., 1985). There was enormous media attention to this event, but the baby's survival of only 20 days led to disappointment. It wasn't until 1992, with the advent of tacrolimus, a now common form of maintenance immunosuppression which is 100 times more potent than previously available cyclosporine, that Starzl reinitiated clinical efforts in the field. Starzl subsequently transplanted baboon livers into two human recipients, who survived for 70 and 26 days post-transplantation, respectively.

Preformed natural antibodies do not impede transplantation between the majority of non-human primates and humans. However, other issues, including the availability of organ donors, ethical concerns associated with the use of any non-human primate donors, and transmission of pathogenic viruses, which are more likely to cross into humans from a closely related species than from a more distant one, prevent further consideration of non-human primates being used as xenogeneic donors.

## Choice of the most appropriate donor species

Although the most successful clinical xenotransplants have been from non-human primates to humans, currently the pig is viewed as the most acceptable source of organs for future xenotransplantation (Sachs, 1994). Pigs have many advantages. First, the supply of pigs is essentially inexhaustible. Biologically, pigs have favourable breeding characteristics, reproducing in 3-month gestation cycles, and are physiologically and anatomically similar to humans. Partially inbred Massachusetts General Hospital (MGH) miniature swine, which were developed by David H. Sachs and pedigree-bred for the past 35 years, are a particularly attractive choice (Sachs, 1994; Mezrich et al., 2003). Their maximum adult weights are approximately 120 kg, which is similar to that of humans, in contrast to domestic swine, which can weigh in excess of 500 kg. Three lines of inbred miniature swine are maintained. Each line is homozygous for a different MHC haplotype represented by the swine leucocyte antigens $SLA^a$, $SLA^c$, and $SLA^d$, which are analogous to HLA in humans. Five lines bearing different intra-MHC recombinant haplotypes are also maintained. One subline, $SLA^{dd}$, was chosen for successive inbreeding. Sequential mating of brother–sister pairs has resulted in an inbred line of miniature swine with a coefficient of inbreeding of > 96%. This high degree of consanguinity permits acceptance of transplants among offspring within the line without immunosuppressive drugs (Mezrich et al., 2003). Further, if immunological tolerance can be induced across a xenogeneic barrier using these inbred swine, these donors (see the section 'Immunological barriers of xenotransplantation in a pig to primate model') should make it possible to exchange a failed organ for another immunologically identical organ, without manipulation of the immune response.

Until recently, hyperacute rejection (HAR) caused by natural preformed xenoreactive antibodies directed against the oligosaccharide galactose α-1,3-galactose (Gal) (Galili et al., 1987, 1988a, 1996; Cooper et al., 1993; Galili, 1993a) was a major hurdle in pig-to-human discordant xenotransplantation. To avoid this problem, in 2002 two groups, including our colleagues, produced galactosyltransferase knockout (GalT-KO) pigs, which do not express the Gal epitope (Phelps et al., 2003; Kolber-Simonds et al., 2004). In the research centres of the authors and our colleagues, the nucleus was taken from a fibroblast cell line derived from the most highly inbred $SLA^{dd}$ subline of MGH miniature swine and this cell line was then subjected to homologous recombination and selection to ablate expression of the α-1,3-GalT gene (Lai et al., 2002; Kolber-Simonds et al., 2004). This process allowed for the production of a GalT-KO animal from our most highly inbred line of miniature swine (Mezrich et al., 2003). This line of inbred swine could be used to replace transplanted organs that have failed due to technical reasons or non-immunological causes with a genetically identical organ. These homozygous GalT-KO animals demonstrated no Gal expression on their cells; in fact, they produced natural anti-Gal antibodies (Dor et al., 2004). We have reported the initial results using GalT-KO animals in a pig to baboon model, demonstrating that HAR was completely eliminated in both kidney and heart models (Kuwaki et al., 2005; Yamada et al., 2005a) (see the section 'Immunological barriers of xenotransplantation in a pig to primate model').

## Immunological barriers of xenotransplantation in a pig to primate model

Because the immune system of a recipient recognizes the antigenic differences of a different species as greater than those within a species, the immunological barriers to xenotransplantation are more powerful than those encountered for allotransplantation. Some of the immunological reactions that characterize major xenograft rejection are described in the following sections.

### Anti-xeno humoral responses

HAR occurs within the first 24 hours and is generally caused by xenoreactive antibodies (predominately of the IgM subclass) (Oriol et al., 1993; Sandrin et al., 1993; McKenzie et al., 1994; Parker et al., 1994; Sandrin and McKenzie 1994; Lin et al., 1997a, 1997b). Antibody binding induces complement-dependent cytotoxicity of target cells. This is a complex and coordinated event that leads to graft loss in seconds–minutes (Platt et al., 1990a, 1990b, 1991, 1994; Kearns-Jonker et al., 1997). In humans and non-human primates the predominating preformed natural antibodies (Nabs) are to Gal, as mentioned earlier (see the section 'Choice of the most appropriate donor species') (Galili et al., 1985; Cooper et al., 1993, 1994; Galili, 1993a, 1993b). It is believed that a frame shift mutation in the gene encoding the enzyme α-1,3-GalT rendered it inactive (Galili et al., 1988b; Galili, 1993a) in primates. Old World primates and humans are presumably sensitized and form antibody to Gal soon after birth by Gal-expressing micro-organisms that colonize the gut. As much as 70–90% of human preformed IgM antibodies to pig are directed against this single sugar epitope (Buonomano et al., 1999; Diaz et al., 2003). The aggregate cytotoxicity of all other human anti-pig Nabs is less than one-tenth that of the anti-Gal Nabs (Parker et al., 1994). As described in the section 'Choice of the most appropriate donor species'), HAR was eliminated by utilizing GalT-KO organs in both kidney and heart models (Kuwaki et al., 2005; Yamada et al., 2005a) (more details in the section 'Anti-xeno cellular responses').

### Anti-xeno cellular responses

Prior to overcoming HAR, xenogeneic T-cellular responses were underappreciated. Studies of discordant xenogeneic reactions originally conducted in mice suggested that responder antigen-presenting cells (APC) were required for T-cell recognition (*indirect pathway*) of xenogeneic antigens (Yamada et al., 1995b; Dorling et al., 1996b; Garrovillo et al., 1999). However, it now appears that the mouse may be unusual in this regard, since human T-cells have been demonstrated to react directly with stimulators of other species (*direct pathway*) (Yamada et al., 1995b; Baker et al., 2001), including pig endothelial cells. T-cell responses are crucial for both xenograft acceptance and/or rejection (Alter and Bach, 1990; Moses et al., 1990, 1992; Auchincloss et al., 1993; Kirk et al., 1993; Kumagai-Braesch et al., 1993; Yamada et al., 1995a, 1995b, 1996; Chan and Auchincloss, 1996; Dorling et al., 1996a).

The same immunosuppressive drugs that were developed to suppress cellular immunity to allografts have been used in xenotransplantation. However, the required doses for these agents are markedly higher than is necessary for allotransplantation (Kozlowski et al., 1999c; Barth et al., 2003; Chen et al., 2005; Hering et al., 2006). Despite higher drug doses, complete inhibition of antidonor T-cell-dependent antibody formation has not been achieved. Therefore the levels of chemical immunosuppression required to avoid rejection of a xenograft are prohibitively high. For these reasons, xenogeneic tolerance represents the 'holy grail' of xenotransplantation (Latinne et al., 1993; Sykes and Sachs, 1997; Alwayn et al., 1999; Kozlowski et al., 1999c; Smith and Mandel 2000; Appel, III et al., 2001a, 2001b; Barth et al., 2003; Lan et al., 2004).

At the Massachusetts General Hospital in Boston two tolerance strategies have been attempted: (1) a *mixed chimerism* (i.e. mixed lymphohaematopoietic reconstitution) approach; and (2) a *thymic tissue transplantation* approach (Auchincloss and Sachs, 1983a, 1983b; Kappler et al., 1987; Marrack et al., 1988; Arnold et al., 1990, 1993; Burkly et al., 1990; Heeg and Wagner 1990; Brombacher et al., 1991; Hoffmann et al., 1992; Tomita et al., 1994; Carrier et al., 1995; Colson et al., 1995, 2000; Eto et al., 1999; Nikolic et al., 1999; Ito et al., 2001; Bhattacharyya et al., 2002; Rodriguez-Barbosa et al., 2002). With the mixed chimerism approach either bone marrow (BM) or cytokine-mobilized peripheral blood progenitor cells (PBPC) are infused into immunocompromised baboons (Kozlowski et al., 1998, 1999a, 1999b) in order to achieve long-term haematopoietic chimerism (Sablinski et al., 1997, 1999; Kozlowski et al., 1999a, 1999b). Although successful tolerance induction has been achieved across an allogeneic barrier, investigators have met limited success with the mixed chimerism approach across a xenogeneic barrier. However, preliminary data from the development of GalT-KO/CD47 transgenic swine as BM donors and ex-vivo transfection of donor BM cells with CD47 have been encouraging (Am J Transplant. 2014 Dec;14(12):2713-22).

The other tolerance strategy is to transplant porcine vascularized thymus to induce tolerance. Thus far this strategy is the most successful in life-supporting kidney transplant models (i.e. cotransplantation of vascularized thymus with kidneys). The author, Yamada, has developed two methods of transplanting vascularized thymic tissue: either by direct vascular anastomosis of the thymic blood supply, so-called vascularized thymic lobe transplantation (LaMattina et al., 2002; Kamano et al., 2004) or as a 'thymokidney' (prepared by injecting autologous thymic tissue under the renal capsule in donors and allowing 2 months for neovascularization prior to transplantation) (Yamada et al., 1999, 2000a) (see Figure 12.1).

Our studies have demonstrated functional thymopoiesis in transplanted thymic grafts and donor-specific tolerance induction across a full MHC mismatch barrier in an allogeneic miniature swine model (Yamada et al., 2000b, 2003; Kamano et al., 2004). By utilizing GalT-KO animals as donors for either vascularized thymic grafts or thymokidneys, our initial attempts have resulted in markedly prolonged renal xenograft survival with normal renal function for > 80 days (Yamada et al., 2005b). Because infection was a concern in the initial group, a modified immunotolerance regimen was designed lacking steroids and whole-body irradiation. The modified regimen led to an improvement in average survival from 34 to > 50 days (Griesemer et al., 2009). Long-term survivors demonstrated donor-specific unresponsiveness in vitro in Cytotoxic T lymphocyte assays along with evidence of thymopoiesis in transplanted porcine thymic grafts, suggesting these baboons were on a path towards tolerance. Recent findings using this vascularized thymus plus kidney model have shown the importance of optimal T-cell depletion in the induction period. We have determined that T-cell depletion (1) was essential for avoidance of rejection, (2) may lead to lethal infection if too extensive, and (3) likely requires maintenance at an optimal level (in our experience 50–150 T-cells/μL in the peripheral blood) during the first 2 weeks following attempted induction of xenotransplantation tolerance of vascularized grafts (Nishimura et al., 2011).

## Delayed xenograft rejection

Delayed xenograft rejection (DXR) is associated with the increased deposition of antipig antibodies in the xenograft and likely involves preformed non-Gal Abs and/or induced antipig Abs, complement, macrophages, and activation of coagulation (Bach et al., 1996; Ierino et al., 1998; Chen et al., 2004; Shimizu et al., 2008, 2011). Morphologically, DXR is characterized by the development of thrombotic microangiopathy, platelet aggregation, and macrophage infiltration (Bach et al., 1996; Candinas et al., 1996; Ierino et al., 1998). It is likely that preformed non-Gal Nabs or newly induced, T-cell-dependent antibodies to other pig determinants mediate this process. In order to avoid DXR, several attempts can be considered, including (1) absorption of anti-non-Gal preformed Nab and (2) transgenic GalT-KO donors with transgenic regulatory proteins such as human decay accelerating factor (hDAF) (CD55), membrane cofactor protein (MCP), CD59 (inhibitor of the

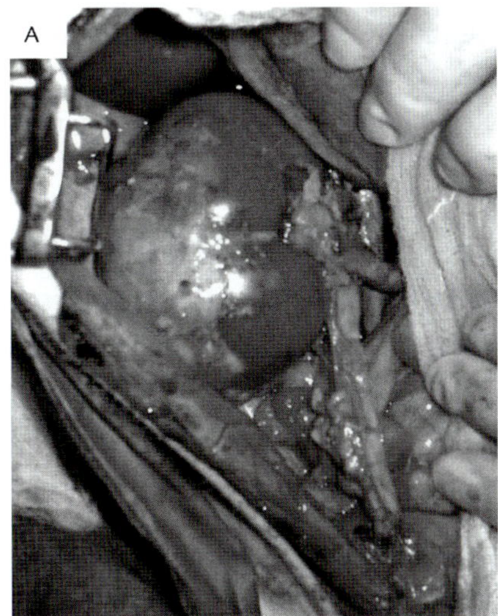


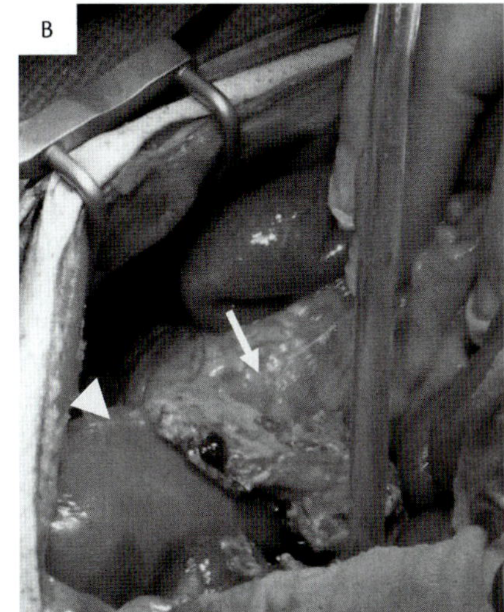


**Fig. 12.1** Gross findings of a GalT-KO porcine thymokidney (A) and a vascularized thymic lobe graft (arrow) with a kidney (arrowhead) simultaneously transplanted (B) in baboon recipients (1 hour after reperfusion)

formation of the membrane attack complex), and human membrane cofactor protein (hMCP) (CD46), and more recently CD39 or CD47 (Bhatti et al., 1999; Buhler et al., 2000, 2001).

## Advantages of xenotransplantation using pig donors

The single most compelling rationale for xenotransplantation is the severe shortage of organs and the tremendous improvement in morbidity and mortality seen with organ transplantation. However, in addition to availability, xenogeneic organs could have a number of benefits over their allogeneic counterparts. Among these are:

- The potential to cure or alleviate diseases caused by human-specific viruses: many human-tropic viruses, including viral hepatitis and HIV (Starzl et al., 1993; Mueller et al., 2002), would be incapable of infecting a pig organ.
- Potential for gene delivery: the transplantation of tissues or organs from genetically engineered animals producing desired gene products (antineoplastic modalities, congenitally absent proteins and enzymes, etc.), either constitutively or under regulation, would be uniquely possible with xenotransplantation (Lin and Platt, 1998; Platt, 2000).
- Avoidance of the risk of human disease transmission to the organ recipient and/or to healthcare personnel: although the risk of infection with endogenous viruses (such as porcine endogenous retrovirus—PERV) has been the subject of considerable interest and investigation (Patience et al., 1998), its relevance has been largely disproven. However, the unfortunate occurrence of transmission of occult tumours and infections, which have been reported following allotransplantation, should be avoidable with the use of xenografts.
- Ease of coordination and cost-effectiveness: the administrative efforts and the multilevel coordination required to perform cadaveric organ transplantation is both time-consuming and costly. Both of these pressing issues would be minimized using xenotransplantation. This is because xenotransplantation would be elective and conveniently timed. The elective nature of the procedures would avoid many of the pressures associated with current cadaver donor selection and distribution. In addition, the costs of donor organ procurement and preservation would be essentially eliminated.
- Capacity for retransplantation: given the essentially unlimited supply of porcine organs, a recipient would be able to receive a replacement organ as needed—whether because of technical failure or loss of function for other reasons. Indeed, using the approach being developed in the laboratory of the authors, the donors will be inbred (i.e. genetically identical) animals and tolerance induction to many of the major antigens will be part of the preparative regimen (Ierino et al., 1999; Utsugi et al., 2001; Mezrich et al., 2003). Under these circumstances, replacement of a failed organ for any reason other than rejection should be possible without need for any additional immunosuppression.

## Surgical approach to xenotransplantation

As described in the section 'Anti-xeno cellular responses', the best results with xenotransplantation have been achieved in preclinical models of life-supporting renal xenotransplantation of GalT-KO kidneys from swine to thymectomized baboons using simultaneous transplantation of the vascularized thymus. For this reason much of this section will be centred on the procedures required to safely and reproducibly perform this complex procedure.

### Donor selection and preparation

Selection and management of the donor are crucial to success of the surgical transplant. First, donor pigs grow to near-full adult weight in 12–18 months, whereas baboons grow much more slowly. In addition, adult baboons are much smaller than adult pigs. Second, the donor (in many cases) must undergo two procedures prior to the actual transplant: (1) placement of the autologous thymus beneath the renal capsule to prepare the 'thymokidney' (Yamada et al., 1999, 2000a) in donors, and (2) donor nephrectomy, immediately prior to xenotransplantation. The authors' laboratory advocates for performing the preparation of the thymokidney 6–8 weeks before the nephrectomy. During this time the thymus is given time to engraft. We have previously demonstrated that in order to induce transplantation tolerance, donor thymus must be transplanted as a vascularized graft (Yamada et al., 2000a). To ensure that the donor is the appropriate weight at the time of thymokidney procurement and transplantation, animals undergo thymokidney preparation (see the section 'Recipient selection and preparation') at 4–6 weeks of age and donation at 10–12 weeks of age.

### Recipient selection and preparation

Selection of the baboon recipient is important from an immunological standpoint. Just as panel reactive antibody (PRA) and cross-match are measured in humans, each baboon is tested pretransplantation for levels of anti-non-Gal antibody. If cytotoxicity against donor cells is greater than 60% at a 1:4 dilution preoperatively, recipients are generally referred to as having 'high cytotoxicity'. Once selected, the baboon, which should be at least 6 kg at the time of transplantation, undergoes preoperative thymectomy (a protocol designed for the induction of tolerance by a donor vascularized thymic graft, either thymokidney or vascularized thymic lobe). This procedure is performed under general anaesthesia and involves the steps outlined in the following sections.

### Sedation with intramuscular ketamine or benzodiazepine

Ketamine is a good choice for baboons as it can be given intramuscularly (IM), through a small-gauge needle, from outside the animal's cage. Should the animal not tolerate ketamine or if ketamine is not available, short-acting benzodiazepines may also be given.

### Shaving in preparation of jacket training

Shaving of the baboon is important both for surgical approach and to avoid pruritis associated with jacket placement. Shaving should be performed on all areas that will be covered by the jacket or where an incision will be performed. As with human surgery, electrical shavers are a better choice than razors, with regard to the avoidance of wound infections.

### Jacket sizing

Selection of the jacket size is important. If the jacket is too large, the animal may be able to inadvertently pull out centrally placed venous and arterial catheters, which are tunnelled to the animal's back. If too small, the jacket may restrict respiratory efforts.

### Induction of anaesthesia with inhaled isoflurane

Generally, in baboons the degree of sedation and appropriateness of intubation is determined by jaw laxity. Bag-mask ventilation is performed with inhaled isoflurane until the jaw is lax and the vocal cords are easily visualized.

### Intubation

Once the animal is appropriately sedated, it should be intubated and the tip of the endotracheal tube should be past the vocal cords but above the carina. Postintubation the animal should have bilateral breath sounds. Once sedated and intubated, the animal is given IM buprenorphine and banamine for pain control intraoperatively.

### Monitoring and setup

Once intubated, leads for cardiac monitoring, a cuff for non-invasive blood pressure, and a sensor for oxygen saturation and carbon dioxide can be placed. In addition the grounding pad for electrocautery should be placed in an area that (1) has been shaved and (2) will be protected from moisture, in order to avoid burns. This pad is usually wrapped around the baboon's calf. A Foley or other urinary catheter is not generally placed for renal transplantation given the small size of the urethra and given the difficulty with management of urinary catheters in baboons.

## Recipient procedures prior to transplantation

### Thymectomy (recipients)

Because the basic principle of the thymokidney approach is that immature T-cells from the recipient will be re-educated in the thymic tissue of the donor after thymokidney transplantation, removal of the recipient thymus is crucial for development of post-transplantation tolerance (Kamano et al., 2004; Rodriguez-Barbosa et al., 2005). Once sedated, animals are prepped and draped with triple scrub: soap plus water, alcohol, and iodine paint. Thereafter a midline sternotomy is performed from the sternal notch to over the xiphoid. Electrocautery is then used to dissect down to the level of the sternum. Heavy scissors or a bone saw are used to split the sternum. The thymus should be immediately apparent and in the baboon is greyish-white in colour. The gland is infiltrated with higher degrees of fat in older animals. The thymus is then dissected free from the pericardium using blunt dissection. The vascular supply of the thymus are clipped or tied. The thymus is then weighed and measured. The chest is closed with interrupted non-absorbable monofilament sutures. Thereafter, the surgical team should reinflate the lungs with bag ventilation (typically with three deep breaths), to (1) confirm lung reinflation and limit atelectasis and (2) confirm there is no lung injury. Next, the skin is closed with absorbable sutures. A fentanyl patch is then placed on the animal's chest or back and the jacket is secured.

### Line placement (recipients)

Because animals will require drug infusions and daily laboratory testing (two- to three-times daily lab draws) central venous and arterial lines are placed. The most common locations are: simultaneous (1) carotid, (2) external jugular (EJ), and (3) internal jugular (IJ) cannulation. The lines are prefitted to the jacket and tether system. Then, once sedated, intubated, and prepped, a transverse incision is made over the animal's left or right neck. The platysma muscles are divided and the EJ is identified first. Because the vessel may go into spasm and will be cannulated last, it is typically tagged with a silk suture or vessel loop. Thereafter the carotid and IJ are dissected out of the carotid sheath by retracting the sternocleidomastoid (SCM) laterally (although it is also reasonable to retract the SCM medially). The artery is then tied cephalad, clamped proximally, and an arteriotomy is performed using a number 11 blade not to exceed 50% of the vessel's diameter. Thereafter proximal ties are placed and the catheter is flushed with heparinized saline. A similar procedure is then done for the IJ and the EJ, respectively. Line-tunnelling is then performed (although it may also be performed prior to cannulation) through the subcutaneous tissues to a position 50% of the distance between the shoulder blades. The neck is closed with absorbable sutures.

## Donor procedures

### Swine anaesthetics and preoperative preparation

#### Sedation with IM ketamine or benzodiazepine

Ketamine or Telazol are also good choices for swine as they can be given IM, through a small-gauge needle. Typically, animals are also premedicated with preoperative IM glycopyrolate to decrease respiratory secretions that may be encountered during intubation. Should the animal not tolerate ketamine or if ketamine is not available, short-acting benzodiazepines may also be given.

### Shaving the surgical area

Shaving of the surgical area is performed before surgery by using electrical shavers, which are a better choice than razors with regard to the avoidance of wound infections.

### Induction of anaesthesia with inhaled isoflurane

In the authors' laboratory the degree of sedation and appropriateness of intubation are determined by jaw laxity and ocular reflex. Bag-mask ventilation is performed with inhaled isoflurane until the jaw is lax, ocular reflexes are absent, and the vocal cords are easily visualized.

### Intubation

Once the animal is appropriately sedated, it should be intubated and the tip of the endotracheal tube should be past the vocal cords but above the carina. Postintubation, the animal should have bilateral breath sounds. Once sedated and intubated, the animal is given IM buprenorphine and banamine for pain control intraoperatively.

### Monitoring and setup

Once intubated, leads for cardiac monitoring, a cuff for non-invasive blood pressure, and a sensor for oxygen saturation and carbon dioxide can be placed. In addition, the grounding pad for electrocautery should be placed in an area that (1) has been shaved and (2) will be protected from moisture, in order to avoid burns. Foley or other urinary catheters are not generally placed for pigs, as the male penis has a tortuous shape and the female urethral orifice is frequently dirty and difficult to access.

## Thymokidney preparation (donors)

Once the donor has been selected, the thymokidney is prepared. The 4- to 6-week-old miniature swine is sedated, intubated, and prepped with triple scrub as detailed in the section 'Recipient procedures prior to transplantation: thymectomy'). Thereafter a 4- to 6-cm longitudinal incision is made from the level of the angle of the mandible to the sternal notch. The soft tissues are dissected with electrocautery and the platysma is divided. A wound retractor is then placed and the thymus is identified, again as a slightly greyish-white organ. A cervical lobe is removed and minced on the back table. Haemostasis is obtained and the wound is irrigated. Thereafter the neck is closed and a dressing is placed. Next the flank is incised transversely, below the costal margin in order to access the retroperitoneum and identify the kidney. In doing so, a small incision is made in the renal capsule and the minced thymic tissue is placed subcapsularly. Then the capsule is closed with interrupted 7-0 prolene sutures. This procedure is performed bilaterally in order to obtain two identical thymokidneys for future use. The advantage of this technique is that should the first xenorenal graft fail for non-immunological reasons, the second kidney can be transplanted without exposure to additional xenogeneic antigens. The swine skin and soft tissues are both closed with running absorbable suture. A fentanyl patch is then placed prior to cessation of the fentanyl drip in order to avoid postoperative pain.

### Renal procurement (donors)

Six to eight weeks after thymokidney preparation, the donor swine is again sedated in anticipation of surgery according to the steps outlined in the section 'Recipient procedures prior to transplantation'). Thereafter the animal is sedated, intubated, and prepped. The animal's abdomen is then opened through a midline incision and the retroperitoneum is accessed. The kidney is removed by isolating the renal artery and vein, at their aortic and caval origins, respectively. The vessels are then ligated and transected, and the graft is removed. Great care must be taken to avoid manipulating the donor vessels, as minor traumatic injury may lead to severe vasospasm once transplanted into the xenogeneic recipient. The ureter is also isolated, ligated, and transected, such that at least 50% of the swine ureter is taken with the renal graft. The kidney is then gently perfused with Euro-Collins solution and placed on ice.

## Recipient procedure on day of xenotransplantation

### Recipient preparation

#### Thymokidney transplantation (recipients)

Once the baboon recipient has been thymectomized and lines are placed, it must undergo a stringent immunological regimen of transplantation induction, which includes both T- and B-cell depletion. Thereafter the animal is sedated (now with intravenous medication), intubated, and prepped as described in the section 'Recipient procedures prior to transplantation'). The thymokidney transplantation procedure is similar to that of paediatric kidney transplantation. A midline abdominal incision is made using a number 10 blade. First, attention is directed to the right kidney, which is removed. This is because, at the MGH, a right-sided renal transplant is typically performed. We usually remove the left kidney as well (i.e. both kidneys are removed). However, the researcher may decide to leave the second kidney in place in order to keep the animal alive should the transplant fail. In this case, in order to determine graft function using this scenario, the ureter from the left native kidney should be ligated. Thereafter the thymokidney graft is brought into the field.

Again, as porcine kidney is subject to vasospasm, the surgeon should be cautious of touching the graft and take all precautions to ensure that the anastomoses are completed as quickly and skillfully as possible (must be within 7–12 minutes each). In the experience of the authors, even minimal trauma to the transplanted vessels may yield severe vasospasm after reperfusion. Similar to human transplantation, the venous anastomosis is typically performed first, followed by the arterial, again using a technique of minimal graft manipulation. This is done because the vena cava lies to the animal's right, and performing the arterial anastomosis first can yield a challenging approach to the, now posterior, venous anastomosis. In addition, performing the arterial anastomosis second avoids clamping the artery for an extended period of time. Thereafter the kidney is perfused. The graft should make urine almost immediately. In animals with a high degree of antidonor, cytotoxic, anti-non-Gal antibody, the graft may also experience severe vasospasm. If this is the case, papavarine can be given directly into (or onto) the renal artery. Heparin (generally 70–100 units/kg) should be given to the animal > 2 minutes prior to revascularization of the graft. The ureteral anastomosis is then performed over a stent, which is left in place postoperatively. The abdomen is closed with either running or interrupted sutures. The skin is closed with absorbable, running, subcuticular stitches. A fentanyl patch is then placed prior to cessation of the fentanyl drip, and the animal is awoken from anaesthesia.

## Postoperative management (recipients)

The major benefits of preoperative placement of indwelling central catheters are two-fold. First, it is important to have adequate perfusion pressure, and the animal's blood pressure can be continuously monitored. Second, the arterial catheter, and possibly the venous catheters, allow the investigator to draw blood for laboratory testing without disturbing the animals. Placement of two central venous lines is preferable, so one catheter can be used for maintenance fluids and the other for drug administration. The protocols require administration of multiple intravenous drugs, which can react and crystallize when administered through the same line. Following the animal's laboratory values, particularly the animal's creatinine and haematocrit, is important postprocedurally. Daily blood draws are also important for monitoring immunosuppression levels as well as T-cell counts.

## Immunosuppression and/or tolerance induction (recipients)

Regardless of whether or not a tolerance approach is attempted, immunosuppression will undoubtedly remain a part of xenotransplantation protocols. The improved efficacy and specificity of immunosuppressive agents have increased survival rates for allografts. These agents include both pharmacological and antibody reagents (Anderson et al., 1984; Bradley et al., 1987; Caralps 1988; Bouchart et al., 1993; Haug et al., 1993; Isobe et al., 1994; Bourdage and Hamlin 1995; Costanzo et al., 1997; Delmonico et al., 1997; Allan et al., 1998; Knoll and Bell, 1999; Matthews et al., 2003). Since most antibody responses to allografts are T-cell-dependent, these same reagents have been effective in avoiding antibody responses to xenografts as well. In most cases, these agents can be titrated to a level at which they are effective in inhibiting the response to the transplant without undue side effects. Unfortunately, for xenografts the level of these agents needed to fully suppress the immune response is greater than for allografts and might be expected to lead to greater complications. *For this reason adoption of a tolerance strategy is imperative to the success of xenotransplantation.* In addition, antibody-mediated responses appear to be more prevalent and more robust in xenograft rejection than in allograft rejection, and even when the major response to Gal has been eliminated by use of GalT-KO donors, it appears likely that low levels of T-cell-dependent antibodies may still form, possibly contributing to the thrombotic complications that are associated with xenograft rejection (Seebach et al., 1997; Cretin et al., 2002).

An approach utilizing tolerance induction, at least to some of the most important xenogeneic antigens, may be capable of avoiding such persistent immune reactivity. Initial results, also from the authors' laboratory, have demonstrated that when cotransplanted with donor vascularized thymic grafts described in the section 'Thymokidney preparation (donors)'), a method for inducing tolerance at the T-cell level, *life-supporting* GalT-KO renal xenografts showed no evidence of rejection for up to 83 days (Yamada et al., 2005b). The 83-day baboon survivor maintained stable renal function until death from another cause, with an essentially normal renal graft. Although immunosuppression was still in the process of being tapered, the animal showed in-vitro evidence for donor-specific unresponsiveness, suggesting that it may have been on a path toward development of tolerance.

## The future of clinical xenotransplantation

Which should be the first organ to transplant across a xenogeneic barrier? Among the most likely candidates are (1) kidney, (2) heart, (3) liver, (4) lung, and (5) pancreas/islets. Each has its proponents and detractors. In favour of the kidney is the fact that failure of the transplant would not be fatal, as the patient could presumably be put back on dialysis. In addition, numerous patients on most waiting lists for kidneys are highly sensitized to potential human donors (i.e. they have high PRA) (Duquesnoy et al., 2003). On the other hand, the availability of living donor transplants and the fact that renal failure is treatable by dialysis argue against its adoption.

Short of extracorporeal membrane oxygenation, one cannot live without a heart and/or lungs. Thus, an alternative source of hearts or lungs is an enticing solution to end-stage heart or lung disease. For this reason some have suggested that xenotransplanted organs might be used as a 'bridge' to allotransplantation. However, others argue that the use of a xenogeneic organ as a bridge does not solve the problem of organ shortage but rather increases the number of people on the waiting list for a human organ. Unlike end-stage kidney disease, end-stage liver disease cannot be treated with dialysis. Regarding xenotransplantation of the liver, some have argued that the complex natural function of the liver (e.g. production of enzymes, coagulation factors, complement components) makes it unlikely that a xenograft would function properly across a species disparity, although some investigators suggest otherwise (Ramirez et al., 2000).

Since porcine insulin is very similar to human insulin, (Galloway, 1980; Schernthaner, 1993; Rayat et al., 1999), it is very likely that the pig pancreas (or islets) would support the insulin needs of a diabetic patient as well as a human cadaver transplant. Porcine-to-human islet cell transplantation has been attempted with variable results. However, with the advent of transgenic pigs with or without the GalT-KO background, it may be reasonable to assume that this will be the next most likely clinical xenograft attempt. Should the tolerance strategy approach by Yamada and colleagues yield continued positive results, it would be reasonable to include islets under the kidney capsule and, much like the thymus, have these tissues engraft prior to transplantation (Korsgren et al., 2003; Rayat and Gill, 2003; Matsumoto et al., 2005). Yamada again attempted a similar approach in what was called the 'islet kidney' across an allogeneic barrier with very encouraging results (Kumagai et al., 2002a, 2002b; Yamada et al., 2011).

## Conclusion

Xenotransplantation remains on the cutting edge of transplantation science and represents the most viable option for a large-scale expansion of the donor pool. In this chapter we have attempted to review briefly the history of this field, to summarize the current state of the art, and to present what we consider to be the most likely areas of future success. The most compelling reason for continuing this pursuit is the large number of patients who continue to die every year while on the waiting list for an organ transplant. The burgeoning fields of stem cell biology and tissue engineering may offer solutions as well, but these technologies for solid organs will likely require many more years of research before clinically applicable protocols are developed. At present, xenotransplantation, despite its hurdles, remains the most encouraging potential solution to the organ shortage.

## References

Allan JS, Slisz JK, Vesga L, et al. (1998) Enhanced efficacy of repeated anti-CD8 monoclonal antibody therapy by high-dose cyclosporine treatment. *Transplant Proc*, **30**(8):4062–4063.

Alter BJ, Bach FH (1990) Cellular basis of the proliferative response of human T cells to mouse xenoantigens. *J Exp Med*, **171**:333–338.

Alwayn IP, Basker M, Buhler L, Cooper DK (1999) The problem of anti-pig antibodies in pig-to-primate xenografting: current and novel methods of depletion and/or suppression of production of anti-pig antibodies. *Xenotransplantation*, **6**(3):157–168.

Anderson CB, Tyler JD, Sicard GA, Anderman CK, Rodey GE, Etheredge EE (1984) Pretreatment of renal allograft recipients with immunosuppression and donor-specific blood. *Transplantation*, **38**:664–668.

Appel JZ III, Alwayn IP, Buhler L, DeAngelis HA, Robson SC, Cooper DK (2001a) Modulation of platelet aggregation in baboons: implications for mixed chimerism in xenotransplantation. I. The roles of individual components of a transplantation conditioning regimen and of pig peripheral blood progenitor cells. *Transplantation*, **72**(7):1299–1305.

Appel JZ III, Alwayn IP, Correa LE, Cooper DK, Robson SC (2001b) Modulation of platelet aggregation in baboons: implications for mixed chimerism in xenotransplantation. II. The effect of cyclophospamide on pig peripheral blood progenitor cell-induced aggregation. *Transplantation*, **72**(7):1306–1310.

Arnold B, Messerle M, Jatsch L, Külbeck G, Koszinowski U (1990) Transgenic mice expressing a soluble foreign H-2 class I antigen are tolerant to allogeneic fragments presented by self class I but not to the whole membrane-bound alloantigen. *Proc Natl Acad Sci USA*, **87**:1762–1766.

Arnold B, Schonrich G, Hammerling GJ (1993) Induction of tolerance in mature peripheral T cells. *Exp Nephrol*, **1**:72–77.

Auchincloss H Jr, Sachs DH (1983a) Mechanisms of tolerance in murine radiation bone marrow chimeras. I. Nonspecific suppression of alloreactivity by spleen cells from early, but not late, chimeras. *Transplantation*, **36**:436–441.

Auchincloss H Jr, Sachs DH (1983b) Mechanisms of tolerance in murine radiation bone marrow chimeras. II. Absence of nonspecific suppression in mature chimeras. *Transplantation*, **36**:442–445.

Auchincloss H Jr, Lee R, Shea S, Markowitz JS, Grusby MJ, Glimcher LH (1993) The role of 'indirect' recognition in initiating rejection of skin grafts from major histocompatibility complex class II-deficient mice. *Proc Natl Acad Sci USA*, **90**(8):3373–3377.

Bach FH, Winkler H, Ferran C, Hancock WW, Robson SC (1996) Delayed xenograft rejection. *Immunol Today*, **17**(8):379–384.

Bailey LL, Nehlsen-Cannarella SL, Concepcion W, Jolley WB (1985) Baboon-to-human cardiac xenotransplantation in a neonate. *JAMA*, **254**(23):3321–3329.

Baker RJ, Hernandez-Fuentes MP, Brookes PA, Chaudhry AN, Cook HT Lechler RI (2001) Loss of direct and maintenance of indirect alloresponses in renal allograft recipients: implications for the pathogenesis of chronic allograft nephropathy. *J Immunol*, **167**(12):7199–7206.

Barth RN, Yamamoto S, LaMattina JC, et al. (2003) Xenogeneic thymokidney and thymic tissue transplantation in a pig-to-baboon model: I. Evidence for pig-specific T-cell unresponsiveness. *Transplantation*, **75**(10):1615–1624.

Bertoye A, Marion P, Mikaeloff P, BolotJF (1969) [Attempt at treatment of various severe acute hepatic insufficiencies by temporary heterotopic heterologous liver graft (baboon liver)]. *Lyon Med*, **222**(33):347–354.

Bhattacharyya S, Chawla A, Smith K, et al. (2002) Multilineage engraftment with minimal graft-versus-host disease following in utero transplantation of S-59 psoralen/ultraviolet a light-treated, sensitized T cells and adult T cell-depleted bone marrow in fetal mice. *J Immunol*, **169**(11):6133–6140.

Bhatti FN, Schmoeckel M, Zaidi A, et al. (1999) Three-month survival of HDAFF transgenic pig hearts transplanted into primates. *Transplant Proc*, 31(1-2):958.

Bouchart F, Gundry SR, van Schaack-Gonzales J, et al. (1993) Methotrexate as rescue/adjunctive immunotherapy in infant and adult heart transplantation. *J Heart Lung Transplant*, **12**(3):427–433.

Bourdage JS, Hamlin DM (1995) Comparative polyclonal antithymocyte globulin and antilymphocyte/antilymphoblast globulin anti-CD antigen analysis by flow cytometry. *Transplantation*, **59**(8):1194–1200.

Bradley JW, Cho SI, Cosimi AB, Monaco AP (1987) Cyclosporine immunosuppression and perfusion preservation of cadaver kidneys. *Transplant Proc*, **19**:2104–2105.

Brombacher F, Köler G, Eibel H (1991) B cell tolerance in mice transgenic for anti-CD8 immunoglobulin m chain. *J Exp Med*, **174**:1335–1346.

Buhler L, Yamada K, Alwayn I, et al. (2000) Miniature swine and hDAF pig kidney transplantation in baboons treated with a nonmyeloablative regimen and CD154 blockade. *Proc 18th International Congress of The Transplantation Society*, 220, (Abstract 0618).

Buhler L, Yamada K, Alwayn I, et al. (2001) Miniature swine and hDAF pig kidney transplantation in baboons treated with a nonmyeloablative regimen and CD154 blockade. *Transplant Proc*, **33**(1–2):716.

Buonomano R, Tinguely C, Rieben R, Mohacsi PJ, Nydegger UE (1999) Quantitation and characterization of anti-Galalpha1-3Gal antibodies in sera of 200 healthy persons. *Xenotransplantation*, **6**(3):173–180.

Burkly LC, Lo D, Flavell RA (1990) Tolerance in transgenic mice expressing major histocompatibility molecules extrathymically on pancreatic cells. *Science*, **248**:1364–1368.

Candinas D, Belliveau S, Koyamada N, et al. (1996) T cell independence of macrophage and natural killer cell infiltration, cytokine production, and endothelial activation during delayed xenograft rejection. *Transplantation*, **62**:1920–1927.

Caralps A (1988) History of immunosuppression in kidney transplantation. *Transplant Proc*, **20**(Suppl 6):3–4.

Carrier E, Lee TH, Busch MP, Cowan MJ (1995) Induction of tolerance in nondefective mice after in utero transplantation of major histocompatibility complex-mismatched fetal hematopoietic stem cells. *Blood*, **86**(12):4681–4690.

Chan DV, Auchincloss H Jr (1996) Human anti-pig cell-mediated cytotoxicity in vitro involves non-T as well as T cell components. *Xenotransplantation*, **3**:158–165.

Chen D, Cao R, Guo H, et al. (2004) Pathogenesis and pathology of delayed xenograft rejection in pig-to-rhesus monkey cardiac transplantation. *Transplant Proc*, **36**(8):2480–2482.

Chen G, Qian H, Starzl T, et al. (2005) Acute rejection is associated with antibodies to non-Gal antigens in baboons using Gal-knockout pig kidneys. *Nat Med*, **11**(12):1295–1298.

Colson YL, Wren SM, Schuchert MJ, et al. (1995) A nonlethal conditioning approach to achieve durable multilineage mixed chimerism and tolerance across major, minor, and hematopoietic histocompatibility barriers. *J Immunol*, **155**(9):4179–4188.

Colson YL, Schuchert MJ, Ildstad ST (2000). The abrogation of allosensitization following the induction of mixed allogeneic chimerism. *J Immunol*, **165**(2):637–644.

Cooper DK, Good AH, Koren E, et al. (1993) Identification of alpha-galactosyl and other carbohydrate epitopes that are bound by human anti-pig antibodies: relevance to discordant xenografting in man. *Transpl Immunol*, **1**:198–205.

Cooper DK, Koren E, Oriol R (1994) Oligosaccharides and discordant xenotransplantation. *Immunol Rev*, **141**:31–58.

Costanzo MR, Koch DM, Fisher SG, Heroux AL, Kao WG, Johnson MR (1997) Effects of methotrexate on acute rejection and cardiac allograft vasculopathy in heart transplant recipients. *J Heart Lung Transplant*, **16**(2):169–178.

Cretin N, Bracy J, Hanson K, Iacomini J (2002) The role of T cell help in the production of antibodies specific for Gal alpha 1-3Gal. *J Immunol*, **168**(3):1479–1483.

Delmonico FL, Cosimi AB, Colvin R, et al. (1997) Murine OKT4A immunosuppression in cadaver donor renal allograft recipients—A cooperative clinical trial in a transplantation pilot study. *Transplantation*, **63**:1087–1095.

Diaz I, Veira P, Valdes F, Alonso C, Sanchez P (2003) Quantitation and comparison of anti-Gal-alpha-1,3-Gal antibodies in sera of healthy individuals and patients waiting for kidney transplantation. *Transplant Proc*, **35**(5):2043–2044.

Dor FJ, Tseng YL, Cheng J, et al. (2004) alpha1,3-Galactosyltransferase gene-knockout miniature swine produce natural cytotoxic anti-Gal antibodies. *Transplantation*, **78**(1):15–20.

Dorling A, Binns R, Lechler RI (1996a) Cellular xenoresponses: Observation of significant primary indirect human T cell anti-pig xenoresponses using co-stimulator-deficient or SLA class II-negative porcine stimulators. *Xenotransplantation*, **3**:112–119.

Dorling A, Lombardi G, Binns R, Lechler RI (1996b) Detection of primary direct and indirect human anti-porcine T cell responses using a porcine dendritic cell population. *Eur J Immunol*, **26**(6):1378–1387.

Duquesnoy RJ, Howe J, Takemoto S (2003) HLAmatchmaker: a molecularly based algorithm for histocompatibility determination. IV. An alternative strategy to increase the number of compatible donors for highly sensitized patients. *Transplantation*, **75**(6):889–897.

Eto M, Kong YY, Uozumi J, Naito S, Nomoto K (1999) Importance of intrathymic mixed chimerism for the maintenance of skin allograft tolerance across fully allogeneic antigens in mice. *Immunology*, **96**(3):440–446.

Galili U (1993a) Evolution and pathophysiology of the human natural anti-alpha- galactosyl IgG (anti-Gal) antibody. *Springer Semin Immunopathol*, **15**:155–171.

Galili U (1993b) Interaction of the natural anti-Gal antibody with alpha-galactosyl epitopes: a major obstacle for xenotransplantation in humans. *Immunol Today*, **14**(10):480–482.

Galili U, Macher BA, Buehler J, Shohet SB (1985) Human natural anti-alpha-galactosyl IgG. II. The specific recognition of alpha (1-3)-linked galactose residues. *J Exp Med*, **162**:573–582.

Galili U, Clark MR, Shohet SB, Buehler J, Macher BA (1987) Evolutionary relationship between the natural anti-Gal antibody and the Gal alpha 1-3Gal epitope in primates. *Proc Natl Acad Sci USA*, **84**:1369–1373.

Galili U, Shohet SB, Kobrin E, Stults CL, Macher BA (1988a) Man, apes, and Old World monkeys differ from other mammals in the expression of alpha-galactosyl epitopes on nucleated cells. *J Biol Chem*, **263**(33):17755–17762.

Galili U, Shohet SB, Kobrin E, Stults CL, Macher BA (1988b) Man, apes, and Old World monkeys differ from other mammals in the expression of alpha-galactosyl epitopes on nucleated cells. *J Biol Chem*, **263**:17755–17762.

Galili U, Gregory CR, Morris RE (1996) New World monkeys as a primate model for xenografts in the absence of anti-Gal. *Transplant Proc*, **28**(2):567–568.

Galloway JA (1980) Insulin treatment for the early 80s: facts and questions about old and new insulins and their usage. *Diabetes Care*, **3**(5):615–622.

Garrovillo M, Ali A, Oluwole SF (1999) Indirect allorecognition in acquired thymic tolerance: induction of donor-specific tolerance to rat cardiac allografts by allopeptide-pulsed host dendritic cells. *Transplantation*, **68**(12):1827–1834.

Giles GR, Boehmig HJ, Amemiya H, Halgrimson CG, Starzl TE (1970) Clinical heterotransplantation of the liver. *Transplant Proc*, **2**(4):506–512.

Green MD, Chen A, Nostro MC, et al. (2011) Generation of anterior foregut endoderm from human embryonic and induced pluripotent stem cells. *Nat Biotechnol*, **29**(3):267–272.

Griesemer AD, Hirakata A, Shimizu A, et al. (2009) Results of gal-knockout porcine thymokidney xenografts. *Am J Transplant*, **9**(12):2669–2678.

Hardy JD, Kurrus FD, Chavez CM, et al. (1964) Heart transplantation in human.developmental studies and report of a case. *JAMA*, **188**:1132–1140.

Haug CE, Colvin RB, Delmonico FL, et al. (1993) A phase I trial of immunosuppression with anti-ICAM-1 (CD54) mAb in renal allograft recipients. *Transplantation*, **55**:766–72.

Heeg K Wagner H (1990) Induction of peripheral tolerance to class I major histocompatibility complex (MHC) alloantigens in adult mice: transfused class I MHC-incompatible splenocytes veto clonal responses of antigen-reactive Lyt-2+ T cells. *J Exp Med*, **172**:719–728.

Hering BJ, Wijkstrom M, Graham ML, et al. (2006) Prolonged diabetes reversal after intraportal xenotransplantation of wild-type porcine islets in immunosuppressed nonhuman primates. *Nat Med*, **12**(3):301–303.

Hoffmann MW, Allison J, Miller JF (1992) Tolerance induction by thymic medullary epithelium. *Proc Natl Acad Sci USA*, **89**(7):2526–2530.

Ierino FL, Kozlowski T, Siegel JB, et al. (1998) Disseminated intravascular coagulation in association with the delayed rejection of pig-to-baboon renal xenografts. *Transplantation*, **66**(11):1439–1450.

Ierino FL, Yamada K, Hatch T, Rembert J, Sachs DH (1999) Peripheral tolerance to class I mismatched renal allografts in miniature swine: donor antigen-activated peripheral blood lymphocytes from tolerant swine inhibit antidonor CTL reactivity. *J Immunol*, **162**(1):550–559.

Isobe M, Suzuki J, Yagita H, et al. (1994) Immunosuppression to cardiac allografts and soluble antigens by anti-vascular cellular adhesion molecule-1 and anti-very late antigen-4 monoclonal antibodies. *J Immunol*, **153**:5810–5818.

Ito H, Kurtz J, Shaffer J, Sykes M (2001) CD4 T cell-mediated alloresistance to fully MHC-mismatched allogeneic bone marrow engraftment is dependent on CD40-CD40 ligand interactions, and lasting T cell tolerance is induced by bone marrow transplantation with initial blockade of this pathway. *J Immunol*, **166**(5):2970–2981.

Kamano C, Vagefi PA, Kumagai N, et al. (2004) Vascularized thymic lobe transplantation in miniature swine: Thymopoiesis and tolerance induction across fully MHC-mismatched barriers. *Proc Natl Acad Sci USA*, **101**(11):3827–3832.

Kappler JW, Roehm N, Marrack P (1987) T cell tolerance by clonal elimination in the thymus. *Cell*, **49**(2):273–280.

Kearns-Jonker MK, Cramer DV, Dane LA, Swensson JM, Makowka L (1997) Human serum reactivity to porcine endothelial cells after antisense-mediated down-regulation of GpIIIa expression. *Transplantation*, **63**:588–593.

Kirk AD, Li RA, Kinch MS, Abernethy KA, Doyle C, Bollinger RR (1993) The human antiporcine cellular repertoire. In vitro studies of acquired and innate cellular responsiveness. *Transplantation*, **55**:924–931.

Knoll GA, Bell RC (1999) Tacrolimus versus cyclosporin for immunosuppression in renal transplantation: meta-analysis of randomised trials. *BMJ*, **318**(7191):1104–1107.

Kobayashi T, Yamaguchi T, Hamanaka S, et al. (2010) Generation of rat pancreas in mouse by interspecific blastocyst injection of pluripotent stem cells. *Cell*, **142**(5):787–799.

Kolber-Simonds D, Lai L, Watt SR, et al. (2004) Production of a-1,3-galactosyltransferase null pigs by means of nuclear transfer with fibroblasts bearing loss of heterozygosity mutations. *Proc Natl Acad Sci USA*, **101**(19):7335–7340.

Korsgren O, Buhler LH, Groth CG (2003) Toward clinical trials of islet xenotransplantation. *Xenotransplantation*, **10**(4):289–292.

Kozlowski T, Monroy R, Xu Y, et al. (1998) Anti-a Gal antibody response to porcine bone marrow in unmodified baboons and baboons conditioned for tolerance induction. *Transplantation*, **66**(2):176–182.

Kozlowski T, Monroy R, Giovino M, et al. (1999a) Effect of pig-specific cytokines on mobilization of hematopoietic progenitor cells in pigs and on pig bone marrow engraftment in baboons. *Xenotransplantation.*, **6**(1):17–27.

Kozlowski T, Monroy R, Giovino M, et al. (1999b) Effect of pig-specific cytokines on mobilization of hematopoietic progenitor cells in pigs and on pig bone marrow engraftment in baboons. *Xenotransplantation*, **6**(1):17–27.

Kozlowski T, Shimizu A, Lambrigts D, et al. (1999c) Porcine kidney and heart transplantation in baboons undergoing a tolerance induction regimen and antibody adsorption. *Transplantation*, **67**(1):18–30.

Kumagai N, LaMattina JC, Kamano C, et al. (2002a) Vascularized islet cell transplantation in miniature Swine: islet-kidney allografts correct the diabetic hyperglycemia induced by total pancreatectomy. *Diabetes*, **51**(11):3220–3228.

Kumagai N, O'Neil JJ, Barth RN, et al. (2002b) Vascularized islet-cell transplantation in miniature swine. I. Preparation of vascularized islet kidneys. *Transplantation*, **74**(9):1223–1230.

Kumagai-Braesch M, Satake M, Korsgren O, Andersson A, Moller E (1993) Characterization of cellular human anti-porcine xenoreactivity. *Clinical Transplantation*, **7**:273–280.

Kuwaki K, Tseng YL, Dor FJ, et al. (2005) Heart transplantation in baboons using α-1,3-galactosyltransferase gene-knockout pigs as donors: initial experience. *Nat Med*, **11**(1):29–31.

Lai L, Kolber-Simonds D, Park K, et al. (2002) Production of a-1,3-Galactosyltransferase Knockout Pigs by Nuclear Transfer Cloning. *Science*, **295**(5557):1089–1092.

LaMattina JC, Kumagai N, Barth RN, et al. (2002) Vascularized thymic lobe transplantation in miniature swine: I. Vascularized thymic lobe allografts support thymopoiesis. *Transplantation*, **73**(5):826–831.

Lan P, Wang L, Diouf B, et al. (2004) Induction of human T cell tolerance to porcine xenoantigens through mixed hematopoietic chimerism. *Blood*, **103**(10):3964–3969.

Latinne D, Gianello P, Smith CV, et al. (1993) Xenotransplantation from pig to cynomolgus monkey: approach toward tolerance induction. *Transplant Proc*, **25**(1):336–338.

Lin SS, Platt JL (1998) Genetic therapies for xenotransplantation. *J Am Coll Surg*, **186**(4):388–396.

Lin Y, VandeputteM, Waer M (1997a) Factors involved in rejection of concordant xenografts in complement-deficient rats. *Transplantation*, **63**:1705–1712.

Lin Y, Vandeputte M, Waer M (1997b) Natural killer cell- and macrophage-mediated rejection of concordant xenografts in the absence of T and B cell responses. *J Immunol*, **158**:5658–5667.

Marrack P, Lo D, Brinster R, et al. (1988) The effect of thymus environment on T cell development and tolerance. *Cell*, **53**:627–634.

Matsumoto S, Okitsu T, Iwanaga Y, et al. (2005) Insulin independence after living-donor distal pancreatectomy and islet allotransplantation. *Lancet*, **365**(9471):1642–1644.

Matthews JB, Ramos E, Bluestone JA (2003) Clinical trials of transplant tolerance: slow but steady progress. *Am J Transplant*, **3**(7):794–803.

McKenzie IFC, Xing PX, Vaughan HA, Prenzoska J, Dabkowski PL, Sandrin MS (1994) Distribution of the major xenoantigen (gal (alpha 1-3)gal) for pig to human xenografts. *Transpl Immunol*, **2**(2):81–86.

Mezrich JD, Haller GW, Arn JS, Houser SL, Madsen JC, Sachs DH (2003) Histocompatible miniature swine: an inbred large-animal model. *Transplantation*, **75**(6):904–907.

Moses RD, Pierson RN III, Winn HJ, Auchincloss H Jr (1990) Xenogeneic proliferation and lymphokine production are dependent on CD4+ helper T cells and self antigen-presenting cells in the mouse. *J Exp Med*, **172**:567–575.

Moses RD, Winn HJ, Auchincloss H Jr (1992) Evidence that multiple defects in cell-surface molecule interactions across species differences are responsible for diminished xenogeneic T cell responses. *Transplantation*, 53:203–209.

Mueller NJ, Barth RN, Yamamoto S, et al. (2002) Activation of cytomegalovirus in pig-to-primate organ xenotransplantation. *J Virol*, **76**(10):4734–4740.

Nikolic B, Gardner JP, Scadden DT, Arn JS, Sachs DH, Sykes M (1999) Normal development in porcine thymus grafts and specific tolerance of human T cells to porcine donor MHC. *J Immunol*, **162**(6):3402–3407.

Nishimura H, Scalea J, Wang Z, et al. (2011) First experience with the use of a recombinant CD3 immunotoxin as induction therapy in pig-to-primate xenotransplantation: the effect of T-cell depletion on outcome. *Transplantation*, **92**(6):641–647.

Oriol R, Ye Y, Koren E, Cooper DK (1993) Carbohydrate antigens of pig tissues reacting with human natural antibodies as potential targets for hyperacute vascular rejection in pig-to-man organ xenotransplantation. *Transplantation*, **56**:1433–1442.

Ott HC, Matthiesen TS, Goh SK, et al. (2008) Perfusion-decellularized matrix: using nature's platform to engineer a bioartificial heart. *Nat Med*, **14**(2):213–221.

Parker W, Bruno D, Holzknecht ZE, Platt JL (1994) Characterization and affinity isolation of xenoreactive human natural antibodies. *J Immunol*, **153**, 3791–3803.

Patience C, Takeuchi Y, Weiss RA (1998) Zoonosis in xenotransplantation. *Curr Opin Immunol*, 10(5):539–542.

Phelps CJ, Koike C, Vaught TD, et al. (2003) Production of alpha 1,3-galactosyltransferase-deficient pigs. *Science*, **299**(5605):411–414.

Platt JL (2000) Xenotransplantation—New risks, new gains. *Nature*, 407(6800):27–30.

Platt JL, Dalmasso AP, Vercellotti GM, Lindman BJ, Turman MA, Bach FH (1990a) Endothelial cell proteoglycans in xenotransplantation. *Transplant Proc*, **22**:1066.

Platt JL, Lindman BJ, Chen H, Spitalnik SL, Bach FH (1990b) Endothelial cell antigens recognized by xenoreactive human natural antibodies. *Transplantation*, **50**:817–822.

Platt JL, Lindman BJ, Geller RL, et al. (1991) The role of natural antibodies in the activation of xenogenic endothelial cells. *Transplantation*, **52**:1037–1043.

Platt JL, Holzknecht ZE, Lindman BJ (1994) Porcine endothelial cell antigens recognized by human natural antibodies. *Transplant Proc*, **26**:1387.

Ramirez P, Chavez R, Majado M, et al. (2000) Life-supporting human complement regulator decay accelerating factor transgenic pig liver xenograft maintains the metabolic function and coagulation in the nonhuman primate for up to 8 days. *Transplantation*, **70**(7):989–998.

Rayat GR Gill RG (2003) Pancreatic islet xenotransplantation: barriers and prospects. *Curr Diab Rep*, **3**(4):336–343.

Rayat GR, Rajotte RV, Korbutt GS (1999) Potential application of neonatal porcine islets as treatment for type 1 diabetes: a review. *Ann N Y Acad Sci*, **875**:175–188.

Reemtsma K, McCracken BH, Schlegel JU (1964) Renal heterotransplantation in man. *Ann Surg*, **160**:384.

Rodriguez-Barbosa JI, Zhao Y, Zhao G, Ezquerra A, Sykes M (2002) Murine CD4 T cells selected in a highly disparate xenogeneic porcine thymus graft do not show rapid decay in the absence of selecting MHC in the periphery. *J Immunol*, **169**(12):6697–6710.

Rodriguez-Barbosa JI, Haller GW, Zhao G, Sachs DH, Sykes M (2005) Host thymectomy and cyclosporine lead to unstable skin graft tolerance after class I mismatched allogeneic neonatal thymic transplantation in mice. *Transpl Immunol*, **15**(1):25–33.

Sablinski T, Gianello PR, Bailin M, et al. (1997) Pig to monkey bone marrow and kidney xenotransplantation. *Surgery*, **121**(4):381–391.

Sablinski T, Emery DW, Monroy R, et al. (1999) Long-term discordant xenogeneic (porcine-to-primate) bone marrow engraftment in a monkey treated with porcine-specific growth factors. *Transplantation*, **67**(7):972–977.

Sachs DH (1994) The pig as a potential xenograft donor. *Vet Immunol Immunopathol*, **43**:185–191.

Sandrin MS, McKenzie IF (1994) Gal alpha (1,3)Gal, the major xenoantigen(s) recognised in pigs by human natural antibodies. *Immunol Rev*, **141**:169–190.

Sandrin MS, Vaughan HA, Dabkowski PL, McKenzie IF (1993) Anti-pig IgM antibodies in human serum react predominantly with Gal(alpha 1-3)Gal epitopes. *Proc Natl Acad Sci USA*, **90**:11391–11395.

Schernthaner G (1993) Immunogenicity and allergenic potential of animal and human insulins. *Diabetes Care*, **16**(Suppl 3):155–165.

Seebach J D, McMorrow IM, Holley C, Sachs DH (1997) IgG subtypes and xenogeneic antibody-dependent cell-mediated cytotoxicity (ADCC) mediated by Gala1,3 Gal and non-Gala1,3Gal reactive natural antibodies (NAbs). *Proc 4th International Congress for Xenotransplantation*, Nantes.

Shimizu A, Hisashi Y, Kuwaki K, et al. (2008) Thrombotic microangiopathy associated with humoral rejection of cardiac xenografts from alpha-1,3-galactosyltransferase gene-knockout pigs in baboons. *Am J Pathol*, **172**(6):1471–1481.

Shimizu A, Yamada K, Robson SC, Sachs DH, Colvin RB (2011) Pathologic Characteristics of Transplanted Kidney Xenografts. *J Am Soc Nephrol*, **23**(2):225–235.

Smith RM, Mandel TE (2000) Pancreatic islet xenotransplantation: the potential for tolerance induction. *Immunol Today*, **21**(1):42–48.

Starzl TE, Marchioro TL, Peters GN (1964) Renal heterotransplantation from baboon to man: experience with six cases. *Transplantation*, **2**:752.

Starzl TE, Ishikawa M, Putnam CW, et al. (1974) Progress in and deterrents to orthotopic liver transplantation, with special reference to survival, resistance to hyperacute rejection, and biliary duct reconstruction. *Transplant Proc*, **6**(4 Suppl 1):129–139.

Starzl TE, Fung J, Tzakis A, et al. (1993) Baboon-to-human liver transplantation. *Lancet*, **341**:65–71.

Sykes M, Sachs DH (1997) Xenogeneic tolerance through hematopoietic cell and thymic transplantation. In: Cooper DKC, et al. (eds) *Xenotransplantation*, 2nd edn, pp. 496–518. Springer, New York.

Takahashi K, Yamanaka S (2006) Induction of pluripotent stem cells from mouse embryonic and adult fibroblast cultures by defined factors. *Cell*, **126**(4):663–676.

Takahashi K, Tanabe K, Ohnuki M, et al. (2007) Induction of pluripotent stem cells from adult human fibroblasts by defined factors. *Cell*, **131**(5):861–872.

Tomita Y, Khan A, Sykes M (1994) Role of intrathymic clonal deletion and peripheral anergy in transplantation tolerance induced by bone marrow transplantion in mice conditioned with a non-myeloablative regimen. *J Immunol*, **153**:1087–1098.

Utsugi R, Barth RN, Lee RS, et al. (2001) Induction of transplantation tolerance with a short course of tacrolimus (FK506): I. Rapid and stable tolerance to two-haplotype fully mhc-mismatched kidney allografts in miniature swine. *Transplantation*, **71**(10):1368–1379.

Yamada K, Sachs DH, DerSimonian H (1995a) Direct and indirect recognition of pig class II antigens by human T cells. *Transplant Proc*, **27**:258–259.

Yamada K, Sachs DH, DerSimonian H (1995b) Human anti-porcine xenogeneic T-cell response. Evidence for allelic specificity of MLR and for both direct and indirect pathways of recognition. *J Immunol*, **155**(11):5249–5256.

Yamada K, Seebach JD, DerSimonian H, Sachs DH (1996) Human anti-pig T-cell mediated cytotoxicity. *Xenotransplantation*, **3**:179–187.

Yamada K, Shimizu A, Ierino FL, et al. (1999) Thymic transplantation in miniature swine—I. Development and function of the 'thymokidney'. *Transplantation*, **68**(11):1684–1692.

Yamada K, Shimizu A, Utsugi R, et al. (2000a) Thymic transplantation in miniature swine. II. Induction of tolerance by transplantation of composite thymokidneys to thymectomized recipients. *J Immunol*, **164**(6):3079–3086.

Yamada K, Shimizu A, Utsugi R, et al. (2000b) Thymic transplantation in miniature swine. II. Induction of tolerance by transplantation of composite thymokidneys to thymectomized recipients. *J Immunol*, **164**(6):3079–3086.

Yamada K, Vagefi PA, Utsugi R, et al. (2003) Thymic transplantation in miniature swine: III. Induction of tolerance by transplantation of composite thymokidneys across fully major histocompatibility complex-mismatched barriers. *Transplantation*, **76**(3):530–536.

Yamada K, Yazawa K, Shimizu A, et al. (2005a) Marked prolongation of porcine renal xenograft survival in baboons through the use of alpha-1,3-galactosyltransferase gene-knockout donors and the cotransplantation of vascularized thymic tissue. *Nat Med*, **11**(1):32–34.

Yamada K, Yazawa K, Shimizu A, et al. (2005b) Marked prolongation of porcine renal xenograft survival in baboons through the use of α-1,3-galactosyltransferase gene-knockout donors and the cotransplantation of vascularized thymic tissue. *Nat Med*, **11**(1):32–34.

Yamada K, Hirakata A, Tchipashvili V, et al. (2011) Composite islet-kidneys from single baboon donors cure diabetes across fully allogenic barriers. *Am J Transplant*, **11**(12):2603–2612.

SECTION 5

# Kidney and kidney–pancreas

# CHAPTER 13

# Indications, selection, and evaluation of the kidney transplant candidate

M. Francesca Egidi and Giuseppe Segoloni

## Indications

Among therapeutic options available to patients diagnosed with ESRD, kidney transplantation (KTx) is the preferred option because it results in better quality of life and less morbidity and mortality as compared to renal replacement therapy (Wolfe et al., 1999; Garcia et al., 2012). Although hundreds of thousands of ESRD patients have received a KTx worldwide, there continues to exist a gap between the number of potential candidates and available kidneys. In fact some suitable candidates may never be listed and others will die waiting (Meier-Krieschu and Kaplan, 2002; Goldfarb-Rumyantzev et al., 2005; Oniscu et al., 2005). The barriers to KTx are multiple, including negligence in referring a patient to a transplant centre, failure to maintain updated candidate lists, and the lack and/or poor quality of organs (Schold et al., 2009; Schold and Segev, 2012).

Evidence suggests that the years living with chronic kidney disease (CKD) and the duration of dialysis affect KTx outcome, so early referral is key to successful KTx (Inrig et al., 2006; de Mattos et al., 2008; Hickson et al., 2008). Pre-emptive transplantation (before dialysis is required) is the preferred option, although seldom realized, mostly due to delays in referring the candidate to a transplant centre (Kasiske et al., 2002; Davis, 2010; Grams et al., 2011; Friedewald and Reese, 2012). Another barrier to pre-emptive transplantation is the shortage of cadaveric and living kidney donors.

In terms of outcome, the best option for a patient with CKD is to receive a kidney from a live donor (LD) and by so doing pre-empting or minimizing the dialysis period, thus avoiding dialysis-associated complications.

LD KTx provides most patients with the best chances of long-term rehabilitation and survival and increases access to cadaver KTx for those without the option of an LD. Moreover, LD KTx enables the scheduling of the procedure at a time when the recipient is in optimum medical and psychological condition and may be the only option for high-risk recipients by allowing pre-transplant treatments in selected categories of high-risk patients (Davis and Delmonico, 2005; Kher and Mandelbrot, 2012; Mandelbrot and Pavlakis, 2012). For example, ESRD patients may develop PRA against HLA (classes I and II) from previous transplants, blood transfusions, or pregnancies and thus may become immune sensitized. PRA is a major obstacle for KTx because of the limited ability for identifying a compatible graft with a negative cross-match (Böhmig et al., 2011; Terasaki, 2012). Sensitized patients with an LD can benefit from therapeutic approaches for desensitization, such as plasma exchange and other therapies aimed at removal of antibodies (Montgomery et al., 2011; Sanoof et al., 2012). Although the temporary immunological quiescence facilitates KTx, the risk of antibody-mediated rejection remains elevated (Terasaki, 2008). In recent years, specific immunological techniques have led to the detection of HLA donor-specific antibodies (DSA) that can induce chronic rejection and consequent graft failure. The pretransplant detection of DSA is a contraindication to KTx and constitutes a barrier also in the case of LD KTx.

Unfortunately DSA can also develop after KTx (de-novo DSA) and to date there are no effective treatments for their prevention or removal (Caro-Oleas et al., 2011; Wiebe et al., 2012). The increasing need for KTx has led to innovations such as donor exchange programmes, which offer transplant recipients with incompatible donors an opportunity to receive a compatible kidney. These programmes also provide an alternative to costly desensitization protocols that have unproven long-term outcomes. Donor exchange programmes afford multiple options, including simple two-pair exchanges, more complicated domino exchanges, and chain donations (Akkina et al., 2011). ABO-incompatible KTx is another option to facilitate LD transplant for incompatible pairs. Although this modality has not yet reached widespread adoption, several centres have reported encouraging results (Fehr and Stussi, 2012; Montgomery et al., 2012).

Although patients with a variety of causes of ESRD may be considered for KTx (see Table 13.1), some aetiologies may have a direct impact on the outcome of the transplant, such as recurrence of the original disease (Ponticelli and Glassock, 2010; Toledo et al., 2011; Canaud et al., 2012). The primary renal diseases that may recur post-KTx are listed in Table 13.2. In most cases transplantation is worthwhile since recurrence is usually very slow to develop. These risks are discussed with patients on a case-by-case basis. For example, among the different types of glomerulonephritis, FSGS has the highest recurrence rate in the new graft. The overall recurrence of FSGS is nearly 30% for the first KTx and can reach 80% for a second KTx if the first KTx was lost to FSGS recurrence (Hwang et al., 2012). Different therapeutic approaches have been

**Table 13.1** Causes of ESRD

**Glomerulonephritis**
- Idiopathic and post-infectious
- Membranous
- Mesangiocapillary (type I and type II (dense-deposit disease))
- IgA nephropathy
- Antiglomerular basement membrane
- Focal glomerulosclerosis
- Henoch–Schönlein

**Chronic pyelonephritis (reflux nephropathy)**

*Hereditary*
- Polycystic kidneys
- Nephronophthisis (medullary cystic disease)
- Nephritis (including Alport's syndrome)
- Tuberous sclerosis

*Metabolic*
- Diabetes mellitus
- Hyperoxaluria
- Cystinosis
- Fabry's disease
- Amyloid
- Gout
- Porphyria

**Obstructive nephropathy**

*Toxic*
- Analgesic nephropathy
- Opiate abuse

*Multisystem diseases*
- Systemic lupus erythematosus
- Vasculitis
- Progressive systemic sclerosis

**Haemolytic–uraemic syndrome**

*Tumours*
- Wilms' tumour
- Renal cell carcinoma
- Incidental carcinoma
- Myeloma

*Congenital*
- Hypoplasia
- Horseshoe kidney

*Irreversible acute renal failure*
- Cortical necrosis
- Acute tubular necrosis

attempted in case of early FSGS recurrence as preventive treatment before LD procedure. Although the pathogenesis of FSGS recurrence is still unknown, the monoclonal antibody Rituximab and plasma exchange are the most commonly used therapies, but results have not always been effective (Audard et al., 2012; Keith, 2012). Patients affected by FSGS should be informed about the risk of losing the kidney graft, in particular in case of LD.

Systemic diseases such as lupus erythematosus, haemolytic–uraemic syndrome, and Wegener's granulomatosis can also recur after KTx. It is crucial to avoid KTx until those diseases have reached a quiescent phase. Patients with primary oxalosis require combined kidney–liver transplantation, since without metabolic correction of oxalosis in liver transplantation recurrent kidney disease could develop very rapidly (Mehrabi et al., 2009).

All candidates for KTx need a pretransplant evaluation to determine if they meet the criteria for the transplant procedure (Kasiske et al., 1995; Fritsche et al., 2000). During the evaluation process the patients will be categorized as low, moderate, or high risk based on surgical risk and medical condition. Apart from the indications, it is important to define the absolute and relative contraindications for KTx (see Table 13.3 and Table 13.4).

## Evaluation process

Once a patient is referred to a transplant centre by the dialysis unit the first step is an information and education session where the entire process is explained not only to the potential recipient but also to the family members. Patients will benefit from a KTx only if carefully evaluated by a multidisciplinary team of transplant surgeons, nephrologists, anaesthesiologists, nurses, and social workers. It is important to understand that potential candidates will have CKD-associated comorbidities that may compromise extrarenal organ function with potential to impact post-KTx outcome. Therefore pre-existing extrarenal disease must be carefully assessed in order to anticipate potential medical problems that may jeopardize KTx. Anaemia is a well-recognized complication in patients with CKD (Kamar et al., 2012; Malyszko et al., 2012; Naci et al., 2012). The extensive use of recombinant erythropoietin has enormously reduced the need for blood transfusions and the consequent risk for infections or anti-HLA-class I antibody development. The uraemic status of ESRD patients induces different abnormalities of the coagulation cascade that can range from platelet dysfunction to hypercoagulable status (Milburn et al., 2011; Phelan et al., 2011). This latter condition can not only affect the arteriovenous grafts but also induce clotting or thrombosis of the graft (Keller et al., 2012).

The upper and lower gastrointestinal tract must be evaluated before KTx as abnormalities such as gastritis, diverticulitis, and/or diverticulosis are very common (Scheff et al., 1980; Parnaby et al., 2012). Hepatic dysfunction related to viral infection, alcohol

**Table 13.2** Primary diseases that can recur in KTx

| Disease | Incidence (%) | Likelihood of graft loss (%) |
|---|---|---|
| Focal segmental glomerulosclerosis | 20–100 | 30–50 |
| MPGN | 20–70 (type I) | 10–40 |
| | 20–50 (type II) | 50–100 |
| Membranous glomerulonephritis | 3–10 | <2 |
| IgA nephropathy | 50–80 | <10 |
| Anti-GBM disease | 25–50 | <2 |

MPGN, Membranoproliferative glomerulonephritis; GBM, glomerular basement membrane.

**Table 13.3** Absolute contraindications to KTx

| |
|---|
| Disseminated or untreated cancer |
| Chronic untreated or active infection |
| Active glomerulonephritis |
| Positive T-cell cross-match |
| Severe irreversible extrarenal disease (heart, liver, lung) |
| Severe psychiatric disease |
| Unsolvable psychosocial problems |
| Persistent substance abuse |
| Severe mental retardation |
| Advanced forms of coronary artery disease, refractory congestive heart failure |
| Primary oxalosis |
| Active systemic disease (Lupus, Goodpasture, Wegener) |

**Table 13.4** Relative contraindications to KTx

| |
|---|
| Treated malignancy: the cancer-free interval required will vary depending on the stage and type of cancer |
| Substance abuse history: patients should be involved in rehabilitation programmes and screened for random toxicological texts |
| Chronic liver disease: candidates with chronic hepatitis B or C or persistently abnormal function testing must have hepatology clearance prior to transplantation |
| Cardiovascular disease, including aorto-iliac abnormalities |
| Morbid obesity |

use, or toxic drugs must be addressed and cleared by a hepatologist (Fabrizi et al. 2010; Butt et al., 2011).

Bone disease secondary to impaired calcium and phosphorus metabolism and elevated parathyroid hormone (PTH) levels are frequently observed in dialysis patients (Moorthi and Moe, 2011; Tanaka et al., 2012). A pretransplant evaluation should be performed also in view of the immunosuppressive regimens (IS), since this may impact the degree of osteopaenia and osteoporosis (Kalantar-Zadeh et al., 2012; Kulak et al., 2012). An important consideration is to determine if the recipient will be able to tolerate IS and related side effects (Srinivas and Kaplan, 2011).

The ability to understand the risks and benefits of the procedure, and compliance with the medical regimen, including routine laboratory tests and clinic appointments, should be addressed with patients and their caregivers. Patients should also be warned that a KTx might not last a lifetime and there exists the possibility of returning to dialysis. For this reason KTx candidates should be informed that pre-existing vascular access (i.e. arteriovenous fistulae) for haemodialysis should be preserved, whereas peritoneal dialysis catheters will be removed during or shortly after the transplant procedure. Pretransplant removal of one or both native kidneys is rarely required. The few exceptions are for oversized, infected, or bleeding polycystic kidneys, intractable hypertension (HTN), chronic infection secondary to stones, or reflux nephropathy (Patel et al., 2011). Bilateral nephrectomy may be indicated also in the case of heavy proteinuria secondary to FSGS. The pretransplant evaluation includes a complete medical/surgical history, a review of systems, and a physical examination. A thorough medical history is essential in determining the candidate's risk profile and informs the remainder of the evaluation. Key information includes the original diagnosis that led to ESRD, history of urologic, cardiovascular (CV), and neoplastic disease, pregnancies, and previous blood transfusions. It is important to identify potential hereditary risk factors, including family history of ESRD, HTN, CV disease, cancer, and diabetes.

Particular attention should be directed at the CV assessment. In KTx, CV disease can be detected at any time interval and is the most common cause of death among patients with ESRD, ranging from 34% to 55% of the overall mortality. Pretransplant CV disease is a major risk factor for developing post-transplant CV events, with an odds ratio varying between 1.55 and 4.59 (Soveri et al., 2012). The problem is that CV disease is often asymptomatic, especially in diabetic patients. Coronary artery disease (CAD) accounts for approximately 50% of the mortality observed in patients with ESRD who have undergone KTx. Therefore prior to transplantation it is mandatory to detect and treat CAD, even if latent, as well as heart failure due to valvular failure or cardiomyopathy.

In contrast, based on evidence indicating that KTx may halt CV progression (Herwig-Ulf et al., 2004), CV morbidity, per se, even in patients with signs of uraemia, should not be considered an absolute contraindication to transplantation. For this reason CV screening (clinical evaluation by transplant cardiologist, EEG, echocardiography with evaluation of the ejection fraction) is recommended for all candidates prior to wait-listing. For those patients who are symptomatic or considered at higher CV risk (diabetics, patients with a history of poorly controlled or chronic severe HTN, smoking, age > 55 years, hyperlipidaemia, etc.) a more specific screening is requested. An analytical evaluation of screening tests to assess cardiac function in KTx candidates is beyond the scope of this chapter (see Chapter 14). However, the routine screening work-up should include the following (Pilmore, 2006):

1. Non-invasive test to evaluate myocardial perfusion in the asymptomatic patient considered at higher CV risk. Because of the high prevalence of non-specific abnormalities, neither the resting nor the exercise electrocardiogram are useful for the screening of KTx candidates undergoing cardiac evaluation.

In general, exercise tests are not feasible in many patients affected by renal failure. Instead, myocardial perfusion studies are commonly used in clinical practice. These include thallium/sestamibi/dipyridamol/scintigraphy-single photon emission computed tomography (SPECT) and dobutamine stress echocardiography.

2. Coronary angiography in symptomatic patients or those with an impaired perfusion scan. If perfusion studies reveal evidence of reversible ischaemia in higher-risk KTx candidates (e.g. diabetic type I with chronic renal disease), then angiography is mandatory.
3. Coronary revascularization for patients with critical CAD: the American College of Cardiology (ACC)/American Heart Association (AHA) (Fleisher et al., , 2014) guidelines do not recommend prophylactic revascularization prior to non-cardiac surgery in stable CAD patients. However, several authors (Karthykeyan and Ananthasubramanian, 2009) believe these guidelines may not be readily extrapolated to KTx candidates. In fact, renal dysfunction may persist after KTx and can be aggravated by the adverse effects of immunosuppressive drugs, which may contribute to the development of a form of accelerated atherosclerosis. Although the debate remains open, in the case of critical coronary lesions most KTx candidates will benefit from the appropriate revascularization procedure, prior to wait-listing.

Finally, for all KTx candidates there is convincing evidence that beta-blockers and statins in the perioperative period may exert a protective effect with a reduction of CV morbidity (Wang and Kasiske, 2010; Jardine et al., 2011). Transplant candidates should be strongly encouraged to stop smoking before and after KTx. An association between the effects of cigarette smoking and reduced patient and graft survival has been reported (Kasiske and Klinger, 2000; Sung et al., 2001). Regardless of the type of KTx, patients undergo immunological screening to include: blood and tissue typing, PRA and DSA, and cross-match (Ayala García et al., 2012). The other relevant components of the pretransplant evaluation are outlined in Table 13.5.

**Table 13.5** Laboratory and diagnostic evaluations for KTx candidates

| |
|---|
| Complete blood chemistry and blood count, coagulation profile, PTH level |
| CMV, EBV, HIV, hepatitis A, B, C, varicella-zoster serologies |
| RPR, PPD |
| Urine analysis and culture |
| Immunological tests in case of glomerulonephritis and/or systemic disease, including C3, C4 Rheumatoid factor, double strain DNA, ANA, anti-GBM, ANCA |
| Immunological profile, blood type (ABO), PRA |
| HLA typing, DSAs |
| Chest X-ray, EKG |
| Gynaecological evaluation (Pap smear) |
| Mammography (family history of, > 40 years of age) |
| Urologic assessment in selected patients (PSA if > 50 years of age) |
| Upper GI endoscopy |
| Abdominal ultrasound, CT if indicated |
| Pulmonary function tests in selected patients |
| Carotid duplex study, peripheral arterial Doppler in selected patients |
| Complete cardiac work-up |
| Dental evaluation and clearance |

PRA, Panel reactive antibody; DSA, donor-specific antibodies; PTH, Parathyroid hormone; CMV, Cytomegalovirus; EBV, Ebstein barr virus; HIV, Human immunodeficiency virus; RPR, Rapid plasma reagin; PPD, Purified protein derivative; PSA, Protein specific antibody.

## Selection

When the transplant evaluation is complete, the transplant team will meet, discuss the results, and make the decision to place the candidate on the transplant waiting list or to request further tests. Generally, patients for whom the KTx is not indicated due to a serious medical condition are notified of such at the first meeting with the transplant team or during the evaluation process. Due to the scarcity of cadaveric organs, previously established patient categories should be deemed suitable for ECD kidney and defined based on donor risk factors such as: age, serum creatinine (Cr) in milligrammes per litre (Cr), cerebrovascular accident (CVA) as a cause of death, and history of HTN, as shown in Table 13.6 (Savoye et al., 2007; Pascual et al., 2008; Mezrich et al., 2012).

Dual kidneys are also allocated to selected patient categories if the donor meets at least two of the following conditions: age > 60 years, estimated serum Cr clearance < 60 mL/min, rising Cr > 2.5%, and abnormal histological findings (i.e. moderate to severe glomerulosclerosis) (Moore et al., 2007). During the wait-listing period, the dialysis centre should actively communicate with the transplant centre any relevant changes in the medical condition of the KTx candidate (Kim et al., 2012). The dialysis centre is responsible for sending the patient's serum to the transplant immunology laboratory for the possible detection of PRA. Patients on the active transplant list should also be re-evaluated yearly and some tests repeated according to patient status and progression of underlying medical conditions.

**Table 13.6** Cardiovascular risk factors and age in the expanded criteria donor

| Donor condition | Age 50–59 years | Age > 60 years |
|---|---|---|
| CVA + HTN + serum CR > 1.5 | X | X |
| CVA + HTN | X | X |
| CVA + serum CR > 1.5 | X | X |
| CVA | – | X |
| HTN | – | X |
| Serum CR > 1.5 | – | X |

## Conclusion

In this chapter we have presented the key points in the selection and evaluation of the kidney transplant recipient. Based on the evidence we have reviewed it is clear that years of life with end-stage kidney disease and the duration of dialysis have a major impact on the outcome following KTx. Therefore we recommend early referral for KTx to ensure successful outcome. Ideally, pre-emptive (before dialysis) LD KTx is the preferred option with the best possible outcome, although seldom realized. This is mostly due to delays in referring candidates to a transplant centre. Finally, a barrier to pre-emptive transplantation is the shortage of cadaveric and living kidney donors.

## References


Akkina SK, Muster H, Steffens E, et al. (2011) Donor exchange programs in kidney transplantation: rationale and operational details from the north central donor exchange cooperative. *Am J Kidney Dis*, **57**:152–158.

Audard V, Kamar N, Sahali D, et al. (2012) Rituximab therapy prevents focal and segmental glomerulosclerosis recurrence after a second renal transplantation. *Transplant Int*, **25**:62–66.

Ayala García MA, González Yebra B, López Flores AL, Guaní Guerra E (2012) The major histocompatibility complex in transplantation. *J Transplant*, 2012: 842141.

Böhmig GA, Wahrmann M, Bartel G (2011) Transplantation of the broadly sensitized patient: what are the options? *Curr Opin Organ Transplant*, **16**:588–593.

Butt AA, Wang X, Fried LF (2011) HCV infection and the incidence of CKD. *Am J Kidney Dis*, **57**:396–407.

Canaud G, Audard V, Kofman T, et al. (2012) Recurrence from primary and secondary glomerulopathy after renal transplant. *Transplant Int*, **25**:812–824.

Caro-Oleas JL, Gonzalez/Escribano MF, Gonzalez/Roncero FM, et al. (2011) Clinical relevance of HLA donor-specific antibodies detected by single antigen assay in kidney transplantation. *Nephrol Dialysis Transplant*, **27**:1231–1238.

Davis CL (2010) Preemptive transplantation and the transplant first initiative. *Curr Opin Nephrol Hypertens*, **19**:592–597.

Davis CL, Delmonico FL (2005) Living-donor kidney transplantation: a review of the current practices for the live donor. *J Am Soc Nephrol*, **16**:2098–2110.

de Mattos AM, Siedlecki A, Gaston RS, et al. (2008) Systolic dysfunction portends increased mortality among those waiting for renal transplant. *J Am Soc Nephrol*, **19**:1191–1196.

Fabrizi F, Martin P, Messa P (2010) Hepatitis B and hepatitis C virus and chronic kidney disease. *Acta Gastroenterol Belg*, **73**: 465–471.

Fehr T, Stussi G (2012) ABO-incompatible kidney transplantation. *Curr Opin Organ Transplant*, **17**:376–385.

Fleisher LA, Fleischmann KE, Auerbach AD, et al. (2014) ACC/AHA guideline on perioperative cardiovascular evaluation and management of patients undergoing noncardiac surgery. *Circulation*, **130**:e278–e333.

Friedewald JJ, Reese PP (2012). The kidney-first initiative: what is the current status of preemptive transplantation? *Adv Chronic Kidney Dis*, **19**:252–256.

Fritsche L, Vanrenterghem Y, Nordal KP, et al. (2000) Practice variations in the evaluation of adult candidates for cadaveric kidney transplantation: a survey of the European Transplant Centers. *Transplantation*, **70**:1492–1497.

Garcia GG, Harden P, Chapman J, World Kidney Day Steering Committee (2012) The global role in kidney transplantation. *Curr Opin Organ Transplant*, **17**:362–367.

Goldfarb-Rumyantzev A, Hurdle JF, et al. (2005) Duration of end-stage renal disease and kidney transplant outcome. *Nephrol Dialysis Transplant*, **20**:167–175.

Grams ME, Massie AB, Coresh J, et al. (2011) Trends in the timing of pre-emptive kidney transplantation. *J Am Soc Nephrol*, **22**:1615–1620.

Herwig-Ulf Meier Kriesche HU, Schold SD, et al. (2004) Kidney transplantation halts cardiovascular disease progression in patient with end stage renal disease. *Am J Transplant*, **4**:1662–1668.

Hickson LJ, Cosio FG, El-Zoghby ZM (2008) Survival of patients on the kidney transplant wait list: relationship to cardiac troponin T. *Am J Transplant*, **8**:2352–2359.

Hwang JH, Han SS, Huh W, et al. (2012) Outcome of kidney allograft in patients with adulthood-onset focal segmental glomerulosclerosis: comparison with childhood-onset FSGS. *Nephrol Dialysis Transplant*, **27**:2559–2565.

Inrig JK, Sun JL, Yang Q, et al. (2006) Mortality by dialysis modality among patients who have end-stage renal disease and are awaiting renal transplantation. *Clin J Am Soc Nephrol*, **1**:774–779.

Jardine AG, Gaston RS, Fellstrom BC, Holdaas H (2011) Prevention of cardiovascular disease in adult recipients of kidney transplants. *Lancet*, **378**:1419–1427.

Kalantar-Zadeh K, Molnar MZ, Kovesdy CP, et al. (2012) Management of mineral and bone disorder after kidney transplantation. *Curr Opin Nephrol Hypertens*, **21**:389–403.

Kamar N, Rostaing L, Ignace S, et al. (2012) Impact of post-transplant anemia on patient and graft survival rates after kidney transplantation: a meta-analysis. *Clin Transplant*, **26**:461–469.

Karthykeyan V, Ananthasubramanian P (2009) *Curr Cardiol Rev*, **5**:177–186.

Kasiske B, Klinger D (2000) Cigarette smoking in renal transplant recipients. *JAMA*, **11**:753–759.

Kasiske BL, Ramos EL, Gaston RS, et al. (1995) The evaluation of renal transplant candidates: clinical practice guidelines. Patient Care and Education Committee of the American Society of Transplant Physicians. *J Am Soc Nephrol*, **6**:1–34.

Kasiske BL, Snyder JJ, Matas AJ, et al. (2002) Preemptive kidney transplantation: the advantage and the advantaged. *J Am Soc Nephrol*, **13**:1358–1364.

Keith DS (2012) Therapeutic apheresis rescue mission: recurrent focal segmental glomerulosclerosis in renal allografts. *Semin Dial*, **25**:190–192.

Keller AK, Jorgensen TM, Jespersen B (2012) Identification of risk factors for vascular thrombosis may reduce early renal graft loss: a review of recent literature. *J Transplant*, 2012:793461.

Kher A, Mandelbrot DA (2012) The living kidney donor evaluation: focus on renal issues *Clin J Am Soc Nephrol*, **17**:366–371.

Kim MG, Ro H, Kim YJ, Park HC, et al. (2012) Management of patients on the waiting list for deceased donor kidney transplantation. *Transplant Proc*, **44**:66–71.

Kulak CA, Borba VZ, Kulak J Jr, et al. (2012) Osteoporosis after transplantation. *Curr Osteop Rep*, **10**:48–55.

Małyszko J, Watschinger B, Przybyłowski P, et al. (2012) Anemia in solid organ transplantation. *Annal Transplant*, **17**:86–100.

Mandelbrot DA, Pavlakis M (2012) Living donor practices in the United States. *Adv Chronic Kidney Dis*, **19**:212–219.

Mehrabi A, Fonouni H, Ayoub E, et al. (2009) A single center experience of combined liver kidney transplantation. *Clin Transplant*, **23**:102–114.

Meier-Kriesche HU, Kaplan B (2002) Waiting time on dialysis as the strongest modifiable risk factor for renal transplant outcomes. *Transplantation*, **74**:1377–1381.

Mezrich JD, Pirsch JD, Fernandez LA, et al. (2012) Differential outcomes of expanded-criteria donor renal allografts according to recipient age. *Clin J Am Soc Nephrol*, **7**:1163–1171.

Milburn JA, Cassar K, Ford I, et al. (2011) Prothrombotic changes in platelet, endothelial and coagulation function following hemodialysis. *Int J Artificial Organs*, **34**:280–287.

Montgomery JR, Berger JC, Warren DS, et al. (2012) Outcomes of ABO-incompatible kidney transplantation in the United States. *Transplantation*, **93**:603–609.

Montgomery RA, Lonze BE, King KE, et al. (2011) Desensitization in HLA-incompatible kidney recipients and survival. *N Engl J Med*, **365**:318–326.

Moore PS, Farney AC, Sundberg AK, et al. (2007) Dual kidney transplantation: a case-control comparison with single kidney transplantation from standard and expanded criteria donors. *Transplantation*, **83**:1551–1556.

Moorthi RN, Moe SM (2011) CKD-mineral and bone disorder: core curriculum 2011. *Am J Kidney Dis*, **58**:1022–1036.

Naci H, de Lissovoy G, Hollenbeak C, et al. (2012) Historical clinical and economic consequences of anemia management in patients with end-stage renal disease on dialysis using erythropoietin stimulating agents versus routine blood transfusions: a retrospective cost- effectiveness analysis. *J Med Econ*, **15**:293–304.

Oniscu GC, Brown H, Forsythe JLR (2005) Impact of cadaveric renal transplantation on survival in patients listed for transplantation *J Am Soc Nephrol*, **16**:1859–1865.

Parnaby CN, Barrow EJ, Edirimanne SB, et al. (2012) Colorectal complications of end-stage renal failure and renal transplantation: a review. *Colorectal Dis*, **14**:403–415.

Pascual J, Zamora J, Pirsch JD (2008) A systematic review of kidney transplantation from expanded criteria donors. *Am J Kidney Dis*, **52**:553–586.

Patel P, Horsfield C, Compton F, Taylor J, et al. (2011) Native nephrectomy in transplant patients with autosomal dominant polycystic kidney disease *Annal R Coll Surg Engl*, **93**:391–395.

Phelan PJ, O'Kelly P, Holian J, et al. (2011) Warfarin use in hemodialysis patients: what is the risk? *Clin Nephrol*, **75**:204–211.

Pilmore H (2006) Cardiac Assessment for renal transplantation. *Am J Transplant*, **6**:659–665.

Ponticelli C, Glassock RJ (2010) Post-transplant recurrence of primary glomerulonephritis. *Clin J Am Soc Nephrol*, **5**:2363–2372.

Sanoff SL, Balogun RA, Lobo PL (2012) The role of therapeutic apheresis in high immunologic risk renal transplantation: a review of current trends. *Semin Dial*, **25**:193–200.

Savoye E, Tamarelle D, Chalem Y, et al. (2007) Survival benefits of kidney transplantation with expanded criteria deceased donors in patients aged 60 years and over. *Transplantation*, **84**:1618–1624.

Scheff RT, Zuckerman G, Harter H, et al. (1980) Diverticular disease in patients with chronic renal failure due to polycystic kidney disease. *Annal Internal Med*, **92**:202–204.

Schold JD, Segev DL (2012) Increasing pool the of deceased donor organs for kidney transplantation. *Natl Rev Nephrol*, **8**:325–331.

Schold J, Srinivas TR, Sehgal AR, et al. (2009) Half of kidney transplant candidates who are older than 60 years now placed on the waiting list will die before receiving a deceased-donor transplant. *Clin J Am Soc Nephrol*, **4**:1239–1245.

Soveri I, Holme I, Holdaas H, et al. (2012) A cardiovascular risk calculator for renal transplant Recipients. *Transplantation*, **94**:57–62.

Srinivas TR, Kaplan B (2011) Transplantation in 2011: new agents, new ideas and new hope. *Nat Rev Nephrol*, **8**:74–75.

Sung RS, Althoen M, Howell TA, et al. (2001) Excess risk of renal allograft loss associated with cigarette smoking. *Transplantation*, **71**:1752–1757.

Tanaka H, Komaba H, Koizumi M, et al. (2012) Role of uremic toxins and oxidative stress in the development of chronic kidney disease—mineral and bone disorder. *J Renal Nutr*, **22**:98–101.

Terasaki P (2012) A personal perspective 100-year history of the humoral theory of transplantation. *Transplantation*, **93**:751–756.

Terasaki P, Cai J (2008) Human leukocyte antigen antibodies and chronic rejection: from association to causation. *Transplantation*, **86**:377–383.

Toledo K, Pérez-Sáez MJ, Navarro MD, et al. (2011) Impact of recurrent glomerulonephritis on renal graft survival. *Transplant Proc*, **43**:2182–2216.

Wang JH, Kasiske B (2010) Screening and management of pretransplant vascular disease. *Curr Opin Nephrol Hypertens*, **19**:586–591.

Wiebe C, Gibson IW, Blydt-Hansen TD, et al. (2012) Evolution and clinical pathologic correlations of de novo donor-specific HAL antibody post kidney transplant. *Am J Transplant*, **12**:1157–1167.

Wolfe RA, Ashby VB, Milford EL, et al. (1999) Comparison of mortality in all patients on dialysis, patients on dialysis awaiting transplantation and recipients of a first cadaveric transplant. *N Engl J Med*, **341**:1725–1730.

# CHAPTER 14

# Kidney transplantation: perioperative cardiovascular risk and anaesthetic management

Livia Pompei, Maria Gabriella Costa, Mauricio Sainz-Barriga, George Burke, and Giorgio Della Rocca

## Perioperative cardiovascular risk screening and evaluation

The overall goal of screening patients with ESRD who are being evaluated for KTx is to reduce perioperative morbidity and mortality from cardiovascular disease (CVD). There are three primary objectives for screening: (1) to determine whether CVD is present; (2) to implement therapies to reduce major adverse cardiac events (MACE) for those with CVD who are considered suitable candidates; and (3) to identify patients with unstable cardiac conditions (unstable angina, decompensated heart failure, critical valvular disease, and severe arrhythmia) who may not be suitable transplant candidates. In this surgical patient population screening makes sense only if the results lead to changes in management that improve outcomes.

Recently, the AHA and ACC together promulgated 'Guidelines on Cardiovascular Evaluation and Care for Non-Cardiac Surgery' (Lentine et al., 2012). These evidence-based guidelines are intended to assist in the evaluation of cardiac risk and management of transplant candidates during the pretransplant decision-making process. Prior to the AHA/ACC guidelines there was no consensus on cardiovascular evaluation in patients with ESRD being considered for KTx; further, there was no agreement regarding the utility of routine screening methods to reliably detect cardiac disease (Lentine et al., 2008; Patel et al., 2008; Poldermans et al., 2009). Other guidelines, such as those from the American Society of Nephrology (ASN) and those of the AST, differ from those of the AHA/ACC (Kasiske et al., 2001; National Kidney Foundation, 2005; Fleisher et al., 2014). Both should be taken into account in the pretransplant period.

Although KTx per se is considered an intermediate-risk procedure for cardiac complications, prospective candidates often have multiple risk factors for CAD, such as advanced age, diabetes mellitus, hypertension, and known ischaemic heart disease, in addition to their ESRD (Boersma et al., 2005). The minimum required investigations include a complete history and physical examination, ECG, and a chest radiograph. A well-executed and thorough history and physical can detect an active cardiac condition. 'Active' conditions include unstable angina, coronary syndrome, decompensated heart failure, significant arrhythmias, and severe valvular disease (Fleisher et al., 2014).

The AHA/ACC 2014 guidelines (Fleisher et al., 2014) were designed to assess cardiovascular risk among a wide age range of patients with a broad spectrum of chronic medical conditions. However, because the transplant population is on average younger than the general population, the use of mean exercise tolerance (MET) to assess functional status may be limited in some patients. Recently, Friedman et al. (2011) in a study of 204 consecutive transplant candidates with no active cardiac conditions found that 80% had good functional status (> 4 MET) but that functional status was not a useful discriminator of the presence of CAD. Importantly, patients scheduled for KTx usually have more than one clinical risk factor for CAD. Azotemia and diabetes mellitus are the most common risk factors in these patients. Although the guidelines focus on short-term risk assessment, both short-term and long-term management of CAD are important considerations among KTx candidates. Few studies have focused on the incidence of major adverse cardiac events during hospitalization or within 30 days of transplant surgery.

One alternative to the use of the AHA/ACC-defined CAD risk factors is to consider those more specific to the transplantation population, as suggested in the 2007 Lisbon Conference report (Abbud-Filho et al., 2007). In contrast to the AHA/ACC approach, this strategy appeared to improve sensitivity and specificity for the identification of CAD and reduced the overall frequency of testing in a single centre (Friedman et al., 2011). The risk factors for CAD deemed relevant to transplantation candidates in the Lisbon Conference report include diabetes mellitus, prior cardiovascular disease, > 1 year on dialysis, left ventricular hypertrophy, age > 60 years, smoking, hypertension, and dyslipidaemia (Abbud-Filho et al., 2007).

In order to simplify the screening process a classification scheme based on risk factors and functional status may be useful, as outlined in the following sections.

### Asymptomatic patients (MET > 4)

There are no definitive data at this time for or against screening for myocardial ischaemia among KTx candidates who are free

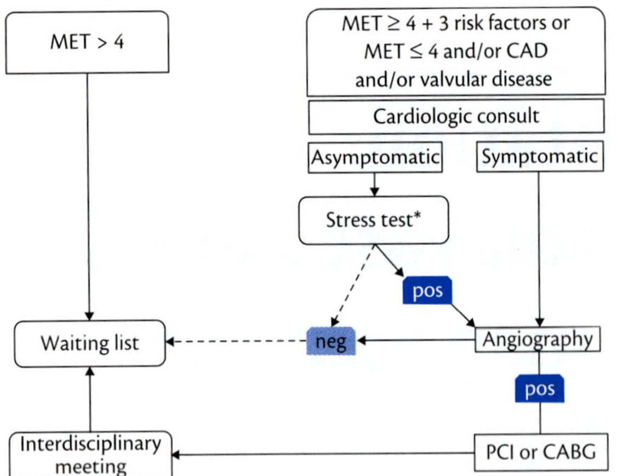


Risk factors = diabetes mellitus, prior cardiovascular disease, more than 1 year on dialysis, left ventricular hypertrophy, age greater than 60 years, smoking, hypertension, and dyslipidemia.
CAD = coronary artery disease
PCI = percutaneous coronary intervention
CABG = coronary artery bypass grafting
*Non invasive stress testing.

**Fig. 14.1** Flowchart for cardiac evaluation in KTx candidates after history, physical examination, ECG, and chest X-ray evaluation

of active cardiac conditions (Lentine et al., 2012; Fleisher et al., 2014). However, until more data are available it may be useful to use aggregate CAD risk factors to target screening of patients with the highest pretest likelihood of 'prognostically significant' CAD (Lentine et al., 2012) (see Figure 14.1).

## Asymptomatic patients (MET ≥ 4) with multiple cardiac risk factors

Non-invasive stress testing may be considered in KTx candidates with no active cardiac conditions but who have multiple CAD risk factors regardless of functional status (Abbud-Filho et al., 2007). As previously reported, relevant risk factors among transplant candidates include diabetes mellitus, prior cardiovascular disease, more than 1 year on dialysis, left ventricular hypertrophy, age > 60 years, smoking, hypertension, and dyslipidaemia. The specific number of risk factors that should be used to prompt testing remains to be determined, but the consensus is three or more as reasonable (Lentine et al., 2012) (see Figure 14.1). It is important for transplant programmes to include a primary cardiology consultant to screen potential kidney transplant candidates with high cardiovascular risk and for coordination of care.

## Symptomatic patients or known patients for CAD

Symptomatic patients with known CAD and poor functional status require additional screening. These include candidates with left ventricular ejection fraction (LVEF) less than 50%, evidence of ischaemic left ventricular dilation, exercise-induced hypotension, angina, or demonstrable ischaemia in the distribution of multiple coronary arteries. These patients require referral to cardiology for comprehensive cardiac evaluation and long-term management and may not be good candidates for transplantation.

Testing for CAD may be performed non-invasively using several modalities including nuclear myocardial perfusion studies and dobutamine stress echocardiography (Herzog et al., 1999; De Lima et al., 2003; Rabbat et al., 2003; Wijeysundera et al., 2010). Even though the studies are conflicting with regard to perioperative predictive value, nuclear imaging and echocardiographic studies are especially useful for screening high-risk patients. The choice of tests depends on the expertise of the personnel performing the study. Non-invasive testing, when positive, should be followed by coronary angiography and revascularization, if indicated, even if potentially harmful (Manske et al., 1992; De Lima et al., 2010; Lentine et al., 2012). Coronary revascularization before transplantation surgery should be considered in patients who meet AHA/ACC guidelines criteria (Hillis et al., 2011). It is recognized that in some asymptomatic transplant candidates the risk of coronary revascularization may outweigh the risk of transplantation, and these risks must be considered on a case-by-case basis by a multidisciplinary transplant team (Lentine et al., 2012). The most uncertainty surrounds high-risk patients with significant coronary disease but who are not candidates for revascularization. In these cases it is reasonable to maximize medical therapy and re-evaluate them on a more frequent basis. Routine prophylactic coronary revascularization before transplant surgery is not recommended in asymptomatic patients with stable CAD (Lentine et al., 2012). Finally, patients with symptomatic CAD who have undergone successful revascularization (bypass or angioplasty) are at lower risk of perioperative ischaemic events and hence can be listed (Herzog et al., 2004).

## Cardiac surveillance on the waiting list

There are limited data on the appropriate level of surveillance for candidates on the waiting list (Danovitch et al., 2002; Matas et al., 2002). The usefulness of periodically screening asymptomatic KTx candidates for myocardial ischaemia while on the transplant waiting list to reduce the risk of MACE is uncertain (Lentine et al., 2012). Nevertheless, clinical assessment should occur at initial evaluation and again immediately before anticipated transplantation to determine whether there has been an interval change in cardiovascular conditions. In addition, there is no evidence for or against repeated left ventricular function testing after listing for KTx.

Re-evaluation should be performed in asymptomatic patients (MET > 4) on a yearly basis. This should include history and physical examination, 12-lead ECG, and chest X-ray. If the patient at any point during re-evaluations shows signs of reduction in cardiorespiratory functional reserve (MET ≤ 4 and/or peripheral capillary oxygen saturation ($SpO_2$) < 94%) the patient should be referred for appropriate treatment and receive more frequent evaluations thereafter (Figure 14.2, arms A and B). Patients with known CAD, even if asymptomatic, should be re-evaluated on a regular basis (every 6 months) (Figure 14.2, arm B); if these patients show changes in their cardiac condition, consultation with a cardiologist should be sought and additional testing considered. The appearance of or worsening of symptoms during the wait-list period should trigger referral to cardiology for follow-up non-invasive and/or invasive stress testing. Based on these results, eligibility for continued listing should be reassessed by a multidisciplinary 'high-risk' committee (Figure 14.2, arm C).

High-risk patients on the transplant waiting list should be treated aggressively with risk-factor reduction strategies. In this regard, the expert consensus statement suggested:

- It is recommended in patients already receiving beta-blockers to continue beta-blocked medication perioperatively to prevent rebound hypertension and tachycardia.

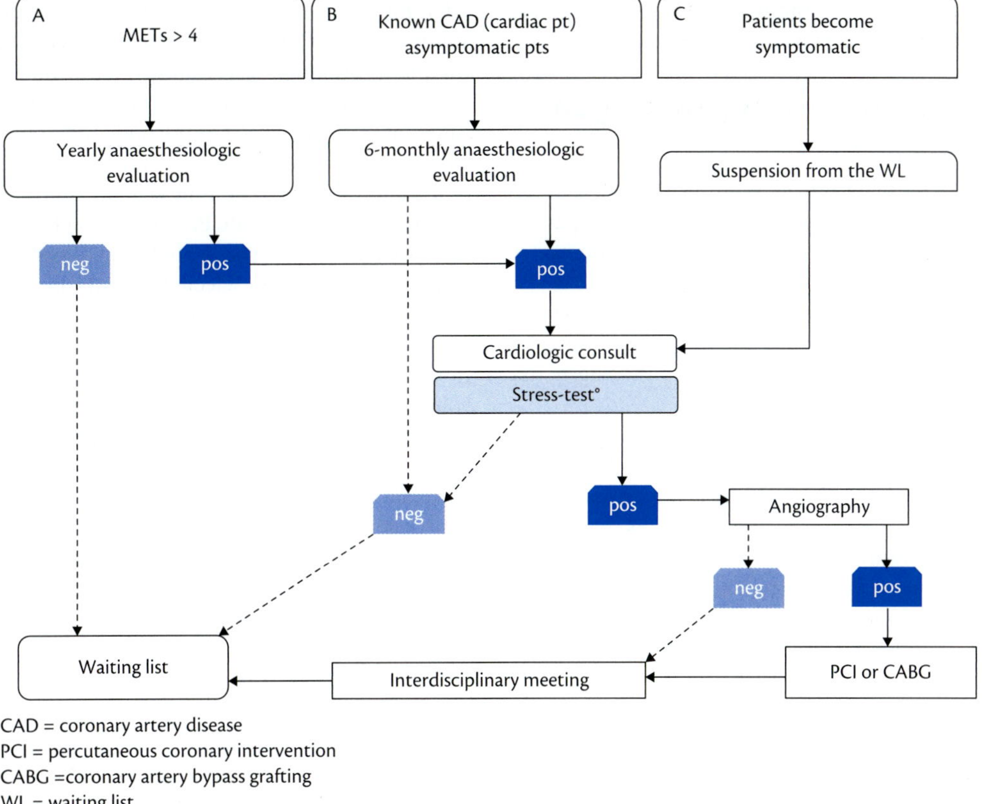


**Fig. 14.2** Flowchart for surveillance on the wait-list in KTx candidates

- It is reasonable to initiate beta-blockers preoperatively and to continue them postoperatively among patients being considered for renal transplantation with clinical markers of cardiac risk and those with unequivocal myocardial ischaemia on preoperative stress testing, provided that dose titration is done carefully to avoid bradycardia and hypotension.
- Perioperative initiation of beta-blockers in beta-blocker-naïve patients may be considered in KTx candidates with established CAD and three or more cardiovascular risk factors to protect against perioperative cardiovascular events if dosing is titrated and monitored.
- It is not recommended to initiate beta-blocker therapy in beta-blocker-naïve patients the day of transplant surgery; it may be reasonable to begin more than 1 day before surgery.
- Continuation of angiotensin-converting enzyme (ACE) inhibitors or angiotensin II receptor antagonists is reasonable before transplant surgery in patients with left ventricular systolic dysfunction.
- When ACE inhibitors and angiotensin II receptor antagonists are prescribed for hypertension their withdrawal may be considered 24 hours before surgery, if there is time. They should be resumed after transplant as soon as blood pressure and volume are stable.
- Administration of dopamine to the kidney transplant recipient is not beneficial for renal allograft function, and administration may be harmful.
- Starting or carrying on aspirin therapy is not beneficial in patients undergoing elective non-cardiac non-carotid surgery without previous coronary stenting.
- It may be reasonable to administer statins to kidney transplant candidates to reduce the risk of vascular disease events.
- It is recommended that statin treatment be continued perioperatively and in patients undergoing renal transplantation who are taking statin therapy.
- It is reasonable to initiate low-to-moderate-dose statin therapy preoperatively and to continue treatment postoperatively in patients undergoing renal transplantation in whom preoperative evaluation established unequivocal evidence of atherosclerosis.

## Pulmonary evaluation

A chest radiograph should be included in the preoperative respiratory assessment of KTx, in addition to routine evaluation with medical history and physical examination. If the patient has an $SpO_2 < 94\%$, additional tests should be ordered such as arterial blood gases and/or pulmonary function tests.

All patients considered for KTx should be strongly encouraged to stop smoking. It must start early (at least 6–8 weeks prior to surgery, 4 weeks minimum). As proposed by the European Society of Anaesthesiologists (ESA) guidelines, incentive spirometry preoperatively can be of benefit in upper abdominal surgery to avoid postoperative pulmonary complications. In addition, correction of a malnutrition state may be beneficial (De Hert et al., 2011).

## Perioperative physiological monitoring and anaesthetic management

Anaesthesia for renal transplant surgery requires a patient-centred perioperative approach based on severity of ESRD and patient comorbidities. Major anaesthetic considerations are maintenance of adequate renal blood flow and avoidance of nephrotoxic drugs. No data are available to determine whether inhalational versus total intravenous techniques are superior for preserving graft renal blood flow or whether haemodynamic monitoring better preserves preload status in these patients.

### Intraoperative period

Anaesthesia monitoring should encompass relevant comorbidities and volume status which can vary during the interval since the last dialysis. Body temperature and neuromuscular transmission monitoring is necessary to avoid postoperative residual muscle relaxation. A non-invasive technique is preferable over invasive techniques for systemic blood pressure monitoring, because any damage to a peripheral artery may preclude its later use for dialysis access, if the need arises. It is also valuable to protect existing vascular routes for dialysis.

We have yet to develop methods to monitor renal perfusion, which would be the ideal monitor for renal transplantation. As such, we are limited to ensuring renal perfusion via indirect measurements and careful maintenance of intravascular volume (preload), cardiac performance, and systemic perfusion as mean systemic arterial pressure (MAP).

#### Invasive haemodynamic monitoring

In patients undergoing renal transplant surgery, assessment of adequate preload has been presumed to be achieved with placement of internal jugular or subclavian vein catheters for preload monitoring or, more seldom, by insertion of pulmonary artery catheter (PAC) for measurement of pulmonary arterial occlusion pressure (PAOP). However, it is controversial to believe that CVP or PAOP are in fact reliable indices of preload, useful for perioperative volume management (Sakka et al., 1999; Della Rocca et al., 2002a, 2002b). Continuous $SvO_2$ monitoring (with near-infrared equipped PAC) or intermittent sampling of mixed venous oxygen saturation are also of questionable value for guiding haemodynamic management, especially during anaesthesia in patients with arteriovenous fistula (Della Rocca and Pompei, 2011).

#### Non-invasive and mini-invasive haemodynamic monitoring

Non-invasive preload assessment can include the monitoring of cardiac output and corrected flow time (FTc) with an oesophageal Doppler monitor. Other techniques employed during anaesthesia to assess intravascular volume status in paralyzed patients on mechanical ventilation include non-invasive measurement of systolic pressure or stoke volume variation using plethysmographic techniques or with transthoracic electrical bioimpedance (TEB). However, values so derived have not been well validated and will, as the name implies, vary widely during positive pressure ventilation. Systolic pressure variation correlates well with left ventricular end-diastolic volume. Stroke volume variation and pulse pressure variation as measured with the LiDCO (LiDCO System, London, UK), PiCCO (Pulsion Medical System, Munich, Germany), and Vigileo system (Edwards Lifesciences Irvine, California, US) and the plethysmographic variability index obtained from Masimo monitor (Masimo Corporation Irvine, California, US) are all indicators of fluid responsiveness (Jones and Tonser, 2002) and hence volume status. Another option may consist of direct measurement of intrathoracic blood volume (ITBV) and/or global end-diastolic volume (GEDV) with the PiCCO system (Reuter et al., 2002). The latter two techniques require both radial and femoral arterial catheterization. Data from selected patients undergoing KTx are lacking. Non-calibrated systems such as the Vigileo cannot be precise and accurate methods of preload evaluation in patients with arteriovenous fistulas. Thus far, data on the accuracy of intravascular volume assessment using these non-invasive techniques sufficient to justify routine use in this group of patients are lacking.

The most direct non-invasive method to clinically monitor for adequate intravascular volume or preload during surgery, especially in patients with altered cardiac function, is assessment of left ventricular end-diastolic area (LVEDA) and all the other data derived with TEE. Table 14.1 lists commonly employed invasive and non-invasive and mini-invasive haemodynamic monitoring modalities.

### Choice of anaesthetics

When selecting anaesthetic agents for renal transplant recipients several important factors must be taken into account. These include the pharmacokinetic profile of the drug, the patient's preoperative volume status, the interval of time since the last dialysis, and comorbid conditions. Muscle relaxants such as pancuronium, atracurium, and succinylcholine, morphine, meperidine, and the non-steroidal analgesics are not suitable for use in patients undergoing KTx because of the kinetics of distribution, elimination, and side effects. Premedication prior to transplantation may be highly desirable. The water-soluble benzodiazepine midazolam is less influenced than diazepam by reduced plasma protein binding and can be more safely administered as a premedicant (Vinik

**Table 14.1** Variables useful to guide fluid therapy in KTx patients

| Preload indices | Monitor | Normal values |
|---|---|---|
| FTc | ED | 330–360 ms |
| ITBVI | PiCCO | 800–1000 mL/m$^2$ |
| GEDVI | PiCCO | 600–800 mL/m$^2$ |
| EDVI | Advanced PAC | 110–130 mL/m$^2$ |
| LVEDAI | TEE | 5.5–10 cm/m$^2$ |
| **Fluid responsiveness indices** | | |
| SVV | PiCCO–LiDCO | < 13% |
| PPV | PiCCO–LiDCO | < 12% |
| SPV | LiDCO | < 13% |
| PVI | Masimo | < 15% |

FTc, Flow time corrected; ED, oesophageal Doppler; ITBVI, intrathoracic blood volume index; GEDVI, global end-diastolic volume index; EDVI, end-diastolic volume index; PAC, pulmonary artery catheter; LVEDAI, left ventricular end-diastolic area index; TEE, transoesophageal echocardiography; SVV, stroke volume variation; PPV, pulse pressure variation; SPV, systolic pressure variation; PVI, plethismography variability index.

et al., 1983). As many patients undergoing renal transplantation may suffer from comorbid conditions such as diabetes, which can further contribute to the functional alteration in gastrointestinal motility, gastric aspiration prophylaxis and rapid sequence induction are frequently required. Succinylcholine is not recommended in patients with ESRD who have concomitant hyperkalaemia (Thapa and Brull, 2000). A non-depolarizing alternative to succinylcholine is rocuronium bromide that is given in a dose of 1.2 mg/kg and can provide optimal intubating conditions in approximately 55 seconds (Magorian et al., 1993). The elimination of this drug is primarily dependent on the hepatobiliary system, so that its clearance is not significantly altered in renal failure (Orko et al., 1987; Beauvoir et al., 1993; Della Rocca et al., 2003; Robertson et al., 2005). The liver also rapidly metabolizes vecuronium bromide, with only a slight increase in the duration of action in patients with renal failure (Beauvoir et al., 1993). However, when large doses are repeatedly administered for maintenance of muscle paralysis, prolongation of neuromuscular block may occur (Orko et al., 1987; Della Rocca et al., 2003).

Cisatracurium besilate is the most commonly used non-depolarizing agent. The elimination half-life of anticholinesterase drugs is prolonged in patients with ESRD, so much so that their plasma clearance tends to match or even to exceed that of non-depolarizing muscle relaxants, making postoperative residual relaxation unlikely. An alternative to anticholinesterase is sugammadex, a modified gamma-cyclodextrin that specifically encapsulates the steroidal neuromuscular blocking agent. When rocuronium or vecuronium bromide are used, neuromuscular block can be more safely reversed with sugammadex, with minimal to no risk of postoperative residual relaxation in patients with creatinine clearance higher than 30 mL/min (Staals et al., 2008). General anaesthesia is usually started with propofol, a drug with a rapid hepatic metabolism and inactive bioproducts excreted by the kidneys. Propofol pharmacokinetics is unaffected by end-stage renal failure, so that a standard induction dose as well as a continuous infusion can be safely administered in patients with renal failure (Ickx et al., 1998).

Thiopental is another agent used in patients undergoing renal transplantation, although in order to prevent undesirable cardiodepressant effects, a dose adjustment is frequently required, in relation to the reduced serum protein levels and hypovolaemia following dialysis (Burch and Stanski, 1982). As these authors have clearly demonstrated, the free fraction of an induction dose of thiopental is almost doubled in chronic renal failure. Although the free fraction of etomidate is increased in end-stage renal failure, the clinical effects of reduced protein binding are marginal, most likely because of the relative lack of depressant effects of the drug on the cardiovascular system (Carlos et al., 1979).

Inhalational anaesthetics appear not to produce significant adverse effects when administered in patients with ESRD. Isoflurane and desflurane are metabolized minimally, and therefore serum fluoride concentration does not rise significantly (Sutton et al., 1991). Although sevoflurane metabolism may result in higher concentrations of fluoride, studies on patients with end-stage renal failure have shown a lack of renal toxicity when sevoflurane is employed (Artru, 1998). The analgesic component of anaesthesia for renal transplant surgery can be achieved with the administration of potent opioids. The older-generation opioids such as morphine, oxycodone, and meperidine should be avoided because decreased clearance may result in accumulation of active metabolites, leading to prolonged postoperative respiratory depression. Remifentanil is rapidly metabolized by esterases in blood and tissues, with production of a weakly active metabolite, GR90291, which is excreted by the kidneys. Although renal failure does not seem to alter the clearance of remifentanil, the elimination of GR90291 is greatly reduced (Hoke et al., 1997a). Despite the potential risk of accumulation in patients with renal insufficiency, studies of pharmacokinetic simulation have shown that even after 24 hours of infusion, the primary metabolite does not reach clinically significant concentrations (Hoke et al., 1997b). Because of the lack of active metabolites of the unaltered free fraction and of the short redistribution phase, fentanyl appears to be an excellent choice for patients with end-stage renal failure (Sear, 1995). Although alfentanil undergoes a reduction in protein binding because of renal failure, it is completely metabolized to inactive compounds, without any significant alteration in its clearance and elimination half-life (Chauvin et al., 1987). Sufentanil may also be suitable for patients undergoing renal transplantation.

Although its unbound fraction is unmodified in ESRD, the pharmacokinetics may vary, and cases of prolonged respiratory depression have been reported (Wiggum et al., 1985). In renal transplant recipients, postoperative analgesia is best achieved by administration of opioid analgesics, since they represent the least risk of altering allograft function. The use of NSAIDs is strongly discouraged, as they are well-known nephrotoxins and induce a reversible inhibition of prostaglandin synthesis. The incidence of NSAID-induced renal dysfunction is highest in patients with coexisting renal vasoconstriction or hypoperfusion, two conditions that can affect renal transplant recipients.

Other risk factors for the development of NSAID-induced acute renal failure are advanced age, hypovolaemia, end-stage hepatic disease, congestive heart failure, sepsis, and major surgery. Ketorolac, a parenterally administered NSAID, has been reported to induce oliguric acute renal failure after a single dose and may predispose critically ill and elderly patients to ischaemic acute renal failure when given in the perioperative period (Quan and Kayser, 1994; Hock and Anderson, 1995). Multimodal analgesia is recommended for acute postoperative pain management to avoid the adverse effects of single-drug opioid analgesics. Among the disposable NSAIDs, acetaminophen seems to be the least kidney-toxic drug when used in this population of patients.

## Maintenance of intravascular volume and haemodynamic management

Once the transplant anastomoses are completed, the early onset of urine output represents the main goal, since it is directly correlated with graft survival. Several measures can be used to stimulate urine production intraoperatively in order to improve organ viability and patient outcome.

The most important intraoperative measure that improves the probability of immediate graft function consists of maintaining an adequate intravascular volume to ensure a sufficient perfusion of the transplanted kidney. Postoperative acute tubular necrosis may in fact result from inadequate hydration. Historically, a CVP of 10–15 mm Hg and a mean pulmonary artery pressure above 20 mm Hg have been recommended as the main intraoperative goal, because they have shown to reduce the likelihood of postoperative acute tubular necrosis (Carlier et al., 1982). So far, no data are available on other intraoperative monitoring parameters such as left ventricular end-diastolic area, intrathoracic blood volume, and FTc during renal transplant surgery. On the other hand, because many recipients display pre-existing cardiovascular disease (CAD, chronic heart failure), careful attention must be paid to signs of fluid overload, to avoid pulmonary oedema. Isotonic crystalloid solutions are the first choice for volume restoration during renal transplantation, but various crystalloid solutions can impact electrolyte and acid-base balance differently. Renal impairment is associated with hyperchloremic metabolic acidosis, which can be exacerbated by saline infusion (Guidet et al., 2010).

O'Malley et al. (2005) showed that lactated Ringer's solution is associated with less hyperkalaemia and acidosis when compared to normal saline, demonstrating that Ringer's lactated solution can be a safe choice for intravenous fluid therapy. If rapid resuscitation of intravascular depletion is needed, low molecular weight 6% hydroxyethyl starch (HES) 130/0.4 is generally used during and after renal transplantation (Hokema et al., 2011). HES 130/0.4 can be safely used in case of bleeding, even if today its use is questionable. No negative effects on renal function with low-dose HES 130/0.4 have been observed (Simon et al., 2012). Intravascular volume expansion with serum albumin has been used to improve graft perfusion and trigger the immediate onset of urine output. Several studies found that aggressive volume expansion with albumin resulted in an improved outcome (Willms et al., 1991; Dawidson et al., 1992). Despite these positive results, when administering albumin for intravascular volume expansion, important untoward effects and costs must be kept in mind (Davidson, 2006). New guidelines tend to discourage albumin administration as plasma expanders and recommend its use only in patients with severe hypoalbuminaemia (< 1.8 g/dL) (Nicholson et al., 2000) (see Table 14.1).

Diuretics, osmotic agents, and dopamine agonists are administered to promote diuresis immediately after reperfusion, but only mannitol, when combined with volume expansion, has been shown to decrease the incidence of acute tubular necrosis after transplantation (Tiggeler et al., 1985; van Valenberg et al., 1987). A randomized controlled trial did not show any benefit for the administration of furosemide for the treatment of renal failure (Cantarovich et al., 2004). There is also no positive effect of furosemide in acute renal failure (van der Voort et al., 2009; Hanif et al., 2011). Although there are no randomized controlled studies investigating the effect of diuretics on the recovery of renal function after transplantation, the use of furosemide in renal transplant surgery seems not to be beneficial.

Dopamine has been administered as therapy for renal failure for years. However, two major meta-analyses showed that dopamine had a detrimental effect on renal function in acute renal failure (Kellum and Decker, 2001; Marik, 2002). Ciapetti et al. (2009) studied 105 patients undergoing KTx and found that low-dose dopamine improved kidney function during neither the postoperative period nor the short term but was associated with an increased heart rate, ICU length of stay, and 6-month mortality. Dopamine decreases serum prolactin concentration, thereby inducing a transient decrease in T-cell function with an increase in the risk of infections (Devins et al., 1992). It decreases growth hormone and thyrotropine release, while other adverse effects include depression of respiratory drive and a pro-arrhythmic effect (Van den Berghe and de Zeager, 1996; ANZICS Clinical Trials Group, 2000; Holmes and Walley, 2003; Debaveye and Van den Berghe, 2004). Therefore the use of dopamine cannot be recommended for renal transplant surgery.

The role of fenoldopam in the transplant population has not been sufficiently evaluated, although the results of few trials seem to suggest a beneficial effect in liver transplantation recipients (Biancofiore et al., 2004; Della Rocca et al., 2004; Sorbello et al., 2007). One study investigated the effect of fenoldopam 0.05 mcg/kg/min for 48 hours vs dopamine 2 mcg/kg/min for 48 hours only in 14 patients undergoing renal transplantation. There were no significant differences in the two groups but with a trend favouring the fenoldopam group (Fontana et al., 2005). The dose-dependent antihypertensive effects associated with an improved renal function along with its favourable pharmacokinetic profile make the drug particularly attractive for the perioperative management of renal transplant recipients.

In this category of patients, other potential benefits may derive from the ability of fenoldopam to prevent cyclosporine-induced renal vasoconstriction in the acute phase and to completely reverse the nephrotoxicity caused by chronic administration of the immunosuppressant, without affecting blood levels of the drug (Brooks et al., 1990; Jorkasky et al., 1992). Although clinical trials are needed to further investigate the ability of fenoldopam to prevent renal injury during renal transplantation, the introduction of this new agent into clinical practice may provide a new pharmacological option for preventing postoperative renal failure.

## Surgical technique

KTx is not a technically complex procedure; however, it requires precise surgical technique. This surgical technique is nowadays standardized, although kidney transplant procedures differ from one another. The KTx candidate is hospitalized and re-evaluated shortly before surgery. At this time, potential infectious or unexpected medical conditions that could contraindicate surgery are excluded.

KTx begins with donor kidney retrieval. There must be good communication between the retrieval and the transplant teams to inform of any anatomical variations or accidental section of kidney vasculature or ureter that may compromise the outcome of KTx. The operation usually takes 2–4 hours. After induction of anaesthesia, a urethral catheter is inserted into the bladder aseptically. A large catheter is necessary due to the possibility of obstruction from blood clots due to the cystotomy. A three-way urinary catheter with a check valve, urine flow port, and a port for bladder irrigation can be used. After preparation of the surgical field, the skin incision is performed. Three incisions have been used: the orthotopic lumbar approach, the lower abdominal (hockey-stick) approach, and the pelvic approach.

Orthotopic placement of the kidney in its normal position is rarely used because the renal pedicle provides a feeble support for the graft. Moreover, the extra length of ureter needed to anastomosis with the bladder may risk ischaemic stenosis and torsion, resulting in difficult access for the performance of cutaneous biopsies or other surgical manipulations. In case occlusion of the IVC is present, orthotopic placement of the kidney is indicated. More commonly, the kidney graft is placed heterotopically in the iliac fossa. The anatomic side for placement of the graft is selected based on areas of vascular disease. If there is no contraindication, the right iliac fossa is generally preferred, since the right common iliac vein is more superficial, nearly vertical in its direction, and ascends behind and then lateral to its corresponding artery. No disadvantage has been proved in positioning the left kidney in the left iliac fossa or the right kidney in the right iliac fossa. Placement of the contralateral kidney in the iliac fossa might render a better alignment when the recipient vein is mobilized laterally to the artery.

The hockey-stick incision can be extended cephalad towards the subcostal margin. This approach has the advantage of minimal muscle splitting and excellent access to the common iliac vessels, aortic bifurcation, and IVC. The more common pelvic approach extends from the midline, approximately two to three fingerbreadths above the symphysis pubis in a curvilinear direction, to a point three fingerbreadths medial to the anterior superior iliac spine. The external oblique muscle is divided in the direction of its fibres, and at the lateral corner the muscle is split. The incision is extended medially into the rectus sheath and, if present, the pyramidalis muscle to facilitate exposure of the bladder. The internal oblique and transversus abdominis muscles are divided and exposure of the iliac fossa is obtained by reflecting the peritoneum medially and cephalad from the undersurface of the transversus abdominis muscle and superior to the level of the common iliac artery. Reflecting it medially preserves the spermatic cord in male patients, while the round ligament in female patients can be ligated and divided. The inferior epigastric vessels can be ligated and divided without adverse consequences.

A self-retaining retractor affords exposure of the iliac vessels. Attention must be paid to avoid compression injury of the lateral femoral cutaneous nerve and the femoral nerve. Traction injuries to these structures can cause sensorimotor deficits on the ipsilateral anterior thigh. These symptoms present within the first postoperative days and resolve within 3–12 months.

The kidney is brought to the operative field and prepared at this time if it has not been already done at the bench-table. During the bench-table surgery, the vascular anatomy is confirmed.

The excess fat surrounding the kidney is removed, taking care to avoid the triangle that contains the ureteral blood supply formed by the renal artery, the lower pole of the kidney, and the ureter. All vessel branches that will not be reconstructed are ligated and the aorta and vena cava patches are prepared. In right kidney grafts harvested with the whole infrahepatic cava, suturing the superior margin of the cava vein and using the inferior margin to perform the anastomosis can serve to elongate the vein.

The kidney is then brought to the abdominal cavity. During the vascular anastomoses the kidney is kept cold by continuous surface irrigation with iced-cold saline and contact with cold sterile gauze pads. The kidney is placed where it lies most naturally within the renal pelvis, with the ureter oriented distally. The site of vascular anastomosis is then chosen according to the vascular anatomy of the graft and the recipient (vessel length and quality). Recipient arterial segments with atherosclerotic disease should be identified and avoided whenever possible. Unless the graft artery is particularly short or the anastomosis deemed difficult, the deeper venous anastomosis is usually performed first. Conventionally, uraemic patients do not require systemic heparinization for the vascular anastomosis. However, pre-uraemic patients should be heparinized. After application of proximal and distal vascular clamps, a venotomy congruent with the graft vein size is performed and the lumen is flushed with 10% heparin solution. The venous anastomosis is constructed with two running sutures of non-absorbable 5-0 or 6-0 monofilament sutures. Traction of the kidney should be avoided to prevent tearing of the vein.

At the selected site for arterial anastomosis a small segment is dissected from the surrounding tissue. Meticulous ligation and division of the lymphatic tissue surrounding the vascular structures is required to reduce the incidence of postoperative lymphocele formation. After proximal and distal vascular clamping, an end-to-side anastomosis between the external or common iliac artery and the aortic Carrel-patch is performed with either an interrupted suture or a continuous 6-0 vascular monofilament suture. Whenever a small graft artery is found, an end-to-end anastomosis with the internal iliac artery might be preferred provided that the hypogastric artery is free of atherosclerosis at its origin. In such case the distal vessel is ligated above its trifurcation into the superior vesicle, pudenda, and deep-gluteal arteries. A clip to reinforce the ligature should be applied. This type of arterial revascularization could be contraindicated in male patients in case there is a previous transplant with anastomosis at the level of the contralateral hypogastric artery, thus avoiding the risk of impotence if both internal iliac arteries are ligated.

After completion of each anastomosis a test to confirm the absence of anastomotic bleeding can be performed by distal renal venous or arterial clamping. The low-pressure vascular clamps are removed (the superior venous clamp and inferior arterial clamp on the external iliac vessels). Then the high-pressure clamps are removed (the inferior venous clamp and superior arterial clamp on the external iliac vessels). Upon verifying a correct haemostasis of the suture line, the renal vein clamp is removed, allowing for revascularization of the renal graft, quickly followed by release of the renal arterial clamp. It is important at this time to ensure that the patient has an adequate circulating blood volume. In absence of complications, the kidney graft should regain its normal colour and consistency (Risaliti et al., 2004). The kidney is irrigated with warm saline and wrapped in warm sterile gauze pads. Haemostasis of the kidney surface and hilum follows. In most cases, urine output is immediately observed through the graft ureter.

Timely identification of technical complications that might compromise the success of KTx is critical at this time, allowing for immediate correction. Although not yet standardized, the use of Doppler or transit-time vascular probes might improve early diagnosis of vascular complications.

After completion of the vascular anastomosis the bladder is filled under gravity to facilitate intraoperative identification; an antiseptic or antibiotic solution is commonly used and the urethral catheter is clamped. There are many surgical techniques for the re-establishment of urinary tract continuity (Politano and Leadbetter, 1958; Lich et al., 1961; Gregoir, 1962; Leadbetter et al., 1996). In all cases, the distal graft ureter is spatulated anteriorly for 2–3 cm to perform a wide-enough anastomosis.

The type of anastomosis varies between urothelial anastomosis and full-thickness sutures. An antireflux technique might be also used or not. In most cases, a double-J-ureteral stent is used to stabilize the anastomosis. Our preferred technique is the Knechtle modification of the Lich–Gregoir technique (Knechtle, 1999) where an incision is made in the bladder wall musculature at the dome for 2–3 cm to expose the mucosa. Careful haemostasis of the rich vascularization of the bladder wall is mandatory. The bladder mucosa protrudes through this opening due to the bladder filling, and a tunnel is made with a straight clamp laterally to the margin of the bladder wall incision, taking care to avoid accidental opening of the mucosa. The spatulated graft ureter is passed through this tunnel, avoiding twisting. The mucosa is then opened and the antibiotic or antiseptic solution removed from the surgical field. One extremity of the double-J-ureteral stent is placed in the renal pelvis and the other in the bladder. The urothelial anastomosis is then performed between the ureter and the bladder mucosa using one or two 4-0 or 5-0 continuous absorbable monofilament sutures. After completion of the anastomosis the detrusor muscle is closed over the anastomosis using single stitches of absorbable 3-0 sutures. In case the tunnel opening is too wide, an extra stitch at this level can be placed.

Other centres favour another extravesical approach to ureteroneocystostomy that also includes an antireflux tunnel but lacks a urothelial anastomosis. The U-stitch technique is where the spatulated ureter is passed through the bladder opening and the sutures taken out through the anterior bladder wall so that the ureteral end is anchored to the inner bladder wall. The tunnelling procedure is achieved by imbricating the seromuscular layer above the graft ureter. The technique described by Schanfield (1972) uses only one stitch for the bladder attachment placed at the distal aspect of the ureter, whereas that described by MacKinnon et al. (1968) uses two stitches at the distal aspect of the ureter. By elimination of the urothelial anastomosis, the U-stitch technique was demonstrated to shorten operative times. Urological complications are similar with both extravesical techniques in most comparative analyses, except for a potentially higher rate of haematuria with the U-stitch method (Kayler et al., 2010).

## Paediatric KTx: surgical aspects

KTx in the paediatric age group (< 18 years of age) presents a number of unique challenges to the transplant team. The aetiology leading to the need for KTx includes genetic, congenital, and acquired defects with kidney, ureter, and/or bladder involvement. The pretransplant condition of the patient may include issues involving nutrition, infection, and weight/size specific to this age group. Considerations include the following:

- A retroperitoneal approach for placement of the transplant is preferred, since it offers a faster recovery period, with ileus less likely, and exposure to the IVC and distal aorta is possible from either the right or the left side.
- Intra-abdominal placement for the kidney transplant may be necessary depending on the need for bilateral nephrectomy (if there are large polycystic kidneys that need to be removed or for treatment of hypertension, reflux/infection risk, or severe protein loss). On occasion, the two-stage procedure with laparoscopic bilateral nephrectomy carried out first may be preferred.
- The donor may be living or deceased, adult size or paediatric, or paediatric en bloc. An adult-size kidney may have an intravascular volume nearly equivalent to that of the patient's own liver, in the case of small babies (< 10 kg), receiving an adult kidney. Therefore allowing for adequate intravascular volume intraoperatively is critical. The CVP should be sufficient so that when the vascular clamps are released and the kidney transplant is perfused, this does not result in hypotension. Generally, a CVP between 12 and 15 mm Hg is sufficient to accommodate the vascular volume of the kidney transplant. On occasion a TEE may be needed to assess intracardiac volume, particularly if there is a cardiac history.
- Possible hypercoagulable state: despite the uraemic effect on platelets, hypercoagulability may be suggested in the context of a number of basic lab results: a reduced prothrombin time (PT), reduced INR, reduced partial thromboplastin time (PTT), higher than normal fibrinogen, higher than normal platelet count, or higher haematocrit. This can be confirmed in the operating room with a TEG (Burke et al., 2004). If in fact severe hypercoagulability is present, then heparin may be necessary intraoperatively. The combination of hypovolaemia with hypotension and unrecognized hypercoagulability can result in thrombosis of the kidney transplant.
- Perioperative immunosuppression includes induction antibody, which generally involves the use of thymoglobulin with or without an anti-CD25 agent. Maintenance immunosuppression generally includes a CNI, for example tacrolimus, as well as mycophenolate mofetil. Steroid-free maintenance immunosuppression is being used by a growing number of centres with good results, specifically regarding kidney transplant allograft survival and improved growth characteristics in this patient population.
- For those patients with FSGS who progress within 3 years from diagnosis to need for therapeutic intervention for their ESRD, the risk of recurrence of proteinuria/FSGS in the kidney transplant can be extremely high. We have reported that the use of rituximab as a single dose perioperatively in this group of patients has been helpful as far as reducing the likelihood of recurrence and rendering those patients who do recur more easily treatable with plasmapheresis (Fornoni et al., 2011).
- Postkidney transplant compliance with medications (immunosuppression/other medications) tends to be a more difficult problem in this age group than in the adult population. The paediatric kidney transplant recipient is not simply a small-for-size adult.

## Postoperative ICU admission criteria

After KTx surgery the patients are generally discharged to the ward. In case of pre-existing respiratory and/or cardiac disease, patients should be admitted to the ICU (or need postoperative ICU admission).

As proposed by the Society of Critical Care Medicine criteria, the patients that will benefit from ICU admission are critically ill, unstable patients in need of intensive treatment and monitoring that cannot be provided outside of the ICU (Task Force of the American College of Critical Care Medicine, Society of Critical Care Medicine, 1999). Usually, these treatments include ventilator support and continuous vasoactive drug infusions. Examples may include postoperative and acute respiratory failure patients requiring mechanical ventilatory support and shock or haemodynamically unstable patients receiving invasive monitoring and/or vasoactive drugs.

## Conclusion

Kidney renal transplant patients present many challenges for the anaesthetist, during the pre-, intra-, and postoperative time.

The optimal approach should be to develop a perioperative plan tailored to the patient's specific conditions. Optimization of the patient's therapy other than the comorbidities in the preoperative period, close intraoperative and postoperative monitoring, optimization of fluid status and haemodynamics, as well as appropriate use of anaesthetic agents are the 'crucial keys' to perioperative renal transplantation success.

## References


Abbud-Filho M, Adams PL, Alberu J, et al. (2007) A report of the Lisbon Conference on the care of the kidney transplant recipient. *Transplantation*, **83**(Suppl):S1–22.

ANZICS Clinical Trials Group (2000) Low-dose dopamine in patients with early renal dysfunction: a placebo-controlled randomized trial. *Lancet*, **356**:2139–2143.

Artru AA (1998) Renal effects of sevoflurane during conditions of possible increased risk. *J Clin Anesth*, **10**:531–538.

Beauvoir C, Peray P, Daures JP, et al. (1993) Pharmacodynamics of vecuronium in patients with and without renal failure: a meta-analysis. *Can J Anesth*, **40**:696–702.

Biancofiore G, Della Rocca G, Bindi L, et al. (2004) Use of fenoldopam to control renal dysfunction early after liver transplantation. *Liver Transplant*, **10**:986–992.

Boersma E, Kertai M, Schouten O, et al. (2005) Perioperative cardiovascular mortality in noncardiac surgery: validation of the Lee cardiac risk index. *Am J Med*, **118**:1134–1141.

Brooks DP, Druds DJ, Ruffolo RR, et al. (1990) Prevention and complete reversal of Cyclosporine A induced renal vasoconstriction and nephrotoxicity in the rat by Fenoldopam. *J Pharmacol Exper Ther*, **254**:375–379.

Burch PG, Stanski DR (1982) Decreased protein binding and thiopental kinetics. *Clin Pharmacol Ther*, **32**:212–217.

Burke III GW, Ciancio G, Figueiro J, et al. (2004) Hypercoagulable state associated with kidney-pancreas transplantation. Thromboelastogram-directed anti-coagulation and implications for future therapy. *Clin Transplant*, **18**:423–428.

Cantarovich F, Rangoonwala B, Lorenz H, et al. (2004) High-dose furosemide for established ARF: a prospective, randomized, double-blind, placebo-controlled, multicenter trial. *Am J Kidney Dis*, **44**:402–409.

Carlier M, Squifflet JP, Pirson Y, et al. (1982) Maximal hydration during anesthesia increases pulmonary arterial pressures and improves early function of human renal transplants. *Transplantation*, **34**:201–204.

Carlos R, Calvo R, Erill S (1979) Plasma protein binding of etomidate in patients with renal failure or hepatic cirrhosis. *Clin Pharmacokin*, **4**:144–148.

Chauvin M, Lebrault C, Levron JC, et al. (1987) Pharmacokinetics of alfentanil in chronic renal failure. *Anesth Analg*, **66**:53–6.

Ciapetti M, di Valvasone S, di Filippo A, et al. (2009) Low-dose dopamine in kidney transplantation. *Transplant Proc*, **41**:4165–4168.

Danovitch GM, Hariharan S, Pirsch JD, et al. (2002) Management of the waiting list for cadaveric kidney transplants: report of a survey and recommendations by the Clinical Practice Guidelines Committee of the American Society of Transplantation. *J Am Soc Nephrol*, **13**:528–535.

Davidson IJ (2006) Renal impact of fluid management with colloids: a comparative study. *Eur J Anesth*, **23**:721–738.

Dawidson I, Sandor ZF, Coorpender L, et al. (1992) Intraoperative albumin administration affects outcome of cadaver renal transplantation. *Transplantation*, **53**:774–782.

Debaveye YA, Van den Berghe GH (2004) Is there still a place for dopamine in the modern intensive care unit? *Anesth Analg*, **98**:461–468.

De Hert S, Imberger G, Carlisle J, et al. (2011) Preoperative evaluation of the adult patient undergoing non-cardiac surgery: guidelines from the European Society of Anaesthesiology. *Eur J Anaesth*, **28**:684–722.

De Lima JJ, Sabbaga E, Vieira ML, et al. (2003) Coronary angiography is the best predictor of events in renal transplant candidates compared with non- invasive testing. *Hypertension*, **42**:263–268.

De Lima JJG, Gowdak LHW, de Paula FJ, et al. (2010) Treatment of coronary artery disease in hemodialysis patients evaluated for transplant: a registry study. *Transplantation*, **89**:845–850.

Della Rocca G, Pompei L (2011) Goal-directed therapy in anesthesia: any clinical impact or just a fashion? *Minerva Anest*, **77**:545–53.

Della Rocca G, Costa MG, Coccia C, et al. (2002a) Preload and haemodynamic assessment during liver transplantation: a comparison between the pulmonary artery catheter and transpulmonary indicator dilution techniques. *Eur J Anaesth*, **19**:868–875.

Della Rocca G, Costa GM, Coccia C, et al. (2002b) Preload index: pulmonary artery occlusion pressure versus intrathoracic blood volume monitoring during lung transplantation. *Anesth Analg*, **95**:835–843.

Della Rocca G, Pompei L, Coccia C, et al. (2003) Atracurium, cisatracurium, vecuronium and rocuronium in patients with renal failure. *Minerva Anest*, **69**:605–615.

Della Rocca G, Pompei L, Costa MG, et al. (2004) Fenoldopam mesylate and renal function in patients undergoing liver transplantation: a randomized, controlled pilot trial. *Anesth Analg*, **99**:1604–1609.

Devins SS, Miller A, Herndon BL, et al. (1992) Effects of dopamine on T-lymphocyte proliferative responses and serum prolactin concentrations in critically ill patients. *Crit Care Med*, **20**:1644–1649.

Fleisher LA, Fleischmann KE, Auerbach AD (2014) 2014 ACC/AHA Guideline on perioperative cardiovascular evaluation and management of patients undergoing noncardiac surgery: a report of the American College of Cardiology/American Heart Association. Task Force on Practice Guidelines. *J Am Coll Cardiol*, **64**(22):e77–e137.

Fontana I, Germi MR, Beatini M, et al. (2005) Dopamine 'renal dose' versus fenoldopam mesylate to prevent ischemia-reperfusion injury in renal transplantation. *Transplant Proc*, **37**:2474–2475.

Fornoni A, Sageshima J, Wei C, et al. (2011) Rituximab targets podocytes in recurrent focal segmental glomerulosclerosis. *Sci Transl Med*, **3**:85–86.

Friedman S, Palac R, Chobanian M, Costa S (2011) A call to action: variability in guidelines for cardiac evaluation before to renal transplantation. *Clin J Am Soc Nephrol*, **6**:1185–1191.

Gregoir W (1962) Congenital vesico-ureteral reflux. *Acta Urol Belg*, **30**:286–300.

Guidet B, Soni N, Della Rocca G et al. (2010) A balanced view of balanced solutions. *Crit Care*, **14**:325.

Hanif F, Macrae AN, Littlejohn MG, et al. (2011) Outcome of renal transplantation with and without intra-operative diuretics. *Int J Surg*, **9**:460–463.

Herzog CA, Marwick TH, Pheley AM, et al. (1999) Dobutamine stress echocardiography for the detection of significant coronary artery disease in renal transplant candidates. *Am J Kidney Dis*, **33**:1080–1090.

Herzog CA, Ma JZ, Collins AJ (2004) Long-term outcome of renal transplant recipients in the united states after coronary revascularization procedures. *Circulation*, **109**:2866–2871.

Hillis LD, Smith PK, Anderson JL, et al. (2011) ACCF/AHA guideline for coronary artery bypass graft surgery: a report of the American College of Cardiology Foundation/American Heart Association Task Force on Practice Guidelines. *J Am Coll Cardiol*, **58**:123–210.

Hock R, Anderson RJ (1995) Prevention of drug induced nephrotoxicity in the intensive care unit. *J Crit Care*, **10**:33–43.

Hoke JF, Shlugman D, Dershwitz M, et al. (1997a) Pharmacokinetics of remifentanil in persons with renal failure compared with healthy volunteers. *Anesthesiology*, **87**:533–541.

Hoke JF, Cunningham F, James MK, et al. (1997b) Comparative pharmacokinetics and pharmacodynamics of remifentanil, its principle metabolite (GR90291), and alfentanil in dogs. *J Pharmacol Exp Ther*, **281**:226–232.

Hokema F, Ziganshyna S, Bartels M, et al. (2011) Is perioperative low molecular weight hydroxyethyl starch infusion a risk factor for delayed graft function in renal transplant recipients? *Nephrol Dial Transplant*, **26**:3373–3378.

Holmes CL, Walley KR (2003) Bad medicine: low-dose dopamine in the ICU. *Chest*, **123**:1266–1275.

Ickx B, Cockshott ID, Barvais L, et al. (1998) Propofol infusion for induction and maintenance of anaesthesia in patients with end-stage renal disease. *Br J Anaesth*, **81**:854–860.

Jones MM, Tanser SJ (2002) Lithium dilution measurement of cardiac output and arterial pulse waveform analysis: an indicator dilution calibrated beat-by-beat system for continuous estimation of cardiac output. *Curr Opin Crit Care*, **3**:257–261.

Jorkasky DK, Audet P, Shusterman N, et al. (1992) Fenoldopam reverses cyclosporine-induced renal vasoconstriction in kidney transplant recipients. *Am J Kidney Dis*, **19**:567–572.

Kasiske BL, Cangro CB, Hariharan S, et al. (2001) The evaluation of renal transplantation candidates: clinical practice guidelines. *Am J Transplant*, **1**(Suppl 2):3–95.

Kayler L, Kang D, Molmenti E, et al. (2010) Kidney transplant ureteroneocystostomy techniques and complications: review of the literature. *Transplant Proc*, **42**:1413–1420.

Kellum JA, M Decker (2001) Use of dopamine in acute renal failure: a meta-analysis. *Crit Care Med*, **29**:1526–1531.

Knechtle SJ (1999) Ureteroneocystostomy for renal transplantation. *J Am Coll Surg*, **188**:707–709.

Leadbetter GW, Monaco AP, Russell PS (1996) A technique for reconstruction of the urinary tract in renal transplantation. *Surg Gynec Obstet*, **123**:839–841.

Lentine KL, Schnitzler MA, Brennan DC, et al. (2008) Cardiac evaluation before kidney transplantation: a practice patterns analysis in Medicare-insured dialysis patients. *Clin J Am Soc Nephrol*, **3**:1115–1124.

Lentine KL, Costa SP, Wir MR, et al. (2012) Cardiac disease evaluation and management among kidney and liver transplantation candidates: a scientific statement from the American Heart Association and the American College of Cardiology Foundation. *J Am Coll Cardiol*, **60**:434–480.

Lich R, Howerton LW, Davis LA (1961) Childhood urosepsis. *J Ky Med Assoc*, 59:1177–1179

MacKinnon KJ, Oliver JA, Morehouse DD, et al. (1968) Cadaver renal transplantation: emphasis on urological aspects. *J Urol*, **99**:486–490.

Magorian T, Flannery KB, Miller RD (1993) Comparison of rocuronium, succinylcholine, and vecuronium for rapid-sequence induction of anesthesia in adult patients. *Anesthesiology*, **79**:913–918.

Manske CL, Wang Y, Rector T, et al. (1992) Coronary revascularization in insulin-dependent diabetic patients with chronic renal failure. *Lancet*, **340**:998–1002.

Marik PE (2002) Low-dose dopamine: a systematic review. *Intens Care Med*, **28**:877–883.

Matas AJ, Kasiske B, Miller L (2002) Proposed guidelines for re-evaluation of patients on the waiting list for renal cadaver transplantation. *Transplantation*, **73**:811–812.

National Kidney Foundation (2005) K/DOQI clinical practice guidelines for cardiovascular disease in dialysis patients. *Am J Kidney Dis*, **45**:S1–S153.

Nicholson JP, Wolmarans MR, Park GR (2000) The role of albumin in critical illness. *Br J Anaesth*, **85**:599–610.

O'Malley CM, Frumento RJ, Hardy MA, et al. (2005) Randomized, double-blind comparison of lactated Ringer's solution and 0.9% NaCl during renal transplantation. *Anesth Analg*, **100**:1518–1524.

Orko R, Heino A, Bjorksten F, et al. (1987) Comparison of atracurium and vecuronium in anaesthesia for renal transplantation. *Acta Anaesth Scand*, **31**:450–453.

Patel RK, Mark PB, Johnston N, et al. (2008) Prognostic value of cardiovascular screening in potential renal transplant recipients: a single-center prospective observational study. *Am J Transplant*, **8**:1673–1683.

Poldermans D, Bax JJ, Boersma E, et al. (2009) Guidelines for preoperative cardiac risk assessment and peri-operative cardiac management in noncardiac surgery. *Eur Heart J*, **30**:2769–2812.

Politano VA, Leadbetter WF (1958) An operative technique for the correction of vesicoureteral reflux. *J Urol*, **79**:932–941.

Quan DJ, Kayser SR (1994) Ketorolac induced renal failure after a single dose. *J Toxicol Clin Toxicol*, **32**:305–309.

Rabbat CG, Treleaven DJ, Russell JD, et al. (2003) Prognostic value of myocardial perfusion studies in patients with end-stage renal disease assessed for kidney or kidney- pancreas transplantation: a meta-analysis. *J Am Soc Nephrol*, **14**:431–439.

Reuter DA, Felbinger TW, Moerstedt K, et al. (2002) Intrathoracic blood volume index measured by thermodilution for preload monitoring after cardiac surgery. *J Cardio-Thorac Vasc Anesth*, **16**:191–195.

Risaliti A, Sainz-Barriga M, Baccarani U, et al. (2004) Surgical complications after kidney transplantation. *G Ital Nefrol*, **21**(Suppl 26):S43–S47.

Robertson EN, Driessen JJ, Vogt M, et al. (2005) Pharmacodynamics of rocuronium 0.3 mg $kg^{-1}$ in adult patients with and without renal failure. *Eur J Anaesthesiol*, **22**:929–932.

Sakka SG, Bredle DL, Reinhart K, et al. (1999) Comparison between intrathoracic blood volume and cardiac filling pressures in the early phase of hemodynamic instability of patients with sepsis or septic shock. *J Crit Care*, **14**:78–83.

Shanfield I (1972) New experimental methods for implantation of the ureter in bladder and conduit. *Transplant Proc*, **4**:637–638.

Sear JW (1995). Kidney transplants: induction and analgesic agents. *Int Anesthesiol Clin*, **33**:45–68.

Simon TP, Schuerholz T, Hüter L, et al. (2012) Impairment of renal function using hyperoncotic colloids in a two hit model of shock: a prospective randomized study. *Crit Care*, **16**:R16.

Sorbello M, Morello G, Paratore A, et al. (2007). Fenoldopam vs dopamine as a nephroprotective strategy during living donor kidney transplantation: preliminary data. *Transplant Proc*, **39**:1794–1796.

Staals LM, Snoeck MM, Driessen JJ, et al. (2008) Multicentre, parallel-group, comparative trial evaluating the efficacy and safety of sugammadex in patients with end-stage renal failure or normal renal function. *Br J Anaesth*, **101**:492–497.

Sutton TS, Koblin DD, Gruenke LD, et al. (1991) Fluoride metabolites after prolonged exposure of volunteers and patients to desflurane. *Anesth Analg*, **73**:180–185.

Task force of the American College of Critical Care Medicine, Society of Critical Care Medicine (1999) Guidelines for intensive care unit admission, discharge, and triage. *Crit Care Med*, **27**:633–638.

Thapa S, Brull SJ (2000) Succinylcholine-induced hyperkalemia in patients with renal failure: an old question revisited. *Anesth Analg*, **91**:237–241.

Tiggeler RG, Berden JH, Hoitsma AJ, Koene RA (1985) Prevention of acute tubular necrosis in cadaveric kidney transplantation by the combined use of mannitol and moderate hydration. *Annal Surg*, **201**:246–251.

van den Berghe G, de Zegher F (1996) Anterior pituitary function during critical illness on dopamine treatment. *Crit Care Med*, **24**:1580–1590.

van der Voort PH, Boerma EC, Koopmans M, et al. (2009) Furosemide does not improve renal recovery after hemofiltration for acute renal failure in critically ill patients: a double blind randomized controlled trial. *Crit Care Med*, **37**:533–538.

van Valenberg PL, Hoitsma AJ, Tiggeler RG, et al. (1987) Mannitol as an indispensable constituent of an intraoperative hydration protocol for the prevention of acute renal failure after renal cadaveric transplantation. *Transplantation*, **44**:784–788.

Vinik HR, Reves JG, Greenblatt DJ, et al. (1983) The pharmacokinetics of midazolam in chronic renal failure patients. *Anesthesiology*, **59**:390–394.

Wiggum DC, Cork RC, Weldon ST, et al. (1985) Postoperative respiratory depression and elevated sufentanil levels in a patient with chronic renal failure. *Anesthesiology*, **63**:708–710.

Wijeysundera D, Beattie WS, Austin PC, et al. (2010) Noninvasive cardiac stress testing before major elective non-cardiac: population based cohort study. *BMJ*, **340**:b5526

Willms CD, Dawidson IHA, Dickerman R, et al. (1991) Intraoperative blood volume expansion induces primary function after renal transplantation: a study of 96 cadaver kidneys. *Transplant Proc*, **23**:1338–1339.

# CHAPTER 15

# Perioperative management of the kidney–pancreas and pancreas transplant recipient

Ugo Boggi, George Burke, and Kumar Belani

## Anatomy and physiology of the pancreas

The pancreas was first described by Herophilus in about 300 BC and was named 'pancreas' from the Greek words '*pan*' and '*krèas*' meaning 'all flesh' by Rufus of Ephesus in about AD 100. The ability of the pancreas to produce exocrine secretions, however, was recognized only in the sixteenth century by Vesalius, and Wirsung and Santorini described the pancreatic ducts in 1642 and 1724, respectively. Knowledge of the endocrine pancreas was not obtained until 1869, thanks to the work of Langerhans, a medical student working in Rudolf Virchow's laboratory in Berlin (Howard, 1994). The significance of Langerhans' discovery was appreciated in 1889 when Minkowski and von Mering showed that if the pancreas was removed from a dog, the animal developed fatal diabetes (Howard, 1994). In 1922 Banting and Best, working in the laboratory of Professor MacLeod, made the historical observation concerning the effect of injecting extracted insulin. Banting and MacLeod received the Nobel Prize for the discovery of insulin in 1923 ( Howard, 1994).

On 17 December 1966, Kelly and Lillehei, working at the University of Minnesota, first reversed type I diabetes, transplanting a duct-ligated, segmental, pancreas graft into a 28-year-old diabetic woman (Kelly, 1967). In 1989 the same result was achieved by islet transplantation at the Washington University in St Louis (Scharp, 1990).

### Gross anatomy

The pancreas is between 18 and 28 cm long and weighs some 80–100 g. It is divided into four portions: the head, including the uncinate process, the neck, the body, and the tail (see Figure 15.1). Because of development from two embryonic primordia, originating on opposite sides of the primitive gut, the pancreas may also be divided into a ventral portion, corresponding to the uncinate process and part of the pancreatic head, and a dorsal portion including the cranial part of the head, the neck, the body, and the tail. Anatomic variants of pancreatic anatomy have their roots in the embryological development of the organ (Trede, 1997). Further, the ventral and dorsal pancreas components have different patterns of lymphatic drainage (Kitagawa et al., 2008). The pancreas lies transversely and somewhat obliquely in the retroperitoneum. The head, nestling within the curve of the duodenum, is located just to the right of the second lumbar vertebra, while the tail reaches the splenic hilum at the level of the twelfth thoracic vertebra. The healthy pancreas is a soft and friable organ, which lacks a firm capsule, being covered by tenuous connective tissue strands which extend between its lobules (Kitagawa et al., 2008). The deep anatomic location of the pancreas makes its anatomic relationships with surrounding organs quite complex.

The typical pancreas graft is a whole pancreatic duodenal graft, composed of the entire pancreas plus a duodenal segment of variable length. If the head of the pancreas or the donor duodenum is damaged or poorly perfused, a segmental graft, made up of the body and the tail, may still be used (Boggi, 2010a). Segmental grafts can produce insulin independence but at the price of a higher rate of technical complications (Boggi, 2010b).

### Blood supply to the pancreas allograft

The native pancreas is a low-flow organ, which parasitizes its blood supply from hepatic, splenic, and intestinal vessels. Since the pancreas allograft is transplanted without spleen, liver, and intestines, a 'new anatomy' for arterial inflow must be created at the back table. In most instances a single arterial pedicle can be fashioned using a Y-bifurcated iliac graft, made up of common, external, and internal iliac arteries. The external iliac artery is anastomosed to the superior mesenteric artery (SMA) and the internal iliac artery to the splenic artery (SA), respectively. When the Y-bifurcated iliac graft is not available or unsuitable, the brachiocephalic trunk and the carotid artery may also be used. Alternatively, the SA may be anastomosed end-to-side to the SA, either directly or using an interposition graft (Boggi, 2010a).

Because of rich intrapancreatic collateral circulation, patency of either the SMA or SA pedicle is enough to supply the entire pancreas and duodenal segment. However, variations in intraparenchymal vasculature and origin of the dorsal pancreatic artery (DPA) may lead to segmental graft ischaemia in the case of thrombosis of one of the two main allograft arteries (Boggi, 2009a). In particular, the DPA acts as a sort of vascular gate between the head and body–tail of the pancreas. When the transverse pancreatic artery is missing (type I vascularization of the body–tail, occurring in 22% of persons) or does not anastomose with other vessels

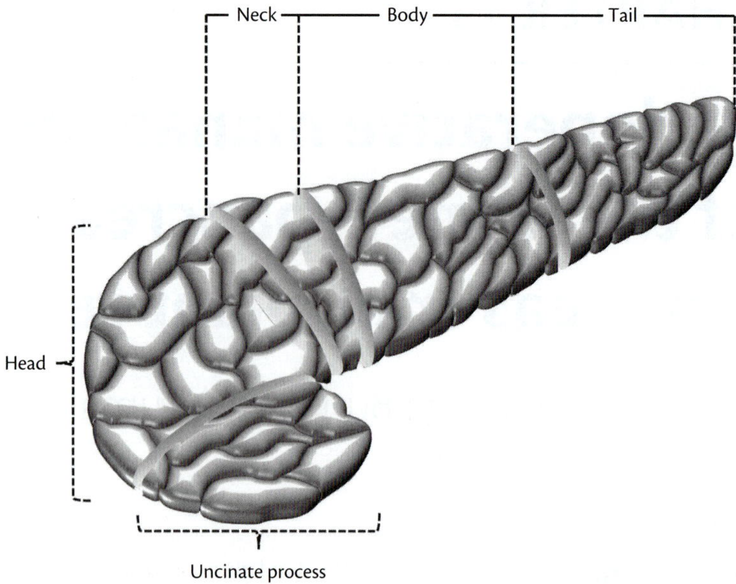


**Fig. 15.1** Pancreas partition

in the body–tail (type II vascularization of the body–tail, occurring in 23% of persons), occlusion of either the SMA or SA may lead to segmental graft ischaemia if the DPA was ligated or is also occluded. The DPA, indeed, must be ligated when it arises from the celiac trunk (28% of persons) or the hepatic artery (17% of persons) and becomes occluded when the main artery from which it arises develops thrombosis (Boggi, 2009a). This anatomical background is one of the main reasons for routine revascularization of the gastroduodenal artery. However, based on back-table angiograms only 7% of pancreas allografts show poor perfusion of the donor duodenum/pancreatic head, which occasionally results in segmental ischaemia (Boggi, 2009a).

## Physiology of the pancreas allograft

Despite pancreas transplantation being pursued solely to restore a critical mass of viable β-cells in insulin-dependent diabetic patients, only 2% of the human pancreas is comprised of endocrine cells. In the native organ, exocrine pancreas secretions significantly contribute to the digestion of complex carbohydrates, proteins, and lipids via enzymatic hydrolysis. The main pancreatic enzymes are α-amylase, trypsin, and chymotrypsin, lipase, and colipase. The most relevant inorganic components of pancreatic juice are water, potassium, chloride, and bicarbonate. The high bicarbonate concentration of pancreatic juice causes its alkaline pH, which protects pancreatic enzymes from acid denaturation and increases their hydrolytic activity (Layer and Keller, 2008). The rate of exocrine secretion starts increasing in response to the cephalic phase of digestion, but the strongest stimulant is duodenal exposure to nutrients. Secretion of pancreatic enzymes is more sustained after a solid meal compared with an identical meal that has been homogenized. Lipids, especially duodenal free fatty acids, are the strongest stimulants of pancreatic enzyme secretion, but also proteins contribute markedly to the induction of the digestive pancreatic enzyme response (Layer and Keller, 2008).

Physiology of exocrine secretion of the pancreas allograft has not been studied extensively. It is, however, known that bladder drainage produces hyperchloremic metabolic acidosis and dehydration as a consequence of urinary loss of pancreatic juice (Egidi, 2007). Enteric drainage of exocrine secretions is clearly more physiological. Ideally, duodenoenteric anastomosis should be created as proximally as possible on the jejunum (40–80 cm distal to the ligament of Treitz) to establish near-normal physiology and prevent discharge of pancreatic graft exocrine secretions into the distal ileum, which can result in diarrhoea (Gruessner, 2004). The islets of Langerhans represent the vast majority of endocrine pancreatic tissue, small clusters of endocrine cells being also dispersed within the exocrine parenchyma (Gallwitz and Fölsch, 2008). Islets contain four major cell types: α-cells secrete glucagon, β-cells secrete insulin and islet amyloid polypeptide, δ-cells secrete somatostatin, and pancreatic polypeptide (PP) cells secrete PP(Robertson, 2004). Insulin is the major regulator of anabolic and metabolic processes. It promotes the uptake of glucose and amino acids into the peripheral tissues and the metabolic reactions resulting in energy storage, such as glycogen synthesis (Gallwitz and Fölsch, 2008). Insulin is formed independently of actual hormone needs. Excess insulin is stored in β-cells until it is released by an appropriate stimulatory signal for secretion (Gallwitz and Fölsch, 2008). The primary stimuli for insulin secretion are glucose and some amino acids (predominantly arginine, lysine, leucine, and phenylalanine) (Gallwitz and Fölsch, 2008).

Glucagon stimulates hepatic glucose production through glycogenolysis, being the primary defence against hypoglycaemia. Somatostatin inhibits the secretion of other hormones, while no convincingly important metabolic function has been associated with pancreatic polypeptide (Robertson, 2004).

Islets have a higher perfusion rate in comparison to exocrine pancreatic tissue and have fenestrated capillaries ensuring rapid exchange of substrates and hormones. Capillaries first reach the β-cell, then the α-cell, and finally the δ-cell, so that insulin may have a direct influence on the other islet cell types, whereas glucagon and somatostatin reach the β-cell via the general circulation. Paracrine interaction between the different cell types, especially between δ-cells and the other endocrine cells, is also possible (Gallwitz and Fölsch, 2008).

Secretion of pancreatic hormones is also influenced by sympathetic and parasympathetic innervation, which is lacking in the pancreas allograft (Gallwitz and Fölsch, 2008). Despite this, technically successful pancreas transplantation consistently induces insulin independence in β-cell-penic diabetic recipients. Response to oral glucose tolerance test is also nearly normal, and intravenous glucose tolerance test produces intact first- and second-phase glucose-induced secretion responses. As assessed by glucose potentiation of arginine-induced insulin secretion, insulin secretory reserve in the transplanted pancreas is less than normal. Further, serum insulin levels are usually more elevated than in healthy subjects, probably as a consequence of the use of diabetogenic immunosuppression and systemic hormone delivery. Insulin is indeed degraded up to 90% in a single pass through the liver. Portal venous drainage restores the first liver pass of insulin and lowers peripheral hormone levels, although there is no convincing proof that this laboratory finding translates into clinically relevant benefits (Robertson, 2004). Glucagon responses are also returned to normal following successful pancreas transplantation (Robertson, 2004).

## Surgical techniques in kidney–pancreas and isolated pancreas transplantation

The pancreas is comprised of both exocrine and endocrine components. The exocrine portion of the pancreas synthesizes and excretes enzymes, including amylase and lipase that are used by the gastrointestinal (GI) tract to digest food. From a transplant standpoint, the duodenal portion of the pancreas transplants and hence the exocrine secretions can be drained into the bladder or into the bowel, the latter being the more physiological approach. Bladder drainage is performed in about 10% of centres in the US (Gruessner, 2011). It allows the measurement of amylase in the urine as another index of pancreatic function and is a safe technique for handling exocrine secretions of the pancreas. Bladder drainage is performed slightly more often in pancreas after kidney (PAK) transplant (11% of patients) and pancreas alone transplant (PAT) (15%) (Gruessner, 2011). Bladder drainage, however, is associated with metabolic derangements including dehydration and acidosis. Primary enteric drainage is physiological and does not result in dehydration or other metabolic derangement; however, it is associated with potential spill of enteric contents into the abdomen at the time of transplantation. Enteric drainage can be performed between the donor duodenum and jejunum or ileum directly or via a Roux-en-Y limb. It can be constructed in an end-to-end, end-to-side, or side-to-side fashion (Linhares, 2012). Enteric drainage into the stomach has also been reported (Linhares, 2012). There does not appear to be a significant benefit with either technique for patient or pancreas graft survival (Gruessner, 2011).

The endocrine pancreas is responsible for glucose homeostasis dependent on islet β-cell recognition of glucose concentrations, and the secretion of insulin into the portal vein in response to rising glucose levels. In addition, the islet α-cells secrete glucagon into the portal vein in response to low glucose levels. The venous drainage options for pancreas transplant include either systemic venous or mesenteric/portal venous drainage. The external or common iliac vein is usually used for systemic venous drainage of the pancreas transplant, and typically when this is performed in the context of bladder drainage (for the exocrine component of the pancreas) the external iliac vein is dissected to the level of the IVC with ligation and division of all the internal iliac venous branches. This allows freedom and flexibility of the external and common iliac venous system to compensate for the unpredictable nature of the ischaemia–reperfusion response of the pancreas, which can result in significant pancreatitis. The enlargement of the pancreas transplant due to pancreatitis can potentially compress the portal vein, compromising flow and resulting in thrombosis.

Typically, systemic venous drainage of the endocrine pancreas results in high levels of C-peptide (hyper C-peptidaemia). It is possible that this could favourably impact the potential side effect of insulin resistance associated with maintenance immunosuppression (CNIs, steroids, and rapamycin). When the endocrine pancreas venous drainage is through the mesenteric/portal system of the recipient, this results in normal C-peptide levels. Interestingly, while this was felt in early trials to confer a physiological advantage, there does not appear to be any significant long-term benefit to one technique over the other for metabolic parameters (HbA1c, lipid profiles, creatinine) or survival (patient, pancreas or kidney transplant) (Bazerbachi, 2012). In view of this, the frequency of portal vein drainage has fallen to 10–18% (Gruessner, 2011).

The arterial in-flow into the pancreas transplant is usually taken from the external or common iliac artery. However, in some patients with long-standing type 1 diabetes there may be significant atherosclerotic disease throughout the iliac arterial system. A number of surgical approaches have been used and devised to address this particular issue. These approaches include the placement of both kidney and pancreas on the ipsilateral side, i.e. one side of the abdomen, making use of the external and common iliac arterial system (Fridell, 2004). Another option includes back-table preparation of the kidney and pancreas, so that there is a common single arterial conduit and single venous conduit of both the kidney and pancreas so that the arterial conduit can be used when there is limited availability of the external/common iliac artery system.

Other options include replacement of the native external iliac artery with donor external iliac artery (Moon et al., 2005); endarterectomy of the recipient native iliac artery; and a long donor patch of the aorta along with the donor artery (patch angioplasty). The distal SMA of the donor pancreas graft placed in the right abdomen can be used along with a segment of donor external iliac artery jump graft to provide inflow to a left-sided kidney transplant when there is severe disease of the left iliac arterial system (Gorin, 2012). For retransplantation, each of these can also be applied, as well as the use of the donor artery from previous transplant, as long as the artery hasn't developed the significant changes of chronic rejection with onion skinning, etc.

In most transplant centres the kidney–pancreas transplant is performed as an intra-abdominal operation with a midline incision and placement of the organs in the intraperitoneal location. The pancreas can also be placed retroperitoneally, behind the caecum, where there is easier access for biopsy (Boggi, 2012). Recently, with great technical innovation, kidney–pancreas transplantation has also been performed using a combined laparoscopic and robotic approach (Boggi, 2011a, 2012b).

Note that in most circumstances the pancreas is transplanted first in order to minimize the cold ischaemia time. This also allows more time to observe the pancreas for possible bleeding sites, which not uncommonly occur sometimes associated with fluctuations in blood pressure during the surgery. On occasion the kidney may be transplanted first in order to establish diuresis. While this delays the performance of the pancreas transplant by an extra 40 minutes, this is ultimately not likely to significantly impact the ischaemia–reperfusion injury to the pancreas transplant. The kidney-first approach may also be useful when the recipient is a Jehovah's Witness, and Cell Saver® can be used to recycle the recipient's own blood, until the duodenum has been opened (contamination), after the pancreas has been reperfused (Figueiro, 2003).

## Perioperative anaesthetic management of the kidney–pancreas and pancreas recipient

### Transplant recipient

Patients scheduled for either kidney, kidney–pancreas, or pancreas transplant alone need preoperative evaluation. The preoperative evaluation must include overall general assessment followed by a focused examination related to the pathology resulting from either kidney or pancreas failure alone or from kidney + pancreas failure together. In the predialysis era, kidney failure was associated with a myriad of systemic problems, posing significant challenge for anaesthesia care providers. However, dialysis is now routinely available in almost all countries and most definitely in centres where kidney transplant will be occurring. Thus these patients need to be dialyzed before surgery. Table 15.1 summarizes the common preoperative problems that require attention before surgery.

**Table 15.1** Common preoperative problems requiring attention before surgery for pancreas + kidney or pancreas alone transplantation

| |
|---|
| *All patients need to undergo standard preoperative evaluation* |
| NPO status |
| Allergies |
| Medications |
| Airway |
| GORD |
| Pulmonary and cardiovascular status |
| Neuromuscular disease |
| *Specially relevant to chronic renal disease and diabetes* |
| Electrolyte and metabolic status |
| Glucose control measures |
| Anaemia |
| Osteodystrophy |
| Coronary artery disease |
| Gastroparesis and autonomic dysfunction |
| Cerebrovascular disease (strokes/TIA) |
| Hypertension |
| Parathyroid function |
| Platelet function |
| Coagulation factor levels, hepatitis, cytochrome P450 abnormalities |
| Intravascular volume status |
| Evaluation of existing AV fistula used for dialysis |

NPO, Nil per os; GORD, gastro-oesophageal reflux disease; AV, arteriovenous.

There are only a few contraindications for renal transplantation. These include active infection, active drug abuse, complete thrombosis of the vena cava and iliac veins, and disseminated malignancies. Relative contraindications include sensitization by previous failed transplants, blood transfusions, and pregnancy. Individual assessment will help evaluate feasibility for transplantation (Dilioglou, 2001). Those that are developmentally delayed may be transplanted provided there is a caregiver responsible for administering immunosuppressive and other medications (Benedetti, 1998).

Patients who are scheduled to undergo pancreas transplantation alone or with kidney transplantation also need special attention with regard to the complications that result from chronic diabetes mellitus. These include a more thorough evaluation of the upper airway, details of cardiovascular disease including cerebrovascular disease involvement (history of stroke, transient ischaemic attack (TIA)), hypertension, gastro-oesophageal reflux disease (GORD) (gastric aparesis), and autonomic dysfunction. In addition, evaluation of their severity of diabetes including diabetes control and insulin dosing is important.

Special investigations are a requirement in those with renal failure or diabetes mellitus. These include a 12-lead ECG for all diabetics undergoing kidney or kidney + pancreas transplantation or pancreas transplantation alone. When diabetes is present and especially if they have been diabetic for > 25 years, have a body mass index of > 25, and have a smoking history, a more thorough cardiovascular evaluation is necessary.

In addition to a 12-lead ECG, an echocardiogram along with a stress test is essential to rule out and define the extent of coronary artery disease.

When these tests are inconclusive, a cardiology evaluation including coronary angiography may be required. Knowledge of the functional performance of the cardiovascular system and extent of coronary artery disease will be helpful to provide for the required intraoperative and immediate postoperative care for transplant recipients. Some of these patients may require coronary artery bypass grafting or coronary angioplasty with or without stenting prior to solid organ transplantation (Ramanathan, 2005).

### Preoperative preparation: surgical aspects

Pancreas transplantation is indicated when, despite insulin therapy, diabetic nephropathy and/or other invalidating chronic complications of diabetes have occurred or when metabolic control is extremely poor. Most recipients have therefore a long-standing history of diabetes. The combination of these facts puts potential pancreas transplant recipients at increased risk for many medical complications in everyday life. When they became actual pancreas transplant recipients the risk of developing life-threatening complications is further compounded by major surgery, the intrinsic propensity of the pancreas allograft to develop surgical complications (e.g. vascular thrombosis, haemorrhage, pancreatitis, duodenal leaks), and the need for vigorous immunosuppression. Pretransplant evaluation is therefore critically important.

Medical, immunological, and surgical evaluations are carried out simultaneously because of reciprocal interactions in the decision-making process. When focusing on surgical issues, the main objective of pretransplant evaluation is not to select only 'ideal', easy-to-transplant recipients but rather to identify technical solutions enabling most patients to receive a pancreas or a pancreas–kidney transplant. This information is important also to triage recipients with respect to their operative needs on the day of transplantation. From a practical point of view, 'ideal' recipients should be able to receive all suitable grafts under standard organizational and operative conditions. 'Less than ideal' recipients could still receive their grafts, but only in the presence of favourable organizational (e.g. short ischaemia time, 'ideal' donor) or operative (e.g. availability of a surgeon with special expertise in vascular surgery) conditions. In uraemic diabetic patients in need of a pancreas and kidney transplant but deemed too fragile to safely receive a simultaneous transplant, an option is to receive a live donor kidney first, followed by a pancreas after kidney transplantation (Boggi, 2012c).

Pancreas and kidney grafts require a site for arterial and venous anastomosis, often on the iliac vessels. Defining the anatomic site for vascular anastomoses, and their anticipated difficulty, is therefore key. For instance, a patient with iliacocaval thrombosis may still be eligible for pancreas transplantation if the superior mesenteric vein (SMV) is suitable for venous anastomosis. In most diabetic patients, however, most concerns regard the site for arterial anastomosis because of the high prevalence of atherosclerotic lesions. Patients with clinically overt peripheral arterial disease should undergo specific work-up and treatment (Khwaja and Humar, 2004; McCauley, 2007). In the other patients, if physical examination or Doppler ultrasound suggest the possibility of extensively calcified vessels, unenhanced computed tomography scan is helpful in defining the site and thickness of calcified vascular plaques.

Anatomy and function of the urinary bladder is also important in pancreas transplant recipients in case of either simultaneous renal transplant or bladder drainage of exocrine pancreatic secretions. Contrast cystography easily defines bladder anatomy and, during the voiding phase, identifies ureteral reflux as well as residual urine volume. Patients with neurogenic bladder may also require urodynamic testing (Khwaja and Humar, 2004). Screening for occult malignancies is also part of surgical/medical pretransplant scrutiny (McCauley, 2007). Assessment of familial and environmental risk factors provides a guide for individualized evaluation. Standard evaluation includes thorough history, physical examination (including skin inspection), pelvic examination and cervical smear for all women, breast examination and mammogram for women over 40, prostate-specific antigen assay for men over 55, faecal occult blood test for all patients, and barium enema or colonoscopy for patients over 50 (Khwaja and Humar, 2004; Wong, 2008). In patients with cancer history the important question is how long to wait before proceeding with the transplant. Although the longer the disease-free interval, the lower the risk of cancer recurrence, waiting too long may not be in the best interest of the patient. Recommendations assist in taking this difficult decision (Khwaja and Humar, 2004), which, however, should be multidisciplinary and individualized.

Sigmoid resection should be considered in patients with history of diverticulitis (Khwaja and Humar, 2004). In patients with asymptomatic gallstones, cholecystectomy is not mandatory (Khwaja and Humar, 2004; McCauley, 2007).

Obesity is a significant risk factor for technical failure of pancreas transplantation and increased postoperative morbidity. Obese transplant candidates should be strongly encouraged to lose weight pretransplant (Khwaja and Humar, 2004). The possibility of pre-emptive bariatric surgery has also been recently reported (Porubsky, 2012). The presence of active infections should be identified and treated to allow subsequent transplantation. Occult infections should also be ruled out, with special attention to dental caries, urinary tract infections, dialysis access site infections, and chronic pulmonary infections. Pulmonary tuberculosis may remain latent, until the patient is immunosuppressed. A purified protein-derivative skin test should be therefore obtained in all transplant candidates. Viral status should also be assessed (i.e. HIV, hepatitis B and C virus, CMV, EBV, and *Herpes simplex* virus, in particular) (Khwaja and Humar, 2004). HIV positivity, in selected patients, is no longer considered an absolute contraindication to pancreas transplantation (Grossi, 2012).

Although not specifically a surgical issue, evaluation of renal function in recipients of solitary pancreas transplantation is of paramount importance. Loss of renal function has indeed ominous prognostic implications in diabetic patients (Boggi, 2012c). In posturaemic patients, renal graft function is usually deemed sufficient if creatinine clearance exceeds 50 mL/min in the presence of 'nephrotoxic' immunosuppression. Higher levels of native renal function are required in patients eligible for a pancreas transplant alone (creatinine clearance usually > 70 mL/min), also because of the possible presence of underlying diabetic nephropathy (McCauley, 2007; Boggi, 2012).

## Intraoperative planning and care

In addition to standard monitoring, the need for an arterial line needs to be determined based upon the preoperative evaluation (Figure 15.2). If there is significant cardiovascular or cerebrovascular disease and for those undergoing simultaneous kidney–pancreas transplantation (SKPT), an arterial line is essential for direct blood pressure monitoring. The anaesthesia care team can effectively provide a rapid response to changes that occur during anaesthesia and surgery, particularly induction, clamping and unclamping of the newly revascularized grafts, and unexpected blood loss. Diabetics with autonomic neuropathy may become severely hypotensive and bradycardic during induction and similarly may be at risk of sudden death in the postoperative period (Usher, 1999). In addition, if the surgery is done laparoscopically, one can evaluate ventilatory status with frequent arterial blood gas monitoring. The arterial pulse wave can also be used to estimate fluid status and cardiac output.

All patients undergoing either kidney or pancreas transplantation or both organs will need placement of a multilumen central venous catheter. Besides providing central venous pressure information, the catheter can be used for administration of drugs, particularly immunosuppressants that need to be given centrally (thymoglobulin). It also provides a route for blood sampling in the absence of an arterial catheter. Those patients that are extreme cardiac risk may benefit from a pulmonary artery catheter and/or transoesophageal echocardiography during surgery.

## Anaesthesia induction

Most patients tolerate standard induction with intravenous agents. Those with gastroparesis or a full stomach will benefit from a rapid sequence induction to minimize aspiration risk

| **Preoperative evaluation** (important issues) | **Intraoperative care** (important issues) |
|---|---|
| Airway | Place CVP multilumen catheter |
| (difficult – yes video laryngoscope or awake) | Place pain block catheters Replace fluid deficits |
| | Fluid loading for reperfusion preparation |
| Gastroparesis or full stomach (RSI or awake if difficult airway) | Normothermia |
| | Administer immunosuppression |
| | Ensure normoglycemia |
| Cardiac disease | Prepare for reperfusion |
| (significant – yes beta blockade/pulmonary artery catheter/TEE) | **Emergence and postoperative care** |
| | Prepare for extubation |
| Arterial line | Ensure hemodynamic stability |
| (yes if cardiac disease and KP transplantation) | Ensure normothermia |
| | Ensure beta-blockade |
| Pain care plan | Monitor for cardiac ischemia |
| (discuss and implement: Transverse abdominis plane block Paravertebral block (continuous catheter technique) I.V. opioid PCA | Ensure normoglycemia |
| | Avoid stress (check pain scores) |
| | Check renal function status frequently |
| | Avoid hypovolemia |
| | Ensure adequate analgesia |

**Fig. 15.2** Summary of anaesthesia care of pancreas and kidney–pancreas transplant recipients. RSI, Rapid sequence induction; TEE, Transeosophageal echocardiography; KP, Kidney-Pancreas; I.V., Intravenous; PCA, patient controlled analgesia; CVP, central venous pressure.

(Usher, 1999). Video-assisted laryngoscopes should be available to help with the unexpected difficult intubation. In those with a known difficult upper airway, endotracheal intubation should be established before induction. If severe cardiovascular disease is present, the agents should be carefully titrated to avoid undue hypotension. Etomidate serves a useful purpose for such patients. Opioids are well tolerated; however, morphine and meperidine need to be avoided in renal failure because of active metabolites requiring renal elimination. Fentanyl, sufentanil, alfentanil, and remifentanil are useful opioids for kidney or pancreas + kidney or pancreas transplant alone (Marik, 2013). Cisatracurium is the muscle relaxant of choice because of Hoffman elimination. Vecuronium and rocuronium have dual hepatic and renal elimination but are acceptable when used in proper doses. Desflurane and isoflurane are well tolerated for the maintenance of general anaesthesia. Unlike sevoflurane, neither is nephrotoxic.

## Regional analgesia techniques

Continuous epidural, combined spinal and epidural analgesia, and spinal analgesia are options that may be used for care of patients undergoing renal transplantation (Boggi, 2011b). However, because of the duration of surgery, general anaesthesia is the preferred option for either pancreas transplantation or combined kidney–pancreas transplantation. Another reason is the intra-abdominal approach of pancreas transplantation when enteral drainage is planned. Also, if a laparoscopic robotic approach is used, the procedure and positioning will often require general endotracheal anaesthesia with controlled ventilation (Boggi, 2012b).

## Fluid and metabolic care

The intraoperative fluid status is difficult to evaluate during kidney and pancreas transplantation and requires clinical judgement along with the use of available monitoring. The central venous pressure provides a rough estimate of fluid balance. More sensitive indices include the use of non-invasive cardiac output and respiratory variation of the arterial waveform (Halpern, 2004a). The goal should be to replace preoperative deficits during the early surgical phase before graft anastomosis begins. Normal saline crystalloid solution is used at our institution, but a recent study suggests that plasmalyte is superior to both normal saline and Ringer's lactate (Dean, 2004). This solution can also be used to replace intraoperative deficits. Serum potassium must be closely followed and it is advisable not to aggressively replace potassium deficits until there is evidence of renal function following reperfusion. Also, since preservative solutions contain potassium, reperfusion hyperkalaemia is better tolerated if serum potassium levels are in the low–normal range. Packed red blood cells are given to maintain haemoglobin levels in the 9–11 g/dL range and are often required during combined pancreas and kidney transplantation and only rarely during renal transplantation.

## Glucose control during pancreas transplantation

The goal during surgical care is to prevent hyperglycaemia and avoid hypoglycaemia during surgery. Since hyperglycaemia > 150 mg/dL may be detrimental to pancreatic graft β-cells, one should monitor blood glucose levels every 30–60 minutes during surgical care and use insulin either as an infusion or as an intermittent bolus dose to keep blood glucose between 100 and 150 mg/dL (see Figure 15.3) (Bhosale, 2008). For control of exocrine function somatostatin may be administered to decrease pancreatic enzyme secretion in pancreas transplant recipients (Biais, 2011). Figure 15.3 is a guide to glucose care during pancreas transplantation.

## Preparation for graft reperfusion

Prior to kidney and/or pancreas graft reperfusion one should ensure that the patient is mildly hypervolaemic, normothermic, and metabolically stable (as indicated by either arterial or venous blood gases and electrolyte levels). There is evidence that using targeted fluid loading is helpful for optimal graft reperfusion (Hadimioglu, 2008). Most centres will request that the patient be loaded with a diuretic for renal unclamping (furosemide, 0.5 mg/kg) and 250 mL of 20% mannitol along with 150 mL of 20% human albumin before pancreas and renal unclamping. The goal should be to prevent and minimize the transient hypotension that usually ensues. As soon as the clamps are released, rapid transfusion (250–500 mL) of either normal saline or 5% albumin is usually required to achieve this. A summary of graft reperfusion is displayed in Figure 15.4.

After reperfusion of the allograft, there should be close monitoring of urine output, fluid balance, and overall circulatory status. Causes for decreased urine output include hypovolaemia, hypotension, acute tubular necrosis, and acute rejection.

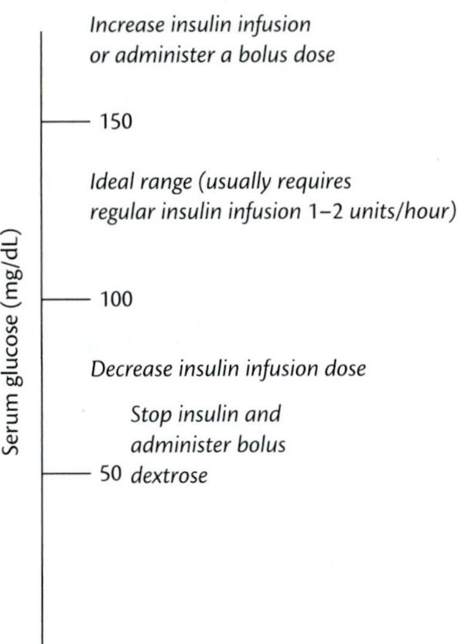


**Fig. 15.3** Guide to care of blood glucose during surgery for pancreas transplantation. The care provider should aim for normoglycaemia and keep blood glucose levels between 100 and 150 mg/dL

A biopsy of the transplanted kidney may be required to diagnose acute tubular necrosis or graft rejection. For pancreas allograft recipients, one needs to ensure stable haemodynamics to prevent graft vessel thrombosis, a common cause of pancreas graft failure. It is best to avoid a hypercoagulable state during the care of pancreas graft recipients. When the kidney is functioning (native or transplanted organ), the use of hydroxyethyl starch as a colloid fluid expander will be helpful in this regard (Halpern, 2004b).

### Emergence from anaesthesia and initial postoperative and pain care

Most patients can be successfully weaned from anaesthesia and successfully extubated either in the operating room or soon after arrival in the postanaesthesia care unit (PACU). Care should be taken to extubate them after complete recovery from neuromuscular blockade. Prior to extubation the patients need to be normothermic and haemodynamically stable. Renal function should be followed closely in all renal transplant recipients. Causes of low urine output should be explored quickly. One common cause in the PACU is urinary catheter obstruction from blood clots. This will require bedside irrigation of the catheter.

Diabetic patients with or without a pancreas transplant will need close monitoring for cardiac ischaemia. This is done with daily monitoring for 3 days of serum troponin levels, along with a 12-lead ECG. In addition, serum glucose needs to be monitored closely to ensure normoglycaemia. Dehydration and hypothermia should be avoided to prevent cardiac stress. Beta-blockers will need to be continued in the perioperative period to reduce episodes of tachycardia. For optimal oxygen delivery it is recommended to keep the blood haemoglobin level to around 10 g/dL.

The analgesic needs of renal recipients are not as serious a concern as they are for pancreas transplant recipients. However, transverse abdominis plane block has been shown to be quite helpful (Stratta, 1993). This can be done bilaterally and also helps pancreas transplant recipients (Othman, 2010). The use of the paravertebral block technique to control pain in this group of patients is being investigated in our institution and appears promising. All patients will need opioid supplements, best administered via a patient-controlled analgesia setup.

## Operative management

During the kidney–pancreas transplant operation, communication between the surgical team and anaesthesia team is important in order to provide a safe transit for the patient, as well as optimizing the physiological conditions for allowing immediate function of both kidney and pancreas. Monitoring of the patient includes placement of the arterial line for continuous evaluation of systemic blood pressure. In addition, a central venous line is placed in either the neck or the chest in order to monitor central venous pressures continuously during the surgery. In patients with a significant cardiac history, a TEE is placed for continuous monitoring of the intracardiac volume and on occasion a Swan–Ganz may be used for evaluation of the wedge pressure, if the TEE is not available.

The blood sugar is checked every 20–30 minutes during the surgery. Generally, the blood glucose is maintained between 100

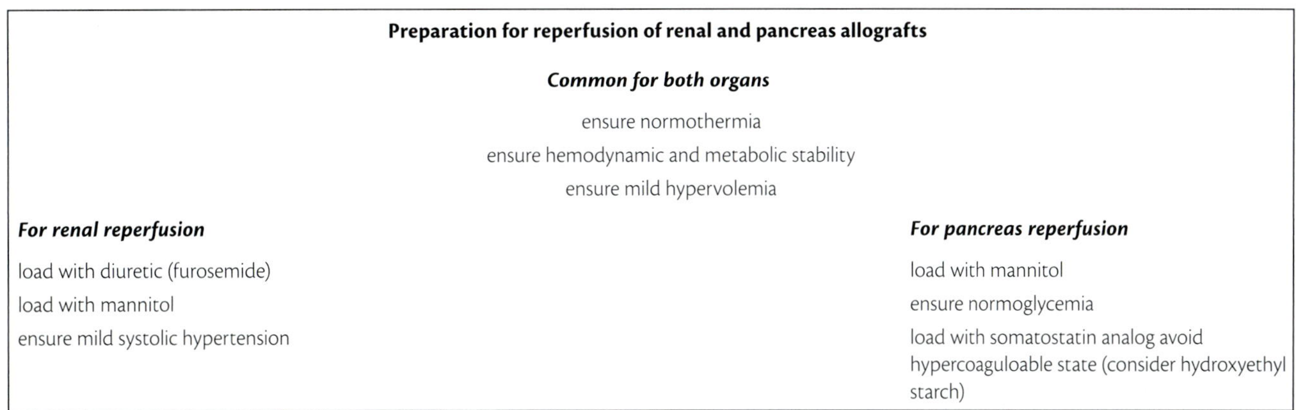


**Fig. 15.4** Summary of important care issues for graft reperfusion of kidney and pancreas allografts

and 150 mg/dL (Figure 15.3). Prior to revascularization of the pancreas transplant, our goal is to maintain blood sugar so as to protect from the possibility of a bolus of insulin release that may result in transient hypoglycaemia. Once the pancreas transplant has been reperfused, the blood glucose will fall towards normal.

Although kidney–pancreas transplant recipients are uraemic with the well-described impact of uraemia on platelet function resulting in a tendency to bleed, many type 1 diabetics with ESRD in fact have a proclivity towards hypercoagulability (Burke, 2004a; Fukazawa, 2011). This is associated with the following commonly obtained blood tests: shortened prothrombin time, INR < 1, shortened PTT, elevated fibrinogen level, elevated hematocrit, and elevated platelet count. The hypercoagulable state is associated with hypertension, dyslipidaemia, and the obesity that may accompany type 1 diabetes with ESRD. A TEG can be helpful to confirm the presence of the hypercoagulable state. Our current approach is to combine both laboratory data and TEG results with assessment of the intraoperative field. If there is minimal bleeding during the dissection, then in the context of the TEG-demonstrated hypercoagulable state, heparin (2,000–5,000 units) is given as an intravenous bolus prior to placing vascular clamps. If the operative field remains pristine with minimal evidence of bleeding by the end of surgery, then the patient is maintained on a continuous heparin drip with a target PTT of 45–50 s (1.5–1.9 times upper normal). In our experience, this approach has led to a low number of pancreas transplant thromboses, as well as minimizing postoperative bleeding (Burke, 2004a). The absence of haematuria (in the bladder-drained pancreas transplant recipient) confirms the appropriate use of anticoagulation when defined in this setting.

In our centre, flushing the pancreas on the back table to assess for possible bleeding is avoided. Instead, once the vascular anastomoses are completed, the vascular clamps are removed in serial fashion starting with the cephalad venous clamp (low pressure) in order to assess haemostasis. Subsequently the distal arterial clamp is removed, which allows for the low-pressure testing of the arterial system. Once haemostasis is obtained, the distal venous vascular clamp is removed and then finally the proximal arterial clamp is removed. Haemostasis is again assured. Once the pancreas has been reperfused, the exocrine pancreas will begin to secrete fluids and the duodenum will begin to expand. It is important that the anastomosis of the duodenum to bladder or bowel is performed in a timely fashion prior to expansion of the duodenum. In the case of bladder-drained pancreas transplants, during the back-table preparation the duodenal segment is made as small as possible and the duodenal contents are drained into the distal duodenum and jejunum, prior to stapling the distal duodenal segment, in order to minimize residual duodenal content. After reperfusion the duodenum begins to fill, and, if allowed to become tense, can contribute to the pancreatitis that has already been initiated with the ischaemia–reperfusion injury to the pancreas transplant.

A culture of the donor duodenum is obtained and the duodenal contents are emptied into the bladder (for bladder-drained transplants). In the case of primary enteric-drained pancreas transplants the duodenal segment is usually longer. However, the same principles apply as far as decompressing the duodenal segment in order to minimize further pancreatitis in the pancreas transplant. The culture of the duodenum may demonstrate yeast, in which case antifungal therapy is recommended (Ciancio, 1996). Intraoperative immunosuppression generally includes steroids and some form of induction antibody; this antibody may include anti-CD25 monoclonal antibody, thymoglobulin, or Campath. In Miami we have used a combination of anti-CD25 and thymoglobulin since 2000 ( Sageshima, 2011). Maintenance immunosuppression generally includes tacrolimus, mycophenolate mofetil, and steroids, although rapamycin may also be effective (Gruessner, 2011; Ciancio, 2012).

## Postoperative care: surgical aspects

Besides all medical interventions needed to ensure optimal liquid/electrolyte balance, pH homeostasis, adequate oxygen delivery to tissues (including adequate haematological parameters), to promote graft function in general and to achieve effective immunosuppression (Boggi, 2011), pancreas transplant recipients need special surgical care since they are at increased risk of post-transplant surgical complications (Boggi, 2010b). Reoperation is indeed needed for between 15 and 25% of recipients, the leading causes for repeat surgery being vascular thrombosis, haemorrhage, intra-abdominal infection, and enteric leak (Boggi, 2010b).

The propensity of the pancreas graft to develop thrombosis and the hypercoagulable state of many recipients makes antithrombotic prophylaxis a main postoperative issue. In most patients, however, there is a combination of early anticoagulant therapy followed by long-term low-dose aspirin administration (Ciancio, 1996; Egidi, 2007).

Antithrombotic prophylaxis increases the risk of postoperative haemorrhage. Close monitoring of coagulation values is therefore recommended, especially during the early days, since the limit between thrombosis and bleeding is poorly defined in this recipient population. Severe bleeding, requiring re-exploration, occurs at an intra-abdominal level usually in a limited percentage of patients. It is preferable to vascular thrombosis, which is often irreversible, but it can be life-threatening and may require urgent reintervention. Patients with enteric drainage may also develop intestinal bleeding, which is typically self-limited but also very tedious to manage (Boggi, 2010b).

To help in the balance between the risk of thrombosis and haemorrhage we prefer to scan pancreas transplant recipients daily by Doppler ultrasound during the early post-transplant course. This policy may be helpful in identifying non-occlusive vascular thrombosis, which is often amenable to resolution with enhanced anticoagulation (Sageshima, 2011). Because of the underlying diabetes and the vigorous immunosuppression, pancreas transplant recipients do need antibacterial, antifungal, and antiviral prophylaxes. CMV prophylaxis seems to be particularly important also because of the possible interactions between CMV infection and increased expression of MHC class I possibly promoting graft rejection (Ciancio, 1996).

The rest of the care of pancreas transplant recipients is similar to that of other solid-organ recipients. However, in patients receiving bladder drainage of exocrine pancreatic secretions, particular attention should be paid to appropriate bicarbonate supplementation, since urinary loss of pancreatic juice may result in hyperchloraemic metabolic acidosis (Egidi, 2007).

### Short- and long-term outcomes

The outcome of kidney and pancreas transplant can be divided into early issues, specifically within the first week, survival for the first year, and long term, up to 10 years. The early outcome, i.e.

during the first week, generally is dependent on the degree of pancreatitis in the pancreas transplant and this is dependent on the cold ischaemia time, warm ischaemia time, as well as preservation fluid used and donor-specific issues, i.e. preterminal events, particularly hypotension and sepsis. Early technical failure of the pancreas transplant continues to occur in about 10% of cases, for all categories, SKPT, PAK transplant, and PAT (Gruessner, 2011).

The incidence of thrombosis of pancreas transplants is the highest of all the solid organ transplants, occurring in between 2 and 15% of cases and on average about 10% (Gruessner, 2011). This can be explained on the basis of (1) the hypercoagulable state identified in type 1 diabetics with ESRD, (2) the endothelial cell damage that occurs with the ischaemia–reperfusion events, and finally (3) the size and capacitance of the venous conduits located in the pancreas (Burke, 2004a). This includes the splenic vein as well as the SMV and portal vein, which provide venous return from the spleen and the small bowel, respectively. While located in the pancreas, the much-reduced flow from the pancreas transplant without the spleen or small bowel results in significantly reduced flow in these large-capacitance veins. These three issues together comprise Virchow's triad and offer a rational explanation for why the pancreas transplant has the highest rate of thrombosis of solid organs (Burke, 2004a; Fukazawa, 2011). The approach to this is reviewed in the operative management.

The 1-year outcome of kidney and pancreas transplantation is typically in the range of patient survival 90–95%, pancreas transplant survival 85–95%, and kidney transplant survival 90–95% (Scharp, 1990; Howard, 1994; Gruessner, 2011). After the issue of thrombosis/technical failure of the pancreas transplant, the next most significant negative impact is due to acute rejection of the kidney or pancreas transplant (Gruessner, 2011). Long-term patient survival following a kidney and pancreas transplant generally depends on the cardiovascular history of the patient, since cardiovascular events are the most frequent cause of death in this patient population (Burke, 2004a; Gruessner, 2011; Ciancio, 2012). Ten-year SKPT patient survival is generally greater than 70% (Burke, 2004b; Gruessner, 2011; Bazerbachi, 2012; Ciancio, 2012). The loss of either pancreas or kidney graft function has a significant negative impact on patient survival, with kidney loss impacting patient survival over five-fold greater than pancreas loss (Gruessner, 2011). However, long-term euglycaemia and kidney function is certainly possible.

Long-term, 10-year pancreas and kidney graft survival has improved since 1995. Many factors impact graft survival, including recipient and donor age, degree of recipient sensitization, preservation time, and immunosuppression, both induction (depleting or non-depleting agent) and maintenance (Burke, 2004b; Gruessner, 2011; Cianco et al., 2012). Pancreas transplant 10-year survival (death-censored) was reported to be 91%, while kidney transplant survival (death-censored) was 72% (Ciancio, 2012). We found an advantage to using rapamycin with tacrolimus and steroids over the use of mycophenolate mofetil, due to better GI tolerance of rapamycin in this patient population with a high incidence of gastroparesis, which led to less rejection over 10 years (Ciancio, 2012).

In our experience, with bladder-drained pancreas transplants, chronic rejection with loss of pancreas transplant C-peptide secretion occurs in approximately 5% of patients over time. Chronic rejection of the pancreas transplant may occasionally be associated with a euglycaemic state ('burnt-out pancreas'), i.e. the exocrine portion of the pancreas transplant has been lost, yet the endocrine portion of the pancreas transplant remains preserved, i.e. C-peptide is preserved, and the HbA1c is normal. Other causes of late graft loss include viral infections, particularly polyomavirus (BK virus) (Akpinar, 2010), which can result in loss of kidney transplant. Viral infections including CMV and EBV, and PTLD, typically due to EBV infection, can result in significant morbidity, graft loss, and occasional mortality, although low incidence over 10 years has been reported (Ciancio, 2012). In our experience, chronic rejection with graft loss occurs more commonly in the kidney transplant than the pancreas transplant over the long term (Ciancio, 2012).

Recurrence of autoimmunity in the pancreas transplant (type 1 diabetes recurrence (T1DR)) occurs in about 5% of SKPT recipients, similar to the rate of chronic rejection in our patient population (Vendrame, 2010; Burke, 2011). Patients with T1DR present with hyperglycaemia 2.5–10 years following SKPT, with normal kidney transplant function and no change in urine amylase. The recurrence of autoimmunity/T1DR has been associated in our experience with the development of autoantibodies in the peripheral blood, along with T-cells specific for autoantigens. The clinical development of hyperglycaemia is associated with either persistent C-peptide secretion or loss of C-peptide. Biopsies of the pancreas transplant demonstrate insulitis with preserved insulin staining in those patients who continue to secrete C-peptide and loss of insulin staining in those patients who no longer secrete C-peptide (Vendrame, 2010; Burke, 2011 ).

## Conclusion

In this chapter we have provided an overview of the care of patients undergoing either a combined kidney and pancreas transplantation or pancreas transplantation alone. Both these organs provide an important historical aspect that led to the initial establishment of kidney transplantation, followed later by pancreas transplantation. Although the endocrine mass of the pancreas is only 2% of the entire organ, it plays an important role in glucose control, and the procedures described are aimed at preserving this endocrine function during transplantation. Endocrine failure of the pancreas leads to renal failure, and thus combined kidney and pancreas transplantation can be carried out along with the same immunosuppression that will be used for either organ alone. A thorough preoperative evaluation along with careful intraoperative and postoperative care, paying attention to minute details, is important for enhancing early and late successful outcomes in these patients. One needs to pay close attention to pancreas ischaemia times and closely monitor and treat the hypercoagulable state in pancreas transplant recipients. The perioperative process has significantly been enhanced to achieve optimal outcomes because of close communication between the primary care provider, anaesthesia care team, surgical care team, and the long-term follow-up care teams involved in the care of these patients. It is important to have the established protocols in place and minimize alterations in care. This will result in improved outcomes in these patients undergoing either pancreas and kidney or pancreas transplantation alone.

## References

Akpinar E (2010) BK virus nephropathy after simultaneous pancreas–kidney transplantation. *Clin Transplant*, **24**:801–806.

Aniskevich S (2011) Bilateral transversus abdominis plane block for managing pain after a pancreas transplant. *Exp Clin Transplant*, **9**:277–278.

Bazerbachi F (2012) Portal venous versus systemic venous drainage of pancreas grafts: Impact on long-term results. *Am J Transplant*, **12**:226–232.

Benedetti E (1998) Kidney transplantation in recipients with mental retardation: clinical results in a single-center experience. *Am J Kidney Dis*, **31**:509–512.

Bhosale G (2008) Combined spinal-epidural anesthesia for renal transplantation. *Transplant Proc*, **40**:1122–1124.

Biais M (2011) The ability of pulse pressure variations obtained with CNAP device to predict fluid responsiveness in the operating room. *Anesth Analg*, **113**:523–528.

Boggi U (2009a) Contribution of contrast-enhanced ultrasonography to non-operative management of segmental graft ischemia of the head of a pancreas graft. *Am J Transplant*, **9**:413–418.

Boggi U (2009b) Contribution of contrast-enhanced ultrasonography to nonoperative management of segmental ischemia of the head of a pancreas graft. *Am J Transplant*, **9**:413–418.

Boggi U (2010a) Surgical techniques of pancreas transplantation. In: Hakim NS, Stratta RJ, Gray D, Friend P, Colman A (eds) *Pancreas, Islet, and Stem Cell Transplantation for Diabetes*, 2nd edn, pp. 111–135. Oxford University Press, New York.

Boggi U (2010b) Surgical techniques for pancreas transplantation. *Curr Opin Organ Transplant*, **15**:102–111.

Boggi U (2011a) Current perspectives on laparoscopic robot-assisted pancreas and pancreas–kidney transplantation. *Rev Diab Stud*, **8**:28–34.

Boggi U (2011b) Results of pancreas transplantation alone with special attention to native kidney function and proteinuria in type 1 diabetes patients. *Rev Diab Stud*, **8**:259–267.

Boggi U (2012a) Long-term (5 years) efficacy and safety of pancreas transplantation alone in type 1 diabetic patient. *Transplantation*, **93**:842–846.

Boggi U (2012b) Laparoscopic robot-assisted pancreas transplantation: First World experience. *Transplantation*, **93**:201–206.

Boggi U (2012c) Transplantation of the pancreas. *Curr Diab Rep*, **12**:568–579.

Burke GW (2004a) Hypercoagulable state associated with kidney–pancreas transplantation. Thromboelastogram-directed anti-coagulation and implications for future therapy. *Clin Transplant*, **18**:423–428.

Burke GW (2004b) Advances in pancreas transplantation. *Transplantation*, **77**:S62–S67.

Burke G (2011) Recurrence of autoimmunity following pancreas transplantation. *Curr Diab Rep*, **11**:413–419.

Ciancio G (1996) Destructive allograft fungal arteritis following simultaneous pancreas–kidney transplantation. *Transplantation*, **61**:172–1175.

Ciancio G, Sageshima G, Chen L (2012) Advantage of rapamycin over mycophenolate mofetil when used with tacrolimus for simultaneous pancreas kidney transplants: randomized, single-center trial at 10 years. *Am J Transplant*, **12**(12):3363–3376.

Dean M (2004) Opioids in renal failure and dialysis patients. *J Pain Sympt Manage*, **28**:497–504.

Dilioglou S (2001) High panel reactive antibody against cross-reactive group antigens as a contraindication to renal allotransplantation. *Exp Molec Pathol*, **71**:73–78.

Egidi MF (2007) Medical management after pancreas transplantation. In: Corry RJ, Shapiro R (eds) *Pancreatic Transplantation*, pp. 83–91. Informa Healthcare, New York.

Figueiro J (2003) Simultaneous pancreas-kidney transplantation in Jehovah's Witness patients. *Clin Transplant*, **17**:140–143.

Fridell JA (2004) Ipsilateral placement of simultaneous pancreas and kidney allografts. *Transplantation*, **78**:1074–1076.

Fukazawa K (2011) Reversal of hypercoagulability with hydroxyethyl starch during transplantation: a case series. *J Clin Anesth*, **23**:61–65.

Gallwitz B, Fölsch UR (2008) Physiology and pathophysiology of endocrine pancreatic secretion. In: Beger HG, Matsuno S, Cameron JL (eds) *Diseases of the Pancreas. Current Surgical Therapy*, pp. 37–48. Springer, Berlin.

Gorin MA (2012) Emergent renal revascularization of a simultaneous pancreas–kidney transplant recipient. *Transplantation*, **93**:16–17.

Grossi PA (2012) Report of four simultaneous pancreas–kidney transplants in HIV-positive recipients with favorable outcomes. *Am J Transplant*, **12**:1039–1045

Gruessner RWG (2004) Recipient procedures. In: Gruessner RWG, Sutherland DER (eds) *Transplantation of the Pancreas*, pp. 150–178. Springer, New York.

Gruessner AC (2011) 2011 Update on pancreas transplantation: comprehensive trend analysis of 25,000 cases followed up over the course of twenty-four years at the International Pancreas Transplant Registry (IPTR). *Rev Diab Stud*, **8**:6–16.

Hadimioglu N (2008). The effect of different crystalloid solutions on acid-base balance and early kidney function after kidney transplantation. *Anesth Analg*, **107**:264–269.

Halpern H (2004a) Anesthesia for pancreas transplantation alone or simultaneous with kidney. *Transplant Proc*, **36**:3105–3106.

Halpern H (2004b) Glycemic control during pancreas transplantation: continous infusion versus bolus. *Transplant Proc*, **36**:984–985.

Howard JM (1994) Notes on the history of pancreatic surgery, anatomy, and physiology. In: Braasch JW, Tompkins RK (eds) *Surgical Disease of the Biliary Tract and Pancreas. Multidisciplinary Management*, pp. 381–406. Mosby-Year Book, St Louis.

Jankovic ZB (2009) Continuous transversus abdominis plane block for renal transplant recipients. *Anesth Analg*, **109**:1710–1711.

Kelly WD (1967) Allotransplantation of the pancreas and duodenum along with the kidney in diabetic nephropathy. *Surgery*, **61**:827–835.

Khwaja K, Humar A (2004) Pretransplant evaluation and cardiac risk assessment. In: Gruessner RWG, Sutherland DER (eds) *Transplantation of the Pancreas*, pp. 103–109. Springer, New York.

Kitagawa H, Ohta T, Makino I, et al. (2008) Carcinomas of the ventral and dorsal pancreas exhibit different patterns of lymphatic spread. *Frontiers Biosci*, **13**:2728–2735.

Layer P, Keller J (2008) Pancreatic exocrine secretion. In: Beger HG, Matsuno S, Cameron JL (eds) *Current Surgical Therapy. Diseases of the Pancreas*, pp. 31–35. Springer, Berlin.

Leone JP, Christensen K (2004) Postoperative management uncomplicated course. In: Gruessner RWG, Sutherland DER (eds). *Transplantation of the Pancreas*, pp. 179–190. Springer, New York.

Linhares MM (2012) Duodenum-stomach anastomosis: a new technique for exocrine drainage in pancreas transplantation. *J Gastrointest Surg*, **16**:1072–1075.

Marik PE (2013) Noninvasive cardiac output monitors: a state-of-the-art review. *J Cardio-Thorac Vasc Anesth*, **27**:121–134.

McCauley (2007) Evaluation of the pancreas transplant recipient. In: Corry RJ, Shapiro R (eds) *Pancreatic Transplantation*, pp. 31–45. Informa Healthcare, New York.

Moon JI, Ciancio G, Burke GW (2005) Arterial reconstruction with donor iliac vessels during pancreas transplantation: an intraoperative approach to arterial injury or inadequate flow. *Clin Transplant*, **19**:286–290.

Othman MM (2010) The impact of timing of maximal crystalloid hydration on early graft function during kidney transplantation. *Anesth Analg*, **110**:1440–1446.

Porubsky M (2012) Pancreas transplantation after bariatric surgery. *Clin Transplant*, **26**(1):E1–E6.

Ramanathan V (2005) Screening asymptomatic diabetic patients for coronary artery disease prior to renal transplantation. *Transplantation*, **79**:1453–1458.

Robertson RP (2004) Endocrine function and metabolic outcomes in pancreas and islet transplantation. In: Gruessner RWG, Sutherland DER (eds) *Transplantation of the Pancreas*, pp. 441–454. Springer, New York.

Sageshima J (2011) Addition of anti-CD25 to thymoglobulin for induction therapy: delayed return of peripheral blood CD25 positive population. *Clin Transplant*, **25**:E132–135.

Scharp DW (1990) Insulin independence after islet transplantation into type I diabetic patient. *Diabetes*, **39**:515–518.

Stratta RJ (1993) Selective use of Sandostatin in vascularized pancreas transplantation. *Am J Surg*, **166**:598–604.

Trede M (1997) Embryology and surgical anatomy of the pancreas. In: Trede M, Carter DC (eds) *Surgery of the Pancreas*, pp. 17–27. Churchill Livingstone, New York.

Usher S (1999) Peri-operative asystole in a patient with diabetic autonomic neuropathy. *Anaesthesia*, **54**:1125.

Vendrame F (2010) Recurrence of type 1 diabetes after simultaneous pancreas–kidney transplantation, despite immunosuppression, is associated with autoantibodies and pathogenic auto reactive CD4 T-cells. *Diabetes*, **59**:947–957

Wong G (2008) Cancer screening in renal transplant recipients: what is the evidence? *Clin J Am Soc Nephrol*, **3**:S87–S100.

# CHAPTER 16

# Critical care of the kidney, pancreas, and kidney–pancreas transplant recipient

Martin Birch, Robby Sikka, and Kumar Belani

## Introduction

Increasing numbers of patients are receiving kidney, pancreas, and kidney–pancreas transplants. Despite advances in care, complications continue to occur and can lead to serious morbidity and increased mortality (Bindi, et al., 2005). The complications can be serious enough that patients may become critically ill, necessitating care in the ICU. This chapter focuses on the care of these patients in the ICU.

The complications are myriad and depend on patient and procedural factors. Recipients of kidney, pancreas, and kidney–pancreas transplants have significant comorbidities: specifically ESRD and/or diabetes mellitus and their subsequent effects on organ function. The surgical procedures are long and complex, placing great stress on the patient. Additionally, the required potent immunosuppressive therapy predisposes them to increased risk of infection.

Physiological stability is a homeostatic concept. Physiological stability does not mean that vital signs do not change. It means that vital signs fluctuate around relatively acceptable set points and will return to these set points when perturbations have ceased. Stable organisms can be modelled as a marble placed in a bowl (see Figure 16.1). If the marble is displaced it will oscillate until it returns to the original set point.

Critically ill patients are different from other patient populations. They are inherently unstable. Their vital signs no longer fluctuate around a set point. They can be modelled as a marble perched precariously on top of an upside-down bowl (see Figure 16.2). If displaced it will not oscillate until the set point is once again attained. It will roll down the side of the bowl, and it can take tremendous effort to place it back in its original position, if that is even possible.

This chapter is divided into several sections. The first discusses infectious complications, including the treatment of sepsis, severe sepsis, and septic shock. The second focuses on respiratory failure, with an emphasis on the importance of ventilation in meeting metabolic demands and how this is closely related to the work of breathing and a patient's acid-base status. Additionally, non-invasive positive pressure ventilation and lung-protective ventilation are discussed, as well as liberation from mechanical ventilation. The third section provides an update on cardiovascular complications, with an emphasis on perioperative myocardial infarction (MI). Finally, vascular catastrophies are discussed, with emphasis placed on the diagnosis and treatment of arterial to enteric fistulas.

## Care of the solid organ transplant recipient

Critically ill patients require tremendous support to keep their vital signs compatible with life, and further perturbations can worsen the situation to such an extent that life is not possible. If further perturbations occur, such as an interruption of vasopressor support, it is not certain that a patient will regain his or her former status even if aggressive support is reinitiated. The final common pathway of continued uncorrected instability is multisystem organ failure, where initially reversible cellular injury occurring in various organs becomes irreversible and death eventually ensues.

### Infections

Infectious complications are an important cause of morbidity and mortality in solid organ transplant recipients (Bassetti et al., 2004; Bindi, et al., 2005; Fishman, 2007; Fontana et al., 2009; Rostambeigi et al., 2010; Ziaja et al., 2011). They decrease the rate of graft survival and can progress to life-threatening sepsis and septic shock. Appropriate treatment of sepsis and septic shock depends upon early recognition and diagnosis, early and appropriate broad-spectrum antimicrobial coverage, infectious source control if possible, and aggressive resuscitation with vasopressor and/or inotropic support, if needed, to restore MAP along with vital organ blood flow and adequate oxygen delivery. Further care is based on supporting the various damaged or stressed organ systems by mechanically ventilating or haemodialysing patients with respiratory or renal failure if needed, while preventing complications such as line infections, ventilator-associated pneumonia, stress ulcers, and venous thromboembolisms. Each aspect of care is important and there are continued problems adequately achieving all aspects of care (Dellinger et al., 2008).

Severe sepsis and septic shock are devastating complications. The pathophysiology is extremely complex and begins with an invading organism and the host response to the invasion. An uncontrolled generalized inflammatory cascade is unleashed

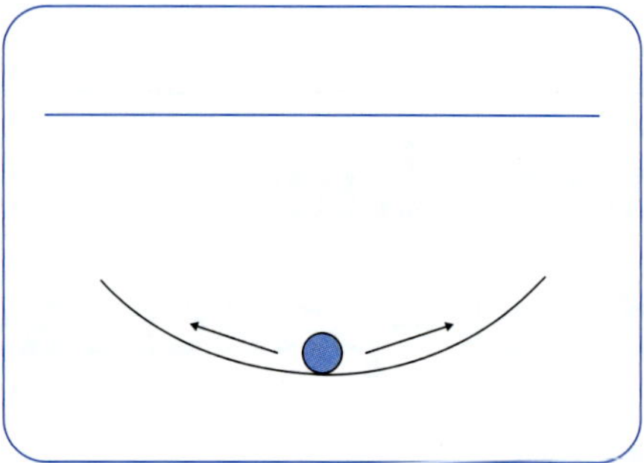

**Fig. 16.1** Physiological stability modelled as a marble in a bowl. As the marble is displaced it oscillates around a stable set point, eventually resting at its original position. Physiological stable organisms have vital signs that vary around relatively stable set points when perturbations occur. When the perturbation ends, vital signs return to their original position

characterized by increased levels of inflammatory cytokines, such as $TNF_{\alpha}$, IL-2, and IL-6. The inflammatory response causes multiple problems including vasodilation, myocardial depression, capillary leak, microvascular dysfunction, and cellular dysfunction especially in relation to oxygen utilization and energy metabolism and apoptosis (Russell, 2006; Singer, 2008). The inflammatory response is followed by the compensatory anti-inflammatory response syndrome (CARS), characterized by increased levels of anti-inflammatory cytokines leading to pronounced immunosuppression (Shubin et al., 20100). The patient can be in the worst of all possible worlds, with severe derangements of organ function resulting from the inflammatory response. This, coupled with profound immunosuppression, predisposes the patient to secondary infections.

Approximately 750,000 cases of severe sepsis occur in the US each year and 36,800 sepsis-related deaths every year in the UK (Martin et al., 2003; Daniels, 2011). The mortality is approximately 35% for severe sepsis and is increased in septic shock. The mortality also increases with the number of organ systems that have failed (Russell, 2006). In comparative terms, the mortality rate is 6–10 times higher than for patients admitted with acute MI and 4–5 times higher than similar patients admitted with acute ischaemic strokes (Daniels, 2011). Despite this, significant problems exist with recognition, diagnosis, and treatment. In order to improve diagnosis and outcome the Surviving Sepsis Campaign was created, and the first set of guidelines was published in 2004 and updated in 2008. The guidelines attempt to standardize initial diagnosis, indicators of organ dysfunction, approach to resuscitation, and the use of adjunctive agents such as corticosteroids (Dellinger et al., 2004, 2008). Though imperfect and recently updated—especially regarding intensive insulin therapy, the use of activated protein C, and vasopressor choice—there has been documented outcome benefit since the publication of the guidelines (Levy et al., 2010; Dellinger et al., 2013). Unfortunately, the vast majority of clinical trials have actively excluded transplant recipients (Kalil et al., 2007). Applying the literature to transplant recipients requires several assumptions, not the least of which is that they will respond to therapy as non-recipients.

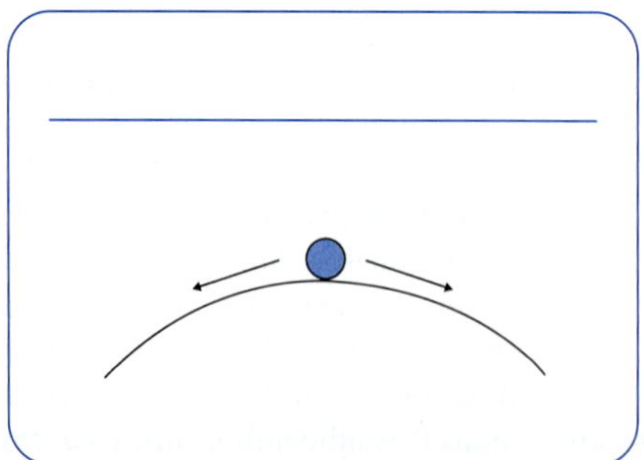

**Fig. 16.2** Physiological instability modelled as a marble perched on top of a bowl. When perturbed, the marble will roll off the bowl and it will not regain its original position. Physiologically unstable organisms are like this marble. When perturbations occur, significant derangements will follow. Regaining the original position is improbable. It can take tremendous work to keep the marble, or organism, in its precarious position

The management of sepsis hinges on appropriate diagnosis. In 2001 a consensus definition was created to aid diagnosis. The definition combined the criteria for SIRS with a source of, or evidence of, infection. The definition was further refined in order to stage the process according to severity based upon end-organ dysfunction and the presence of shock. Severe sepsis requires evidence of end-organ dysfunction, such as an acutely increased creatinine or a metabolic acidosis. Septic shock requires continued hypotension despite what should be adequate volume resuscitation (see Table 16.1) (Levy et al., 2003).

Immunosuppressed transplant recipients may not show classical signs of infection, such as fever or leucocytosis. Clinicians require a very high index of suspicion regarding these patients, and indicators of organ dysfunction and hypoperfusion may be more sensitive indicators of infection (Kalil et al., 2007). Newer markers of sepsis and septic shock, such as procalcitonin, may be of use, although prospective data in transplant recipients are lacking (Schuetz et al., 2011). The types of infection and the infecting organisms are variable and depend on multiple factors, including the organ transplanted and the time since transplantation

**Table 16.1** Criteria for defining SIRS and sepsis

| **SIRS criteria** |
|---|
| *Requires two or more of the following:* |
| ◆ Temperature > 38°C or < 36°C |
| ◆ Heart rate > 90 bpm |
| ◆ Respiratory rate > 20/min or $PaCO_2$ < 32 mm Hg |
| ◆ White blood count > 12,000 or < 4,000/μL |
| **Sepsis** |
| *Sepsis* |
| ◆ SIRS + infection |
| *Severe sepsis* |
| ◆ Sepsis + organ dysfunction |
| *Septic shock* |
| ◆ Sepsis + cardiovascular collapse despite adequate fluid resuscitation (systolic blood pressure < 90 mm Hg, MAP 65 mm Hg, or ≥ 40 mm Hg decrease from baseline) |

Data from 'American College of Chest Physicians/Society of Critical Care Medicine Consensus Conference: Definitions of sepsis and organ failure and guidelines for the use of innovative therapies in sepsis', Critical Care Medicine, 20, 6, 1992.

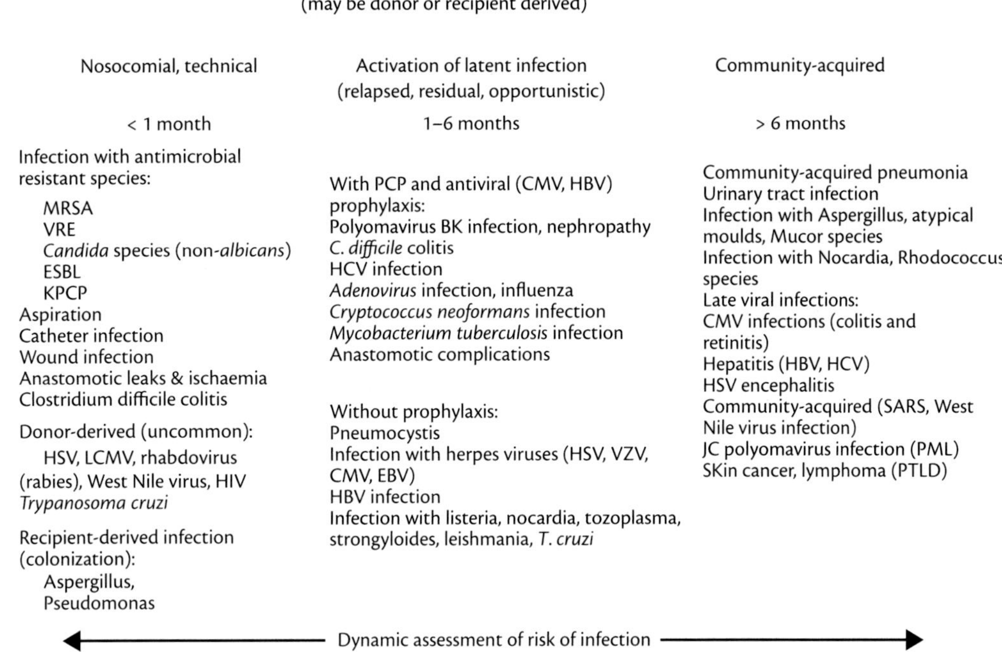


**Fig. 16.3** Common infections that occur in solid organ recipients as they relate to the time period following transplantation

(Fishman, 2007). Figure 16.3 describes the time course of common infections occurring in solid organ transplant recipients. A full microbiological work-up is imperative, including blood, urine, sputum cultures, and viral and fungal cultures, as well as appropriate imaging studies to look for intra-abdominal pathology.

Bacteria are the most common source of infection in kidney, pancreas, and kidney–pancreas transplant recipients, followed by viral, fungal, and polymicrobial infections. The greatest risk appears to be within the first 3–6 months following transplant, and this decreases relatively quickly afterwards (Bassetti et al., 2004; Singh et al., 2008; Fontana et al., 2009; Rostambeigi et al., 2010). The infection rate is higher with pancreas transplantation than renal transplantation (Moreno et al., 2007). There are conflicting data regarding the infection rate among the various types of pancreas transplants. There are data demonstrating increased rates of infections for simultaneous kidney–pancreas transplants compared to pancreas after kidney and solitary pancreas transplants. There are data demonstrating no difference in infection rates between the three types of pancreas transplant (Bassetti et al., 2004; Rostambeigi et al., 2010). The sources of infection are multiple, originating from the urinary tract, abdomen, surgical site, indwelling venous catheters, bloodstream, and lung. The rates of infection originating from the myriad sources can vary based on the type of transplant. The infecting organisms vary based on their source. Urinary tract infections (UTIs) are the most common type of infection occurring following renal transplantation, pancreas transplantation alone, and simultaneous kidney–pancreas transplantation. Rates can range from 35% to 79% following kidney transplant, and approximately 14% to 89% following simultaneous kidney–pancreas transplant. The data are conflicting regarding the difference in UTIs following bladder or enteric drainage. Gram-negative organisms are most common, particularly *E. coli*, followed by *Candida* species and Gram-positive organisms such as *Enterococcus* (Bassetti et al., 2004; Saemann and Hori, 2008; Hlava et al., 2009; Kawecki et al., 2009; Rostambeigi et al., 2010; Yacoub and Akl, 2011; Ziaja et al., 2011).

Intra-abdominal infections are more common following pancreas transplantation and kidney–pancreas transplantation than after kidney transplantation alone (Moreno et al., 2007). They are the most common cause of graft loss and death in pancreas transplant recipients. Rates range from 8% to approximately 20%. They are associated with increased amounts of red cell transfusions, early perioperative re-exploration (laparotomy), and postoperative dialysis therapy. The most common organisms are enteric Gram-negative bacteria and *Candida* species. Multi-organism infections can be common (Rivera-Sanchez et al., 2010; Rostambeigi et al., 2010). Treatment requires appropriate antimicrobial therapy coupled with source control. There are multiple ways to achieve source control. Abscesses may be amenable to radiological drainage or may require surgery. Anastomotic problems can require surgical repair. Close consultation with the transplant surgeons is exceptionally important. The rates of documented bloodstream infection are high, approaching 5–25% for pancreas and kidney–pancreas transplant patients and approximately 4–7% in kidney transplant. Most bloodstream infections are related to infections at other sites, especially UTIs, as well as central venous catheters. The most frequent organisms are *E. coli*, *Pseudomonas aeruginosa*, coagulase-negative *Staphylococcus* species, and *Klebsiella pneumonia*. Coagulase-negative *Staphylococcus* is particularly associated with catheter-related bloodstream infections (Moreno et al., 2007; Linares et al., 2009). Multidrug-resistant organisms have been frequently isolated. One study demonstrated that 39% of the organisms isolated from bacteraemic pancreas transplant recipients were multidrug resistant (Singh et al., 2008).

Patients should receive appropriate antimicrobial coverage within 1 hour of presentation. Although obtaining cultures is important, it should not delay the initiation of antimicrobial therapy (Dellinger et al., 2008). Delayed administration of appropriate antimicrobial treatment has been shown to increase mortality in multiple studies (Ibrahim et al., 2000; Garnacho-Montero et al., 2003; Kumar et al., 2006; Paul et al., 2010). Delayed or inadequate antimicrobial coverage increases mortality in transplants as it does in the general population (Hamandi et al., 2009; Lupei et al., 2010). Broad-spectrum empiric coverage should be started and narrowed following the return of cultures. As stated previously, the rate of fungal infections can be high (Pappas et al., 2010). Given the high rate of fungal infections, especially among pancreas transplant recipients, empiric antifungal therapy may be warranted. Infectious disease consultation can be useful.

Transplant recipients require potent immunosuppressive therapy to prevent rejection, but these medications decrease the ability of patients to fight infection. Doses may need to be adjusted, especially of purine analogues which can cause leucopaenia. CNI doses may need to be adjusted, especially in patients with sepsis-induced acute kidney injury. The appropriate administration of immunosuppressive medication requires close coordination between the transplant and critical care teams. The role of steroids in the treatment of severe sepsis and septic shock remains controversial. The work of Annane et al. (2002) demonstrated significantly improved survival in patients with septic shock, with documented evidence of adrenal deficiency if they were treated with both low-dose hydrocortisone and fludrocortisone. This was a small study, and a large-scale attempt to replicate this result but using hydrocortisone alone as opposed to hydrocortisone and fludrocortisones proved to have no benefit on mortality, though patients were weaned from vasopressors more quickly (Sprung et al., 2008). This was underpowered, with patients less sick than the patients in the Annane studies. How to apply these results to the transplant population is difficult, especially if the patients were taking steroids as part of their immunosuppressive regimen. It is reasonable to begin empiric stress dose steroids in septic patients who chronically take steroids for immunosuppression.

The cause of organ dysfunction in sepsis is complex, multifactorial, and incompletely understood. Decreased organ perfusion and global tissue hypoxia are considered a key process in the development of organ failure (Balk, 2000). Prior to the development of haemodynamic instability, signs of impaired organ perfusion are seen. Lactate levels can be elevated and central and mixed venous oxygen saturation can be decreased. Many argue that these are signs of global tissue hypoxia and cryptic shock (Otero et al., 2006). Lactate levels > 4 mg/dL are particularly concerning and are a marker for increased mortality (Shapiro et al., 2005).

Although surrogate measures of oxygen delivery can be markedly abnormal, it is not clear that this is due to decreased oxygen delivery. The animal data are contradictory, with some studies demonstrating decreased organ blood flow and others demonstrating increased flow. Many animal models have used boluses of endotoxin or $TNF_\alpha$ to mimic septic shock, but these are extremely potent myocardial depressants. Using a model that creates a hypodynamic state will invariably lead to decreased blood flow and oxygen delivery.

Though myocardial depression is frequently seen in septic shock, the circulatory system is generally hyperdynamic and accompanied by significant systemic vasodilation (Holmes et al., 2001). Rinaldo Bellomo developed a model that better mimics the more clinically encountered condition. His model entailed surgically implanting Doppler flow probes in various vital organ beds of sheep, and then making them septic by infusing *E. coli*. The sheep developed clear signs of sepsis but were hyperdynamic and severely vasodilated. Measures of organ blood flow mirrored cardiac output, but organ function worsened (Giantomasso et al., 2006). Hyperlacticaemia and renal dysfunction developed despite significant increases in the blood flow to the vascular beds of these organs (Giantomasso et al., 2006). Although it is not clear that organ failure is caused by decreased oxygen delivery, the early goal-directed therapy (EGDT) resuscitation protocol, described in the landmark randomized controlled study conducted by Rivers et al. (41), significantly decreased mortality. The study randomized patients during the first 6 hours of presentation. Patients in the EGDT group were treated with crystalloid fluid resuscitation until a goal CVP of 8–12 mmHg was achieved. Norepinephrine was started if the patient remained hypotensive, titrated to an MAP of 65 mm Hg. Central venous oxygen saturation was measured, and if less than 70% red cells were transfused to achieve a haematocrit of 30%. If that failed to increase venous oxygenation then dobutamine was started. Patients in the EGDT group had an improved 28-day and 60-day mortality (Rivers et al., 2001).

The role of insulin therapy and glucose control was revolutionized by the work of Van den Berghe and ushered in a radical change in glucose management (Van den Berghe et al., 2001, 2006). Aiming for normoglycaemia became the standard of care. There were significant problems with the studies, including the large amounts of glucose given to the surgical patients, the fact that there was no overall mortality difference in medical ICU patients with or without tight glucose control, and the inability to replicate the results in other studies, along with unacceptably high rates of hypoglycaemia (Bellomo and Egi, 2005; Arabi et al., 2008; Brunkhorst et al., 2008). In medical ICU patients who stayed in the ICU longer than 3 days there was an improvement in mortality, though no one was able to predict who would stay in the ICU for more than 3 days prior to starting treatment. More importantly, a survival benefit was found with subgroup analysis, which is hypothesis generating at best. The results of the NICE-SUGAR trial (NICE-SUGAR Study Investigators, 2009), the largest intensive care study ever conducted, contradicted the Van den Berghe studies (2001, 2006).

Patients were randomized to a group receiving intensive insulin therapy titrated to achieve normoglycaemia verses a group where blood glucose was targeted to be below 180 mg/dL. Mortality was increased in the patients receiving tight glucose control (NICE-SUGAR Study Investigators, 2009).

Although targeting normoglycaemia with intensive insulin therapy is inappropriate as a general rule, pancreas transplant recipients benefit from insulin therapy and glucose control in the acute perioperative period. Insulin administration and the prevention of hyperglycaemia decrease the stress placed on the new graft.

## Respiratory failure

Respiratory failure can occur following solid organ transplantation, and aetiology ranges from infection to acute lung injury (ALI) and acute respiratory distress syndrome (ARDS) to heart failure to renal failure with subsequent volume overload. A thorough work-up is necessary, including imaging, examination of the patient's volume status, and especially a full microbiological examination. Sputum sampling is essential, especially for viruses and fungi. Sometimes this requires bronchoscopy. If a patient's condition is severe, bronchoscopy may not be possible unless the patient is intubated for the procedure. This creates a dilemma, as clinicians attempt to avoid intubation but desire appropriate sampling at the same time.

Starting broad-spectrum empiric coverage for bacteria, viruses, and fungi is an option, but having a definitive diagnosis is useful. In the opinion of the authors, intubating the patient to perform an important diagnostic procedure may be the better option, though there are no clear data to precisely guide the clinical decision-making process. If a patient continues to decline and requires intubation, a bronchoscopy may be performed at that time, though the sample may not show anything as the patient has already received treatment.

Very frequently patients in respiratory failure require support. Patients who are critically ill are frequently hypoxaemic, hypermetabolic, and catabolic. The surgical stress response can increase basal metabolic rate by approximately 10%. Fever can increase it by approximately 5–7% for every 0.5°C increase. Finally, SIRS progressing to sepsis can increase basal metabolic rate by an additional 10–20% (Kinney et al., 1970; Moriyama et al., 1991). These patients need to increase minute ventilation to meet metabolic demands. An examination of the alveolar air equation demonstrates this necessity clearly. The equation states:

$$PAO_2 = FiO_2\left(PB - PH_2O\right) - PaCO_2 / RQ$$

where RQ = $CO_2$ produced/$O_2$ consumed.

Mathematically, $PaCO_2$/RQ = $O_2$ consumption/alveolar ventilation. As $O_2$ consumption increases, effective alveolar ventilation must increase or metabolic demands will not be met (Reade and Storey, 2009). Consequently, $PaCO_2$ will increase. The increase in $PaCO_2$ can cause a significant respiratory acidosis unless metabolic compensation ensues. Unfortunately, a concurrent metabolic acidosis is frequently found in critically ill patients, and these patients can have a very high mortality (Jung et al., 2011). A combined acidosis can develop quickly and be very severe as there is no compensatory mechanism available. The end result is acute hypoxaemia, combined with a respiratory and metabolic acidosis. These patients need prompt intervention. These critically ill patients have a greatly increased work of breathing. Work of breathing can be calculated using a pressure–time product. The pressure–time product is the average difference between intrathoracic inspiratory pressures and intrathoracic end expiratory pressures multiplied by the amount of time during which these pressure differences occur. In respiratory failure, work of breathing can be increased by as much as a factor of six and can account for more than 20% of basal energy expenditure (Franco and Tobin, 2006). Unless the process of decline can be interrupted, patients will not be able to breathe well enough on their own and will need mechanical support. If not recognized early, these declining patients will suffer from a respiratory arrest and possible subsequent cardiac arrest. Data describing in-hospital cardiac arrests illustrate this phenomenon. The vast majority of patients admitted to the hospital with a non-cardiac diagnosis who suffered a cardiac arrest first had a declining physiological status that was not recognized, and then had a respiratory arrest leading to the cardiac arrest. The majority of arrests were asystolic or pulseless electrical activity, not ventricular tachycardia or ventricular fibrillation (Peberdy et al., 2003).

Respiratory support can be either non-invasive or invasive. The use of non-invasive positive pressure ventilation has advantages in the setting of chronic obstructive pulmonary disease (COPD) exacerbations (Ram et al., 2004; Quon et al., 2008). The data regarding the use of non-invasive positive pressure ventilation in the setting of respiratory failure in a solid organ transplant recipient are less clear, but there are two small studies demonstrating decreased intubation rates and lower mortality (Antonelli et al., 2000; Hilbert et al., 2001). These data are promising, but the sample sizes were small, 52 and 40 patients, respectively, and one study (Esteban et al., 2002) contained a very mixed population of immunosuppressed patients, the majority of whom were bone marrow transplant recipients. Further studies are needed to demonstrate if a trial of non-invasive positive pressure ventilation should be the standard of care in solid organ transplant recipients suffering from acute respiratory failure.

Prior to deciding whether or not to initiate non-invasive ventilation (NIV) certain questions should be answered. First, can the patient protect his or her airway? If the answer is no, then the patient should be intubated. Second, is the process causing the respiratory failure one that will reverse quickly? If the answer is no, then non-invasive positive pressure ventilation may not be the right choice. Third, if non-invasive positive pressure ventilation is started, then what determines treatment failure? When should a patient be intubated following the initiation of non-invasive positive pressure ventilation? This question should be answered prior to the start of non-invasive positive pressure ventilation. As a patient's condition worsens, the danger of intubation increases. It is much safer to intubate a patient receiving bilevel positive airway pressure (BiPAP) support of 12/5 and 50% $FiO_2$ than the same patient receiving BiPAP of 20/12 and 100% $FiO_2$. One retrospective observational study did show that patients intubated after receiving non-invasive positive pressure ventilation had a higher mortality than those intubated without having received non- invasive positive pressure ventilation (Esteban et al., 2002).

Mechanical ventilation may be necessary. In the setting of ALI or ARDS a lung-protective strategy should be used. The ARDSNET demonstrated clearly that patients ventilated with a tidal volume of 6 cc/kg of ideal body weight had a significantly reduced mortality compared to similar patients randomized to receive a tidal volume of 10–12 cc/kg of ideal body weight (Acute Respiratory Distress Syndrome Network, 2000). Low tidal volume ventilation can lead to hypercapnia, a concept known as permissive hypercapnia. Hypercapnia does not necessarily need to be treated, unless the subsequent acidaemia is severe. If the academia is severe, then buffering agents can be utilized to treat the academia, though the use of buffering agents is controversial (Kallet et al., 2003; Dellinger et al., 2008). Administration of sodium bicarbonate can cause hypernatraemia and volume overload. Additionally, it may worsen intracellular acid-base balance, as $CO_2$ will be produced as bicarbonate is given. $CO_2$ easily crosses cell membranes. Once inside the cell it can combine with $H_2O$, forming carbonic acid, thereby decreasing intracellular pH. This theoretical problem is compounded in difficult-to-ventilate patients. These patients already have difficulty in eliminating $CO_2$. Adding bicarbonate can improve the arterial pH, but the $CO_2$ will increase, and these increases are difficult to treat by increasing the patient's minute ventilation, as this may not be tolerated or possible (Thomas and Schmidt, 2009). Increasing minute ventilation would entail increasing either tidal volume or respiratory rate. Both strategies can cause intolerable increases in tidal volume or airway pressures, worsening ventilator-induced lung injury (Kallet et al., 2000, 2003).

Tromethamine (THAM) is another possible buffer that has certain advantages. Unlike sodium bicarbonate, THAM use will not increase sodium. Additionally, THAM may actually decrease $CO_2$, as THAM directly binds $H^+$, eventually causing a subsequent decrease in $CO_2$ as the following reaction moves to the right as THAM binds $H^+$ and decreases its concentration, thus:

$$H_2O + CO_2 \leftrightarrow H_2CO3 \leftrightarrow H^+HCO_3^- \ [60,\ 63]$$

(according to Kallet et al., 2003; Hoste et al., 2005).

Considerable debate exists regarding the appropriate use of PEEP during mechanical ventilation for ALI/ARDS. PEEP has two purposes. The first is to improve oxygenation. The second is to theoretically decrease ventilator-induced lung injury, known as the open lung concept. PEEP protects the lung by decreasing the cyclic opening and closing of small airways and alveoli, which can cause what is known as 'atelectrauma'. As stated by Lachman (1992), 'Open up the lung and keep the lung open.' There have been multiple studies examining the use of PEEP in ALI/ARDS and no clear benefit in outcome was demonstrated in the high PEEP groups, defined as a PEEP > 15 cm $H_2O$, as opposed to < 10 cm $H_2O$ in the low PEEP groups (National Heart, Lung, and Blood Institute ARDS Clinical Trials Network, 2004; Meade et al., 2008; Mercat et al., 2008). Unfortunately, these studies included patients with both ALI and ARDS, even though ALI is a much milder phenomenon than ARDS. Three meta-analyses have examined the use of PEEP in ALI/ARDS and the conclusions are similar. Though there is no overall outcome benefit seen using high PEEP in ALI/ARDS, there appears to be an outcome benefit if ARDS is solely examined (Phoenix et al., 2009; Putensen et al., 2009; Briel et al., 2010).

Careful fluid management is critical in managing ALI/ARDS. Although ALI/ARDS are the archetypal examples of non-cardiogenic pulmonary oedema, volume overload can increase pulmonary oedema significantly, even if the pulmonary capillary wedge pressure is not high enough to meet criteria for a cardiogenic cause of pulmonary oedema. As pulmonary capillary permeability increases, oedema formation increases dramatically as the pulmonary hydrostatic pressure increases (see Figure 16.4). As a patient reaches the flat portion of his/her Starling curve, oedema formation can be pronounced (Brown et al., 2009). At least one randomized clinical trial has shown improvement in oxygenation, decreased days of mechanical ventilation, and shorter ICU length of stay if a protocolized conservative fluid replacement strategy is used compared to a liberal fluid replacement strategy. Importantly, the vast majority of included patients were haemodynamically stable and there was no overall difference in mortality (National Heart, Lung, and Blood Institute ARDS Clinical Trials Network, 2006).

When the patient begins to improve, achieves haemodynamic stability, and his/her reasons for mechanical ventilation start to resolve, liberation from mechanical ventilation should be attempted. Liberation is the key point, as this term has very different connotation from ventilator weaning. Weaning implies a deliberate staged decrease in the amount of respiratory support given to the patient. Liberation implies an abrupt decrease in ventilator support and assessing the patient's respiratory function in a way that models how the patient will perform after the cessation of mechanical support.

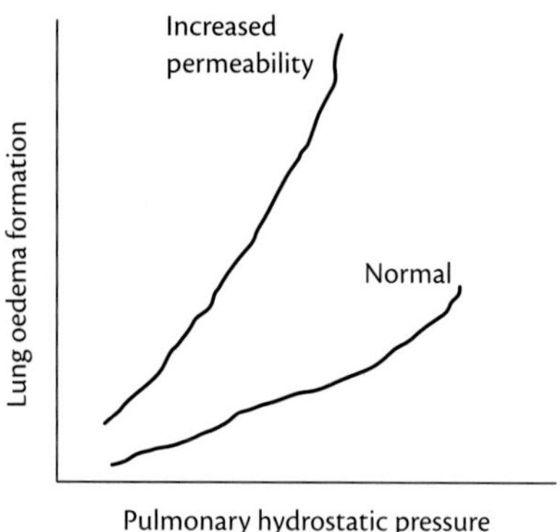


**Fig. 16.4** Relationship between lung oedema formation and pulmonary capillary permeability. Lung oedema formation is increased with increased pulmonary capillary permeability. The same pulmonary capillary hydrostatic pressure will cause significantly more oedema if permeability is increased

Esteban's (Esteban et al., 1995) classic paper conclusively proved the superiority of liberation as opposed to weaning. His group compared four different 'weaning' strategies. One group was weaned by gradually decreasing the number of mandatory breaths given by synchronized intermittent mandatory ventilation (SIMV). When they received minimal support they were then extubated. The second group was weaned by placing the patients on a relatively high level of pressure support ventilation. The level of pressure support was gradually decreased, and the patients were extubated when they received minimal support. Patients in the third and fourth groups took part in a daily spontaneously breathing trial. They were placed on a t-piece either once a day or multiple times during the day. Thus they received no ventilator support during the spontaneous breathing trials. They were extubated if they met predefined criteria for extubation. The third and fourth groups spent significantly less time receiving mechanical ventilation, on average 3 days less than the SIMV group. There were no significant differences between the once-daily and the multiple-times-a-day spontaneous breathing trial groups (Esteban et al., 1995).

Using spontaneous breathing trials decreases the average length of time spent receiving mechanical ventilation, but there are patients who continue to have difficulty meeting criteria for extubation. Up to 20% of patients can require 7 days or more of mechanical ventilation after failing their first spontaneous breathing trial (Epstein, 2008). One can consider extubating these patients directly to non-invasive positive pressure ventilation, using non-invasive positive pressure ventilation as a bridge between full ventilatory support and breathing without support. Theoretical advantages of this approach include decreased time receiving mechanical ventilation, lower rates of ventilator-associated pneumonia, decreased need for sedation, improved mobility, and improved haemodynamics. Data do exist supporting this approach but come almost exclusively from patients with chronic respiratory disorders, especially COPD (Agarwal et al., 2007; Burns et al., 2010).

How to apply these data to the solid organ transplant recipient suffering from hypoxaemic respiratory failure is not clear. Data supporting the use of non-invasive positive pressure ventilation as a bridge have led some to argue that it can be used as rescue therapy for patients who have failed a trial of extubation. As one group argued, '(T)he recognized risk of reintubation and the particular characteristics of post-transplantation respiratory impairment make noninvasive ventilation (NIV) worth trying before reintubation' (Feltracco et al., 2008).

Unfortunately there is no evidence that using NIV for the treatment of postextubation respiratory failure reduces rates of reintubation. On the contrary, the only published study adequately powered to examine mortality does not favour its use. The study was an international, multicentre, randomized controlled trial involving 221 patients in 37 centres, and compared the use of NIV as a rescue compared to standard treatment without NIV. The results clearly demonstrated that using non-invasive positive pressure ventilation to prevent reintubation in patients with postextubation respiratory failure did not decrease the rate of reintubation but did cause a dramatic increase in mortality. The rate of reintubation was 48% in both groups.

There was, on average, a delay of approximately 10 hours to reintubate patients in the NIV group. The trial was stopped prematurely because of the mortality data. The mortality in the standard care group was 14%, contrasted with 25% in the non-invasive positive pressure ventilation group (Esteban et al., 2004). Although this study did not exclude transplant recipients, and there is no information provided to show if recipients were included, it would behove any clinician to carefully consider making an intervention that has been shown to cause a dramatic increase in mortality without demonstrating any decrease in the outcome one is trying to prevent.

## Cardiac complications

Cardiovascular complications are a frequent cause of post-transplant morbidity and mortality. They account for as much as 30% of post-transplant mortality, with nearly 40% of renal transplant recipients experiencing a cardiovascular complication, often within 3 months of transplantation. Boschiero et al. (2009) noted a bimodal distribution of cardiovascular events at 1 year and at 8 years after renal transplantation. They hypothesized that later cardiovascular complications may be due to the cumulative effects of traditional and non-traditional risk factors. The most common causes are MI and CVA (Kasiske, 1988). For patients undergoing SKPT, the cardiovascular mortality rates vary between 8.9% and 14.9% (Kasiske, 1988; Kasiske et al., 1996). Recent data suggest that renal and pancreatic transplant candidates have a significantly higher prevalence of risk factors for obstructive CAD than the general population, with a higher mortality rate. Moreover, silent MI is typical of type 1 diabetes mellitus and left ventricular hypertrophy is common in SKPT candidates. Left ventricular systolic dysfunction has significant prognostic implications independent of CAD, including decreased median survival, increased wait-list mortality, increased risk of cardiac death, and increased risk of cardiac complications.

Some studies have suggested that patients with left ventricular hypertrophy with diabetes for > 25 years and patients who are older than 45 years are at increased risk of perioperative cardiac events (de Mattos et al., 2008; Diaz and O'Connor, 2011). Currently there is no consensus on pretransplant screening for CAD or determination of perioperative risk in candidates. As recipient criteria change, the importance of pretransplant cardiovascular evaluation becomes more important. Cardiac evaluation should begin with screening for CAD and typically includes structural and physiological assessment. Exercise stress testing should be performed for evaluation of ischaemic heart disease, although SKPT recipients often have comorbidities that decrease the utility of the examination. In a systematic review Wang et al. (2011) found that data were highly variable and inconclusive. Hypertension is frequently noted, with an increased prevalence of cardiomyopathy, valvular lesions, calcific vascular disease, and peripheral vascular disease (Diaz and O'Connor, 2011). Additionally, uraemia may reduce exercise capacity such that some candidates may not achieve the necessary heart rate to complete the evaluation. Thus exercise stress testing is not a reliable predictor of CAD or cardiovascular complications in abdominal solid organ transplant recipients (Sharma et al., 2005).

Most studies conducted on stress scintigraphy have been limited to orthotopic liver transplants and report a low sensitivity (37%) and specificity (63%) versus coronary angiography. The sensitivity decreased in candidates with more than three cardiac risk factors (Davidson et al., 2002). Limitations in SPECT have been thought to arise from decreased arterial vascular resistance in chronic liver disease, thus limiting coronary artery response to vasodilatory agents in patients undergoing liver transplant. However, a retrospective study by Ruparelia et al. (2011) suggests that in patients with SKPT, scintigraphy may be useful in evaluating cardiovascular risk prior to transplantation. In a study of 167 consecutive patients, they noted a high sensitivity and 1-year cardiovascular outcomes comparable to those managed with more invasive and risky testing. They suggest that scintigraphy can be used as a first-line test in evaluating cardiovascular function prior to transplant. However, there are no current level I or II studies elaborating this, and thus additional research is needed to evaluate the role of scintigraphy in patients undergoing SKPT.

Limitations on exercise stress testing and myocardial stress scintigraphy restrict diagnostic evaluation to dobutamine stress echocardiography (DSE) or coronary angiography. Eschertzhuber et al. (2005) compared patients who underwent SKPT with those who underwent only kidney transplant. The patients who underwent SKPT were more likely to suffer a perioperative cardiac event. Coronary angiography was performed in 69/84 (79.76%) of patients undergoing SKPT and revealed or confirmed significant CAD (> 50% stenosis) in 37/84 (44%) of patients; the remaining 17 patients underwent echocardiography (ECHO), exercise stress test, or scintigraphy. Ten percent of patients underwent angioplasty and 3/84 underwent coronary artery bypass grafting (CABG) before listing for SKPT. The authors reported avoiding contrast angiography in candidates with residual kidney function in order to avoid contrast load and preserve urinary output. Pretransplant routine screening for CAD in candidates for renal transplant without a history of diabetes includes echocardiography and scintigraphy or stress test, and angiography can be reserved for those at high coronary risk, whereas those patients who have ESRD and a history of diabetes should routinely undergo echocardiography and coronary angiography.

Pretransplant revascularization and invasive perioperative monitoring together with aggressive medical treatment and careful intraoperative monitoring minimize the cardiac risk in these patients and improve outcomes (Medina-Polo et al., 2010). These authors evaluated the incidence of cardiovascular events after functioning SKPT. Eighty-nine patients were retrospectively reviewed and 9/89 had cardiovascular events, including CVA in four patients. When comparing various groups of kidney recipients, it is clear that patients with significant coronary stenosis benefit most from invasive pretransplant diagnostics and treatment (Medina-Polo et al., 2010). Patients with significant stenosis and no pretransplant treatment are at great risk.

Improvement in glucose concentration may reduce the risk of cardiovascular complications in patients with diabetes. Some studies have suggested that SKPT may reduce cardiovascular mortality associated with diabetes. Successful SKPT may be protective against progression of cardiovascular disease because recipients demonstrate better survival rates compared with patients who have undergone only kidney transplantation and those continuing to receive dialysis therapy. However, immunosuppressive agents and inflammatory cytokines associated with rejection may augment the risk of cardiovascular disease. Some studies have suggested that chronic immunosuppression, despite its adverse effects, has a less harmful influence on the cardiovascular system compared with combination insulin and dialysis therapy (Szmidt et al., 2003). It is thought that renal transplantation alone may improve intravascular volume distribution (Alvares et al., 1998). Echocardiograms performed postoperatively have shown improvement to normal in most cases after renal transplantation and may be due to lower total intravascular volume and physiologically uniform fluid removal, as opposed to the cycles of increased hypervolaemia followed by rapid volume removal as in haemodialysis. Although such volume cycles are not as prominent in patients on peritoneal dialysis, there were no significant associations of dialysis modality with acute coronary syndrome in a study by Hypolite et al. (2002).

Renal transplantation will also correct many of the metabolic abnormalities associated with ESRD, some of which may worsen CAD. Calcific arterial disease increases systemic vascular resistance. This may be worsened by calcium supplementation that is administered in ESRD (Guerin et al., 2000). Although severe hyperparathyroidism does not resolve as often as previously supposed after transplantation, improvement does occur and it is unusual for patients to require supplemental calcium after kidney transplant (Dennis and Robinson, 1996; Wang et al., 2011). Homocysteine levels are an independent risk factor for cardiovascular events in ESRD; however, they do not predict patient or graft survival or graft function, as do other risk factors such as hypercholesterolaemia (Dennis and Robinson, 1996). Hypolite et al. (2002) reported that for patients who had experienced acute coronary syndrome prior to renal transplant, none had intensification of their symptoms after transplant. They further noted that patients with renal transplant had an incidence of acute coronary syndrome of 0.79% per patient year compared to 1.67% per patient year prior to transplant. In comparison to maintenance dialysis, renal transplantation was associated with a lower risk for acute coronary syndrome (hazard ratio 0.38, 95% confidence interval 0.30–0.49). Patients with ESRD due to diabetes on the renal transplant waiting list were much less likely to be hospitalized for acute coronary syndrome after renal transplant (Hypolite et al., 2002).

Graft loss represents a possible intersection between immunosuppression and renal insufficiency and is associated with an increased risk of acute coronary syndrome. Abbott et al. (2002) noted an incidence of acute coronary syndrome that was twice as high after graft loss. Other risk factors associated with this syndrome included diabetes, older recipients, and male gender. Allograft rejection, through renal insufficiency and volume overload, may raise blood pressure and alter lipid levels, both risk factors for acute coronary syndrome. Two or more rejection episodes in the first transplant year were associated with increased risk of ischaemic heart disease outcomes (Abbott et al., 2002). Staging of transplantation for patients with type 1 diabetes mellitus may reduce the risk of cardiovascular events in the perioperative period. Ideal candidates for pancreas transplant alone are those with poorly controlled glycaemic levels, hypoglycaemic episodes, good renal function with a creatinine clearance > 80 mL/min, proteinuria < 3 g/24 hours, and simultaneous presence of at least two early diabetes-related complications such as neuropathy, retinopathy, or vascular disease. Patients in whom SKPT is recommended are those whose diabetes has led to severe kidney damage resulting in chronic renal insufficiency, regardless of whether they are treated conservatively (creatinine clearance < 30 mL/min) or with dialysis. Bindi et al. (2005) showed that pancreas transplant alone recipients experienced fewer postoperative complications than those undergoing SKPT. This can be related to the more severe preoperative condition of SKPT patients, who often have a more severe renal dysfunction. In Bindi and colleague's series, SKPT recipients needed more frequent medication to control hypertension and they had a higher risk of infection, as measured by the degree of colonization. SKPT patients also showed a higher incidence of cardiac complications (15.8% vs 2.8%, $P = 0.04$) and haemodynamic instability (17% vs 5.5%, $P = 0.006$). However, graft function was not affected by the severity of diabetes (Bindi et al., 2005).

The treatment of myocardial ischaemia in the renal transplant, pancreas transplant, or kidney–pancreas transplant recipient is not terribly different from the treatment of myocardial ischaemia in the population at large, although there are some important considerations especially relating to contrast administration and arterial access during revascularization. Diagnosis may be difficult, especially in diabetic patients, as well as in the postoperative period. Most perioperative patients with a myocardial event will not experience ischaemic symptoms (Deveraux et al., 2011). Myocardial ischaemia can be conveniently divided into two basic types. Type I MI refers to acute plaque rupture within a coronary artery causing an acute interruption of flow. Type II refers to a general mismatch between myocardial oxygen delivery and myocardial oxygen demand. Supply–demand mismatch can be caused by decreased delivery due to hypotension, hypoxia, and/or anaemia; or by increased demand due to tachycardia or hypertension (Thygesen et al., 2007). Considerable debate exists as to which process is primarily involved in perioperative myocardial events (Landesberg, 2003; Deveraux et al., 2005).

The distinction is crucial because treatment differs. The treatment of type II MI consists of correcting the mismatch. The treatment of type I MI is more extensive. In addition to the standard care consisting of pain control with morphine and nitroglycerin, antiplatelet administration with aspirin, beta-blockade in haemodynamically stable patients, and systemic anticoagulation with heparin, it is imperative to attempt revascularization. Revascularization is not without complications, not limited to contrast administration to a recipient with a fresh graft, arterial dissection, thrombosis, and access limitations. Arterial canalization should not be attempted on the side upon which the graft is located. Duvall et al. (2012) conducted an elegant retrospective review in an attempt to determine the relative frequency of type I and II MI occurring in the perioperative period. They retrospectively reviewed all angiograms performed on patients following a diagnosis of perioperative MI. They then attempted to determine the cause of the myocardial event in terms of demand-related ischaemia with a fixed lesion, whether the patient was thrombotic, or demand without an obstructive lesion; 54.5% of the 66 patients reviewed suffered a demand-related event with a fixed lesion, 25.8% were thrombotic, and 19.7 were non-obstructive (Duvall et al., 2012).

### Vascular catastrophies

Vascular complications can be due to thrombosis or haemorrhage. Thrombotic complications, though devastating to graft survival, generally are not acutely life-threatening. Complications arising from the breakdown of the arterial anastomosis are acutely life-threatening. These can include arterial aneurysms, pseudoaneurysms, and the development of arterial to enteric fistulas. Life-threatening bleeding can ensue. Severe haemorrhage from fistula development can be preceded by a sentinel bleed. As appropriate treatment hinges on early recognition, clinicians must have a very high index of suspicion when a kidney, pancreas, or kidney–pancreas transplant recipient presents with a GI bleed. Treatment requires prompt recognition, large-bore intravenous access, replacement of intravascular volume, transfusions of red cells, and plasma and platelets if coagulopathy ensues. Control of the bleeding is imperative. This may require a surgical approach. Endovascular placement of a covered stent may provide immediate control (Fridell et al., 2012).

## Conclusion

For successful outcomes in patients undergoing kidney, kidney–pancreas, and pancreas transplants, it is important to recognize and treat common perioperative critical care issues in order to protect transplanted grafts and prevent early mortality. These patients are at increased risk because of their inherent pre-existing organ failure and multisystem involvement, particularly those with diabetes mellitus. The need for immunosuppression predisposes recipients to infection that requires dynamic monitoring for early diagnosis and treatment. Critical care has played a major role in improving outcomes in transplant recipients.

## References


Abbott KC, Bucci JR, Taylor AJ, et al. (2002) Graft loss and acute coronary syndromes after renal transplantation in the United States. *J Am Soc Nephrol*, **13**:2560–2569.

Acute Respiratory Distress Syndrome Network (2000) Ventilation with lower tidal volumes as compared with traditional tidal volumes for acute lung injury and the acute respiratory distress syndrome. *N Engl J Med*, **342**:1301–1308.

Agarwal R, Aggarwal AN, et al. (2007) Role of noninvasive positive-pressure ventilation in postextubation respiratory failure: a meta-analysis. *Respiratory Care*, **52**:1472–1479.

Alvares S, Mota C, Soares L, et al. (1998) Cardiac consequences of renal transplantation changes in left ventricular morphology. *Revista Portug Cardiol*, **17**:145–152.

Annane D, Sebille V, Charpentier C, et al. (2002) Effect of treatment with low doses of hydrocortisone and fludrocortisones on mortality in patients with septic shock. *JAMA*, **288**:862–871.

Antonelli, M, Conti G, Bufi M, et al. (2000) Noninvasive ventilation for treatment of acute respiratory failure in patients undergoing solid organ transplantation. A randomized trial. *JAMA*, **283**:235–241.

Arabi YM, Dabbagh OC, Tamim HM, et al. (2008) Intensive versus conventional insulin therapy: A randomized controlled trial in medical and surgical critically ill patients. *Crit Care Med*, **36**:3190–3197.

Balk RA (2000) Pathogenesis and management of multiorgan dysfunction and failure in severe sepsis and septic shock. *Crit Care Clinic*, **16**:337–352.

Bassetti M, Salvalaggio PRO, Topal J, et al. (2004) Incidence, timing and site of infections among pancreas transplant recipients. *J Hospital Inf*, **56**:184–190.

Bellomo R, Egi M. (2005) Glycemic control in the intensive care unit: why we should wait for NICE-SUGAR. *Mayo Clinic Proc*, **80**:1546–1548.

Bindi ML, Biancofiore G, Meacci L, et al. (2005) Early morbidity after pancreas transplantation. *Transplant Int*,**18**:1356–1360.

Boschiero L, Fior F, Nacchia F (2009) Bimodal distribution of major cardiovascular events in kidney allograft recipients. *Transplant Proc*, **41**:1183–1186.

Briel M, Meade M, Mercat A, et al. (2010) Higher vs lower positive end-expiratory pressure in patient with acute lung injury and acute respiratory distress syndrome systematic review and meta-analysis. *JAMA*, **303**:865–873.

Brown LM, Liu KD, Matthay M (2009) Measurement of extravascular lung water using the single indicator method in patients: research and potential clinical value. *Am J Physiol Lung Cell Molec Physiol*, **297**:L547–L558.

Brunkhorst FM, Engel C, Bloos F, et al. (2008) Intensive insulin therapy and pentastarch resuscitation in severe sepsis. *N Engl J Med*, **358**:125–139.

Burns KEA, Adhikari NKJ, Keenan SP, Meade MO (2010) Noninvasive positive pressure ventilation as a weaning strategy for intubated adults with respiratory failure. *Cochrane Lib*, **8**:1–53.

Daniels R (2011) Surviving the first hours in sepsis: getting the basics right (an intensivist's perspective). *J Antimicrobial Chemother*, **66**:ii11–ii23

Davidson C, Gheorghiade M, Flaherty J, et al. (2002) Predictive value of stress myocardial perfusion imaging in liver transplant candidates. *Am J Cardiol*, **89**:359–360.

Dellinger RP, Carlet JM, Masur H, et al. (2004) Surviving sepsis campaign guidelines for management of sever sepsis and septic shock. *Crit Care Med*, **32**:858–873.

Dellinger PR, Levy MM, Carlet JM (2008) Surviving sepsis campaign: international guidelines for management of severe sepsis and septic shock: 2008. *Crit Care Med*, **36**:296–327.

Dellinger RP, Rhodes A, Levy MM, et al. (2013) Surviving sepsis campaign: International guidelines for management of severe sepsis and septic shock: 2012. *Crit Care Med*, **41**:580–637

de Mattos A, Siedlecki A, Gaston R, et al. (2008) Systolic dysfunction portends increased mortality among those waiting for renal transplant. *J Am Soc Nephrol*, **19**:1191–1196.

Dennis VW, Robinson K (1996) Homocysteinemia and vascular disease in end-stage renal disease. *Kidney Int*, **57**:S11–S17.

Deveraux PJ, Goldman L, Cook DJ, et al. (2005) Perioperative cardiac events in patients undergoing noncardiac surgery: a review of the magnitude of the problem, the pathophysiology of the events and methods to estimate and communicate risk. *Can Med Assoc J*, **173**:627–634.

Deveraux PJ, Xavier D, Guyatt, et al. (2011) Characteristics and short-term prognosis of perioperative myocardial infarction in patients undergoing noncardiac surgery: a cohort study. *Annal Internal Med*, **154**:523–8.

Diaz G, O'Connor M (2011) Cardiovascular and renal complications in patients receiving a solid organ transplant. *Curr Opin Crit Care*, **17**:382–389.

Duvall WA, Sealove B, Pungoti C, et al (2012) Angiographic investigation of the pathophysiology of perioperative myocardial infarction. *Cathet Cardiovasc Intervention*, **80**:768–776.

Epstein SK (2008) Size of the problem, what constitutes prolonged mechanical ventilation, natural history, epidemiology. In: Ambrosino N, Goldstein RS (eds) *Ventilatory Support in Chronic Respiratory Failure*, pp. 39–57. Informa Healthcare, New York.

Eschertzhuber S, Hohlrieder M, Boesmueller C, et al. (2005) Incidence of coronary heart disease and cardiac events in patients undergoing kidney and pancreas transplantation. *Transplant Proc*, **37**:1297–1300.

Esteban A, Frutos F, Tobin MJ, et al. (1995) A comparison of four methods of weaning patients from mechanical ventilation. *N Engl J Med*, **332**:345–350.

Esteban A, Anzueto A, Frutos F, et al. (2002) Characteristics and outcomes in adult patients receiving mechanical ventilation a 28-day international study. *JAMA*, **287**:345–355.

Esteban A, Frutos-Vivar F, Ferguson ND, et al. (2004) Noninvasive positive-pressure ventilation for respiratory failure after extubation. *N Engl J Med*, **350**:2452–2460.

Feltracco P, Serra E, Barbieri S, et al. (2008) Noninvasive ventilation in adult liver transplantation. *Transplantation Proceedings*, **8**:1979–1982.

Fishman JA (2007) Infection in solid-organ transplant recipients. *N Engl J Med*, **357**:2601–2614.

Fontana I, Bertocchi M, Diviacco P, et al. (2009) Infections after simultaneous pancreas and kidney transplantation: a single-center experience. *Transplant Proc*, **41**:1333–1335.

Franco L, Tobin M (2006) Indications for mechanical ventilation. In: Tobin M (ed) *Principles and Practice of Mechanical Ventilation*, 2nd edn, pp. 129–162. McGraw-Hill, New York.

Fridell JA, Johnson MS, Goggins WC, et al. (2012) Vascular catastrophes following pancreas transplantation: an evolution in strategy at a single center. *Clin Transplant*, **26**:164–172.

Garnacho-Montero J, Garcia-Garmendia JL, Barrero-Almodovar A, et al. (2003) Impact of adequate empirical antibiotic therapy on the outcome of patients admitted to the intensive care unit with sepsis. *Crit Care Med*, **31**:2742–2751.

Giantomasso DD, May CN, Bellomo R. (2006) Vital organ blood flow during hyperdynamic sepsis. *Chest*, **124**:1053–1059.

Guerin AP, London GM, Marchais SJ, et al. (2000) Arterial stiffening and vascular calcifications in end-stage renal disease. *Nephrol Dial Transplant*, **15**:1014–1021.

Hamandi B, Holbrook AM, Humar A, et al. (2009) Delay of adequate empiric antibiotic therapy is associated with increased mortality among solid-organ patients. *Am J Transplant*, **9**:1657–1665.

Hilbert G, Gruson D, Vargas F, et al. (2001) Noninvasive ventilation in immunosuppressed patients with pulmonary infiltrates, fever and acute respiratory failure. *N Eng J Med*, **344**:481–487.

Hlava N, Niemann CU, Gropper MA, Melcher ML (2009) Postoperative infectious complications of abdominal solid organ transplantation. *J Intensive Care Med*, **24**:3–17.

Holmes CL, Walley KR, Chitock DR, et al. (2001) The effect of vasopressin on hemodynamics and renal function in severe septic shock: a case series. *Inten Care Med*, **27**:1416–1421.

Hoste EA, Colpaert K, Vanholder RC, et al. (2005) Sodium bicarbonate versus THAM in ICU patients with mild metabolic acidosis. *J Nephrol*, **18**:303–307.

Hypolite IO, Bucci J, Hsheieh P, et al. (2002) Acute coronary syndromes after Renal transplantation in patients with end-stage renal disease resulting from diabetes. *Am J Transplant*, **2**:274–281.

Ibrahim EH, Sherman G, Ward S, et al. (2000) The influence of inadequate antimicrobial treatment of bloodstream infections on patient outcomes in the ICU setting. *Chest*, **118**:146–155.

Jung B, Rimmele T, Le Goff C, et al. (2011) Severe metabolic or mixed acidemia on intensive care unit admission: incidence, prognosis and administration of buffer therapy. A prospective, multiple-center study. *Crit Care*, **15**:1–9.

Kalil AC, Dakroub J, Freifeld AG (2007) Sepsis and solid organ transplantation. *Curr Drug Target*, **8**:533–541.

Kallet RH, Jasmer RM, Luce JM, et al. (2000) The treatment of acidosis in acute lung injury with trishydroxymethyl aminomethane (THAM). *Am J Resp Crit Care Med*, **161**:1149–1153.

Kallet RH, Liu K, Tang J (2003) Management of acidosis during lung-protective ventilation in acute respiratory distress syndrome. *Resp Care Clin N Am*, **9**:437–456.

Kasiske BL (1988) Risk factors for accelerated atherosclerosis in renal transplant patients. *Am J Med*, **84**:985.

Kasiske BL, Guijarro C, Massy ZA, et al. (1996) Cardiovascular disease after renal transplantation. *J Am Soc Nephrol*, 7:158.

Kawecki D, Kwiatkowski A, Michalak G (2009) Etiologic agents of bacteremia in the early period after simultaneous pancreas-kidney transplantation. *Transplant Proc*, **41**:3151–3153.

Kinney JM, Duke JF, JR, Long CL, Gump FE (1970) Tissue fuel and weight loss after injury *J Clin Pathol*, **4**:65–72.

Kumar A, Roberts D, Wood KE, et al. (2006) Duration of hypotension before initiation of effective antimicrobial therapy is the critical determinant of survival in human septic shock. *Crit Care Med*, **34**:1589–1596.

Lachmann B (1992) Open up the lungs and keep the lung open. *Intensive Care Med*, **18**:319–321.

Landesberg G (2003) The pathophysiology of perioperative myocardial infarction: Facts and perspectives. *J Cardio-Thorac Vasc Anesth*, **17**:90–100.

Levy MM, Fink MP, Marshall JC, et al. (2003) 2001 SCCM/ESICM/ACCP/ATS/SIS International sepsis definitions conference. *Crit Care Med*, **31**:1250–1356.

Levy MM, Dellinger RP, Townsend SR, et al. (2010) The surviving sepsis campaign: results of an international guideline-based performance improvement program targeting severe sepsis. *Crit Care Med*, **38**:367–374.

Linares L, Garcia-Goez JF, Almela M et al. (2009) Early bacteremia after solid organ transplantation. *Transplant Proc*, **41**:2262–2264.

Lupei MI, Mann HJ, Beilman GJ, et al. (2010) Inadequate antibiotic therapy in solid organ transplant recipients is associated with a higher mortality rate. *Surg Infection*, **11**:33–39.

Martin GS, Mannino DM, Eaton S, Moss M (2003) The epidemiology of sepsis in the United States from 1979 through 2000. *N Engl J Med*, **348**:1546–1554.

Meade MO, Cook DJ, Guyatt GH, et al. (2008) Ventilation strategy using low tidal volumes, recruitment maneuvers, and high positive end-expiratory pressure for acute lung injury and acute respiratory distress syndrome. A randomized controlled trial. *JAMA*, **299**:637–645.

Medina-Polo J. Dominguez-Esteban M, Morales JM, et al. (2010) Cardiovascular events after simultaneous pancreas-kidney transplantation. *Transplant Proc*, **42**:2981–2983.

Mercat A, Richard JCM, Vielle B (2008) Positive end-expiratory pressure setting in adults with acute lung injury and acute respiratory distress syndrome a randomized controlled trial. *JAMA*, **299**:646–655.

Moreno A, Cervera C, Gavalda J (2007) Bloodstream infections among transplant recipients: results of a nationwide surveillance in Spain. *Am J Transplant*, 7:2579–2586.

Moriyama S, Okamoto K, Tabira Y, et al. (1991) Evaluation of oxygen consumption and resting energy expenditure in critically ill patients with systemic inflammatory response syndrome. *Crit Care Med*, **27**:2133–2136.

National Heart, Lung, and Blood Institute ARDS Clinical Trials Network (2004) Higher versus lower positive end-expiratory pressures in patients with the acute respiratory distress syndrome. *N Engl J Med*, **351**:327–336.

National Heart, Lung, and Blood Institute ARDS Clinical Trials Network (2006) Comparison of two fluid-management strategies in acute lung injury. *N Engl J Med*, **345**:2564–2575.

NICE-SUGAR Study Investigators (2009) Intensive care conventional glucose control in critically ill patients. *N Engl J Med*, **360**:1283–1297.

Otero RM, Nguyen B, Huang DT, et al. (2006) Early goal-directed therapy in severe sepsis and septic shock revisited. *Chest*, **130**:1579–1595.

Pappas PG, Alexander BD, Andes DR, et al. (2010) Invasive fungal infection among organ transplant recipients: results of the transplant-associated infection surveillance network (TRANSNET). *Clin Infectious Dis*, **50**:1101–1111.

Paul M, Shani V, Muchtar E, Kariv G, et al. (2010) Systematic review and meta-analysis of the efficacy of appropriate empiric antibiotic therapy for sepsis. *Antimicrob Agents Chemother*, **54**:4851–4863.

Peberdy MA, Kaye W, Ornato JP, et al. (2003) Cardiopulmonary resuscitation of adults in the hospital: a report of 14720 cardiac arrests from the national registry of cardiopulmonary resuscitation. *Resuscitation*, **58**:297–308.

Phoenix SI, Paravastu S, Columb M, et al. (2009) Does a higher positive end expiratory pressure decrease mortality in acute respiratory distress syndrome? A systematic review and meta-analysis. *Anesthesiology*, **110**:1098–1106.

Putensen C, Theuerkauf, Zinserling J, et al. (2009) Meta-analysis: ventilation strategies and outcomes of the acute respiratory distress syndrome and acute lung injury. *Annal Internal Med*, **151**:566–576.

Quon BS, Gan WQ, Sin DD (2008) Contemporary management of acute exacerbations of COPD: a systematic review and metaanalysis. *Chest*, **133**:756–766.

Ram FS, Picot J, Lightowler J, Wedzicha JA (2004) Non-invasive positive pressure ventilation for treatment of respiratory failure due to exacerbations of chronic obstructive pulmonary disease. *Cochrane Database Syst Rev*, **1**:CD004104.

Reade MC, Storey DA (2009) Respiratory acid-base physiology. In: Bellomo R, Kellum JA, Ronco C (eds) *Crit Care Nephrology*, pp. 592–596. Elsevier, Philadelphia.

Rivera-Sanchez R, Delgado-Ochoa D, Flores-Paz RR, et al. (2010) Prospective study of urinary tract infection surveillance after kidney transplantation. *BMC Infectious Dis*, **10**:1–6.

Rivers E, Nguyen B, Havstad S, et al. (2001) Early goal-directed therapy in the treatment of severe sepsis and septic shock. *N Engl J Med*, **345**:1368–1377.

Rostambeigi N, Kudva YC, John S, et al. (2010) Epidemiology of infections requiring hospitalization during long-term follow-up of pancreas transplantation. *Transplantation*, **89**:1126–1133.

Ruparelia N, Bhindi R, Sabharwal N, et al. (2011) Myocardial perfusion is a useful screening test for the evaluation of cardiovascular risk in patients undergoing simultaneous pancreas kidney transplantation. *Transplant Proc*, **43**:1797–1800

Russell J (2006) Management of sepsis. *N Engl J Med*, **355**:1699–1713.

Saemann M, Hori WH (2008) Urinary tract infection in renal transplant recipients. *Eur J Clin Investigation*, **38**:58–65.

Schuetz P, Chiappa V, Briel M, Greenwald JL (2011) Procalcitonin algorithms for antibiotic therapy decisions. A systematic review of randomized controlled trials and recommendations for clinical algorithms. *Arch Internal Med*, **171**:1322–1330.

Shapiro NI, Howell MD, Talmor D, et al. (2005) Serum lactate as a predictor of mortality in emergency department patients with infections. *Annal Emerg Med*,**1**:75–80.

Sharma R, Pellerin D, Gaze D, et al. (2005) Dobutamine stress echocardiography and the resting by not exercise electrocardiograph predict severe coronary artery disease in renal transplant candidates. *Nephrol Dial Transplant*, **20**:2207–2214.

Shubin NJ, Monaghan SF, Ayala A (2011) Anti-inflammatory mechanisms of sepsis. *Contrib Microbiol*, **17**:108–124.

Singer M (2008) Cellular dysfunction in sepsis. *Clin Chest Med*, **29**:655–660.

Singh RP, Farney AC, Rogers J, et al. (2008) Analysis of bacteremia after pancreatic transplantation with enteric drainage. *Transplant Proc*, **40**:506–509.

Sprung CL, Annane D, Keh D, et al. (2008) Hydrocortisone therapy for patients with septic shock. *N Engl J Med*, **358**:111–124.

Szmidt J, Grochowiecki T, Galazka Z, et al. (2003) Influence of pancreas and kidney transplant function on recipient survival. *Transplant Proc*, **25**:2019.

Thomas KW, Schmidt GA (2009) Alkalinizing therapy in the management of acid-base disorders. In: Bellomo R, Kellum JA, Ronco C (eds) *Critical Care Nephrology*, pp. 685–688. Elsevier, Philadelphia.

Thygesen K, Alpert JS, White HD, et al. (2007) Universal definition of myocardial infarction. *Circulation*, **116**:2634–2653.

Van den Berghe G, Wouters P, Weekers F, el al. (2001) Intensive insulin therapy in critically ill patients. *N Engl J Med*, **345**:1359–1367.

Van den Berghe G, Wilmer A, Hermans G, et al. (2006) Intensive insulin therapy in the medical ICU. *N Engl J Med*, **354**:449–461.

Wang L, Fahim M, Hayen A, et al. (2011) Cardiac testing for coronary artery disease in potential kidney transplant recipients: a systematic review of test accuracy studies. *Am J Kidney Dis*, **57**:476–487.

Yacoub R, Akl NK (2011) Urinary tract infections and asymptomatic bacteriuria in renal transplant recipients. *J Global Infectious Dis*, **3**:383–389

Ziaja J, Krol R, Chudek J, et al. (2011) Intra-abdominal infections and simultaneous pancreas-kidney transplantation. *Annal Transplant*, **16**:36–43.

# CHAPTER 17

# Diabetes mellitus: epidemiology, pathophysiology, and treatment

Piero Marchetti, Margherita Occhipinti, Gabriella Amorese, and Ugo Boggi

## The burden of diabetes mellitus

Nearly four million deaths in the 20–79 age group were attributable to diabetes in 2010, accounting for 6.8% of global all-cause mortality in this age group and corresponding to a 5.5% increase over the estimates for the year 2007. Diabetes mellitus is a group of metabolic diseases characterized by hyperglycaemia resulting from defects in insulin secretion, insulin action, or both (American Diabetes Association, 2012a). On the basis of aetiology and clinical presentation, it is classified into four types: type 1 (caused by autoimmune destruction of the insulin-producing β-cells in the pancreas, and representing 5–10% of all cases), type 2 (characterized by relative insulin deficiency and insulin resistance, very often associated with obesity, and accounting for approximately 90% of cases), gestational diabetes (with onset or first recognition during pregnancy), and a heterogeneous group identified as other specific types (that includes forms due to monogenic defects leading to β-cell failure, genetic defects in insulin action, diseases of the exocrine pancreas, endocrinopathies, drugs or chemicals, infections, uncommon forms of autoimmunity, and other genetic syndromes sometimes associated with diabetes) (American Diabetes Association, 2012a, 2012b).

The disease can be diagnosed by the use of the following criteria (American Diabetes Association, 2012b): (1) presence of classic symptoms of hyperglycaemia or hyperglycaemic crisis and a random plasma glucose value ≥ 200 mg/dL (11.1 mmol/L); (2) fasting plasma glucose (FPG) value ≥ 126 mg/dL (7.0 mmol/L), with fasting defined as no caloric intake for at least 8 hours before the test; (3) glycated haemoglobin (HbA1c) value ≥ 6.5% (provided the test is performed in a laboratory using a method that is National Glycohemoglobin Standardization Program (NGSP) certified and standardized to the Diabetes Control and Complications Trial (DCCT) assay); (4) 2-hour plasma glucose level ≥ 200 mg/dL (11.1 mmol/L) during an oral glucose tolerance test (OGTT), performed as described by the WHO using a glucose load containing the equivalent of 75 g anhydrous glucose dissolved in water (American Diabetes Association, 2012a). In the absence of clear symptoms of hyperglycaemia, criteria (2)–(4) should be confirmed by repeat testing. In addition, three categories of increased risk for diabetes have been identified: impaired fasting glycaemia (IFG) (FPG values of 100–125 mg/dL (5.6–6.9 mmol/L)); impaired glucose tolerance (IGT) (2-hour plasma glucose on the 75-g OGTT between 140 and 199 mg/dL (7.8–11.0 mmol/l)); and the situation when HbA1c value is 5.7–6.4%. For all three conditions, risk is continuous, extending below the lower limit of the range and becoming greater at higher ends of the range.

Diabetes is one of the most common chronic diseases in nearly all countries and it continues to increase in number and significance (according to the International Diabetes Federation (IDF) and WHO). The augmenting incidence of the disease appears to be mainly due to changes in lifestyle leading to decreased physical activity and obesity. In addition, the disease is associated with high morbidity and mortality, mediated by the development of vascular chronic complications. Eventually, all this leads to an enormous socio-economic burden, which is increasing as the 'epidemic' grows. There are several reports on the prevalence, numerical estimates, and projections of the disease (Wild et al., 2004; Shaw et al., 2010; Danaei et al., 2011). The WHO published data for the years 2000 and 2030 using information from 40 countries that were extrapolated to the 191 WHO member states (Wild et al., 2004). It was reported that the total number of individuals with diabetes was expected to rise from 171 million in 2000 to 366 million in 2030. Other estimates have been produced by the IDF, which have been updated recently (Shaw et al., 2010) and now include all 216 countries of the United Nations. From these data it is concluded that the prevalence of diabetes among adults aged 20–79 years in the world was 6.4% in 2010 (corresponding to 284 million people) and will be 7.7% in 2030 (corresponding to 438 million people), representing a 54% increase in 20 years.

Lifestyle interventions focused on dietary habits and physical activity are fundamental components of diabetes management. In type 1 diabetes (caused by autoimmune destruction of pancreatic β-cells) this must be associated with appropriate insulin treatment regimens. In type 2 diabetes (due to both insulin resistance and reduced β-cell functional mass) several oral agents and non-insulin injectable drugs are available, and insulin is needed in 20–30% of patients in late stages.

As mentioned above, morbidity and mortality are dramatically high in diabetes (American Diabetes Association, 2012a, 2012b). The disease increases the risk of heart disease and stroke three- to five-fold, and 50–70% of people with diabetes die of these events. Diabetic retinopathy is a major cause of blindness that occurs in approximately 2% of patients after 15 years of diabetes; moreover, about 40–50% of patients develop severe visual impairment over the years. Despite improved therapies, diabetes remains the leading cause of kidney failure, and 10–20% of people with diabetes die of kidney failure. Diabetic neuropathy, in one or more of its several forms, affects up to 50% of people with diabetes, and, in combination with reduced blood flow, neuropathy in the feet increases the chance of foot ulcers up to 25-fold and eventual limb amputation several fold.

## The pathophysiology of diabetes

Pancreatic β-cell dysfunction and failure is key to the onset and development of diabetes (Ferrannini and Mari, 2004; Marchetti et al., 2008). In a normal pancreas there are approximately 1,000,000 islets of Langerhans, which contain several different types of endocrine cells (Table 17.1). The insulin-secreting β-cells represent the majority of islet endocrine cells, and their mass is regulated by four major mechanisms: apoptosis (programmed cell death), size modification, replication (division of existing β-cells), and neogenesis (development from precursor cells) (Ferrannini and Mari, 2004; Cnop et al., 2005; Johnson and Luciani, 2010). At any given moment, the amount of β-cell mass is represented by the sum of replication, size, and neogenesis, minus the rate of apoptosis, a form of programmed cell death. The contribution made by each of the above-mentioned mechanisms is variable and may change with species as well as at different stages of life or metabolic demand. It is accepted that, in humans, right after birth there is a transient burst of β-cell replication, followed by a transitory rise in neogenesis, since in this phase the rate of apoptosis is low, and the net effect is a marked increase in β-cell growth early in life. Then, during childhood and adolescence, the rates of β-cell replication, neogenesis, and apoptosis decrease, to reach a balance, which guarantees the adequate β-cell mass through adulthood.

In type 1 diabetes there is a selective loss of insulin-producing β-cells in the pancreatic islets in genetically susceptible subjects, triggered and driven by autoimmune processes (Ounissi-Benkalha and Polychronakos, 2008; Rich et al., 2009; van Belle et al., 2011; American Diabetes Association, 2012a, 2012b). There are genes contributing to disease susceptibility, of which the most important ones are located in the *HLA* class II locus on chromosome 6. Other additional genes or genetic regions have been observed to be associated with this form of diabetes (Ounissi-Benkalha and Polychronakos, 2008; Rich et al., 2009; van Belle et al., 2011). Nevertheless, only a relatively small proportion (less than 10%) of individuals with *HLA*-conferred diabetes susceptibility progress to clinical disease. This implies that additional factors, presumably linked to the environment but still to be clearly identified, are needed to determine β-cell destruction in genetically predisposed subjects. It is generally accepted that the destruction of the β-cells is mediated by cellular immune responses, as supported by the presence of T-cells in the islets (insulitis), the delay of disease progression by immunosuppressive drugs directed specifically against T-cells, and the presence of circulating autoreactive T-cells in patients at clinical presentation (Knip and Siljander, 2008; Roep and Peakman, 2011; Todd et al., 2011; van Belle et al., 2011). The activation of T-cells requires the presentation of autoantigenic determinants to self-reactive T-cells by MHC II molecules that might be induced on the surface of the β-cells by the combined effect of cytokines. In addition, and probably more importantly, islet autoantigens could be presented to naïve autoreactive T-cells by APC, which primarily express MHC II molecules. The activated T-cells are capable of invading the islets, where they become reactivated by encountering cognate β -cell autoantigens and thereby initiate insulitis.

**Table 17.1** Main endocrine components of pancreatic islets

| Cell type | Main hormone(s) | Size of secretory granule (nm) | Percentage of islet cells |
|---|---|---|---|
| β-cell | Insulin, amylin | 250–350 | 60–80 |
| Alpha-cell | Glucagon | 200–250 | 15–20 |
| Delta-cell | Somatostatin | 300–350 | 5–10 |
| PP cell | Pancreatic polypeptide | 120–160 | 10–15 |

Type 2 diabetes is associated with impaired β-cell function and reduced tissue insulin sensitivity (insulin resistance) (American Diabetes Association, 2012a, 2012b). However, there is growing evidence that β-cell failure is the crucial defect for the development and progression of this form of diabetes, as shown by several cross-sectional and, more stringently so, prospective studies (Wajchenberg, 2007; Meier, 2008; Marchetti et al., 2009). This applies to subjects with high risk of developing diabetes, as well as patients after the diagnosis of hyperglycaemia. The role of reduced β-cell mass in human type 2 diabetes, the primary importance of β-cell apoptosis, and the insufficiency of replication/neogenesis have been studied by several authors, and decreased islet mass, reduced β-cell mass, and diminished β-cell insulin secretory granules have been generally reported (Wajchenberg, 2007; Marchetti et al., 2008, 2009; Meier, 2008). The study of pancreatic samples from non-diabetic subjects and type 2 diabetic patients has consistently shown an approximately 30–40% decrease of β-cell amount in the latter. This is probably due to a significantly increased frequency of apoptosis in type 2 diabetic β-cells not compensated for by adequate regeneration. In addition, quantitative and qualitative alterations of insulin release have been described in type 2 diabetes. Commonly found abnormalities include reduced or absent first-phase insulin secretion to intravenous glucose, delayed or blunted responses to mixed meal ingestion, and, with time, reduced second-phase release and diminished responses to non-glucose stimuli (Ferrannini and Mari, 2004; Choi et al., 2012). Additional qualitative defects of insulin release are represented by alterations of oscillatory patterns and increased pro-insulin release.

## The therapy of diabetes: an overview

It is largely accepted that the recommendation of lowering HbA1c (a major marker of glycaemic control) to < 7.0% in most diabetic patients reduces the incidence of microvascular disease (American Diabetes Association, 2012a; Inzucchi et al., 2012). Accordingly, intensive diabetes management can lower the incidence of macrovascular complications in type 1 diabetic patients (DCCT/EDIC Research Group et al., 2011), which is, however, more questionable in the case of type 2 diabetes (Holman et al., 2008; ACCORD Study Group et al., 2011). More stringent HbA1c targets (e.g. 6.0–6.5%) might be considered in patients with short disease duration, long life expectancy, or no significant CVD, provided this could be achieved without significant hypoglycaemia or other adverse effects of treatment (Inzucchi et al., 2012). On the other hand, HbA1c levels of 7.5–8.0% or even slightly higher may be appropriate for patients at risk of severe hypoglycaemia and/or with limited life expectancy, advanced vascular complications, or extensive comorbid conditions (Inzucchi et al., 2012).

Lifestyle interventions focused, in particular, on dietary habits and physical activity are fundamental components of diabetes management (American Diabetes Association, 2012a; Inzucchi et al., 2012). When needed (and this is the case in the majority of type 2 diabetic patients), weight reduction should be pursued in order to improve glycaemic control and other cardiovascular risk factors. Even relatively modest weight loss (5–10%) contributes in this regard significantly. Dietary recommendations should be personalized and patients encouraged to eat healthy foods according to personal preferences and culture. Foods high in fibre, low-fat dairy products, and fresh fish should be encouraged, whereas high-energy foods, including those rich in saturated fats, should be eaten seldom and in lower amounts. Physical activity should be promoted, aiming at least at 150 minutes/week of moderate activity including aerobic, resistance, and flexibility training.

In type 1 diabetic patients all this must be necessarily coupled with appropriate insulin treatment regimens, to be started at diagnosis (Daneman, 2006; American Diabetes Association, 2012a). Several types of insulin and insulin analogues are available, which essentially differ in terms of pharmacokinetics and can be used to try to mimic the endogenous secretion of the hormone. Insulin therapy is also needed in about 20–30% of patients with late stages of type 2 diabetes to ensure appropriate glycaemic control. In this form of diabetes, however, several oral agents and non-insulin injectable drugs are available (Tahrani et al., 2011; American Diabetes Association, 2012b; Inzucchi et al., 2012). A position statement of the American Diabetes Association (ADA) and the European Association for the Study of Diabetes (EASD) has been recently published on how to better manage the hyperglycaemia in type 2 diabetic patients, where further details are available (Inzucchi et al., 2012).

## Diabetes and surgery

Patients with diabetes undergo surgical procedures at a higher rate than non-diabetic subjects (Root, 1966; Alberti, 1990; Siegelaar et al., 2011). In addition, diabetes is associated with increased morbidity, longer length of hospital stay, and enhanced perioperative mortality in the surgical ICU (Frisch et al., 2010; Siegelaar et al., 2011; Dhatariya et al., 2012). This is due to several reasons including hyper- or hypoglycaemia, multiple comorbidities (in particular microvascular and macrovascular complications), complex polypharmacy (including insulin), risk of management errors when converting from the intravenous insulin infusion to usual medication, higher rate of perioperative infection, failure to identify patients with diabetes, and sometimes limited knowledge of diabetes in the setting of surgical delivery care.

Typically, surgery causes a pronounced metabolic stress response, leading to the release of the catabolic hormones epinephrine, norepinephrine, cortisol, glucagon, and growth hormone, and inhibition of insulin secretion and anabolic action (Alberti, 1990; Dhatariya et al., 2012). Some of the important anabolic actions of insulin that may be negatively affected by the stress of surgery include stimulation of glucose uptake and glycogen storage, stimulation of amino acid uptake and protein synthesis by skeletal muscle, and stimulation of fatty acid synthesis in the liver and storage in adipocytes. In addition, insulin has anticatabolic effects, such as inhibition of glycogenolysis, lipolysis and proteolysis, inhibition of fatty acid oxidation and ketone body formation, and inhibition of amino acid oxidation. Therefore the combination of excessive catabolism from the action of counter-regulatory hormones, relative hypoinsulinaemia, and insulin resistance is a serious threat to glucose homeostasis in all patients with diabetes undergoing surgery, in particular when preoperative glycaemic control is defective.

Due to this very complex scenario, over the years several recommendations have been made available on the management of the diabetic patient undergoing surgery (Meneghini, 2009; Kadoi, 2010; Pichardo-Lowden and Gabbay, 2012). Recently published guidelines (Dhatariya et al., 2012) identify and discuss seven stages: primary care referral, surgical outpatients, preoperative assessment, hospital admission, surgery, and postoperative care and discharge. Each stage involves different groups of healthcare professionals with specific responsibilities, and two key recommendations are given: first, that the management of elective adult surgery patients should be with modification to their usual diabetes treatment if the fasting is minimized, rather than the routine use of a variable-rate intravenous insulin infusion; and second, that poor preoperative glycaemic control leads to poor postoperative outcomes and thus, where appropriate, needs to be addressed prior to referral for surgery. However, intravenous insulin therapy is needed in all patients who are expected to miss more than one meal (i.e. in the majority of patients), and when so, a few protocols have been proposed (reviewed in Dhatariya et al., 2012).

A major issue is how strictly should the degree of hyperglycaemia be regulated in the ICU surgical population. Whereas the occurrence of hyperglycaemia, in particular severe hyperglycaemia, is associated with increased morbidity and mortality in a variety of groups of critically ill patients, trials examining the effects of tighter glucose control have had conflicting results, and systematic reviews and meta-analyses have also led to differing conclusions (Wiener et al., 2008; Griesdale et al., 2009; Lipshutz and Gropper, 2009; NICE-SUGAR Study Investigators, 2009). A randomized trial examined the effects of intensive glucose control (target: 81–108 mg/dL) versus conventional glucose control (target: 180 mg/dL or less) in a series of 6,104 patients admitted to an ICU (NICE-SUGAR Study Investigators, 2009). The authors found that a blood glucose target of 180 mg/dL or less resulted in lower mortality than did a target of 81–108 mg/dL, possibly due to reduced incidence of hypoglycaemic episodes. While waiting for a more definitive consensus on this issue, it appears safe to recommend a glucose range of 140–180 mg/dL for the majority of critically ill diabetic patients (American Diabetes Association, 2012b).

## Indication, evaluation, and selection of diabetic patients for pancreas or kidney–pancreas transplantation

The pathophysiology and medical and surgical considerations of diabetes, discussed above, fully apply to the issue of transplantation, which undoubtedly represents a major surgical situation.

Pancreas transplantation, in its different options (see Table 17.2), is intuitively performed with the aim of replenishing the lost β-cell mass and hence restoring a condition of normoglycaemia. In addition, diabetic patients may need kidney transplantation due to the damage caused by diabetic nephropathy.

Pancreas transplantation, when technically successful, is expected to restore insulin independence in diabetic patients, but at the expense of significant surgical morbidity and life-long immunosuppression (Orlando et al., 2011; Boggi et al., 2012a). Therefore pancreas transplantation is indicated in selected patients with complicated diabetes, in whom the risks of surgery and immunosuppression are deemed to be lower than those of ineffective insulin therapy (Sutherland, 2004; Orlando et al., 2011; Boggi et al., 2012a), which may be also influenced by genetic factors (Freedman et al., 2007). Once a favourable risk:benefit balance has been established, additional benefits of pancreas transplantation can also be appreciated on the side of improved quality of life (Gross et al., 2004).

Since the primary goal of pancreas transplantation is restoring a critical mass of viable β-cells, the prototype recipient for this transplant is a type 1 diabetic patient without detectable C-peptide. Recent evidence suggests that some patients with type 2 diabetes but requiring high-dose insulin and having low to mild insulin resistance (usually non- or mildly obese) may also regain insulin independence with pancreas transplantation and enjoy benefits similar to those experienced by prototype recipients (Sutherland, 2004; Orlando et al., 2011; Boggi et al., 2012a).

Because pancreas transplantation is convenient only in patients in whom insulin-based therapies have failed, most recipients become transplant candidates after some 20–25 years of history of diabetes. By this time, many of them have developed clinically relevant diabetic nephropathy and are often in ESRD. Ideally, these patients should receive an SKPT. Since nephropathy is a grim prognosticator in diabetic patients (Borch-Johnsen and Kreiner, 1987; Wolfe et al., 1999; Allen and Walker 2003), SKPT is the therapy of choice for insulin-dependent diabetic patients with ESRD. Seventy-five percent of insulin-dependent diabetic patients do not survive longer than 5 years while receiving dialysis (Wolfe et al., 1999). However, SKPT improves patient survival compared to dialysis treatment of deceased donor kidney transplant (Tydén et al., 2000; Ojo et al., 2001; White et al., 2009).

When a live renal donor is available, a further option is to proceed with the kidney transplant first and then correct diabetes with a PAK transplant (Sutherland, 2004; Orlando et al., 2011; Boggi et al., 2012a). Actually, a live donor kidney and a deceased donor pancreas may be transplanted simultaneously, but this option has high organizational needs and has not been practised frequently (Sutherland, 2004; Orlando et al., 2011; Boggi et al., 2012a). Sequential kidney and PAK transplantation require two surgical operations and a dual course of induction therapy; correcting uraemia is key in these patients, and the chance of a kidney transplant should not be denied simply because of the wish to pursue the 'ideal' SKPT path. Further, the excellent renal function provided by a live donor kidney is especially rewarding in the fragile diabetic and uraemic recipient. The rationale for PAK transplantation is to prevent the recurrence of diabetic nephropathy in the renal graft in the long term. PAK, however, is associated with all the typical complications of pancreas transplantation, which, paradoxically, may jeopardize renal function in the short term. Although there is no agreed cut-off of renal function to safely proceed with PAK, a stable renal function with a creatinine clearance of at least 60 mL/min/1.73 m$^2$ and a negative urine analysis are all very much welcome (Sutherland, 2004; Orlando et al., 2011; Boggi et al., 2012a).

**Table 17.2** Options in pancreas transplantation

| Option | Indication | Comment |
|---|---|---|
| Simultaneous pancreas and kidney | Diabetes and ESRD (uraemic or pre-uraemic) | Kidney may be from live donor |
| Pancreas after kidney | Brittle diabetes and/or diabetes complications | Demonstrated functioning kidney graft |
| Pancreas alone | Brittle diabetes and/or diabetes complications | Demonstrated maintained native kidney function |

Selected diabetic patients may also be considered for PAT when native renal function is normal or 'acceptable'. According to the ADA, patients with brittle diabetes, suffering from frequent unawareness hypoglycaemic events and/or having medical or psychological problems with insulin therapy are eligible for PAT (Robertson et al., 2006). Recent evidence suggests that also patients having progressive diabetic complications (i.e. reversible nephropathy, progressive retinopathy, and severe neuropathy) may significantly benefit from PAT (Boggi et al., 2011, 2012b). Whereas the impact of PAT on patient survival is still debated (Venstrom et al., 2003; Gruessner et al., 2004), in suitable recipients PAT improves the course of diabetic retinopathy (Giannarelli et al., 2006), diabetic neuropathy (Boggi et al., 2012b), and diabetic nephropathy (Fioretto et al., 1998; Coppelli et al., 2005; Boggi et al., 2012b), and reduces the level of cardiovascular risk (Coppelli et al., 2003; Boggi et al., 2012b). Regarding native renal function, the anticipated long-term improvement of diabetic nephropathy is thought to exceed the yet concrete risk of accelerated deterioration of renal function, which is mostly caused by the nephrotoxic effects of immunosuppressants (Fioretto et al., 1998; Coppelli et al., 2005; White et al., 2009).

The evaluation of pancreas transplant candidates is presented in detail in Chapter 16. Briefly, all diabetic patients potentially eligible for pancreas transplantation are at high risk for cardiovascular disease, making cardiac and vascular work-up key in this transplant population. In PAK and PAT recipients great attention should be paid to the level of grafted and native renal function, respectively. The indication to proceed with a solitary pancreas transplant (either PAK or PAT) should be well balanced against the inherent risk of a complex procedure such as pancreas transplantation. On the contrary, there is no good medical reason to contraindicate an SKPT in diabetic patients with ESRD excluding the usual absolute contraindications to any type of transplant. These patients, if left on insulin and dialysis, do really poorly and die soon. Thus the evaluation process should focus on exploring all possible venues for each patient to receive his or her 'life-saving' SKPT. Sometimes, despite all efforts, a diabetic patient with ESRD may be felt to be too sick to undergo any kind of transplant (including kidney transplant alone) with a reasonable chance of success.

These are simply the patients in whom the transplant evaluation was started too late in the natural course of the disease or in whom the disease pursued a really high-grade biological course, with virtually no chance of rescue at any time.

Finally, some diabetic patients may benefit from pancreas transplant procedure, either alone or combined with a kidney if renal failure has developed. Restoration of insulin independence and rescue from the uraemic condition are commonly achieved at the expense of significant surgical morbidity and life-long immunosuppression. Therefore pancreas transplantation is indicated in selected patients with complicated diabetes, in whom the risks of surgery and immunosuppression are deemed to be lower than those of ineffective insulin therapy.

## Conclusion

Diabetes mellitus is one of the foremost chronic diseases in the world today, and its incidence continues to increase. It is associated with high morbidity and mortality, causing an estimated 4 million deaths annually or 6.8% of global all-cause mortality among people aged 20–79. Diabetes mellitus is a metabolic disease characterized by hyperglycaemia resulting from defects in insulin secretion, and/or insulin action, with defects of the pancreatic β-cells playing a key role. In this chapter we have reviewed advances in the treatment of diabetes. However, treatment options have not demonstrated a clear improvement in morbidity and mortality, perhaps because they are based on the principle that medical therapy should aim at attaining tight metabolic control in order to prevent long-term complications. Tight control may delay the progression of complications but also contributes to increased occurrence of severe hypoglycaemic episodes that may be life-threatening, especially in individuals who lost autonomic response. We look forward to additional studies focused on the therapeutic benefits of tight glucose control delivered by more advanced glucose delivery in conjunction with advanced glucose monitoring systems.

## References


ACCORD Study Group, Gerstein HC, Miller ME, et al. (2011) Long-term effects of intensive glucose lowering on cardiovascular outcomes. *N Eng J Med*, **364**:818–828.

Alberti KGMM (1990) Diabetes and surgery. In: Porte D, Sherwin RS (eds) *Ellenberg and Rifkin's Diabetes Mellitus*, pp. 623–633. Elsevier, New York.

Allen KV, Walker JD (2003) Microalbuminuria and mortality in long-duration type 1 diabetes. *Diabetes Care*, **26**:2389–9231.

American Diabetes Association (2012a) Standards of medical care in diabetes—2012. *Diabetes Care*, **35**(Suppl 1):11–63.

American Diabetes Association (2012b) Diagnosis and classification of diabetes mellitus. *Diabetes Care*, **35**(Suppl l):s64–71.

Boggi U, Vistoli F, Amorese G, et al. (2011) Results of pancreas transplantation alone with special attention to native kidney function and proteinuria in type 1 diabetes patients. *Rev Diab Stud*, **8**:259–267.

Boggi U, Vistoli F, Egidi FM, et al. (2012a) Transplantation of the pancreas. *Curr Diab Rep*, **12**(5):568–579.

Boggi U, Vistoli F, Amorese G, et al. (2012b) Long-term (5 years) efficacy and safety of pancreas transplantation alone in type 1 diabetic patients. *Transplantation*, **93**:842–846.

Borch-Johnsen K, Kreiner S (1987) Proteinuria: value as predictor of cardiovascular mortality in insulin dependent diabetes mellitus. *BMJ*, **294**:1651–1654.

Choi CS, Kim MY, Han K, Lee MS (2012) Assessment of beta-cell function in human patients. *Islets*, **4**:79–83.

Cnop M, Welsh N, Jonas JC, et al (2005) Mechanisms of pancreatic beta-cell death in type 1 and type 2 diabetes: many differences, few similarities. *Diabetes*, **54**:S97–S107.

Coppelli A, Giannarelli R, Mariotti R, et al. (2003) Pancreas transplant alone determines early improvement of cardiovascular risk factors and cardiac function in type 1 diabetic patients. *Transplantation*, **76**:974–976.

Coppelli A, Giannarelli R, Vistoli F, et al. (2005) The beneficial effects of pancreas transplant alone on diabetic nephropathy. *Diabetes Care*, **28**:1366–1370.

Danaei G, Finucane MM, Lu Y, et al. (2011) Global Burden of Metabolic Risk Factors of Chronic Diseases Collaborating Group (Blood Glucose). National, regional, and global trends in fasting plasma glucose and diabetes prevalence since 1980: systematic analysis of health examination surveys and epidemiological studies with 370 country-years and 2.7 million participants. *Lancet*, **378**:31–40.

Daneman D (2006) Type 1 diabetes. *Lancet*, **367**:847–858.

DCCT/EDIC Research Group, de Boer IH, Sun W, et al. (2011) Intensive diabetes therapy and glomerular filtration rate in type 1-diabetes. *N Engl J Med*, **365**:2366–2376.

Dhatariya K, Levy N, Kilvert A, et al. (2012) NHS Diabetes guideline for the perioperative management of the adult patient with diabetes. *Diabetic Med*, **29**:420–433.

Ferrannini E, Mari A (2004) Beta cell function and its relation to insulin action in humans: a critical appraisal. *Diabetologia*, **47**: 943–956.

Fioretto P, Steffes MW, Sutherland DE, et al. (1998) Reversal of lesions of diabetic nephropathy after pancreas transplantation. *N Engl J Med*, **339**:69–75.

Freedman BI, Bostrom M, Daeihagh P, Bowden DW (2007) Genetic factors in diabetic nephropathy. *Clin J Am Soc Nephrol*, **2**:1306–1316.

Frisch A, Chandra P, Smiley D, et al. (2010) Prevalence and clinical outcome of hyperglycemia in the perioperative period in noncardiac surgery. *Diabetes Care*, **33**:1783–1788.

Giannarelli R, Coppelli A, Sartini MS, et al. (2006) Pancreas transplant alone has beneficial effects on retinopathy in type 1 diabetic patients. *Diabetologia*, **49**:2977–2982.

Griesdale DE, de Souza RJ, van Dam RM, et al. (2009) Intensive insulin therapy and mortality among critically ill patients: a meta-analysis including NICE-SUGAR study data. *Can Med Assoc J*, **180**:821–827.

Gross CR, Gruessner AC, Treesak C (2004) Quality of life for pancreas recipients. In: Gruessner RWG, Sutherland DER (eds) *Transplant Pancreas*, pp. 509–519. Springer, New York.

Gruessner RW, Sutherland DE, Gruessner AC (2004) Mortality assessment for pancreas transplants. *Am J Transplant*, **4**:2018–2026.

Holman RR, Paul SK, Bethel MA, et al (2008) 10-year follow-up of intensive glucose control in type 2 diabetes. *N Eng J Med*, **359**:1577–1589.

Inzucchi SE, Bergenstal RM, Buse JB, et al. (2012) Management of hyperglycemia in type 2 diabetes: a patient-centered approach: position statement of the American Diabetes Association (ADA) and the European Association for the Study of Diabetes (EASD). *Diabetes Care*, **35**:1364–1379.

Johnson JD, Luciani DS (2010) Mechanisms of pancreatic beta-cell apoptosis in diabetes and its therapies. *Adv Exp Med Biol*, **654**:447–462.

Kadoi Y (2010) Anesthetic considerations in diabetic patients. Part II: intraoperative and postoperative management of patients with diabetes mellitus. *J Anesth*, **24**:748–756.

Kansagara D, Fu R, Freeman M, et al. (2011) Intensive insulin therapy in hospitalized patients: a systematic review. *Annal Intern Med*, **154**:268–282.

Knip M, Siljander H (2008) Autoimmune mechanisms in type 1 diabetes. *Autoimmun Rev*, **7**:550–557.

Lipshutz AK, Gropper MA (2009) Perioperative glycemic control: an evidence-based review. *Anesthesiology*, **110**(2):408–421.

Maerz LL, Akhtar S (2011) Perioperative glycemic management in 2011: paradigm shifts. *Curr Opin Crit Care*, **17**:370–375.

Marchetti P, Dotta F, Lauro D, Purrello F (2008) An overview of pancreatic beta-cell defects in human type 2 diabetes: implications for treatment. *Regulatory Peptides*, **146**:4–11.

Marchetti P, Lupi R, Del Guerra S, et al. (2009) Goals of treatment for type 2 diabetes: beta-cell preservation for glycemic control. *Diabetes Care*, **32**:S178–S183.

Marchetti P, Lupi R, Del Guerra S, et al. (2010) The beta-cell in human type 2 diabetes. *Adv Exp Med Biol*, **654**:501–514.

Meier JJ (2008) Beta cell mass in diabetes: a realistic therapeutic target? *Diabetologia*, **51**:703–713.

Meneghini LF (2009) Perioperative management of diabetes: translating evidence into practice. *Cleve Clin J Med*, **76**:S53–S59.

NICE-SUGAR Study Investigators (2009) Intensive versus conventional glucose control in critically ill patients. *N Engl J Med*, **360**(13):1283–1297.

Ojo AO, Meier-Kriesche HU, Hanson JA, et al. (2001) The impact of simultaneous pancreas-kidney transplantation on long-term patient survival. *Transplantation*, **71**:82–90.

Orlando G, Stratta RJ, Light J (2011) Pancreas transplantation for type 2 diabetes mellitus. *Curr Opin Organ Transplant*, **16**:10–115.

Ounissi-Benkalha H, Polychronakos C (2008) The molecular genetics of type 1 diabetes: new genes and emerging mechanisms. *Trend Molec Med*, **14**:268–725.

Pichardo-Lowden A, Gabbay RA (2012) Management of hyperglycemia during the perioperative period. *Curr Diabetes Rep*, **12**:108–118.

Rich SS, Akolkar B, Concannon P, et al. (2009) Overview of the Type I Diabetes Genetics Consortium. *Genes Immuol*, **10**:S1–S4.

Robertson RP, Davis C, Larsen J, et al. (2006) Pancreas and islet transplantation in type 1 diabetes. *Diabetes Care*, **29**:935.

Roep BO, Peakman M (2011) Diabetogenic T lymphocytes in human type 1 diabetes. *Curr Opin Immunol*, **23**:746–753.

Root HF (1966) Preoperative medical care of the diabetic patient. *Postgrad Med*, **40**:439–444.

Shaw JE, Sicree RA, Zimmet PZ (2010) Global estimates of the prevalence of diabetes for 2010 and 2030. *Diabetes Res Clin Prac*, **87**:4–14.

Siegelaar SE, Hickmann M, Hoekstra JB, et al. (2011) The effect of diabetes on mortality in critically ill patients: a systematic review and meta-analysis. *Crit Care*, **15**:R205.

Sutherland DER (2004) Pancreas and islet transplant population. In: Gruessner RWG, Sutherland DER (eds) *Transplant Pancreas*, pp. 91–102. Springer, New York.

Tahrani AA, Bailey CJ, Del Prato S, Barnett AH (2011) Management of type 2 diabetes: new and future developments in treatment. *Lancet*, **378**:182–197.

Todd JA, Knip M, Mathieu C (2011) Strategies for the prevention of autoimmune type 1 diabetes. *Diabetic Med*, **28**:1141–1143.

Tydén G, Tollemar J, Bolinder J (2000) Combined pancreas and kidney transplantation improves survival in patients with end-stage diabetic nephropathy. *Clin Transplant*, **14**:505–508.

van Belle TL, Coppieters KT, von Herrath MG (2011) Type 1 diabetes: etiology, immunology, and therapeutic strategies. *Physiol Rev*, **91**:79–118.

Venstrom JM, McBride MA, Rother KI, et al. (2003) Survival after pancreas transplantation in patients with diabetes and preserved kidney function. *JAMA*, **290**:2817–2823.

Wajchenberg BL (2007) Beta-cell failure in diabetes and preservation by clinical treatment. *Endocrinol Rev*, **28**:187–218.

White SA, Shaw JA, Sutherland DE (2009) Pancreas transplantation. *Lancet*, **373**:1808–1817.

Wild S, Roglic G, Green A, Sicree R, King H (2004) Global prevalence of diabetes: estimates for the year 2000 and projections for 2030. *Diabetes Care*, **27**:1047–1053.

Wiener RS, Wiener DC, Larson RJ (2008) Benefits and risks of tight glucose control in critically ill adults: a meta-analysis. *JAMA*, **300**:933–944.

Wolfe RA, Ashby VB, Milford EL, et al. (1999) Comparison of mortality in all patients on dialysis, patients on dialysis awaiting transplantation, and recipients of a first cadaveric transplant. *N Engl J Med*, **341**:1725–1730.

## Further reading

International Diabetes Federation: <http://www.idf.org>.

World Health Organization: <http://www.who.int/en>.

# CHAPTER 18

# Islet cell transplantation

Antonello Pileggi and Camillo Ricordi

## Introduction

Diabetes mellitus is a growing, global medical problem. Diet, exercise, and insulin therapy remain the primary choice for diabetes treatment, thought mostly inadequate to attain tight control in the majority of diabetics. Current medical management of diabetes has greatly benefitted from technological improvements in insulin formulations, infusion pumps, and continuous glucose monitoring systems. It has been recognized that medical therapy should aim at attaining tight metabolic control throughout the day to prevent the development of progressive diabetes complications affecting the neural, vascular, retinal, and renal systems. Progression of diabetes complications can be delayed or prevented via intensive insulin therapy, though via increased occurrence of severe hypoglycaemic episodes that may be life-threatening, especially in individuals who have lost autonomic response (hypoglycaemia awareness) (Skyler, 2006).

Restoration of β-cells represents an appealing therapeutic approach to attain ideal metabolic control and treat and prevent progressive diabetes complications. Since the 1980s there has been steady progress in clinical trials of islet transplantation as isolated islet cells or vascularized pancreas, demonstrating the reproducible achievement of physiological release of endocrine hormones in subjects with diabetes (Marzorati et al., 2007).

## Indications, evaluation, and selection of patients for islet cell transplantation

Islet cell transplantation represents a therapeutic option for conditions associated with loss of β-cell function (Piemonti and Pileggi, 2013) (see Table 18.1).

Islets for transplant may be obtained from the patient's own pancreas (*autologous* or *autotransplant*) mainly when surgical removal of the gland is required (i.e. palliative treatment of chronic pain for recurrent pancreatitis or severe trauma of the gland) (Table 18.1) (reviewed in Bellin et al., 2012a). After total pancreatectomy, *surgery-induced (iatrogenic) insulin-requiring diabetes* is induced, requiring life-long exogenous insulin therapy. Since the early 1970s (Najarian et al., 1979) islet autotransplantation has been performed to attain adequate metabolic control, which has been reportedly achieved in approximately 70% of cases with insulin independence when adequate numbers (generally > 250,000 islet equivalents) could be recovered from the gland. Nonetheless, even when lower numbers of islets have been transplanted that were inadequate attain insulin-independence, stable metabolic control and can be achieved in most subjects receiving autologous islet transplantation (Teuscher et al., 1998; Robertson et al., 2001, 2004; Blondet et al., 2007; Bellin and Sutherland, 2010, 2011a; Bellin et al., 2011b). Importantly, islet autotransplantation is currently reimbursed by health insurance in the US.

The only option currently available to subjects who have lost islet function (type 1 diabetes or, more rarely, previous total pancreatectomy) is *allogeneic* islet transplantation, generally from the pancreas of multi-organ donors (donation after cerebral death) following ABO blood-type matching. While it is possible to use a segment of the pancreas from living-related donors (Matsumoto et al., 2005, 2004), this is not preferred for islet transplantation currently, considering the limited duration of graft function when suboptimal islet numbers are transplanted under conventional immunosuppressive protocols, as well as due to the intrinsic risks for the donor (i.e. morbidity and risk of developing diabetes). Non-uraemic subjects may receive islet transplant alone (ITA) for the treatment of iatrogenic (surgery-induced) and type 1 diabetes, while individuals with ESRD may receive simultaneous islet–kidney (SIK) or islet after kidney (IAK) transplantation. In particular situations, islets may be transplanted along with other organs (i.e. in the context of multivisceral transplantation following exenteration comprising the pancreas) (Tzakis et al., 1990).

Type 1 diabetes, which is characterized by the selective destruction of islet β-cells due to an autoimmune process, is considered the main indication for an allogeneic islet transplant at the present time. The primary goal of islet transplantation is to correct the high susceptibility to severe hypoglycaemia and glycaemic imbalance which are associated with high mortality (8% in non-uraemic subjects on the waiting list for 4 years to receive pancreas transplantation). Further indications include progressive complications of diabetes and psychological problems with insulin therapy that may compromise adherence to the therapeutic regimen. Moreover, islet transplantation is indicated also for cases of subcutaneous insulin resistance requiring intraperitoneal or intravenous infusions, which are associated with high morbidity and render challenging clinical management. The criteria for inclusion in current allogeneic islet transplantation clinical trials (see Table 18.2) include sex with brittle type 1 diabetes; 18–65 years of age; characterized by frequent metabolic instability requiring medical treatment (hypo-/hyperglycaemia, ketoacidosis) despite intensive insulin therapy; hypoglycaemia unawareness (< 54mg/dL); and severe metabolic lability (mean amplitude of glycaemic excursion > 11.1 mmol/L or 200 mg/dL). The inadequate efficacy of medical therapy to attain desirable metabolic control in this

**Table 18.1** Indications for islet cell transplantation

| Condition | Technique | Type of transplant |
|---|---|---|
| *Diabetes mellitus* | | |
| Type 1 | ITA, SIK, IAK | Allogeneic |
| Type 2 | ITA, SIK, IAK | Allogeneic |
| *Surgery-induced diabetes* | | |
| Chronic pancreatitis | ITA | Autologous/allogeneic |
| Trauma | ITA | Autologous/allogeneic |
| Cystic fibrosis | ITA<br>Liver–islet transplantation | Autologous/allogeneic<br>Allogeneic |
| Benign enucleable tumours | ITA | Autologous |
| Multi-organ transplantation | Liver–islet transplantation, bowel–liver–islet transplantation, heart–islet transplantation, or other combinations | Allogeneic |

ITA, Islet transplant alone; SIK, simultaneous islet–kidney; IAK, islet after kidney.

specific patient population with unstable diabetes justifies the use of transplantation of pancreatic islets (isolated cell clusters or whole pancreas transplantation).

## Isolation, processing, and implantation of pancreatic islet cells

Pancreatic islets are highly vascularized endocrine cell clusters ranging from < 50 μm to ~ 800 μm in diameter and accounting for ~1% of total pancreatic tissue (approximately $10^6$ islets scattered throughout a healthy gland). Each cluster comprises thousands of specialized endocrine cells that establish intimate relationship with each other and with intra-insular capillaries. The function of islet cells derives from complex cell–cell interactions between different cell subsets, innervation, incretins, and metabolites in the blood and interstitial space, which all contribute to the finely tuned control of glucose homeostasis (Cabrera et al., 2006). That is why preservation of the cluster integrity is essential to achieve optimal performance of islets after isolation. The aim of cell isolation and the purification process is to obtain the largest number of islets from a donor pancreas while preserving their 3-D morphological structure and functional integrity. The isolation phase aims at freeing islets from the pancreatic tissue through a combined mechanically enhanced enzymatic digestion. The gland is perfused via the pancreatic duct with an enzymatic buffer and then cut into large pieces that are transferred with marbles to the dissociation chamber (Ricordi et al., 1988). After dissociation of the gland, purification is performed by centrifugation on density gradients of the pancreatic digest (slurry) to enrich for the endocrine fraction (Alejandro et al., 1990; Ichii et al., 2005). Generally, after the purification step, islet clusters with different degrees of purity are obtained and cultured separately until the time of transplant. The final cellular product contains the highest number of endocrine clusters in the smaller volume (≤ 10 mL of tissue) derived by combining different purity fractions. An animation of the islet isolation and transplant procedures is available online at <http://www.youtube.com/watch?v=amnku-zvuls>.

## Islet transplantation techniques

The primary technique for pancreatic islet transplantation utilized at the present time consists of their embolization into the hepatic sinusoids by portal vein infusion (Piemonti and Pileggi, 2013). The final cellular product in suspension is loaded into gas-permeable infusion bags and infused by gravity into the recipient's hepatic portal system (Baidal et al., 2003) through a minimally invasive, percutaneous, transhepatic catheterization of the portal vein under ultrasound and fluoroscopic guidance while monitoring portal pressure to prevent and detect portal hypertension and thrombosis (Alejandro and Mintz, 1988; Owen et al., 2003). After infusion, the tract is sealed using fibrin-based plugs to prevent haemorrhage (Casey et al., 2002; Froud et al., 2004). In high-risk subjects with vascular anatomical variations or requiring anticoagulation therapy, access to a mesenteric vein tributary of the hepatic portal system via minilaparotomy may be preferable (Tzakis et al., 1990). Cannulation of the umbilical vein via mini-invasive laparoscopic approach may also provide an alternative access to the portal system (Casavilla et al., 1992).

In recent years there has been a renewed interest in developing alternative, extrahepatic sites for islet grafts (reviewed in Cantarelli and Piemonti, 2011). Encouraging data from pilot clinical studies have demonstrated the engraftment of autologous islets into an intramuscular site in the forearm (Weber et al., 1978; Rafael et al., 2008). Other pilot clinical studies have shown different degrees of function of immuno-isolated allogeneic or xenogeneic islets into biocompatible polymers that were implanted in the peritoneal cavity (free floating) (Basta and Calafiore, 2011; Basta et al., 2011). Other approaches, biodevices, and alternative sites are being actively explored in preclinical models (Pileggi et al., 2006b; Dufrane et al., 2010; Cantarelli and Piemonti, 2011; Perez et al., 2011; Pedraza et al., 2013).

## Immunosuppression

Different immunosuppressive protocols are utilized in ongoing allogeneic islet transplantation trials. Generally, the immunosuppressive drugs are administered before the transplant (induction) and then maintained based on trough levels monitoring in the peripheral blood to achieve the targeted therapeutic dose. At induction, lymphodepleting agents are generally utilized (i.e. antilymphocyte serum; monoclonal antibody targeting CD3 or CD52 expressing cells; or anti-CD25 antibody), particularly combined with adjuvant anti-inflammatory treatment (i.e. anti-TNF-α antibody and anti-IL1R) (Pileggi et al., 2004; Frank et al., 2005; Hering et al., 2005; Marzorati et al., 2007; Alejandro et al., 2008; Bellin et al., 2008; Froud et al., 2008; Gerber et al., 2008; Tan et al., 2008).

Maintenance regimens rely generally on the synergy obtained by combinatorial use of different classes of immunosuppressants, allowing lowering doses to avoid side effects. Amongst them are CNI (cyclosporine-A and tacrolimus), inhibitors of the mTOR (sirolimus and everolimus), and purine synthesis inhibitors (mycophenolic acid) (Shapiro et al., 2000; Froud et al., 2005; Hering et al., 2005; Vantyghem et al., 2009). Steroid avoidance or

**Table 18.2** Inclusion and exclusion criteria for islet transplantation in T1DM. (Modified from the Clinical Islet Transplant Consortium Adapted with kind permission from the Clinical Islet Transplant Consortium (www.citisletstudy.org/; http://clinicaltrials.gov/ct2/show/NCT00434811).

| **Criteria for inclusion** |
|---|
| Mentally stable and able to comply with study procedures |
| Clinical history compatible with type 1 diabetes with onset of disease at < 40 years of age, insulin dependence for at least 5 years at study entry, and a sum of age and insulin-dependent diabetes duration of at least 28 |
| Absent stimulated C-peptide (< 0.3 ng/mL) 60 and 90 minutes post-mixed-meal tolerance test |
| Involvement of intensive diabetes management, defined as: |
| ◆ Self-monitoring of glucose values no less than a mean of three times each day averaged over each week |
| ◆ Administration of three or more insulin injections each day or insulin pump therapy |
| ◆ Under the direction of an endocrinologist, diabetologist, or diabetes specialist, with at least three clinical evaluations during the past 12 months prior to study enrolment |
| At least one episode of severe hypoglycaemia in the past 12 months, defined as an event with one of the following symptoms: memory loss; confusion; uncontrollable behaviour; irrational behaviour; unusual difficulty in awakening; suspected seizure; seizure; loss of consciousness or visual symptoms, compatible with hypoglycaemia in which the individual requires assistance of another subject and is unable to treat him-/herself and which is associated with either a blood glucose level < 54 mg/dL or prompt recovery after oral carbohydrate, intravenous glucose, or glucagon administration in the 12 months prior to study enrolment |
| Reduced awareness of hypoglycaemia |
| **Reasons for exclusion** |
| Body mass index (BMI) > 30 kg/m$^2$ or weight ≤ 50 kg |
| Insulin requirement of > 1.0 IU/kg/day or < 15 units/day |
| HbA1c > 10% |
| Untreated proliferative diabetic retinopathy |
| Systolic blood pressure > 160 mm Hg or diastolic blood pressure > 100 mm Hg |
| Measured glomerular filtration rate using iohexol of < 80 mL/min/1.73 mm$^2$ |
| Presence or history of macroalbuminuria (> 300 mg/g creatinine) |
| Presence or history of panel-reactive anti-HLA antibody levels greater than background by flow cytometry |
| Pregnant, breastfeeding, or unwilling to use effective contraception throughout the study and 4 months after study completion |
| Presence or history of active infection, including hepatitis B, hepatitis C, HIV, or tuberculosis |
| Negative for EBV by IgG determination |
| Invasive *Aspergillus*, histoplasmosis, or coccidioidomycosis infection in the past year |
| History of malignancy except for completely resected squamous or basal cell carcinoma of the skin |
| Known active alcohol or substance abuse |
| Baseline haemoglobin (Hgb) below the lower limits of normal, lymphopaenia, neutropaenia, or thrombocytopaenia |
| History of factor V deficiency |
| Any coagulopathy or medical condition requiring long-term anticoagulant therapy after transplantation or individuals with an INR > 1.5 |
| Severe coexisting cardiac disease, characterized by any one of the following conditions: |
| ◆ Heart attack within the last 6 months |
| ◆ Evidence of ischaemia on functional heart examination within the year prior to study entry |
| ◆ Left ventricular ejection fraction < 30% |
| Persistent elevation of liver function tests at the time of study entry |
| Symptomatic cholecystolithiasis |
| Acute or chronic pancreatitis |
| Symptomatic peptic ulcer disease |
| Severe unremitting diarrhoea, vomiting, or other gastrointestinal disorders that could interfere with the ability to absorb oral medications |
| Hyperlipidaemia despite medical therapy, defined as fasting LDL cholesterol > 130 mg/dL (treated or untreated) and/or fasting triglycerides > 200 mg/dL |
| Currently receiving treatment for a medical condition that requires chronic use of systemic steroids except for the use of 5 mg or less of prednisone daily, or an equivalent dose of hydrocortisone, for physiological replacement only |
| Treatment with any antidiabetic medication other than insulin within the past 4 weeks |
| Use of any study medications within the past 4 weeks |
| Received a live attenuated vaccine(s) within the past 2 months |
| Any medical condition that, in the opinion of the investigator, might interfere with safe participation in the trial |
| Treatment with any immunosuppressive regimen at the time of enrolment |
| A previous islet transplant |
| A previous pancreas transplant, unless the graft failed within the first week due to thrombosis, followed by pancreatectomy and the transplant occurred more than 6 months prior to enrolment |

reduced regimen is preferred due to the potential diabetogenic effects (Kaufman et al., 2002; Toso et al., 2003; Toso et al., 2006; Cure et al., 2008b). New anti-inflammatory agents that target cytokines (Hering et al., 2005; Alejandro et al., 2008; Faradji et al., 2008; Matsumoto et al., 2011; Rickels et al., 2013) or chemokines (Citro et al., 2012) involved in the amplification of the innate immune response post implant, as well as biologics that target costimulation pathways and/or adhesion molecules (cytotoxic T-lymphocyte-associated protein 4 (CTLA4-Ig) or leucocyte function antigen (LFA)-1, respectively), are currently being evaluated for their potential synergy and, importantly, lower islet cell and organ toxicity profiles (Badell et al., 2010; Posselt et al., 2010a, 2010b; Turgeon et al., 2010; Fotino and Pileggi, 2011).

## Concomitant therapy and clinical monitoring

Therapy comprises conventional antibiotic prophylaxis for *Pneumocystis carinii* (trimethoprim and sulfamethoxazole) and antiviral prophylaxis to reduce the risk or treat CMV infections and reactivation of EBV infection (vanglancyclovir daily for the first trimester post-transplant). Monitoring of viraemia in peripheral blood samples by PCR is routinely performed in transplant recipients (Hafiz et al., 2004; Cure et al., 2008a). Heparin is generally administered with the islet infusion, while low-molecular-weight heparin injections are given as maintenance in the post-transplant period. This regimen is implemented to enhance islet engraftment in the hepatic portal system while reducing the risk of portal thrombosis. To avoid high workload for newly implanted islets, basal insulin therapy is administered in the immediate peritransplant period, while strictly monitoring glycaemic control to prevent hypoglycaemia.

Clinical monitoring includes routine cell blood counts (erythrocytes, white blood cells, and differential), haemoglobin, platelets, and coagulation markers, to assess the myelosuppressive effects of immunosuppression. Anaemia may require iron supplementation and erythropoietin treatment for more severe cases. Marrow stimulation with granulocyte-colony stimulating factor (G-CSF) is promptly implemented for severe neutropaenia. Monitoring also includes standard serological tests (serum creatinine, azotaemia), urine tests (spot and 24-hour collections), and glomerular filtration rates (GFR) estimated using different algorithms (i.e. modification of diet in renal disease (MDRD)) to assess the impact of restoring β-cell function on the progression of diabetic nephropathy, and timely correct nephrotoxicity of immunosuppressants (i.e. CNI and mTOR inhibitors). Standard nephroprotective therapy with ACE inhibitors and of antagonists of angiotensin-receptor (ARB) should be considered in transplant recipients treated with immunosuppressive drugs known for their negative effects on renal function (Senior et al., 2005; Maffi et al., 2007; Warnock et al., 2008; Leitao et al., 2009, 2010b). Elevations of blood pressure above the range 130/80 mm Hg are promptly treated pharmacologically. Lipids are monitored and dyslipidaemia is promptly treated (i.e. statins targeting low-density lipoprotein (LDL) cholesterol levels < 100 mg/dL) in transplanted patients, particularly since immunosuppressive drugs (i.e. mTOR inhibitors and CNIs) may contribute to dyslipidaemia, which may be toxic to β-cells (Leitao et al., 2010a).

Transient and self-limited transaminitis is common following islet embolization in the liver sinusoids (Barshes et al., 2005; Hafiz et al., 2005) and associates with the ultrasound hyperechoic pattern of the liver parenchyma. Ultrasound evaluation of the liver and abdominal cavity in the days post-transplant may help in identifying procedural complications (i.e. portal thrombosis, peritoneal haemorrhage) and alterations of echogeneicity of hepatic parenchyma. PRA titres are performed to determine sensitization against HLA class I and II of the histocompatibility complex of transplanted tissue. Achievement of adequate immunosuppressive levels generally prevents allosensitization (Lobo et al., 2005; Rickels et al., 2006; Cardani et al., 2007). However, alloreactivity against donor or non-specific antigens may develop whenever there is reduction (i.e. during infections, toxicity, and drug conversion, amongst other causes) or suspension (i.e. after complete graft loss) of immunosuppression (Campbell et al., 2007; Cardani et al., 2007). Autoantibody titres (towards glutamic acid decarboxylase (GAD), zinc finger protein IA-1 (IA-1), insulin, and zinc transporter 8 (ZnT8)) are monitored in patients with type 1 diabetes as they may enable the detection of a reactivation of the autoimmune process (i.e. positive values in previously negative subjects, or increased titres), which is associated with lower rates of insulin independence and shorter duration of islet allograft function (Shapiro et al., 2006). New assays for the evaluation of autoreactive T-cells using tetramers are underway to help refine immune monitoring of transplant recipients (Bosi et al., 1989; Vendrame et al., 2010; Burke et al., 2011).

## Monitoring islet graft function

Metabolic monitoring of transplanted islets includes several readouts (see Table 18.3). Subjects with type 1 diabetes who have undetectable stimulated C-peptide (< 0.3 ng/dL) before transplant are currently considered for islet transplantation, so that monitoring of basal and stimulated C-peptide can be used as a biomarker of graft function, even if exogenous insulin is administered. Several algorithms and indices that combine multiple parameters have been proposed to help with the functional assessment of islet transplant recipients (Ryan et al., 2001, 2002, 2005b; Faradji et al., 2007; Matsumoto et al., 2009; Takita et al., 2011) and identify early signs of graft dysfunction. The response to stimulation with secretagogues (i.e. glucose, arginine, or mixed-meal test) is performed at baseline and periodically throughout post-transplant follow-up

**Table 18.3** Monitoring of islet graft function

| Standard | Stimulation | Indices |
|---|---|---|
| Glycosylated Hb (A1c) | Mixed meal | Hypo score |
| Fasting glycaemia | Intravenous glucose | Liability index |
| Postprandial glycaemia | Intravenous arginine | Beta score |
| MAGE | | Basal C-peptide/ glucose ratio |
| CGMS | | HOMA-B |
| Basal C-peptide | | HOMA-IR |
| Daily insulin requirement | | |

MAGE, Mean amplitude of glucose excursions; CGMS, continuous glucose monitoring system; HOMA-B, homeostasis model assessment—functional β-cell mass; HOMA-IR, homeostasis model assessment—insulin-resistance.

to evaluate the potency of the transplanted islets. Exogenous insulin therapy (generally at much fewer doses than before transplant) is promptly introduced when graft dysfunction is detected (based on random glycaemic sampling demonstrate on three subsequent occasions within the same week with fasting values > 140 mg/dL and postprandial values > 180 mg/dL, or after two consecutive weeks with A1c values > 6.5%.

## Clinical outcomes of islet cell transplantation

Insulin independence is achieved reproducibly after transplantation of an adequate islet mass (≥ 10,000 islet equivalents (IEq)/kg of recipient's body weight), generally obtained from one or more donor pancreas. Data from the centres reporting to the Clinical Islet Transplant Registry and from trial reports show insulin independence at 1 year from completion of the transplant in > 70% of cases, with virtually 100% of graft function (measurable C-peptide) if patients maintain adequate immunosuppression regimens (Alejandro et al., 2008). The impact of islet transplantation on metabolic control has been quite reproducible in recent clinical trials (see Table 18.4). Optimal glycaemic control is generally achieved soon after islet transplantation. Insulin independence can be observed when adequate islet numbers are implanted. However, even when islet numbers are suboptimal, the much-reduced than baseline exogenous insulin doses are required to attain tight metabolic control with reduction of mean amplitude of glycaemic excursions (MAGE) throughout the day and normalization of A1c < 6.5% (Shapiro et al., 2000; Froud et al., 2005).

One of the most important effects of islet transplantation is the prevention of severe hypoglycaemic events (Johnson et al., 2004; Poggioli et al., 2006; Leitao et al., 2008; Tharavanij et al., 2008). This phenomenon is confirmed by the means of the Hypo Score and Liability Index, which showed significantly reduced incidence of severe hypoglycaemia over a 4-year follow-up period in islet transplant recipients, suggesting the achievement of a better and more physiological metabolic control than medical therapy (Ryan et al., 2004, 2005a).

**Table 18.4** Benefits of islet transplantation

| |
|---|
| **Metabolic control** |
| ◆ Reduction of exogenous insulin requirements or insulin independence |
| ◆ Reduction of MAGE |
| ◆ Reduction or normalization of A1c |
| ◆ Absence of severe hypoglycaemia |
| **Quality of life** |
| ◆ Reduced fear of hypoglycaemia |
| ◆ Improvement of diabetes QOL |
| **Diabetes complications** |
| ◆ Improvement of micro- and macro-angiopathy |
| ◆ Improvement of cardiovascular and endothelial function |
| ◆ Reduced incidence of acute cardiovascular events |
| ◆ Reduced nephropathy progression |
| ◆ Stabilization/slower neuropathy progression |
| ◆ Stabilization/slower retinopathy progression |

The prevention of severe hypoglycaemia observed after islet transplantation persists long term, as far as C-peptide is measurable, even after exogenous insulin is reintroduced to help maintain optimal glycaemic control (i.e. suboptimal islet mass implant or development of graft dysfunction) (Pileggi et al., 2004; Alejandro et al., 2008). From the metabolic standpoint (reviewed in Rickels, 2012), transplantation of islet cells is associated with (1) restoration of β-cell responses to secretagogue stimulation leading to (2) improved 'first phase' insulin secretion in response to intravenous glucose, and (3) increased C-peptide secretion in response to oral glucose. These effects associate with (4) normalization of glycaemic threshold triggering the release of counter-regulatory hormones during hypoglycaemic clamp studies, (5) partial normalization of the magnitude of the vegetative response, and (6) quasinormalization of glucagon secretion in response to hypoglycaemia (Paty et al., 2002, 2006; Rickels et al., 2005a, 2005b, 2007). Collectively, these observations help explain the improvements in metabolic control and recovery of hypoglycaemia awareness observed after islet transplantation persisting several months after loss of detectable C-peptide (graft failure). The absence of severe hypoglycaemic events following islet transplantation is likely the reason for the significant positive effects on the fear score, gained sense of independence from insulin therapy, and overall quality of life (QOL) assessed by standardized psychometric instruments and interviews carried out by psychologists (Johnson et al., 2004; Poggioli et al., 2006; Toso et al., 2007; Leitao et al., 2008; Tharavanij et al., 2008).

Based on the recognition that the improvement of metabolic control, absence of severe hypoglycaemic events, amelioration of diabetes complications, and sustained QOL improvements outweigh the drawbacks of islet transplantation in this selected population with unstable diabetes, insulin independence, although desirable, is no longer considered the primary objective of islet transplantation.

## Impact on diabetes complications

Proof-of-concept of the beneficial impact of restoring β-cell function by islet transplantation on diabetes complications is mostly based on the results of non-randomized pilot studies and should be cautiously interpreted (reviewed in Bassi and Fiorina, 2011). Nonetheless, several benefits (Table 18.4), including improved micro- and macro-angiopathy (the main causes of diabetic nephropathy) and stabilization/reduced progression of retinopathy and neuropathy, amelioration of cardiovascular and endothelial function, and reduction of atherothrombotic profile paralleled by reduced incidence of cardiovascular accidents and higher survival rates, have been reported in IAK recipients (Fiorina et al., 2003a, 2003b, 2005a; Del Carro et al., 2007). Improved longevity of allogeneic renal transplants has been reported after islet transplantation (Fiorina et al., 2005b).

## Adverse events

The most frequent adverse events (AEs) observed are mainly related to the transplant procedure and immunosuppression therapy (see Table 18.5). Procedural AEs include portal thrombosis and bleeding, which have become rare thanks to the introduction of technical improvements that have contributed to reducing the morbidity associated with the islet transplant procedure (i.e. using

**Table 18.5** Frequent complications in islet transplant recipients

| |
|---|
| **Procedure-related** |
| ◆ Haemorrhage |
| ◆ Portal thrombosis |
| ◆ Transient transaminitis |
| **Immunosuppression-related** |
| ◆ Anaemia |
| ◆ Leucopaenia |
| ◆ Neutropaenia |
| ◆ Dyslipidaemia |
| ◆ Oral ulcers (sirolimus) |
| ◆ Diarrhoea (mycophenolic acid) |
| ◆ CMV colitis |
| ◆ Upper respiratory infections |
| ◆ Interstitial pneumonitis (sirolimus) |
| ◆ Neurotoxicity (tacrolimus) |
| ◆ Urinary infections |
| ◆ Ovarian cysts |
| ◆ Dysmenorrhoea |
| ◆ Nephropathy |
| ◆ Proteinuria |
| ◆ Cutaneous infections |
| ◆ Skin cancer |

gas-permeable bags and infusion by gravity to reduce clumping and sudden rise of portal pressure during the embolization procedure; antithrombotic prophylaxis; ultrasound-guided portal vein cannulation; monitoring of portal pressure; and sealing of the trans-hepatic catheter tract with fibrin plugs (Alejandro and Mintz, 1988; Casey et al., 2002; Baidal et al., 2003; Froud et al., 2004). Known untoward side effects of immunosuppressive drugs are observed also after islet transplantation (Table 18.5) (Hafiz et al., 2005), including opportunistic infections (urinary tract, upper respiratory tract, and skin), myelosuppression (neutropaenia), and gastrointestinal effects (buccal ulcers, diarrhoea). Generally, these adverse events are not severe and are successfully controlled with medical treatment. CMV and EBV viraemia in the presence of overt clinical symptoms (i.e. de-novo infection or reactivation in seropositive subjects) should prompt timely implementation of antiviral therapy and reduction of immunosuppressive drug dose (Cure et al., 2008a), which may result in resolution of symptoms without compromising graft survival. Immunosuppressive drugs may result in neuro- and/or nephrotoxicity, which may require modifications of the therapeutic regimens (i.e. dose reduction or conversion to a different combination) (Molinari et al., 2005; Ponte et al., 2007).

## Current challenges and future developments

Among the many challenges currently limiting islet cell transplantation (Pileggi et al., 2006a; Mineo et al., 2009) is the progressive loss of insulin independence reported in approximately 90% of type 1 diabetes recipients who required reintroduction of exogenous insulin despite persistence of detectable C-peptide under the 'Edmonton protocol' (induction with anti-IL2R antibody; maintenance with sirolimus and tacrolimus) and variations trials (Shapiro et al., 2000, 2006; Hering et al., 2005; Ryan et al., 2005a; Vantyghem et al., 2009; Bellin et al., 2012b). The use of potent lymphodepletion (i.e. thymoglobulin, anti-CD3 or anti-CD52 antibodies) and/or biologics (anti-IL2R, anti-TNF, anti-LFA-1 antibody, or CTLA-4 Ig) improved the outcome to approximately 50% of insulin independence at 5 years after islet transplantation, which is comparable to some of the data in whole pancreas transplantation in subjects with type 1 diabetes (Froud et al., 2008; Tan et al., 2008; Vantyghem et al., 2009; Posselt et al., 2010a, 2010b; Bellin et al., 2012b).

Another challenge is the cost of the procedure. Dedicated infrastructures and specialized personnel are needed, which impose a significant financial burden on the Clinical Islet Transplant Program. The team's experience in cell processing and management of immunosuppression can impact the success of an islet transplantation clinical trial (Shapiro et al., 2006). The development of regional consortia of distant transplant centres supported by a single cell-processing centre represents a practical and cost-effective strategy, as shown by European and US trials (Benhamou et al., 2001; Goss et al., 2002, 2004). In the US, healthcare providers currently reimburse only islet autotransplantation, while a validation multicentre trial is close to completion to obtain a Biological License Application approved by the FDA. In European countries and Canada, where the health system covers the costs of the procedure, clinical islet programmes are moving at a faster pace than in the US.

Great efforts are currently focused on improvement of donor selection and organ allocation, in order to increase pancreas utilization for transplantation. These include development of novel cytoprotective strategies to enhance the recovery of islets with uncompromised potency reproducibly from deceased donor pancreata, and enhancing their resilience from hypoxia and oxidative stress at the time of transplantation.

Meanwhile, encouraging progress has been made in the use of unlimited alternative sources of transplantable islets, including xenogeneic cells (i.e. porcine) (reviewed in Marigliano et al., 2011) and those derived from human stem cells (reviewed in Baiu et al., 2011). The potential choice of pigs as islet donors derives from the fact that they may be available in plentiful amounts, from 'specific pathogen-free' herds. The recent progress of genetic engineering has rendered available pigs lacking or overexpressing specific molecules that may reduce their immunogenicity for transplantation into humans, leading to long-term function under conventional immunosuppressive regimens that are used for allogeneic cells or facilitating the induction of immune tolerance to xenogeneic islet cells.

Regenerative medicine approaches using human stem cells from embryonic or adult sources are also showing encouraging results toward generation of insulin-producing cells from human multipotent stem cells; main efforts are currently concentrating on the optimization of the differentiation protocols to provide consistently cellular products with adequate potency and safety profiles (Ricordi and Edlund, 2008; Dominguez-Bendala et al., 2011). Moreover, alternative transplantation sites (reviewed in Cantarelli and Piemonti, 2011) are being considered to enhance islet engraftment and allow for sustained graft function long term, including through novel bioengineering approaches (reviewed in Hallé et al., 2009) to create a favourable micro-environment and/

or immune isolated islets to reduce/avoid life-long immunosuppression needs (reviewed in Hallé et al., 2009; Basta and Calafiore, 2011)].

## Conclusion

We are living in very exciting times in the field of β-cell replacement therapies for the treatment of diabetes. Transplantation of pancreatic islet cells represents a viable option to achieve stable metabolic control in the most severe manifestation of type 1 diabetes, which cannot be matched by conventional medical treatments. The steady progress of clinical islet transplantation and the promising emerging new approaches to modulate immunity and overcome β-cell paucity justify great optimism for the potential of β-cell replacement in all cases of insulin-dependent diabetes in the near future.

## Acknowledgements

This work was partially supported by the National Institutes of Health (NIDDK 5R01 DK25802, 5R01 DK56953, 1U01 DK70460, 1R21 DK076098, 5R01 DK059993, 1DP2 DK083096, NCRR-ICR5, U42 RR016603, NCRR-GCRC MO1RR16587, NBI 1R01 EB008009), the Cooperative Study Group for Autoimmune Disease Prevention Formation and History (NIH—5U19AI050864-10), the Juvenile Diabetes Research Foundation International (JDRFI) (under grants 4-2000-946, 4-2000-947, 4-2004-361, 4-2008-811, and 17-2012-361), the Leona M. and Harry B. Helmsley Charitable Trust (managed by the JDRFI), the American Diabetes Association (7-13-IN-32), the state of Florida, the University of Miami (Interdisciplinary Research Development Initiative), and the Diabetes Research Institute Foundation (<http://www.diabetesresearch.org>). A contract for support of this research, sponsored by US Congressman Bill Young and funded by a special congressional out of the US Navy Bureau of Medicine and Surgery, is presently managed by the Naval Health Research Center, San Diego. The authors alone are responsible for reporting and interpreting these data; the views expressed herein are those of the authors and not necessarily those of the funding agencies or of the US government.

## References

Alejandro R, Mintz DH (1988) Experimental and clinical methods of islet transplantation. In: van Schilfgaarde R, Hardy MA (eds) *Transplantation of the Endocrine Pancreas in Diabetes Mellitus*. Elsevier, Amsterdam.

Alejandro R, Barton FB, Hering BJ, Wease S (2008) 2008 Update from the Collaborative Islet Transplant Registry. *Transplantation*, **86**:1783–1788.

Alejandro R, Strasser S, Zucker PF, Mintz DH (1990) Isolation of pancreatic islets from dogs. Semiautomated purification on albumin gradients. *Transplantation*, **50**:207–210.

Badell IR, Russell MC, Thompson PW, et al. (2010) LFA-1-specific therapy prolongs allograft survival in rhesus macaques. *J Clin Invest*, **120**:4520–4531.

Baidal DA, Froud T, Ferreira JV, Khan A, Alejandro R, Ricordi C (2003) The bag method for islet cell infusion. *Cell Transplant*, **12**:809–813.

Baiu D, Merriam F, Odorico J (2011) Potential pathways to restore beta-cell mass: pluripotent stem cells, reprogramming, and endogenous regeneration. *Curr Diab Rep*, **11**:392–401.

Barshes NR, Lee TC, Goodpastor SE, et al. (2005) Transaminitis after pancreatic islet transplantation. *J Am Coll Surg*, **200**:353–361.

Bassi R, Fiorina P (2011) Impact of islet transplantation on diabetes complications and quality of life. *Curr Diab Rep*, **11**:355–363.

Basta G, Calafiore R (2011) Immunoisolation of pancreatic islet grafts with no recipient's immunosuppression: actual and future perspectives. *Curr Diab Rep*, **11**:384–391.

Basta G, Montanucci P, Luca G, et al. (2011) Long-term metabolic and immunological follow-up of nonimmunosuppressed patients with type 1 diabetes treated with microencapsulated islet allografts: four cases. *Diabetes Care*, **34**:2406–2409.

Bellin MD, Kandaswamy R, Parkey J, et al. (2008) Prolonged insulin independence after islet allotransplants in recipients with type 1 diabetes. *Am J Transplant*, **8**:2463–2470.

Bellin MD, Sutherland DE (2010) Pediatric islet autotransplantation: indication, technique, and outcome. *Curr Diab Rep*, **10**:326–331.

Bellin MD, Freeman ML, Schwarzenberg SJ, et al. (2011a) Quality of life improves for pediatric patients after total pancreatectomy and islet autotransplant for chronic pancreatitis. *Clin Gastroenterol Hepatol*, **9**:793–799.

Bellin MD, Sutherland DE, Beilman GJ, et al. (2011b) Similar islet function in islet allotransplant and autotransplant recipients, despite lower islet mass in autotransplants. *Transplantation*, **91**:367–372.

Bellin M, Balamurugan AN, Pruett TL, Sutherland DER (2012a) No islets left behind: islet autotransplantation for surgery-induced diabetes. *Curr Diab Rep*, **12**(5):580–586.

Bellin MD, Barton FB, Heitman A, et al. (2012b) Potent induction immunotherapy promotes long-term insulin independence after islet transplantation in type 1 diabetes. *Am J Transplant*, **12**:1576–1583.

Benhamou PY, Oberholzer J, Toso C, et al. (2001) Human islet transplantation network for the treatment of type I diabetes: first data from the Swiss-French GRAGIL consortium (1999–2000). Groupe de Recherche Rhin Rhjne Alpes Geneve pour la Transplantation d'Ilots de Langerhans. *Diabetologia*, **44**:859–864.

Blondet JJ, Carlson AM, Kobayashi T, et al. (2007) The role of total pancreatectomy and islet autotransplantation for chronic pancreatitis. *Surg Clin N Am*, **87**:1477–1501.

Bosi E, Bottazzo GF, Secchi A, et al. (1989) Islet cell autoimmunity in type I diabetic patients after HLA-mismatched pancreas transplantation. *Diabetes*, **38**(Suppl 1):82–84.

Burke GW 3rd, Vendrame F, Pileggi A, et al. (2011) Recurrence of autoimmunity following pancreas transplantation. *Curr Diab Rep*, **11**:413–419.

Cabrera O, Berman DM, Kenyon NS, Ricordi C, Berggren PO, Caicedo A (2006) The unique cytoarchitecture of human pancreatic islets has implications for islet cell function. *Proc Natl Acad Sci USA*, **103**:2334–2339.

Campbell PM, Senior PA, Salam A, et al. (2007) High risk of sensitization after failed islet transplantation. *Am J Transplant*, **7**:2311–2317.

Cantarelli E, Piemonti L (2011) Alternative transplantation sites for pancreatic islet grafts. *Curr Diab Rep*, **11**:364–374.

Cardani R, Pileggi A, Ricordi C, et al. (2007) Allosensitization of islet allograft recipients. *Transplantation*, **84**:1413–1427.

Casavilla A, Rilo HL, Julian TB, Fontes PA, Starzl TE, Ricordi C (1992) Laparoscopic approach for islet cell transplantation. *Transplant Proc*, **24**:2800.

Casey JJ, Lakey JR, Ryan EA, et al. (2002) Portal venous pressure changes after sequential clinical islet transplantation. *Transplantation*, **74**:913–915.

Citro A, Cantarelli E, Maffi P, et al. (2012) CXCR1/2 inhibition enhances pancreatic islet survival after transplantation. *J Clin Invest*, **122**:3647–3651.

Cure P, Froud T, Leitao CB, et al. (2008a) Late Epstein Barr virus reactivation in islet after kidney transplantation. *Transplantation*, **86**:1324–1325.

Cure P, Pileggi A, Froud T, et al. (2008b) Improved metabolic control and quality of life in seven patients with type 1 diabetes following islet after kidney transplantation. *Transplantation*, **85**:801–812.

del Carro U, Fiorina P, Amadio S, et al. (2007) Evaluation of polyneuropathy markers in type 1 diabetic kidney transplant patients and effects of islet transplantation: neurophysiological and skin biopsy longitudinal analysis. *Diabetes Care*, **30**:3063–3069.

Dominguez-Bendala J, Pileggi A, Ricordi C (2011) Islet cell therapy and pancreatic stem cells. In: Atala A, Lanza R, Thomson JA, Nerem RM (eds) *Principles of Regenerative Medicine*, 2nd edn. Academic Press, New York.

Dufrane D, Goebbels RM, Gianello P (2010) Alginate macroencapsulation of pig islets allows correction of streptozotocin-induced diabetes in primates up to 6 months without immunosuppression. *Transplantation*, **90**:1054–1062.

Faradji RN, Monroy K, Messinger S, et al. (2007) Simple measures to monitor beta-cell mass and assess islet graft dysfunction. *Am J Transplant*, **7**:303–308.

Faradji RN, Tharavanij T, Messinger S, et al. (2008) Long-term insulin independence and improvement in insulin secretion after supplemental islet infusion under exenatide and etanercept. *Transplantation*, **86**:1658–1665.

Fiorina P, Folli F, Bertuzzi F, et al. (2003a) Long-term beneficial effect of islet transplantation on diabetic macro-/microangiopathy in type 1 diabetic kidney-transplanted patients. *Diabetes Care*, **26**:1129–1136.

Fiorina P, Folli F, Maffi P, et al. (2003b) Islet transplantation improves vascular diabetic complications in patients with diabetes who underwent kidney transplantation: a comparison between kidney-pancreas and kidney-alone transplantation. *Transplantation*, **75**:1296–1301.

Fiorina P, Gremizzi C, Maffi P, et al. (2005a) Islet transplantation is associated with an improvement of cardiovascular function in type 1 diabetic kidney transplant patients. *Diabetes Care*, **28**:1358–1365.

Fiorina P, Venturini M, Folli F, et al. (2005b) Natural history of kidney graft survival, hypertrophy, and vascular function in end-stage renal disease type 1 diabetic kidney-transplanted patients: beneficial impact of pancreas and successful islet cotransplantation. *Diabetes Care*, **28**:1303–1310.

Fotino C, Pileggi A (2011) Blockade of leukocyte function antigen-1 (LFA-1) in clinical islet transplantation. *Curr Diab Rep*, **11**:337–344.

Frank AM, Barker CF, Markmann JF (2005) Comparison of whole organ pancreas and isolated islet transplantation for type 1 diabetes. *Adv Surg*, **39**:137–163.

Froud T, Yrizarry JM, Alejandro R, Ricordi C (2004) Use of D-STAT to prevent bleeding following percutaneous transhepatic intraportal islet transplantation. *Cell Transplant*, **13**:55–59.

Froud T, Ricordi C, Baidal DA, et al. (2005) Islet transplantation in type 1 diabetes mellitus using cultured islets and steroid-free immunosuppression: Miami experience. *Am J Transplant*, **5**:2037–2046.

Froud T, Baidal DA, Faradji R, et al. (2008) Islet transplantation with alemtuzumab induction and calcineurin-free maintenance immunosuppression results in improved short- and long-term outcomes. *Transplantation*, **86**:1695–1701.

Gerber PA, Pavlicek V, Demartines N, et al. (2008) Simultaneous islet-kidney vs pancreas-kidney transplantation in type 1 diabetes mellitus: a 5 year single centre follow-up. *Diabetologia*, **51**:110–119.

Goss JA, Schock AP, Brunicardi FC, et al. (2002) Achievement of insulin independence in three consecutive type-1 diabetic patients via pancreatic islet transplantation using islets isolated at a remote islet isolation center. *Transplantation*, **74**:1761–1766.

Goss JA, Goodpastor SE, Brunicardi FC, et al. (2004) Development of a human pancreatic islet-transplant program through a collaborative relationship with a remote islet-isolation center. *Transplantation*, **77**:462–466.

Hafiz MM, Poggioli R, Caulfield A, et al. (2004) Cytomegalovirus prevalence and transmission after islet allograft transplant in patients with type 1 diabetes mellitus. *Am J Transplant*, **4**:1697–1702.

Hafiz MM, Faradji RN, Froud T, et al. (2005) Immunosuppression and procedure-related complications in 26 patients with type 1 diabetes mellitus receiving allogeneic islet cell transplantation. *Transplantation*, **80**:1718–1728.

Hallé JP, Devos P, Rosenberg L (2009) *The Bioartificial Pancreas and Other Biohybrid Therapies*. Transworld Research Network, Kerala, India.

Hering BJ, Kandaswamy R, Ansite JD, et al. (2005) Single-donor, marginal-dose islet transplantation in patients with type 1 diabetes. *JAMA*, **293**:830–835.

Ichii H, Pileggi A, Molano RD, et al. (2005) Rescue purification maximizes the use of human islet preparations for transplantation. *Am J Transplant*, **5**:21–30.

Johnson JA, Kotovych M, Ryan EA, Shapiro AM (2004) Reduced fear of hypoglycemia in successful islet transplantation. *Diabetes Care*, **27**:624–625.

Kaufman DB, Baker MS, Chen X, Leventhal JR, Stuart FP (2002) Sequential kidney/islet transplantation using prednisone-free immunosuppression. *Am J Transplant*, **2**:674–677.

Leitao CB, Tharavanij T, Cure P, et al. (2008) Restoration of hypoglycemia awareness after islet transplantation. *Diabetes Care*, **31**:2113–2115.

Leitao CB, Cure P, Messinger S, et al. (2009) Stable renal function after islet transplantation: importance of patient selection and aggressive clinical management. *Transplantation*, **87**:681–688.

Leitao CB, Bernetti K, Tharavanij T, et al. (2010a) Lipotoxicity and decreased islet graft survival. *Diabetes Care*, **33**:658–660.

Leitao CB, Froud T, Cure P, et al. (2010b) Nonalbumin proteinuria in islet transplant recipients. *Cell Transplant*, **19**:119–125.

Lobo PI, Spencer C, Simmons WD, et al. (2005) Development of anti-human leukocyte antigen class 1 antibodies following allogeneic islet cell transplantation. *Transplant Proc*, **37**,3438–3440.

Maffi P, Bertuzzi F, de Taddeo F, et al. (2007) Kidney function after islet transplant alone in type 1 diabetes: impact of immunosuppressive therapy on progression of diabetic nephropathy. *Diabetes Care*, **30**:1150–1155.

Marigliano M, Bertera S, Grupillo M, Trucco M, Bottino R (2011) Pig-to-nonhuman primates pancreatic islet xenotransplantation: an overview. *Curr Diab Rep*, **11**:402–412.

Marzorati S, Pileggi A, Ricordi C (2007) Allogeneic islet transplantation. *Expert Opin Biol Ther*, **7**:1627–1645.

Matsumoto S, Tanaka K, Strong DM, Reems JA (2004) Efficacy of human islet isolation from the tail section of the pancreas for the possibility of living donor islet transplantation. *Transplantation*, **78**:839–843.

Matsumoto S, Okitsu T, Iwanaga Y, et al. (2005) Insulin independence of unstable diabetic patient after single living donor islet transplantation. *Transplant Proc*, **37**:3427–3429.

Matsumoto S, Noguchi H, Hatanaka N, et al. (2009) SUITO index for evaluation of efficacy of single donor islet transplantation. *Cell Transplant*, **18**:557–562.

Matsumoto S, Takita M, Chaussabel D, et al. (2011) Improving efficacy of clinical islet transplantation with iodixanol-based islet purification, thymoglobulin induction, and blockage of IL-1beta and TNF-alpha. *Cell Transpl*, **20**:1641–1647.

Mineo D, Pileggi A, Alejandro R, Ricordi C (2009) Point: steady progress and current challenges in clinical islet transplantation. *Diabetes Care*, **32**:1563–1569.

Molinari M, Al-Saif F, Ryan EA, et al. (2005) Sirolimus-induced ulceration of the small bowel in islet transplant recipients: report of two cases. *Am J Transplant*, **5**:2799–2804.

Najarian JS, Sutherland DE, Matas AJ, Goetz FC (1979) Human islet autotransplantation following pancreatectomy. *Transplant Proc*, **11**:336–340.

Owen RJ, Ryan EA, O'Kelly K, et al. (2003) Percutaneous transhepatic pancreatic islet cell transplantation in type 1 diabetes mellitus: radiologic aspects. *Radiology*, **229**:165–170.

Paty BW, Ryan EA, Shapiro AM, Lakey JR, Robertson RP (2002) Intrahepatic islet transplantation in type 1 diabetic patients does not restore hypoglycemic hormonal counterregulation or symptom recognition after insulin independence. *Diabetes*, **51**:3428–3434.

Paty BW, Senior PA, Lakey JR, Shapiro AM, Ryan EA (2006) Assessment of glycemic control after islet transplantation using the continuous glucose monitor in insulin-independent versus insulin-requiring type 1 diabetes subjects. *Diabetes Technol Ther*, **8**:165–173.

Pedraza E, Brady AC, Fraker CA, et al. (2013). Macroporous three dimensional PDMS scaffolds for extrahepatic islet transplantation. *Cell Transplant*, **22**(7):1123–1135.

Perez VL, Caicedo A, Berman DM, et al. (2011) The anterior chamber of the eye as a clinical transplantation site for the treatment of diabetes: a study in a baboon model of diabetes. *Diabetologia*, **54**:1121–1126.

Piemonti L, Pileggi A. (2013) 25 Years of the Ricordi Automated Method for Islet Isolation. *CellR4* **1**: e128

Pileggi A, Ricordi C, Kenyon NS, et al. (2004) Twenty years of clinical islet transplantation at the Diabetes Research Institute—University of Miami. *Clin Transplant*, 2004:177–204.

Pileggi A, Cobianchi L, Inverardi L, Ricordi C (2006a) Overcoming the challenges now limiting islet transplantation: a sequential, integrated approach. *Ann N Y Acad Sci*, 1079:383–398.

Pileggi A, Molano RD, Ricordi C, et al. (2006b) Reversal of diabetes by pancreatic islet transplantation into a subcutaneous, neovascularized device. *Transplantation*, **81**:1318–1324.

Poggioli R, Faradji RN, Ponte G, et al. (2006) Quality of life after islet transplantation. *Am J Transplant*, **6**:371–378.

Ponte GM, Baidal DA, Romanelli P, et al. (2007) Resolution of severe atopic dermatitis after tacrolimus withdrawal. *Cell Transplant*, **16**:23–30.

Posselt AM, Bellin MD, Tavakol M, et al. (2010a) Islet transplantation in type 1 diabetics using an immunosuppressive protocol based on the anti-LFA-1 antibody efalizumab. *Am J Transplant*, **10**:1870–1880.

Posselt AM, Szot GL, Frassetto LA, et al. (2010b) Islet transplantation in type 1 diabetic patients using calcineurin inhibitor-free immunosuppressive protocols based on T-cell adhesion or costimulation blockade. *Transplantation*, **90**:1595–1601.

Rafael E, Tibell A, Ryden M, et al. (2008) Intramuscular autotransplantation of pancreatic islets in a 7-year-old child: a 2-year follow-up. *Am J Transplant*, **8**:458–462.

Rickels MR (2012) Recovery of endocrine function after islet and pancreas transplantation. *Curr Diab Rep*, **12**(5):587–596.

Rickels MR, Schutta MH, Markmann JF, Barker CF, Naji A, Teff KL (2005a) {beta}-Cell function following human islet transplantation for type 1 diabetes. *Diabetes*, **54**:100–106.

Rickels MR, Schutta MH, Mueller R, et al. (2005b) Islet cell hormonal responses to hypoglycemia after human islet transplantation for type 1 diabetes. *Diabetes*, **54**:3205–3211.

Rickels MR, Kearns J, Markmann E, et al. (2006) HLA sensitization in islet transplantation. *Clin Transplant*, 2006:413–420.

Rickels MR, Naji A, Teff KL (2007) Acute insulin responses to glucose and arginine as predictors of beta-cell secretory capacity in human islet transplantation. *Transplantation*, **84**:1357–1360.

Rickels MR, Liu C, Shlansky-Goldberg RD, et al. (2013) Improvement in beta-cell secretory capacity following human islet transplantation according to the CIT07 protocol. *Diabetes*, **62**(8):2890–2897.

Ricordi C, Edlund H (2008) Toward a renewable source of pancreatic beta-cells. *Nat Biotechnol*, **26**:397–398.

Ricordi C, Lacy PE, Finke EH, Olack BJ, Scharp DW (1988) Automated method for isolation of human pancreatic islets. *Diabetes*, **37**:413–420.

Robertson RP (2004) Consequences on beta-cell function and reserve after long-term pancreas transplantation. *Diabetes*, **53**:633–644.

Robertson RP, Lanz KJ, Sutherland DE, Kendall DM (2001) Prevention of diabetes for up to 13 years by autoislet transplantation after pancreatectomy for chronic pancreatitis. *Diabetes*, **50**:47–50.

Ryan EA, Lakey JR, Rajotte RV, et al. (2001) Clinical outcomes and insulin secretion after islet transplantation with the Edmonton protocol. *Diabetes*, **50**:710–719.

Ryan EA, LakeyJR, Paty BW, et al. (2002) Successful islet transplantation: continued insulin reserve provides long-term glycemic control. *Diabetes*, **51**:2148–2157.

Ryan EA, Shandro T, Green K, et al. (2004) Assessment of the severity of hypoglycemia and glycemic lability in type 1 diabetic subjects undergoing islet transplantation. *Diabetes*, **53**:955–962.

Ryan EA, Paty BW, Senior PA, et al. (2005a) Five-year follow-up after clinical islet transplantation. *Diabetes*, **54**:2060–2069.

Ryan EA, Paty BW, Senior PA, Lakey JR, Bigam D, Shapiro AM (2005b) Beta-score: an assessment of beta-cell function after islet transplantation. *Diabetes Care*, **28**:343–347.

Senior PA, Paty BW, Cockfield SM, Ryan EA, Shapiro AM (2005) Proteinuria developing after clinical islet transplantation resolves with sirolimus withdrawal and increased tacrolimus dosing. *Am J Transplant*, **5**:2318–2323.

Shapiro AM, Lakey JR, Ryan EA, et al. (2000) Islet transplantation in seven patients with type 1 diabetes mellitus using a glucocorticoid-free immunosuppressive regimen. *N Engl J Med*, **343**:230–238.

Shapiro AM, Ricordi C, Hering BJ, et al. (2006) International trial of the Edmonton protocol for islet transplantation. *N Engl J Med*, **355**:1318–1330.

Skyler JS (2006) *Atlas of Diabetes*, 3rd edn. Current Medicine Inc, Philadelphia.

Takita M, Matsumoto S, Qin H, et al. (2011) Secretory unit of islet transplant objects (SUITO) index can predict severity of hypoglycemic episodes in clinical islet cell transplantation. *Cell Transplant*, **21**(1):91–98.

Tan J, Yang S, Cai J, et al. (2008) Simultaneous islet and kidney transplantation in seven patients with type 1 diabetes and end-stage renal disease using a glucocorticoid-free immunosuppressive regimen with alemtuzumab induction. *Diabetes*, **57**:2666–2671.

Teuscher AU, Kendall DM, Smets YF, Leone JP, Sutherland DE, Robertson RP (1998) Successful islet autotransplantation in humans: functional insulin secretory reserve as an estimate of surviving islet cell mass. *Diabetes*, **47**:324–330.

Tharavanij T, Betancourt A, Messinger S, et al. (2008) Improved long-term health-related quality of life after islet transplantation. *Transplantation*, **86**:1161–1167.

Toso C, Morel P, Bucher P, et al. (2003) Insulin independence after conversion to tacrolimus and sirolimus-based immunosuppression in islet-kidney recipients. *Transplantation*, **76**:1133–1134.

Toso C, Baertschiger R, Morel P, et al. (2006) Sequential kidney/islet transplantation: efficacy and safety assessment of a steroid-free immunosuppression protocol. *Am J Transplant*, **6**:1049–1058.

Toso C, Shapiro AM, Bowker S, et al. (2007) Quality of life after islet transplant: impact of the number of islet infusions and metabolic outcome. *Transplantation*, **84**:664–666.

Turgeon NA, Avila JG, Cano JA, et al. (2010) Experience with a novel efalizumab-based immunosuppressive regimen to facilitate single donor islet cell transplantation. *Am J Transplant*, **10**:2082–2091.

Tzakis AG, Ricordi C, Alejandro R, et al. (1990) Pancreatic islet transplantation after upper abdominal exenteration and liver replacement. *Lancet*, **336**:402–405.

Vantyghem MC, Kerr-Conte J, Arnalsteen L, et al. (2009) Primary graft function, metabolic control, and graft survival after islet transplantation. *Diabetes Care*, **32**:1473–1478.

Vendrame F, Pileggi A, Laughlin E, et al. (2010) Recurrence of type 1 diabetes after simultaneous pancreas-kidney transplantation, despite immunosuppression, is associated with autoantibodies and pathogenic autoreactive CD4 T-cells. *Diabetes*, **59**:947–957.

Warnock GL, Thompson DM, Meloche RM, et al. (2008) A multi-year analysis of islet transplantation compared with intensive medical therapy on progression of complications in type 1 diabetes. *Transplantation*, **86**:1762–1766.

Weber CJ, Hardy MA, Pi-Sunyer F, Zimmerman E, Reemtsma K (1978) Tissue culture preservation and intramuscular transplantation of pancreatic islets. *Surgery*, **84**:166–174.


## Further reading

Clinical Islet Transplant Consortium: <http://www.citisletstudy.org/>.
Collaborative Islet Transplant Registry

Diabetes Research Institute Foundation
Health Resources and Services Administration
International Pancreas and Islet Transplant Association
National Institute of Diabetes and Digestive and Kidney Diseases (NIDDK)
Organ Procurement and Transplantation Network
The Cell Transplant Society
Scientific Registry of Transplant Recipients
United States Department of Health and Human Services
United Network for Organ Sharing (UNOS)
American Diabetes Association
American Society of Transplantation
American Society of Transplant Surgeons
Beta Cell Biology Consortium
European Pancreas Club
European Society for Organ Transplantation
International Pancreas Transplant Registry
International Xenotransplantation Association
Juvenile Diabetes Research Foundation
The Cure Focus Research Alliance

SECTION 6

# Liver

# CHAPTER 19

# Liver disease: epidemiology, pathophysiology, and medical management

Andre De Wolf, Paul Martin, and Hui-Hui Tan

## Epidemiology of liver disease

The true epidemiology and incidence of liver disease is difficult to ascertain, as most liver diseases are insidious, with a latent period between disease occurrence and detection (Kim, 2002). Hence, population-based studies are often used as surrogates to estimate disease burden.

### The United States

A population-based study by the CDC reported the incidence of newly diagnosed chronic liver disease in adults to be 63.9 per 100,000 population as seen by gastrointestinal specialists. The most common aetiology of chronic liver disease was hepatitis C (hepatitis C virus (HCV)) (42%), followed by hepatitis C combined with alcohol-related liver disease (22%), non-alcoholic fatty liver disease (NAFLD) (9%), alcoholic liver disease alone (8%), and hepatitis B (hepatitis B virus (HBV)) (3%). Other aetiologies (primary sclerosing cholangitis, primary biliary cirrhosis, hereditary haemochromatosis, autoimmune hepatitis, α1-antitrypsin deficiency, and hepatocellular carcinoma (HCC)) accounted for less than 3% of all newly diagnosed cases of chronic liver disease (Bell, 2008).

The prevalence of antibodies against HCV (anti-HCV) was 1.8% in the third National Health and Nutrition Examination Survey (NHANES III) study, which corresponds to approximately 3.9 million Americans infected with HCV. Of these, approximately 70%, or 2.7 million, had evidence of chronic infection as determined by the presence of the viral RNA in serum (Alter, 1999). By 2007, HCV mortality had superseded that of HIV in the US, with HCV and HBV deaths occurring disproportionately in middle-aged persons (Ly, 2012).

The prevalence of aminotransferase elevation in the general population in the NHANES III study was 7.9%—the majority of which could not be explained by alcohol consumption, viral hepatitis, or haemochromatosis. Aminotransferase elevation was more common in men compared to women (9.3% vs 6.6%), in Mexican Americans (14.9%), and in non-Hispanic blacks compared to non-Hispanic whites (8.1% vs 7.1%). Unexplained aminotransferase elevation (69.0%) was strongly associated with adiposity (higher body mass index, higher waist circumference) and other features of the metabolic syndrome (higher triglycerides, higher fasting insulin, lower high-density lipoprotein (HDL); and type 2 diabetes and hypertension in women) and thus may represent NAFLD (Clark, 2003). Other studies based on histological sources (liver biopsy, autopsy, and postmortem series) indicate that 10–40% (median ~ 20%) of the general population may have NAFLD (including steatosis alone) and 2–5% have non-alcoholic steatohepatitis (NASH) (Falk-Ytter et al., 2001).

Based on NHANES III data, the seroprevalence of HBV surface antigen (HBsAg) or antibodies to HBV core antigen is 4.9% (McQuillan, 1999). HBV infection is more prevalent in non-whites than whites, regardless of age. As the NHANES samples only civilian, non-institutionalized persons living in households, the true prevalence of disease may be underestimated (Kim, 2002). Approximately 240,000 new HBV infections occurred annually between 1988 and 1994 (Coleman, 1998), but in 1997 the estimated number of incident HBV cases was only 185,000.

In both Europe and the US the incidence of primary biliary cirrhosis (PBC) among adults (aged > 20 years) has been estimated to be between 2 and 3 per 100,000 persons per year, with a strong female predominance. While the incidence has remained unchanged since 1995, the prevalence has risen, suggesting that the survival is longer, which may be due to early diagnosis (Kim, 2002).

The incidence of fulminant hepatic failure is estimated to be 2,300–2,800 cases per year in the US. In earlier reports from the 1980s, viral hepatitis (hepatitis A virus (HAV), HBV, non-A non-B hepatitis) was the most common aetiology of fulminant hepatic failure in the US. By the 1990s, drug-induced (especially acetaminophen) causes had become the most common cause of fulminant hepatic failure (Rakela, 1985; McCashland, 1996; Schiodt, 1999).

Age-adjusted incidence rate of HCC increased from 1.4 per 100,000 during 1976–1980 to 4.7 per 100,000 during 1996–1997 (El-Serag and Mason, 1999). Asian-Americans have the highest incidence rates of HCC (up to 23 per 100,000 in Asian men > 60 years of age), followed by African-Americans, whose incidence is two to three times that of whites (El-Serag and Mason, 1999).

Chronic liver disease in 2008 was the twelfth commonest cause of mortality in the US, accounting for nearly 34,000 deaths annually (Kim, 2002; Kochanek, 2011).

### Europe

In the EU an estimated 29 million people have chronic liver disease. Alcohol consumption, viral hepatitis B and C, and the metabolic syndrome are reported to be leading causes of liver cirrhosis and primary liver tumours. Liver cirrhosis is responsible for around 170,000 deaths in Europe annually, with wide variations between countries—ranging from about 1 per 100,000 Greek women to 103 per 100,000 Hungarian men dying each year. The mortality rate from alcohol-related liver diseases is as high as 47 per 100,000 inhabitants. Liver cancer is responsible for almost 47,000 deaths in Europe annually, according to the WHO mortality database (Blachier, 2013). The mortality rate of primary liver cancer is very close to its incidence because of the lack of curative options for most patients (Blachier, 2013). The prevalence of NAFLD in the European population is 2–44% in the general population and 42.6–69.5% in patients with type 2 diabetes. The prevalence of chronic hepatitis C in the European population is 0.13–13.26%, whilst that of chronic hepatitis B is 0.5–0.7% (Anonymous, 2013; Blachier, 2013).

## Liver anatomy and physiology

The liver is the largest internal organ of the human body. It has a dual blood supply: the hepatic artery supplies oxygenated blood to the liver and the portal vein brings venous blood rich in the products of digestion that have been absorbed from the gastrointestinal tract, and also blood from the spleen and pancreas. Under normal circumstances the portal vein supplies approximately 70% of the liver's blood supply and the hepatic artery is responsible for the remaining 30%. Blood from the hepatic artery and portal vein perfuse the liver sinusoids and is conducted to the central vein of each liver lobule. Resistance to blood flow in the sinusoids is low under normal circumstances. The central veins drain into hepatic veins that drain into the inferior vena cava. The endothelial lining of the hepatic sinusoids is fenestrated and discontinuous. Beneath this lining is a very narrow space between the endothelial cells and the hepatic cells called the space of Disse, where hepatic stellate cells (Ito cells) are found. The spaces of Disse connect with lymphatic vessels in the interlobular septa, allowing excess fluid to be removed.

The liver plays a major role in metabolism, including plasma protein synthesis, carbohydrate homeostasis, lipid metabolism, and metabolism of toxins and drugs.

## Pathophysiology of chronic liver disease

### Liver cirrhosis

Chronic liver injury results in fibrosis and, if unchecked, liver cirrhosis, defined as the histological development of regenerative nodules, surrounded by fibrotic tissue that replaces normal hepatocytes. Fibrosis represents an excessive healing response to injured liver tissue and is thought to be mediated by activation of hepatic stellate cells (Ito cells); activated stellate cells proliferate, contract, and secrete collagen. The collagen deposits (forming fibrotic tissue: liver fibrosis) separate isolated hepatocyte islands and portal vessels, resulting in impaired hepatocyte function. Liver fibrosis may progress to cirrhosis when the hepatic vasculature is significantly disrupted. The intrahepatic resistance to blood flow is increased by fibrosis and regenerative nodules, and portal hypertension develops. Thus the portal pressure increases as a result of an increased resistance to outflow through the liver (Gatta, 2008; Schuppan and Afdhal, 2008; Bosch, 2010; Thabut and Shah, 2010) (see Figures 19.1 and 19.2).

Besides this disruption of hepatic architecture, there is a dynamic component of increased vascular resistance. There is an intrahepatic decrease in the production of NO and an increase in the production of vasoconstrictors, both a result of endothelial dysfunction (Iwakiri and Groszmann, 2007; Poordad, 2009; Bosch, 2010). This results in vasoconstriction of smooth muscle cells in the wall of hepatic and portal veins and venules and of myofibroblasts located around the sinusoids and hepatic venules. Myofibroblasts are derived from stellate cells under cirrhotic conditions. It is estimated that about 30% of the increased portal resistance is the result of hepatic vasoconstriction and impaired response to vasodilators. Finally, cirrhosis results in an increase in splanchnic circulation (including splenic blood flow), and this large increase in inflow contributes to portal hypertension. The main mechanism of this increased splanchnic circulation is the dramatic increase in NO production in the intestinal microcirculation in the presence of portal hypertension; other vasodilators may contribute. This vasodilation persists even when all vasoconstrictor systems are activated; this could be the result of changes in receptor affinity or downregulation of receptors.

Patients with cirrhosis have an increased risk of developing hepatocellular carcinoma, probably the result of the development of regenerative nodules with small-cell dysplasia (D'Amico, 2006).

### Hepatocellular dysfunction

The consequences of cirrhosis include hepatocellular insufficiency and/or failure (ESLD) and portal hypertension. Hepatocellular dysfunction results in hyperbilirubinaemia, reduced synthesis of proteins such as albumin and coagulation factors, and reduced clearance of toxins or intestinal vasoactive substances. In addition, drugs that undergo hepatic metabolism will have altered pharmacokinetics. Portosystemic collateral circulation with portosystemic shunting contributes to the reduced clearance. Other direct consequences of hepatocellular dysfunction are discussed later in this chapter.

### Circulatory changes

The pathophysiology of haemodynamic changes in cirrhosis is shown in Figure 19.3. The abnormalities in intrahepatic blood flow influence not only regional circulation (splanchnic blood flow) but also overall haemodynamics and specific organ blood flow. Patients with cirrhosis have a hyperdynamic circulation (sometimes called hyperdynamic circulatory syndrome), i.e. peripheral vasodilation, reduced arterial blood pressure, and increased heart rate and cardiac output (Møller and Henriksen, 2008; Henriksen and Møller, 2009). Mild liver dysfunction may result in circulatory changes that are clinically not readily apparent. Vasodilation is the result of increased plasma concentrations of NO, prostacyclin, oestrogen, bradykinin, and vasoactive intestinal peptide, all a consequence of reduced metabolic activity by the liver and blood bypassing the liver through collateral vessels. In addition, there may be an increased sensitivity to these substances, while there also is a reduced sensitivity to vasoconstrictors such as norepinephrine, vasopressin, and endothelin-1 (decreased number of receptors and postreceptor defects).

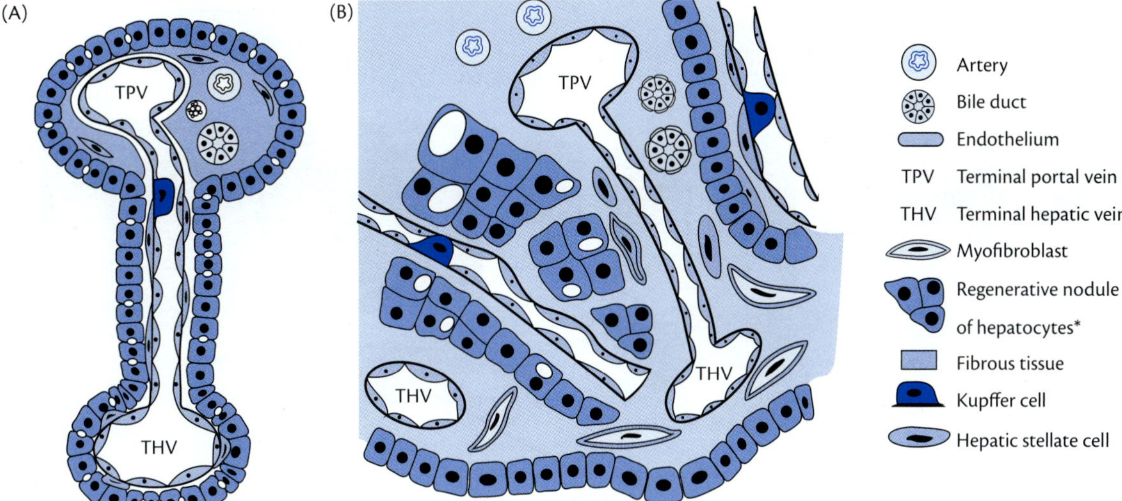


**Fig. 19.1** Vascular and architectural alterations in cirrhosis. Mesenteric blood flows via the portal vein and hepatic artery that extend branches into terminal portal tracts. (A) Healthy liver: terminal portal tract blood runs through hepatic sinusoids where fenestrated sinusoidal endothelia that rest on loose connective tissue (space of Disse) allow for extensive metabolic exchange with the lobular hepatocytes; sinusoidal blood is collected by terminal hepatic venules that disembogue into one of the three hepatic veins and finally the caval vein. (B) Cirrhotic liver: activated myofibroblasts that derive from perisinusoidal hepatic stellate cells and portal or central-vein fibroblasts proliferate and produce excess extracellular matrix (ECM). This event leads to fibrous portal-tract expansion, central-vein fibrosis, and capillarization of the sinusoids, characterized by loss of endothelial fenestrations, congestion of the space of Disse with ECM, and separation or encasement of perisinusoidal hepatocyte islands from sinusoidal blood flow by collagenous septa. Blood is directly shunted from terminal portal veins and arteries to central veins, with consequent (intrahepatic) portal hypertension and compromised liver synthetic function. (Reprinted from *The Lancet*, 371, Detlef Schuppan and Nezam H Afdhal, 'Liver cirrhosis', pp. 838–851, 2008, with permission from Elsevier.)

It has recently been suggested that bacterial translocation with increased production of proinflammatory cytokines may contribute to the hyperdynamic circulation. However, a large part of the reduced peripheral vascular resistance is the result of the reduction in splanchnic vascular resistance (the result of a massive increase in NO production in the splanchnic circulation). The disturbance of microcirculatory function causes arteriovenous shunting, increased cardiac output, and abnormal blood volume distribution, all in proportion to the severity of the underlying hepatic disease. Not all the vascular beds are affected to the same degree, and there may even be areas with vasoconstriction as the result of compensatory mechanisms. Despite the fact that total blood volume is increased, there is redistribution of total blood volume away from the circulation, mainly towards the splanchnic circulation (Møller and Henriksen, 2008; Møller, 2011). This central hypovolaemia is perceived by baroreceptors, and this leads to the activation of compensatory mechanisms to increase blood volume. These compensatory mechanisms include activation of the sympathetic nervous system (including the release of norepinephrine from the adrenal glands), activation of the ADH–arginine–vasopressin pathway, activation of the renin–angiotensin–aldosterone system (RAAS), and increased concentrations of circulating endothelin. The stimulation of these compensatory systems in combination with the low systemic vascular resistance (SVR) results in an increase in stroke volume and cardiac output. With worsening liver failure, the compensatory mechanisms are maximally stimulated, and the increase in cardiac output and vasoconstriction in some vascular beds becomes insufficient to maintain an adequate central blood volume and effective cardiac output. Blood pressure and effective tissue perfusion will progressively decrease, ultimately resulting in end-organ failure.

## Assessing severity and prognosis in chronic liver disease

The severity of liver disease has been assessed by the Child–Turcotte–Pugh (CTP) score (see Table 19.1) and more recently by the MELD score (see Table 19.2) (Wiesner, 2003).

$$\text{MELD} = [9.57 \times \log_e \text{creatinine (mg/dL)} + 3.78 \times \log_e \text{bilirubin (mg/dL)} + 11.2 \times \log_e \text{INR} + 6.43 \times (\text{constant for liver disease aetiology})]$$

Prognostic tools in patients with chronic liver diseases, apart from CTP and MELD scoring, include disease-specific indices for primary biliary cirrhosis and sclerosing cholangitis and the impact of specific complications of cirrhosis on patient survival.

The CTP score is as effective as quantitative liver function tests in determining short-term prognosis among groups of patients awaiting liver transplantation (Oellerich, 1991). Although its limitations have been well described, the CTP score has been widely adopted for risk-stratifying patients before transplantation because of its simplicity and ease of use (Conn, 1981).

The MELD was originally developed to assess short-term prognosis in patients undergoing transjugular intrahepatic portosystemic shunts (TIPS). Among patients who had undergone this procedure, serum bilirubin, INR of PT, and serum creatinine seemed to be the best predictors of 3-month postoperative survival (Malinchoc, 2000). Subsequent studies of this model demonstrated its usefulness as an effective tool for determining the prognosis of groups of patients with chronic liver disease (Kamath, 2001). A modification of this model is now used to prioritize patients for donor allocation in the US and has been shown to be useful in predicting both short-term survival in groups of patients on the waiting list for liver transplantation and the risk of postoperative mortality (Wiesner, 2003; Freeman, 2004). A similar model

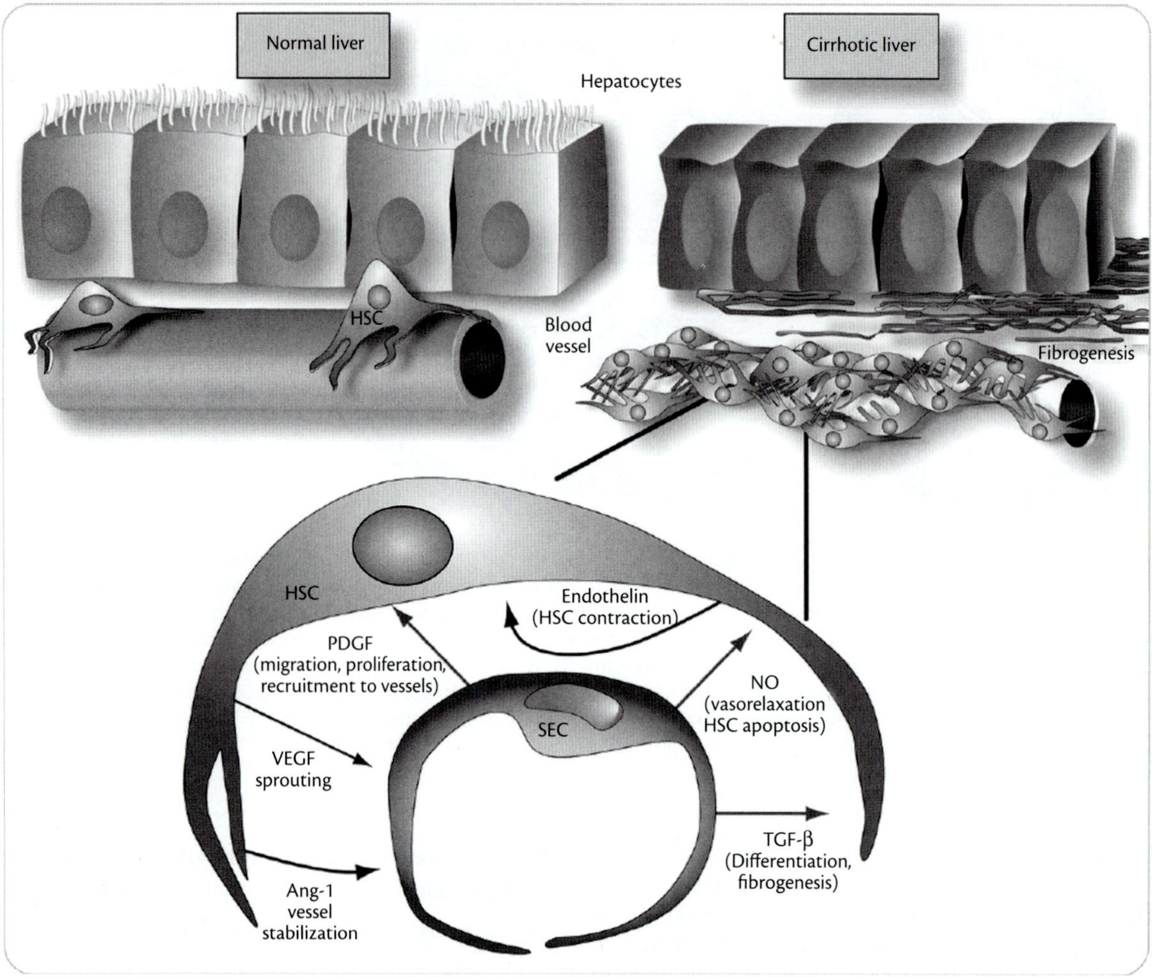


**Fig. 19.2** Pathological sinusoidal remodelling in cirrhosis and portal hypertension. Hepatic stellate cells (HSC) align themselves around the sinusoidal lumen in order to induce contraction of the sinusoids. While in normal physiological conditions HSC contractility and coverage of sinusoids is sparse, in cirrhosis increased numbers of HSC with increased cellular projections wrap more effectively around sinusoids, thereby contributing to a high-resistance, constricted sinusoidal vessel. At the cellular level a number of growth factor molecules contribute to this process through autocrine and paracrine signalling between HSC and sinusoidal endothelial cells (SEC). A number of these molecules are depicted, along with their proposed role in paracrine function. PDGF, Platelet-derived growth factor; VEGF, vascular endothelial growth factor; Ang-1, angiopoietin-1; NO, nitric oxide; TGF-β, transforming growth factor β. (This figure was published in *Journal of Hepatology*, 53, Dominique Thabut, Vijay Shah, 'Intrahepatic angiogenesis and sinusoidal remodeling in chronic liver disease: New targets for the treatment of portal hypertension', pp. 976–980, Copyright © 2010 Elsevier and the European Association for the Study of the Liver (EASL).)

has been developed for paediatric end-stage liver disease (PELD) (Wiesner, 2001; McDiarmid, 2002). This model has been useful in predicting deaths of paediatric patients waiting for transplantation (Freeman, 2001). Calculation of individual MELD or PELD scores for patients can be determined at <http://www.unos.org/resources/meldpeldcalculator.asp>.

## Management of chronic liver disease complications

### Portal hypertension and varices

Portal hypertension is defined as a pressure >5 mm Hg higher than central venous pressure; once the gradient is >10 mm Hg, complications associated with cirrhosis become more prevalent (Toubia and Sanyal, 2008; Garcia-Tsao, 2009; Sass and Chopra, 2009). Portal hypertension can be classified as prehepatic, intrahepatic, and post-hepatic; others classify it as presinusoidal, sinusoidal, and postsinusoidal. In the western world, liver cirrhosis is the cause in 90% of cases. An example of prehepatic portal hypertension is portal vein thrombosis, while post-hepatic portal hypertension can be caused by Budd–Chiari syndrome or congestive heart failure. Once the portal pressure–central venous pressure gradient increases above 10 mm Hg, collaterals will develop. Indeed, portal hypertension results in the dilatation of pre-existing vascular channels between the portal circulation and the vena cava, while the release of vascular endothelial growth factor (VEGF) and PDGF promotes the development of new portosystemic collaterals (Poordad, 2009; Bosch, 2010).

Varices are formed at the distal oesophagus/proximal stomach, retroperitoneum, umbilicus, and rectum (Garcia-Tsao and Bosch, 2010; Mehta, 2010). Thus one of the consequences of portal hypertension is the formation of *gastro-oesophageal varices*, which can result in life-threatening bleeding. About one-third of patients with varices will develop variceal bleeding, and this is associated with a

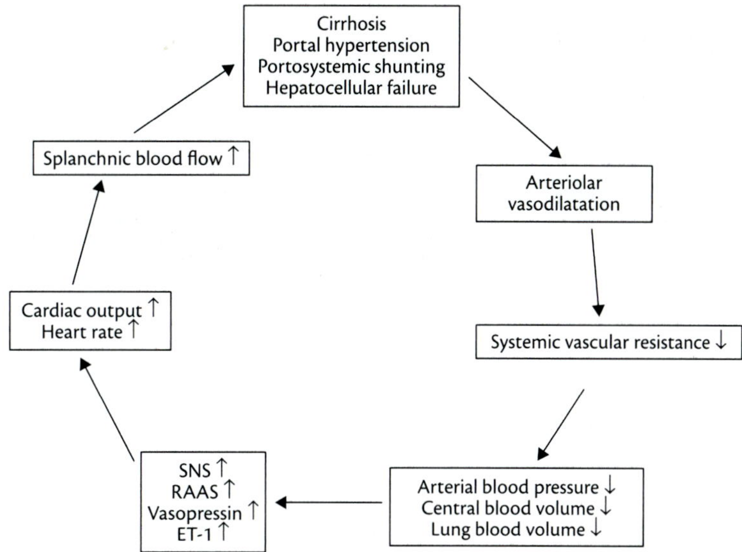


**Fig. 19.3** Pathophysiology of haemodynamic changes in cirrhosis. Peripheral arteriolar vasodilatation in cirrhosis is caused by portosystemic shunting or impaired hepatic degradation of vasodilators. Reduced systemic and splanchnic vascular resistance leads to reduced central and pulmonary blood volumes and hence to activation of vasoconstrictor systems. The haemodynamic and clinical consequences are increases in cardiac output, heart rate, and plasma volume, and decreased renal blood flow, low arterial blood pressure, and fluid and water retention. SNS, Sympathetic nervous system; RAAS, renin–angiotensin–aldosterone system; ET-1, endothelin-1. (Reproduced from Liver Anesthesiology and Critical Care Medicine, 'The patient with severe co-morbidities: cardiac disease', 2012, pp. 243–253, Shayan C and De Wolf AM, © Springer Science+Business Media New York 2012, with kind permission of Springer Science+Business Media.)

**Table 19.1** Child–Turcotte–Pugh (CTP) classification of cirrhosis. (From *The New England Journal of Medicine*, Garcia-Tsao G and Bosch J, 'Management of Varices and Variceal Hemorrhage in Cirrhosis', 362, 9, pp. 823–832. Copyright © 2010 Massachusetts Medical Society. Reprinted with permission from Massachusetts Medical Society.)

| Clinical and biochemical criteria | Points[a] | | |
|---|---|---|---|
| | 1 | 2 | 3 |
| Encephalopathy | None | Mild to moderate (grade 1 or 2) | Severe (grade 3 or 4) |
| Ascites | None | Mild to moderate | Large or refractory to diuretics |
| Bilirubin (mg/dL) | < 2 | 2–3 | > 3 |
| Albumin (g/dL) | > 3.5 | 2.8–3.5 | < 2.8 |
| Prothrombin time[b] | | | |
| Seconds prolonged | < 4 | 4–6 | > 6 |
| INR | < 1.7 | 1.7–2.3 | > 2.3 |

[a]In the CTP classification system, class A (5–6 points) indicates least severe liver disease; class B (7–9 points) indicates moderately severe liver disease; and class C (10–15 points) indicates most severe liver disease. To convert the values for bilirubin to micromoles per litre, multiply by 17.1.

[b]Either seconds prolonged or the INR is used.

**Table 19.2** Three-month mortality based on MELD score ('Mortality + too sick' means 'mortality or too sick to undergo liver transplantation'). (Reprinted from *Gastroenterology*, 124, 1, Wiesner et al, 'Model for end-stage liver disease (MELD) and allocation of donor livers', pp. 91–96, Copyright 2003, with permission from Elsevier and the AGA Institute.)

| | MELD score | | | | |
|---|---|---|---|---|---|
| | < 9 | 10–19 | 20–29 | 30–39 | > 40 |
| Number of patients | 124 | 1,800 | 1,098 | 295 | 120 |
| Mortality (%) | 1.9 | 6.0 | 19.6 | 52.6 | 71.3 |
| Mortality + too sick (%) | 2.9 | 7.7 | 23.5 | 60.2 | 79.3 |

mortality risk of 40% at 1 year (Stokkeland, 2006). Although these portosystemic collaterals could be expected to result in a decompression of the portal circulation, portal hypertension persists because there is an increasing NO-mediated vasodilation of the spanchnic arterioles, resulting in an accelerating increase in portal blood flow (see Figure 19.4) (Poordad, 2009). Another similar consequence of portal hypertension is portal hypertensive gastropathy.

Portal hypertension results in splenomegaly through the increase in splenic venous pressure. Sequestration of platelets followed by their destruction frequently results in thrombocytopaenia. Intrasplenic production of autoantibodies may contribute to this complication.

Prophylaxes against and treatment of oesophageal variceal bleeding include non-selective β-blockers, endoscopic sclerotherapy or ligation, TIPS placement, and the creation of a surgical shunt (see Table 19.3) (Garcia-Tsao and Bosch, 2010; Mehta, 2010). Variceal ligation and non-selective β-blockers are probably equivalent in their efficacy and have been used in combination (Mehta, 2010). Non-selective β-blockers (propranolol, nadolol, timolol) reduce portal pressure by reducing cardiac output (β1-blockade effect) and by reducing portal blood inflow through splanchnic vasoconstriction (β2-blockade effect). However, non-selective

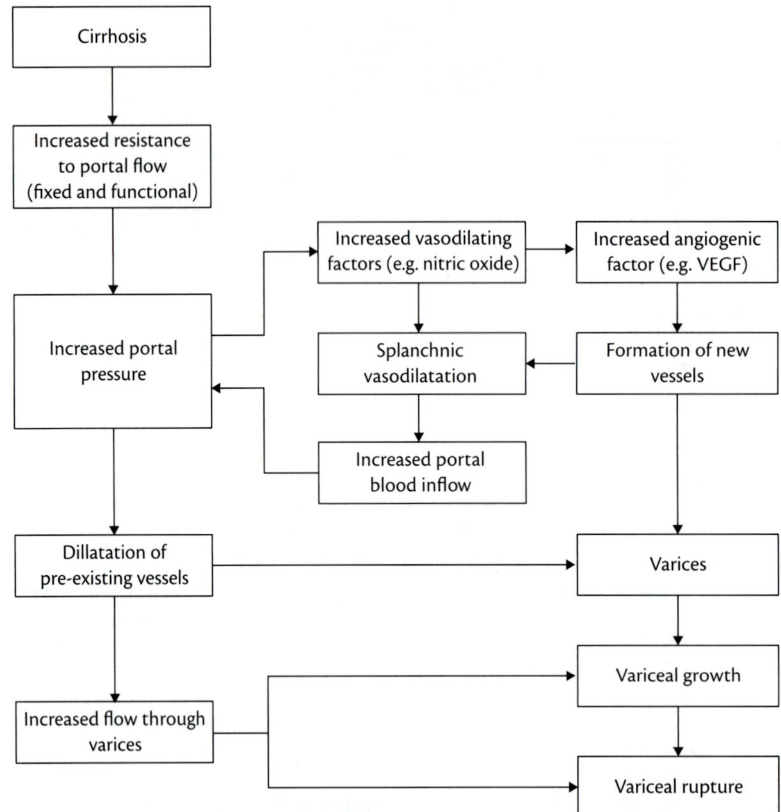


**Fig. 19.4** Pathogenesis of portal hypertension, varices, and variceal haemorrhage. The initial mechanism in development of portal hypertension in cirrhosis is an increase in vascular resistance to portal flow. Subsequent increase in portal venous inflow maintains the portal hypertensive state. Portal hypertension leads to formation of portosystemic collaterals, of which the most clinically relevant are gastroesophageal varices. Increase in flow through these collaterals, enhanced by presence of splanchnic vasodilatation and increased portal blood inflow, leads to variceal growth and rupture. This process is modulated by angiogenic factors. (From *The New England Journal of Medicine*, Garcia-Tsao G and Bosch J, 'Management of Varices and Variceal Hemorrhage in Cirrhosis', 362, 9, pp. 823–832. Copyright © 2010 Massachusetts Medical Society. Reprinted with permission from Massachusetts Medical Society)

**Table 19.3** Effect on portal flow, resistance, and pressure with different therapies for varices/variceal haemorrhage. (Reproduced with permission from Garcia-Tsao et al., 'Prevention and management of gastroesophageal varices and variceal hemorrhage in cirrhosis', *Hepatology*, 46, 3, pp. 922–938. Copyright © 2007 American Association for the Study of Liver Diseases.)

| Treatment | Portal flow | Portal resistance | Portal pressure |
|---|---|---|---|
| Vasoconstrictors (β-blockers) | ↓↓ | ↑ | ↓ |
| Venodilators (nitrates) | ↓ | ↓ | ↓ |
| Endoscopic therapy (band ligation/ sclerotherapy) | — | — | — |
| TIPS/shunt therapy | ↑ | ↓↓↓ | ↓↓↓ |

β-blockers do not prevent the formation of oesophageal varices and are associated with side effects (Groszmann, 2005; Sersté, 2010; Wong and Salerno, 2010). Selective β1-blockers (tenolol, metoprolol) are less effective in reducing portal pressure because they lack the β2-blockade effect.

Although non-selective β-blockers reduce the risk of variceal bleeding, in sicker patients (refractory ascites) their use may be associated with a higher mortality, possibly by reducing the capacity of the cardiovascular system to compensate (see Figure 19.5) (Sersté, 2010; Wong and Salerno, 2010). Nitrates in combination with non-selective β-blockers may further reduce the incidence of variceal haemorrhage (Mehta, 2010). Other interventions during acute variceal bleeding include the administration of vasopressin, terlipressin, somatostatin, octreotide, and the placement of a Sengstaken–Blakemore tube (Krag, 2008; Garcia-Tsao and Bosch, 2010). Ultimately the only definitive therapy is liver transplantation.

## Ascites, hydrothorax, and spontaneous bacterial peritonitis

*Ascites* is one of the most frequent complications of cirrhosis. It results from the combination of increased splanchnic capillary pressure and sodium retention; sodium retention is caused by the activation of neurohumoral systems (see the section 'Circulatory changes'). Initial medical treatment consists of diuretics and sodium restriction. Despite sodium retention, hyponatraemia is frequently seen because there is even more water retention due to the release of vasopressin (Krag, 2010a). Massive ascites commonly results in dyspnoea and abdominal discomfort. Refractory ascites is frequently associated with hepatorenal syndrome (HRS) type 2, spontaneous bacterial peritonitis, dilutional hyponatraemia, muscle wasting, and pleural effusion. Refractory ascites, an independent

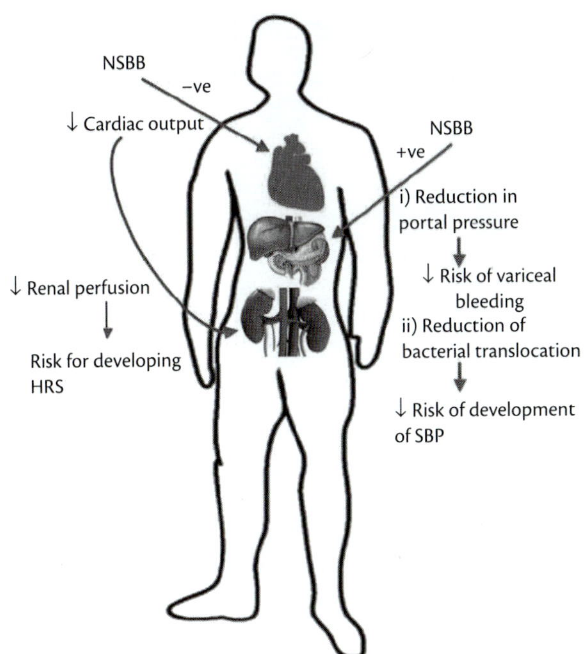


**Fig. 19.5** Proposed mechanisms of beneficial (*right*) and deleterious (*left*) effects of non-selective β-blockers (NSBB) in patients with advanced cirrhosis. HRS, Hepatorenal syndrome; SBP, spontaneous bacterial peritonitis. (Reproduced with permission from Wong and Salerno, 'Beta-Blockers in Cirrhosis: Friend and Foe?', *Hepatology*, 52, 3, pp. 811–813. Copyright © 2010 American Association for the Study of Liver Diseases.)

predictor of short-term survival, requires large-volume paracentesis for control accompanied by albumin infusion in an effort to reduce the incidence of renal failure (Ginès, 1996; Salerno, 2010). Alternatively, drugs to reduce splanchnic blood flow have been used (terlipressin, octreotide, midodrine).

A *TIPS* can be placed but this increases the risk of hepatic encephalopathy and congestive heart failure (Salerno, 2010). Still, TIPS results in better elimination of persistent ascites, improved renal function, and better nutritional status. In patients with recurrent ascites it may actually improve survival (Salerno, 2010). A new type of drug has been used in this situation: vaptans, selective antagonists of vasopressin-2 receptors. Definitive therapy is obviously liver transplantation.

*Hepatic hydrothorax*, defined as a pleural effusion of 500 mL, occurs in about 5–12% of patients with advanced cirrhosis (Kiafar and Gilani, 2008). It is virtually always seen in patients who already have ascites, and it occurs predominantly on the right side (85%). It reflects diaphragmatic defects that allow fluids to shift from the peritoneal cavity to the pleural cavity. These defects may be microscopic, may be created by stretching of the diaphragm (due to ascites), and are more prevalent in the right hemidiaphragm. Symptoms include dyspnoea and chest pain. Therapy is the same as for ascites, including TIPS, but there are a few additional options available: thoracentesis, thoracoscopic repair of diaphragmatic defects, and pleurodesis.

*Spontaneous bacterial peritonitis (SBP)* is the result of intestinal oedema that disrupts the gut mucosal barrier that normally prevents the crossing of enteric bacteria. SBP caused by Gram-negative bacteria can result in the release of endotoxins in the bloodstream; this may induce monocytes to produce the cytokine TNF-α. TNF-α reduces cardiac function, stimulates further release of NO, and reduces vascular reactivity to vasopressors. Bacterial translocation in the gut is thought to result in complications such as SBP and HRS. Proper treatment includes the use of selected antibiotics, and prophylactic antibiotics reduce the recurrence of SBP. Non-selective β-blockers increase intestinal transit and decrease bacterial translocation (Senzolo, 2009; Mehta, 2010). Ascites but especially SBP frequently precipitates HRS (Venkat and Venkat, 2010).

## Hepatorenal syndrome

The compensatory systems (⇑RAAS, ⇑ADH–arginine–vasopressin pathway, sympathetic nervous system activation, increased concentrations of circulating endothelin) result in vasoconstriction of the coronary, cerebral, and renal arterioles. This is especially apparent in the kidneys and may result in the development of HRS (Wong, 2008) (see Figure 19.6). Cytokines (TNF-α, endogenous cannabinoids) contribute to renal injury. Renal blood flow is reduced, despite activation of prostaglandin-mediated protective mechanisms in the kidney; there are no discernible structural changes in the kidneys. Sudden decreases in preload (bleeding, vomiting, diarrhoea) can result in further reduction in effective renal perfusion, and bacterial infections (such as SBP) can result in additional renal injury through release of cytokines. Also, NSAIDs impair renal function by decreasing the intrarenal synthesis of vasodilating prostaglandins. HRS results in fluid and sodium retention and ascites formation.

Diagnosis of HRS is usually based on excluding other causes of renal failure. Serum creatinine concentration does not necessarily inversely correlate with the significant reduction in glomerular filtration rate, because there is decreased creatinine generation by skeletal muscle due to wasting seen in severe liver disease. Type 1 HRS is the acute, rapid progressive form of renal failure and type 2 HRS is associated with a more moderate and slow loss of renal function (Wong, 2008). Still, the prognosis is poor for both types: 80% 2-week mortality for type 1 and a median survival of type 2 of 3–6 months.

In decompensated cirrhosis, renal vasodilators do not improve renal perfusion, but splanchnic vasoconstrictors such as terlipressin, midodrine, octreotide, and norepinephrine in combination with volume restoration (albumin) do (Møller, 2005; Krag, 2008; Wong, 2008). Other management options include paracentesis combined with volume expansion with intravenous albumin, treatment of SBP, TIPS (mainly in the presence of refractory ascites), and renal replacement therapy. Ultimately the only curative therapy is liver transplantation; if prolonged (> 8–12 weeks), pretransplant dialysis is required and simultaneous liver–kidney transplantation is likely indicated. Alternatively, renal dysfunction can be the result of overtreatment with diuretics (prerenal effect), and acute tubular necrosis may be seen in patients with acute hepatic failure or sepsis. Renal impairment is a strong predictor of sepsis and mortality.

## TIPS

TIPS was used for the first time by Rösch and colleagues in 1969 in dogs and in a cirrhotic patient by Colapinto in 1982 (Rösch, 1969; Colapinto, 1982). It is an expandable flexible metal shunt prosthesis that is placed through the internal jugular vein and connects the portal vein with a hepatic vein. This results in a

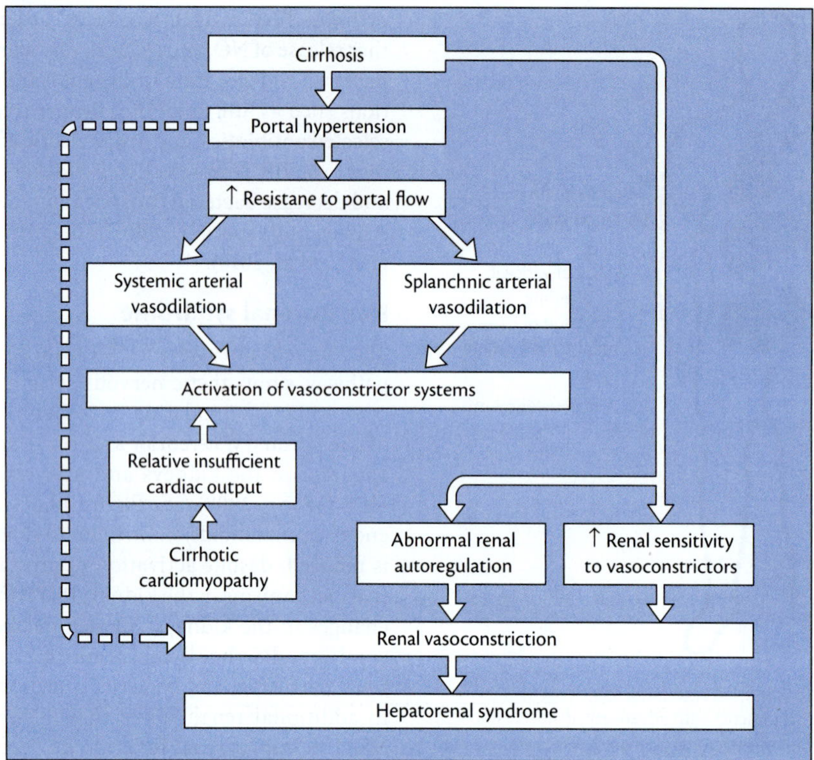


**Fig. 19.6** Pathophysiology of hepatorenal syndrome. (Reproduced from *Current Gastroenterology Reports*, 10, 2008, 'Hepatorenal syndrome: Current management', pp. 22–29, Florence Wong, with kind permission from Springer Science and Business Media.)

portacaval intrahepatic shunt that functions as a side-to-side portacaval shunt (Wong, 2006). Over the years, polytetrafluoroethylene (PTFE)-covered stents have replaced bare metal stents as they markedly improved the long-term patency of the shunt and also prevent portobiliary fistulae (Cejna, 2001; Angermayr, 2003; Bureau, 2007).

One of the main complications of TIPS placement is new or worsening hepatic encephalopathy (20–30%). Other complications include worsening liver function, cardiac failure (especially in patients with cirrhotic cardiomyopathy) due to the sudden increase in venous return to the heart, and HRS, despite the fact that TIPS has been successfully used in the treatment for type 1 HRS. Absolute contraindications to TIPS procedure include right-sided heart failure, biliary tract obstruction, uncontrolled infection, pulmonary hypertension, recurrent chronic hepatic encephalopathy (in the absence of known precipitants), and hepatocellular carcinoma involving the hepatic veins. Relative contraindications include severe liver failure (CTP score > 12), portal vein thrombosis, and multiple hepatic cysts (Pomier-Layrargues, 2012).

TIPS has typically been used as treatment for uncontrolled oesophageal variceal bleeding (Sanyal, 1996; Azoulay, 2001; D'Amico and Luca, 2008). However, a recent randomized controlled trial evaluating the use of emergent TIPS as compared to standard medical therapy in patients with severe portal hypertension found that early TIPS was associated with less treatment failure and better survival rates (García-Pagán, 2010). This approach could justify the use of TIPS early after bleeding episodes in patients with moderate or severe liver failure and severe portal hypertension. Meta-analyses have demonstrated that TIPS was more efficient than β-blockers or variceal band ligation in preventing variceal rebleeding, but it was more frequently followed by episodes of encephalopathy, and survival was not different between groups (Papatheodoridis, 1999; Burroughs and Vangeli, 2002; Zheng, 2008). Therefore TIPS is not recommended as a first-line therapy for secondary prophylaxis of oesophageal variceal bleeding.

The first-line treatment for bleeding gastric varices is endoscopic sclerotherapy with cyanoacrylate (Irani, 2011), although TIPS has been used successfully in patients in whom endoscopic therapy failed (Chau, 1998; Barange, 1999). TIPS is more efficient than obturation of the varices through cyanoacrylate (glue) injection in secondary prophylaxis of bleeding from large gastric varices (Lo, 2007) and has also been shown to be effective treatment for ectopic varices (Vangeli, 2004; Vidal, 2006).

TIPS has been used successfully to treat medically refractory ascites (Lebrec, 1996; Rössle, 2000; Ginès, 2002; Sanyal, 2003; Salerno, 2004; Narahara, 2011). Although hepatic encephalopathy is observed more frequently, and survival is not improved in the majority of trials (Albillos, 2005; D'Amico, 2005; Deltenre, 2005), a meta-analysis showed different results after analysing individual patient data (Salerno, 2007).

The risks of severe hepatic encephalopathy and/or liver failure following TIPS for patients with hepatic hydrothorax are similar to those observed in ascitic patients (Gordon, 1997; Siegerstetter, 2001; Dhanasekaran, 2010).

TIPS is effective treatment for type 2 HRS. TIPS has no role in type 1 HRS, except for highly selected cases as a bridge to liver transplantation, as it may aggravate the liver insufficiency (Spahr, 1995; Guevara, 1998a; Brensing, 2000).

TIPS has been reported to improve oxygenation in some patients with hepatopulmonary syndrome (HPS) (Riegler, 1995; Lasch, 2001; Paramesh, 2003).

## Hepatic encephalopathy

There are several theories on the pathogenesis of hepatic encephalopathy. As the clearance of ammonia produced by intestinal bacteria is reduced, increased serum ammonia concentrations result in glutamine accumulation in cerebral astrocytes, causing swelling and dysfunction. Hyponatraemia may make this situation worse. Another hypothesis of hepatic encephalopathy is based on false neurotransmitters, while the systemic inflammatory response contributes. Treatment includes the use of oral lactulose or lactitol enemas that increase faecal elimination of ammonia; oral antibiotics such as neomycin in the past and now rifaximin which decrease the bacterial flora have been used in patients who do not tolerate lactulose.

Hepatic encephalopathy occurs in both chronic liver disease and acute liver failure (ALF); in ALF it can lead to dramatic increases in intracranial pressure. In ALF initially there is reduced cerebral blood flow and reduced metabolism of the brain (metabolic autoregulation). In the second stage there is further increased cerebrovascular resistance, consistent with the hyperdynamic circulation, resulting in compensatory mechanisms that give rise to vasoconstriction in certain vascular beds (Guevara, 1998b). In the next stage there is significant hyperaemia (caused by oxidative stress) which results in an increase in intracranial pressure.

## Cardiac and pulmonary complications

### Cirrhotic cardiomyopathy

The sympathetic stimulation caused by central hypovolaemia does not result in an improved cardiac function. Instead, cirrhotic cardiomyopathy is not uncommonly seen in these patients. It is defined as systolic and diastolic dysfunction in combination with electrophysiological abnormalities (Møller and Henriksen, 2010). Repolarization abnormalities such as prolonged QT interval may be seen and reduced inotropic and chronotropic responses to β-agonists are observed. Although cardiac output is much increased, there is echocardiographic evidence of systolic and diastolic dysfunction.

The cause of cirrhotic cardiomyopathy is complex and includes downregulation of β-receptors, abnormal excitation–contraction coupling, circulating myocardial depressant factors, and areas of fibrosis and subendothelial oedema (see Figure 19.7). Cirrhotic cardiomyopathy may not be apparent at rest (mainly because of the reduced afterload) but becomes more noticeable during cardiac stress (increase in preload after TIPS, increase in afterload during vasopressin or terlipressin therapy, or after liver transplantation) (Krag, 2010b). On echocardiography, left atrial enlargement is frequently seen, and diastolic dysfunction is reflected by a decreased

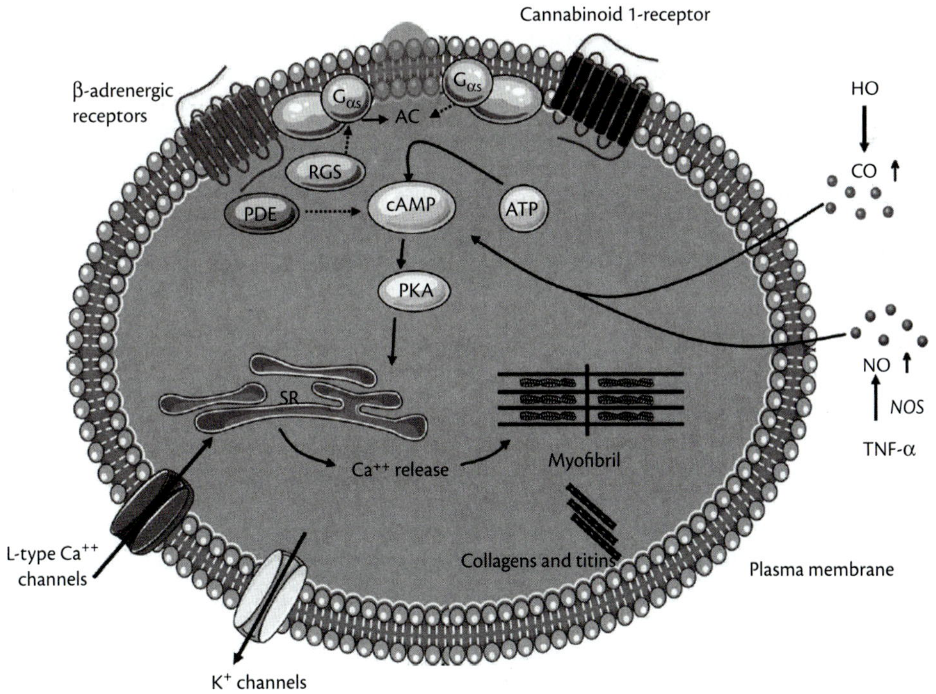


**Fig. 19.7** Potential mechanisms involved in impaired contractile function of cardiomyocyte in cirrhotic cardiomyopathy: downregulation of β-adrenergic receptors with decreased content of G-protein ($G_{\alpha i}$, inhibitory G-protein; $G_{\alpha s}$, stimulatory G-protein); upregulation of cannabinoid 1-receptor stimulation; increased inhibitory effects of cardiodepressant substances such as haemoxygenase (HO), carbon monoxide (CO), nitric oxide synthase (NOS)-induced nitric oxide (NO) release, and tumour necrosis factor-α (TNF-α). Many post-receptor effects are mediated by adenylcyclase (AC) inhibition or stimulation (RGS, regulator of G-protein signalling; PDE, phosphodiesterase; PKA, protein kinase A). Sarcoplasmatic reticulum (SR), altered function and reduced conductance of potassium channels, inhibition of L-type calcium channels, and increased fluidity of plasma membrane (increased cholesterol/phospholipid ratio) also contribute to reduced calcium release and contractility, together with altered ratio of collagens and titins. ATP, Adenosine triphosphate; cAMP, cyclic adenosine monophosphate. (This figure was published in *Journal of Hepatology*, 53, Søren Møller et al, 'Cirrhotic cardiomyopathy', pp. 179–190, Copyright © 2010 Elsevier and the European Association for the Study of the Liver (EASL).)

E/A ratio across the mitral valve: the E wave reflects passive flow through the mitral valve, while the A wave is the result of atrial contraction. The decreased E/A ratio indicates diastolic dysfunction caused mainly by abnormal relaxation of the myocardium. Finally, mild left ventricular hypertrophy is common.

Cirrhotic cardiomyopathy is reversed after liver transplantation (Torregrosa, 2005). Patients with alcoholic cirrhosis, amyloidosis, and Wilson's disease may have overt cardiomyopathy; a left ventricular ejection fraction < 40–45% is considered by many to be a contraindication for liver transplantation.

## Portopulmonary hypertension

Pulmonary hypertension has a higher incidence in patients with liver disease (0.73–2%) than in the general population (0.13%) and is called portopulmonary hypertension (PPHTN). Portal hypertension is a prerequisite, but the degree of PPHTN is unrelated to the degree of portal hypertension or to the severity of liver disease. PPHTN is defined as a mean pulmonary artery pressure (PAP) > 25 mm Hg with a normal PCWP and an increased calculated pulmonary vascular resistance (PVR) > 240 dynes/s/$cm^{-5}$). True PPHTN has to be distinguished from pulmonary hypertension (usually mild or moderate) as a result of high left atrial pressure, caused by volume overload and/or left ventricular diastolic dysfunction; in this situation the pulmonary vascular resistance is not significantly increased.

The cause of PPHTN is unknown, but likely shear stress from increased pulmonary blood flow results in endothelial dysfunction, resulting in endothelial cell proliferation and humoral imbalance, causing smooth muscle hypertrophy, plexiform lesions, and non-specific intimal fibrous thickening. Metabolic mediators probably also play a role (kinins, serotonin, toxins, NO, endothelin) (Pellicelli, 2010; Tsiakalos, 2011). There is also an active component of vasoconstriction in the pulmonary vasculature. Pathologically, PPHTN is indistinguishable from primary pulmonary hypertension. Clinical manifestations range from asymptomatic to non-specific signs and symptoms such as fatigue, dyspnoea on exertion, chest pain, and haemoptysis. Eventually right ventricular failure results in hypoxaemia and cyanosis.

Screening tests for PPHTN include ECG, CXR, and echocardiography; this latest test has the advantage that it allows estimation of right ventricular systolic pressure based on the tricuspid regurgitation test (Kim, 2000). Patients with an estimated peak right ventricular (RV) pressure > 45 mm Hg should undergo further evaluation. Definitive diagnosis is made through right heart catheterization. PPHTN can be classified as mild (mean PAP 25–35 mm Hg), moderate (35–45 mm Hg), or severe (> 45 mm Hg). Patients with severe PPHTN are not considered to be acceptable candidates for liver transplantation because of the excessively high perioperative mortality (Krowka, 2000; Ramsay, 2010). Patients with moderate PPHTN may be transplanted only if right ventricular function is good and if there is no significant disease in the right coronary artery. Even then, perioperative mortality is increased (Krowka, 2000).

Pulmonary vasodilators are used in an attempt to reduce mean PAP by reducing PVR. Earlier, this management was based on chronic intravenous administration of prostaglandins, but recently a combination of inhaled prostaglandins (iloprost), phosphodiesterase-5 inhibitors such as sildenafil, and endothelin antagonists such as bosentan has been used (Austin, 2008; Bandara, 2010; Melgosa, 2010). If this reduces severe PPHTN to moderate and if RV function is good, liver transplantation could be considered. In exceptional cases, combined liver–heart–lung transplantation has been performed (Scouras, 2011). In addition to the mentioned pulmonary vasodilators, inhaled NO should be available perioperatively. PPHTN may be reversible after liver transplantation, but very rarely PPHTN has developed after successful liver transplantation.

## Hepatopulmonary syndrome

HPS is defined as hypoxaemia (usually $PaO_2$ < 80 mm Hg) associated with intrapulmonary vascular dilatations in the presence of liver disease; there is no intrinsic pulmonary disease. These intrapulmonary vasodilations are located predominantly at precapillary and capillary levels (type 1 HPS, more common) or consist mainly as arteriovenous communications (type 2 HPS, less common, more severe hypoxaemia) (Rodriguez-Roisin and Krowka, 2008). The hypoxaemia in type 1 HPS is caused by ventilation/perfusion mismatch and diffusion problems caused by the dilated capillaries (perfusion–diffusion defect: oxygen insufficiently diffuses to the centre of the dilated capillaries), while in type 2 HPS the main cause is right to left shunt (see Figure 19.8). Thus hypoxaemia in type 1 HPS could be considered to be the result of an oxygen diffusion problem (difficulty of oxygen transfer to the whole capillary; increasing $FiO_2$ can overcome this problem), while decreased intrapulmonary transit time may contribute to hypoxaemia. In type 2 HPS, hypoxaemia is not much improved by inhaling high concentrations of oxygen.

The intrapulmonary vascular dilatations are documented by echocardiography: after intravenous injection of echogenic contrast (agitated saline), microbubbles are quickly observed in the right atrium and ventricle and 3–5 heart beats later can be seen in the left atrium (microbubbles do not pass through normal pulmonary capillaries) (Hopkins, 1992). Contrast-enhanced echocardiography can exclude right-to-left shunt at the atrial level as the cause of hypoxaemia. Also left atrial volume > 50 mL is associated with HPS (Zamirian, 2007). A 99Tc-macroaggregated albumin scan has also been used to document intrapulmonary vascular

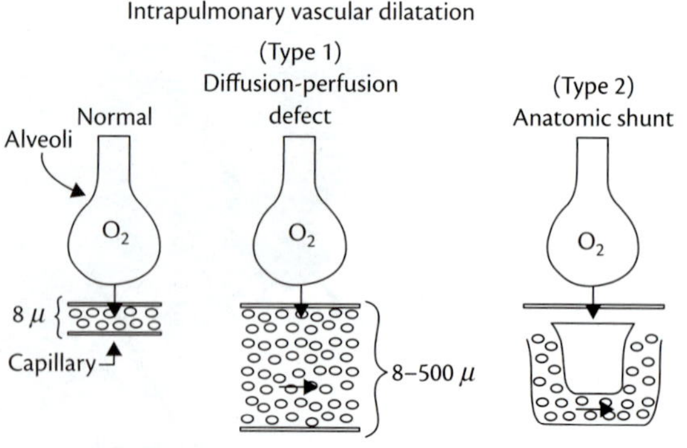


**Fig. 19.8** Pathophysiology of hypoxaemia in hepatopulmonary syndrome. Red blood cells (open discs) pass through diffuse dilated channels (type I) and/or discrete arteriovenous communications (type II). In both cases, oxygen molecules from alveoli are unable to completely diffuse into the passing blood below. Depending on the size of the dilatations and proportion of inspired oxygen, varying degrees of hypoxaemia occur. (Reprinted from *Journal of Hepatology*, 34, 5, Michael J. Krowka, 'Caveats concerning hepatopulmonary syndrome', pp. 756–758, Copyright 2001, with permission from Elsevier and the European Association for the Study of the Liver (EASL).)

dilatations, but this test does not differentiate between intrapulmonary and intracardiac shunt. Overall, echocardiography provides more information and there rarely is a need for pulmonary angiography (Rodriguez-Roisin and Krowka, 2008).

A long list of mediators could result in the vascular dilatations; among these are endotoxins, TNF, VEGF, NO, and endothelin. There likely is an imbalance between pulmonary vasodilators and vasoconstrictors, while an altered sensitivity to vasodilators and vasoconstrictors is quite likely too. Nevertheless, factors other than vasodilators have a role to play since the up to ten-fold dilation of capillaries, which have little or no smooth muscle, cannot be explained simply by vasodilators.

The incidence of intrapulmonary vascular dilatations is high: up to 47% of patients with liver disease have a positive contrast-enhanced echocardiogram, but not all of these patients have hypoxaemia and therefore have HPS. In addition, because the threshold for defining hypoxaemia varies, the reported incidence of HPS ranges widely from 5% to 32%. Because the intrapulmonary vascular dilatations are predominantly located at the bases of the lungs, hypoxaemia is more severe in the standing position (more pulmonary blood flow through the bases of the lungs) than in the supine position (orthodeoxia). Similarly there is more dyspnoea in the standing position (platypnoea). Because of the predominantly basal location of these vascular dilatations, CXR frequently shows increased markings at the bases. Besides dyspnoea in virtually all patients with HPS, there may be clubbing of the fingers and cyanosis, depending on the degree of hypoxaemia.

Without liver transplantation, survival in patients with cirrhosis and HPS is much less than in those without HPS. HPS is reversible after liver transplantation, but especially patients with type 2 HPS can have a complicated postoperative course. Coiling of large arteriovenous (AV) communications is an option in refractory hypoxaemia (Poterucha, 1995; Saad, 2007). Patients with HPS have a higher incidence of stroke and cerebral abscesses, probably as a result of embolic events through the pulmonary circulation. Also there is an increased incidence of biliary and vascular complications, probably related to hypoxaemia. High levels of PEEP should not be used to treat perioperative hypoxaemia because it cannot improve the pathophysiology of hypoxaemia in HPS. Although some consider severe HPS to be a contraindication for liver transplantation, others have obtained good results (Gupta, 2010).

### Other complications

HPS and PPHTN have been observed very rarely to exist in one patient (Shah, 2005; Pham, 2010). Patients with severe liver disease are more susceptible to pneumonia, and frequently the massive ascites results in a reduction of the functional residual capacity of the lungs, resulting in shortness of breath, sometimes even at rest. Finally, autoimmune liver diseases may be associated with immune-mediated lung disease.

## Haematological complications

Traditional coagulation tests suggest profound abnormalities in the haemostatic system in patients with cirrhosis. Thrombocytopaenia, platelet dysfunction, and decreased concentration of coagulation factors (resulting in prolonged PT and activated partial thromboplastin time (aPTT)) are commonly seen, and as a result a bleeding diathesis is expected. However, inhibitors of the coagulation cascade (antithrombin III, protein C, protein S) also have low concentrations, as well as proteins involved in fibrinolysis (actually both pro- and antifibrinolytic factors may be decreased in cirrhosis). Then again, factor VIII and platelet adhesive protein von Willebrand factor (vWF) are increased and at least to some degree compensate for thrombocytopaenia and platelet dysfunction (Warnaar, 2008; Tripodi and Mannucci, 2011).

The basic laboratory tests of coagulation (i.e. measurement of the PT and aPTT) correlate poorly with the onset and duration of bleeding after liver biopsy or other potentially haemorrhagic procedures (Ewe, 1981; McGill, 1990; Terjung, 2003; Grabau, 2004; Segal, 2005) and the occurrence of gastrointestinal bleeding in patients with ESLD (Boks, 1986; Vieira da Rocha, 2009). There is also evidence that a thromboprotective glycocalyx on endothelial cells is degraded quickly, resulting in enhanced platelet adhesion and aggregation. Finally, there is resistance to the action of thrombomodulin that normally activates protein C. The result is that the haemostatic system is actually in a delicate balance, and this despite the abnormal PT, aPTT, and low platelet count (Lisman and Porte, 2010). The relative deficiency of both coagulation-system drivers makes the balance unstable in patients with liver disease and may tip it toward haemorrhage or thrombosis, depending on the prevailing circumstantial risk factors (Tripodi and Mannucci, 2011).

Anaemia and thrombocytopaenia are also common complications of liver cirrhosis. Anaemia is the result of impaired haematopoiesis and gastrointestinal bleeding, while thrombocytopaenia is related to impaired production in bone marrow (reduced synthesis of thrombopoietin in the liver), bleeding, and hypersplenism (Afdhal, 2008). Frequent transfusion of platelets may result in refractoriness, febrile non-haemolytic transfusion reaction, and transfusion-associated infections. Plasma concentrations of erythropoietin are reduced, and synthetic erythropoietin has been used in patients with cirrhosis.

## Infectious complications

Bacterial infections are very frequent in advanced cirrhosis and are the leading cause of death in these patients (Fernández and Gustot, 2012). These are more frequent in patients with decompensated cirrhosis than in those with compensated disease (Borzio, 2001). Risk factors associated with occurrence of bacterial infections in cirrhosis are high CTP score, variceal bleeding, low ascitic protein levels, and prior episode of SBP (Ginès, 1990; Llach, 1992; Yoshida, 1993; Bernard, 1999). Bacterial infections frequently lead to the development of severe sepsis and septic shock in the cirrhotic population, resulting in hospital mortality rates of up to 70% (Tandon and Garcia-Tsao, 2008; Gustot, 2009). Sepsis is known to rapidly worsen liver function in patients with cirrhosis. This acute deterioration, called acute-on-chronic liver failure, is associated with poor short-term prognosis (Sanchez and Kamath, 2008).

The most common infection in cirrhotic patients is SBP, followed by urinary tract infection, pneumonia, bacteraemia following a therapeutic procedure, cellulitis, and spontaneous bacteraemia (Fernández, 2002). Fungal infections (*Candida* spp.) are involved in up to 15% of cases of severe sepsis in cirrhosis (Plessier, 2003).

Early diagnosis and treatment of infection is key in the management of patients with decompensated cirrhosis (Rimola, 2000;

Tandon and Garcia-Tsao, 2008). Prompt admission to the ICU is also essential in the management of these patients. Resuscitation with albumin is associated with a decrease in mortality compared to other solutions in non-cirrhotic patients with sepsis (Delaney, 2011). Broad-spectrum antibiotics should be started as early as possible and always within the first hour of recognizing severe sepsis or septic shock (Rivers, 2001; Kumar, 2006, 2010; Dellinger, 2008). De-escalation to the most appropriate single antibiotic may be done once the susceptibility profile of the responsible bacteria is known (Dellinger, 2008).

Renal failure may be associated with sepsis in a cirrhotic patient. Common causes include prerenal failure, type 1 HRS (Ruiz-del-Arbol, 2005), and ischaemic acute tubular necrosis. Every care should be taken to prevent renal failure in the cirrhotic patient with infection (e.g. diuretic withdrawal, intravenous albumin supplementation, avoidance of large-volume paracentesis, avoidance of aminoglycoside use) (Cabrera, 1982).

Antibiotic prophylaxis is recommended in all cirrhotic patients with gastrointestinal haemorrhage, independent of the presence or absence of ascites (Runyon, 2009; de Franchis, 2010; European Association for the Study of the Liver, 2010). Oral norfloxacin (400 mg every 12 hours) is the first choice suggested since it is simple to administer and has a low cost. The Baveno V Consensus Conference recommends that antibiotics are instituted from admission, ideally before or immediately after endoscopy (de Franchis, 2010).

Patients with low protein ascites (<15 g/L) and advanced liver failure (CTP score ≥ 9 with serum bilirubin ≥ 3 mg/dL) or impaired renal function (serum creatinine ≥ 1.2 mg/dL, blood urea nitrogen (BUN) ≥ 25 mg/dL, or serum sodium ≤ 130 mEq/L) are at risk of developing SBP and HRS. Quinolones like norfloxacin (400 mg/day) or oral ciprofloxacin (500 mg/day) are effective as primary or secondary prophylaxis of SBP and improve short-term survival (Ginès, 1990; Llach, 1992; Bauer, 2002; Fernández, 2007; Terg, 2008).

## Electrolyte changes

Renal sodium retention increases as cirrhosis progresses, due to the gradually worsening systemic and portal haemodynamics and the associated compensatory mechanisms. Hyponatraemia may be caused by diuretic therapy, secondary hyperaldosteronism, and other, poorly understood renal abnormalities. It predicts worse outcomes. Correction is not always possible.

Hyperkalaemia is uncommon but should be treated aggressively. It may be associated with renal failure, treatment with spironolactone, or transfusion. Treatment of hyperkalaemia includes glucose/insulin administration and, if necessary, continuous venovenous haemofiltration (CVVH) or dialysis.

## Nutritional management

Up to 50–90% of cirrhotic patients have malnutrition, which is also an important poor prognostic factor (Kalaitzakis, 2006; Merli, 2010; Cheung, 2012). Complications such as infections, hepatic encephalopathy, ascites, and HRS are increased with malnourished cirrhotic patients, who also have longer hospital stays and a two-fold increase in in-hospital mortality compared with well-nourished patients (Alvares-da-Silva, 2005; Sam and Nguyen, 2009).

Aetiological factors for malnutrition include hypermetabolism, malabsorption, altered nutrient homeostasis, and anorexia. Hypermetabolism in cirrhotic patients may result from sympathetic overactivity (Braillon, 1986, 1992; Müller, 1999), infection, or immune compromise. Portosystemic shunting in cirrhosis causes nutrients to bypass the liver, without metabolic processing (Dudrick and Kavic, 2002; Tsiaousi, 2008). This shunting, coupled with impaired fat absorption and glucose–glycogen metabolism, results in increased insulin resistance in cirrhotic patients (Badley, 1970; Kalaitzakis, 2007). Alcoholic cirrhotics may also have chronic pancreatitis, which further contributes to malabsorption.

Anorexia can occur from the mechanical effects of ascitic fluid resulting in early satiety (Aqel, 2005), upregulation of inflammation and appetite mediators, including leptin (Le Moine, 1995; McCullough, 1998; Kalaitzakis, 2007; Peng, 2007; Grossberg, 2010), and poor socioeconomic status leading to poor and irregular feeding (Levine and Morgan, 1996; Bergheim et al., 2003).

It is a challenge to optimize nutrition in cirrhotic patients because of alterations to metabolic and storage functions of the liver. The energy recommendation, based on the American Society of Parenteral and Enteral Nutrition (ASPEN) and European Society for Clinical Nutrition and Metabolism (ESPEN) guidelines, ranges from 25 to 40 kcal/kg/day, depending on the presence or absence of encephalopathy or malnutrition (Plauth, 2006; Delich, 2007). Patients with oedema and ascites are usually placed on sodium-restricted diets (< 2 g/day) (Moore and Aithal, 2006). For patients with advanced liver disease, diet supplementation with fat-soluble vitamins (A, D, E, and K), zinc, and selenium is recommended (Delich, 2007; Lindor, 2009). Patients with alcohol abuse should receive folic acid and thiamine supplementation (Delich, 2007).

## Pharmacology and drug metabolism in end-stage liver disease

Patients with liver disease have altered drug pharmacokinetics because of an increased volume of distribution, decreased cytochrome P450 enzyme metabolism, decreased serum drug binding due to low protein/albumin levels, and sometimes decreased biliary drug excretion. The increased portal pressure results in the compensatory formation of portosystemic shunts, impairing the efficiency of hepatic extraction and reducing the extraction ratio of drugs. Cirrhotic patients also have a hypoproteinaemic and hypoalbuminaemic state that may reduce drug binding to plasma proteins (Garcia-Morillas, 1984). The volume of distribution of drugs, especially those that are highly protein bound (> 90%), is increased in patients with chronic liver disease who exhibit hypoalbuminaemia or ascites (Lewis and Jusko, 1975; Branch, 1976; Howden, 1989). As cirrhosis progresses, extensive fibrosis causes a reduction in liver size, resulting in a marked reduction of total P450 concentrations (Brodie, 1981; Murray, 1992; George, 1996). This limits and decreases drug metabolism and hepatic clearance of most drugs. However, not all P450 activities are decreased uniformly in severe liver disease (Farrell, 1979; Elbekai, 2004). Commonly used drugs that may have altered metabolism in this setting include theophylline (CYP1A2), alcohol (CYP2E1), acetaminophen (CYP2E1), CNIs (CYP3A4), HMG-CoA reductase inhibitors (CYP3A4), and warfarin (CYP2C9). NADPH-cytochrome P450 reductase activity is normal even in severe liver disease (George, 1995). The effect of hepatic clearance or metabolism of a drug in cirrhosis depends on the net result of changes of various factors. Active metabolite formation also complicates drug response and dose adjustments.

Drug dosing in patients with liver disease requires the consideration of the nature and severity of the liver disease, haemodynamic factors, and the drug's pharmacokinetics. Even then, predicting drug metabolism in patients with liver disease can be challenging as most clinical trials only enrol patients with mild or moderate liver disease.

## Liver transplantation

### Indications

Liver transplantation is the treatment of choice for patients with ESLD, acute liver failure, or small HCCs (Lucey, 2013). As it is a major undertaking with its associated risks and complications, the natural history of the patient's disease must be carefully weighed against the anticipated survival after liver transplantation (Murray and Carithers, 2005).

### Types

An orthotopic liver transplantation is performed using a whole liver from a deceased donor, where the donor liver is placed in the orthotopic position in the recipient. However, depending on circumstances, it may be feasible for a split liver transplantation to be performed, where the donor liver is divided and transplanted into two different recipients (Keeffe, 2001). For example, the left lobe of an adult donor organ can be transplanted into a child and the remaining right lobe transplanted into an adult (Otte, 1998; Malagó, 2002; Gridelli, 2003; Renz, 2004) or, rarely, the split grafts can be transplanted into two adult recipients (Renz, 2004). The same techniques are used with living donors, where only a portion of the donor liver is removed for transplantation. Living donor transplantation for children, using a portion of the left lobe, is a well-established procedure (Otte, 1998; Malagó, 2002). Living donor transplantation for adults, in which the donor right lobe is transplanted, also is performed at many transplant centres (Surman, 2002; Trotter, 2002). Although perioperative complications are more common with split grafts, long-term patient survival is comparable with that of deceased whole liver transplantation (Renz, 2004; Settmacher, 2004).

### Outcomes and prognosis

Current survival rates 1, 3, and 5 years after liver transplantation in the US are 88%, 80%, and 75%, respectively (<http://www.optn.org/latestdata/step2.asp>). Hence, patients with a MELD score ≥ 15 and a CTP score ≥ 7 are likely to have improved survival with liver transplantation (Lucey, 1997; Wiesner, 2003; Freeman, 2004).

The causes of death and graft loss differ according to the time from transplantation. Infection, intraoperative, and perioperative causes account for nearly 60% of deaths and graft losses in the first post-transplant year. After the first year death due to acute infections declines, whereas malignancies and cardiovascular causes account for a greater proportion of mortality. Cardiovascular disease and renal failure are the leading non-hepatic causes of morbidity and mortality late after liver transplantation. Long-term immunosuppression use increases the risk of bacterial, viral, and fungal infections, metabolic complications such as hypertension, diabetes mellitus, hyperlipidaemia, obesity and gout, and hepatobiliary or extrahepatic de-novo cancers (including post-transplant lymphoproliferative disorder). Longer patient survival post-transplant is also associated with complications of recurrence of the primary disease (e.g. chronic HCV, autoimmune liver disease, alcoholic liver disease). Death or retransplantation for allograft rejection is now uncommon in the first 10 years after transplantation (Lucey, 2013).

## Conclusion

Severe liver disease affects the whole body. Liver cirrhosis results in portal hypertension, ascites, and the creation of gastro-oesophageal varices. But since the liver plays a central role in the body's physiological homeostasis, the whole body becomes affected. There are major changes in systemic and pulmonary circulation, and other organ systems will become affected as well. The most important resulting complications are encephalopathy, cirrhotic cardiomyopathy, hepatopulmonary syndrome, portopulmonary hypertension, hepatorenal syndrome, and malnutrition. Liver transplantation remains the only viable option in the treatment of severe liver disease.

## References


Afdhal N, McHutchison J, Brown R, et al. (2008) Thrombocytopenia associated with chronic liver disease. *J Hepatol*, **48**(6):1000–1007.

Albillos A, Banares R, Gonzalez M, Catalina MV, Molinero LM (2005) A meta-analysis of transjugular intrahepatic portosystemic shunt versus paracentesis for refractory ascites. *J Hepatol*, **43**(6):990–996.

Alter MJ, Kruszon-Moran D, Nainan OV, et al. (1999) The prevalence of hepatitis C virus infection in the United States, 1988 through 1994. *N Engl J Med*, **341**(8):556–562.

Alvares-da-Silva MR, Reverbel da Silveira T (2005) Comparison between handgrip strength, subjective global assessment, and prognostic nutritional index in assessing malnutrition and predicting clinical outcome in cirrhotic outpatients. *Nutrition*, **21**(2):113–117.

Angermayr B, Cejna M, Koenig F, et al. (2003) Survival in patients undergoing transjugular intrahepatic portosystemic shunt: ePTFE-covered stentgrafts versus bare stents. *Hepatology*, **38**(4):1043–1050.

Anonymous (2013) Liver disease in Europe (editorial). *Lancet*, **381**(9866):508–509.

Aqel BA, Scolapio JS, Dickson RC, Burton DD, Bouras EP (2005) Contribution of ascites to impaired gastric function and nutritional intake in patients with cirrhosis and ascites. *Clin Gastroenterol Hepatol*, **3**(11):1095–1100.

Austin MJ, McDougall NI, Wendon JA, et al. (2008) Safety and efficacy of combined use of sildenafil, bosentan, and iloprost before and after liver transplantation in severe portopulmonary hypertension. *Liver Transplant*, **14**(3):287–291.

Azoulay D, Castaing D, Manjo P, et al. (2001) Salvage transjugular intrahepatic portosystemic shunt for uncontrolled variceal bleeding in patients with decompensated cirrhosis. *J Hepatol*, **35**(5):590–597.

Badley BW, Murphy GM, Bouchier IA, Sherlock S (1970) Diminished micellar phase lipid in patients with chronic nonalcoholic liver disease and steatorrhea. *Gastroenterology*, **58**(6):781–789.

Bandara M, Gordon FD, Sarwar A, et al. (2010) Successful outcomes following living donor liver transplantation for portopulmonary hypertension. *Liver Transplant*, **16**(8):983–989.

Barange K, Péron JM, Imani K, et al. (1999) Transjugular intrahepatic portosystemic shunt in the treatment of refractory bleeding from ruptured gastric varices. *Hepatology*, **30**(5):1139–1143.

Bauer TM, Follo A, Navasa M, et al. (2002) Daily norfloxacin is more effective than weekly rufloxacin in prevention of spontaneous bacterial peritonitis recurrence. *Dig Dis Sci*, **47**(6):1356–1361.

Bell BP, Manos MM, Zaman A, et al. (2008) The epidemiology of newly diagnosed chronic liver disease in gastroenterology practices in the United States: results from population-based surveillance. *Am J Gastroenterol*, **103**(11):2727–2736.

Bergheim I, Parlesak A, Dierks C, Bode JC, Bode C (2003) Nutritional deficiencies in German middle-class male alcohol consumers: relation to dietary intake and severity of liver disease. *Eur J Clin Nutr*, **57**(3):431–438.

Bernard B, Grangé JD, Khac EN, Amiot X, Opolon P, Poynard T (1999) Antibiotic prophylaxis for the prevention of bacterial infections in cirrhotic patients with gastrointestinal bleeding: a meta-analysis. *Hepatology*, **29**(6):1655–1661.

Blachier M, Leleu H, Peck-Radosavljevic M, Valla DC, Roudot-Thoraval F (2013) The burden of liver disease in Europe: a review of available epidemiological data. *J Hepatol*, **58(3)**:593–608.

Boks AL, Brommer EJ, Schalm SW, VanVliet HH (1986) Hemostasis and fibrinolysis in severe liver failure and their relation to hemorrhage. *Hepatology*, **6**(1):79–86.

Borzio M, Salerno F, Piantoni L, et al. (2001) Bacterial infection in patients with advanced cirrhosis: a multicentre prospective study. *Dig Liver Dis*, **33**(1):41–48.

Bosch J, Abraldes JG, Fernández M, García-Pagán JC (2010) Hepatic endothelial dysfunction and abnormal angiogenesis: new targets in the treatment of portal hypertension. *J Hepatol*, **53**(3):558–567.

Braillon A, Cales P, Valla D, Gaudy D, Geoffroy P, Lebrec D (1986) Influence of the degree of liver failure on systemic and splanchnic haemodynamics and on response to propranolol in patients with cirrhosis. *Gut*, **27**(10):1204–1209.

Braillon A, Gaudin C, Poo JL, Moreau R, Debaene B, Lebrec D (1992) Plasma catecholamine concentrations are a reliable index of sympathetic vascular tone in patients with cirrhosis. *Hepatology*, **15**(1):58–62.

Branch RA, James J, Read AE (1976) A study of factors influencing drug disposition in chronic liver disease, using the model drug (+)-propranolol. *Br J Clin Pharmacol*, **3**(2):243–249.

Brensing KA, Textor J, Perz J, et al. (2000) Long term outcome after transjugular intrahepatic portosystemic stent-shunt in non-transplant cirrhotics with hepatorenal syndrome: a phase II study. *Gut*, **47**(2):288–295.

Brodie MJ, Boobis AR, Bulpitt CJ, Davies DS (1981) Influence of liver disease and environmental factors on hepatic monooxygenase activity *in vitro*. *Eur J Clin Pharmacol*, **20**(1):39–46.

Bureau C, Garcia Pagan JC, Layrargues GP, et al. (2007) Patency of stents covered with polytetrafluoroethylene in patients treated by transjugular intrahepatic portosystemic shunts: long-term results of a randomized multicentre study. *Liver Int*, **27**(6):742–747.

Burroughs AK , Vangeli M (2002). Transjugular intrahepatic portosystemic shunt versus endoscopic therapy: randomized trials for secondary prophylaxis of variceal bleeding: an updated meta-analysis (editorial). *Scand J Gastroenterol*, **37**(3):249–252.

Cabrera J, Arroyo V, Ballesta AM, et al. (1982) Aminoglycoside nephrotoxicity in cirrhosis. Value of urinary beta 2-microglobulin to discriminate functional renal failure from acute tubular damage. *Gastroenterology*, **82**(1):97–105.

Cejna M, Peck-Radosavljevic M, Thurnher SA, Hittmair K, Schoder M, Lammer J (2001) Creation of transjugular intrahepatic portosystemic shunts with stent-grafts: initial experiences with a polytetrafluoroethylene-covered nitinol endoprosthesis. *Radiology*, **221**(2):437–446.

Chau TN, Patch D, Chan YW, Nagral A, Dick R, Burroughs AK (1998) "Salvage" transjugular intrahepatic portosystemic shunts: gastric fundal compared with esophageal variceal bleeding. *Gastroenterology*, **114**(5):981–987.

Cheung K, Lee SS, Raman M (2012) Prevalence and mechanisms of malnutrition in patients with advanced liver disease, and nutrition management strategies. *Clin Gastrenterol Hepatol*, **10**(2):117–125.

Clark JM, Brancati FL, Diehl AM (2003) The prevalence and etiology of elevated aminotransferase levels in the United States. *Am J Gastroenterol*, **98**(5):960–967.

Colapinto RF, Stronell RD, Birch JS, et al. (1982) Creation of an intrahepatic portosystemic shunt with a Grüntzig balloon catheter. *Can Med Assoc J*, **126**(1):267–268.

Coleman PJ, McQuillan GM, Moyer LA, Lambert SB, Margolis HS (1998). Incidence of hepatitis B virus infection in the United States, 1976–1994: estimates from the National Health and Nutrition Examination Surveys. *J Infect Dis*, **178**(4):954–959.

Conn HO (1981) A peek at the Child–Turcotte classification. *Hepatology*, **1**(6):673–676.

D'Amico G, Luca A, Morabito A, Miraglia R, D'Amico M (2005) Uncovered transjugular intrahepatic portosystemic shunt for refractory ascites: a meta-analysis. *Gastroenterology*, **129**(4):1282–1293.

D'Amico G, Garcia-Tsao G, Pagliaro L (2006) Natural history and prognostic indicators of survival in cirrhosis: a systematic review of 118 studies. *J Hepatol*, **44**(1):217–231.

D'Amico G, Luca A (2008) TIPS is a cost effective alternative to surgical shunt as a rescue therapy for prevention of recurrent bleeding from esophageal varices. *J Hepatol*, **48**(3):387–390.

de Franchis R, on behalf of the Baveno V Faculty (2010) Revising consensus in portal hypertension: report of the Baveno V Consensus Workshop on methodology of diagnosis and therapy in portal hypertension. *J Hepatol*, **53**(4):762–768.

Delaney AP, Dan A, McCaffrey J, Finfer S (2011) The role of albumin as a resuscitation fluid for patients with sepsis: a systematic review and meta-analysis. *Crit Care Med*, **39**(2):386–391.

Delich PC, Siepler JK, Parker P (2007) Liver disease. In: Gottschlich MM (ed) *The A.S.P.E.N. Nutrition Support Core Curriculum: A Case Based Approach–the Adult Patient*, pp. 540–547. American Society for Parenteral and Enteral Nutrition, Silver Spring, Maryland.

Dellinger RP, Levy MM, Carlet JM, et al. (2008) Surviving Sepsis Campaign: international guidelines for management of severe sepsis and septic shock. *Crit Care Med*, **36**(1):296–327.

Deltenre P, Mathurin P, Dharancy S, et al. (2005) Transjugular intrahepatic portosystemic shunt in refractory ascites: a meta-analysis. *Liver Int*, **25**(2):349–356.

Dhanasekaran R, West JK, Gonzales PC et al. (2010) Transjugular intrahepatic portosystemic shunt for symptomatic refractory hepatic hydrothorax in patients with cirrhosis. *Am J Gastroenterol*, **105**(3):635–641.

Dudrick SJ, Kavic S (2002) Hepatobiliary nutrition: history and future. *J Hepatobil Pancreat Surg*, **9**(4):459–468.

El-Serag HB, Mason AC (1999) Rising incidence of hepatocellular carcinoma in the United States. *N Engl J Med*, **340**(10):745–750.

Elbekai RH, Korashy HM, El-Kadi AO (2004) The effect of liver cirrhosis on the regulation and expression of drug metabolizing enzymes. *Curr Drug Metab*, **5**(2):157–167.

European Association for the Study of the Liver (2010) EASL clinical practice guidelines on the management of ascites, spontaneous bacterial peritonitis, and hepatorenal syndrome in cirrhosis. *J Hepatol*, **53**(3):397–417.

Ewe K (1981) Bleeding after liver biopsy does not correlate with indices of peripheral coagulation. *Digest Dis Sci*, **26**(5):388–393.

Falck-Ytter Y, Younassi ZM, Marchesini G, McCullough AJ (2001) Clinical features and natural history of nonalcoholic steatosis syndromes. *Semin Liver Dis*, **21**(1):17–26.

Farrell GC, Cooksley WG, Powell LW (1979) Drug metabolism in liver disease: activity of hepatic microsomal metabolizing enzymes. *Clin Pharmacol Ther*, **26**(4):483–492.

Fernández J, Gustot T (2012) Management of bacterial infections in cirrhosis. *J Hepatol*, **56**(Suppl 1):S1–S12.

Fernández J, Navasa M, Gómez J, et al (2002) Bacterial infections in cirrhosis: epidemiological changes with invasive procedures and norfloxacin prophylaxis. *Hepatology*, **35**(1):140–148.

Fernández J, Navasa M, Planas R, et al (2007) Primary prophylaxis of spontaneous bacterial peritonitis delays hepatorenal syndrome and improves survival in cirrhosis. *Gastroenterology*, **133**(3):818–824.

Freeman RB, Rohrer RJ, Katz E, et al. (2001) Preliminary results of a liver allocation plan using a continuous medical severity score that de-emphasizes waiting time. *Liver Transplant*, **7**(3):173–178.

Freeman RB, Wiesner RH, Edwards E, et al. (2004) Results of the first year of the new liver allocation plan. *Liver Transpl*, **10**(1):7–15.

Garcia-Morillas M, Gil-Extremera B, Caracuel-Ruiz MD (1984) Differential effects of hepatic cirrhosis on the plasma protein binding of drugs. *Int J Clin Pharmacol Res*, **4**(5):327–333.

García-Pagán JC, Caca K, Bureau C, et al. (2010) Early use of TIPS in patients with cirrhosis and variceal bleeding. *N Engl J Med*, **362**(25):2370–2379.

Garcia-Tsao G, Bosch J (2010) Management of varices and variceal hemorrhage in cirrhosis. *N Engl J Med*, **362**(9):823–832.

Garcia-Tsao G, Lim J, Members of the Veterans Affairs Hepatitis C Resource Center Program (2009) Management and treatment of patients with cirrhosis and portal hypertension: recommendations from the Department of Veterans Affairs Hepatitis C Resource Center Program and the National Hepatitis C Program. *Am J Gastroenterol*, **104**(7):1802–1829.

Gatta A, Bolognesi M, Merkel C (2008) Vasoactive factors and hemodynamic mechanisms in the pathophysiology of portal hypertension in cirrhosis. *Mol Aspects Med*, **29**(1-2):119–129.

George J, Murray M, Byth K, Farrell GC (1995) Differential alterations of cytochrome P450 proteins in livers from patients with severe chronic liver disease. *Hepatology*, **21**(1):120–128.

George J, Byth K, Farrell GC (1996) Influence of clinicopathological variables on CYP protein expression in human liver. *J Gastroenterol Hepatol*, **11**(1):33–39.

Ginès A, Fernández-Esparrach G, Monescillo A, et al. (1996) Randomized trial comparing albumin, dextran 70, and polygeline in cirrhotic patients with ascites treated by paracentesis. *Gastroenterology*, **111**(4):1002–1010.

Ginès A, Uriz J, Calahorra B, et al. (2002) Transjugular intrahepatic portosystemic shunting versus paracentesis plus albumin for refractory ascites in cirrhosis. *Gastroenterology*, **123**(6):1839–1847.

Ginès P, Rimola A, Planas R, et al. (1990) Norfloxacin prevents spontaneous bacterial peritonitis recurrence in cirrhosis: results of a double-blind, placebo-controlled trial. *Hepatology*, **12**(4):716–724.

Gordon FD, Anastopoulos HT, Crenshaw W, et al (1997) The successful treatment of symptomatic, refractory hepatic hydrothorax with transjugular intrahepatic portosystemic shunt. *Hepatology*, **25**(6):1366–1369.

Grabau CM, Crago S, Hoff LK, et al. (2004) Performance standards for therapeutic abdominal paracentesis. *Hepatology*, **40**(2):484–488.

Gridelli B, Spada M, Petz W, et al (2003) Split-liver transplantation eliminates the need for living-donor liver transplantation in children with end-stage cholestatic liver disease. *Transplantation*, **75**(8):1197–1203.

Grossberg AJ, Scarlett JM, Marks DL (2010) Hypothalamic mechanisms in cachexia. *Physiol Behav*, **100**(5):478–489.

Groszmann RJ, Garcia-Tsao G, Bosch J, et al. (2005) Beta-blockers to prevent gastroesophageal varices in patients with cirrhosis. *N Engl J Med*, **353**(21):2254–2261.

Guevara M, Ginès P, Bandi JC, et al. (1998a) Transjugular intrahepatic portosystemic shunt in hepatorenal syndrome: effects on renal function and vasoactive systems. *Hepatology*, **28**(2):416–422.

Guevara M, Bru C, Ginès P, et al. (1998b) Increased cerebrovascular resistance in cirrhotic patients with ascites. *Hepatology*, **28**(1):39–44.

Gupta S, Castel H, Rao RV, et al. (2010) Improved survival after liver transplantation in patients with hepatopulmonary syndrome. *Am J Transplant*, **10**(2):354–363.

Gustot T, Durant F, Lebrec D, Vincent JL, Moreau R (2009) Severe sepsis in cirrhosis. *Hepatology*, **50**(6):2022–2033.

Henriksen JH, Møller S (2009) Cardiac and systemic hemodynamic complications of liver cirrhosis. *Scan Cardiovasc J*, **43**(4):218–225.

Hopkins WE, Waggoner AD, Barzilai B (1992) Frequency and significance of intrapulmonary right-to-left shunting in end-stage hepatic disease. *Am J Cardiol*, **70**(4):516–519.

Howden CW, Birnie GG, Brodie MJ (1989) Drug metabolism in liver disease. *Pharmacol Ther*, **40**(3):439–474.

Irani S, Kowdley K, Kozarek R (2011) Gastric varices: an updated review of management. *J Clin Gastroenterol*, **45**(2):133–148.

Iwakiri Y, Groszmann RJ (2007) Vascular endothelial dysfunction in cirrhosis. *J Hepatol*, **46**(5):927–934.

Kalaitzakis E, Simrén M, Olsson R, et al. (2006) Gastrointestinal symptoms in patients with liver cirrhosis: associations with nutritional status and health-related quality of life. *Scand J Gastroenterol*, **41**(12):1464–1472.

Kalaitzakis E, Bosaeus I, Öhman L, Björnsson E (2007) Altered postprandial glucose, insulin, leptin, and ghrelin in liver cirrhosis: correlations with energy intake and resting energy expenditure. *Am J Clin Nutr*, **85**(3):808–815.

Kamath PS, Wiesner RH, Malinchoc M, et al (2001) A model to predict survival in patients with end-stage liver disease. *Hepatology*, **33**(2):464–470.

Keeffe EB (2001) Liver transplantation: current status and novel approaches to liver replacement. *Gastroenterology*, **120**(3):749–762.

Kiafar C, Gilani N (2008) Hepatic hydrothorax: current concepts of pathophysiology and treatment options. *Ann Hepatol*, **7**(4):313–320.

Kim WR, Krowka MJ, Plevak DJ, et al. (2000) Accuracy of Doppler echocardiography in the assessment of pulmonary hypertension in liver transplant candidates. *Liver Transpl*, **6**(4):453–458.

Kim WR, Brown RS Jr, Terrault NA, El-Serag H (2002) Burden of liver disease in the United States: summary of a workshop. *Hepatology*, **36**(1):227–242.

Kochanek KD, Xu J, Murphy SL, Miniño AM, Kung HC (2011) Deaths: final data for 2009. *Natl Vital Stat Rep*, **60**(4)(3):1–116.

Krag A, Borup T, Møller S, Bendtsen F (2008) Efficacy and safety of terlipressin in cirrhotic patients with variceal bleeding and hepatorenal syndrome. *Adv Ther*, **25**(11):1105–1140.

Krag A, Møller S, Pedersen EB, Henriksen JH, Holstein-Rathlou NH, Bendtsen F (2010a) Impaired free water excretion in Child C cirrhosis and ascites: relations to distal tubular function and the vasopressin system. *Liver Int*, **30**(9):1364–1370.

Krag A, Bendtsen F, Mortensen C, Henriksen JH, Møller S (2010b) Effect of a single terlipressin administration on cardiac function and perfusion in cirrhosis. *Eur J Gastroenterol Hepatol*, **22**(9):1085–1092.

Krowka MJ, Plevak DJ, Findlay JY, Rosen CB, Wiesner RH, Krom RAF (2000) Pulmonary hemodynamics and perioperative cardiopulmonary-related mortality in patients with portopulmonary hypertension undergoing liver transplantation. *Liver Transpl*, **6**(4):443–450.

Kumar A, Roberts D, Wood KE, et al. (2006) Duration of hypotension before initiation of effective antimicrobial therapy is the critical determinant of survival in human septic shock. *Crit Care Med*, **34**(6):1589–1596.

Kumar A, Zarychanski R, Light B, et al. (2010) Early combination antibiotic therapy yields improved survival compared with monotherapy in septic shock: a propensity-matched analysis. *Crit Care Med*, **38(9)**:1773–1785.

Lasch HM, Fried MW, Zacks SL, et al. (2001) Use of transjugular intrahepatic portosystemic shunt as a bridge to liver transplantation in a patient with severe hepatopulmonary syndrome. *Liver Transpl*, **7**(2):147–149.

Le Moine O, Marchant A, De Groote D, Azar C, Goldman M, Deviere J (1995) Role of defective monocyte interleukin-10 release in tumor necrosis factor-alpha overproduction in alcoholics cirrhosis. *Hepatology*, **22**(5):1436–1439.

Lebrec D, Giuily N, Hadengue A, et al. (1996) Transjugular intrahepatic portosystemic shunts: comparison with paracentesis in patients with cirrhosis and refractory ascites: a randomized trial. *J Hepatol*, **25**(2):135–144.

Levine JA, Morgan MY (1996) Weighed dietary intakes in patients with chronic liver disease. *Nutrition*, **12**(6):430–435.

Lewis GP, Jusko WJ (1975) Pharmacokinetics of ampicillin in cirrhosis. *Clin Pharmacol Ther*, **18**(4):475–484.

Lindor KD, Gershwin ME, Poupon R, Kaplan M, Bergasa NV, Heathcote EJ (2009) Primary biliary cirrhosis. *Hepatology*, **50**(1):291–308.

Lisman T, Porte RJ (2010) Rebalanced hemostasis in patients with liver disease: evidence and clinical consequences. *Blood*, **116**(6):878–885.

Llach J, Rimola A, Navasa M, et al. (1992) Incidence and predictive factors of first episode of spontaneous bacterial peritonitis in cirrhosis with ascites: relevance of ascitic fluid protein concentration. *Hepatology*, **16**(3):724–727.

Lo GH, Liang HL, Chen WC, et al. (2007) A prospective, randomized controlled trial of transjugular intrahepatic portosystemic shunt versus cyanoacrylate injection in the prevention of gastric variceal rebleeding. *Endoscopy*, **39**(8):679–685.

Lucey MR, Brown KA, Everson GT, et al. (1997) Minimal criteria for placement of adults on the liver transplant waiting list: a report of a national conference organized by the American Society of Transplant Physicians and the American Association for the Study of Liver Diseases. *Liver Transplant Surg*, **3**(6):628–637.

Lucey MR, Terrault N, Ojo L, et al. (2013) Long-term management of the successful adult liver transplant: 2012 practice guideline by the American Association for the Study of Liver Diseases and the American Society of Transplantation. *Liver Transplant*, **19**(1):3–26.

Ly KN, Xing J, Klevens RM, Jiles RB, Ward JW, Holmberg SD (2012) The increasing burden of mortality from viral hepatitis in the United States between 1999 and 2007. *Ann Intern Med*, **156**(4):271–278.

Malagó M, Hertl M, Testa G, Rogiers X, Broelsch CE (2002) Split-liver transplantation: future use of scarce donor organs. *World J Surg*, **26**(2):275–282.

Malinchoc M, Kamath PS, Gordon FD, Peine CJ, Rank J, ter Borg PC (2000) A model to predict poor survival in patients undergoing transjugular intrahepatic portosystemic shunts. *Hepatology*, **31**(4):864–871.

McCashland TM, Shaw BW Jr, Tape E (1996) The American experience with transplantation for acute liver failure. *Semin Liver Dis*, **16**(4):427–433.

McCullough AJ, Bugianesi E, Marchesini G, Kalhan SC (1998) Gender-dependent alterations in serum leptin in alcoholic cirrhosis. *Gastroenterology*, **115**(4):947–953.

McDiarmid SV, Anand R, Lindblad AS, and the principal investigators and institutions of the Studies of Pediatric Liver Transplantation (SPLIT) research group (2002) Development of a pediatric end-stage liver disease score to predict poor outcome in children awaiting liver transplantation. *Transplantation*, **74**(2):173–181.

McGill DB, Rakela J, Zinsmeister AR, Ott BJ (1990) A 21-year experience with major hemorrhage after percutaneous liver biopsy. *Gastroenterology*, **99**(5):1396–1400.

McQuillan GM, Coleman PJ, Kruszon-Moran D, Moyer LA, Lambert SB, Margolis HS (1999) Prevalence of hepatitis B virus infection in the United States: the National Health and Nutrition Examination Surveys, 1976 through 1994. *Am J Public Health*, **89**(1):14–18.

Mehta G, Abraldes JG, Bosch J (2010) Developments and controversies in the management of oesophageal and gastric varices. *Gut*, **59**(6):701–705.

Melgosa MT, Ricci GL, García-Pagan JC, et al. (2010) Acute and long-term effects of inhaled iloprost in portopulmonary hypertension. *Liver Transplant*, **16**(3):348–356.

Merli M, Giusto M, Gentili F, et al. (2010) Nutritional status: its influence on the outcome of patients undergoing liver transplantation. *Liver Int*, **30**(2):208–214.

Møller S, Bendtsen F, Henriksen JH (2005) Pathophysiological basis of pharmacotherapy in the hepatorenal syndrome. *Scand J Gastroenterol*, **40**(5):491–500.

Møller S, Henriksen JH (2008) Cardiovascular complications of cirrhosis. *Gut*, **57**(2):268–278.

Møller S, Henriksen JH (2010) Cirrhotic cardiomyopathy. *J Hepatol*, **53**(1):179–190.

Møller S, Hobolth L, Winkler C, Bendtsen F, Christensen E (2011) Determinants of the hyperdynamic circulation and central hypovolaemia in cirrhosis. *Gut*, **60**(9):1254–1259.

Moore KP, Aithal GP (2006) Guidelines on the management of ascites in cirrhosis. *Gut*, **55**(Suppl 6):1–12.

Müller MJ, Böttcher J, Selberg O, et al. (1999) Hypermetabolism in clinically stable patients with liver cirrhosis. *Am J Clin Nutr*, **69**(6):1194–1201.

Murray KF, Carithers RL Jr (2005) AASLD practice guidelines: evaluation of the patient for liver transplantation. *Hepatology*, **41**(6):1407–1432.

Murray M (1992) P450 enzymes. Inhibition mechanisms, genetic regulation and effects of liver disease. *Clin Pharmacokinet*, **23**(2):132–146.

Narahara Y, Kanazawa H, Fukuda T, et al. (2011) Transjugular intrahepatic portosystemic shunt versus paracentesis plus albumin in patients with refractory ascites who have good hepatic and renal function: a prospective randomized trial. *J Gastroenterol*, **46**(1):78–85.

Oellerich M, Burdelski M, Lautz HU, Binder L, Pichlmayr R (1991) Predictors of one-year pretransplant survival in patients with cirrhosis. *Hepatology*, **14**(6):1029–1034.

Otte JB, de Ville de Goyet J, Reding R, et al. (1998) Pediatric liver transplantation: from the full-size liver graft to reduced, split, and living related liver transplantation. *Pediatr Surg Int*, **13**(5-6):308–318.

Papatheodoridis GV, Goulis J, Leandro G, Patch D, Burroughs AK (1999) Transjugular intrahepatic portosystemic shunt compared with endoscopic treatment for prevention of variceal rebleeding: a meta-analysis. *Hepatology*, **30**(3):612–622.

Paramesh AS, Husain SZ, Shneider B, et al. (2003) Improvement of hepatopulmonary syndrome after transjugular intrahepatic portasystemic shunting: case report and review of literature. *Pediatr Transplant*, **7**(2):157–162.

Pellicelli AM, Barbaro G, Puoti C, et al. (2010) Plasma cytokines and portopulmonary hypertension in patients with cirrhosis waiting for orthotopic liver transplantation. *Angiology*, **61**(8):802–806.

Peng S, Plank LD, McCall JL, Gillanders LK, McIlroy K, Gane EJ (2007) Body composition, muscle function, and energy expenditure in patients with liver cirrhosis: a comprehensive study. *Am J Clin Nutr*, **85**(5):1257–1266.

Pham DM, Subramanian R, Parekh S (2010) Coexisting hepatopulmonary syndrome and portopulmonary hypertension. Implications for liver transplantation. *J Clin Gastroenterol*, **44**(7):e136–e140.

Plauth M, Cabré E, Riggio O, et al. (2006) ESPEN guidelines on enteral nutrition: liver disease. *Clin Nutr*, **25**(2):285–294.

Plessier A, Denninger MH, Consigny Y, et al. (2003) Coagulation disorders in patients with cirrhosis and severe sepsis. *Liver Int*, **23**(6):440–448.

Pomier-Layrargues G, Bouchard L, Lafortune M, Bissonnette J, Guérette D, Perreault P (2012) The transjugular intrahepatic portosystemic shunt in the treatment of portal hypertension: current status. *Int J Hepatol*, 2012(2012):1–12.

Poordad FF, Sigal SH, Brown RS Jr (2009) Pathophysiologic basis for the medical management of portal hypertension. *Expert Opin Pharmacother*, **10**(3):453–467.

Poterucha JJ, Krowka MJ, Dickson ER, Cortese DA, Stanson AW, Krom RA (1995) Failure of hepatopulmonary syndrome to resolve after liver transplantation and successful treatment with embolotherapy. *Hepatology*, **21**(1):96–100.

Rakela J, Lange SM, Ludwig J, Baldus WP (1985) Fulminant hepatitis: Mayo Clinic experience with 34 cases. *Mayo Clin Proc*, **60**(5):289–292.

Ramsay M (2010) Portopulmonary hypertension and right heart failure in patients with cirrhosis. *Curr Opin Anaesthesiol*, **23**(2):145–150.

Renz JF, Emond JC, Yersiz H, Ascher NL, Busuttil RW (2004) Split-liver transplantation in the United States: outcomes of a national survey. *Annal Surg*, **239**(2):172–181.

Riegler JL, Lang KA, Johnson SP, Westerman JH (1995) Transjugular intrahepatic portosystemic shunt improves oxygenation in hepatopulmonary syndrome. *Gastroenterology*, **109**(3):978–983.

Rimola A, García-Tsao G, Navasa M, et al. (2000) Diagnosis, treatment and prophylaxis of spontaneous bacterial peritonitis: a consensus document. *J Hepatol*, **32**(1):142–153.

Rivers E, Nguyen B, Havstad S, et al. (2001) Early goal-directed therapy in the treatment of severe sepsis and septic shock. *N Engl J Med*, **345**(19):1368–1377.

Rodriguez-Roisin R, Krowka MJ (2008) Hepatopulmonary syndrome—a liver-induced lung vascular disorder. *N Engl J Med*, **358**(22):2378–2387.

Rösch J, Hanafee WN, Snow H (1969) Transjugular portal venography and radiologic portacaval shunt: an experimental study. *Radiology*, **92**(5):1112–1114.

Rössle M, Ochs A, Gülberg V, et al. (2000) A comparison of paracentesis and transjugular intrahepatic portosystemic shunting in patients with ascites. *N Engl J Med*, **342**(23):1701–1707.

Ruiz-del-Arbol L, Monescillo A, Arocena C, et al. (2005) Circulatory function and hepatorenal syndrome in cirrhosis. *Hepatology*, **42**(2):439–447.

Runyon BA (2009) Management of adult patients with ascites due to cirrhosis: an update. *Hepatology*, **49**(6):2087–2107.

Saad NEA, Lee DE, Waldman DL, Saad WEA (2007) Pulmonary arterial coil embolization for the management of persistent type I hepatopulmonary syndrome after liver transplantation. *J Vasc Interv Radiol*, **18**(12):1576–1580.

Salerno F, Merli M, Riggio O, et al. (2004) Randomized controlled study of TIPS versus paracentesis plus albumin in cirrhosis with severe ascites. *Hepatology*, **40**(3):629–635.

Salerno F, Camma C, Enea M, Rössle M, Wong F (2007) Transjugular intrahepatic portosystemic shunt for refractory ascites: a meta-analysis of individual patient data. *Gastroenterology*, **133**(3):825–834.

Salerno F, Guevara M, Bernardi M, et al. (2010) Refractory ascites: pathogenesis, definition and therapy of a severe complication in patients with cirrhosis (review) *Liver Int*, **30**(7):937–947.

Sam J, Nguyen GC (2009) Protein-calorie malnutrition as a prognostic indicator of mortality among patients hospitalized with cirrhosis and portal hypertension. *Liver Int*, **29**(9):1396–1402.

Sanchez W, Kamath PS (2008) Prevention and treatment of acute liver failure in patients with chronic liver disease. In: Arroyo V, Sanchez-Fueyo A, Fernandez-Gomez J, Forns X, Ginès P, Rodés J (eds) *Advances in the Therapy of Liver Diseases*, pp 73–79. Ars Medica, Barcelona.

Sanyal AJ, Freedman AM, Luketic VA, et al. (1996) Transjugular intrahepatic portosystemic shunts for patients with active variceal hemorrhage unresponsive to sclerotherapy. *Gastroenterology*, **111**(1):138–146.

Sanyal AJ, Genning C, Reddy KR, et al. (2003) The North American study for the treatment of refractory ascites. *Gastroenterology*, **124**(3):634–641.

Sass DA, Chopra KB (2009) Portal hypertension and variceal hemorrhage. *Med Clin N Am*, **93**(4):837–853.

Schiodt FV, Atillasoy E, Shakii AO, et al. (1999. Etiology and outcome for 295 patients with acute liver failure in the United States. *Liver Transplant Surg*, **5**(1):29–34.

Schuppan D, Afdhal NH (2008) Liver cirrhosis. *Lancet*, **371**(9615):838–851.

Scouras NE, Matsusaki T, Boucek CD, et al. (2011) Portopulmonary hypertension as an indication for combined heart, lung, and liver or lung and liver transplantation: literature review and case presentation. *Liver Transplant*, **17**(2):137–143.

Segal JB, Dzik WH, on behalf of the Transfusion Medicine/Hemostasis Clinical Trials Network (2005) Paucity of studies to support that abnormal coagulation test results predict bleeding in the setting of invasive procedures: an evidence-based review. *Transfusion*, **45**(9):1413–1425.

Senzolo M, Cholongitas E, Burra P, et al. (2009) β-blockers protect against spontaneous bacterial peritonitis in cirrhotic patients: a meta-analysis. *Liver Int*, **29**:(8)1189–1193.

Sersté T, Melot C, Francoz C, et al. (2010) Deleterious effects of beta-blockers on survival in patients with cirrhosis and refractory ascites. *Hepatology*, **52**(3):1017–1022.

Settmacher U, Theruvath T, Pascher A, Neuhaus P (2004) Living-donor liver transplantation—European experiences. *Nephrol Dial Transplant*, **19**(Suppl 4):iv16–iv21.

Shah T, Isaac J, Adams D, Kelly D, Liver Units (2005) Development of hepatopulmonary syndrome and portopulmonary hypertension in a paediatric liver transplant patient. *Pediatr Transplant*, **9**(1):127–131.

Siegerstetter P, Deibert P, Ochs A, Olschewski M, Blum HE, Rössle M (2001) Treatment of refractory hepatic hydrothorax with transjugular intrahepatic portosystemic shunt: long-term results in 40 patients. *Eur J Gastroenterol Hepat*, **13**(5):529–534.

Spahr L, Fenyves D, N'Guyen W, et al. (1995) Improvement of hepatorenal syndrome by transjugular intrahepatic portosystemic shunt. *Am J Gastroenterol*, **90**(7):1169–1171.

Stokkeland K, Brandt L, Ekbom A, Hultcrantz R (2006) Improved prognosis for patients hospitalized with esophageal varices in Sweden 1969–2002. *Hepatology*, **43**(3):500–505.

Surman OS (2002) The ethics of partial-liver donation. *N Engl J Med*, **346**(14):1038.

Tandon P, Garcia-Tsao G (2008) Bacterial infections, sepsis, and multiorgan failure in cirrhosis. *Semin Liver Dis*, **28**(1):26–42.

Terg R, Fassio E, Guevara M, et al. (2008) Ciprofloxacin in primary prophylaxis of spontaneous bacterial peritonitis: a randomized, placebo-controlled study. *J Hepatol*, **48**(5):774–779.

Terjung B, Lemnitzer I, Dumoulin FL, et al. (2003) Bleeding complications after percutaneous liver biopsy. An analysis of risk factors. *Digestion*, **67**(3):138–145.

Thabut D, Shah V (2010) Intrahepatic angiogenesis and sinusoidal remodeling in chronic liver disease: new targets for the treatment of portal hypertension? *J Hepatol*, **53**(5):976–980.

Torregrosa M, Aguadé S, Dos L, et al. (2005) Cardiac alterations in cirrhosis: reversibility after liver transplantation. *J Hepatol*, **42**(1):68–74.

Toubia N, Sanyal AJ (2008) Portal hypertension and variceal hemorrhage. *Med Clin N Am*, **92**(3):551–574.

Tripodi A, Mannucci PM (2011) The coagulopathy of chronic liver disease. *N Engl J Med*, **365**(2):147–156.

Trotter JF, Wachs M, Everson GT, Kam I (2002) Adult-to-adult transplantation of the right hepatic lobe from a living donor. *N Engl J Med*, **346**(14):1074–1082.

Tsiakalos A, Hatzis G, Moyssakis I, Karatzaferis A, Ziakas PD, Tzelepis GE (2011) Portopulmonary hypertension and serum endothelin levels in hospitalized patients with cirrhosis. *Hepatobil Pancreat Dis Int*, **10**(4):393–398.

Tsiaousi ET, Hatzitolios AI, Trygonis SK, Savopoulos CG (2008) Malnutrition in end stage liver disease: recommendation and nutritional support. *J Gastroenterol Hepatol*, **23**(4):527–533.

Vangeli M, Patch D, Terreni N, et al. (2004) Bleeding ectopic varices—treatment with transjugular intrahepatic porto-systemic shunt (TIPS) and embolisation. *J Hepatol*, **41**(4):560–566.

Venkat D, Venkat KK (2010) Hepatorenal syndrome. *South Med J*, **103**(7):654–659.

Vidal V, Joly L, Perreault P, Bouchard L, Lafortune M, Pomier-Layrargues G (2006) Usefulness of transjugular intrahepatic portosystemic shunt in the management of bleeding ectopic varices in cirrhotic patients. *Cardiovasc Interv Radiol*, **29**(2):216–219.

Vieira da Rocha EC, D'Amico EA, Caldwell SH, et al. (2009) A prospective study of conventional and expanded coagulation indices in predicting ulcer bleeding after variceal band ligation. *Clin Gastroenterol Hepatol*, 7(9):988–993.

Warnaar N, Lisman T, Porte RJ (2008) The two tales of coagulation in liver transplantation. *Curr Opin Organ Transplant*, **13**(3):298–303.

Wiesner RH, McDiarmid SV, Kamath PS, et al. (2001) MELD and PELD: application of survival models to liver allocation. *Liver Transplant*, 7(7):567–580.

Wiesner R, Edwards E, Freeman R, et al. (2003) Model for end-stage liver disease (MELD) and allocation of donor livers. *Gastroenterology*, **124**(1):91–96.

Wong F (2006) The use of TIPS in chronic liver disease. *Ann Hepatol*, **5**(1):5–15.

Wong F (2008) Hepatorenal syndrome: current management. *Curr Gastroenterol Rep*, **10**(1):22–29.

Wong F, Salerno F (2010) Beta-blockers in cirrhosis: friend and foe? *Hepatology*, **52**(3):811–813.

Yoshida H, Hamada T, Inuzuka S, Ueno T, Sata M, Tanikawa K (1993) Bacterial infection in cirrhosis, with and without hepatocellular carcinoma. *Am J Gastroenterol*, **88**(12):2067–2071.

Zamirian M, Aslani A, Shahrzad S (2007) Left atrial volume: a novel predictor of hepatopulmonary syndrome. *Am J Gastroenterol*, **102**(7):1392–1396.

Zheng M, Chen Y, Bai J, et al. (2008) Transjugular intrahepatic portosystemic shunt versus endoscopic therapy in the secondary prophylaxis of variceal rebleeding in cirrhotic patients: meta-analysis update. *J Clin Gastroenterol*, **42**(5):507–516.

# CHAPTER 20

# Liver transplantation: patient selection, organ allocation, and outcomes

Vishal C. Patel and John O'Grady

## Introduction

Advanced liver disease has a wide range of causes and survival is usually limited, measured in months to a few years. It has enormous implications in terms of disease burden in the population and expense to healthcare systems. Liver transplantation is the only life-prolonging therapeutic option for most patients with acute or chronic liver failure, offering many of them extended survival and greatly improved quality of life (Belle et al., 1997).

The aim of this chapter is to provide an overview of patient selection and indications for liver transplantation, how potential recipients are evaluated and prioritized, how organs are allocated, the importance of comorbidity, and disease-related outcomes. Consideration will also be given to retransplantation and to relevant ethical issues.

## Timing of referral

Several authorities have made recommendations on the timing of referral of patients with acute liver failure and chronic liver disease for assessment at transplant units (Devlin and O'Grady, 2000; BASL Liver Transplant Guidelines, 2012). These emphasize the need to allow a reasonable period for comprehensive evaluation investigation and for potential recipients to make informed decisions about their clinical options. These guidelines are intended to be flexible and should not override local clinical judgement.

It is clear that late referral has detrimental effects on post-transplant outcomes, since these are affected by pretransplant disease severity. Earlier referral may provide an opportunity to optimize the patient in terms of both the underlying hepatic disease and many comorbidities and gives time for alternative treatments that may benefit the potential transplant candidate. Even when it is considered too early for transplant, early referral permits better planning of transfer in the future if deterioration occurs. This cautious approach to referral has assumed greater importance as waiting times have increased, since listing as soon as a candidate becomes eligible improves the likelihood of obtaining a graft in time.

Clarification of eligibility for transplantation is essential to ensure that disparities in access to such a vital health resource are minimized, particularly in view of geographical differences in disease prevalence and referral for transplantation. National selection criteria for listing should provide a uniform set of guidelines, minimizing variation between transplant units.

## Indications and selection criteria for liver transplantation

In most jurisdictions, minimum listing criteria have been agreed and implemented by all transplant units. In the UK these fall into four categories:

1. Acute liver failure
2. End-stage chronic liver disease
3. Variant syndromes
4. Individual cases not covered by these groupings

### Acute liver failure

The indications for listing for super-urgent liver transplantation are broadly based on the King's College Criteria (KCC) (O'Grady et al., 1989). Although first described in 1989, they are still effective in assessing prognosis in the majority of patients. A strength of the KCC has been specificity and a weakness has been lack of sensitivity, especially in patients with paracetamol-related acute liver failure. This was the basis for adding section 4 to the standard KCC, as outlined in Table 20.1.

The effectiveness of this modification is currently under review. The other modification has been the addition of listing criteria for patient cohorts not included in the original KCC study (e.g. Wilson's disease, Budd–Chiari syndrome) and early hepatic artery thrombosis or graft failure requiring urgent retransplantation.

### Chronic liver disease

In order to be registered on the elective liver transplant list a candidate must meet one of two criteria:

(1) Chronic liver disease due to an accepted aetiology and/or

(2) HCC within transplant criteria

Adult patients (17 years or older) with chronic liver disease and no HCC should have a clinical indication and a qualifying United

**Table 20.1** Selection criteria for super-urgent liver transplantation. (Adapted with kind permission from Liver Advisory Group, NHS Blood and Transplant Liver Selection Policy, Copyright 2014, policy version POL195/4, updated February 2015, http://www.odt.nhs.uk/pdf/liver_selection_policy.pdf.)

| **Paracetamol hepatotoxicity** |
|---|
| ◆ pH < 7.25 > 24 hours after overdose and after fluid resuscitation |
| ◆ Serum lactate > 3.5 mmol/L > 24 hours after overdose on admission or > 3.0 mmol/L after fluid resuscitation |
| ◆ PT > 100 s (INR > 6.5) + creatinine > 300 µmol/L anuria, + grade 3–4 encephalopathy |
| ◆ Two criteria from above plus evidence of clinical deterioration (increased ICP, $FiO_2$ > 50%, increasing inotrope requirements) in the absence of clinical sepsis |
| **Other aetiologies** |
| ◆ Seronegative hepatitis, hepatitis A, hepatitis B, drug-induced liver failure: INR > 6.5 or PT > 100 s |
| ◆ Seronegative hepatitis, hepatitis A, hepatitis B, drug-induced liver failure. Any three from: |
| ◆ unfavourable aetiology |
| ◆ age > 40 years; jaundice–encephalopathy (J–E) > 7 days |
| ◆ bilirubin > 300 mmol/L |
| ◆ INR > 3.5 |
| ◆ Acute presentation of Wilson's disease or Budd–Chiari syndrome: a combination of coagulopathy and any grade of encephalopathy |
| ◆ Hepatic artery thrombosis on days 0–21 after liver transplantation |
| ◆ Early graft dysfunction on days 0–7 after liver transplantation with at least two of the following: |
| ◆ AST > 10,000 |
| ◆ INR > 3.0 |
| ◆ serum lactate > 3 mmol/L |
| ◆ absence of bile production |
| ◆ The total absence of liver function (e.g. after total hepatectomy) |
| ◆ Any patient who has been a live liver donor (NHS entitled) who develops severe liver failure within 4 weeks of the donor operation |

AST, Aspartate aminotransferase.

Kingdom Model for End-Stage Liver Disease (UKELD) score of 49 or greater (Barber et al., 2011). Of these, patients who are clinically well should not be listed for transplantation simply because of the presence of a qualifying UKELD score but should be kept under surveillance. The UKELD threshold was chosen to reflect a similar likelihood of dying within 1 year from either the underlying liver disease or liver transplantation (9% at time of analysis). Those with HCC are subject to separate criteria which do not take liver dysfunction into account (see Table 20.2).

### Variant syndromes

About 25% of patients have clinical manifestations of liver disease that will benefit from transplantation but do not have qualifying UKELD scores. Many of these patients have cirrhosis and diuretic-resistant ascites, chronic hepatic encephalopathy, intractable pruritis (e.g. in primary biliary cirrhosis), recurrent

**Table 20.2** Selection criteria for elective liver transplantation—chronic liver disease and hepatocellular carcinoma. (Adapted with kind permission from Liver Advisory Group, NHS Blood and Transplant Liver Selection Policy, Copyright 2014, policy version POL195/4, updated February 2015, http://www.odt.nhs.uk/pdf/liver_selection_policy.pdf.)

| |
|---|
| **Chronic liver disease or failure—**the patient has a projected 1-year liver disease mortality without transplantation of > 9%, predicted by UKELD score of 49 or greater. UKELD score is derived from the patient's serum sodium, creatinine, and bilirubin, and INR of prothrombin time |
| **Hepatocellular carcinoma—**size is assessed by the widest dimensions on either MDCT or MRI scan. A tumour (for the purposes of counting numbers) is identified as an arterialized focal abnormality with portal phase washout. Other lesions are considered indeterminate and do not count. Tumour rupture and AFP > 10,000 IU/mL are absolute contraindications to transplantation, as are extrahepatic spread and macroscopic vascular invasion. The following are criteria for listing:<br>◆ A single tumour ≤ 5 cm diameter, or<br>◆ Up to five tumours all ≤ 3 cm, or<br>◆ A single tumour > 5 cm and ≤ 7 cm diameter where there has been no evidence of tumour progression (volume increase by < 20%), no extrahepatic spread, and no new nodule formation over a 6-month period. Locoregional therapy +/– chemotherapy may be given during that time. Candidates' waiting-list place may be considered from the time of their first staging scan. |

MDCT, Multidector computed tomography; AFP, alpha-fetoprotein.

cholangitis, or hepatopulmonary syndrome, despite optimal medical management. The other categories are for rare diseases in patients without cirrhosis and include conditions such as familial amyloidosis, primary hyperlipidaemias, and polycystic liver disease. To date, the UKELD points system has not been adjusted to guide these patients through the allocation system, as is done in France and the US (Francoz et al., 2011) (see Table 20.3).

### Individual cases

It is recognized that not all patients can be assessed within the framework in Table 20.3, and so patients need to be evaluated on a case-by-case basis. The mechanism for doing this in the UK is the National Appeals Process. A clinical summary is distributed to each of the seven transplant centres and a patient can be listed if at least four centres support the application.

## Selection criteria and evaluation of potential recipients

Evaluation for liver transplantation requires comprehensive assessment in an accredited liver transplant unit. It should confirm that all other treatment options have been exhausted, that transplantation is necessary, and that the potential recipient is an appropriate candidate from both clinical and psychosocial perspectives. Candidates should be assessed on the basis of presenting complications of liver disease and on the severity of known comorbidities, weighing prognosis and quality of life with and without liver transplantation. Potential contraindications, not all of which are absolute, should also be sought and considered because these may predict poorer outcomes than would be expected without a transplant.

As emphasized above, referral should occur before the development of severe complications, to allow timely assessment and,

**Table 20.3** Selection criteria for elective liver transplantation—variant syndromes (Adapted with kind permission from Liver Advisory Group, NHS Blood and Transplant Liver Selection Policy, Copyright 2014, policy version POL195/4, updated February 2015, http://www.odt.nhs.uk/pdf/liver_selection_policy.pdf)

| |
|---|
| **Diuretic resistant ascites**—ascites unresponsive to or intolerant of maximum diuretic dosage and non-responsive to TIPS or where TIPS deemed impossible or contraindicated. |
| **Hepatopulmonary syndrome**—arterial $PO_2$ < 7.8, alveolar arterial oxygen gradient > 20 mm Hg, calculated shunt fraction > 8% (brain uptake following Tc macroaggregated albumen), pulmonary vascular dilatation documented by positive contrast-enhanced transthoracic echo, in the absence of overt chronic lung disease. |
| **Chronic hepatic encephalopathy**—confirmed by EEG or trail-making tests, with at least two admissions in 1 year due to exacerbations in encephalopathy, not manageable by standard therapy. Structural neurological disease must be excluded by appropriate imaging and, if necessary, psychometric testing. |
| **Persistent and intractable pruritus**—consequent on cholestastic liver disease which is intractable after therapeutic trials. Exclude psychiatric comorbidity that might contribute to the itch. Lethargy is not an accepted primary indication for orthotopic liver transplantation. |
| **Familial amyloidosis**—confirmed transthyretin gene mutation in the absence of significant debilitating cardiac involvement, or autonomic neuropathy. |
| **Primary hyperlipidaemia**—homozygous familial hypercholesterolaemia, absent LDL receptor expression, and LDL receptor gene mutation. |
| **Polycystic liver disease**—intractable symptoms due to mass of liver or pain unresponsive to cystectomy, or severe complications secondary to portal hypertension. |
| **Recurrent cholangitis**—recurrent significant cholangitis not responsive to medical, surgical, or endoscopic therapy. |
| **Hepatic haemangioendothelioma**—histological confirmation; not a single lesion amenable to resection; extrahepatic spread confined to abdominal lymph nodes; minimum observation period of 3 months. |

Tc, Technitium; LDL, low density lipoprotein.

if appropriate, the earliest opportunity to list for transplantation. These complications, some of which may complicate or even preclude transplantation, include musculoskeletal deconditioning, recurrent hepatic encephalopathy requiring hospital admissions, intractable ascites (by virtue of diuretic resistance or intolerance), spontaneous bacterial or fungal peritonitis, hepatorenal syndrome, and variceal haemorrhage. Malnutrition in particular is common in chronic liver disease, especially in alcohol-related cirrhosis and primary sclerosing cholangitis, and is associated with both late referral and worse post-transplant outcomes (Shaw et al., 1989; McCullough and Tavill, 1991; Harrison et al., 1997).

The need for liver transplantation must be determined by considering the natural history of the patient's disease process and how this may be altered by liver transplantation, in particular the effect on anticipated survival. Several clinical tools are used to determine prognosis in patients with both acute liver failure syndromes and chronic liver disease, and these are expanded upon below. The overall impact of specific complications on patient survival, some of which are outlined above, should also be taken into consideration with respect to the potential benefit and timing of liver transplantation. Although transplantation can transform and prolong life, it can be associated with higher mortality and long-term morbidity than alternative treatments for some patients with chronic liver disease. This is in part related to the need for long-term immunosuppression, which accelerates the progression of cardiovascular disease and increases the risk of some forms of malignancy.

Accordingly, all therapeutic options should be carefully explored for each individual, in a multidisciplinary setting, and involving transplant-trained hepatologists. However, in critically ill patients with advanced liver disease and where the outcome of another medical therapy is uncertain or limited it may be appropriate to begin evaluation for transplantation whilst initiating and assessing alternative disease-specific treatments.

Once it has been established that patients have reached a threshold where liver transplantation is likely to best serve them, given their disease trajectory, and that other alternative treatment options have been exhausted, careful evaluation should occur. These should address some fundamental questions (Murray and Carithers, 2005):

1. Is the patient expected to meet the 50% 5-year survival threshold operative in the UK based on assessment of comorbidity and potential for recurrent disease?
2. Is the patient likely to survive the operation and the immediate postoperative period?
3. Is the patient able to comply with the complex medical regimen required after liver transplantation?

Assuming the above can be satisfied with a degree of confidence, the potential recipient should be evaluated formally in a dedicated transplant unit. Various processes and investigations must be followed and performed to assess the current disease severity to allow prognostication, assessment of other organ function and overall fitness, and ensure that no contraindications exist that would preclude transplantation. A summary of the procedures involved in a typical evaluation is shown in Table 20.4, but whilst the timelines and processes are more applicable to 'elective' liver transplantation where there is adequate time to perform all the required investigations, there will be some difference between this and presentations of acute liver failure due to, for example, acetaminophen-induced hepatotoxicity, where rapid assessment and super-urgent listing are required. Whilst the overall time frames may differ, the actual recipient assessment processes are similar in cases of acute liver failure, with all the vital investigations still needing to be performed, albeit over a period of usually 24–48 hours.

## Contraindications to liver transplantation

Contraindications to transplantation are listed in Table 20.5. The number of conditions considered absolute contraindications has declined since 1990 as expertise and experience have grown and as novel treatments have been introduced. Acquired immunodeficiency syndrome (AIDS), extrahepatic malignancy, and severe cardiorespiratory disease remain absolute contraindications based on their predictable adverse effects on post-transplant outcomes.

It can be argued that 'relative contraindications' represent challenges to successful transplantation that are sometimes overcome.

**Table 20.4** Evaluation of the potential liver transplant recipient at the transplant unit

| **Thorough history and physical examination** |
|---|
| **Laboratory studies**:<br>◆ Evaluation of aetiology and severity of liver disease<br>◆ Assessment for presence of cofactors for liver disease<br>◆ Blood typing<br>◆ Status of current or previous HBV, HCV, EBV, CMV, and HIV infections<br>◆ Assessment of renal function with 24-hour urine collection for creatinine clearance and protein excretion<br>◆ Liver biopsy may be required to evaluate histologically the extent and underlying aetiology, and may need to be undertaken by a transjugular route if a percutaneous route is precluded or contraindicated |
| **Cardiopulmonary evaluation**<br>◆ Arterial blood gas analysis<br>◆ Chest radiograph<br>◆ Pulmonary function testing<br>◆ Electrocardiogram<br>◆ Echocardiography—may be contrast-enhanced with microbubbles to evaluate for hepatopulmonary syndrome<br>◆ Cardiopulmonary exercise testing<br>◆ Coronary angiography—may be necessary, particularly if significant risk factors present for cardiovascular disease |
| **Radiological evaluation** to determine patency and anatomy of major hepatic vasculature (hepatic artery, portal vein, and hepatic venous drainage), presence of HCC, evidence of biliary abnormalities, as well as any other incidental findings that may affect the transplant procedure itself or represent contraindications such as malignancy. Modalities will include ultrasound, CT with contrast, MRI (including magnetic resonance cholangiopancreatography), and occasionally positron emission tomography and bone scintigraphy |
| **Endoscopic evaluation** to assess for presence of varices and exclude inflammatory disease or neoplastic lesions, particularly in conditions such as primary sclerosing cholangitis. Endoscopic retrograde cholangiopancreatography (ERCP) may be required to evaluate and treat for biliary strictures and where there is a high suspicion for cholangiocarcinoma |
| **Additional evaluations**<br>Together with medical tests, transplant evaluation requires additional assessments, which include the following:<br>◆ *Psychosocial assessment*: psychologist and social worker teams help recipients develop coping mechanisms for stress they will encounter throughout the transplant process<br>◆ *Substance misuse assessment*: where prior alcohol and substance abuse are identified, substance misuse specialists undertake a detailed analysis of the situation and can develop strategies to minimize recrudescence of the problem after transplantation<br>◆ *Nutritional assessment*: an integral component of the transplant evaluation process, given that malnutrition is known to adversely affect recovery following transplant. Nutrient deficiencies need to be identified and nutritional supplementation implemented where required, and this may include nasogastric feeding. What is becoming increasingly common is patients with high body mass indices being evaluated for transplant—this group requires intensive education as to calorific reduction and exercise regimens to produce sustained weight loss and an improvement in physiological reserve |

**Table 20.5** Absolute and relative contraindications to liver transplantation (Reproduced with permission from Devlin J and O'Grady J', 'Indications for referral and assessment in adult liver transplantation: a clinical guideline', Gut, 45, supplement 6. Copyright © 1999 BMJ Publishing Group Ltd.)

| **Absolute contraindications** |
|---|
| ◆ AIDS<br>◆ Advanced cardiopulmonary disease<br>◆ Extrahepatic malignancy[a]<br>◆ Cholangiocarcinoma[b] |
| **Relative contraindications** |
| ◆ HIV positivity<br>◆ Age > 70 years<br>◆ Significant sepsis outside the extrahepatic biliary tree<br>◆ Active alcohol/substance misuse<br>◆ Severe psychiatric disorder<br>◆ Pulmonary hypertension<br>◆ ?Extremes of body mass index (>40, <18) |

[a] Haemangioendothelioma and neuroendocrine malignancy are an exception in some units.

[b] Relative contraindication in some centres in conjunction with experimental approaches.

This argument is best made for specific issues that increase the complexity or risk of the procedure but not necessarily to a prohibitive level, e.g. extensive but incomplete portomesenteric vein thrombosis. However, the concept of 'relative contraindication' remains strong when multiple conditions exist that cumulatively tip the balance towards futility. Increasingly this scenario is encountered in older candidates with multiple comorbidities. To illustrate this point, when does the perceived risk for a 69-year-old patient with metabolic syndrome and cirrhosis change from 'acceptable' to 'prohibitive' as the following co-existing problems are considered: glomerular filtration rate of 44 mL/min, body mass index 33, occlusive coronary artery disease suitable for stenting, exercise tolerance of 500 m, and $pO_2$ of 9.2 kPa? This paradigm of summative risk quantification related to comorbidities is one of the greatest challenges in transplant candidate assessment and is poorly underpinned by current evidence.

## Age

There is no defined upper age limit to successful liver transplantation, although advanced age is relevant and cannot be ignored. In the past, an age of over 60 years was considered to be a contraindication to listing, but current data from the European Liver Transplant Registry show that 20% of transplant recipients are now over 60 years old (<http://www.eltr.org>), and it is now accepted that all potential recipients should be considered up to the age of 65 years. Those who are older with good functional capacity and no significant comorbidities should also be considered on the premise that they have a 50% likelihood of being alive 5 years post-transplantation.

However, when advanced age is linked with certain comorbidities the likelihood of a poor outcome is much higher, which should preclude listing. This has become clearer on review of data looking at predictors of outcome after liver transplantation in individuals over the age of 60. In addition to in-patient factors (in particular, mechanical ventilation), diabetes mellitus, renal dysfunction, and HCV seropositivity independently predicted a worse outcome (Aloia et al., 2010). On the other hand, an earlier study of recipients aged 65 and over found that correlates of disease severity did not appear to predict survival. These included the presence of ascites and spontaneous bacterial peritonitis, previous variceal haemorrhage, serum bilirubin levels, prothrombin time, malnutrition, and underlying aetiology (Markmann et al., 2001).

Thus severity of liver disease may have little impact on post-transplant outcome in older patients except in very advanced disease, while organ failure, in particular the need for mechanical ventilation and renal replacement therapy, are much more relevant as age increases.

## Obesity and malnutrition

Significant obesity is increasingly prevalent in the context of liver transplantation and has a direct impact on surgical fitness, as well as potentially aggravating liver disease by contributing to hepatic steatosis. Although poor long-term outcomes reported in the US literature in the 1990s suggested that a body mass index of > 40 should be a contraindication to liver transplantation (Murray and Carithers, 2005), later observations did not support this conclusion (Pelletier et al., 2007; Dick et al., 2009). It is clear, however, that obesity is associated with higher short-term morbidity and with higher prevalences of cardiovascular disease and diabetes mellitus, which are independently associated with worse outcomes. At the other end of the spectrum, very low body mass index (< 16–18) indicates severe nutritional impairment and musculoskeletal deconditioning and is associated with marked increase in early post-transplant mortality (Dawwas et al., 2008; Dick et al., 2009). In these patients, aggressive supplemental nutrition and weight gain are needed if listing is to be considered.

## Cardiovascular disease

Assessment of cardiovascular fitness and reserve is very important in relation to both short- and long-term outcomes after transplantation. However, the development of evidence-based protocols has proved challenging and a wide range of methodologies have been employed. Multivessel coronary artery disease has been shown to predict significantly worse outcomes 1 year after transplant (Yong et al., 2010), but it is less clear whether revascularization modifies this risk. There is also no consistency in defining the population that should be subjected to direct coronary angiography based on risk factors such as age, diabetes mellitus, family history, and smoking history. Echocardiography offers both anatomical and functional data, but its value as a stress test is uncertain because of the pre-existing hyperdynamic state in many patients with ESLD. Most recently, integrated functional cardiorespiratory fitness evaluation through exercise has been applied, but this approach also lacks validation.

## Diabetes mellitus

Diabetes confirmed during pretransplant assessment is an independent predictor of worse outcome after liver transplantation (Pageaux et al., 2009), especially when insulin-requiring and when evidence of end-organ damage exists. Although well-controlled diabetes is not a contraindication to transplant, the presence of cofactors such as age (Aloia et al., 2010), cardiac disease (Plotkin et al., 1996; Bilbao et al., 2008), and renal dysfunction (Fabrizi et al., 2011) may compromise long-term survival and contribute to a decision not to list. Assessment of adherence to prescribed treatment also gives some insight into how patients will cope with even more demanding regimens after transplantation.

## Alcohol misuse

Less than 5% of the population at risk of dying from alcohol-related liver disease are actively considered for liver transplantation (O'Grady, 2006). There remains a stigma attached to the condition, which is seen as 'self-inflicted' and therefore less deserving of liver transplantation, when the views of healthcare professionals and the public are gauged (Neuberger, 2007). Nevertheless, carefully selected patients do well after liver transplantation. The following key issues should be addressed (Devlin and O'Grady, 2000):

1. Is there potential for reversibility and recompensation of alcohol-related liver disease, including alcoholic hepatitis, following a period of abstinence?
2. Is the disease associated with ongoing alcohol dependence and can sustained abstinence be achieved?
3. Are there other comorbid alcohol-related conditions that could jeopardize post-transplant outcome?

In the acutely decompensated patient it is vital to evaluate the degree to which a superimposed and potentially reversible acute alcoholic hepatitis is present, since with abstinence and supportive medical therapy, recovery is possible. However, the risk of early death from this condition remains high (Forrest et al., 2005; Mathurin et al., 2011a) and the role of transplantation is the subject of much debate. Although not usually considered for transplant because of the presence of multi-organ failure and the limited ability to assess comorbid medical and psychiatric conditions, a recent series has challenged this view, showing that early liver transplantation in selected patients greatly improves survival (Mathurin et al., 2011b).

All transplant candidates with a history of alcohol misuse are at risk of a return to drinking, which will compromise outcome. Therefore the risk of relapse and the patient's ability to comply with post-transplant treatment are routinely evaluated in a multidisciplinary process. It is important to differentiate candidates who suffer from alcoholism from those who have engaged in moderate but non-dependent alcohol use. Those who demonstrate a clear ability to control their alcohol use have a good prognosis following transplantation, but when a diagnosis of alcohol dependency is established, future sobriety is more difficult to predict. Prediction is currently based on a rating scale (Beresford, 1994) comprising favourable and non-favourable factors identified in seminal early studies of recidivism (Strauss and Bacon, 1951; Vaillant et al., 1983). Concomitant psychiatric illness, drug dependency, social instability, and high-risk drinking patterns have to be considered alongside favourable prognostic factors, which include activity that structures time, a rehabilitation relationship, a source of hope or self-esteem, and noxious consequences of ongoing use.

To this end, the '6-month rule' defining a minimum period of alcohol abstinence is widely quoted, although sometimes misconstrued as an absolute prior to being listed for liver transplantation. This is not specified in current guidelines but is still applied by many healthcare professionals and may limit access to transplantation. The evidence that attaining a 6-month period of abstinence predicts sobriety post-transplant remains inconsistent, and factors other than any specific duration are likely to be more important (Beresford and Everson, 2000; Pfitzmann et al., 2007; Gedaly et al., 2008; Karimet al., 2010).

Nonetheless, there is a strong rationale for encouraging and mandating a period of abstinence prior to transplantation: first, to evaluate the scope for recompensation when alcohol is removed as the major aetiological factor, such that transplantation is no longer indicated; and second, to allow time for the potential candidates to demonstrate their motivation to modify their lifestyle and achieve the best possible outcome after transplantation.

Recommendations were established in the UK in 2005 (Bathgate, 2006), allowing transplant centres to use similar approaches in the assessment of patients with alcohol-related liver disease and defining listing criteria and contraindications. Factors precluding liver transplantation were agreed as follows:

1. Alcoholic hepatitis—clinical syndrome as opposed to histological diagnosis
2. Repetitive episodes (more than two) of non-adherence to medical care—not necessarily related only to hepatological care
3. Return to drinking after full professional assessment and advice (this advice should have been clearly documented)
4. Current or consecutive illicit drug misuse (except occasional cannabis use)

Organ damage caused by alcohol is a significant concern and must be identified to ensure it does not preclude listing. This includes cerebral atrophy and cerebellar disease or Korsakoff's syndrome. These often result in functional impairment that correlates poorly with findings on imaging and electroencephalography. There can be difficulty distinguishing these processes from hepatic encephalopathy. Clinical cardiomyopathy attributable to alcohol must also be excluded, given the impact cardiac reserve has on early post-transplant outcome and keeping in mind that myocardial dysfunction may indicate ongoing alcohol use (Estruch et al., 1995). Musculoskeletal deconditioning due to alcohol-related myopathy usually improves with abstinence and is rarely of importance in selection unless very debilitating. More challenging is assessment and optimization of impaired nutrition, found in over half of candidates with alcoholic cirrhosis. Precise evaluation of nutritional indices is often complicated by the presence of ascites and the oedema. Intensive, specialist dietetic input is needed to manage appropriate supplementation, including, in severe cases, long-term nasogastric feeding (Masuda et al., 2012).

## Substance misuse

Psychosocial issues and a history of illicit drug use require careful evaluation in potential liver transplant recipients. Intravenous drug abuse, HCV, alcohol abuse, psychiatric disorders, and social isolation are all closely correlated, and graft loss from non-compliance with immunosuppressive and other treatments post-transplant presents a substantial risk.

Although cigarette smoking is not a contraindication to transplantation, it should be actively discouraged, given the known harmful effects it has on post-transplant outcomes. A key early risk is that of hepatic artery thrombosis, which returns to baseline in candidates who discontinue cigarette use 2 years before transplantation (Pungpapong et al., 2002). Long-term post-transplant survival is also decreased in smokers, who have a much higher risk of cardiovascular events and de-novo malignancy than non-smoking controls (Chandok and Watt, 2012).

## Concomitant HIV infection

Well-controlled HIV infection per se is not a barrier to successful liver transplantation (O'Grady, 2012; Brook et al., 2010). This reflects changes in the natural history of the disease with use of highly active antiviral therapy (HAART), which often achieves long-term viral suppression and has contributed to satisfactory post-transplant outcomes. However, transplantation in the setting of HIV–HCV co-infection yields inferior results, with 3-year graft survival rates of 53% in a recent prospective study (O'Grady, 2012; Terrault et al., 2012). Patients with a preserved CD count (>100–200 cells/mm$^3$, depending on portal pressure), low HIV-1 RNA viral load, and absence of viral resistance profile are considered suitable for transplant from the HIV perspective. Referral should occur early, as the progression of both chronic liver disease and HCC is accelerated in these patients (Merchante et al., 2006).

## Previous malignancy

Patients with previous extrahepatic malignancy are at increased risk of recurrent disease after liver transplantation due to the need for immunosuppression. It is therefore recommended that consideration should be conditional on a recurrence-free period of 2–5 years, especially in the context of breast, colonic, and melanoma-related cancer, although the safe intervals between diagnosis of different types of extrahepatic malignancy and transplantation are not well defined. An oncologist should be consulted to confirm the nature and stage of the tumour and the disease-free interval and to give an estimate of prognosis.

## Renal dysfunction

The presence of renal dysfunction is an important and consistent predictor of post-transplant renal failure and mortality (Lafayette et al., 1997; Bilbao et al., 1998; Nair et al., 2002; Thuluvath, 2002), highlighting the importance of a thorough assessment and optimization of renal reserve before transplant. Studies have demonstrated that given the same MELD score, serum creatinine is inversely associated with survival benefit, and renal replacement therapy at the time of liver transplantation predicts significantly decreased transplant benefit (Sharma et al., 2009). However, serum creatinine is a poor indicator of renal dysfunction in many patients with ESLD because of decreased muscle mass; these patients require more accurate methods to better stratify risk, such as calculation of creatinine clearance, radionuclide techniques, and measurement of urinary protein:creatinine ratio. In a large study of non-renal transplant recipients, increased risk of chronic renal failure was associated with increasing age, pretransplantation hepatitis C infection, hypertension, diabetes mellitus, and post-operative acute kidney injury (Ojo et al., 2003). Chronic renal failure increased the risk of death at 5 years more than four-fold, but early kidney transplant greatly reduced this risk compared to dialysis. Thus combined liver and renal transplantation is an attractive option for selected patients with pre-existing renal disease who develop liver failure.

## Recipient prioritization and organ allocation

Organ allocation can be based on need, benefit, or utility, prioritizing those who need a transplant most to prevent imminent death, those who would gain the longest survival relative to the natural history of their condition, and those whose condition and status favour the longest absolute survival. There is significant common ground in these parameters, but they reflect conflicting positions on how organs should be used. Allocation based on need, using simplified severity scoring (MELD and UKELD), is currently the norm in most systems. These scores were developed to make prioritization more objective and accurately predict mortality risk in 70–75% of patients with chronic liver disease. However, need-based allocation may not translate into acceptable medium- or long-term survival, especially in older recipients with comorbidities. When these are prioritized over younger, less-debilitated patients who might gain many more years of life from a graft, the net gain in life-years from a graft may be reduced.

In patients in whom liver dysfunction per se is not the reason for transplant and those with defined atypical presentations ('variant syndromes'), MELD scores are disregarded or supplemented with extra 'points' to achieve transplantation in a timely manner. The most common use of such points is in patients with HCC. All allocation systems prioritize patients with acute liver failure and some give equivalent status to patients with chronic liver disease in intensive care facilities.

The allocation system in the UK is in transition at the time of writing. There is a national allocation policy to prioritize patients with acute liver failure or those in need of emergency retransplantation. Thereafter, most organs are allocated to centres based on geography, and the recipient is selected according to local protocols that tend to balance time spent on the waiting list with need as determined by UKELD scores (UKELD is similar to MELD-sodium). One advantage of the current system is the ability to better match patients and donors with respect to parameters that influence outcome. However, the system is not completely transparent and there have been disparities between centres with respect to mortality on waiting lists.

**Table 20.6** Indications for referral in acute liver failure. (Data from Liver Advisory Group, NHS Blood and Transplant Liver Selection Policy, Copyright 2014, http://www.odt.nhs.uk/pdf/liver_selection_policy.pdf)

| **Paracetamol ingestion** | | |
|---|---|---|
| **Day 2** | **Day 3** | **Day 4** |
| Arterial pH < 7.30 | Arterial pH < 7.30 | |
| INR > 6 or PT > 100 s | | |
| INR > 3.0 or PT > 50 s | INR > 4.5 or PT > 75 s | |
| Progressive rise in PT to any level | | |
| Oliguria | Oliguria | Oliguria |
| Creatinine > 200 μmol/L | Creatinine > 200 μmol/L | Creatinine > 300 μmol/L |
| Hypoglycaemia | Encephalopathy | Encephalopathy |
| | Severe thrombocytopaenia | Severe thrombocytopaenia |
| **Non-paracetamol aetiologies** | | |
| **Hyperacute** | **Acute** | **Subacute** |
| Encephalopathy | Encephalopathy | Encephalopathy |
| Hypoglycaemia | Hypoglycaemia | Hypoglycaemia (less common) |
| PT > 30 s | PT >30 s | PT > 20 s |
| INR > 2.0 | INR > 2.0 | INR > 1.5 |
| Renal failure | Renal failure | Renal failure |
| Hyperpyrexia | | Serum sodium < 130 μmol/L |
| | | Shrinking liver volume |

## Specific referral guidance: acute liver failure

The guiding principle is that if in doubt a case should be discussed with a transplant centre. The specific thresholds outlined in Table 20.6 for different categories of patients are extrapolated backwards in the clinical course from the corresponding values in a historical cohort with poor outcomes and have not been formally validated. The subset of patients in whom the impact of delayed referral is most apparent is those with subacute liver failure. In this group the classical indicators of acute liver failure—encephalopathy and coagulopathy—are less significant until a relatively late stage. Furthermore, when clinical deterioration occurs it is often triggered by sepsis, which may contraindicate liver transplantation. Age is more relevant in these patients and of those successfully transplanted most are under age 60. Thus the upper age threshold is about 10 years younger than in patients having elective transplants.

## Specific referral guidance: chronic liver disease (including primary liver cancer)

All patients with severe liver disease should undergo a primary screen to meet the following criteria:

- The patient has a clinical condition that could benefit from transplantation
- MELD > 14 or UKELD > 49, or there are criteria for an exceptional indication
- There are no clear contraindications
- The patient has social support
- The patient has an appropriate attitude to transplantation

UKELD scores in isolation should not determine a decision to list for transplantation but could influence the timing of referral because of differing waiting times, which depend on blood group and patient size. This consideration may be obviated by future changes in organ allocation.

It is now good practice for all patients with HCC to be discussed within a multidisciplinary network that includes input from a transplant centre. Therefore the assessment of suitability for transplantation should be initiated at an early stage. At present, the criteria determining suitability are largely based on tumour bulk as determined by the number and size of the tumours. This may change to give more weight to tumour biology, both inherent and as modified by other therapies.

## Outcomes

The outcomes of liver transplantation are now generally good. In adults, 1-year survival rates for primary elective transplants are

88–92% as compared with 78–80% for emergency transplantation. The outcome for patients with chronic liver disease who are in intensive care at the time of the transplant is less good at 60–65%. Survival is lower for retransplants and falls progressively the higher the number of previous transplants. Disease recurrence has a variable effect on long-term outcomes. This is most significant in hepatitis C and HCC. Non-alcoholic fatty liver disease may also recur but is also associated with increased cardiovascular risk. Alcoholic liver disease recurs in recipients who return to heavy drinking, but a more common cause of death is malignancy of the upper gastrointestinal tract and lung. Primary biliary cirrhosis recurs, but this has little long-term impact. Donor factors and comorbidities are very relevant to short- and medium-term outcomes, in particular severe nutritional impairment, cardiovascular disease, renal dysfunction, and diabetes mellitus.

Transplant registries provide excellent data on demographics and survival based on age, indication, and numerous other variables. However, confidence limits for survival are wide and registry figures may understate what can be achieved in the best units. At present they collect too little relevant data to evaluate the role of comorbidities or to characterize disease recurrence and other complications in the medium and long term.

## Liver–kidney transplantation

The management of pre- and post-transplant renal dysfunction remains a formidable problem in liver transplantation. Serum creatinine, despite its limitations, is a powerful predictor of post-transplant outcome, and kidney injury is the greatest determinant of mortality (Nair et al., 2002; Davis et al., 2007). With the widespread adoption of MELD-based allocation, powerfully influenced by serum creatinine, the number of combined liver–kidney transplants has increased substantially since 2005. A major challenge is to achieve a balance between benefit and utility, by ensuring that patient and graft survival are optimized while limiting unnecessary transplants, particularly when the kidney donor pool is constrained. A consensus conference in the US established guidelines for evaluation and transplantation of patients with ESLD and renal failure (Eason et al., 2008).

It was agreed that the following groups should be routinely considered as candidates for combined liver–kidney transplantation:

1. ESRD patients with cirrhosis and symptomatic portal hypertension, or hepatic vein wedge pressure with gradient > 10 mm Hg
2. Patients with advanced liver disease and stage IV or V chronic kidney disease with GFR ≤ 30 mL/min
3. Patients with acute kidney injury including hepatorenal syndrome with creatinine ≥ 200 mg/L and dialysis ≥ 8 weeks (given evidence for a survival advantage in this situation)
4. Patients with advanced liver disease and evidence of chronic kidney disease with kidney biopsy demonstrating > 30% glomerulosclerosis or 30% fibrosis

Other criteria supporting consideration of combined liver–kidney transplantation included the presence of diabetes, hypertension, and other pre-existing renal disease; proteinuria; kidney size; and duration of elevated serum creatinine ≥ 200 mg/L.

## Retransplantation

Retransplantation accounts for 10% of all liver transplants performed, and this is likely to increase as the use of marginal and non-heart-beating donors increases and as patients live long enough to develop graft failure from recurrent disease. Whilst retransplantation is associated with significantly diminished survival (20% lower than for primary transplantation) and increased costs, it cannot be abandoned as a life-saving therapeutic modality. Recommendations in this potentially controversial area therefore require the development of prognostic models that can identify subsets of patients for whom retransplantation outcomes are comparable to those associated with primary transplantation, whilst balancing ethical considerations (Biggins et al., 2002).

The most frequent indications for retransplantation are primary graft non-function, allograft rejection, hepatic artery thrombosis, and recurrent disease. Hepatitis C recurrence is common, but retransplantation in this context is associated with poor outcomes (Neff et al., 2004). This may change with the advent of newer and more potent antiviral therapies.

## Conclusion

Timely referral and careful selection of candidates for liver transplantation are essential, both to achieve the best possible outcome for the individual patient and to ensure optimal use of available organs. This chapter has outlined the key clinical features and investigations that determine prognosis in severe liver disease and indications for transplant. The specific contexts of acute and chronic liver failure, variant syndromes, combined liver–kidney failure, and graft failure requiring retransplantation have been described. Comorbidities and how they affect both perioperative risk and long-term outcomes have also been highlighted, along with contraindications to transplant and challenges in organ allocation.

## References


Aloia TA, Knight R, Gaber AO, Ghobrial RM, Goss JA (2010) Analysis of liver transplant outcomes for United Network for Organ Sharing recipients 60 years old or older identifies multiple model for end-stage liver disease-independent prognostic factors. *Liver Transplant*, **16**(8):950–959.

Barber K, Madden S, Allen J, et al. (2011) Elective liver transplant list mortality: development of a United Kingdom end-stage liver disease score. *Transplantation*, **92**(4):469–476.

Bathgate AJ, UK Liver Transplant Units (2006) Recommendations for alcohol-related liver disease. *Lancet*, **367**(9528):2045–2046.

Belle SH, Porayko MK, Hoofnagle JH, Lake JR, Zetterman RK (1997) Changes in quality of life after liver transplantation among adults. National Institute of Diabetes and Digestive and Kidney Diseases (NIDDK) Liver Transplantation Database (LTD). *Liver Transplant Surg*, **3**:93–104.

Beresford TP (1994) Psychiatric assessment of alcoholic liver transplant candidates. In: Lucey MR, Merion RM, Beresford TP (eds) *Liver Transplantation and the Alcoholic Patient*. Cambridge University Press, Cambridge.

Beresford TP, Everson GT (2000) Liver transplantation for alcoholic liver disease: bias, beliefs, 6-month rule, and relapse—but where are the data? *Liver Transplant*, **6**(6):777–778.

Biggins SW, Beldecos A, Rabkin JM, Rosen HR (2002) Retransplantation for hepatic allograft failure: prognostic modeling and ethical considerations. *Liver Transplant*, **8**(4):313–322.

Bilbao I, Charco R, Balsells J, et al. (1998) Risk factors for acute renal failure requiring dialysis after liver transplantation. *Clin Transplant*, **12**(2):123–129.

Bilbao I, Dopazo C, Lazaro JL, et al. (2008) Our experience in liver transplantation in patients over 65 yr of age. *Clin Transplant*, **22**:82–88.

Brook G, Main J, Nelson M, et al. (2010) British HIV Association guidelines for the management of coinfection with HIV-1 and hepatitis B or C virus 2010. *HIV Med*, **11**:1–30.

Chandok N, Watt KD (2012) The burden of de novo malignancy in the liver transplant recipient. *Liver Transplant*, **18**(11):1277–1289.

Davis CL, Feng S, Sung R, et al. (2007) Simultaneous liver-kidney transplantation: evaluation to decision making. *Am J Transplant*, 7(7):1702–1709.

Dawwas MF, Gimson AE, Watson CJ, Allison ME (2008) Modelling the impact of recipient body mass index on post-liver transplant survival: A fractional polynomial approach. *Hepatology*, **48**:554A

Devlin J, O'Grady J (2000) *Indications for referral and assessment in adult liver transplantation: a clinical guideline.* <http://www.bsg.org.uk/clinical-guidelines/liver/indications-for-referral-and-assessment-in-adult-liver-transplantation-a-clinical-guideline.html >.

Dick AA, Spitzer AL, Seifert CF, et al. (2009) Liver transplantation at the extremes of the body mass index. *Liver Transplant*, **15**(8):968–977.

Eason JD, Gonwa TA, Davis CL, Sung RS, Gerber D, Bloom RD (2008) Proceedings of Consensus Conference on Simultaneous Liver Kidney Transplantation (SLK). *Am J Transplant*, **8**(11):2243–2251.

Estruch R, Fernández-Solá J, Sacanella E, Paré C, Rubin E, Urbano-Márquez A (1995) Relationship between cardiomyopathy and liver disease in chronic alcoholism. *Hepatology*, **22**(2):532–538.

Fabrizi F, Dixit V, Martin P, Messa P (2011) Pre-transplant kidney function predicts chronic kidney disease after liver transplant: meta-analysis of observational studies. *Dig Dis Sci*, **56**(5):1282–1289.

Forrest EH, Evans CD, Stewart S, et al. (2005) Analysis of factors predictive of mortality in alcoholic hepatitis and derivation and validation of the Glasgow alcoholic hepatitis score. *Gut*, **54**(8):1174–1179.

Francoz C, Belghiti J, Castaing D, et al. (2011) Model for end-stage liver disease exceptions in the context of the French model for end-stage liver disease score-based liver allocation system. *Liver Transplant*, **17**(10):1137–1151.

Gedaly R, McHugh PP, Johnston TD, et al. (2008) Predictors of relapse to alcohol and illicit drugs after liver transplantation for alcoholic liver disease. *Transplantation*, **86**(8):1090–1095.

Harrison J, McKiernan J, Neuberger JM (1997) A prospective study on the effect of recipient nutritional status outcome in liver transplantation. *Transplant Int*, **10**:369–374.

Karim Z, Intaraprasong P, Scudamore CH, et al. (2010) Predictors of relapse to significant alcohol drinking after liver transplantation. *Can J Gastroenterol*, **24**(4):245–250.

Lafayette RA, Pare G, Schmid CH, King AJ, Rohrer RJ, Nasraway SA (1997) Pre-transplant renal dysfunction predicts poorer outcome in liver transplantation. *Clin Nephrol*, **48**:159–164.

Liver Advisory Group (2007) *UK Liver Transplant Group recommendations for liver transplant assessment in the context of illicit drug use, V1.* <http://www.organdonation.nhs.uk/ ukt/about_transplants/organ_allocation/pdf/uk_ liver_transplant_group_ recommendations_for_liver_ transplant_assessment_ illict_drug_use-2007.pdf>.

Markmann JF, Markmann JW, Markmann DA, et al. (2001) Preoperative factors associated with outcome and their impact on resource use in 1148 consecutive primary liver transplants. *Transplantation*, **72**(6):1113–1122.

Masuda T, Shirabe K, Yoshiya S, et al. (2012) Nutrition support and infections associated with hepatic resection and liver transplantation in patients with chronic liver disease. *J Parenter Enteral Nutr*, **37**(3):318–326.

Mathurin P, O'Grady J, Carithers RL, et al. (2011a) Corticosteroids improve short-term survival in patients with severe alcoholic hepatitis: meta-analysis of individual patient data. *Gut*, **60**:255–260.

Mathurin P, Moreno C, Samuel D, et al. (2011b) Early liver transplantation for severe alcoholic hepatitis. *N Engl J Med*, **365**(19):1790–1800.

McCullough AJ, Tavill AS (1991) Disordered energy and protein metabolism in liver disease. *Semin Liver Dis*, **11**:265–277.

Merchante N, Giron-Gonzalez J, Gonzalez-Serrano M, et al. (2006) Survival and prognostic factors of HIV-infected patients with HCV-related end stage liver disease. *AIDS*, **20**:49–57.

Murray KF, Carithers RL Jr (2005) *AASLD Practice Guidelines: evaluation of the patient for liver transplantation.* <www.aasld.org/practiceguidelines/documents/bookmarked%20practice%20guidelines/liver%20transplant.pdf>.

Nair S, Verma S, Thuluvath PJ (2002) Pre-transplant renal function predicts survival in patients undergoing orthotopic liver transplantation. *Hepatology*, **35**(5):1179–1185.

Neff GW, O'Brien CB, Nery J, et al. (2004) Factors that identify survival after liver retransplantation for allograft failure caused by recurrent hepatitis C infection. *Liver Transplant*, **10**(12):1497–1503.

Neuberger J (2007) Public and professional attitudes to transplanting alcoholic patients. *Liver Transplant*, **13**(11 Suppl 2):S65–68.

O'Grady JG (2006) Liver transplantation alcohol related liver disease: (deliberately) stirring a hornet's nest! *Gut*, **55**(11):1529–1531.

O'Grady J (2012) Liver transplantation in human immunodeficiency virus/hepatitis C virus-coinfected patients: response needed! *Liver Transplant*, **18**:617–618.

O'Grady JG, Alexander GJ, Hayllar KM, Williams R (1989) Early indicators of prognosis in fulminant hepatic failure. *Gastroenterology*, **97**:439–445.

O'Grady J, Taylor C, Brook G (2005) Guidelines for liver transplantation in patients with HIV infection (2005). *HIV Med*, **6**(Suppl 2):149–153.

Ojo AO, Held PJ, Port FK, et al. (2003) Chronic renal failure after transplantation of a non-renal organ. *N Engl J Med*, **349**(10):931–940.

Pageaux GP, Faure S, Bouyabrine H, Bismuth M, Assenat E (2009) Long-term outcomes of liver transplantation: diabetes mellitus. *Liver Transplant*, **15**(Suppl 2):S79–S82.

Pelletier SJ, Schaubel DE, Wei G, et al. (2007) Effect of body mass index on the survival benefit of liver transplantation. *Liver Transplant*, **13**:1678–1683.

Pfitzmann R, Schwenzer J, Rayes N, Seehofer D, Neuhaus R, Nüssler NC (2007) Long-term survival and predictors of relapse after orthotopic liver transplantation for alcoholic liver disease. *Liver Transplant*, **13**(2):197–205.

Plotkin JS, Scott VL, Pinna A, et al. (1996) Morbidity and mortality in patients with coronary artery disease undergoing orthotopic liver transplantation. *Liver Transplant*, **2**:426–430.

Pungpapong S, Manzarbeitia C, Ortiz J, et al. (2002) Cigarette smoking is associated with an increased incidence of vascular complications after liver transplantation. *Liver Transplant*, **8**(7):582–587.

Sharma P, Schaubel DE, Guidinger MK, Merion RM (2009) Effect of pretransplant serum creatinine on the survival benefit of liver transplantation. *Liver Transplant*, **15**(12):1808–1813.

Shaw BW Jr, Wood RP, Stratta RJ, Pillen TJ, Langnas AN (1989) Stratifying the causes of death in liver transplant recipients. An approach to improving survival. *Arch Surg*, **124**:895–900.

Strauss R, Bacon SD (1951) Alcoholism and social stability. *Q J Study Alcohol*, **12**:231–260.

Terrault NA, Roland ME, Schiano T, et al. (2012) Outcomes of liver transplant recipients with hepatitis C and human immunodeficiency virus coinfection. *Liver Transplant*, **18**:716–726.

Thuluvath PJ (2002) Pre-transplant renal function predicts survival in patients undergoing orthotopic liver transplantation. *Hepatology*, **35**:1179–1185.

Vaillant GE, Clark W, Cyrus C, et al. (1983) Prospective study of alcoholism treatment. Eight-year follow-up. *Am J Med*, 75(3):455–463.

Yong CM, Sharma M, Ochoa V, et al. (2010) Multivessel coronary artery disease predicts mortality, length of stay, and pressor requirements after liver transplantation. *Liver Transplant*, **16**(11):1242–1248.

Zalewska K (2014) *UK Blood and Transplant Liver Selection Policy 2014, document ref POL 195.3.* <http://www.odt.nhs.uk/pdf/liver_selection_policy.pdf>.

# CHAPTER 21

# Critical care of the patient with liver disease

Andrea De Gasperi, James Y. Findlay, and John R. Klinck

## Introduction

### Critical care in chronic liver disease

Decompensated chronic liver disease accounts for a substantial and rising proportion of intensive care admissions (Saliba, 2006). Admission is usually precipitated by acute complications of chronic liver disease (Olson and Kamath, 2011; Karvellas et al., 2013a). These include variceal haemorrhage, sepsis from spontaneous bacterial peritonitis or pneumonia, portomesenteric thrombosis, and aggravated encephalopathy related to infection, dehydration, or hepatorenal failure. A significant proportion of admissions, however, follow an 'unrelated' clinical event, including trauma, a surgical procedure, or any acute medical condition, while others follow an acute exacerbation of underlying chronic liver disease, as in alcoholic or reactivated viral hepatitis.

Although organ failure is more likely in these patients because of their limited physiological reserve, impaired nutritional state, and compromised immunity, an altered inflammatory response analogous to that seen in patients presenting with sepsis also appears to be an important factor in prognosis. This has been described as acute-on-chronic liver failure (ACLF), seen in patients with stable chronic liver disease who suffer deteriorating liver function and extrahepatic organ failure associated with a marked SIRS, with or without an identifiable cause (Saliba et al., 2013b). Differing definitions exist but that proposed by a recent EASL/AASLD symposium and based on the presence of organ failure indicates that it may affect up to one-third of acute hepatology hospital admissions and a much higher proportion of those needing intensive care (Olson and Kamath, 2011; Jalan et al., 2012). Prospective studies to identify diagnostic and prognostic markers and to create a uniform definition are ongoing. This is of interest because ACLF often develops rapidly in patients not sick enough to be listed for transplant, yet mortality is high and the potential for both reversibility and benefit from transplantation may be significant.

Outcome in the setting of ESLD and ACLF is related to the number of extrahepatic systems affected, and mortality is 50% or higher when mechanical ventilation, renal replacement therapy, or vasopressors are needed. In patients already listed for transplant, a rapid response to initial measures means that they can remain on the waiting list. In others, although a life-threatening complication of ESLD may constitute an indication for transplant, referral to a transplant centre for formal assessment is only undertaken when they recover enough to be discharged from the ICU. More often, multi-organ failure (MOF) makes immediate transplant futile. However, transplant in an ICU-dependent patient with decompensated ESLD or ACLF may not be clearly contraindicated, and good results have been reported (Bahirwani et al., 2011; Finkenstedt et al., 2013; Karvellas et al., 2013a). A clear consensus on suitability for transplant in this setting awaits further experience

### Critical care in acute liver failure

Mortality is also high in the setting of ALF, which requires aetiology-specific treatment and early transfer to a specialist unit offering liver transplantation. The onset of extrahepatic organ failure, especially deepening encephalopathy, should be managed with the full support of a liver transplant ICU. The aim of intensive care is to optimize hepatic oxygen delivery, preserving residual hepatocyte function and enabling regeneration. The prevention and treatment of complications such as sepsis, cerebral oedema, renal and cardiorespiratory failure, and haemorrhage are described in the section 'Critical care management of liver failure'.

In the event of worsening liver failure, when prognostic scoring indicates that recovery is unlikely, liver transplant should be undertaken as soon as an acceptable organ can be found. However, when transplant is indicated but the patient deteriorates before an organ can be secured, the signs associated with near-certain peritransplant mortality or severe neurological injury should be heeded to prevent the waste of a valuable graft.

## Acute liver failure

### Background

ALF is characterized by new-onset, generalized liver injury leading rapidly to encephalopathy, cerebral oedema, coagulopathy, systemic inflammation, and MOF. It has a range of aetiologies, mainly toxic and infectious, but a cause may not be identifiable. It is associated with elevated transaminases, hyperbilirubinaemia, encephalopathy, and coagulopathy in the absence of pre-existing hepatic disease, and is differentiated from more indolent conditions by the occurrence of encephalopathy within 8 weeks of the onset of jaundice. Hyperacute, acute, and subacute types are also defined (< 7 days, 8–28 days, 29 days to 8 weeks, respectively; see Table 21.1). The J–E interval, which also depends on aetiology, is fundamental to prognosis (Bernal and Wendon, 2013; Bernal et al., 2013).

**Table 21.1** Classification of acute liver failure. (Data from O'Grady, 'Acute Liver Failure', 2005, *Postgraduate Medical Journal*, 81, pp. 148-154..)

| | Hyperacute | Acute | Subacute |
|---|---|---|---|
| Jaundice–encephalopathy interval | 0–1 week | 1–4 weeks | 4–8 weeks |
| Coagulopathy extent | +++ | ++ | + |
| Jaundice extent | + | ++ | +++ |
| Intracranial hypertension | ++ | ++ | +/– |
| Survival without orthotropic liver transplantation (OLT) | Good (> 60%) | Moderate (50%) | Low (10–20%) |

Each year about 2,000 cases of ALF are treated in the US (Ostapowicz et al., 2002; Khashab et al., 2007). Acetaminophen overdose, hepatitis A, B, and E, seronegative and drug-induced hepatitis, and Wilson's disease are common causes in adults, but geographic variability is prominent. In seronegative ALF an autoimmune aetiology may be suspected but can be difficult to confirm. Less frequent causes include Budd–Chiari syndrome, HELPP syndrome (haemolysis, elevated liver enzymes, and low platelets), and acute fatty liver of pregnancy. Rare causes include haemophagocytic syndrome, malignant infiltration, and heatstroke.

Diffuse hepatic necrosis results from direct cytotoxic, immune, or ischaemic mechanisms (Stravitz et al., 2007). A direct effect on hepatocytes occurs in the setting of hepatitis A, drug toxicity (acetaminophen, nimesulide, flutamide, cyproterone, amphetamines), the mushroom toxin *Amanita phalloides*, and carbon tetrachloride (De Carlis et al., 2001). An immune-mediated cytopathic effect is seen in hepatitis B-induced necrosis and the drug-related eosinophilic syndrome (DRESS). Acute ischaemic injury may occur in critically ill patients with cardiovascular or respiratory failure, often but not exclusively associated with severe sepsis (Finfer and Vincent, 2013).

In the 1970s, mortality in ALF was 70–90%, but modern intensive care and liver transplantation have transformed the prognosis. Even without liver transplant, improved management has seen mortality in the developed world fall to less than 40% for some forms of ALF, in particular those associated with hepatitis A, acetaminophen toxicity, ischaemic injury, and pregnancy. Nonetheless, the impact of liver transplantation is beyond doubt, and this treatment has also steadily improved since 1990. In this interval, 1-year survival post transplant for ALF has improved from less than 50% to better than 80% in patients with the most common indications. Five-year survival after transplantation approaches 70%.

Prognosis varies depending on aetiology and age. It is most favourable in ALF linked to hepatitis A or E, acetaminophen overdose, and pregnancy and worse in the setting of idiosyncratic drug reactions, Wilson's disease, hepatitis B infection, and seronegativity. The grade of encephalopathy is highly relevant (grade 1–2, 70% survival vs grade 3–4, 54% survival) (Stravitz et al., 2007; Bernal et al., 2010). Death in ALF is frequently due to cerebral herniation secondary to cerebral oedema and intracranial hypertension. Most other deaths are related to refractory septic shock and MOF (Jalan, 2005).

## Pathogenesis and presentation

The pathogenesis of ALF is linked to impaired hepatocyte synthetic and excretory function. There is a rise in concentrations of inflammatory cytokines, of hydrosoluble toxins (ammonia and mercaptan), and of hydrophobic substances bound to albumin (bilirubin, aromatic amino acids, endogenous benzodiazepines, bile salts, short-chain fatty acids), some of which are implicated in hepatic encephalopathy (HE) and cerebral oedema. The close relationship between arterial ammonia concentrations and both encephalopathy and intracranial hypertension is particularly well recognized. Inflammatory mediators may trigger or worsen encephalopathy by altering cerebral blood flow or endothelial permeability to neurotoxins. High levels of NO and cytokines are associated with renal injury and with observed cardiocirculatory alterations. Finally, increasing concentrations of free radical oxidants may cause increased capillary permeability and altered immune competence (Auzinger and Wendon, 2008).

ALF presents with progressive jaundice and encephalopathy, accompanied by transaminase elevation, rising blood lactate, and prolongation of prothrombin time (INR). The onset of oliguria, hypotension, impaired gas exchange, hypoglycaemia, or pancytopaenia, especially a rapidly falling platelet count, indicates significant deterioration and impending MOF. Management is optimal when guided by or provided in a specialist unit offering liver transplantation, whose experience may enhance the prevention and management of MOF and where rapid evaluation for liver transplant is possible. Criteria for referral to a specialist liver unit (O'Grady, 2005) and listing for transplant are shown in Table 21.2. Admission to intensive care from a ward or high-dependency area is usually associated with the transition from grade 2 to grade 3 encephalopathy, the onset of sepsis, or respiratory failure.

## Prognostic scoring and selection for liver transplantation

In developed countries, emergency liver transplantation is routine for selected cases of ALF and has improved prognosis dramatically. Outcome is predominantly determined by the underlying cause, the patient's age (> 50 years doubles mortality), the severity of MOF, and the quality of the graft. The decision to transplant must be taken as soon as it is clear that the probability of spontaneous recovery is low, but before severe organ failure or cerebral injury make transplantation unsurvivable or futile.

The most widely used prognostic scoring system for ALF was developed in the 1980s at King's College Hospital in London, based on outcomes in the era before liver transplantation. The parameters used, given that they are associated with a low chance of spontaneous recovery, have also been adopted as criteria for urgent transplantation (King's College Criteria, Table 21.2) (O'Grady et al., 1989; Bernal et al., 2010). The Clichy criteria, based on data from patients with fulminant hepatitis B, use encephalopathy grade, factor V concentration, and age, but appear to be less sensitive, even with the introduction of additional variables (Bernal et al., 2010). A recent proposal employs a version of the MELD in which bilirubin concentration is replaced with that of CK18/M65, a cytoskeleton protein filament which is a marker of cell death. This appears to correlate with the absence of cellular potential for spontaneous recovery (Bechmann et al., 2010). However, neither spontaneous recovery nor successful

**Table 21.2** Selection criteria for super-urgent liver transplantation. (Adapted with kind permission from Liver Advisory Group, NHS Blood and Transplant Liver Selection Policy, Copyright 2014, http://www.odt.nhs.uk/pdf/liver_selection_policy.pdf.)

| Acetaminophen hepatotoxicity |
|---|
| 1. pH < 7.25 > 24 hours after overdose and after fluid resuscitation |
| 2. Serum lactate > 3.5 mmol/L >24 hours after overdose on admission or >3.0 mmol/L after fluid resuscitation |
| 3. PT > 100 s (INR > 6.5) + creatinine >300 μmol/L anuria, + grade 3–4 encephalopathy |
| 4. Two criteria from above plus evidence of clinical deterioration (increased ICP, $FiO_2$ > 50%, increasing inotrope requirements) in the absence of clinical sepsis |
| **Other aetiologies** |
| 1. Seronegative hepatitis, hepatitis A, hepatitis B, drug-induced liver failure: **INR > 6.5 or PT > 100 s** |
| 2. Seronegative hepatitis, hepatitis A, hepatitis B, drug-induced liver failure. Any three from: |
| i. **unfavourable aetiology** |
| ii. **age > 40 years; J–E > 7 days** |
| iii. **bilirubin > 300 mmol/L** |
| iv. **INR > 3.5** |
| 3. Acute presentation of Wilson's disease or Budd–Chiari syndrome: **a combination of coagulopathy and any grade of encephalopathy** |
| 4. Hepatic artery thrombosis on days 0–21 after liver transplantation |
| 5. Early graft dysfunction on days 0–7 after liver transplantation, with at least two of the following: |
| i. **AST > 10,000** |
| ii. **INR > 3.0** |
| iii. **serum lactate > 3 mmol/L** |
| iv. **absence of bile production** |
| 6. The total absence of liver function (e.g. after total hepatectomy) |
| 7. Any patient who has been a live liver donor who develops severe liver failure within 4 weeks of the donor operation |

transplant can be accurately predicted by any scoring system currently in use. The rarity of ALF makes it difficult to test predictive scores, but new markers and multicentre data collection make enhancements in the near future likely (Bernal et al., 2010; Samuel and Ichai, 2010).

# Critical care management of liver failure

## General considerations

Management stratagems in ALF, ACLF, and ESLD in the critical care setting have much in common. Close monitoring of conscious level and cardiorespiratory and renal function and frequent evaluation of metabolic and coagulation parameters (blood glucose, sodium, lactate, INR, and platelet count in particular) are essential. Liver-specific monitoring, especially in ALF, is enhanced in some units by indocyanine green (ICG) clearance (LiMon Pulsion) (Jalan et al., 1994; Hetz et al., 2001, 2002). ICG clearance levels lower than 8–10% per minute are considered pathological. However, very low values may be misleading in the presence of hyperbilirubinaemia (> 6 mg/dL), since bilirubin competes for the ICG carrier (Mazza et al., 2008).

Initial management of ALF should also include tests to identify a treatable cause, since some conditions respond to early targeted treatment. These include assays for acetaminophen, illicit drugs, urine and serum copper, viral markers, and autoantibodies. Ultrasound and computed tomography (CT) imaging are also indicated to exclude arterial or venous thrombosis and malignancy. ALF may present as MOF, especially when hyperacute, so accidental acetaminophen overdose should be considered when MOF presents with disproportionate liver dysfunction and no clear cause (Steadman et al., 2010).

The ESLD patient presenting to the ICU will more often require urgent volume resuscitation and targeted management of bleeding or sepsis. Acute encephalopathy may be associated with these conditions and require airway management and mechanical ventilation. Although reported, dangerous increases in ICP are uncommon (Jalan et al., 2012). A source of infection should always be sought, including peritonitis, cholangitis, bronchopneumonia, lower limb cellulitis, and urinary tract infection. If suspected, medical or surgical conditions not directly attributable to chronic liver disease should be excluded. These might include alcohol withdrawal, drug intoxication, trauma, pulmonary embolus, gastroenteritis, hernia with bowel obstruction, and intracranial haemorrhage.

## Encephalopathy and intracranial hypertension: pathophysiology and monitoring

Encephalopathy is a hallmark of both ALF and ESLD, but other causes of altered sensorium must be excluded, both on diagnosis and when deterioration occurs. These include hypoglycaemia, sedative drugs, and intracranial haemorrhage. The pathogenesis of HE and cerebral oedema appears to be multifactorial but is clearly associated with increased blood concentrations of ammonia, which is generated by intestinal flora and normally metabolized to urea in the liver. Ammonia is a precursor of glutamine synthesis in astrocytes, and raised levels typical of ALF lead to glutamine accumulation, astrocyte swelling, and intracranial hypertension (Bernal et al., 2007; Frontera and Kalb, 2011). These effects may be attenuated in chronic liver disease by compensating mechanisms at cellular level and by the presence of cerebral atrophy, which may increase intracranial compliance.

A limited correlation between ammonia concentrations and severity of encephalopathy and intracranial hypertension suggests a role for other factors, which may include cerebral hyperaemia (impaired autoregulation of blood flow), inflammatory mediators, and false transmitters. Inflammation associated with infection appears to intensify the cerebral effects of ammonia, and both hyponatraemia and hyperglycaemia are well-recognized aggravating factors (Stravitz, 2008).

Encephalopathy is monitored clinically (Table 21.3), but assessment may be difficult in ventilated patients. Stopping sedation for a period each day to evaluate conscious level may be helpful. EEG can also be of value in these patients by identifying significant progression of encephalopathy, subclinical seizures, and responses to treatment, for example when barbiturates are given (Trotter, 2009; Frontera and Kalb, 2011).

**Table 21.3** Modified Parsons–Smith scale of hepatic encephalopathy. (Reproduced from *Postgraduate Medical Journal*, O'Grady J, 'Acute liver failure', 81, 953, pp. 148–154, copyright 2005, with permission from BMJ Publishing Group Ltd..)

| Grade | Clinical features | Neurological signs | Glasgow Coma Scale |
|---|---|---|---|
| 0/Subclinical | Normal | Only seen on neuropsychometric testing | 15 |
| 1 | Trivial lack of awareness, shortened attention span | Tremor, apraxia, incoordination | 15 |
| 2 | Lethargy, disorientation, personality change | Asterixis, ataxia, incoordination | 11–14 |
| 3 | Confusion, somnolence to semistupor, responsive to stimuli, fits of rage | Asterixis, ataxia | 8–10 |
| 4 | Coma | ± Decerebration | < 8 |

In ALF, increasing grade of encephalopathy is associated with an increased prevalence of intracerebral hypertension and the risk of uncal herniation and death (Wijdicks et al., 1995). ICP monitoring is advocated in some centres, with supporters arguing that monitoring allows targeted therapeutic intervention. Groups that use this monitor report that prolonged periods of brain hypoperfusion, with ICP > 40 mm Hg or cerebral perfusion pressure (CPP) < 50 mm Hg, are linked to unfavourable outcome (Frontera and Kalb, 2011). Intracerebral haemorrhage is a concern, although uncommon (7% of monitored patients) (Karvellas et al., 2013b). However, there are no data showing improved outcomes nor any consensus on risk versus benefit (Stravitz et al., 2007; Auzinger and Wendon, 2008; Stravitz, 2008; Larson, 2010; Frontera and Kalb, 2011; Karvellas et al., 2013b).

An indirect and less invasive monitor of brain perfusion, jugular bulb oxygen saturation ($SjO_2$), is used in some units. A decreasing difference between arterial and jugular venous saturations suggests cerebral hyperaemia and impending intracranial hypertension. Thus it may help identify a subgroup of patients who could benefit from direct monitoring, although improved outcomes have not been demonstrated (Stravitz, 2008).

Transcranial Doppler is also used in some units. Algorithms to estimate ICP have been derived and the flow contour of the middle cerebral artery may provide a subjective indicator of intracerebral compliance, but this method has not been widely tested (Frontera and Kalb, 2011). Ultrasound evaluation of the optic nerve may also prove useful once better defined. Brain scans such as CT, magnetic resonance imaging (MRI), and positron emission tomography (PET) have limited value in this setting. They reflect intracranial hypertension poorly and much later than direct monitoring. Transfer of the patient and positioning in the scanner also present hazards in the critically ill patient (Shawcross and Wendon, 2012).

## Treatment of intracranial hypertension in ALF

Intracranial hypertension should be suspected in ALF patients with new-onset systemic hypertension, progression of HE, alterations in pupillary reactivity, abnormal oculovestibular reflexes, and signs of decerebration. However, most of these signs are neither specific nor sensitive and patients with grade IV encephalopathy without intracranial hypertension may be observed (Mohsenin, 2013). Initial management should involve supportive measures and correction of any precipitating or aggravating conditions. Brain CT is indicated to rule out other potential causes of high ICP, especially bleeding.

In grades 3 and 4 HE, intracranial hypertension should be assumed to be present and factors known to aggravate it carefully avoided. The patient should be intubated and mechanically ventilated to protect the airway and to maintain oxygenation and normocapnia. Positioning with a 20–30° head-up tilt and minimal neck rotation is routine. Hyperventilation and hypocapnia are used only to treat episodes of refractory intracranial hypertension. The endotracheal tube should be secured with adhesive tape in a way that reduces the risk of jugular venous obstruction, and PEEP is typically minimized, although low levels do not adversely affect ICP (Huynh et al., 2002). Sedation can be maintained with propofol (3–5 mg/kg/hour), reducing the neuroendocrine stress response and associated surges in cerebral blood flow, oxygen consumption, and ICP (Mohsenin, 2013). Long-term maintenance may also include the administration of pentobarbital, titrated against burst-suppression on EEG (Steadman et al., 2010; Frontera and Kalb, 2011).

Treatment for raised ICP is based on clinical status or, where ICP is monitored, is typically commenced for a persistent ICP > 25 mm Hg. Mannitol is administered in boluses of 0.5–1 g/kg to reduce brain oedema; if regular administration is necessary, serum osmolality should be followed and kept < 320 mmol/L. Hypertonic saline is an alternative, given as 20 mL of 30% sodium chloride or 200 mL of 3% sodium chloride, keeping serum sodium at < 150 mmol/L (Frontera and Kalb, 2011). Normoglycaemia should be maintained. Moderate hypothermia (32–34°C) decreases ICP and has been advocated (Frontera and Kalb, 2011), but a recent randomized trial has not confirmed benefit. Although a core temperature < 33°C resulted in a greater fall in ammonia production, the side effects of this level of hypothermia, including worsened coagulopathy, altered drug metabolism, and greater susceptibility to infections, appeared to outweigh potential advantages (Stravitz and Larsen, 2009; Larsen et al., 2011). A temperature range of 34–36°C is therefore recommended (Bernal and Wendon, 2013). In cases where the increased ICP is resistant to therapy, intravenous indomethacin may be useful (Tofteng and Larsen, 2004).

Maintenance of systemic arterial pressure is essential to avoid cerebral hypoperfusion. When ICP is monitored, a CPP (MAP – ICP) of > 50 mm Hg is an important therapeutic goal. Noradrenaline remains the vasopressor of choice (vide infra) (Stravitz et al., 2007; Auzinger and Wendon, 2008; Stravitz, 2008; Frontera and Kalb, 2011). Terlipressin has been used but was initially reported to increase cerebral blood flow and ICP. Other reports, however, contradict this experience (Jalan, 2005; Eefsen et al., 2007). One describes increased cerebral blood flow without alteration of ICP, accompanied by signs of restoration of blood flow autoregulation and improved neuronal metabolism (lactate and lactate/pyruvate ratio). Further studies of this agent's utility in ALF are needed.

Possibly the most significant factors in the management of intracranial hypertension are early recognition and treatment. From an historical perspective, the early use of NAC when indicated, prompt administration of appropriate fluids and antibiotics, and timely renal replacement therapy may have lowered the risk of intracranial hypertension in ALF, by modulating key contributory factors and limiting the severity of hepatotoxicity and MOF (Bernal et al., 2013).

## Treatment of hepatic encephalopathy in ESLD

Significant intracranial hypertension is uncommon in ESLD and the focus is on the correction of encephalopathy. Again, underlying and aggravating factors should be treated, including infection, gastrointestinal bleeding, hypoventilation, hypoglycaemia, hyponatraemia, and acid-base disturbance. Brain imaging should be considered, especially if focal neurological signs are present, and lumbar puncture if CNS infection is suspected.

Drug treatments of proven benefit include lactulose, which lowers colonic pH and inhibits both urea absorption and urease-producing bacteria, and rifaxamin, a minimally absorbed antibiotic active against urea-producing organisms. Rifaxamin tends not to induce bacterial resistance and has few toxic effects, in contrast to neomycin and metronidazole. It may also exert an effect by reducing gut translocation of pathogenic bacteria and the associated chronic inflammatory state, known to aggravate encephalopathy. Zinc supplementation also appears to be of value. Zinc is needed in the hepatic detoxification of ammonia, and correction of deficiency reduces ammonia concentrations and improves psychometric scores in cirrhotic patients. Protein restriction, once a mainstay of HE treatment, is now seen as potentially harmful, since positive nitrogen balance promotes hepatic regeneration and muscle detoxification of ammonia (Blei et al., 2001; Córdoba et al., 2004). Other recently reported therapies include administration of flumazenil, ammonia-lowering amino acids, and albumin dialysis (Molecular Adsorbent Recirculating System (MARS®)). All have a strong rationale and have produced short-term improvement in HE patients, but more data are needed to establish any effect on survival. These findings are summarized in Table 21.4.

## Cardiovascular monitoring and haemodynamic support

The haemodynamic profile of a patient with both acute and chronic liver failure is hyperkinetic, with an elevated cardiac index (often > 5 L/min/m$^2$), low arterial pressure, low systemic and pulmonary vascular resistance, and medium or low cardiac filling pressures (< 600–800 dynes/s/cm$^{-5}$/m). Increased cardiac output is associated with both increased stroke volume and increased heart rate (Jalan, 2005; Stravitz et al., 2007; Auzinger and Wendon, 2008; Stravitz, 2008; Trotter, 2009), although the latter is not always present. Some data suggest minor differences between the two conditions (Table 21.5), with ALF patients prone to more extreme vasodilation, but the broad pattern is similar and resembles a state of compensated sepsis.

In ALF, the primary cause of hypotension is vasodilation, especially splanchnic, reflecting SIRS. This is linked to increased release and reduced clearance of cytokines by the liver (Stravitz, 2008) and causes relative hypovolaemia. This induces a significant neuroendocrine response that ultimately leads to a reduction of renal, musculocutaneous, and cerebral blood flow mediated by vasoconstriction (Jalan, 2005). In the later stages and in ESLD the relevant vasodilating mediators appear to be NO and cyclic guanosine monophosphate (cGMP); the mechanisms of initial vasodilation are not yet completely understood (Jalan, 2005).

Cardiac function is almost always maintained and signs of heart failure are only evident in the final stages when prolonged hypotension reduces diastolic filling. Heart rhythm changes (bradyarrhythmia, AV block, ectopy, supraventricular tachyarrhythmia, or repolarization changes) may occur but appear to be linked to hypoxia, hypovolaemia, or cerebral oedema and not to inherent cardiac disease or liver failure per se.

ALF guidelines share the common target of maintaining MAP between 55 and 65 mm Hg, both to achieve adequate brain perfusion and to avoid hyperperfusion and baroreceptor-mediated reflexes (Jalan, 2005; Stravitz et al., 2007; Auzinger and Wendon, 2008; Stravitz, 2008; Trotter, 2009). This requires the administration of both fluids and vasopressors. Volume resuscitation is accomplished with crystalloids and colloids guided by fluid responsiveness. The latter can be assessed in terms of filling pressures, central venous oxygen saturation (Scv$O_2$), or stroke volume improvement using measures derived from thermodilution (modified pulmonary artery catheter) or calibrated pulse contour (PiCCO Pulsion®, EV 1000 Edwards). The latter also allows estimation of intrathoracic blood volume index (ITBVi) and extravascular lung water index (EVLWi).

**Table 21.4** Treatment of hepatic encephalopathy. (Reproduced with permission from Findlay et al., 'Critical care of the end-stage liver disease patient awaiting liver transplantation', *Liver Transplantation*, 17, pp. 496–510. Copyright © 2011 American Association for the Study of Liver Diseases.)

| | |
|---|---|
| Proven benefit | Lactulose<br>Rifaximin<br>Zinc<br>Portosystemic shunt occlusion<br>Liver transplantation |
| Unproven or limited benefit | L-Ornithine-L-aspartate (LOLA)<br>L-Ornithine phenylacetate (OP)<br>Flumazenil<br>Extracorporeal albumin dialysis |
| Possibly harmful | Neomycin<br>Metronidazole<br>Protein restriction |

**Table 21.5** Cardiovascular profile in acute and chronic liver disease. (Reprinted from *Journal of Hepatology*, 42, 1, R. Jalan, 'Acute liver failure: current management and future prospects', pp. 115–123, Copyright 2005, with permission from Elsevier and the European Association for the Study of the Liver (EASL).)

| | Acute liver failure | Chronic liver disease |
|---|---|---|
| Systemic vascular resistance | ↓↓ | ↓↓ |
| Cardiac output | ↑↑↑ | ↑↑ |
| Mean arterial pressure | ↓↓↓ | ↓ |
| Muscle blood flow | ↓↑ | ↓ |
| Renal blood flow | ↓↑ | ↓ |
| Splanchnic blood flow | ↑ | ↑↑ |
| Critical hypotension and vascular collapse | ++ | – |

Volumetric preload parameters have long been shown to be more reliable than static filling pressures, despite common use of the latter in guidelines. Fluid challenge and dynamic parameters such as stroke volume variation (SVV) and pulse pressure variation (PPV) during controlled ventilation are more meaningful (Pinsky and Payen, 2005; Trotter, 2009). Other correlates of hypovolaemia include response to passive leg raising, even in non-ventilated patients, and transthoracic echocardiography used to detect IVC diameter.

After initial volume resuscitation, and the implementation of invasive hemodynamic monitoring, administration of vasoconstrictor is recommended. Noradrenaline is usually given first, and vasopressin or terlipressin added if arterial pressure is not improved. In the presence of hypotension of uncertain etiology, further delineation of cardiac status may be helpful, using pulmonary artery or transpulmonary thermodilution (Swan–Ganz catheter or PiCCO Pulsion®, EV 1000 Edwards), or lithium dilution device (LiDCOPlus®) (Pinsky and Payen, 2005; Auzinger and Wendon, 2008; Stravitz, 2008; Trotter, 2009). Transthoracic echocardiography may also be used, providing information on cardiac contractility, chamber filling, and changes in IVC diameter with ventilation (Pinsky and Payen, 2005).

Recent data suggest that latent adrenal insufficiency responding to steroid treatment may be present in ALF. In one report a dose of 200–300 mg hydrocortisone daily for 5–7 days was associated with reduced vasopressor doses, as may be seen in severe sepsis. Others argue that adrenal depression should be confirmed by a tetracosactide (Synacthen®) stimulation test before steroids are given. No survival benefit has been proven (Harry et al., 2002; Jalan, 2005; Stravitz et al., 2007; Auzinger and Wendon, 2008; Stravitz, 2008; Trotter, 2009).

## Haemodynamic management of sepsis in ESLD

Given the presence of a chronically vasodilated state in most patients with ESLD, those with sepsis present with more marked haemodynamic changes than those without chronic liver disease and mortality is high. The high prevalence of chronic structural and functional changes in the heart, recently defined as cirrhotic cardiomyopathy, may contribute (Wong, 2009). This condition is characterized by impairment of the left ventricular contractile response to stress, diastolic dysfunction, and electrophysiological abnormalities, in particular QT prolongation. There are few published data that relate specifically to the haemodynamic management of sepsis in ESLD, but large trials have included ESLD patients and appear relevant.

Early goal-directed treatment is advised, aiming to achieve MAP of 65 mm Hg, central venous pressure of 8–12 mm Hg, central venous oxygen saturation of at least 70%, and urine output of 0.5 mL/kg/hour (Rivers et al., 2001). This requires insertion of central venous and arterial catheters concurrent with initial volume resuscitation. Serum lactate is widely used in liver transplant centres and may supplement the published goals described above.

The specifics of fluids and vasopressors used may vary according to local experience, given the prominence of vasoplegia and lack of published evidence in this group. In the general ICU population, a large trial has shown that resuscitation with colloid is no less effective than with 0.9% sodium chloride (Finfer et al., 2011). However, other data have suggested that ESLD patients with bacterial peritonitis treated with albumin achieve better outcomes, and thus use of albumin-containing solutions may be appropriate in this setting (Sort et al., 1999; Fernández et al., 2005). Trials have suggested that norepinephrine and vasopressin are the most reliable vasopressors for initial use, although in patients given steroids vasopressin appears the more effective single agent. A vasopressin dose of up to 0.04 units/min appears to be safe. Use of both vasopressin plus norepinephrine titrated to effect may be needed.

The use of low-dose steroids in sepsis remains controversial. However, the prevalence of adrenal insufficiency in ESLD may be as high as 68% (Fernández et al., 2006; Jalan et al., 2012) and observational data suggesting a beneficial interaction between steroid and vasopressin may support this treatment. The role of albumin dialysis remains unclear. Haemodynamic improvement in patients with ACLF has been reported (Heemann et al., 2002), but a multicentre randomized trial of the Prometheus® device in patients with ACLF has shown no significant survival benefit at 28 days. Similar results were obtained in the recent RELIEF trial using MARS® (Bañares et al., 2013; Saliba et al., 2013a).

## Respiratory failure, mechanical ventilation, and sedation

Hypoxaemic respiratory failure often accompanies ALF and acute complications of ESLD. Hypoventilation, airway obstruction, and aspiration pneumonitis may result from encephalopathy, while atelectasis, infection, fluid overload, and SIRS-associated interstitial pulmonary oedema are common in all forms of liver failure (Auzinger and Sizer, 2004; Jalan, 2005; Rifai et al., 2005; Stravitz et al., 2007; Auzinger and Wendon, 2008; Stravitz, 2008; Trotter, 2009). Several of these factors may be present and may be compounded by pulmonary shunting (subclinical hepatopulmonary syndrome), pleural effusion, abdominal distention, sarcopaenia, and reduced muscle blood flow.

Continuous monitoring of oxygen saturation and regular blood gas analysis are the standard of care, with capnography, chest X-ray, CT, thoracic ultrasonography, and bronchoscopy used when needed. If PiCCO or EV 1000 systems are used, EVLWi estimation may assist diagnosis and management of interstitial pulmonary oedema (Malbrain, 2004; Jalan, 2005; Stravitz et al., 2007; Auzinger and Wendon, 2008; Stravitz, 2008; Trotter, 2009).

There are few published data on optimization of mechanical ventilation in acute and chronic liver failure and most strategies are derived from trials in mixed populations. The use of protocolized 'ventilator bundles' is recommended, having been shown to decrease complications, including ventilator-associated pneumonia, and improve outcomes (Dodek et al., 2004; Resar et al., 2005; Rello et al., 2010). They typically include head-up positioning (20–30°), infection control measures, sedation management, and gastric ulcer prophylaxis. A lung-protective ventilation strategy with tidal volumes of 6 mL/kg (ideal body weight), plateau pressures < 30 cm $H_2O$, and PEEP has been advocated, since it reduces mortality in ARDS and chest infections after major abdominal surgery (England, 2000; Futier et al., 2013). However, if intracranial hypertension is suspected, hypercarbia should be avoided and PEEP minimized or titrated against ICP and CPP.

Many other modalities have been studied, including high-frequency ventilation, pressure-release ventilation, prone positioning, inhaled NO, and recruitment manoeuvres, but liver failure patients have typically been excluded from these trials.

Although most improve oxygenation, none has reduced mortality. NIV has been successfully applied in the management of both COPD and congestive heart failure, reducing complications of intubation and associated sedation. Use of NIV has also been described following liver transplant or resection, but there are no data on patients with liver failure, in whom encephalopathy, gastrointestinal bleeding, and overt sepsis often would make this approach impractical if not contraindicated.

Sedation is typically required in mechanically ventilated patients except those with the most severe encephalopathy. Shorter-acting drugs such as propofol, dexmedetomidine, remifentanil, and midazolam are now widely used, but all have adverse effects. Again, the literature specific to patients with ESLD and ALF is limited. However, studies in other ICU populations have shown that close, systematic monitoring and goal-directed management of sedation, analgesia, and delirium reduce the duration of ventilation, ventilator-associated pneumonia, and ICU stay (Kress et al., 2000).

Since altered drug kinetics and effects in this group predispose them to harmful oversedation, this individualized approach is strongly recommended. Monitoring of the bispectral index (BIS) to assess conscious level in both ALF and ACLF has been reported, although its utility is not established (Hwang et al., 2010; Kang et al., 2013).

## Prevention and management of renal failure

Renal insufficiency is common in both ALF and ACLF (Cholongitas et al., 2009) and has an important role in prognosis. GFR calculated from creatinine concentrations in ESLD may underestimate renal dysfunction in the presence of sarcopaenia. New criteria using percentage change from baseline creatinine or GFR have been demonstrated to correlate better with outcomes but have not been validated in renal injury associated with ESLD (Cruz et al., 2009). Renal dysfunction may be functional, related to the pathological renal vasoconstriction of ESLD (HRS), or frankly ischaemic with acute tubular necrosis. Underlying renal disease and drug toxicity are also sometimes implicated (Moore, 1999; Jalan, 2005; O'Grady, 2005; Rifai et al., 2005; Stravitz et al., 2007; Auzinger and Wendon, 2008; Stravitz, 2008; Trotter, 2009; Bernal et al., 2010). Monitoring includes hourly urine flow and frequent measurement of urine sodium and chloride. Chloride excretion has been described as particularly sensitive to intravascular volume and renal perfusion pressure (Caironi et al., 2010). Low urinary sodium is typical in HRS, although this finding may be absent in the presence of diuretic therapy. Since ascites, haemoperitoneum, and abdominal wall or intestinal oedema are common, estimation of renal perfusion pressure (MAP minus intra-abdominal pressure) has been advocated if raised intra-abdominal pressure is suspected (Malbrain, 2004; Brochard et al., 2010).

Treatment of HRS and impending acute kidney injury (AKI) consists of optimizing volume status and administration of vasopressors to increase glomerular perfusion pressure (Jalan, 2005; Stravitz et al., 2007; Auzinger and Wendon, 2008; Stravitz, 2008; Trotter, 2009; Frontera and Kalb, 2011). Retrospective studies in ESLD suggest that volume expansion with human albumin solution (1 g/kg followed by 20–40 g/day) combined with an alpha-agonist (midodrine, norepinephrine, or terlipressin) and octreotide is effective in HRS. Although terlipressin is justified in HRS associated with ESLD (Hadengue et al., 1998; Uriz et al., 2000; Duvoux et al., 2002), its value in ALF is unproven (Eefsen et al., 2007; Auzinger and Wendon, 2008; Stravitz, 2008). Although its $V_1$ receptor effects induce vasoconstriction in both splanchnic and efferent glomerular arterioles, increasing both systemic arterial and glomerular filtration pressures, there has been concern that its $V_2$ effects may increase cerebral blood flow and raise ICP (Hadengue et al., 1998; Uriz et al., 2000; Duvoux et al., 2002; Stravitz, 2008). However, some data suggest that there is no adverse effect on ICP (Eefson et al., 2007). No evidence supports the use of dopamine, fenaldopam, or other agents in this setting.

Continuous renal replacement therapy (CRRT) is preferred to intermittent dialysis in both ALF and ESLD because it is better tolerated haemodynamically and is associated with a more stable ICP (Davenport et al., 1993). It must be initiated early and it is an integral part of treatment aimed at reducing cerebral oedema (Jalan, 2005; Stravitz et al., 2007; Auzinger and Wendon, 2008;Stravitz, 2008; Trotter, 2009). Current practice is to reinfuse at 30–35 mL/kg/hour (Ronco et al., 2000; Mehta, 2005). Recent experience of high volume exchange (90 mL/kg/hour) is promising, but this technique is clinically very labour-intensive and remains experimental (Auzinger and Wendon, 2008). Bicarbonate-based replacement solutions are preferred, since lactate administration increases plasma lactate concentration and undermines its utility as a marker of liver function (Stravitz et al., 2007; Auzinger and Wendon, 2008; Stravitz, 2008).

Anticoagulation is achieved with heparin or citrate, depending on local experience. Regional citrate anticoagulation requires close monitoring of ionized calcium and appropriate calcium replacement to avoid hypocalcaemia and hypotension. Alternatively, when thrombocytopaenia and coagulopathy are present, heparin can be replaced with epoprostenol sodium (2–6 ng/kg/min) (Fiaccadori et al., 2002; Jalan, 2005; Auzinger and Wendon, 2008; Stravitz, 2008; Trotter, 2009).

## Diagnosis and management of infection

Patients with both ALF and ESLD are more susceptible to bacterial and fungal infections than the general population (Rolando et al., 1993, 1996, 2000; Vaquero et al., 2003; Jalan, 2005; Antoniades et al., 2006; Stravitz et al., 2007; Auzinger and Wendon, 2008; Stravitz, 2008; Trotter, 2009). Infection is common and both incidence and severity are proportionate to severity of liver disease. Further, any infection is more likely to be associated with sepsis, septic shock, and MOF. SBP, urinary tract infection, and pneumonia are the most common, followed by bacteraemia associated with endoscopic procedures, cellulitis, and indeterminate cause. In a recent series, pneumonia and SBP occurred in 20% and 40% of patients with ESLD admitted to ICU, respectively (Das et al., 2010). Catheter-related and fungal sepsis are also common, especially later in the course of the acute illness.

Immunoparesis accompanied by an excessive inflammatory response has been demonstrated in both ALF and ESLD/ACLF. There is a reduction in opsonization capability (reduced complement levels), functional deactivation of monocytes, and impairment of neutrophil phagocytic function, among other defects (Antoniades et al., 2006; Gustot et al., 2009). The cell-based pro-inflammatory response to both hepatocyte injury and infection is exaggerated, while the compensatory anti-inflammatory response is impaired. This imbalance may be pivotal in the pathogenesis of septic shock and organ failure. Survival decreases markedly in the presence of SIRS (Rolando et al., 1993, 1996, 2000; Vaquero et al., 2003; Jalan, 2005; Antoniades et al., 2006; Auzinger and Wendon, 2008; Stravitz, 2008; Trotter, 2009).

Appropriate nutritional support, maintenance of near-normal blood glucose concentrations, careful oral and airway hygiene, 30° head-up position in ventilated patients, strict asepsis in the insertion and daily use of intravascular devices, and protocol-driven clinical examination and surveillance cultures are well-established infection control measures. These have reduced the incidence and delayed the onset of hospital-acquired bacteraemias, which are now more commonly Gram-negative (Karvellas et al., 2009).

Prompt antimicrobial treatment and source control remain the key elements of treatment, along with rapid haemodynamic resuscitation, as described in the section 'Haemodynamic management of sepsis in ESLD'. Systematic surveillance is essential to identify colonization with pathogens, allow eradication when possible, and aid targeted treatment of infection. Multiresistant bacterial strains, such as methicillin-resistant *Staphylococcus aureus* (MRSA), vancomycin-resistant *Enterococcus* (VRE), and carbapenem-resistant *Klebsiella* species, are becoming more common in liver transplant candidates and colonization has been linked to poorer outcomes. Early empiric treatment of suspected fungal infection is also critical (Rolando et al., 1996). Fluconazole has been used in this context for many years, but new data suggest that an echinocandin or liposomal amphotericin should be considered in the severely compromised candidate (Karvellas et al., 2009; Cornely et al., 2012).

Empirical antibacterial and antifungal treatment is indicated when sepsis is suspected, as with the onset of SIRS, with the identification of likely pathogens in routine cultures, or when there is deepening encephalopathy and/or the onset of refractory hypotension (Stravitz et al., 2007). To date there are no data to support any specific antibacterial or antifungal therapy. However, surveillance cultures, local microbiological trends, and the patient's risk profile should all be considered and dosing adjusted as required to allow for concurrent renal replacement therapy, therapeutic hypothermia, and immunoparesis (Pea et al., 2005, 2007; Stravitz et al., 2007; Auzinger and Wendon, 2008; Stravitz, 2008). Negative cultures in a stable patient or continuing deterioration should prompt re-evaluation of anti-infective therapy.

## Monitoring and treatment of coagulopathy

Changes in coagulation associated with severe liver disease are described in Chapter 19. There is reduced hepatic synthesis of factors II, V, VII, IX, and X (Bernuau et al., 1986, 1991; Elinav et al., 2005), often accompanied by dysfibrinogenaemia, defective platelet function (Stravitz et al., 2007; Munoz et al., 2008, 2009; De Gasperi et al., 2009), pathological fibrinolysis, and thrombocytopaenia. However, in both ALF and ESLD, a concomitant reduction in synthesis of anticoagulant proteins, impaired reticuloendothelial clearance of activated coagulation factors and their inhibitors, and elevated levels of factor VIII and vWF often lead to preservation of clinical coagulation, or even a prothrombotic state (Munoz et al., 2009; Tripodi and Mannucci, 2011). Since the PT measures the activity of factors V, VII, and X without reflecting procoagulant influences, it may be prolonged even when thrombin generation is normal. Moreover, especially in ESLD, a depressed platelet count may be associated with well-maintained or enhanced platelet function and normal clinical haemostasis. Although the short half-lives of factors V and VII make PT a valuable marker of liver function, its correlation with clinical coagulation in liver disease is weak.

Nonetheless, with increasing severity of liver failure and the onset of SIRS, complex coagulopathy and bleeding are common. In ALF an initially preserved platelet count tends to fall as severity of the underlying disease and associated inflammatory response increase, with an increased risk of bleeding. Both disseminated intravascular coagulation (DIC) and hyperfibrinolysis may occur (Munoz et al., 2009) and both are associated with raised fibrin degradation products. Fibrinolysis is distinguished by its characteristic trace on thromboelastogram, which many units now use to supplement standard coagulation screening tests.

Parenteral administration of vitamin K is routine to optimize synthesis of dependent factors (Munoz et al., 2008). Use of blood products for management of coagulopathy in both ALF and ESLD should be limited to treatment of serious bleeding or prophylaxis for insertion of an ICP monitoring device (Jalan, 2005; Stravitz et al., 2007; Auzinger and Wendon, 2008; Munoz et al., 2008, 2009; Stravitz, 2008; Trotter, 2009). In ALF, although spontaneous bleeding is uncommon, events requiring treatment may be seen in 30% of patients (Munoz et al., 2009). However, potential benefits must be balanced against the effect on PT as an indicator of prognosis and need for liver transplant. The risks of volume overload, transfusion-related acute lung injury (TRALI), and aggravated cerebral oedema should also be considered (Munoz et al., 2008, 2009). If indicated, FFP is usually given at an arbitrary dose of 15–20 mL/kg, although this will rarely correct PT. Platelets are given for counts < 75,000 and cryoprecipitate when fibrinogen level is < 100 mg/dL (Pittet et al., 1994; Jonge et al., 2003; Pea et al., 2005, 2007; Rifai et al., 2005; Koeman et al., 2006; Stravitz et al., 2007; Munoz et al., 2009). The use of prothrombin complex, fibrinogen concentrate, and activated recombinant factor VII have also been advocated when available, although evidence of benefit is limited and the cost of these treatments is high (Shami et al., 2003; Munoz et al., 2008, 2009). Antifibrinolytics (tranexamic acid, aminocaproic acid) appear to reduce bleeding during liver transplantation and in trauma, but their use to treat acute bleeding in ALF and ACLF has not been reported.

## Artificial liver support

Severe liver failure results in reduced plasma concentrations of albumin and increased concentrations of many albumin-bound substances, some of which undoubtedly contribute to extrahepatic organ failure. These include bilirubin, aromatic amino acids, bile salts, endogenous benzodiazepines, prostacyclin, tryptophan, and NO, among others. Renal replacement therapies remove free hydrophilic molecules by convection, but clearance of ammonia and albumin-bound toxins is not enough to produce clinical benefit. Commercially available liver support systems combine conventional dialysis with adsorptive removal of molecules bound to albumin by carbon-containing media (McKenzie et al., 2008; Bernal et al., 2010). Bioartificial modalities incorporate living hepatocytes; at present these are under development and licensed only for clinical trials.

Albumin dialysis systems include MARS®, Prometheus®, and SPAD® (Single Pass Albumin Dialysis). MARS® is based on whole-blood dialysis across an albumin-coated membrane. Toxins are removed by filtration and by transfer between blood and membrane-bound and exogenous albumin in the dialysate, which is then purified by adsorption and recycled. In Prometheus®, native albumin is first separated from whole blood by plasmapheresis using a 100-kDa polysulphone filter, then purified and returned to the patient. In simpler SPAD®, albumin is added to dialysis solution in special containers, which are used with standard dialysis equipment and discarded with the dialysate. Comparative study of MARS® and SPAD® showed little difference in detoxification capacity (Saliba, 2006).

These systems have all been shown to improve jaundice, haemodynamic status, encephalopathy, and ICP in a range of settings. However, a recent multicentre randomized trial in ACLF failed to demonstrate a significant improvement in survival (Bañares et al., 2013). Data in ALF are limited and not yet conclusive, since randomized trials are lacking (Liu et al., 2004; McKenzie et al., 2008). Similarly, plasmapheresis has not produced consistent results despite favourable early reports in paediatric patients (Singer et al., 2001).

Bioartificial or hybrid support systems (BAL®, ELAD®) require the use of freshly procured or cryopreserved human or porcine liver cells to replace the functions of the failing liver. The cells are deployed in a hollow-fibre matrix (Rifai et al., 2003; McKenzie et al., 2008). The patient's plasma is passed through the bioreactor chamber, separated from the exogenous hepatocytes by a semipermeable membrane with a maximum pore size sufficient to allow passage of toxins and albumin (66 kDa) but not immunoglobulins (100–900 kDa), complement (200 kDa), viruses, or cells. A cell mass of 6–36 billion hepatocytes appears to be sufficient. This modality may be supplemented by albumin dialysis and haemofiltration. Small studies of these systems in ALF have thus far reported improved clinical parameters and positive trends but no significant difference in survival compared to conventional care. One randomized study using the HepatAssist-BAL® reported better survival in patients with a known cause of ALF in a post-hoc subgroup analysis (Rifai et al., 2005; Stravitz and Kramer, 2009). This system, using porcine hepatocytes, has since been altered with a three-fold increase in the number of cells and is being investigated in a further randomized trial. Recently it has been argued that use of all extracorporeal devices should now be restricted to randomized controlled trials (Bernal and Wendon, 2013).

## Removal of the critically ill patient from the transplant waiting list

Since the number of donated livers falls far short of demand, this limited resource must be managed fairly and to maximize benefit. Futile transplants in the setting of ALF are uncommon, since clinicians broadly agree on the signs of a hopeless prognosis, and the rarity of the condition assures few wasted grafts. Estimation of mortality risk in ESLD patients transplanted from the ICU is more complex and arbitrary. Registry and other published information on outcomes in this context is limited and is constrained by the tendency of most units not to attempt transplantation in patients perceived to be at extreme risk.

However, the number of extrahepatic organs requiring support is clearly the dominant determinant of post- as well as pretransplant mortality, with 1-year survival falling below 60% if two systems are affected. Mechanical ventilation and vasopressor support are particularly powerful adverse predictors, but other factors have been shown to be relevant and should be considered. These include age, race, type of liver disease, previous liver transplant, insulin-dependent diabetes mellitus, and renal dysfunction (Desai et al., 2004; Merion, 2004; Aloia et al., 2010). Nutritional status has not been adequately studied in this setting but is widely held to be another important marker of risk.

Although recent retrospective reports on transplant outcomes in patients with ACLF and extrahepatic organ failure indicate that results are acceptable in selected patients, varying definitions of ACLF and the absence of data on pretransplant cardiorespiratory status limit their utility (Bahirwani et al., 2011). Only one report gives data on selection, finding that 25% of candidates considered appropriate for evaluation received a transplant, and these not necessarily from the ICU (Finkenstedt et al., 2013). In most units, ESLD patients on mechanical ventilation and vasopressor support are not considered for transplant, while renal replacement therapy, at least as the only extrahepatic organ failure, is considered much less ominous. Barring other contraindications or, more frequently, multiple factors contributing to a prohibitive aggregate risk, transplant is considered only after these patients are resuscitated and weaned from cardiorespiratory support.

In a patient already listed, whether in the setting of ALF, ACLF, or ESLD, some conditions should prompt careful re-evaluation of suitability for transplant. These include the following (Steadman et al., 2010; Findlay et al., 2011):

- Severe ischaemic heart disease with a recent acute coronary event or low ejection fraction (< 40%)
- Uncontrolled pulmonary hypertension (mean PA pressure > 40 mm Hg) with elevated pulmonary vascular resistance.
- Circulatory collapse with high-dose vasopressors (norepinephrine infusion > 1 μg/kg/min), especially when associated with patchy peripheral cyanosis
- Respiratory failure requiring intubation (in ESLD), or $FiO_2$ > 0.60, PEEP > 12 cm $H_2O$ (in ALF)
- Persistent stage III–IV encephalopathy (in ESLD); sustained intracranial hypertension with fixed pupillary dilatation or CPP < 40 mm Hg lasting more than 2 hours; new-onset stroke
- Necrotizing pancreatitis
- Systemic sepsis associated with fungi or resistant bacteria
- Hepatocellular cancer outside criteria, or new diagnosis of malignancy
- Adverse psychosocial conditions: failed abstinence, pretransplant non-compliance, loss of social support

Identification of candidates in whom transplant is futile and their removal from the transplant waiting list is essential if the benefits of liver transplantation are to be maximized. However, risk in the individual patient is a matter of probability, estimated on the basis of historical data and clinicians' experience. Nonetheless, a professional consensus exists regarding an acceptable balance between individual need, whatever the odds of survival, and the greatest gain in life-years for the available grafts: predicted survival should be at least 40–60% at 5 years (Murray and Carithers, 2005). Although data predicting survival are inevitably flawed, by failing to take account of recent advances, by uncertainty about comparability between health systems, and by the small number of clinical parameters included, such an estimate is a useful starting point for any case-by-case assessment (Thuluvath et al., 2003; Aloia et al., 2010). Most clinicians will evaluate all factors, with full multidisciplinary input, and attempt to make a judgement on this basis. If intraoperative or early post-transplant mortality risk is likely to exceed 40–50%, there is a strong argument that transplant should not be undertaken.

## Conclusion

Mortality from ALF remains high despite important improvements in treatment. ALF requires early diagnosis, aetiology-specific treatment, and transfer to a specialist unit offering liver transplantation. The onset of extrahepatic organ failure, typically with progression to grade 3 encephalopathy, requires intubation, ventilation, and the full support of a liver transplant ICU. The principal aim of intensive care is to optimize hepatic oxygen delivery, to preserve residual hepatocyte function and facilitate regeneration. Complications such as sepsis, cerebral oedema, renal and cardiorespiratory failure, and haemorrhage must be prevented or treated to support recovery or survival to transplant. When prognostic scoring indicates that recovery is unlikely, liver transplantation should be undertaken as soon as an acceptable organ can be found.

Although these measures have transformed the prognosis in ALF, there is scope for better prediction of spontaneous recovery and avoidance of the risks associated with unnecessary transplantation. Equally, when transplant is indicated but severe cardiorespiratory failure or neurological injury supervene, a decision not to proceed is appropriate. Multicentre studies of ALF prognostic indices and of bioartificial liver support are likely to yield the next major advances in the treatment of this rare and dangerous condition.

The recent emergence of the concept of ACLF, although not yet consistently defined, suggests that patients with chronic liver disease presenting to the ICU may be distinguishable as two broad groups: those with very advanced disease suffering a preterminal event and those with mild or well-compensated liver disease presenting with acute deterioration in liver function accompanied by extrahepatic organ failure. A predisposition to SIRS, or impairment of the compensatory anti-inflammatory response, characterizes ACLF, precipitating a need for mechanical ventilation and/or vasopressors following a triggering event such as surgery. While both conditions have a poor prognosis, ACLF may have greater potential for reversibility with treatment and benefit from transplantation. A clear consensus on the definition of this condition, differentiating it from terminal decompensation, may have implications for intensive care admission policy and clinical management in future.

Treatments based on current concepts in the pathophysiology of severe liver disease have been outlined in this chapter. These aim to maintain a state in which successful transplantation can be performed or to restore the potential recipient to this state as rapidly as possible. The evaluation of perioperative and long-term risks in the critically ill transplant candidate remains a challenge. A sound approach to this increasingly common dilemma will require both an ethical consensus on what constitutes an acceptable predicted mortality risk and much more data from which to estimate this risk in each patient.

## References


Amodio P, Montagnese S, Gatta A, Morgan M (2004) Characteristics of minimal hepatic encephalopathy. *Metabol Brain Dis*, **19**(3–4):253–267.

Aloia TA, Knight R, Gaber AO, Ghobrial RM, Goss JA (2010) Analysis of liver transplant outcomes for United Network for Organ Sharing recipients 60 years old or older identifies multiple model for end-stage liver disease-independent prognostic factors. *Liver Transplant*, **16**:950–959.

Antoniades C, Berry PA, Davies ET, Hussain M, Bernal W, Vergani D, et al. (2006) Reduced monocyte HLA-DR expression: a novel biomarker of disease severity and outcome in acetaminophen-induced acute liver failure. *Hepatology*, **44**(1):34–43.

Auzinger G, Wendon J (2008) Intensive care management of acute liver failure. *Curr Opin Crit Care*, **14**(2):179–188.

Auzinger G, Sizer EBW, et al. (2004) Incidence of lung injury in acute liver failure: diagnostic role of extravascular lung water index. *Crit Care Med*, **8** (Suppl 1):40.

Bahirwani R, Shaked O, Bewtra M, Forde K, Reddy KR (2011) Acute-on-chronic liver failure before liver transplantation: impact on posttransplant outcomes. *Transplantation*, **92**:952–957.

Bañares R, Nevens F, Larsen FS, et al. (2013) Extracorporeal albumin dialysis with the molecular adsorbent recirculating system in acute-on-chronic liver failure: the RELIEF trial. *Hepatology*, **57**(3):1153–1162.

Bechmann LP, Jochum C, Kocabayoglu P, et al. (2010) Cytokeratin 18-based modification of the MELD score improves prediction of spontaneous survival after acute liver injury. *J Hepatol*, **53**(4):639–647.

Bernal W, Wendon J (2013) Acute liver failure. *N Engl J Med*, **369**(26):2525–2534.

Bernal W, Hall C, Karvellas CJ, Auzinger G, Sizer E, Wendon J (2007) Arterial ammonia and clinical risk factors for encephalopathy and intracranial hypertension in acute liver failure. *Hepatology*, **46**(6):1844–1852.

Bernal W, Hyyrylainen A, Gera A, et al (2013) Lessons from look-back in acute liver failure? A single centre experience of 3300 patients. *J Hepatol*, **59**(1):74–80.

Bernuau J, Goudeau A, Poynard T, et al (1986) Multivariate analysis of prognostic factors in fulminant hepatitis B. *Hepatology*, **6**(4):648–651.

Bernuau J, Samuel D, Durand F, et al. (1991) Criteria for emergency liver transplantation in patients with acute viral hepatitis and factor V below 50% of normal: a prospective study. *Abstr Hepatol*, **14**(49A).

Blei AT, Córdoba J, Practice Parameters Committee of the American College of Gastroenterology (2001) Hepatic encephalopathy. *Am J Gastroenterol*, **96**(7):1968–1976.

Brochard L, Abroug F, Brenner M, et al. (2010) An official ATS/ERS/ESICM/SCCM/SRLF statement: prevention and management of acute renal failure in the ICU patient: an international consensus conference in intensive care medicine. *Am J Resp Crit Care Med*, **181**(10):1128–1155.

Caironi P, Langer T, Taccone P, et al. (2010) Kidney instant monitoring (K.IN.G): a new analyzer to monitor kidney function. *Minerva Anestesiol*, **76**(5):316–324.

Cholongitas E, Senzolo M, Patch D, Shaw S, O'Beirne J, Burroughs AK (2009) Cirrhotics admitted to intensive care unit: the impact of acute renal failure on mortality. *Eur J Gastroenterol Hepatol*, **21**:744–750.

Córdoba J, López-Hellín J, Planas M, et al. (2004) Normal protein diet for episodic hepatic encephalopathy: results of a randomized study. *J Hepatol*, **41**:38–43.

Cornely OA, Bassetti M, Calandra T (2012) ESCMID* guideline for the diagnosis and management of Candida diseases

2012: non-neutropenic adult patients. *Clin Microbiol Infect*, **18**(Suppl 7):19–37.

Cruz DN, Ricci Z, Ronco C (2009) Clinical review: RIFLE and AKIN—time for reappraisal. *Crit Care*, **13**:211.

Das V, Boelle PY, Galbois A, et al. (2010) Cirrhotic patients in the medical intensive care unit: early prognosis and long-term survival. *Crit Care Med*, **38**:2108–2116.

Davenport A, Will EJ, Davidson AM (1993) Improved cardiovascular stability during continuous modes of renal replacement therapy in critically ill patients with acute hepatic and renal failure. *Crit Care Med*, **21**(3):328–338.

De Carlis L, De Gasperi A, Slim AO, et al. (2001) Liver transplantation for ecstasy-induced fulminant hepatic failure. *Transplant Proc*, **33**(5):2743–2744.

De Gasperi A, Corti A, Mazza E, Prosperi M, Amici O, Bettinelli L (2009) Acute liver failure: managing coagulopathy and the bleeding diathesis. *Transplant Proc*, **41**(4):1256–1259.

Desai NM, Mange KC, Crawford MD, et al. (2004) Predicting outcome after liver transplantation: utility of the model for end-stage liver disease and a newly derived discrimination function.

Dodek P, Keenan S, Cook D, et al. (2004) Evidence-based clinical practice guideline for the prevention of ventilator-associated pneumonia. *Annal Intern Med*, **141**(4):305–313.

Duvoux C, Zanditenas D, Hézode C, et al. (2002) Effects of noradrenalin and albumin in patients with type I hepatorenal syndrome: a pilot study. *Hepatology*, **36**(2):374–380.

Eefsen M, Dethloff T, Frederiksen HJ, Hauerberg J, Hansen BA, Larsen FS (2007) Comparison of terlipressin and noradrenalin on cerebral perfusion, intracranial pressure and cerebral extracellular concentrations of lactate and pyruvate in patients with acute liver failure in need of inotropic support. *J Hepatol*, **47**(3):381–386.

Elinav E, Ben-Dov I, Hai-Am E, Ackerman Z, Ofran Y (2005) The predictive value of admission and follow up factor V and VII levels in patients with acute hepatitis and coagulopathy. *J Hepatol*, **42**(1):82–86.

England TN (2000) Ventilation with lower tidal volumes as compared with traditional tidal volumes for acute lung injury and the acute respiratory distress syndrome. The Acute Respiratory Distress Syndrome Network. *N Engl J Med*, **342**:1301–1308.

Fernández J, Monteagudo J, Bargallo X, et al. (2005) A randomized unblinded pilot study comparing albumin versus hydroxyethyl starch in spontaneous bacterial peritonitis. *Hepatology*, **42**(3):627–634.

Fernández J, Escorsell A, Zabalza M, et al. (2006) Adrenal insufficiency in patients with cirrhosis and septic shock: effect of treatment with hydrocortisone on survival. *Hepatology*, **44**(5):1288–1295.

Fiaccadori E, Maggiore U, Rotelli C, et al. (2002) Continuous haemofiltration in acute renal failure with prostacyclin as the sole anti-haemostatic agent. *Intens Care Med*, **28**(5):586–593.

Findlay JY, Fix OK, Paugam-Burtz C, et al. (2011) Critical care of the end-stage liver disease patient awaiting liver transplantation. *Liver Transplant*, **17**:496–510.

Finfer S, Vincent J-L (2013) Critical care—an all-encompassing specialty. *N Engl J Med*, **369**(7):669–670.

Harry R, Auzinger G, Wendon J (2002) The clinical importance of adrenal insufficiency in acute hepatic dysfunction. *Hepatology*, **36**(2):395–402.

Jalan R (2005) Acute liver failure: current management and future prospects. *J Hepatol*, **42**(Suppl 1):S115–S123.

Jalan R, Plevris JN, Jalan AR, Finlayson ND, Hayes PC (1994) A pilot study of indocyanine green clearance as an early predictor of graft function. *Transplantation*, **58**(2):196–200.

Jalan R, Gines P, Olson JC, et al. (2012) Acute-on chronic liver failure. *J Hepatol*, **57**:1336–1348.

Jonge E, Schultz MJ, Spanjaard L, et al. (2003) Effects of selective decontamination of digestive tract on mortality and acquisition of resistant bacteria in intensive care: a randomised controlled trial. *Lancet*, **362**(9389):1011–1016.

Kang SH, Hwang S, Jung BH (2013) Post-transplant assessment of consciousness in acute-on-chronic liver failure patients undergoing liver transplantation using bispectral index monitoring. *Transplant Proc*, **45**(8):3069–3071.

Karvellas CJ, Pink F, McPhail M, et al. (2009) Predictors of bacteraemia and mortality in patients with acute liver failure. *Intens Care Med*, **35**:1390–1396.

Karvellas CJ, Lescot T, Goldberg P, et al. (2013a) Liver transplantation in the critically ill: a multicenter Canadian retrospective cohort study. *Crit Care*, **17**(1):R28.

Karvellas C, Fix O, Battenhouse H, et al. (2013b) Outcomes and complications of intracranial pressure monitoring in acute liver failure: a retrospective cohort study. *Crit Care Med*, **42**(5):1157–1167.

Khashab M, Tector A, Kwo P (2007) Epidemiology of acute liver failure. Curr Gastroenterol Rep, **9**(1):66–73.

Koeman M, van der Ven AJ, Hak E, et al. (2006) Oral decontamination with chlorhexidine reduces the incidence of ventilator-associated pneumonia. Am J Resp Crit Care Med, **173**(12):1348–1355.

Kress JP, Pohlman AS, O'Connor MF, Hall JB (2000) Daily interruption of sedative infusions in critically ill patients undergoing mechanical ventilation. N Engl J Med, **342**(20):1471–1477.

Larsen FS, Murphy N, Bernal W, et al. (2011) Prophylactic effect of mild hypothermia to prevent brain edema in patients with acute liver failure: results of a multicenter randomized, controlled trial. J Hepatol, **54**(Suppl):S26.

Larson A (2010) Diagnosis and management of acute liver failure. Curr Opin Gastroenterol, **26**(3):214–221.

Liu JP, Gluud LL, Als-Nielsen B, Gluud C (2004) Artificial and bioartificial support systems for liver failure. Cochrane Database Syst Rev, **1**:CD003628.

Malbrain ML, Cheatham ML (2004) Cardiovascular effects and optimal preload markers in intra-abdominal hypertension. In: Vincent JL (ed) *Yearbook of Intensive Care and Emergency Medicine*, pp. 519–543. Springer, Berlin.

Mazza E, Prosperi M, De Gasperi, et al. (2008) PDR ICG after liver transplantation: always a reliable tool to predict graft function and outcome? *Liver Transplant*, **14**:476.

McKenzie T, Lillegard J, Nyberg S (2008) Artificial and bioartificial liver support. *Semin Liver Dis*, **28**(2):210–217.

Mehta R (2005) Continuous renal replacement therapy in the critically ill patient. *Kidney Intern*, **67**(2):781–795.

Merion RM (2004) When is a patient too well and when is a patient too sick for a liver transplant? *Liver Transplant*, **10**(Suppl2):S69–S73.

Mohsenin V (2013) Assessment and management of cerebral edema and intracranial hypertension in acute liver failure. *J Crit Care*, **28**(5):783–791.

Moore K (1999) Renal failure in acute liver failure. *Eur J Gastroenterol Hepatol*, **11**(9):967–975.

Munoz S, Reddy K, Lee W (2008) The coagulopathy of acute liver failure and implications for intracranial pressure monitoring. *Neurocrit Care*, **9**(1):103–107.

Munoz S, Stravitz R, Gabriel D (2009) Coagulopathy of acute liver failure. *Clin Liver Dis*, **13**(1):95–107.

Murray KF, Carithers RJ (2005) AASLD practice guidelines: evaluation of the patient for liver transplantation. *Hepatology.*, **41**(6):1407–1432.

O'Grady J (2005) Acute liver failure. *Postgrad Med J*, **81**(953):148–154.

O'Grady JG, Alexander GJ, Hayllar KM, Williams R (1989) Early indicators of prognosis in fulminant hepatic failure. *Gastroenterology*, **97**(2):439–445.

Olson J, Kamath P (2011) Acute-on-chronic liver failure: concept, natural history, and prognosis. *Curr Opin Crit Care*, **17**(2):165–169.

Ostapowicz G, Fontana RJ, Schiødt FV, et al. (2002). Results of a prospective study of acute liver failure at 17 tertiary care centers in the United States. *Annal Intern Med*, **137**(12):947–954.

Pea F, Viale P, Furlanut M (2005) Antimicrobial therapy in critically ill patients: a review of pathophysiological conditions responsible for altered disposition and pharmacokinetic variability. *Clin Pharmacokin*, **44**(10):1009–1034.

Pea F, Viale P, Pavan F, Furlanut M (2007) Pharmacokinetic considerations for antimicrobial therapy in patients receiving renal replacement therapy. *Clin Pharmacokin*, **46**(12):997–1038.

Pinsky M, Payen D (2005) Functional hemodynamic monitoring. *Crit Care*, **9**(6):566–572.

Pittet D, Monod M, Suter PM, Frenk E, Auckenthaler R (1994) Candida colonization and subsequent infections in critically ill surgical patients. *Annal Surg*, **220**(6):751–758.

Rello J, Lode H, Cornaglia G, Masterton R, VAP Care Bundle Contributors (2010) A European care bundle for prevention of ventilator-associated pneumonia. *Intensive Care Med*, **36**(5):773–780.

Resar R, Pronovost P, Haraden C, Simmonds T, Rainey T, Nolan T (2005) Using a bundle approach to improve ventilator care processes and reduce ventilator-associated pneumonia. *Jt Comm J Qual Patient Saf*, **31**(5):243–248.

Rifai K, Ernst T, Kretschmer U, et al. (2003) Prometheus—a new extracorporeal system for the treatment of liver failure. *J Hepatol*, **39**(6):984–990.

Rifai K, Ernst T, Kretschmer U, et al. (2005) The Prometheus device for extracorporeal support of combined liver and renal failure. *Blood Purific*, **23**(4):298–302.

Rivers E, Nguyen B, Havstad S, et al. (2001) Early goal-directed therapy in the treatment of severe sepsis and septic shock. *N Engl J Med*, **345**:1368–1377.

Rolando N, Gimson A, Wade J, Philpott-Howard J, Casewell M, Williams R (1993) Prospective controlled trial of selective parenteral and enteral antimicrobial regimen in fulminant liver failure. *Hepatology*, **17**(2):196–201.

Rolando N, Philpott-Howard J, Williams R (1996) Bacterial and fungal infection in acute liver failure. *Semin Liver Dis*, **16**(4):389–402.

Rolando N, Wade J, Davalos M, Wendon J, Philpott-Howard J, Williams R (2000) The systemic inflammatory response syndrome in acute liver failure. *Hepatology*, **32**(4 Pt 1):734–739.

Ronco C, Belomo R, Homel P, et al. (2000) Effects of different doses in continuous veno-venous haemofiltration on outcomes of acute renal failure: a prospective randomised trial. *Lancet*, **356**(9223):26–30.

Saliba F, Camus C, Durand F, et al. (2013a) Albumin dialysis with a non-cell artificial liver support device in patients with acute liver failure: a randomized, controlled trial. *Ann Intern Med*, **159**:522–531.

Saliba F, Ichai P, Levesque E, Samuel D (2013b) Cirrhotic patients in the ICU: prognostic markers and outcome. *Curr Opin Crit Care*, **19**(2):154–160.

Saliba F (2006) The Molecular Adsorbent Recirculating System (MARS) in the intensive care unit: a rescue therapy for patients with hepatic failure. *Crit Care*, **10**(1):118.

Samuel D, Ichai P (2010) Prognosis indicator in acute liver failure: Is there a place for cell death markers? *J Hepatol*, **53**(4):593–595.

Shami VM, Caldwell SH, Hespenheide EE, Arseneau KO, Bickston SJ, Macik BG (2003) Recombinant activated factor VII for coagulopathy in fulminant hepatic failure compared with conventional therapy. *Liver Transplant*, **9**(2):138–143.

Shawcross D, Wendon J (2012) The neurological manifestations of acute liver failure. *Neurochem Int*, **60**(7):662–671.

Singer AL, Olthoff KM, Kim H, Rand E, Zamir G, Shaked A (2001) Role of plasmapheresis in the management of acute hepatic failure in children. *Annal Surg*, **234**(3):418–424.

Sort P, Navasa M, Arroyo V, et al. (1999) Effect of intravenous albumin on renal impairment and mortality in patients with cirrhosis and spontaneous bacterial peritonitis. *N Engl J Med*, **341**(6):403–409.

Steadman RH, Van Rensburg A, Kramer DJ (2010) Transplantation for acute liver failure: perioperative management. *Curr Opin Organ Transplant*, **15**:368–373.

Stravitz R (2008) Critical management decisions in patients with acute liver failure. *Chest*, **134**(5):1092–1102.

Stravitz R, Kramer D (2009) Management of acute liver failure. *Nat Rev Gastroenterol Hepatol*, **6**(9):542–553.

Stravitz RT, Larsen FS (2009) Therapeutic hypothermia for acute liver failure. *Crit Care Med*, **37**:S258–S264.

Stravitz RT, Kramer AH, Davern T, et al. (2007) Intensive care of patients with acute liver failure: recommendations of the U.S. Acute Liver Failure Study Group. *Crit Care Med*, **35**(11):2498–2508.

Thuluvath PJ, Yoo HY, Thompson RE (2003) A model to predict survival at one month, one year, and five years after liver transplantation based on pretransplant clinical characteristics. *Liver Transplant*, **9**:527–532.

Tofteng F, Larsen F (2004) The effect of indomethacin on intracranial pressure, cerebral perfusion and extracellular lactate and glutamate concentrations in patients with fulminant hepatic failure. *J Cerebr Blood Flow Metab*, **24**(7)798–804.

Tripodi A, Mannucci PM (2011) The coagulopathy of chronic liver disease. *N Engl J Med*, **365**:147–156.

Trotter J (2009) Practical management of acute liver failure in the intensive care unit. *Curr Opin Crit Care*, **15**(2):163–167.

Uriz J, Ginès P, Cárdenas A, et al. (2000) Terlipressin plus albumin infusion: an effective and safe therapy of hepatorenal syndrome. *J Hepatol*, **33**(1):43–48.

Vaquero J, Polson J, Chung C, et al. (2003) Infection and the progression of hepatic encephalopathy in acute liver failure. *Gastroenterology*, **125**(3):755–764.

Wijdicks EF, Plevak DJ, Rakela J, Wiesner RH (1995) Clinical and radiologic features of cerebral edema in fulminant hepatic failure. *Mayo Clinic Proc*, **70**:119–124.

Wong F (2009) Cirrhotic cardiomyopathy. *Hepatol Int*, **3**(1):294–304.

# CHAPTER 22

# Liver transplantation: anaesthesia and perioperative care

John R. Klinck and Andre De Wolf

## Preoperative evaluation and management (pathophysiology and relevant comorbidity)

A detailed description of the pathophysiology of severe liver disease is presented in Chapter 19. This chapter begins with an overview of the physiological alterations and co-morbid conditions that are most relevant to management in the perioperative period.

Chronic liver disease causes many systemic abnormalities, including portal hypertension, impaired hepatic synthetic function, ascites, hepatic hydrothorax, hyperdynamic circulatory syndrome, cirrhotic cardiomyopathy, peripheral and pulmonary microvascular shunting, hepatorenal syndrome, hepatic encephalopathy, PPHTN, electrolyte abnormalities, and malnutrition. Life-threatening complications are common, including variceal haemorrhage and sepsis from bacterial peritonitis or pneumonia. ESLD eventually results in circulatory collapse with end-organ failure (Henriksen and Møller, 2009). Relevant pathophysiological disturbances and their management in the perioperative period are summarized in Table 22.1. Although some interventions may improve quality of life and/or improve short-term outcome to some degree, only liver transplantation is a viable option in severe liver disease.

Liver cirrhosis results in portal hypertension and when associated with hypoalbuminaemia leads to severe ascites and hepatic hydrothorax. Sodium restriction and diuretic therapy are usually effective, but some patients need regular paracenteses with infusions of albumin for relief of shortness of breath and abdominal discomfort (Møller et al., 2009). Varices are managed with sclerotherapy or ligation, non-selective beta-blockers such as propranolol, or interventions to reduce portal pressure (distal splenorenal shunt, TIPS) (Garcia-Tsao and Bosch, 2010). Treatment of acutely bleeding varices includes variceal ligation, vasopressin, somatostatin, or a Sengstaken–Blakemore tube.

Coagulation defects caused by reduced concentrations of vitamin K-dependent clotting proteins are well documented. However, liver disease has complex effects on haemostasis and on the balance between pro- and antihaemostatic processes (see Figure 22.1), and the traditional coagulations tests do not predict bleeding. PT or INR, APTT, and platelet count all highlight procoagulant functions, while the effects of anticoagulant proteins, such as protein C and antithrombin, are not measured. Similarly, although platelet numbers and function may be reduced, high levels of factor VIII and vWF in cirrhosis may compensate. The fibrinolytic system is also affected, as both pro- and antifibrinolytic factors may be decreased in cirrhosis. The net effect of these imbalances is unpredictable and sensitivity of the coagulation system to factors promoting both bleeding and thrombosis is probably increased (Warnaar et al., 2008). Routine preoperative administration of FFP, platelets, and other products is disputed because such interventions increase portal and systemic venous pressure and may increase bleeding (Massicotte et al., 2008). Treatment may be better based on clinical findings, such as bleeding from puncture sites, an oozy operative field, or the absence of clots in pooled blood in the surgical wound.

Anaemia is common, from impaired haematopoiesis, gastrointestinal bleeding, hypersplenism, or malnutrition (Gonzalez-Casas et al., 2009). Varices should be treated and iron deficiency corrected, but transfusion is only indicated for active bleeding or in the presence of symptoms clearly caused by low haemoglobin.

Hyponatraemia may be caused by diuretic therapy, secondary hyperaldosteronism, increased release of antidiuretic hormone, and other, still uncharacterized renal abnormalities (Ginès and Guevara, 2008). Low serum sodium concentration predicts worse outcomes, with or without transplant. Because of the risk of a rapid rise in sodium concentration during liver transplantation, from use of blood products or sodium bicarbonate, many but not all units suspend patients from the transplant waiting list when values fall below 122–125 mmol/L and attempt correction. Correction is not always possible, however, and with longer waiting times and lower operative blood losses the risk of disequilibrium myelinolysis may now be lower than that of dying on the waiting list. Patients with sodium < 122 mmol/L are considered on an individual basis according to the risks of major operative blood loss. Factors such as anaemia, retransplant, portal vein thrombosis, and ECD may favour deferral in the patient with plasma sodium below this threshold.

Preoperative hyperkalaemia is uncommon but should be treated aggressively, since fatal intraoperative hyperkalaemic arrest, usually at reperfusion of the liver, still occurs. It may be associated with renal failure, treatment with spironolactone, or transfusion. Preoperative values > 5.5 mmol/L should be treated with haemofiltration (Meltzer and Brentjens, 2010). Some continue haemofiltration into the intraoperative phase if it does not fall to < 5.0; others prefer treatment with insulin (De Wolf et al., 1993b).

Renal impairment develops easily because of underlying circulatory and hormonal disturbances. Hepatorenal syndrome, a

**Table 22.1** Pathophysiology of ESLD and perioperative management of the liver recipient

| System | Disorder | Perioperative management |
|---|---|---|
| Cardiovascular: cardiac function, systemic and splanchnic circulations | ◆ Increased ejection fraction and cardiac output, often with impaired diastolic function and contractile response to increased afterload<br>◆ Increased chamber sizes<br>◆ Prolonged QTc<br>◆ Cardiomyopathy (esp. alcohol, amyloid, Wilson's, haemochromatosis)<br>◆ Increased splanchnic blood volume +/− flow<br>◆ Reduced systemic blood volume +/− flow<br>◆ Activation of compensatory responses (SNS, RAAS, endothelin)<br>◆ Intrahepatic vasoconstriction aggravates portal hypertension and varices<br>◆ Autonomic neuropathy (mild in cirrhosis, marked in amyloid) | ◆ PA catheter and/or transoesophageal echo<br>◆ Balance preload + vasoconstrictors (vasopressin, terlipressin, or norepinephrine)<br>◆ If renal or cardiac dysfunction, consider caval preservation technique or venovenous bypass<br>◆ Pacing wire if amyloid polyneuropathy |
| Cardiovascular: pulmonary circulation | ◆ PPHTN: PA mean > 25 mm Hg, PVR > 250 dyn/s/cm$^{-5}$<br>◆ HPS: hypoxaemia from pulmonary micro- or macrovascular shunting | ◆ PPHTN: preop right heart catheter if Doppler PAsystolic > 40 mm Hg (to differentiate from high-flow state/overload); defer transplant and treat if PA mean > 35 mm Hg (and PVR raised) or RV impaired; intraoperative PA catheter +/− TEE essential if pulmonary hypertension suspected<br>◆ HPS: bubble echo to exclude atrial shunt, chest CT to exclude other causes and treatable macrovascular lesion; increase $FiO_2$; 'lung-protective' ventilation (see below) |
| Respiratory | ◆ Restrictive defect (ascites and/or hydrothorax)<br>◆ Flow-related or anatomical intrapulmonary shunting (HPS)<br>◆ Non-cardiogenic pulmonary oedema (fulminant hepatic failure)<br>◆ Obstructive airways disease (esp. cystic fibrosis, alpha-1 antitrypsin deficiency)<br>◆ Interstitial lung disease (primary biliary cirrhosis) | ◆ $FiO_2$ >= 0.5, 'lung-protective' ventilation (tidal volume 6–8 mL/kg, PEEP 4–6 cm $H_2O$, regular recruitment manoeuvres<br>◆ Drain large effusion early intraop (beware re-expansion pulmonary oedema, especially at reperfusion) |
| Renal | ◆ HRS (prerenal failure from neuroendocrine activation: splanchnic 'steal')<br>◆ Acute tubular necrosis from sepsis, hypovolaemia<br>◆ Tacrolimus/ciclosporin-related renal impairment<br>◆ Renal tubular acidosis | ◆ Preoperative renal replacement therapy if $K^+ > 5.5$; stand-by otherwise<br>◆ Maintain arterial pressure: adequate volume plus norepinephrine, vasopressin, or terlipressin<br>◆ Maintain haemoglobin > 9 g/L (haematocrit > 27)<br>◆ Caval preservation technique or venovenous bypass |
| Electrolytes/metabolic | ◆ Hyponatraemia<br>◆ Hypomagnesaemia<br>◆ Hyperkalaemia<br>◆ Metabolic acidosis<br>◆ Hypoglycaemia in fulminant liver failure<br>◆ Hyperglycaemia and insulin resistance common after reperfusion | ◆ Defer transplant if high surgical risk *and* Na < 122<br>◆ Treat hyperkalaemia if pre-anhepatic > 5.0 or rapid anhepatic rise<br>◆ Wash bank blood using red cell salvage device if pre-existing renal failure or $K^+ > 5.0$<br>◆ $MgSO_4$ if any arrhythmia<br>◆ Consider THAM; intraoperative haemodiafiltration if acidosis severe<br>◆ Close monitoring and treatment of hypo-/hyperglycaemia |

*(Continued)*

**Table 22.1** Continued

| System | Disorder | Perioperative management |
|---|---|---|
| Haematological/coagulation | ◆ Anaemia, thrombocytopaenia, leucopaenia (hypersplenism and marrow depression)<br>◆ Impaired vitamin K absorption<br>◆ Reduced liver synthesis of clotting factors<br>◆ Hyperfibrinolysis<br>◆ Reduced synthesis of anticoagulants (proteins C and S, antithrombin) and reduced clearance pro-coagulants (extrahepatic Factor VIII and vWF) often preserve haemostasis and may cause pathological thrombosis | ◆ Consider prophylactic tranexamic acid or EACA if high bleeding risk and no prothrombotic history<br>◆ Assess coagulation clinically before treatment (cannulation sites, surgical field)<br>◆ Treat clinical coagulopathy according to thromboelastography and laboratory data (plasma, platelets, cryoprecipitate, factor concentrates, antifibrinolytic)<br>◆ Maintain normothermia<br>◆ If loss > 2 blood volumes, consult haematologist and activate massive transfusion protocol |
| Central nervous system | ◆ Encephalopathy<br>◆ Cerebral oedema with intracranial hypertension | ◆ Avoid/minimize benzodiazepines<br>◆ In fulminant liver failure with grade III/IV encephalopathy consider ICP monitoring; maintain cerebral perfusion pressure > 60 mm Hg (norepinephrine) +/– mannitol/hypertonic saline/ thiopental to control ICP |

SNS, Sympathetic nervous system; RAAS, renin–angiotensin–aldosterone system; EACA, ε-aminocaproic acid.

form of prerenal failure occurring in the absence of clinical hypovolaemia or intrinsic renal disease, is also common. This may respond to vasopressor treatment combined with volume loading and resolves after transplantation. However, renal impairment is a strong predictor of both pre- and postoperative sepsis and mortality (Guevara and Arroyo, 2011).

Cardiovascular function in liver failure is characterized by a disturbance of microcirculatory function causing arteriovenous shunting, increased cardiac output, and abnormal blood volume distribution, in proportion to the severity of the underlying hepatic disease. There is marked splanchnic vasodilatation resulting in increased splanchnic blood flow. On the other hand, there is vasoconstriction of other vascular beds, especially in the kidneys, leading to decreased renal perfusion. Central blood volume is reduced, inducing increased sympathetic and hormonal vasoconstrictor activity (Henriksen and Møller, 2009). Both reduced renal perfusion and hormonal changes result in renal dysfunction with water and salt retention. Subtle functional and structural changes occur in the heart, now described as cirrhotic cardiomyopathy. These include impaired responses to increases in preload and afterload and conduction abnormalities. Left atrial enlargement, mild left ventricular hypertrophy, and diastolic dysfunction are common findings on resting echocardiography (Møller and Henriksen, 2010). New, sophisticated methods to diagnose cirrhotic cardiomyopathy based on detection of diastolic dysfunction, including tissue Doppler-estimated mitral valvular velocity and left atrial volume measurements, may better predict complications such as post-transplant cardiac failure (Dowsley et al., 2012).

Liver transplantation is a major challenge to the cardiovascular system: severe changes in preload, fluctuating afterload, prolonged episodes of tachycardia and hypotension, and hyperkalaemic events all increase the possibility of severe cardiac dysfunction and perioperative myocardial infarction. Any evidence of significant cardiac disease must be taken seriously in view of the major insults imposed during and after surgery.

The incidence of ischaemic heart disease (IHD) in patients with liver disease is now known to be as high as in the general population and is likely to be higher in patients with non-alcoholic fatty liver disease (Bhatia et al., 2012). In addition, the proportion of liver transplant candidates over 55 years old is increasing and screening for IHD is extremely important. Good exercise tolerance is reassuring, but many patients with ESLD are unable to exercise due to gross ascites or hydrothorax, lethargy, encephalopathy, or muscle wasting. Therefore screening is based on the presence of risk factors for IHD, including age > 55, diabetes, hypertension, smoking, and obesity.

The most commonly used screening tests are DSE and myocardial perfusion scintigraphy. Most centres prefer DSE because, unlike radionuclide perfusion imaging, it provides information on overall left ventricular function and regional wall motion, valvular function, asymmetrical septal hypertrophy, pericardial effusion, pulmonary hypertension, and HPS. However, in some patients the target heart rate is not achieved, reducing its sensitivity as a screening tool. While DSE has an acceptable positive predictive value for IHD (~ 35%), it has a very good negative predictive value (~ 88%): a negative DSE is highly predictive of absence of IHD (Ehtisham et al., 2010). When the screening test suggests the presence of IHD or when the patient has symptoms compatible with IHD, coronary angiography is indicated, despite the potential for renal dysfunction caused by the angiography dye. While coronary angiography identifies the extent and severity of obstructive lesions and the potential for revascularization, it has its own limitations. It may not identify areas of at-risk myocardium that only become apparent under stress and it cannot characterize obstructive plaques in terms of their risk of rupture. CT angiography may prove more sensitive to the latter, but its value at this moment is unclear.

Outcome after liver transplantation in patients with IHD has improved over the years. In the 1990s the reported 3-year post-transplant mortality was about 50%, even with aggressive preoperative investigation and management (Plotkin et al., 1996).

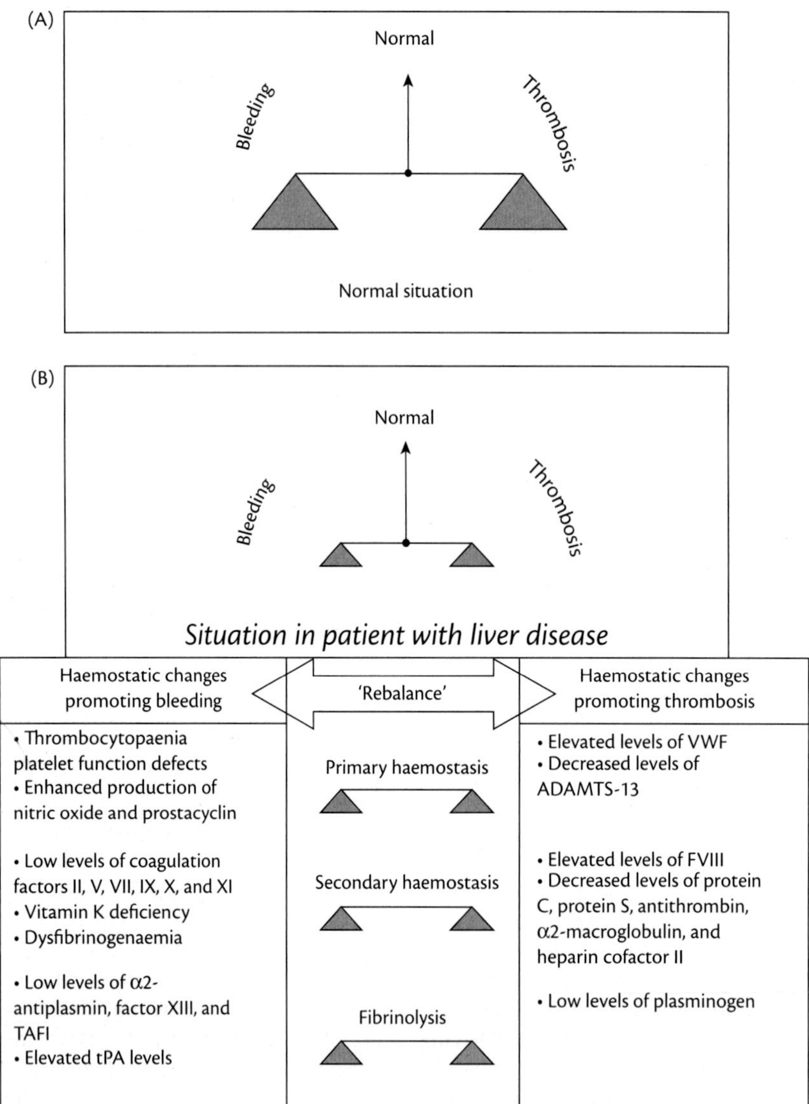


**Fig. 22.1** Coagulation changes in liver disease. TAFI, Thrombin activatable fibrinolysis inhibitor; tPA, tissue-type plasminogen activator; VWF, von Willebrand factor; ADAMTS-13, a disintegrin-like and metalloproteinase with thrombospondin type-1 motif, member 13; FVIII, factor VIII. (Reproduced with permission from Lippincott Williams and Wilkins/Wolters Kluwer Health: *Current Opinion in Organ Transplantation*, Warnaar N et al., 'The two tales of coagulation in liver transplantation', 13, 3, pp. 298–303, 2008.)

Diedrich et al. in 2008 reported a 26% 3-year mortality. A recent multicentre study by Wray et al. (2013) revealed that appropriately treated coronary artery disease resulted in only slightly worse outcomes after liver transplantation, although it remains unclear what 'appropriately treated' means, since 47% of their patients with moderate and severe coronary artery disease did not receive coronary intervention before liver transplantation.

Patients with myocardium at risk should undergo revascularization (stent or coronary artery bypass graft). Since outcomes after on-pump coronary artery bypass grafting in patients with severe liver disease are poor, usually as a result of severe bleeding or multi-organ failure, other options should be considered (Filsoufi et al., 2007). These include stent placement, off-pump bypass grafting, and simultaneous coronary artery bypass grafting and liver transplantation (Axelrod et al., 2004; Ben Ari et al., 2006). Management is influenced by the severity of coronary artery disease and willingness of the cardiac surgery team to participate in a combined procedure whenever a graft becomes available.

Overt cardiomyopathy, usually defined as a left ventricular ejection fraction < 40–45%, is generally considered to be a contraindication to liver transplantation, although there are no data to support or refute this. Left ventricular dysfunction is believed to reduce the chance of surviving liver transplantation, as it does in other settings. Survivors of the perioperative period may still be at risk of progressive biventricular failure and graft loss, as afterload gradually increases after a successful transplant. Alcoholic cirrhosis, amyloidosis, Wilson's disease, and IHD may cause cardiomyopathy.

Although no outcome data are available for severe aortic or mitral stenosis, it is likely to be poor in these patients. Like IHD, valvular aortic stenosis is increasingly common in older patients referred for liver transplantation and remains an important cause of perioperative death in all major surgery. A peak Doppler gradient < 40 mm Hg is usually benign, providing left ventricular function is normal, but higher values should be assessed by exercise testing and/or left heart catheterization. A mean gradient > 50 mm Hg, valve area < 1 $cm^2$, or left ventricular dysfunction contraindicate transplant without prior or simultaneous valve replacement. Mild functional mitral, tricuspid, and aortic regurgitation are frequently found on echocardiography but are usually attributable to the hyperdynamic state and do not appear to predict adverse outcomes.

The hyperdynamic circulation of ESLD makes patients with hypertrophic obstructive cardiomyopathy susceptible to left ventricular outflow tract obstruction. This may vary from mild asymmetric hypertrophy to severe dynamic obstruction involving systolic anterior motion (SAM) of the anterior leaflet of the mitral valve. Although not a contraindication to liver transplantation, it requires meticulous intraoperative monitoring and management and should be fully evaluated and treated by a cardiologist preoperatively. Treatment with a beta-blocker may reduce the gradient significantly, but if outflow tract obstruction is symptomatic, further intervention should be considered, including sequential pacing, myomectomy, and alcohol ablation (Cywinski et al., 2005).

Pulmonary hypertension, defined as mean pulmonary artery pressure (mPAP) > 25 mm Hg, is seen in up to 20% of adult liver transplant candidates. In most cases this is caused by volume overload and/or diastolic left heart dysfunction with normal PVR. In ≤ 6% of patients the cause is an abnormal pulmonary vasculature, including medial hypertrophy and plexiform arteriopathy, resulting in increased PVR and 'true' PPHTN (Ramsay, 2010). Screening is performed by Doppler echocardiography, estimating right ventricular systolic pressure from the peak velocity of the tricuspid regurgitant jet. Estimated pressures > 45–50 mm Hg require confirmation with right heart catheterization. Mild elevation of pulmonary artery pressures (mPAP 25–35 mm Hg) is usually well tolerated, but moderate PPHTN (mPAP 35–45 mm Hg) has a reported 50% perioperative mortality. Severe PPHTN (mPAP > 45 mm Hg) results in a mortality rate approaching 100%, especially if associated with right ventricular dysfunction. Effective treatments include prostenoids, endothelin-1 inhibitors, and phosphodiesterase-5 inhibitors, and these appear to reduce perioperative risk if mPAP can be reduced. Candidacy for liver transplantation is determined by not only the degree of PPHTN but also right ventricular function and the presence of comorbidities (for example, coronary artery disease, especially of the right coronary artery). In most patients, pulmonary hypertension resolves after liver transplantation, although in some it may persist in a stable form for years. Rarely it progresses despite treatment.

HPS is characterized by hypoxaemia associated with intrapulmonary vascular dilatations in the presence of liver disease (Rodriguez-Roisin and Krowka, 2008). Because vascular shunting is gravity-dependent and the largest shunts are in the bases of the lungs, hypoxaemia and dyspnoea are worse in the standing position (orthodeoxia and platypnoea, respectively). For diagnosis, intrinsic pulmonary disease must be absent or too mild to account for the observed signs and symptoms. Hypoxaemia is considered to be the result of a perfusion–diffusion defect (type I—dilated capillaries) or true right to left shunt (type II—dilated arterioles). Contrast-enhanced echocardiography documents the presence of intrapulmonary dilatations and also serves to exclude a right-to-left shunt at the atrial level as the cause of hypoxaemia. Type I HPS is very responsive to high concentrations of inspired oxygen, while type II is not. A preoperative $PaO_2$ < 50 mm Hg has been associated with increased 90-day mortality, although this is not prohibitive. Some centres, with intensive specialist respiratory input, have obtained very good results even with severely hypoxaemic patients (Gupta et al., 2010). Although intraoperative problems with oxygenation are rarely observed, weaning from mechanical ventilation may be prolonged and these patients are more vulnerable to sepsis and other post-transplant complications.

Obstructive airways disease, usually related to smoking but occasionally to familial emphysema or alpha-1 antitrypsin deficiency, is seen in up to 18% of adults presenting for liver transplant (Krowka, 2011). Recurrent chest infections may be a feature, but history and clinical signs are often minimal. Flow-volume measurements show an obstructive pattern, often mixed with the restriction of vital capacity seen in the presence of severe ascites. There are no data on the effect of obstructive lung disease on liver transplant outcome. Forced expiratory volumes (FEV1) as low as 30% of predicted are associated with good outcomes in young recipients with cystic fibrosis, but in older patients values below 40–50% in the absence of pleural effusion or ascites require a cautious approach.

Other causes of respiratory impairment include ascites and ascitic hydrothorax, poorly controlled asthma, aspiration, and pulmonary infection. Primary biliary cirrhosis is occasionally associated with interstitial lung disease, which causes disproportionate dyspnoea and a restrictive defect on pulmonary function testing.

Nutritional impairment and sarcopaenia are severe in up to 30% of patients, resulting from anorexia, malabsorption, impaired protein synthesis, and chronic catabolism. Nutritional reserve is further depleted by accelerated catabolism during infection and surgery (Periyalwar and Dasarathy, 2012). Poorer outcomes are seen in low body mass index (BMI) patients and most centres would not list at BMI < 15. BMIs above this value but with low measured nutritional indices (e.g. grip strength, triceps skin-fold thickness, mid–upper arm circumference < 5th percentile) are common but not regarded as contraindications to transplant. BMI < 18.5 associated with other major comorbidities would be regarded as potentially prohibitive. Calorie, protein, and vitamin supplementation is routinely pursued.

Morbid obesity (BMI > 35) is increasingly common in patients presenting for liver transplantation. It may affect ICU length-of-stay and long-term outcomes but is not regarded as prohibitive in most centres. An abdominal ('apple-shaped') pattern of obesity affects surgical access, perioperative respiratory parameters, and ventilator weaning much more than a pelvic ('pear-shaped') pattern, although this has not been formally investigated. Marked abdominal obesity (BMI > 40) in the presence of one or more major comorbidities would contraindicate transplant in many units (Thuluvath, 2007).

Special problems are encountered in patients with multiorgan dysfunction caused by acute liver failure, primary non-function of a liver graft, or terminal decompensation in chronic liver failure. These patients usually have severe coagulopathy and encephalopathy. Non-cardiogenic pulmonary oedema, renal insufficiency, and/or sepsis may also be present. Raised intracranial pressure is common in fulminant hepatic failure with encephalopathy and may progress to fatal brainstem compression if untreated. Intracranial pressure monitoring is advocated in this setting, although fatal haemorrhagic complications occasionally occur and no consensus on the balance of risks has emerged. Paralysis, ventilation, and 30° head-up tilt are essential, supplemented by mannitol and pentobarbital if needed. Moderate hypothermia is now used in many units to control severe intracranial hypertension. Continuous venovenous haemofiltration may be needed to correct hyperkalaemia and control metabolic acidosis.

Although there are well-recognized indications for liver transplantation in acute liver failure, these tend to be cautious, favouring transplant at the risk of performing this in some patients who might have recovered spontaneously. At the opposite end of the scale of severity, however, there are no data to help identify patients in whom transplant is futile: those who are likely to die or sustain permanent neurological injury even if transplanted. The following criteria have been suggested to preclude liver transplantation: severe intracranial hypertension (CPP < 40 mm Hg for > 2 hours); tonsillar herniation (fixed dilated pupils and CT evidence); cardiorespiratory failure, with norepinephrine infusion > 1 mcg/kg/min, $FiO_2$ > 0.60, PEEP > 12 cm $H_2O$, mPAP > 40 mm Hg; and bedbound > 10 days (Steadman et al., 2010).

Sepsis may complicate acute or chronic hepatic failure. In fulminant liver failure it may be difficult to diagnose, as many of its clinical manifestations are mimicked in terminal hepatic decompensation. However, fever, hypotension, and dependence on vasopressors clearly suggest its presence and the risks of proceeding with transplantation at this stage may be prohibitive. In chronic liver failure, sepsis is a frequent terminal event, usually associated with bacterial peritonitis, pneumonia, or urinary infection. Transplant is contraindicated if there is decompensation with vasopressor dependency and organ failure at the time of the offer. However, in many units, 24–48 hours of appropriate antimicrobial treatment of a known site of infection, with a favourable response to treatment, would allow consideration for transplant.

## Surgical techniques and procedures

Major cardiovascular and biochemical changes are directly related to operative events. The procedure consists of three main phases: dissection, the anhepatic phase, and reperfusion/postreperfusion.

First is the dissection phase, during which the liver and its vessels are isolated from the surrounding tissues. Venous collaterals in the abdominal wall and mesentery may be extensive and will bleed heavily during this stage unless careful attention is paid to surgical haemostasis. After initial exposure of the liver, the structures of the porta hepatis are isolated and the bile duct and hepatic artery divided. Following this, either the plane separating the liver from the anterior wall of the vena cava or the posterior wall of the retrohepatic vena cava itself is carefully dissected (see below). Adhesions from any chronic inflammatory processes involving the liver, previous peritonitis, upper abdominal surgery, or a previous liver transplant may cause major technical problems and substantially increase blood loss. A migrated TIPS also adds to the difficulty of dissection: if the proximal shunt tip is high in the inferior vena cava, there may be the need for supradiaphragmatic dissection; if the distal shunt tip is in the extrahepatic portal vein, there may be the need for peripancreatic dissection. This initial phase of the procedure varies in length (about 1–6 hours). The risk of rapid bleeding is greatest during its final stages, when dissection around the upper retrohepatic vena cava and hepatic veins may be particularly challenging. In some centres, a temporary mesocaval shunt is inserted before clamping of the portal vein, to decompress the portal circulation once the portal vein is clamped.

Following mobilization of the liver, clamps are placed on the portal vein and inferior vena cava. This begins the anhepatic phase. In the *'classical' or caval replacement technique* (see Figures 22.2 and 22.3), the inferior vena cava is clamped both at the level of the diaphragm and above the renal veins. The diseased liver is then removed along with the hepatic veins and retrohepatic length of the vena cava. Anastomoses of the suprahepatic cava, portal vein, and infrahepatic cava are performed. Before completing the caval anastomosis, the graft is flushed with colloid or saline through a cannula in the portal vein to wash out storage perfusate and entrained air, which escape via the incomplete lower caval anastomosis. After flushing and completion of the anastomoses, both caval clamps are released, followed by unclamping of the portal vein. Blood flow to the donor liver is thereby restored.

An alternative approach, the *'piggyback' or caval preservation technique* (see Figure 22.4), leaves the recipient vena cava intact. Although this avoids a full mobilization of the cava, it requires a dissection of the plane between the liver and anterior wall of the cava, which can be more difficult than posterior caval dissection because of dense adhesions caused by direct contact with a chronically inflamed liver. After this dissection the vena cava is side-clamped at the level of the hepatic veins while the donor hepatic veins–vena cava confluence is anastomosed to it, preserving some caval blood flow during the anhepatic phase. A variant of this technique involves creation of a large side-to-side anastomosis between the donor vena cava and the recipient's (*cava-cavaplasty*,

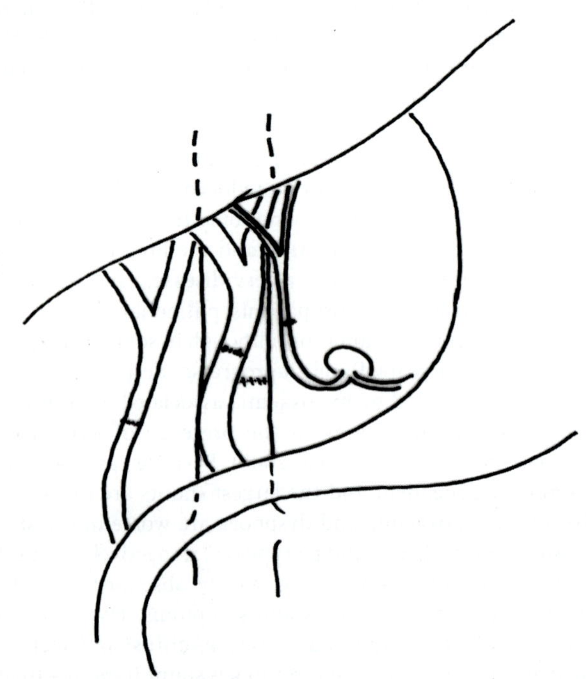

**Fig. 22.2** Anterior view of classical liver transplant anastomoses, including infrahepatic inferior vena cava, portal vein, hepatic artery, and common bile duct

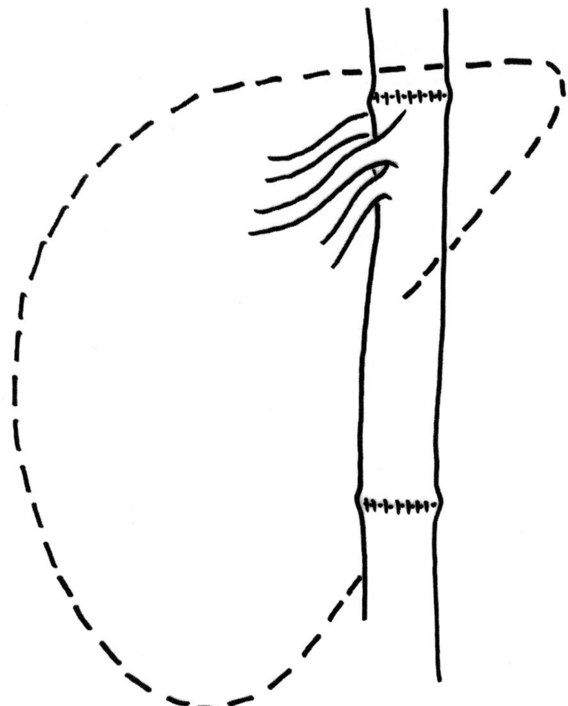

**Fig. 22.3** Lateral view of classical (caval replacement) technique of hepatic venous drainage

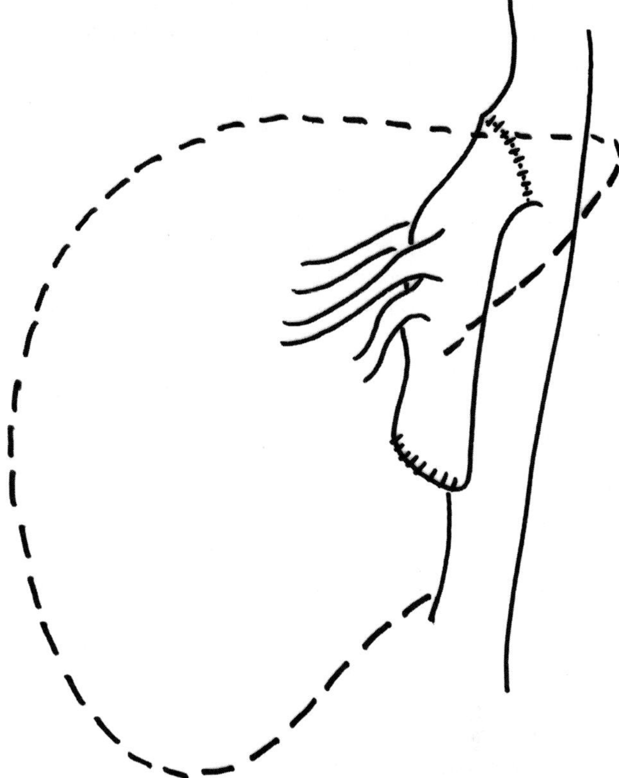

**Fig. 22.4** Lateral view of 'piggyback' caval preservation technique, with end-to-side caval anastomosis

see Figure 22.5). After flushing of the graft (performed as above), the caval side-clamp is removed, followed by unclamping of the portal vein. Lobar implants from living donors are done similarly, without resection of the recipient cava. Restoration of portal blood flow to the liver marks the beginning of the reperfusion phase of the operation. This may be associated with haemodynamic instability, bleeding, or both.

Once the patient is stabilized and any bleeding controlled, the hepatic artery and biliary anastomoses are performed. Arterial reperfusion usually occurs without haemodynamic implications, although side clamping of the aorta is sometimes needed for creation of an arterial conduit. A conduit (iliac artery graft) may be used to take flow directly from the aorta when the standard hepatic-to-hepatic arterial anastomosis appears inadequate. Biliary drainage may be accomplished by a donor–recipient end-to-end anastomosis or by a Roux-en-Y choledochojejunostomy, depending on the recipient's biliary anatomy.

Details of surgical technique vary between centres, particularly in the unclamping sequence of the vascular anastomoses and the use of venovenous bypass (see below) and of a temporary portocaval shunt to decompress the portal circulation during the anhepatic phase. Duration of surgery also varies widely, from 4 to > 12 hours depending on the patient and surgical technique.

*Venovenous bypass* (see Figure 22.6) is a pumped extracorporeal shunt taking blood from the femoral and (in some units) portal vein to the axillary or internal jugular vein, intended to decompress the portal system and maintain venous return during the anhepatic phase (Shaw et al., 1984). Heparin-bonded tubing and non-occlusive pumps allow its use without systemic heparinization. Use of bypass has declined as the caval preservation (piggyback) technique has become more widespread and because many centres have demonstrated good results without it. It is now used selectively in most liver transplant programmes and in some units never (Reddy et al., 2005).

Advocates of bypass cite physiological advantages during the final stages of dissection and during the anhepatic period, at least

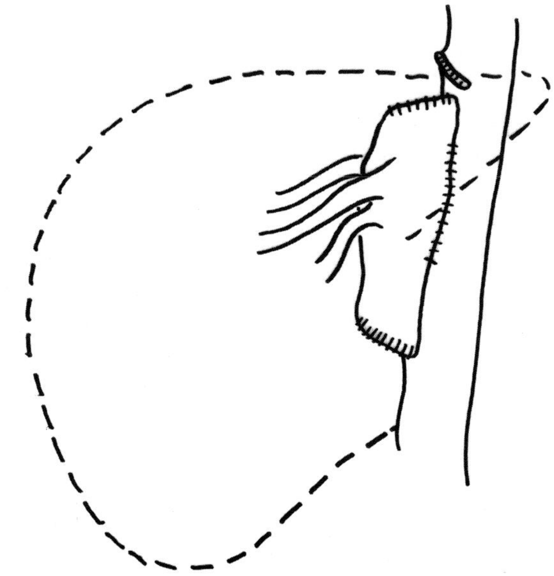

**Fig. 22.5** Lateral view of cava-cavaplasty, an alternative caval preservation technique using side-to-side caval anastomosis

when the implantation technique involves full clamping of the cava. These include decompression of the portal, lower caval, and renal venous systems and better maintenance of cardiac output, thus preserving splanchnic and renal blood flow. Haemodynamic stability and acid-base balance are improved, and control of surgical bleeding is easier since venous pressure in portosystemic collaterals is reduced. However, evidence that bypass improves results is lacking and a comprehensive evaluation of its complications has yet to be published.

The most serious hazards of bypass are perforation of central vessels during insertion of large-bore percutaneous catheters, and embolization of air or thrombus, all of which have caused fatalities. Body temperature decreases during bypass unless a heat exchanger is used, which may carry an added risk of thromboembolism. Local complications at access sites also occur, including nerve injury, haematoma, lymphocele, and infection. Most units now reserve the technique for patients most likely to gain from its use. Indications may include severe cardiac impairment and vasopressor-dependency, and hypotension on trial clamping of the cava.

*Living-donor liver transplantation* originated from the urgent need of grafts for paediatric recipients. A left lateral segment is resected in the donor and transplanted into the paediatric recipient (Strong et al., 1990). A larger graft is needed for adult recipients, but resection of a right lobe is more complicated than a left lateral segmentectomy (Ito et al., 2003). Most donors have mild abnormalities of liver function tests for several days, especially after right lobectomy. Although standard coagulation tests show hypocoagulability (Schumann et al., 2004; Siniscalchi et al, 2004), thromboelastography suggests that coagulation system is normal or even hypercoagulable (Cerutti et al, 2004). Serious postoperative complications, including liver failure, sepsis, and death, are relatively uncommon but devastating (Vastag, 2003; Akabayashi et al., 2004; Miller et al., 2004).

## Anaesthetic management

### Immediate preoperative preparation

Full multisystem assessment should be performed before listing and the patient's condition should be reassessed when a liver becomes available. It is important to exclude untreated infection (e.g. incipient bacterial peritonitis and bronchopneumonia), hyperkalaemia, and severe hyponatraemia. If unusual risks are identified, a discussion between the transplant anaesthesiologist, hepatologist, and surgeon is essential. Although cold ischaemia times should be kept as short as possible, retrieval times and liver preservation techniques typically allow adequate time for reassessment and intervention. The patient's usual proton pump inhibitor should be given, along with antibiotic prophylaxis according to local protocol.

Routine preoperative correction of abnormal coagulation tests (PT, fibrinogen concentration, platelet count) with FFP, fibrinogen, and platelets is no longer recommended unless the patient is actively bleeding or has clinical signs of impaired clotting such as prolonged bleeding from needle-sticks or mucosal abrasions (Massicotte et al., 2008, 2009). Ten units of blood are routinely cross-matched and at least 20 additional group-specific units should be available if needed. Predictors of transfusion requirement include preoperative haemoglobin concentration, renal impairment, and previous transplantation. FFP and platelets must be available irrespective of the preoperative coagulation values, because of the possibility of dilutional or fibrinolytic coagulopathy during surgery.

### Anaesthetic technique

Careful preoxygenation and a rapid sequence induction with propofol and succinylcholine are recommended; if succinylcholine is contraindicated, a modified rapid sequence induction should be used. An orogastric or nasogastric tube and urinary catheter are placed. In our units, anaesthesia is maintained with isoflurane or desflurane in oxygen/air and supplemented with opioids (fentanyl, remifentanil, or sufentanil). The choice of muscle relaxant is arbitrary; most units use atracurium or cis-atracurium. Rocuronium should be avoided because of its hepatic metabolism. If early postoperative extubation is planned, short-acting agents are advocated.

### Vascular access

Large-bore intravenous access is vital. There is a wide choice of cannulae, which may be placed in the arms and/or central veins according to unit preference. A large-bore catheter and a pulmonary artery catheter introducer can both be placed in the right or left internal jugular vein; some prefer to place such catheters under ultrasound guidance. Two 10F cannulae or a single 18F can be used as the return limb of a venovenous bypass circuit (see Figure 22.6). Caution is always advisable when bypass cannulae are used, especially in the left internal jugular vein: large catheters are less flexible and the risk of a venous tear or perforation may be higher. Femoral vessels are not routinely used for volume administration because the vena cava is clamped intraoperatively and because surgical access for venovenous bypass may be required. In some centres the femoral vein is cannulated percutaneously for venovenous bypass and it may also provide a convenient site for a dual-lumen catheter for intraoperative renal replacement therapy. It is prudent always to discuss use of the femoral vessels with the surgical team. Subclavian cannulation has a higher risk of arterial injury, pneumothorax, and haemothorax and in some institutions is avoided or performed only under ultrasound and fluoroscopic guidance in an angiography suite.

### Monitoring

Arterial and central venous pressure monitoring are essential, while pulmonary artery flotation catheters are used routinely in most but not all centres (De Wolf, 2008). Radial artery pressure monitoring may underestimate aortic pressure in hypotensive states, especially when vasopressors are used and after reperfusion (see Figure 22.7); therefore many prefer to use the femoral artery (Arnal et al., 2005; Shin et al., 2007). Pulmonary artery pressures, thermodilation cardiac output, and mixed venous oxygen saturation measurements help in the assessment and management of hypotension, which may arise unpredictably because of changes in venous return, altered systemic vascular resistance, temporary cardiac dysfunction, or embolic events. A pulmonary artery catheter is essential if pulmonary hypertension is present or suspected. Alternative methods to determine cardiac output or oxygen saturation in the superior vena cava are used infrequently because of reduced accuracy (Dahmani et al., 2010; Krejci et al.,

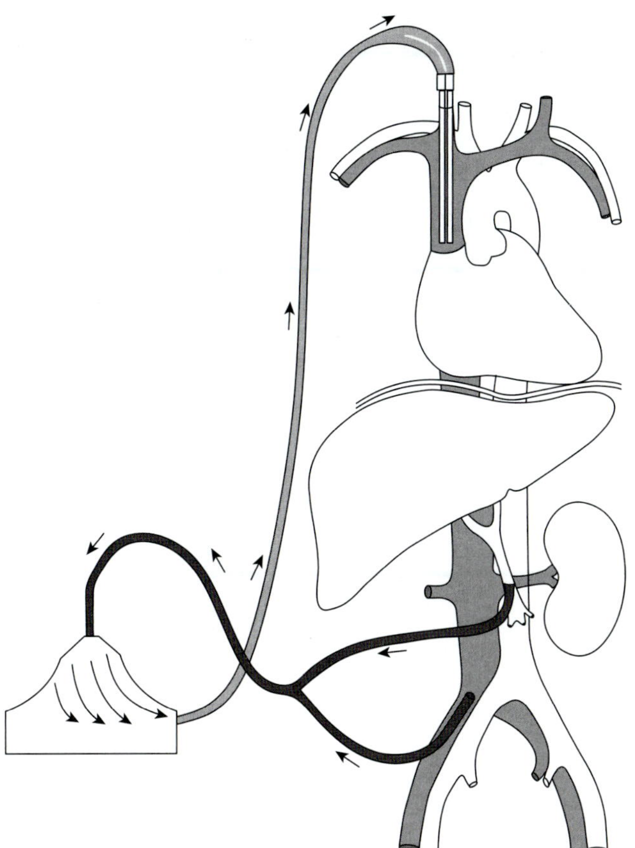

**Fig. 22.6** Venovenous bypass circuit. Outflow is through a femoral venous cannula, with or without a second cannula in the portal or inferior mesenteric vein. Blood is returned via the axillary or internal jugular vein (IJV). In Cambridge, two thin-walled 10F cannulae are placed percutaneously in the right IJV; the femoral cannula may also be placed percutaneously, obviating the need for surgical cutdown. (Reproduced from *Anesthesia and Intensive Care for Organ Transplantation*, Klinck et al., 1998, Figure 13.5, p. 191, with permission.)

2010; Tsai et al., 2012). Modified pulmonary artery catheters allow continuous cardiac output measurements and a volumetric index of preload (right ventricular end-diastolic volume), which provides more valuable information than filling pressures (De Wolf et al., 1993a).

Cardiovascular monitoring is further enhanced by the use of transoesophageal echocardiography, which gives continuous information on ventricular function and volume status and allows the immediate diagnosis of embolization of air or thrombus (De Wolf, 1999). It provides additional information regarding overall contractility, valvular function, and vascular pathology (e.g. migrated portosystemic shunt device) and allows intraoperative diagnosis of pericardial or pleural effusion (Burtenshaw and Isaac, 2006). It is an essential tool in the clinical management of hypertrophic obstructive cardiomyopathy (Cywinski et al., 2005). The risks of this modality appear to be low and the major obstacle to wider use is the significant training requirement and capital cost in units without local cardiac anaesthetic expertise.

Measurement of arterial blood gases, sodium, potassium, glucose, lactate, ionized calcium, and haematocrit should be performed at frequent intervals, at least hourly during the initial and closing phases of the operation and more often if necessary during the anhepatic period. Rapid availability of results is essential, making the availability of quality-assured, multiparameter, point-of-care equipment a standard of care.

Coagulation monitoring practices vary widely. In many centres, routine coagulation screening tests, including PT, PTT, fibrinogen, and platelet count, are supplemented by thromboelastography (TEG) or rotational thromboelastometry (ROTEM®) (Kang, 1995; Roullet et al., 2010). Both TEG and ROTEM assess the viscoelastic properties of whole blood, allowing determination of clot initiation, formation, and stability (Nielsen, 2007). TEG and ROTEM provide prompt global assessment of coagulation function, including hypercoagulability. They also reliably detect fibrinolysis, and targeted sample treatment allows demonstration of heparin effect. Not surprisingly there are only weak relationships between TEG/ROTEM parameters and conventional laboratory coagulation tests, mainly because of the very different nature of these tests. In addition, abnormal results in both conventional and TEG/ROTEM testing are poorly correlated with visually apparent coagulopathy (an oozy surgical field and/or lack of visible clot) and their main value may be to indicate the appropriate treatment when coagulopathy is a clinical problem. Bedside PT monitors are also available but, again, often reflect clinical coagulation poorly in the setting of liver disease.

## Cardiovascular changes

Intraoperative haemodynamic goals include maintenance of an acceptable blood pressure to perfuse the essential organs while keeping the cardiac output elevated, because maldistribution of flow can result in organ hypoperfusion at normal cardiac output values. Preload may be reduced dramatically by surgical bleeding and clamping of major vessels. More subtle changes in cardiac filling occur during the dissection phase by surgical manipulation of the liver and inferior vena cava or by direct compression of the diaphragmatic surface of the heart. Anaesthetic agents and ionized hypocalcaemia will amplify these effects (Marquez et al., 1986).

The responses to clamping of the inferior vena cava for hepatectomy and to unclamping when the grafted liver is reperfused depend on several factors. One important determinant is whether the cava is side-clamped for a piggyback implantation or cross-clamped for the conventional procedure (De Wolf, 1997). During the anhepatic phase, cross-clamping of the cava produces a marked (40–50%) decrease in venous return and cardiac output. Although systemic vascular resistance increases, a decrease in blood pressure is expected (De Wolf et al., 1993a). Fluids should be administered, but there should not be an attempt to reach normovolaemia, since volume overload may occur after graft reperfusion, resulting in congestion of the graft. Therefore to maintain adequate blood pressure vasoconstrictors and/or inotropic agents are frequently required. An inadequate response to these agents or severe hypotension on trial cross-clamping of the inferior vena cava necessitate the initiation of venovenous bypass. When a piggyback technique or venovenous bypass is used the decrease in cardiac output is less (20–30%) and arterial pressure is usually well maintained. However, even bypass and the piggyback technique fall short of maintaining a normal circulatory state and there is a progressive decline in cardiac output during the anhepatic phase, reflected in worsening metabolic acidosis.

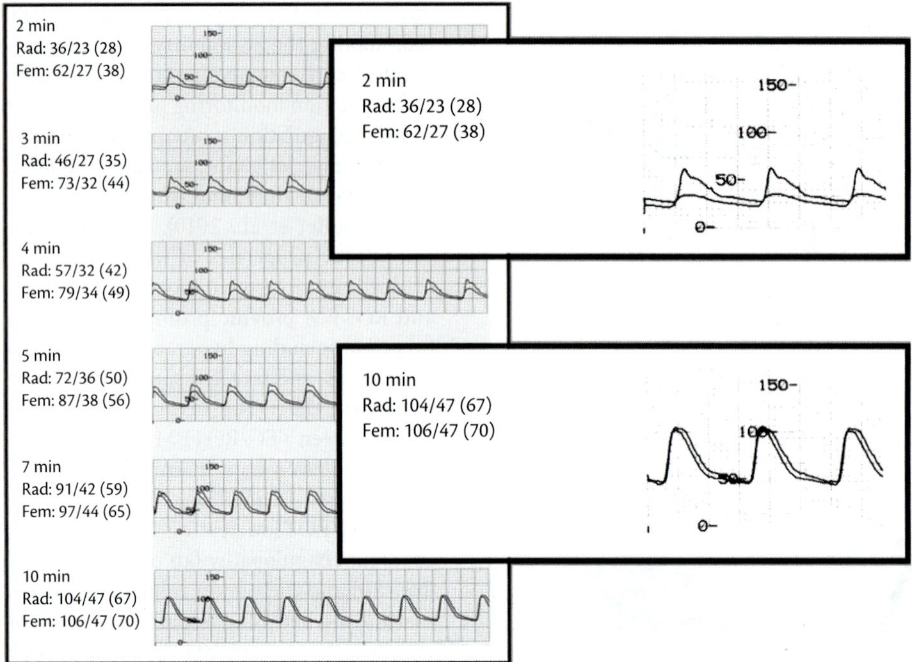


**Fig. 22.7** Printouts showing marked difference between radial and femoral arterial pressures after reperfusion. This may also be observed when vasopressors are used to reduce volume loading during dissection. In the absence of a femoral artery catheter, non-invasive cuff measurements may prevent overtreatment with vasopressor and/or fluid

Unclamping of the vena cava and portal vein results in a range of haemodynamic effects of varying severity. There is a usually significant increase in venous return and cardiac output, tempered by filling of capacitance vessels in the liver. However, significant bleeding from one of the anastomoses may rapidly cause hypovolaemia. Portal vein unclamping allows blood from the splanchnic circulation into the liver, where it mixes with preservation fluid, some of which remains despite routine flushing. On leaving the liver to enter the central circulation, this blood contains high concentrations of potassium, inflammatory mediators, and peptides generated during splanchnic stasis and graft ischaemia and is also cold. Although in some patients the main effect of reperfusion is an increase in blood pressure as a result of increased venous return, it is much more common to observe transient slowing of the heart, arteriolar vasodilatation, and a variable decrease in blood pressure. Blood pressure is usually restored within minutes, aided by bolus vasopressor treatment if necessary, and cardiac output increases above baseline.

In some patients, typically those with a marginal graft or pre-existing vasopressor dependency, reperfusion is associated with severe bradycardia and myocardial depression, sometimes followed by asystole. Bolus epinephrine is very effective in this situation. In others, a poor quality graft may be associated with severe reperfusion hyperkalaemia, rapidly leading to ventricular tachycardia or fibrillation requiring cardioversion or defibrillation. Prophylactic and/or therapeutic administration of calcium chloride, epinephrine, and sodium bicarbonate are advocated as well as treatments to control serum potassium if hyperkalaemia is sustained. Persistent hypotension, associated with a lower than baseline systemic vascular resistance and requiring sustained vasopressor support, is occasionally seen. This is the 'postreperfusion syndrome' and is associated with poorer graft and patient outcomes.

Transient pulmonary hypertension may be seen at reperfusion as central blood volume increases; transpulmonary pressure gradient and PVR remain normal. In patients with pre-existing true PPHTN (mPAP > 25 mm Hg, PVR > 240 dyn.s.cm$^{-5}$, transpulmonary gradient > 15 mm Hg), an exacerbation of PPHTN is common on graft reperfusion and may result in right ventricular failure, especially in those with preoperative mPAP >35 mm Hg (Ramsay, 2010). Monitoring with transoesophageal echocardiography is essential. Administration of potent pulmonary vasodilators (e.g. inhaled nitric oxide, intravenous prostaglandins) is required and is continued in the immediate postoperative period.

## Renal function

Intraoperative changes in renal function are related to marked alterations in cardiac output and renal blood flow. Urine flow is diminished and markers of renal injury raised during caval clamping, when cardiac output is reduced and renal venous pressure acutely raised. This response may be attenuated when venovenous bypass or a piggyback implantation is used. Pre-existing renal impairment, prolonged hypotension, and high transfusion volumes are associated with a high risk of postoperative renal failure. No measures have yet been shown to prevent intraoperative renal injury, although a rationale for the use of low-dose vasopressors including vasopressin and norepinephrine exists, given the pathophysiology of the hepatorenal syndrome. However, concerns about the effects of these on perfusion of the newly implanted liver remain.

## Fluid management, blood replacement, and autotransfusion

Keeping the patient normovolaemic is essential in maintaining haemodynamic stability. Since bleeding during liver transplantation is not usually caused by problems with the major anastomoses but more often by dissection involving portosystemic collateral veins, fluid management, portal hyperaemia, and blood loss may be linked (Massicotte et al., 2006). Patients with cirrhosis and portal hypertension have splanchnic hypervolaemia, which is further exacerbated by volume loading. They also have smaller increases in cardiac output with infusion, so the larger volumes needed to improve systemic perfusion may have a disproportionate effect on portal venous pressure and flow. Aggressive administration of crystalloid and colloid may also have an exaggerated effect on clotting through dilution because concentrations of clotting factors are reduced. The conventional approach of administering blood products pre-emptively and optimizing cardiac output by generous fluid loading has been questioned. Coagulopathy is frequently not as severe as suggested by traditional coagulation tests (Warnaar et al., 2008), while fluid restriction with vasopressor infusion during the dissection and anhepatic phases has been associated with very low blood product use (Massicotte et al., 2008). On the other hand, volume restriction requires liberal use of vasopressors, potentially with adverse effects on systemic and especially renal perfusion. Although some reports suggest this is well tolerated (Schwartz et al., 2001; Massicotte et al., 2010), the optimal approach to volume management remains to be determined.

Fluids that can be administered include packed red blood cells, FFP, crystalloids, and colloids (5% albumin or synthetic colloid). Albumin appears to be safe and has no effects on coagulation apart from dilution but is costly. Gelatin solutions are inexpensive and have been used in high volumes in liver recipients in Europe for many years but are more allergenic. A new hydroxyethyl starch solution (HES 130/0.4) has been reported to be safe in terms of effects on renal function (Mukhtar et al., 2009), but there appear to be some effects on coagulation (Hartog et al., 2011) and a recent randomized study in sepsis has shown increased mortality, so caution is advised (Perner et al., 2012).

Blood product use during liver transplantation has declined over the last 20 years, although there is significant institutional variability (Ozier et al., 2003). The current median red cell requirement is 2–5 units, with a substantial proportion of recipients avoiding blood products altogether. Refinement in surgical techniques, better understanding of haemostasis, and improved anaesthetic management have all contributed to the reduction in transfusion requirements. Autotransfusion techniques are widely used and safe, but effects on coagulation and even on total use of bank blood are still unproven. Cell-salvage is contraindicated in patients with hepatic malignancy and abdominal infections. Although observational studies in patients undergoing resection for hepatic malignancy suggest that long-term outcomes are not worse with cell salvage and cell filtration techniques have been shown to reduce numbers of malignant cells in infusates, many would consider that data are still too limited to support this approach (Liang et al., 2010; Foltys et al., 2011; Kim et al., 2013).

When surgical bleeding occurs, many now accept a transfusion threshold of 7.0 g/dL of haemoglobin (haematocrit about 20–22%). Transfusion at a higher value may be prudent in patients with renal impairment, given the sensitivity of renal oxygen consumption to haemoglobin concentration in experimental models.

## Management of coagulopathy

New concepts in the interpretation of coagulation tests in liver disease, outlined above, should be considered when managing intraoperative coagulation problems (Warnaar et al., 2008). In general, correction of coagulopathy at the start of the liver transplant procedure should not be routine because the resulting increases in portal venous pressure may paradoxically increase blood loss (Massicotte et al., 2008). Rather, correction should be initiated during surgery, once coagulopathy becomes clinically evident or blood loss occurs, and should be guided by coagulation monitoring. Coagulation changes imposed by the procedure include dilution, pathological fibrinolysis, effects of synthetic colloids, and release of heparinoids and inflammatory mediators from the graft. Prophylactic antifibrinolytics (tranexamic acid, ε-aminocaproic acid) are used in some but not all centres (Xia and Steadman, 2005). Fibrinolysis associated with clinical coagulopathy and bleeding can be treated with low doses of ε-aminocaproic acid (250–500 mg); mild fibrinolysis does not necessarily require intervention because it is usually self-limiting. Heparin effect, again in the presence of continuing blood loss, can be treated with low doses of protamine (25–50 mg). Otherwise, platelets, FFP, and cryoprecipitate remain the mainstay of treatment, with frequent assessment of the surgical field to minimize the number of units given. Although data in liver recipients are limited, virally deactivated factor concentrates, including fibrinogen and prothrombin preparations, appear safe and effective and are increasingly used to treat established coagulopathy. Normothermia and a pause in the procedure (after full reperfusion) to allow the liver to recover from surgical handling may also help. Prophylactic administration of recombinant factor VIIa has no beneficial effect on blood loss, but it has been used to correct uncontrollable bleeding as a 'rescue' agent (Planinsic et al., 2005; Porte and Caldwell, 2005).

A growing number of case reports indicate that hypercoagulability and thromboembolism may cause serious or fatal complications during liver transplantation (Gologorsky et al., 2001). The incidence of thrombus formation, including intracardiac thrombosis (ICT) (see Figure 22.8), has been estimated at 1–1.5%. Neither antifibrinolytics nor venovenous bypass nor pulmonary artery catheterization have been firmly implicated.

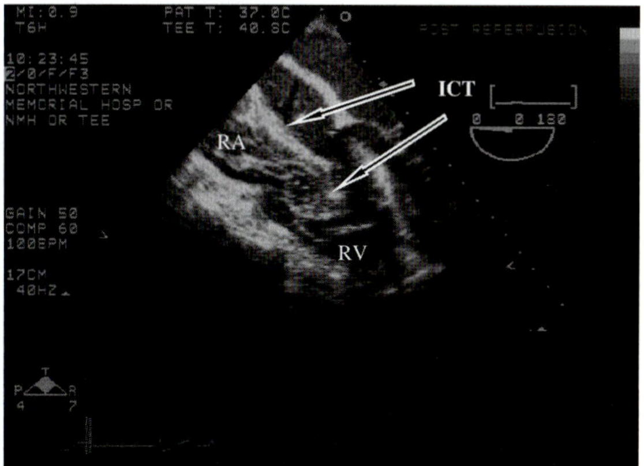


**Fig. 22.8** Transoesophageal echocardiogram showing intracardiac thrombus formation after liver reperfusion. (Reproduced with permission from Lippincott Williams and Wilkins/Wolters Kluwer Health and International Anesthesia Research Society: *Anesthesia & Analgesia*, Boone et al., 'The Successful Use of Low-Dose Recombinant Tissue Plasminogen Activator for Treatment of Intracardiac/Pulmonary Thrombosis During Liver Transplantation', 112, 2, pp. 319–321, 2011.)

Hypercoagulability is demonstrable on thromboelastography and other tests in a significant number of liver recipients, particularly those with primary sclerosing cholangitis and hepatocellular carcinoma, but its importance as a cause of intraoperative thrombosis is unclear. ICT and thromboembolism may occur at any stage of the procedure and overall mortality is probably greater than 50%. Aggressive therapy with thrombectomy or thrombolysis has been successful in very few cases. Early recognition of ICT with transoesophageal echocardiography followed by low-dose tissue plasminogen activator may be the best approach (Boone et al., 2011).

## Electrolyte and acid-base changes

The infusion of large volumes of blood products and reperfusion of the donor liver cause marked changes in plasma biochemistry. Hyponatraemia is present in many recipients, but serum sodium tends to increase during surgery. Rises of more than 12 mmol/L in 24 hours have been associated with central pontine myelinolysis and neurological injury, and these conditions can occur with smaller rises, especially in very debilitated patients (Yu et al., 2004). The use of tris-buffer (tris(hydroxymethyl)aminomethane or THAM) instead of or in combination with sodium bicarbonate moderates these changes.

Hyperkalaemia may complicate rapid transfusion, especially in the presence of renal impairment. Plasma potassium concentrations in stored blood increase with storage time and are often > 20 mmol/L. When hyperkalaemia becomes a concern, red blood cells can be washed using cell salvage equipment and glucose/insulin administered (see Figure 22.9) (De Wolf et al., 1993b). Nebulized or intravenous salbutamol and sodium bicarbonate should also be considered. Plasma potassium increases on reperfusion of the liver, mainly as a result of potassium release from the graft despite flushing. Characteristic ECG changes are seen, including peaked T waves, widening QRS complex, bradycardia, and asystole. Many anaesthesiologists give 500–1,000 mg of calcium chloride prophylactically at reperfusion; others prefer treatment with epinephrine. In most patients, redistribution follows within seconds and a progressive decrease is subsequently seen. However, pre-existing renal failure, residual beta-blockade, and a relatively large, fatty or marginal graft may be associated with prolonged and life-threatening hyperkalaemia and/or hypotension.

Trisodium citrate in transfused blood products reduces ionized calcium concentration, which should be maintained to preserve myocardial function. Calcium chloride or calcium gluconate is given to correct ionized hypocalcaemia (Marquez et al., 1986; Martin et al., 1990). A less marked effect is seen on magnesium concentrations, although supplementation in the absence of either arrhythmias or availability of rapid measurement is not routine (Scott et al., 1996).

Metabolic acidosis is usually absent or minimal at first, unless there is renal impairment or haemodynamic decompensation requiring vasopressor support. However, metabolic acidosis develops rapidly for several reasons. Transfused blood introduces a substantial quantity of exogenous lactic acid into the circulation, while liver lactate metabolism is impaired. Acid metabolites associated with venous stasis in the portal and lower body circulations, as well as those that accumulate in the graft during storage, are released into the general circulation on reperfusion, causing a further increase in acidosis. Worsening lactic acidosis after graft reperfusion is a typical sign of graft failure. Metabolic acidosis is treated with modest hyperventilation. The role of sodium bicarbonate in the management of acidosis remains controversial. Evidence that global circulatory function is impaired by moderate metabolic acidosis is slight, while detrimental effects on oxygen delivery and intracellular pH and plasma lactate associated with bicarbonate therapy have been described. Alternative buffers producing less or no carbon dioxide, including dichloroacetate and tris-buffer (THAM), may be of value but remain to be fully

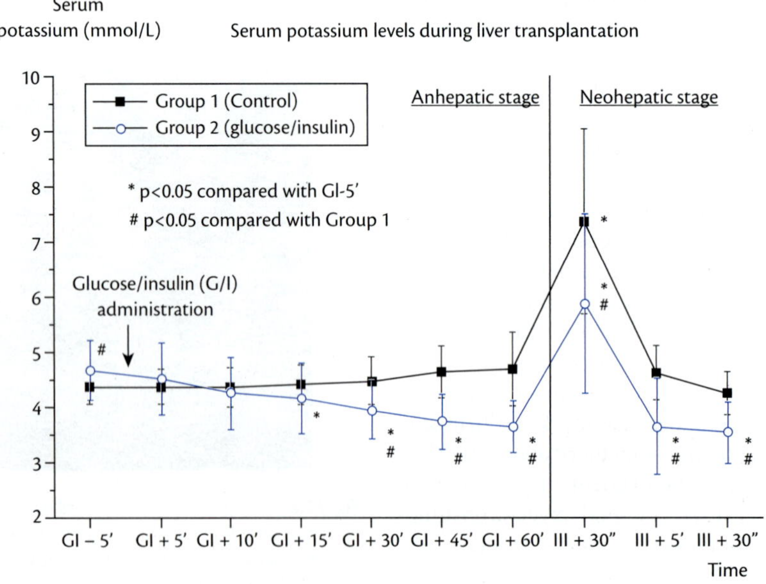


**Fig. 22.9** Serum potassium response to glucose/insulin administration in liver recipients. (Reproduced with permission from Lippincott Williams and Wilkins/Wolters Kluwer Health and the American Society of Anesthesiologists: *Anesthesiology*, De Wolf A et al., 'Insulin decreases the serium potassium concentration during the anhepatic stage of liver transplantation', 78, 4, pp. 677–682, 1993.)

assessed. Intraoperative renal replacement therapy may be implemented if acidosis is severe, especially if hyperkalaemia is present or anticipated. If liver and cardiovascular functions are adequate after reperfusion there is a tendency for metabolic acidosis to clear. Complete correction of metabolic acidosis intraoperatively will result in metabolic alkalosis postoperatively and should be avoided.

### Glucose control

In most patients, blood glucose concentration is normal before surgery but increases during the procedure because of administration of acid-citrate-dextrose blood and stress-related insulin resistance. This may be compounded by glucose released from the graft after reperfusion. Hypoglycaemia, though seen preoperatively in patients with fulminant hepatic failure, is rarely observed intraoperatively even when normal hepatic glucose release is interrupted during the anhepatic phase.

Recent literature has highlighted the association between poor glucose control and adverse outcomes in the perioperative and critical care settings, but a clear causal relationship has not been established and hypoglycaemia is a significant hazard when tight control is attempted, especially in the unconscious patient. Insulin infusions, ranging from 2–10 units/hour, have been advocated to control blood glucose concentrations and prevent hyperkalaemia, but even higher doses are often ineffective after reperfusion. Blood glucose and electrolyte checks, at least hourly, are essential when this is done.

### Respiratory function and early extubation

Changes in respiratory function caused by liver disease have been described (see the section 'Preoperative evaluation and management'). Further respiratory problems arising during surgery are not common. Rapid desaturation readily occurs after induction of anaesthesia, even with preoxygenation, since functional residual capacity (FRC) is often reduced by ascites or hydrothorax. Pulmonary oedema presents a more important hazard and may be the result of overtransfusion, reduced plasma oncotic pressure, or abnormal vascular permeability, especially after reperfusion and if graft function is poor. Intraoperative drainage of a large pleural effusion (hepatic hydrothorax) can cause re-expansion pulmonary oedema. Atelectasis is common but easily treated, while tension pneumothorax and pulmonary embolism are rare. Patients with HPS and cystic fibrosis present few problems intraoperatively, although these conditions may prove challenging in the postoperative period.

With the use of short-acting agents for anaesthesia in the liver recipient, extubation in the operating room or within a few hours of admission to ICU is usually possible and has been advocated as safe and cost-effective (Mandell et al., 2007). However, this depends on recipient comorbidity, the complexity of the surgery, and especially on adequate initial graft function. To be extubated the patient must be awake, haemodynamically stable, and normothermic. Gas exchange must be excellent and there should be no bleeding or significant acidosis. The skills and equipment needed for rapid reintubation must also be immediately available.

## Conclusion

The perioperative care of the liver transplant recipient is a highly specialized undertaking. It demands the skills of an experienced anaesthesiologist with a comprehensive knowledge of the pathophysiology of ESLD, the surgical procedure and its potential pitfalls, and the key haemodynamic, biochemical, and haematological hazards routinely encountered. The anaesthesiologist needs to be supported at all times by a skilled operating-room technical team able to ensure that the modalities used to monitor, maintain and resuscitate the patient are fully effective. Good communication between the anaesthetic and surgical teams is also critical, as is the support of an efficient transfusion service. Under these conditions, even the sickest of liver recipients can undergo this complex life-saving operation and experience a return to excellent health.

## References


Akabayashi A, Slingsby BT, Fujita M (2004) The first donor death after living-related liver transplantation in Japan. *Transplantation*, **77**(4):634.

Arnal D, Garutti I, Perez-Peña J, Olmedilla L, Tzenkov IG (2005) Radial to femoral arterial blood pressure difference during liver transplantation. *Anesthesia*, **60**(8): 766–771.

Axelrod D, Koffron A, De Wolf A, et al. (2004) Safety and efficacy of combined orthotopic liver transplantation and coronary artery bypass grafting. *Liver Transpl*, **10**(11):1386–1390.

Ben Ari A, Elinav E, Elami A, Matot I (2006) Off-pump coronary artery bypass grafting in a patient with Child class C liver cirrhosis awaiting liver transplantation. *Br J Anesth*, **97**(4):468–472.

Bhatia LS, Curzen NP, Byme CD (2012) Nonalcoholic fatty liver disease and vascular risk. *Curr Opin Cardiol*, **27**(4):420–428.

Boone JD, Sherwani SS, Herborn JC, Patel KM, De Wolf AM (2011) The successful use of low-dose recombinant tissue plasminogen activator for treatment of intracardiac/pulmonary thrombosis during liver transplantation. *Anesth Analg*, **112**(2):319–321.

Burtenshaw AJ, Isaac JL (2006) The role of trans-oesophageal echocardiography for perioperative cardiovascular monitoring during orthotopic liver transplantation. *Liver Transpl*, **12**(11):1577–1583.

Cerutti E, Stratta C, Romagnoli R, et al. (2004) Thromboelastogram monitoring in the perioperative period of hepatectomy for adult living liver donation. *Liver Transplant*, **10**(2):289–294.

Cywinski JB, Argalious M, Marks TN, Parker BM (2005) Dynamic left ventricular outflow tract obstruction in an orthotopic liver transplant recipient. *Liver Transplant*, **11**(6):692–695.

Dahmani S, Paugam-Burtz C, Gauss T, et al. (2010) Comparison of central and mixed venous saturation during liver transplantation in cirrhotic patients: a pilot study. *Eur J Anesthesiol*, **27**(8):714–719.

De Wolf A (1997) Monitoring and handling of reperfusion. *Liver Transpl Surg*, **3**(4):459–461.

De Wolf A (1999) Transesophageal echocardiography and orthotopic liver transplantation: general concepts. *Liver Transplant Surg*, **5**(4):339–340.

De Wolf AM (2008) Pulmonary artery catheter: rest in peace? Not just quite yet . . . *Liver Transplant*, **14**(7):917–918.

De Wolf AM, Begliomini B, Gasior TA, Kang Y, Pinsky MR (1993a) Right ventricular function during orthotopic liver transplantation. *Anesth Analg*, **76**(3):562–568.

De Wolf A, Frenette L, Kang Y, Tang C (1993b) Insulin decreases the serium potassium concentration during the anhepatic stage of liver transplantation. *Anesthesiology*, **78**(4):677–682.

Diedrich DA, Findlay JY, Harrison BA, Rosen CB (2008) Influence of coronary artery disease on outcomes after liver transplantation. *Transplant Proc*, **40**(10):3554–3557.

Dowsley TF, Bayne DB, Langnas AN, et al. (2012) Diastolic dysfunction in patients with end-stage liver disease is associated with development of heart failure early after liver transplantation. *Transplantation*, **94**(6):646–651.

Ehtisham J, Altieri M, Salamé E, et al. (2010) Coronary artery disease in orthotopic liver transplantation: pretransplant assessment and management. *Liver Transplant*, **16**(5):550-557

Filsoufi F, Salzberg SP, Rahmanian PB, et al. (2007) Early and late outcome of cardiac surgery in patients with liver cirrhosis. *Liver Transplant*, **13**(7):990–995.

Foltys D, Zimmermann, Heise M, et al. (2011) Liver transplantation for hepatocellular carcinoma—is there a risk of recurrence caused by intraoperative blood salvage autotransfusion? *Eur Surg Res*, **47**:182–187.

Garcia-Tsao G, Bosch J (2010) Management of varices and variceal hemorrhage in cirrhosis. *N Engl J Med*, **362**(9):822–832.

Ginès P, Guevara M (2008) Hyponatremia in cirrhosis: pathogenesis, clinical significance, and management. *Hepatology*, **48**(3):1002–1010.

Gologorsky E, De Wolf AM, Scott V, Aggarwal S, Dishart M, Kang Y (2001) Intracardiac thrombus formation and pulmonary thromboembolism immediately after graft reperfusion in 7 patients undergoing liver transplantation. *Liver Transplant*, **7**(9):783–789.

Gonzalez-Casas R, Jones EA, Moreno-Otero R (2009) Spectrum of anemia associated with chronic liver disease. *World J Gastroenterol*, **15**(37):4653–4658.

Guevara M, Arroyo V (2011) Hepatorenal syndrome. *Expert Opin Pharmacother*, **12**(9):1405–1417.

Gupta S, Castel H, Rao RV, et al. (2010) Improved survival after liver transplantation in patients with hepatopulmonary syndrome. *Am J Transplant*, **10**(2):354–363.

Hartog CS, Reuter D, Loesche W, Hofmann M, Reinhart K (2011) Influence of hydroxyethyl starch (HES) 130/0.4 on hemostasis as measured by viscoelastic device analysis: a systematic review. *Intens Care Med*, **37**(11):1725–1737.

Henriksen JH, Møller JH (2009) Cardiac and systemic hemodynamic complications of liver cirrhosis. *Scand Cardiovasc J*, **43**(4):218–225.

Ito T, Kiuchi T, Egawa H (2003) Surgery-related morbidity in living donors of right-lobe liver graft: lessons from the first 200 cases. *Transplantation*, **76**(1):158–163.

Kang Y (1995) Thromboelastography in liver transplantation. (Review.) *Sem Thromb Hemost*, **21**(Suppl):4:34–44.

Kim JM, Kim GS, Joh JW, et al. (2013) Long-term results for living donor liver transplant recipients with hepatocellular carcinoma using intraoperative blood salvage with leukocyte depletion filter. *Transplant Int*, **26**(1):84–89.

Krejci V, Vannucci A, Abbas A, Chapman W, Kangrga IM (2010) Comparison of calibrated and uncalibrated arterial pressure-based cardiac output monitors during orthotopic liver transplantation. *Liver Transplant*, **16**(6):773–782.

Krowka MJ (2011) Management of pulmonary complications in pretransplant patients. *Clin Liver Dis*, **15**(4):765–777.

Liang TB, Li JJ, Li DL, Liang L, Bai XL, Zheng SS (2010) Intraoperative blood salvage and leukocyte depletion during liver transplantation with bacterial contamination. *Clin Transplant*, **24**(2):265–272.

Mandell MS, Stoner TJ, Barnett R, et al. (2007) A multicenter evaluation of safety of early extubation in liver transplant recipients. *Liver Transplant*, **13**(11):1557–1563.

Marquez J, Martin D, Virji MA, et al. (1986) Cardiovascular depression secondary to ionin hypocalcemia during hepatic transplantation in humans. *Anesthesiology*, **65**(5):457–461.

Martin TJ, Kang Y, Robertson KM, Virji MA, Marquez JM (1990) Ionization and hemodynamic effects of calcium chloride and calcium gluconate in the absence of hepatic function. *Anesthesiology*, **73**(1):62–65.

Massicotte L, Lenis S, Thibeault L, Sassine MP, Seal RF, Roy A (2006) Effect of low central venous pressure and phlebotomy on blood product transfusion requirements during liver transplantations. *Liver Transplant*, **12**(1):117–123.

Massicotte L, Beaulieu D, Thibeault L, et al. (2008) Coagulation defects do not predict blood product requirements during liver transplantation. *Transplantation*, **85**(7):956–962.

Massicotte L, Beaulieu D, Roy JD, et al. (2009) MELD score and blood product requirements during liver transplantation: no link. *Transplantation*, **87**(11):1689–1694.

Massicotte L, Perrault MA, Denault AY, et al. (2010) Effects of phlebotomy and phenylephrine infusion on portal venous pressure and systemic hemodynamics during liver transplantation. *Transplantation*, **89**(8):920–927.

Meltzer J, Brentjens TE (2010) Renal failure in patients with cirrhosis: hepatorenal syndrome and renal support strategies. *Curr Opin Anesth*, **23**(2):139–144.

Miller C, Florman S, Kim-Schluger L, et al. (2004) Fulminant and fatal gas gangrene of the stomach in a healthy live liver donor. *Liver Transplant*, **10**(10):1315–1319.

Møller S, Henriksen JH (2010) Cirrhotic cardiomyopathy. *J Hepatol*, **53**(1):179–190.

Møller S, Henriksen JH, Bendtsen F (2009) Ascites: pathogenesis and therapeutic principles. *Scan J Gasteoenterol*, **44**(8):902–911.

Mukhtar A, Aboulfetouh F, Obayah G, et al. (2009) The safety of modern hydroxyethyl starch in living donor liver transplantation: a comparison with human albumin. *Anesth Analg*, **109**(3):924–930.

Nielsen VG (2007) A comparison of the thromboelastograph and the ROTEM. *Blood Coag Fibrinolysis*, **18**(3):247–252.

Ozier Y, Pessione F, Samain E, Courtois F, French Study Group on Blood Transfusion in Liver Transplantation (2003) Institutional variability in transfusion practice for liver transplantation. *Anesth Analg*, **97**(3):671–679.

Periyalwar P, Dasarathy S (2012) Malnutrition in cirrhosis: contribution and consequences of sarcopenia on metabolic and clinical responses. (Review.) *Clin Liver Dis*, **16**(1):95–131.

Perner A, Haase N, Guttormsen AB, et al. (2012) Hydroxyethyl starch 130/0.42 versus Ringer's acetate in severe sepsis. *N Engl J Med*, **367**(2):24–134.

Planinsic RM, van der Meer J, Testa G (2005) Safety and efficacy of a single bolus administration of recombinant factor VIIa in liver transplantation due to chronic liver disease. *Liver Transplant*, **11**(8):895–900.

Plotkin JS, Scott VL, Pinna A, Dobsch BP, De Wolf AM, Kang Y (1996) Morbidity and mortality in patients with coronary artery disease undergoing orthotopic liver transplantation. *Liver Transplant*, **2**(6):426–430.

Porte RJ, Caldwell SH (2005) The role of recombinant factor VIIa in liver transplantation. (Editorial.) *Liver Transplant*, **11**(8):872–874.

Ramsay M (2010) Portopulmonary hypertension and right heart failure in patients with cirrhosis. *Curr Opin Anesthesiol*, **23**(2):145–150.

Reddy K, Mallett S, Peachey T (2005) Venovenous bypass in orthotopic liver transplantation: time for a rethink? *Liver Transplant*, **11**(7):741–749.

Rodriguez-Roisin R, Krowka MJ (2008) Hepatopulmonary syndrome—a liver-induced lung vascular disorder. *N Engl J Med*, **358**(22):2378–2387.

Roullet S, Pillot J, Freyburger G, et al. (2010) Rotation thromboelastometry detects thrombocytopenia and hypofibrinogenemia during orthotopic liver transplantation. *Br J Anesth*, **104**(4):422–428.

Schumann R, Zabala L, Angelis M, Bonney I, Tighiouari H, Carr DB (2004) Altered hematologic profiles following donor right hepatectomy and implications for perioperative analgesic management. *Liver Transplant*, **10**(3):363–368.

Schwarz B, Pomaroli A, Hoermann C, Margreiter R, Mair P (2001) Liver transplantation without venovenous bypass: morbidity and mortality in patients with greater than 50% reduction in cardiac output after vena cava clamping. *J Cardio-Thorac Vasc Anesth*, **15**:460–462.

Siniscalci A, Begliomini B, De Pietri L, et al. (2004) Increased prothrombin time and platelet counts in living donor right hepatectomy: implications for epidural anesthesia. *Liver Transplant*, **10**(9):1144–1149.

Scott VL, De Wolf AM, Kang Y, et al. (1996) Ionized hypomagnesemia in patients undergoing orthotopic liver transplantation: a complication of citrate intoxication. *Liver Transplant Surg* **2**(5):343–347.

Shaw BW Jr, Martin DJ, Marquez JM, et al. (1984) Venous bypass in clinical liver transplantation. *Ann Surg*, **200**(4):524–534.

Shin BS, Kim GS, Ko JS, et al. (2007) Comparison of femoral arterial blood pressure with radial arterial blood pressure and noninvasive upper arm blood pressure in the reperfusion period during liver transplantation. *Transplant Proc*, **39**(5):1326–1328.

Siniscalci A, Begliomini B, De Pietri L, et al. (2004) Increased prothrombin time and platelet counts in living donor right hepatectomy: implications for epidural anesthesia. *Liver Transplant*, **10**(9):1144–1149.

Steadman RH, Van Rensburg A, Kramer DJ (2010) Transplantation for acute liver failure: perioperative management. *Curr Opin Organ Transplant*, **15**(3):368–373.

Strong RW, Lynch SV, Ong TH, Matsunami H, Koido Y, Balderson GA (1990) Successful liver transplantation from a living donor to her son. *N Engl J Med*, **322**(21):1505–1507.

Thuluvath PJ (2007) Morbid obesity with one or more other serious comorbidities should be a contraindication to liver transplantation (editorial). *Liver Transplant*, **13**(12):1627–1629.

Tsai YF, Su BC, Lin CC, Liu FC, Lee WC, Yu HP (2012) Cardiac output derived from arterial pressure waveform analysis: validation of the third-generation software in patients undergoing orthotopic liver transplantation. *Transplant Proc*, **44**(2):433–437.

Vastag B. (2003) Living-donor transplants reexamined: experts cite growing concerns about safety of donors. *JAMA*, **290**(2):181–182.

Warnaar N, Lisman T, Porte RJ (2008) The two tales of coagulation in liver transplantation. *Curr Opin Organ Transplant*, **13**(3):298–303.

Wray C, Scovotti JC, Tobis J, et al. (2013) Liver transplantation outcome in patients with angiographically proven coronary artery disease: a multi-institutional study. *Am J Transplant*, **13**(1):184–191.

Xia VW, Steadman RH (2005) Antifibrinolytics in orthotopic liver transplantation: current status and controversies. *Liver Transplant*, **11**(1):10–18.

Yu J, Zheng SS, Liang TB, Shen Y, Wang WL, Ke QH (2004) Possible causes of central pontine myelinolysis after liver transplantation. *World J Gastroenterol*, **10**(17):2540–2543.

# CHAPTER 23

# Critical care of the liver transplant recipient

Samantha Vizzini, Anurag Johri, Faisal Anis, Ernesto A. Pretto, Jr., and William Peruzzi

## The routine transplant and early extubation

During the early transplantation experience, it was universally accepted that patients would be transported to the ICU, intubated, and maintained with positive pressure ventilation for 24–48 hours. The rationale for this was to allow for a smooth emergence from anaesthesia and reduce the physical stresses associated with the procedure and recovery. Since the 1990s studies have focused on the safety and feasibility of early extubation. Fortunately, with improvements in surgical technique, the development of shorter-acting anaesthetics, and an overall decrease in transfusion requirements, early extubation has become a viable option (Biancofiore et al., 2005).

Several studies have shown that early discontinuation of mechanical ventilation in the postoperative period is beneficial, not only for the patient's pulmonary status but also for graft viability. Positive pressure ventilation increases intrathoracic pressure, decreases venous return, and increases venous congestion, which in turn decreases splanchnic blood flow. Splanchnic blood flow is obviously critical for graft survival and compromise of this factor at a crucial time when the graft is recovering from ischaemic–reperfusion injury may lead to early graft failure and increased morbidity and mortality. Studies using postoperative aspartate aminotransferase (AST) levels as an indicator of reperfusion injury demonstrated consistently higher levels in those patients extubated later (outside of the operating room) and especially in those patients who underwent mechanical ventilation for more than 24 hours. However, several factors must be taken into consideration prior to such a conclusion. The degree of liver disease before transplantation, the intraoperative course, the level of residual anaesthetic, plus the standard extubation criteria (e.g. normothermia, normocapnia with spontaneous ventilation, haemodynamic stability, and adequate recovery from anaesthetics and muscle relaxants) must be assured before extubation should even be considered.

Although it has been demonstrated that early extubation is beneficial, not all patients are candidates for such intervention. Preoperative factors such as acute liver failure, preoperative mechanical ventilation, and retransplantation are more frequently associated with patients requiring mechanical ventilation for more than 24 hours in the ICU (Glanemann et al., 2001). Elevated TNF was observed in long-term graft storage leading to tissue injury of both the lungs and liver, which resulted in elevated AST, alveolar oedema, haemorrhage, and leucocyte sequestration. These patients were at higher risk for prolonged intubation and mechanical ventilation postoperatively (Glanemann et al., 2001). Other predictors of failure to meet extubation criteria include both a BMI of 34 or higher and uncontrolled preoperative encephalopathy. No correlation has been found with UNOS scores, CTP scores, age, or alcoholic liver disease (Mandell, 2007). Intraoperative factors such as red blood cell transfusion > 6 units have been associated with increased risk of prolonged postoperative mechanical ventilation (Glanemann et al., 2007). Patients who meet any of the above criteria should not be extubated in the early postoperative period.

The benefits of early discontinuation of mechanical ventilation and extubation are not limited to clinical endpoints. Optimal resource utilization, including ventilators and ICU beds, is important on several levels. In one study, on average 1 ICU day per patient was saved when patients were extubated in the operating room and this equated with a 13% overall reduction in costs (Mandell, 2002). The social benefits of such care improvements should be obvious and encouraged. It has also been demonstrated that it is possible to bypass ICU care altogether by sending extubated patients to the surgical ward from the postoperative recovery room when proper protocols are followed and there are no complications associated with the procedure. While these results were possible in a large transplant centre where staff were trained to manage the complex liver transplant patients, this may not be feasible everywhere, at least not currently (Taner, 2012).

## Infection prophylaxis

According to a 2012 consensus statement by the American Society of Transplantation and the American Association for the Study of Liver Diseases, the interval from 3–6 months post-transplant is the highest risk period for opportunistic infections, including *Herpes* viruses, fungi, and atypical bacterial infections such as *Nocardia*, *Listeria*, and *Mycobacteria*. After the sixth post-transplantation month the risk of infection decreases due to the reduction in immunosuppressive therapy. In order to prevent these opportunistic infections, prophylactic antimicrobial therapy, avoidance of high-risk exposures, and minimization of immunosuppression as soon as possible are recommended (Lucey, 2013).

CMV is the most significant opportunistic infection seen in post-transplant patients and often presents with viraemia, bone marrow suppression, and involvement of the GI tract and liver. This statement recommends prophylaxis with either oral valganciclovir 900 mg/day or intravenous ganciclovir 5 mg/kg/day for 3–6 months after transplantation if the recipient is negative and the donor is positive; however, only 3 months of treatment are necessary if both the donor and recipient are positive (Lucey, 2013). Valganciclovir is not FDA-approved for liver transplant patients and its use is controversial; however, it is approved for use in heart and kidney transplant patients. A 2010 study at the University of Maryland published in *HPB: The Official Journal of the International Hepato-Pancreato-Biliary Association* found valganciclovir to be equally effective as ganciclovir and safe in postliver transplant patients. Additional benefits include higher oral bioavailability and lower pill burden when compared to ganciclovir (Fayek, 2010). At the same time, a study from the University of Nebraska found a higher risk of neutropaenia, late-onset CMV disease, and CMV tissue-invasive disease with valganciclovir as opposed to other less expensive therapies and cautioned against its use (Kalil, 2009).

EBV is rarely associated with a post-transplant lymphoproliferative disease (incidence 0.0–2.9%) that manifests with lymphadenopathy, cytopaenia, fever, and disturbances of the GI tract, lungs, spleen, and CNS. The initial treatment of this condition is reduction of immunosuppressive therapy; if there is no response within 2–4 weeks then either surgery, radiation, or cytotoxic chemotherapy may be required. Antiviral therapy has not been proven to affect outcomes (Lucey, 2013).

Fungal infections have shifted since the mid-1990s, with a decrease in overall *Candida* infections and an increase in *Aspergillus* infections and occasional cryptococcal infections. Diagnosis of *Aspergillus* is difficult and may require biopsy, given that sensitivity and specificity of galactomannan testing in the blood or bronchoalveolar lavage (BAL) are variable. Serum and cerebrospinal fluid (CSF) cryptococcal antigen testing is much more sensitive and a rapid tool for diagnosis of CNS infection. Urinary antigens for histoplasmosis and blastomyces have been useful for the diagnosis of disseminated infection. Prophylaxis for fungal infections is recommended with fluconazole 100–400 mg daily, itraconazole 200 mg twice daily, caspofungin 50 mg daily, or liposomal amphotericin 1 mg/kg/day for 4–6 weeks; the optimal duration is unknown and therapy is often reserved for high-risk patients (pretransplant colonization, retransplant, dialysis patients, and those with hepatic iron overload) (Lucey, 2013). A Cochrane Review in 2003 found no overall decrease in mortality with antifungal prophylaxis but did demonstrate a decrease in both proven and suspected fungal infections with fluconazole prophylaxis by about 75%. Similar results were not seen in studies that used other prophylactic regimens such as itraconazole and amphotericin B. When compared within the same study, the reductions in fungal infections were similar. This study also cautions against future development of azole-resistant *Candida* species and moulds such as *C. glabarata*, *C. krusie*, and *Aspergillus* species, which were seen in previous studies but with very low incidence (Playford, 2004).

*Pneumocystis jirovecii* (formerly known as *Pneumocystis carinii*) usually presents with respiratory symptoms including hypoxaemia and fever. It is not commonly seen in liver transplant patients due to widespread prophylaxis after surgery with trimethoprim sulfamethoxazole (single strength given daily or double strength three times per week), or for those with allergy to sulfa, dapsone 100 mg daily or atovaquone 1,500 mg daily for 6 months up to 1 year. A longer duration of therapy is recommended for patients on augmented immunosuppressive therapy and life-long treatment is recommended for patients with HIV. It must be noted that dapsone may increase the occurrence of methaemoglobinaemia in this patient population and this should be monitored (Lucey, 2013).

A study published in 2012 by researchers from the University of British Columbia (Wang et al., 2012) noted that liver recipients who did not receive prophylaxis for pneumocystis pneumonia (PCP), caused by *P. jirovecii*, did in fact become infected, usually around 7 months post-transplant. This study demonstrated that PCP is not an infection of the past and prophylaxis is still crucial in this patient population. Also in this study Wang and colleagues noted late PCP infection more than 1 year post-transplant, usually coinciding with an episode of rejection and increased immunosuppression. Their take-away from this was that perhaps PCP prophylaxis should be reinstated during periods of increased immunosuppression. Another study by Sarwar et al. (2013) in Ireland discussed the possibility of target prophylaxis in patient populations such as theirs, which are low risk. In their centre, they did not give any PCP prophylactic agents and only saw seven cases in their 687 liver transplants, arguing that targeted prophylaxis rather than universal may be beneficial.

Tuberculosis (TB) has several risk factors associated with its development in post-transplant patients, including prior infection, intensified immunosuppression, diabetes, and coinfection with CMV, *Pneumocystis*, mycoses, or *Nocardia*. Diagnosis is often difficult due to atypical presentations, especially those outside of the respiratory system. Prophylaxis with isoniazid (INH) is recommended for the first 9 months after surgery in patients with latent TB. INH is hepatotoxic and liver function tests should be monitored closely for signs of rejection (Lucey, 2013).

Bacterial sepsis and wound infections increase morbidity and mortality after liver transplant, as well as increasing cost and length of hospital stay (Azevedo, 2013). Several preoperative interventions such as selective bowel decontamination and prebiotic/probiotic therapy have been studied in an attempt to reduce such infections; however, they show little benefit to the patient. Selective bowel decontamination may actually increase the risk of infection and incidence of *Clostridium difficile* leading to pseudomembranous colitis; therefore, at this time, such interventions cannot be recommended. The use of prebiotics and probiotics together did show some decrease in infection, but the results were not statistically significant (Gurusamy, 2008).

All liver transplant recipients should receive the following immunizations before transplantation: influenza, pneumococcus, hepatitis A, hepatitis B, tetanus, human papilloma virus, and *Varicella*. After transplantation they should receive an annual influenza vaccine and the pneumococcal vaccine every 3–5 years (Lucey, 2013).

## Perioperative assessment of graft function

Liver graft function following an OLT can be assessed during the reperfusion phase of surgery by visual inspection (a well-perfused graft turns from rather grey to purplish-pink) and/or by monitoring the recovery of the hepatocellular metabolic as well as synthetic functions. The survival of the graft after OLT depends on a number of factors, which are related to donor and recipient conditions as well as surgical technique. These factors are described in detail in different parts of this book, but we will summarize them here so as to help identify the patients who are at highest risk of graft dysfunction and failure.

Donor risk factors influencing postoperative graft survival include:

- Donor age > 60 years (50 in some studies) is associated with poor graft and poor patient survival, while donor age < 30 results in more favourable graft outcomes (Totsuka, 2000, 2004).
- History of cardiac arrest in the donor as the initiating event for brain death is associated with worse graft function.
- Moderate to severe steatosis in the donor allograft frozen section is associated with worse graft function (Nanashima, 2002; Ferraz-Neto, 2007).
- Haemodynamic instability in the donor prior to harvesting requiring large-dose infusions of vasopressor (i.e. dopamine > 10 μg/kg/min) is associated with poor graft survival. This is due to compromise of the mesenteric and portal circulation, which may lead to hepatocyte injury (Avolio et al., 1991).
- Preharvest donor alanine transaminase (ALT) level > 65 units/L signifies initial insult to the hepatocytes and is associated with poor graft survival (Sirivatanauksorn, 2012).
- Preharvest donor serum sodium level > 155 mEq/L is believed to cause intracellular water accumulation. Sudden shifts in serum osmolarity in the neohepatic stage may cause hepatocellular injury and is associated with poor graft survival. Donor serum sodium levels should be managed and maintained below 150 mEq/L prior to graft harvest to diminish this additional risk.
- Small-for-size syndrome (SFSS) occurs primarily in living donor or reduced-size liver transplantation. The principal pathogenesis of SFSS is the imbalance between accelerated liver regeneration and the increased demand for liver function, leading to severe graft dysfunction with prolonged hyperbilirubinaemia and increased ascites.

Several of the above conditions are reviewed under ECD in Chapter 3.

Recipient risk factors influencing postoperative graft survival include:

- UNOS status of the patient. UNOS status 1 candidates for OLT require life-support systems prior to transplantation. These patients have worse graft survival compared to higher UNOS status patients who are more stable.
- A history of cardiopulmonary arrest prior to OLT in the recipient is associated with poor graft survival.
- Smoking and alcohol history in the recipient is associated with poor graft survival.
- Initial aetiology for OLT as described elsewhere in the book is also important in determining postoperative performance of the graft.
- The presence of renal insufficiency and hepatorenal syndrome in the recipient before transplant are independent risk factors for poor graft outcome (Gonwa, 1991).

The CTP classification and MELD score, though very popular in classifying patients in need of transplantation, have limited value in predicting graft survival.

Surgical factors influencing postoperative graft survival are as follows:

- Cold ischaemia time (CIT) is one of the major predictors for the quality of graft and CIT > 12 hours is associated with poor graft survival.
- Warm ischaemia time (WIT) > 45 minutes is associated with poor graft survival.
- Venovenous bypass technique or piggyback technique with inferior vena caval preservation, used during anastomosis, are associated with better graft survival than the conventional technique.

During the initial few hours following OLT, it is not uncommon to see serum levels of lactate dehydrogenase, AST, and ALT elevated, and platelets and coagulation factors lower than normal (Avolio et al., 1991). The important aspect is that the values trend in the right direction.

Liver enzyme values should start trending down by day 2–7, with AST levels reaching values < 2,000 IU/L and PT < 16 s (Ploeg et al., 1993). Other authors favour using AST/ALT < 1,500 units/L within 72 hours after transplantation as a positive sign for ongoing liver function improvement (Nanashima, 2002).

Platelets may remain low for a longer period of time due to active sequestration. This does not necessarily signify the need for platelet transfusion unless active bleeding is present. Platelet values usually return to normal within a couple of days. PT should start normalizing within the first 24 hours following the transplantation, though full recovery may take up to 2–3 days. Any rise in PT following the downward trend or failure to trend downwards should be viewed with concern and investigated aggressively.

Once the anastomosis of the new graft is completed, urine output should start to improve; this should continue during the postoperative phase and should reach the acceptable volume and quality within the first few days after the transplant, depending on the preoperative renal status of the donor, and the serum value of urea and creatinine should reflect the same. Any rise in the serum urea and creatinine or decrease in urine output should be investigated.

In an adequately functioning liver graft the mental status of the recipient should start to improve, indicating adequate urea and nitrogen metabolism. As such, following surgery the patient's mental status should recover enough to allow extubation within the first 6–12 hours (this is discussed further in the section 'Routine transplant and early extubation'). Any disturbance in the mental status (which usually follows rising liver enzymes) should alert the physician to investigate the graft function further.

The arterial ketone body ratio (AKBR; acetoacetate divided by β-hydroxybutyrate) has been shown to correlate with the oxidative status of the graft and its mitochondrial energy production. A falling AKBR is associated with hypoperfusion of the graft liver and may indicate hepatic artery embolization, other vascular compromise, or warm ischaemic injury (Shaked, 1997).

Clinically improving bilirubin, normalizing PT, resolving acidosis, normal glucose metabolism, haemodynamic stability, resolution of hypothermia, adequate urine output, and improving mental status are indicators of good graft function, while graft dysfunction is usually associated clinically with persistent tachycardia, worsening renal failure shutdown, and disturbances in mental status, which may ultimately culminate in hepatic coma. We will discuss the different types of graft failure in the next section.

## Primary graft dysfunction and failure

Primary graft dysfunction is subclassified by different authors based on the time period since the initial transplant and the level of biochemical markers. Unfortunately there is often considerable disparity in the definition of the terms, but most of the authors agree to the classification described by Ploeg et al. (1993). In this work they divided primary liver dysfunction (PDF) into primary non-function (PNF) and initial poor function (IPF). PNF is the more serious form of PDF and means that the graft never functioned following transplantation (Kemmer et al., 2007). The graft, therefore, is non-life-sustaining and must be retransplanted within 7 days or death of the patient will ensue.

IPF was described as AST > 2,000 IU/L and PT > 16 s on post-operative day 2–6. These patients either recover or worsen and require retransplantation. If retransplantation is not available, patients succumb similarly within 7 or more days from their initial transplantation, depending upon the rapidity and severity of the graft failure.

Sirivatanauksorn et al. (2012) further divided PDF into non-primary dysfunction (non-PDF) and PNF/IPF, in which they defined the non-PDF group as the one that had immediate function.

Silberhumer et al. (2007) proposed four grades of initial graft function over the first postoperative 5 days as:

(1) Good function: AST maximal 1,000 IU/L and spontaneous PT > 50%

(2) Fair function: AST 1,000–2,500 IU/L, clotting factor support < 2 days

(3) IPF: AST > 2,500 IU/L, clotting factor support > 2 days

(4) PGNF: retransplantation required within 7 days

According to UNOS (<www.unos.org>), PDF is defined as non-recoverable graft function needing urgent liver replacement during the first 10 days after OLT. UNOS characterizes this by an AST > 5,000 IU/L, INR > 3.0, and acidosis (pH < 7.3 and/or lactate concentration > 2 times normal).

One of the practical problems in IPF with the UNOS and Ploeg et al. definitions is that they encompass a time period of 2–7 days for dysfunction to develop or evolve; thus it becomes difficult to plan for retransplantation earlier in the graft failure process. Hence, different authors have developed variable clinical definitions based on these time frames. Chui et al. (2000) described IPF as the graft with AST or ALT > 2,500 IU/L within the first 24 hours of the surgery and Ardite et al. (1999) defined IPF as occurring within the first 3 days of transplant. The variability in these definitions greatly affects the reported incidence of primary graft dysfunction from various centres. Nevertheless, the estimated incidence seems to be anywhere between 5 and 10% by even the most conservative estimates.

### Causes of early graft dysfunction

The early dysfunction of the graft can be due to:

Vascular issues:

- Hepatic artery thrombosis
- Portal vein thrombosis
- Poor drainage of the suprahepatic veins

Problems of the graft itself:

- Primary dysfunction/malfunction
- Rejection

Biliary drainage issues:

- Biliary fistula
- Biliary leak
- Biliary obstruction (can occur in the setting of anastomotic stenosis)
- Intrahepatic stenosis and choledocholithiasis

Other causes:

- Drug-related liver toxicity (e.g. cyclosporine)
- Infections (CMV, bacterial)

### Clinical features of primary graft dysfunction and assessment

Whatever the cause of the PDF, the clinical picture of PNF is characterized by post-transplantation encephalopathy, coagulopathy, minimal bile output, and progressive renal and multisystem failure, with increasing serum lactate and rapidly rising liver enzyme levels and histological evidence of hepatocyte necrosis in the absence of any vascular compromise (Lock et al., 2010). It should be differentiated from complete hepatic artery thrombosis (HAT) that usually occurs in the very early stages after liver transplantation as well. Any major alteration in liver function should initiate a series of studies, which may include Doppler ultrasound to evaluate vascular patency, bile duct studies (e.g. T-tube cholangiography, ERCP, percutaneous transhepatic cholangiography) to evaluate any abnormality of the biliary system (e.g. stricture, bile leak, obstruction), and liver biopsy to rule out rejection. The management of the PDF will be based on the results of the above studies and will be discussed in the individual sections of this chapter.

## Molecular mechanisms of the hepatocyte injury

Ischaemia–reperfusion (I/R) injury is the underlying mechanism of early graft dysfunction. Reoxygenation liberates endothelin-1, activates Ito cells (perisinusoidal fat-storing cells), constricts hepatic sinusoids (with subsequent decreased hepatic blood flow), and activates Kupffer cells, all simultaneously. Activation of Kupffer cells and T-cells causes increased expression of adhesion molecules with liberation of chemokines and mediation of the neutrophil inflammatory response. Activated neutrophils infiltrate the injured liver in parallel with platelet aggregation and apoptosis of sinusoidal endothelial cells. I/R injury thus creates an inflammation milieu. The mechanisms involved in liver I/R include the Toll-like receptor system, the haem oxygenase system, metalloproteinase-9, the membrane attack complex (C5b-9), and tissue anoxia with depletion of adenosine triphosphate and subsequent mitochondrial dysfunction (Shaked, 1997).

## Predictors of primary graft dysfunction

Although graft function after OLT can be monitored with daily measurements of various liver function tests and biological markers (outlined in the section 'Primary graft dysfunction and failure'), these indicators are often lagging in the evolution of molecular mechanisms of I/R injury. A LiMax (maximal enzymatic liver function capacity) test can be calculated easily and has been shown to be an early predictor of PDF. It is based on the fact that $^{13}$C-methacetin is demethylated by the hepatocytic microsomal cytochrome P450 1A2 system. This reaction results in excretion of $^{13}CO_2$ through the lungs, which subsequently can be detected as a change in the $^{13}CO_2/^{12}CO_2$ ratio (delta over baseline (DOB)) by non-dispersive, isotope-selective infrared spectrometry.

$$\mathrm{Li}_{\mathrm{Max}} = \frac{\left( \begin{array}{l} (\mathrm{DOBmax}) \times (\mathrm{Standard\ CO_2\ /\ CO_2\ ratio}) \\ \times (\mathrm{CO_2\ production}) \times (\mathrm{Molar\ mass\ of\ C\text{-}methacetin}) \end{array} \right)}{\mathrm{Body\ weight}}$$

In multiple studies, it has been observed that LiMax values < 64 μg/kg/hour immediately after liver transplantation are associated with initial graft dysfunction. Lock et al. (2010) used multivariate analysis to compare the LiMax scores with other routine biochemical essays (e.g. bilirubin, ammonia, INR) obtained in the postliver transplant period and concluded that the LiMax test was the single independent predictor of graft dysfunction. LiMax scores also identified patients with impending graft failure before these biochemical tests became clinically significant, thus allowing physicians to identify the patients at risk earlier. Table 23.1 from the study of Lock et al. (2010) looks at the different predictors of graft dysfunction after liver transplant.

Primary graft dysfunction carries a uniformly high mortality unless retransplantation is available soon after the diagnosis is made. The condition usually progresses to multi-organ system failure within 24–48 hours. Once multi-organ failure sets in following PDF there is a mortality rate of over 50% in most studies.

## Seventh day syndrome

Although most patients of OLT do well if they have no issues within the first few days, Memon et al. (2001) described an early rare form of liver failure occurring about 7 days following transplantation (known as seventh day syndrome (7DS)). This syndrome is characterized by the extremely high levels of liver hepatocyte apoptosis, liver or multi-organ failure without any evidence of acute rejection, vascular compromise, infection, or other surgical complications in patients who seem to be doing well otherwise. The phenomenon is associated with a high mortality rate unless retransplantation occurs. Zhongwei et al. (2012) studied the syndrome and postulated the cause to be related to coagulation necrosis and Fas receptor activation which leads to apoptosis of the cell. They also found that extending the intravenous methylprednisolone course from 8 days to 11 days postoperatively may prevent or delay the recurrence of 7DS and reduces mortality (Zhongwei, 2012).

**Table 23.1** Different predictors of initial graft dysfunction directly after liver transplantation. (Reproduced with permission from Lock et al., 'Early Diagnosis of Primary Nonfunction and Indication for Reoperation After Liver Transplantation', *Liver Transplantation*, 16, pp. 172–180. Copyright © 2010 American Association for the Study of Liver Diseases.)

| | Normal range | Initial graft dysfunction (*n* = 8) | Control (*n* = 91) | Univariate P value | Multivariate P value | Receiver operating characteristics | | | |
|---|---|---|---|---|---|---|---|---|---|
| | | | | | | AUROC | 95% = CI | P value | Best cutoff |
| LiMax (μg/kg/hour) | > 315 | 43 ± 18 | 184 ± 98 | < 0.001 | 0.008 | 0.960 | 0.921–0.998 | < 0.001 | 64 |
| ICG-PDR (%/minute) | > 18 | 11.8 ± 6.1 | 15.5 ± 6.4 | 0.200 | | 0.659 | 0.413–0.905 | 0.195 | 8.3 |
| AST (units/L) | < 35 | 2921 ± 1962 | 1629 ± 1823 | 0.110 | | 0.756 | 0.599–0.912 | 0.017 | 1,371 |
| ALT (units/L) | < 34 | 1083 ± 523 | 857 ± 776 | 0.290 | | 0.684 | 0.530–0.838 | 0.086 | 648 |
| GLDH (units/L) | < 4.8 | 736 ± 713 | 351 ± 481 | 0.041 | Excluded | 0.676 | 0.473–0.879 | 0.101 | 233 |
| Bilirubin (mg/dL) | < 1 | 8.8 ± 11.7 | 4.9 ± 3.58 | 0.026 | Excluded | 0.650 | 0.505–0.795 | 0.161 | 4.6 |
| Ammonia (μmol/L) | 10–50 | 83 ± 53 | 46 ± 32 | 0.004 | Excluded | 0.756 | 0.575–0.937 | 0.017 | 82 |
| Albumin (g/dL) | 3.6–5.0 | 3.13 ± 0.56 | 3.21 ± 0.49 | 0.675 | | 0.563 | 0.339–0.786 | 0.560 | 3.25 |
| INR | 0.9–1.25 | 1.94 ± 0.55 | 1.69 ± 0.31 | 0.047 | Excluded | 0.615 | 0.390–0.839 | 0.284 | 1.74 |
| Factor II (%) | 70–130 | 51.5 ± 9.4 | 54.0 ± 13.2 | 0.503 | | 0.552 | 0.360–0.744 | 0.628 | 48.5 |
| Factor VII (%) | 70–130 | 50.6 ± 11.2 | 51.8 ± 15.8 | 0.785 | | 0.506 | 0.343–0.669 | 0.956 | 46.5 |

Note: all parameters were compared by univariate analysis (Student *t* test for independent samples), multivariate analysis (forward and backward logistic regression), and receiver operating characteristics. The best cutoff was chosen at the maximum sum of sensitivity and specificity. *P* value in receiver operating characteristic analysis represents the probability that the true AUROC is 0.5 in this population. A *P* value < 0.05 indicates that the AUROC is significantly different from 0.5 and thus the diagnostic test has the potential to distinguish between the diseased and non-diseased.

ICG, ; PDR, ; GLDH, .AUROC, .

The usual ICU stay for the uncomplicated liver transplant patient is about 3–4 days and discharge to home typically occurs about 2 weeks after surgery.

## Nutritional management

Chronic malnutrition is a common problem in ESLD patients who present for transplant. Nutritional support for patients awaiting liver transplant often includes supplementation of fats, protein, and carbohydrates as well as several liver-specific formulations which contain branched-chain amino acids (BCAAs), omega-3 fatty acids, and arginine.

Postoperative nutrition is a major determinant of surgical outcomes and graft survival and is often suboptimal due to poor preoperative nutritional status, the stress of surgery, immunosuppressive therapy, and, in some patients, renal failure and sepsis (Langer, 2012). There are three issues to consider regarding feeding in the post-transplant period: (1) the timing of nutrition institution, (2) the method of feeding administration, and (3) the composition of the feeding (formulas).

Postoperative support is either enteral, with a feeding tube, or parenteral, as patients often remain intubated after surgery and are unable to tolerate oral nutrition for several days. Recent studies have addressed the benefit of enteral versus parenteral feeding, with arguments favouring early enteral feeding (Ikegami, 2012); in this study those patients who were started on enteral feeding within 48 hours of surgery had a decreased incidence of bacterial sepsis. The authors of this study found that the major pathogens leading to sepsis originated from the gut, specifically Gram-negative bacteria. They argued that enteral nutrition can stimulate bile flow and portal blood flow, thus preventing intestinal mucosal atrophy and preserving the immune functions of the gut.

Another study investigated the benefit of combining enteral and parenteral feeding in reference to overall length of hospital stay and cost of medical care (Jiang, 2007). In this study the authors combined intravenous glutamine-dipeptide with standard parenteral nutrition formulations while, at the same time, feeding the gut via a nasal–jejunal tube. Despite the decreased length in overall hospital stay, there was no strong evidence for improved clinical outcomes such as mortality, transplant rejection, infection, and ventilator dependence.

When deciding which formulation of enteral or parenteral nutrition is best for the post-transplant patient, several new studies have been done on their various components. Such studies have focused on BCAAs and their advantage over dextrose solution in postoperative parenteral nutrition leading to decreased length of ICU stay (Reilly, 1990; Qui et al., 2009). These authors found improved nutritional status and increased levels of pre-albumin in those patients receiving alanylglutamine over those receiving standard total parenteral nutrition (TPN). AST levels were also lower in those patients receiving the amino acid formula, demonstrating a decreased level of hepatocellular damage. Another study focused on parenteral omega-3 fatty acids in the first 6 days after transplantation, which also demonstrated a decrease in length of ICU care and overall hospital stay (Jiang, 2011).

A newer study with early enteral feeding containing hydrolyzed whey peptides showed promising effects in decreasing bacterial sepsis when compared to those patients receiving standard elemental diet. The conclusions that ensued are that these peptides may prevent infection via their anti-inflammatory properties, while also preventing hyperglycaemia, without increasing graft rejection (Kaido, 2012). The exact mechanism by which these peptides exert their salutary effects is poorly understood. The authors believed that, because whey protein contains lactoferrin, beta-lactoglobulin, alpha-lactalbumin, glycomacropeptide, and immunoglobulins, it can enhance immune function. The main carbohydrate in this formulation was isomaltose, which may help prevent hyperglycaemia when compared with standard enteral feeding. Insulin requirements in these patients were less than those receiving standard formulations on postoperative day 7; however, the difference was not statistically significant. Regardless, decreased insulin requirements and a decreased incidence of hyperglycaemia lead to improved wound healing and may be significant in decreasing ICU requirements in post-transplant patients.

A Cochrane Review in 2012 highlighted that the small size sample of these studies introduced a risk of bias and called the statistical validity of some of these studies into question (Langer, 2012). Despite their small sample size and lack of prospective research, these findings will pave the way for future studies on the optimum nutritional support for postliver transplant patients.

## Neurological complications of liver failure

HE or portosystemic encephalopathy (PSE) constitutes an impairment of brain function that occurs in patients with severe liver failure. The mechanisms of CNS dysfunction in liver failure are not well defined and it is clear that the dysfunction is multifactorial, including reversible metabolic encephalopathy, cerebral oedema, brain atrophy, or any combination thereof. In models of acute liver failure these issues overlap. In severe hepatic coma the effects of cerebral oedema, impaired cerebral perfusion, and reversible impairment of neurotransmitter systems are not distinguishable (Ferenci, 1994; Córdoba and Blei, 1996).

The metabolic factors involved in HE include: ammonia, which is clearly implicated; inhibitory neurotransmission, through gamma-aminobutyric acid (GABA) receptors; and changes in CNS neurotransmitters and circulating amino acids (Bassett, 1987). None of these mechanisms is mutually exclusive and it is more likely than not that multiple factors are present simultaneously.

Concurrent pathology that can contribute to the development of brain failure includes:

- Decreased oxygen delivery, which can result from a variety of factors including GI bleeding, sepsis, the effects of cytokines, or compounds released from necrotic liver tissue. In particular, proinflammatory cytokines may have a pivotal role in impairing several brain functions (O'Beirne, 2006). The effects of hypotension on cerebral perfusion may be magnified in liver failure because of an associated impairment in the autoregulation of cerebral blood flow (Strauss, 1997).
- Functional and structural changes in cerebral function independent of the liver failure, as in alcoholics, intravenous drug users, and patients with Wilson's disease (Larsen, 1997).
- Creation of a portosystemic shunt to treat portal hypertension, as with a TIPS, precipitates HE in approximately 30% of patients (Vogels et al., 1997a).

- Other events can precipitate HE such as the administration of sedatives, hypokalaemia, and hyponatraemia (Artz, 1966). The effects of hypokalaemia are believed to be mediated by potassium movement out of the cells, to replenish extracellular stores, while intracellular electroneutrality is maintained largely by migration of extracellular hydrogen into the intracellular space. This creates an extracellular metabolic alkalosis and an intracellular acidosis. In renal tubular cells, this acidosis increases the production of ammonia. Concurrently, the metabolic alkalosis may promote the conversion of the ammonium ion ($NH_4^+$), a charged particle that cannot cross the blood–brain barrier, into uncharged ammonia ($NH_3$) that enters the brain easily (Gabduzda and Hall, 1966).

## Neurotoxins

### Ammonia

Ammonia is the best known neurotoxin associated with HE. The arterial concentration of ammonia is increased in about 90% of patients with HE. The pathogenetic role of ammonia in HE is apparent from the clinical improvements in HE with various therapies aimed at lowering plasma ammonia levels in affected patients (Weissenborn, 2007).

The GI tract is the primary source of ammonia. Ammonia is produced by enterocyte metabolism of glutamine, colonic bacterial catabolism of ingested proteins, and secreted urea digested by *H. pylori* in the stomach (Blei, 2001). Ammonia enters the circulation via the portal vein. The intact liver clears virtually all portal-vein ammonia, by converting it into glutamine, and prevents entry into the systemic circulation. However, glutamine is metabolized in mitochondria, yielding glutamate and ammonia, and glutamine-derived ammonia may interfere with mitochondrial function, leading to astrocyte dysfunction (Albrecht and Norenberg, 2006).

The increase in blood ammonia in advanced liver disease is a consequence of multiple factors. In addition to impaired metabolic function of the liver there is shunting of blood around the liver due to portal hypertension. Since muscle wasting is common in patients with hepatic failure, this contributes to ammonia accumulation because muscle is an important site for extrahepatic ammonia removal (Zieve, 1974).

Ammonia interferes with brain function at several sites, each of which can contribute to the development of encephalopathy. Hyperammonaemia may increase the cerebral uptake of neutral amino acids by enhancing the activity of the L-amino acid transporter at the blood–brain barrier. This hypothesis is supported by the observation that transport of tryptophan into the brain is increased by ammonia infusions. Elevated cerebral concentrations of the neutral amino acids (tyrosine, phenylalanine, and tryptophan) may affect the synthesis of other neurotransmitters such as dopamine, norepinephrine, and serotonin (James, 1979).

### Oxindole

Oxindole is a tryptophan metabolite formed by gut bacteria (via indol) that can cause sedation, muscle weakness, hypotension, and coma. Similar to ammonia, it is produced in the intestine and cleared by the liver. Cerebral concentrations of oxindole are increased 200 times in rats with acute liver failure, but this increase is ameliorated by treatment with oral neomycin (Carpenedo, 1998). Human studies demonstrate indole levels that are significantly higher in patients with overt HE and/or cirrhosis compared with controls. Additional work shows that indole and ammonia levels increase after placement of a TIPS. A small number of patients with deteriorating psychometric performance were demonstrated to have higher indole plasma concentrations compared with patients whose psychometric performance remained stable (Moroni, 1998; Riggio, 2010).

### Neurosteroids

Neurosteroids (allopregnanolone and tetrahydrodeoxycorticosterone) are endogenous neuroactive compounds that are metabolites of progesterone that exert potent selective positive allosteric effects on the GABA-A receptor complex (Ahboucha, 2006). Administration of these steroids induces behavioural effects, including sedation, which is obviously a property consistent with the neuronal inhibition associated with HE. Allopregnanolone levels, comparable to those found in brains with hepatic coma, are pathophysiologically relevant. In one report, allopregnanolone and pregnenolone (a neurosteroid precursor) concentrations were increased in the brains of patients with hepatic coma. Additionally, TGR5 (Gpbar-1) is a G-protein-coupled receptor typically found in the GI tract and immune cells; recent studies show that this receptor is also found in the brain and responds to allopregnanolone. The number of these receptors is decreased in the presence of ammonia and they may be involved in the pathogenesis of HE (Keitel, 2010).

### Catecholamine

Catecholamine-level derangements have been linked to altered amino acid metabolism in subjects with HE. In chronic liver failure, the plasma and brain concentrations of aromatic amino acids (AAAs) (phenylalanine, tryptophan, and tyrosine) are increased, while those of the BCAAs (valine, leucine, and isoleucine) are reduced (Morgan, 1978). Because these amino acids share a common carrier at the blood–brain barrier, decreases in plasma BCAA concentrations may result in an increase in AAA transport into the brain. A low molar ratio of plasma BCAA to AAA is a consistent finding in patients with cirrhosis and HE but is also observed in patients without encephalopathy. This ratio closely correlates with other indices of liver function and a decreased ratio implies seriously impaired hepatocellular function (Ferenci and Wewalka, 1978). Thus it appears unlikely that changes in the plasma concentrations of neutral amino acids contribute to the development of HE.

Cerebral dopamine concentrations in HE are usually within the normal range in both experimental animals and humans and depletion of brain dopamine in rats does not result in the induction of coma. Thus there is no firm evidence that impaired dopaminergic neurotransmission contributes to any appreciable extent to HE. However, some of the extrapyramidal symptoms that cirrhotic patients experience may be due to altered dopaminergic function (Cuilleret, 1980). Finally, another fairly consistent finding in animal models of acute and chronic liver failure is reduced norepinephrine concentrations in the brain. This decreased brain norepinephrine content is related to overactivity of noradrenergic neurotransmission, possibly induced by hyperammonaemia (Zieve, 1977). *Serotonin*, in elevated quantities, has been identified in animal models of HE; studies in rat models of liver failure using serotonin agonists or antagonists to alter hepatic encephalopathic progression have not supported a pathophysiological role for serotoninergic tone in the development of HE (Yurdaydin, 1990).

### Histamine

Histamine is well known to play a role in wakefulness and regulation of circadian rhythms. In autopsy studies of patients with cirrhosis and HE, H1 receptors in brain tissue demonstrated a higher density and lower affinity than those in control subjects. Upregulation of H1 receptors in the brain could contribute significantly to the clinical picture of HE. This raises the interesting question of whether treatment with selective H1 receptor antagonists could be of value in ameliorating the severity or progression of encephalopathy in liver failure (Lozeva, 2001).

### Melatonin

Melatonin has been implicated in abnormal sleep patterns which are common in patients with liver failure and are likely due to the presence of subclinical HE. There is good evidence that peak melatonin levels are displaced to later hours and overall levels are higher during daytime than in subjects with normal liver function (Steindl, 1995). This obviously has implications for the development and severity of HE.

## Impairment of neurotransmission

HE is characterized by biochemically induced alterations in neural membrane function (Raabe, 1992). These altered functional properties result in changes in the uptake of neurotransmitters, enzymatic activity, and expression of neurotransmitter receptors. A possible explanation for these changes may be alterations in neural membrane properties. Gross alterations in cerebral cortical membrane lipid composition (including a decrease in cholesterol, phosphatidylserine, sphingomyelin, and mono- and polyunsaturated fatty acids) and the annular membrane fluidity were documented in rats with experimentally induced HE (Swapna et al., 2006a, 2006b). Ammonia also can directly affect neuronal electrical activity by inhibiting the generation of both excitatory and inhibitory postsynaptic potentials.

### The GABA-A–benzodiazepine neurotransmitter system

A role has been proposed for increased tone of the inhibitory GABA-A–benzodiazepine neurotransmitter system in the development of HE (Schaffer, 1982). Multiple studies have looked at this neurotransmitter system in liver failure; however, in contrast to initial reports of an increase in GABA and benzodiazepine receptors on cortical membranes, subsequent studies yielded conflicting results. In most studies, GABA and benzodiazepine receptors and cerebral GABA concentrations are not significantly altered in subjects with HE.

## Oxidative stress

Oxidative stress plays a major role in cerebral ammonia toxicity and the pathogenesis of HE. Elevated oxidative stress markers (tyrosine-nitrated proteins, heat shock protein-27, and 8-hydroxyguanosine) have been identified in the brains of patients with cirrhosis and severe HE (Görg, 2010). Some studies have suggested a role of ammonia-induced oxidative stress and changes in mitochondrial permeability in the development of cellular swelling (Reinehr, 2007).

## Neurobehavioural studies

Memantine is a non-competitive N-methyl-D-aspartate (NMDA) receptor antagonist. Studies in rats with portacaval shunts that received ammonia infusions and in rats with acute hepatic failure due to liver ischaemia demonstrated that memantine was capable of improving clinical grading and EEG activity (Vogels et al., 1997b). Additionally, there were salutary effects on CSF glutamate concentrations, intracranial pressure, and brain water content. Memantine had no effect on ammonia concentrations in either animal model. In another study, different NMDA receptor antagonists, acting on different sites of NMDA receptors, prevented death in mice that underwent injection of ammonium acetate (Hermenegildo, 1996). These results suggest that NMDA receptor activation might be involved in the development of HE.

## Genetics

Certain patients appear to be more prone to HE than others, despite similar severity of liver disease. The reasons for such differences in susceptibility are not well understood. One study suggested that variation in the glutaminase gene may in part be responsible (Romero-Gómez, 2010). Patients who had a variant of the promoter region of the glutaminase gene associated with increased enzymatic activity were at greater risk of HE.

## Blood–brain barrier dysfunction

In patients with chronic liver disease without HE, studies have demonstrated an intact blood–brain barrier; however, there were significant changes in blood–brain transport in patients with HE (Horowitz, 1983). This is especially true of amino acid transport (see the section 'Catecholamine'). This alteration in the transport of amino acids, some of which are active neurotransmitters, may play a role in the development of HE (Chan, 2000). In addition, studies have demonstrated increased CNS uptake of various tracer substances in animal studies of liver failure. This non-specific change in blood–brain barrier permeability may permit exposure of the brain to many neurotoxins that would not normally pass into the CNS and may partially account for the development of HE and/or brain oedema.

Cerebral oedema occurs with acute hyperammonaemia in both animal models of HE and patients with cirrhosis and HE. Animal experiments have shown that portacaval shunted rats, but not control rats, developed encephalopathy associated with a significant increase in intracranial pressure after infusions with ammonium acetate (Jover, 2006). While both groups had equal elevations in blood and brain ammonia concentrations, brain and CSF concentrations of glutamine and AAAs were higher in the portacaval shunted rats. Inhibition of glutamine synthetase prevents brain swelling in rats infused with ammonia and inhibits cellular swelling in cultures of astrocytes incubated with ammonia (Blei and Larsen, 2004). Hence, brain oedema is likely related to an increase in intracellular osmolarity resulting from the metabolism of ammonia in astrocytes to form glutamine. These animal data were corroborated in human cirrhotic patients by in-vivo measurements using proton magnetic resonance spectroscopy to demonstrate a depletion of brain myoinositol (a sign of increased osmolarity) and increased brain glutamine concentrations (Häussinger, 2000).

It appears that vasodilatation may also contribute to the increase in intracranial pressure in acute liver failure. Elevated glutamate levels may excessively activate NMDA receptors which, in turn, may trigger nitric oxide synthetase (n-NOS) induction followed by increased NO production and subsequent vasodilation (Larsen, 2001).

Mild hypothermia may help prevent brain oedema in experimental acute liver failure by reducing the blood–brain transfer of ammonia and/or reduction of extracellular brain glutamate concentrations (Rose, 2000).

## References


Avolio AW, Agnes S, Peliosi G, et al. (1991) Intraoperative trends of oxygen consumption and blood lactate as predictors of primary dysfunction after liver transplantation. *Transplant Proc*, **23**:2263–2265.

Ahboucha S, Pomier-Layrargues G, Mamer O, Butterworth RF (2006) Increased levels of pregnenolone and its neuroactive metabolite allopregnanolone in autopsied brain tissue from cirrhotic patients who died in hepatic coma. *Neurochem Int*, **49**:372.

Álamo JM, Gómez MA, Pareja F, et al. (2006) Morbidity and mortality in liver retransplantation original research article. *Transplant Proc*, **38**(8):2475–2477.

Albrecht J, Norenberg MD (2006) Glutamine: a Trojan horse in ammonia neurotoxicity. *Hepatology*, **44**:788.

Allert N, Köller H, Siebler M (1998) Ammonia-induced depolarization of cultured rat cortical astrocytes. *Brain Res*, **782**:261.

Ardite E, Ramos C, Rimola A, et al. (1999) Hepatocellular oxidative stress and initial graft injury in human liver transplantation. *J Hepatol*, **31**:921.

Artz SA, Paes IC, Faloon WW (1966) Hypokalemia-induced hepatic coma in cirrhosis. Occurrence despite neomycin therapy. *Gastroenterology*, **51**:1046.

Azevedo LDLS, Stucchi RSB, d. Ataíde EC, Boin IFDF (2013) Assessment of causes of early death after twenty years of liver transplantation original research article. *Transplant Proc*, **45**(3):1116–1118.

Bassett ML, Mullen KD, Skolnick P, Jones EA (1987) Amelioration of hepatic encephalopathy by pharmacologic antagonism of the GABAA-benzodiazepine receptor complex in a rabbit model of fulminant hepatic failure. *Gastroenterology*, **93**:1069.

Biancofiore G, Bindi ML, Romanelli AM, et al. (2005) Fast track in liver transplantation: 5 years' experience. *Eur J Anaesthesiol*, **22**:584–590.

Bergqvist PB, Hjorth S, Apelqvist G, Bengtsson F (1997a) Potassium-evoked neuronal release of serotonin in experimental chronic portal-systemic encephalopathy. *Metab Brain Dis*, **12**:193.

Bergqvist PB, Hjorth S, Wikell C, et al. (1997b) p-Chloroamphetamine- and d-fenfluramine-induced brain serotonin release in experimental portal-systemic encephalopathy. *Metab Brain Dis*, **12**:229.

Blei AT (2001) *Helicobacter pylori*, harmful to the brain? *Gut*, **48**:590–591.

Blei AT, Larsen FS (1999) Pathophysiology of cerebral edema in fulminant hepatic failure. *J Hepatol*, **31**:771.

Carpenedo R, Mannaioni G, Moroni F (1998) Oxindole, a sedative tryptophan metabolite, accumulates in blood and brain of rats with acute hepatic failure. *J Neurochem*, **70**:1998.

Cauli O, Rodrigo R, Piedrafita B, et al. (2007) Inflammation and hepatic encephalopathy: ibuprofen restores learning ability in rats with portacaval shunts. *Hepatology*, **46**:514–519.

Chan H, Hazell AS, Desjardins P, Butterworth RF (2000) Effects of ammonia on glutamate transporter (GLAST) protein and mRNA in cultured rat cortical astrocytes. *Neurochem Int*, **37**:243.

Chui AKK, Shi LW, Rao ARN, et al. (2000) Primary graft dysfunction after liver transplantation Original Research Article. *Transplantation Proc*, **32**(7): 2219–2220.

Córdoba J, Blei AT (1996) Brain edema and hepatic encephalopathy. *Semin Liver Dis*, **16**:271–280.

Cuilleret G, Pomier-Layrargues G, Pons F, et al. (1980) Changes in brain catecholamine levels in human cirrhotic hepatic encephalopathy. *Gut*, **21**:565.

Fayek S, Mantipisitkul W, Rasetto F, Munivenkatappa R, Barth R, Philosophe B (2010) Valgancyclovir is and effective prophylaxis for cytomegalovirus disease in liver transplant recipients. *HPB*, **12**(10):657–663

Ferenci P (1994) Brain dysfunction in fulminant hepatic failure. *J Hepatol*, **21**:487.

Ferenci P, Wewalka F (1978) Plasma amino acids in hepatic encephalopathy. *J Neural Transm*, Suppl 1978:87.

Ferraz-Neto BH, Zurstrassen MPVC, Hidalgo R, et al. Donor liver dysfunction: application of a new scoring system to identify the marginal donor original research article. *Transplant Proc*, **39**(8):2516–2518.

Gabduzda GJ, Hall PW 3rd (1966) Relation of potassium depletion to renal ammonium metabolism and hepatic coma. *Medicine*, **45**:481.

Glanemann M, Langrehr J, Kaisers U (2001) Postoperative tracheal extubation after orthotopic liver transplantation. *Acta Anaesthesiol Scand*, **45**:333–339.

Glanemann M, Hoffmeister R, Neumann U (2007) Fast tracking in liver transplantation: which patient benefits from this approach? *Transplant Proc*, **39**:535–536.

Gonwa TA, Morris CA, Goldstein RM, Husberg BS, Klintmalm GB (1991) Long-term survival and renal function following liver transplantation in patients with and without hepatorenal syndrome—experience in 300 patients. *Transplantation*, **51**:428–430.

Görg B, Qvartskhava N, Bidmon HJ, et al. (2010) Oxidative stress markers in the brain of patients with cirrhosis and hepatic encephalopathy. *Hepatology*, **52**:256.

Gurusamy KS, Kumar Y, Davidson BR (2008) Methods of preventing bacterial sepsis and wound complications for liver transplantation. *Cochrane Database Syst Rev*, **4**:CD006660.

Häussinger D, Kircheis G, Fischer R, et al. (2000) Hepatic encephalopathy in chronic liver disease: a clinical manifestation of astrocyte swelling and low-grade cerebral edema? *J Hepatol*, **32**:1035.

Hermenegildo C, Marcaida G, Montoliu C, et al. (1996) NMDA receptor antagonists prevent acute ammonia toxicity in mice. *Neurochem Res*, **21**:1237.

Horowitz ME, Schafer DF, Molnar P, et al. (1983) Increased blood–brain transfer in a rabbit model of acute liver failure. *Gastroenterology*, **84**:1003.

Ikegami T (2012) Bacterial sepsis after living donor liver transplantation: the impact of early enteral nutrition. *J Am Coll Surg*, **214**(3):288–295

James JH, Ziparo V, Jeppsson B, Fischer JE (1979) Hyperammonaemia, plasma amino acid imbalance, and blood–brain amino acid transport: a unified theory of portal-systemic encephalopathy. *Lancet*, **2**:772.

Jiang H, Li B, Yan LN, Lu SC, Wen TF, Zhao JC (2007) Effect of intravenous glutamine-dipeptide fortified enteral nutrition on clinical outcomes in patients after liver transplantation: a prospective randomized controlled study. *Chin J Clin Nutr*, **15**(1):21–25.

Jiang T, Wang X, Yang AZ, Lu L, Zhang DH, Zhang RS (2011) Effects of omega-3 fish oil emulsion on changes in serum cytokines after liver transplantation. *J Clin Rehab Tissue Eng Res*, **15**(31):5726–5730.

Jover R, Rodrigo R, Felipo V, et al. (2006) Brain edema and inflammatory activation in bile duct ligated rats with diet-induced hyperammonemia: a model of hepatic encephalopathy in cirrhosis. *Hepatology*, **43**:1257.

Kaido T, Ogura Y, Ogawa K (2012) Effects of post-transplant enteral nutrition with an immunomodulating diet containing hydrolyzed whey peptide after liver transplantation. *World J Surg*, **36**(7):1666–1671.

Kalil AC, Freifeld AG, Lyden ER, Stoner JA (2009) Valganciclovir for *Cytomegalovirus* prevention in solid organ transplant patients: an evidence-based reassessment of safety and efficacy. *PLoS ONE*, **4**(5):e5512.

Kemmer N, Secic M, Zacharias V, Kaiser T, Neff GW (2007) Long-term analysis of primary nonfunction in liver transplant recipients original research article. *Transplant Proc*, **39**(5):1477–1480.

Keitel V, Görg B, Bidmon HJ, et al. (2010) The bile acid receptor TGR5 (Gpbar-1) acts as a neurosteroid receptor in brain. *Glia*, **58**:1794.

Langer G, Großmann K, Fleischer S, et al. (2012) Nutritional interventions for liver-transplanted patients. *Cochrane Database Syst Rev*, **8**:CD007605.

Larsen FS, Knudsen GM, Hansen BA (1997) Pathophysiological changes in cerebral circulation, oxidative metabolism and blood-brain barrier in patients with acute liver failure. Tailored cerebral oxygen utilization. *J Hepatol*, **27**:231.

Larsen FS, Gottstein J, Blei AT (2001) Cerebral hyperemia and nitric oxide synthase in rats with ammonia-induced brain edema. *J Hepatol*, **34**:548.

Lock JF, Schwabauer E, Martus P, et al. (2010) Early diagnosis of primary nonfunction and indication for reoperation after liver transplantation. *Liver Transplant*, **16**:172–180.

Lozeva V, Tuomisto L, Sola D, et al. (2001) Increased density of brain histamine H(1) receptors in rats with portacaval anastomosis and in cirrhotic patients with chronic hepatic encephalopathy. *Hepatology*, **33**:1370.

Lucey MR, Terrault N, Ojo L (2013) Long-term management of the successful adult liver transplant: 2012 practice guideline by the American Association for the Study of Liver Diseases and the American Society of Transplantation. *Liver Transpl*, **19**:3–26.

Mandell MS, Lezotte D, Kam I, Zamudio S (2002) Reduced use of intensive care after liver transplantation: influence of early extubation. *Liver Transplant*, **8**:676–681.

Mandell MS, Stoner TJ, Barnett R (2007) A multicenter evaluation of safety of early extubation in liver transplant recipients. *Liver Transplant*, **13**:1557–1563.

Morgan MY, Milsom JP, Sherlock S (1978) Plasma ratio of valine, leucine and isoleucine to phenylalanine and tyrosine in liver disease. *Gut*, **19**:1068.

Moroni F, Carpenedo R, Venturini I, et al. (1998) Oxindole in pathogenesis of hepatic encephalopathy. *Lancet*, **351**:1861.

Nanashima A, Pillay P, Verran DJ (2002) Analysis of initial poor graft function after orthotopic liver transplantation: experience of an Australian single liver transplantation center original research article. *Transplant Proc*, **34**(4):1231–1235.

O'Beirne JP, Chouhan M, Hughes RD (2006) The role of infection and inflammation in the pathogenesis of hepatic encephalopathy and cerebral edema in acute liver failure. *Nat Clin Pract Gastroenterol Hepatol*, **3**:118.

Playford EG, Webster AC, Craig JC, Sorrell TC (2004) Antifungal agents for preventing fungal infections in solid organ transplant recipients. *Cochrane Database Syst Rev*, **3**:CD004291.

Ploeg RJ, D'Alessandro AM, Knechtle SJ, et al. (1993) Risk factors for primary dysfunction after liver transplantation—a multivariate analysis. *Transplantation*, **55**:807–813.

Qiu Y, Zhu X, Wang W, Xu Q, Ding Y (2009) Nutrition support with glutamine dipeptide in patients undergoing liver transplantation. *Transplant Proc*, **41**(10):4232–4237

Raabe W (1992) Ammonium ions abolish excitatory synaptic transmission between cerebellar neurons in primary dissociated tissue culture. *J Neurophysiol*, **68**:93.

Raabe W (1993) Effects of hyperammonemia on neuronal function: $NH4^+$, IPSP and $Cl^{(-)}$-extrusion. *Adv Exp Med Biol*, **341**:71.

Reilly J, Mehta R, Teperman L, et al. (1990) Nutritional support after liver transplantation: a randomized prospective study. *J Parenteral Enteral Nutr*, **14**(4):386–391.

Reinehr R, Görg B, Becker S, et al. (2007) Hypoosmotic swelling and ammonia increase oxidative stress by NADPH oxidase in cultured astrocytes and vital brain slices. *Glia*, **55**:758.

Riggio O, Mannaioni G, Ridola L, et al. (2010)Peripheral and splanchnic indole and oxindole levels in cirrhotic patients: a study on the pathophysiology of hepatic encephalopathy. *Am J Gastroenterol*, **105**:1374.

Romero-Gómez M, Jover M, Del Campo JA, et al. (2010) Variations in the promoter region of the glutaminase gene and the development of hepatic encephalopathy in patients with cirrhosis: a cohort study. *Ann Intern Med*, **153**:281.

Rose C, Michalak A, Pannunzio M, et al. (2000) Mild hypothermia delays the onset of coma and prevents brain edema and extracellular brain glutamate accumulation in rats with acute liver failure. *Hepatology*, **31**:872.

Sarwar S, Carey B, Hegarty JE, McCormick PA (2013) Low incidence of *Pneumocystis jirovecii* pneumonia in an unprophylaxed liver transplant cohort. *Transplant Infect Dis*, **15**(5):510–515.

Shaked A, Nunes FA, Olthoff KM, Lucey MR (1997) Assessment of liver function: pre- and peritransplant evaluation. *Clin Chem*, **43**:8(B):1539–1545.

Silberhumer GR, Pokorny H, Hetz H, et al. (2007) Combination of extended donor criteria and changes in the Model for End-Stage Liver Disease score predict patient survival and primary dysfunction in liver transplantation: a retrospective analysis. *Transplantation*, **83**(5): 588–592.

Sirivatanauksorn Y, Taweerutchana V, Limsrichamrern S, et al. (2012) Analysis of donor risk factors associated with graft outcomes in orthotopic liver transplantation original research article. *Transplant Proc*, **44**(2):320–323.

Steindl PE, Finn B, Bendok B, et al. (1995) Disruption of the diurnal rhythm of plasma melatonin in cirrhosis. *Ann Intern Med*, **123**:274.

Strauss G, Hansen BA, Kirkegaard P, et al. (1997) Liver function, cerebral blood flow autoregulation, and hepatic encephalopathy in fulminant hepatic failure. *Hepatology*, **25**:837.

Swapna I, Kumar KV, Reddy PV, et al. (2006a) Phospholipid and cholesterol alterations accompany structural disarray in myelin membrane of rats with hepatic encephalopathy induced by thioacetamide. *Neurochem Int*, **49**:238.

Swapna I, Sathyasaikumar KV, Murthy ChR, et al. (2006b) Changes in cerebral membrane lipid composition and fluidity during thioacetamide-induced hepatic encephalopathy. *J Neurochem*, **98**:1899.

Taner CB, Willingham DL, Bulatao IG, et al. (2012) Is a mandatory intensive care unit stay needed after liver transplantation? Feasibility of fast-tracking to the surgical ward after liver transplantation. *Liver Transpl*, **18**:361–369.

Totsuka E, Fung JJ, Ishii T, et al. (2000). Influence of donor condition on postoperative graft survival and function in human liver transplantation; *Transplant Proc*, **32**:332–336.

Totsuka E, Fung U, Hakamada K, et al. (2004) Analysis of clinical variables of donors and recipients with respect to short-term graft outcome in human liver transplantation original research article. *Transplant Proc*, **36**(8):2215–2218.

Vogels BA, van Steynen B, Maas MA, et al. (1997a) The effects of ammonia and portal-systemic shunting on brain metabolism, neurotransmission and intracranial hypertension in hyperammonaemia-induced encephalopathy. *J Hepatol*, **26**:387.

Vogels BA, Maas MA, Daalhuisen J, et al. (1997b) Memantine, a noncompetitive NMDA receptor antagonist improves hyperammonemia-induced encephalopathy and acute hepatic encephalopathy in rats. *Hepatology*, **25**:820.

Wang EHZ, Patovi N, Levy RD, Shapiro RJ, Yoshida EM, Greanya ED (2012) Pneumocystis pneumonia in solid organ transplant recipients: not yet an infection of the past. *Transplant Infect Dis*, **14**:519–525.

Weissenborn K, Ahl B, Fischer-Wasels D, et al. (2007) Correlations between magnetic resonance spectroscopy alterations and cerebral ammonia and glucose metabolism in cirrhotic patients with and without hepatic encephalopathy. *Gut*, **56**:1736.

Yurdaydin C, Hörtnagl H, Steindl P, et al. (1990) Increased serotoninergic and noradrenergic activity in hepatic encephalopathy in rats with thioacetamide-induced acute liver failure. *Hepatology*, **12**:695.

Zhongwei Z, Lili C, Bo W, Xiaodong W, Goupeng L (2012) Newly defined clinical features and treatment experience of seventh day syndrome following living donor liver transplantation original research article. *Transplant Proc*, **44**(2):494–499.

Zieve L, Olsen RL (1977) Can hepatic coma be caused by a reduction of brain noradrenaline or dopamine? *Gut*, **18**:688.

Zieve L, Doizaki WM, Zieve J (1974) Synergism between mercaptans and ammonia or fatty acids in the production of coma: a possible role for mercaptans in the pathogenesis of hepatic coma. *J Lab Clin Med*, **83**:16.

## Suggested Reading

Baraldi M, Zeneroli ML, Ventura E, et al. (1984) Supersensitivity of benzodiazepine receptors in hepatic encephalopathy due to fulminant hepatic failure in the rat: reversal by a benzodiazepine antagonist. *Clin Sci*, **67**:167.

Basile AS, Gammal SH, Mullen KD, et al. (1988) Differential responsiveness of cerebellar Purkinje neurons to GABA and benzodiazepine receptor ligands in an animal model of hepatic encephalopathy. *J Neurosci*, **8**:2414.

Basile AS, Pannell L, Jaouni T, et al. (1990) Brain concentrations of benzodiazepines are elevated in an animal model of hepatic encephalopathy. *Proc Natl Acad Sci USA*, **87**:5263.

Basile AS, Hughes RD, Harrison PM, et al. (1991) Elevated brain concentrations of 1,4-benzodiazepines in fulminant hepatic failure. *N Engl J Med*, **325**:473.

Blei AT, Olafsson S, Therrien G, Butterworth RF (1994) Ammonia-induced brain edema and intracranial hypertension in rats after portacaval anastomosis. *Hepatology*, **19**:1437.

Bosman DK, Deutz NE, De Graaf AA, et al. (1990) Changes in brain metabolism during hyperammonemia and acute liver failure: results of a comparative 1H-NMR spectroscopy and biochemical investigation. *Hepatology*, **12**:281.

Bosman DK, van den Buijs CA, de Haan JG, et al. (1991) The effects of benzodiazepine-receptor antagonists and partial inverse agonists on acute hepatic encephalopathy in the rat. *Gastroenterology*, **101**:772.

Brokelman W, Stel AL, Ploeg RJ (1999) Risk factors for primary dysfunction after liver transplantation in the University of Wisconsin solution era original research article. *Transplant Proc*, **31**(5):2087–2090.

Butterworth RF (2000) The astrocytic ('peripheral-type') benzodiazepine receptor: role in the pathogenesis of portal-systemic encephalopathy. *Neurochem Int*, **36**:411.

Cangiano C, Cardelli-Cangiano P, James JH, et al. (1983) Brain microvessels take up large neutral amino acids in exchange for glutamine. Cooperative role of $Na^+$-dependent and $Na^+$-independent systems. *J Biol Chem*, **258**:8949.

Cauli O, Rodrigo R, Llansola M, et al. (2009) Glutamatergic and GABAergic neurotransmission and neuronal circuits in hepatic encephalopathy. *Metab Brain Dis*, **24**:69.

Chu CJ, Wang SS, Lee FY, et al. (2001) Detrimental effects of nitric oxide inhibition on hepatic encephalopathy in rats with thioacetamide-induced fulminant hepatic failure. *Eur J Clin Invest*, **31**:156.

Córdoba J, Cabrera J, Lataif L, et al. (1998) High prevalence of sleep disturbance in cirrhosis. *Hepatology*, **27**:339.

de Knegt RJ, Schalm SW, van der Rijt CC, et al. (1994) Extracellular brain glutamate during acute liver failure and during acute hyperammonemia simulating acute liver failure: an experimental study based on in vivo brain dialysis. *J Hepatol*, **20**:19.

Donovan JP, Schafer DF, Shaw BW Jr, Sorrell MF (1998) Cerebral oedema and increased intracranial pressure in chronic liver disease. *Lancet*, **351**:719.

Fan P, Szerb JC (1993) Effects of ammonium ions on synaptic transmission and on responses to quisqualate and N-methyl-D-aspartate in hippocampal CA1 pyramidal neurons in vitro. *Brain Res*, **632**:225.

Ferenci P, Pappas SC, Munson PJ, Jones EA (1984) Changes in glutamate receptors on synaptic membranes associated with hepatic encephalopathy or hyperammonemia in the rabbit. *Hepatology*, **4**:25.

Ferenci P, Püspök A, Steindl P (1992) Current concepts in the pathophysiology of hepatic encephalopathy. *Eur J Clin Invest*, **22**:573.

Fischer JE, Baldessarini RJ (1971) False neurotransmitters and hepatic failure. *Lancet*, **2**:75.

Goldbecker A, Buchert R, Berding G, et al. (2010) Blood–brain barrier permeability for ammonia in patients with different grades of liver fibrosis is not different from healthy controls. *J Cereb Blood Flow Metab*, **30**:1384.

Gonzalez FX, Rimola A, Grande L, et al. (1994) Predictive factors of early postoperative graft function in human liver transplantation. *Hepatology*, **20**:565.

Görg B, Qvartskhava N, Keitel V, et al. (2008) Ammonia induces RNA oxidation in cultured astrocytes and brain in vivo. *Hepatology*, **48**:567.

Grippon P, Le Poncin Lafitte M, Boschat M, et al. (1986) Evidence for the role of ammonia in the intracerebral transfer and metabolism of tryptophan. *Hepatology*, **6**:682.

Häussinger D, Roth E, Lang F, Gerok W (1993) Cellular hydration state: an important determinant of protein catabolism in health and disease. *Lancet*, **341**:1330.

Howard TK (1996) Postoperative intensive care management of the adult. In: Busuttil RW, Klintmalm GB (eds) *Transplantation of the Liver*, pp. 551–563. Saunders, Philadelphia.

James JH, Escourrou J, Fischer JE (1978) Blood–brain neutral amino acid transport activity is increased after portacaval anastomosis. *Science*, **200**:1395.

Jellinger K, Riederer P, Kleinberger G, et al. (1978) Brain monoamines in human hepatic encephalopathy. *Acta Neuropathol*, **43**:63.

Knecht K, Michalak A, Rose C, et al. (1997) Decreased glutamate transporter (GLT-1) expression in frontal cortex of rats with acute liver failure. *Neurosci Lett*, **229**:201.

Koller J, Wiesner C, Furtwangler W, et al. (1991) Orthotopic liver trans-plantation and perioperative clearance of lactate metabolism. *Transplant Proc*, **23**:1989–1990.

Krieger D, Krieger S, Jansen O, et al. (1995) Manganese and chronic hepatic encephalopathy. *Lancet*, **346**:270.

Laubenberger J, Häussinger D, Bayer S, et al. (1997) Proton magnetic resonance spectroscopy of the brain in symptomatic and asymptomatic patients with liver cirrhosis. *Gastroenterology*, **112**:1610.

Lockwood AH, Ginsberg MD, Rhoades HM, Gutierrez MT (1986) Cerebral glucose metabolism after portacaval shunting in the rat. Patterns of metabolism and implications for the pathogenesis of hepatic encephalopathy. *J Clin Invest*, **78**:86.

Mans AM, Biebuyck JF, Davis DW, et al. (1983) Regional cerebral glucose utilization in rats with portacaval anastomosis. *J Neurochem*, **40**:986.

Michalak A, Butterworth RF (1997) Selective loss of binding sites for the glutamate receptor ligands [3H]kainate and (S)-[3H]5-fluorowillardiine in the brains of rats with acute liver failure. *Hepatology*, **25**:631.

Michalak A, Rose C, Butterworth J, Butterworth RF (1996) Neuroactive amino acids and glutamate (NMDA) receptors in frontal cortex of rats with experimental acute liver failure. *Hepatology*, **24**:908.

Michalak A, Chatauret N, Butterworth RF (2001) Evidence for a serotonin transporter deficit in experimental acute liver failure. *Neurochem Int*, **38**:163.

Montes S, Alcaraz-Zubeldia M, Muriel P, Ríos C (2001) Striatal manganese accumulation induces changes in dopamine metabolism in the cirrhotic rat. *Brain Res*, **891**:123.

Moriyama M, Jayakumar AR, Tong XY, Norenberg MD (2010) Role of mitogen-activated protein kinases in the mechanism of oxidant-induced cell swelling in cultured astrocytes. *J Neurosci Res*, **88**:2450.

Moroni F, Lombardi G, Moneti G, Cortesini C (1983) The release and neosynthesis of glutamic acid are increased in experimental models of hepatic encephalopathy. *J Neurochem*, **40**:850.

Mousseau DD, Butterworth RF (1994) The [3H]tryptamine receptor in human brain: kinetics, distribution, and pharmacologic profile. *J Neurochem*, **63**:1052.

Nair S, Eustace J, Thuluvath PJ (2002) Effect of race on outcome of orthotopic liver transplantation: a cohort study original research article. *Lancet*, **359**(9303):287–293.

Norenberg MD (1996) Astrocytic-ammonia interactions in hepatic encephalopathy. *Semin Liver Dis*, **16**:245.

Norenberg MD, Huo Z, Neary JT, Roig-Cantesano A (1997) The glial glutamate transporter in hyperammonemia and hepatic encephalopathy: relation to energy metabolism and glutamatergic neurotransmission. *Glia*, **21**:124.

Oppong KN, Bartlett K, Record CO, al Mardini H (1995) Synaptosomal glutamate transport in thioacetamide-induced hepatic encephalopathy in the rat. *Hepatology*, **22**:553.

Otero-Raviña F, Rodríguez-Martínez M, Sellés CF (2005) Analysis of survival after liver transplantation in Galicia, Spain original research article. *Transplant Proc*, **37**(9):3913–3915.

Panickar KS, Jayakumar AR, Rama Rao KV, Norenberg MD (2007) Downregulation of the 18-kDa translocator protein: effects on the ammonia-induced mitochondrial permeability transition and cell swelling in cultured astrocytes. *Glia*, **55**:1720.

Park CS, Hwang S, Park HW (2012) Role of plasmapheresis as liver support for early graft dysfunction following adult living donor liver transplantation original research article. *Transplant Proc*, **44**(3):749–751.

Platz KP, Mueller AR, Schäfer C, Jahns S, Guckelberger O, Neuhaus P (1997) Influence of warm ischemia time on initial graft function in human liver transplantation original research article. *Transplant Proc*, **29**(8):3458–3459.

Püspök A, Herneth A, Steindl P, Ferenci P (1993) Hepatic encephalopathy in rats with thioacetamide-induced acute liver failure is not mediated by endogenous benzodiazepines. *Gastroenterology*, **105**:851.

Rama Rao KV, Jayakumar AR, Norenberg DM (2003) Ammonia neurotoxicity: role of the mitochondrial permeability transition. *Metab Brain Dis*, **18**:113.

Rao VL, Butterworth RF (1994) Alterations of [3H]8-OH-DPAT and [3H] ketanserin binding sites in autopsied brain tissue from cirrhotic patients with hepatic encephalopathy. *Neurosci Lett*, **182**:69.

Rao VL, Giguère JF, Layrargues GP, Butterworth RF (1993) Increased activities of MAOA and MAOB in autopsied brain tissue from cirrhotic patients with hepatic encephalopathy. *Brain Res*, **621**:349.

Remiszewski P, Kalinowski P, Dudek K, et al. (2011) Influence of selected factors on survival after liver retransplantation original research article. *Transplant Proc*, **43**(8):3025–3028.

Rose C, Butterworth RF, Zayed J, et al. (1999) Manganese deposition in basal ganglia structures results from both portal-systemic shunting and liver dysfunction. *Gastroenterology*, **117**:640.

Saija A, Princi P, Lanza M, et al. (1995) Systemic cytokine administration can affect blood-brain barrier permeability in the rat. *Life Sci*, **56**:775.

Saransaari P, Oja SS, Borkowska HD, et al. (1997) Effects of thioacetamide-induced hepatic failure on the N-methyl-D-aspartate receptor complex in the rat cerebral cortex, striatum, and hippocampus. Binding of different ligands and expression of receptor subunit mRNAs. *Mol Chem Neuropathol*, **32**:179.

Schafer DF, Jones EA (1982) Hepatic encephalopathy and the gamma-aminobutyric-acid neurotransmitter system. *Lancet*, **1**:18.

Schafer DF, Pappas SC, Brody LE, et al. (1984) Visual evoked potentials in a rabbit model of hepatic encephalopathy. I. Sequential changes and comparisons with drug-induced comas. *Gastroenterology*, **86**:540.

Steindl P, Püspök A, Druml W, Ferenci P (1991) Beneficial effect of pharmacological modulation of the GABAA-benzodiazepine receptor on hepatic encephalopathy in the rat: comparison with uremic encephalopathy. *Hepatology*, **14**:963.

Stockmann M, Lock JF, Riecke B, et al. (2009) Prediction of postoperative outcome after hepatectomy with a new bedside test for maximal liver function capacity. *Annal Surg*, **250**:119–125.

Suto H, Azuma T, Ito S, et al. (2001) *Helicobacter pylori* infection induces hyperammonaemia in Mongolian gerbils with liver cirrhosis. *Gut*, **48**:605.

Taner CB, Bathala V, Nguyen JH (2008) Primary nonfunction in liver transplantation: a single-center experience original research article. *Transplant Proc*, **40**(10):3566–3568.

Tisone G, Vennarecci G, Pisani F (1998) Reduced acute rejection and side effects with neoral in liver transplantation original research article. *Transplant Proc*, **30**(4):1430–1431.

Vardanian AJ, Busuttil RW, Kupiec-Weglinski JW (2008) Molecular mediators of liver ischemia and reperfusion injury: a brief review. *Mol Med*, **14**:337.

Wright G, Soper R, Brooks HF, et al. (2010) Role of aquaporin-4 in the development of brain oedema in liver failure. *J Hepatol*, **53**:91.

Yurdaydin C, Gu ZQ, Nowak G, et al. (1993) Benzodiazepine receptor ligands are elevated in an animal model of hepatic encephalopathy: relationship between brain concentration and severity of encephalopathy. *J Pharmacol Exp Ther*, **265**:565.

Yurdaydin C, Herneth AM, Püspök A, et al. (1996) Modulation of hepatic encephalopathy in rats with thioacetamide-induced acute liver failure by serotonin antagonists. *Eur J Gastroenterol Hepatol*, **8**:667.

Zimmermann C, Ferenci P, Pifl C, et al. (1989) Hepatic encephalopathy in thioacetamide-induced acute liver failure in rats: characterization of an improved model and study of amino acid-ergic neurotransmission. *Hepatology*, **9**:594.

# CHAPTER 24

# Perioperative management in live liver donor transplantation

Anand Sharma, Gyu-Sam Hwang, and Stuart Andrew McCluskey

## Introduction

Centres throughout the world have developed live liver donor programmes to offer a viable alternative or adjunct to deceased donor liver transplantation as the need for organs has increased well beyond supply. This innovative approach to organ procurement may be a tremendous benefit to the recipient population, but the very real risk of perioperative morbidity and mortality with donor hepatectomy must always be respected (Middleton et al., 2006). Donor safety is an ethically mandated necessity for live liver donor programmes and may be a major limiting factor in programme development and expansion (Trotter, 2005). Our objective in this chapter is to outline the perioperative management of the live liver donor for adult-to-adult transplantation. We will delineate the postoperative complications, identify areas where management has been changed based on clinical experience, and suggest areas for future investigation. Numerous international centres and the American National Institute of Health-sponsored Adult-to-Adult Living Donor Liver Transplantation Consortium in the US and Canada underscore the importance of this area of active investigation (Shah et al., 2005; Trotter, 2005; Barr et al., 2006; Hwang et al., 2006; Middleton et al., 2006).

## Donor assessment

Donors undergo a technically complex procedure with high risk and no direct benefit. This raises serious ethical issues such as first do no harm and non-maleficence (Gordon et al., 2011). Donor surgery carries a mortality risk of 0.15% (Trotter et al., 2006); hence thorough preparation is essential. Before potential donors are seen in the anaesthesia preadmission clinic they will have undergone extensive assessment and investigations by the liver transplant team, including health screening surveys, blood tests, viral serology, imaging studies, and independent medical and psychiatric assessments. In some centres, a BMI > 35 is a relative contraindication to surgery as it is associated with increased postoperative morbidity (Shah et al., 2006). Donor weight reduction has been found to be helpful to alleviate excessive hepatic steatosis.

Possible exclusion criteria include any medical condition that is considered to increase the risk of perioperative complications, ABO incompatibility, positive hepatic serology, underlying liver disease, inadequate graft size, steatosis > 10–15%, and abnormal anatomy making surgical resection impossible (Shah et al., 2006). However, ABO-incompatible live donor liver transplantation is now a feasible option in Asia after the outcomes in adults have noticeably improved with application of retuximab, an anti-CD20 antibody terminating B lymphocytes (Ikegami et al., 2009). In addition, the use of paired donor exchange allows for incompatible donor–recipient pairs to avoid the complications associated with ABO mismatches (Hwang et al., 2010). The liver resection plane is chosen to ensure that the residual weight to total liver weight is anticipated to be > 30%. While magnetic resonance imaging is very useful in the preoperative assessment of biliary anatomy, an intraoperative cholangiogram is repeated before the liver resection.

Anaesthesia management involves good communication with the surgical, physiotherapy, and rehabilitation teams for best results. It is important that, as anaesthesiologists, we understand the roles of other members of the team and try to complement their work while keeping the information we provide clear and understandable. Contradictions in patient assessment, management, or estimation of perioperative risk will only serve to confuse and frustrate donor candidates. Anaesthesiologists play an important role in patient care if donor outcome and donor satisfaction are to be improved to allow the greater utilization of this valuable resource.

Donors have reported shortcomings in the provision of medical information, particularly on postoperative recovery and potential complications (Cole et al., 1953; Gordon et al., 2011). In their systematic review of the available evidence Middleton et al. (2006) reported that 85% of donors felt that the information available to them was at least adequate, but at least one-third of patients felt that postoperative pain was worse than expected, the recovery longer, and the scar larger than expected based on the information provided to them preoperatively. This has encouraged the use of alternative techniques to disseminate the required information, including the use of websites compliant with international standards for quality of donor information. Consent forms should be written in a reading level of grade 5–8 to facilitate comprehension (Gordon et al., 2011, 2012).

Donors tend to be highly motivated and altruistic and may downplay information on risks (Gordon et al., 2011; Dimartini et al., 2012). While this may be a coping strategy, they should be given sufficient time and emotional space to deal with the information given to them (Weng et al., 2012). Individuals who seem unconcerned about the procedure during evaluation may be more severely traumatized by complications experienced by themselves or their recipients (Simpson et al., 2011). However, donor anxiety may contribute to delay in recovery. Preliminary data from Toronto suggest that the greater preoperative expectations for pain unpleasantness were correlated with greater postsurgical pain intensity and a longer hospital stay (Holtzman, personal communication, 2012).

Subjects who are ambivalent about donation or selected in a de-facto pattern may be at higher risk of adverse postoperative psychosocial outcomes (Simpson et al., 2011; Uehara et al., 2011; Dimartini et al., 2012; Simpson and Pomfret, 2012; Weng et al., 2012). These risks may be less in liver donors who receive a large amount of positive reinforcement (Simpson et al., 2011). However, more intense preoperative psychological evaluation is recommended to assess factors contributing to hesitancy to donate (Gordon et al., 2011). In addition, donors must undergo counselling and education, with possible postponement of the procedure until the issues are resolved (Dimartini et al., 2012).

## Preoperative anaesthesia assessment

The preoperative anaesthesia assessment should remain at arm's length from the donor selection process to ensure that the donor's best interests are served. While this independence from the live donor selection team can offer a potential donor access to unbiased information, it can also lead to donor anxiety and frustration if there are strong differences of opinion held by several groups involved in the preoperative assessment.

Some centres advocate extensive blood tests and investigations to rule out malignancies, abnormalities of coagulation, and lipid disorders (Kaneko et al., 2005; Nadalin et al., 2005; Bustelos et al., 2009). Certainly, direct relatives of recipients with inherited hepatic disorders should be carefully scrutinized. For example, ceruloplasmin levels should be measured in related donors for a patient with Wilson's disease.

## Intraoperative management

### Prophylactic therapy

An integral part of the anaesthetic management is ensuring that appropriate antibiotic and venous thromboembolic (VTE) prophylactic protocols are followed closely. Antibiotic prophylaxis includes a third-generation cephalosporin (e.g. Cefazolin) and metronidazole to cover potential anaerobic infections (Miller et al., 2004) administered at least 20 minutes before skin incision. VTE protocols include subcutaneous heparins or low-molecular-weight heparin with pneumatic compression stockings. There is very limited evidence for the effectiveness of these therapies in this population and both infection and VTE make up a considerable portion of the morbidity after hepatic resection (see Table 24.1). Some programmes have extended VTE prophylaxis well into the recovery period after discharge from hospital to decrease the rate of late VTE complications (Shah et al., 2005).

Intravenous heparin (1,000–5,000 IU) is administrated prior to donor graft perfusion and is used to prevent thrombosis in the liver graft (Adachi, 2003; Shah et al., 2005). Reversal of this heparin is often not required.

### Anaesthetic drugs

Anaesthetic agents are known to influence hepatic blood flow and this may influence the intraoperative management. Volatile anaesthetic agents may reduce hepatic blood flow as a result of reduced cardiac output and are themselves metabolized by the liver to varying degrees. While alternations in liver and renal function have been detected in patients undergoing liver resection for donation with various inhalational agents, no difference has been demonstrated in terms of clinical outcomes (Ko et al., 2010, 2012). The breakdown of volatile agents resulting in the production of hepatotoxic metabolites must also be kept in mind (Ko et al., 2010). The injury resulting from these effects is commonly manifested as an elevation of liver enzymes, an effect that is difficult to detect post-liver resection, given the usual rise in the enzymes with surgical dissection. However, desflurane has been reported to have less of an effect on the release of liver enzymes and synthetic function, but these results require further clarification and study (Ko et al., 2010). In contrast, similar to their effects on the heart, volatile agents have been shown to promote pharmacological preconditioning of the liver. This effect is theorized to be mediated by nitric oxide and is more pronounced in steatotic organs. Preconditioning is thought to attenuate liver injury and improves clinical outcome (Beck-Schimmer et al., 2008).

Though total intravenous anaesthesia (TIVA) with propofol is a safe technique to anaesthetize liver donors, hepatic elimination of the drug imposes a burden on the remaining liver. Patients anaesthetized using this method have higher bilirubin, PT, and creatinine in the postoperative period (Ko et al., 2008). In addition, more bleeding was noted during TIVA with propofol, possibly due to increased hepatic blood flow (Ko et al., 2008).

### Monitoring

Intraoperative monitoring routinely includes invasive arterial pressure monitoring. The use of a radial arterial catheter allows for repeat assessment of arterial blood and cardiac output assessment. Several monitors are available, including the PiCCO System (Pulsion Medical System, Munich, Germany), LiDCO plus System (LiDCO, Cambridge, UK), and Flotrac/Vigileo Monitor (Edwards Lifesciences, Irvine, California, US). The use of these monitors to guide fluid administration has not as yet been reported in this population; however, fluid therapy guided by non-invasive cardiac output monitoring has been reported in liver resection surgery (Solus-Biguenet et al., 2006). It may be possible to develop protocols using non-invasive cardiac output monitors for donor resection that improve patient outcome as they have been developed for other major abdominal surgery (Abbas and Hill, 2008). The use of cardiac output monitoring to guide fluid administration in the post-hepatectomy period may be particularly important to optimize cardiac output and preload while avoiding fluid overload and liver congestion.

Central venous access offers a number of advantages, including multiple ports for the administration of medication and electrolytes and careful management of CVP. CVP is often kept low (< 5 mmHg) during liver resection to reduce blood loss; however, the evidence to support this management is limited (see Table 24.2). In addition, the efficacy of 'low CVP technique' to

**Table 24.1** Postoperative complications in live liver adult-to-adult donors. Neurological complications include depression, neuropraxia, and postdural puncture headache; respiratory complications include aletectasis, pleural effusions, and pulmonary oedema; other infections include wound infections, urinary tract infections, and pneumonia; 'Other' relates to pressure sores, bowel obstruction, and prolonged ileus

| Reference | Number of patients | Overall number of complications | Severe [a] | LOS (days) | Mortality | Biliary | VTE | Neurological | Respiratory | Other infections | Other |
|---|---|---|---|---|---|---|---|---|---|---|---|
| Kim et al. 2012 | 500 | 108 (21.6%) | 47 (9.4%) | 12.5 ± 3.1 | 0 | 53 (11%) | | | | | |
| Abecassis et al. 2012 | 760 | 557 (73.2%) | 277 (36.4%) | | 3 | 62 (8%) | 13 (2%) | 26 (3%) | 99 (13%) | 121 (15.9%) | 51 |
| Salah et al. 2012 | 100 | 38 (38%) | 23 (23%) | 12.4 ± 9.1 | 1 | 20 (20%) | 1 (1%) | 2 (2%) | 9 (9%) | 10 (10%) | 15 (15%) |
| Salvalaggio et al. 2009 | 35 | 18 (51%) | 0 | 4.2 ± 1 | 0 | 5 (15%) | | 6 (18%) | 1 (3%) | | 6 (18%) |
| Marsh et al. 2009 | 121 | 24 (20%) | 13 (10.7%) | | 0 | 7 (5.8%) | 3 (3%) | | | 6 (5%) | 8 (7%) |
| Ghobrial et al. 2008 | 393 | 81 (21%) | 8 (2%) | | 3 (0.8%) | 36 (9%) | 2 (0.5%) | 16 (4%) | 21 (5%) | 71 (18%) | 21 (5%) |
| Patel et al. 2007 | 433 | 18 (51%) | 0 | 4.2 ± 1 | 1 (0.23%) | 5 (15%) | 0 | 6 (18%) | 3 (9%) | 0 | 3 (9%) |
| Chhibber et al. 2007[b] | 100 | 13 (13%) | 0 | 7.0 ± 1.5 | 0 | | | 5 (5%) | 3 (3%) | | 5 (5%) |
| Ozkardesler et al. 2008 | 101 | 24 (24%) | 11 (11%) | | 1 | 0 | 2 | 4 | 11 | 7 | 1 |
| Gruttadauria et al. 2008 | 75 | 23 (30.6%) | 23 (30.6%) | | | 7 | | | | | |
| Shah et al. 2005 | 100 | 37 (37%) | 0 | | 0 | 3 (3%) | 2 (2%) | | | 11 (11%) | 5 (5%) |
| Chan et al. 2006 | 30 | 5 (16.7%) | 0 | | | | | | 1 (3%) | 3 (9%) | 1 (3%) |
| Hwang et al. 2006 | 591 | | 29 (4.9%) | | 0 | 16 (2.7%) | | | | | 13 (2%) |
| Lo et al. 2004 | 100 | 27 (27%) | 10 (10%) | | 0 | 6 | 1 | 1 | 1 | 14 | 4 |
| Middleton et al. 2006 | 2,500 | (16.1%) | | | 10 (0.4%) | | | | | (5.8%) | |

[a] Severe complication is defined either by the authors or by the modified Clavien grade of > 2. Modified Clavien classification: grade 1, minor complications; grade 2, potentially life threatening; grade 3; life threatening; grade 4; leading to death.

[b] Limited to anaesthesia-related complications.

LOS, Length of hospital stay; VTE, venous thromboembolic.

minimize blood loss has recently been challenged in this otherwise healthy population. Kim et al. (2009) retrospectively reviewed nearly 1,000 liver donors and looked for predictors of blood loss. The only variables associated with intraoperative blood loss were patient gender, body weight, and fatty changes in the liver. Furthermore, Niemann et al. (2007) demonstrated that CVP monitoring did not appear to reduce blood loss when compared with patients without CVP monitoring and suggested that, in centres with extensive experience, CVP monitoring may not be necessary.

It should also be kept in mind that central venous access via the internal jugular or the subclavian vein is associated with its own morbidity such that placement of a peripheral central line may be a better option. A good correlation between centrally and peripherally placed CVP monitors has been reported, but others have questioned whether peripheral CVP lines can be placed precisely without the use of fluoroscopy (Choi et al., 2007a). External jugular venous measurement via a 16-gauge peripheral cannula has been shown to correlate well with CVP and display a clinically acceptable range (Abdullah et al., 2011).

## Fluid management

Dynamic preload indices (i.e. changes in cardiac output) are known to be more reliable than static measurements of preload to evaluate the fluid responsiveness in mechanically ventilated patients. SVV calculated using peripheral arterial waveforms represents cyclical variations in venous return. These indices of fluid responsiveness might also be used in the management of intraoperative fluids to minimize blood loss in much the same way as low CVP has been used to limit blood loss from the cut edge of the resected liver. Kim et al. (2011) demonstrated that a cutoff value of less than 6% for SVV represents increased intravascular volume status and was associated with increased blood loss during donor hepatectomy. This technique is promising as it relies on routine arterial access and may obviate the need for central access and its associated complications.

**Table 24.2** Evidence for the relationship between CVP and blood loss in liver resection (hepatectomy) and liver donation (donor)

| Reference | Study design | *n* | Population | Groups | Estimated blood loss (mL) (range) | RBC Tx n (%) |
|---|---|---|---|---|---|---|
| Niemann et al. 2007 | Observational, retrospective | 50 | Donor | CVP monitored (*n* = 31)<br>No CVP (*n* = 19) | 533 ± 337<br>357 ± 163 | 0<br>0 |
| Chhibber et al. 2007 | Observational, retrospective | 100 | Donor | CVP ≤ 5 $cmH_2O$ (*n* = 39)<br>CVP 5–10 $cmH_2O$ (*n* = 61) | 545 ± 320<br>550 ± 434 | |
| Wang et al. 2006 | RCT | 50 | HCC | CVP < 5<br>CVP control | 903.9 ± 180.8<br>2329.4 ± 2538.4[a] | 8 (32%)<br>14 (56%)[a] |
| Smyrniotis et al. 2004 | Observational, retrospective | 102 | Hepatectomy | CVP ≤ 5 $cmH_2O$ (*n* = 42)<br>CVP > 5 $cmH_2O$ (*n* = 60) | 420 (150–3100)<br>1150 (150–2850) | |
| Chen et al. 2000 | Observational, retrospective | 30 | Donor | 7.7 ± 2.8 $cmH_2O$<br>(4.1–14.5 $cmH_2O$) | 72.0 ± 58.9 (20–300)<br>No correlation with CVP | 0 |
| Jones et al. 1998 | Observational, retrospective | 100 | Hepatectomy | CVP ≤ 5 $cmH_2O$ (*n* = 40)<br>CVP > 5 $cmH_2O$ (*n* = 52) | 200 ml (median)<br>1000 ml (median)* | 2 (5%)<br>25 (48%)[a] |
| Johnson et al. 1998 | Observational, retrospective | 20 | Hepatectomy | CVP ≤ 5 $cmH_2O$ (*n* = 5)<br>CVP 6–12 $cmH_2O$ (*n* = 11)<br>CVP >12 $cmH_2O$ (*n* = 4) | 363 (305–465) ml<br>1259 (415–1789) ml*<br>2703 (2360–3450) ml* | |
| Melendez et al. 1998 | Observational, retrospective | 496 | Hepatectomy | CVP < 5 $cmH_2O$ | 848 ± 972 ml | (25%) |

[a] Statistically significant.

RBC Tx, Red blood cell transfusion.

As important as the amount of intravenous fluid is the type of fluid administered. The use of normal saline is known to be associated with a hyperchloraemic metabolic acidosis, but there is no compelling evidence that this has a detrimental effect on postoperative outcomes (Scheingraber et al., 1999; Williams et al., 1999). The use of Ringer's lactate is relatively contraindicated in liver surgery as lactate is metabolized mainly by the liver and its metabolism is impaired with liver resection and the disruption of hepatic blood flow. Serum lactate levels increase after hepatic resection and the addition of an exogenous racaemic lactate mixture in Ringer's lactate would seem inadvisable (Chhibber et al., 2007). Plasmalyte™, a buffer salt solution containing acetate and gluconate instead of lactate, may be used to avoid provocation of hyperlactaemia and hyperchloraemia. Shin et al. (2011) demonstrated lower donor postoperative lactate levels with Plasmalyte™ compared to Ringer's lactate, though no donor developed lactic acidosis. Interestingly, donors who received Plasmalyte™ had higher magnesium concentrations. A high postoperative lactate was shown not to be associated with hepatic dysfunction. However, those with insufficient liver volume who receive larger volumes of Ringer's lactate may well be at risk of complications associated with an exogenous lactate (D- and L-lactate) load.

Hydroxyethyl starch solutions have not been reported to be associated with adverse outcomes in the live liver donor and have displayed favourable outcomes in acute phase response in hepatectomies for cancer (Waters et al., 2012). However, caution with the use of hydroxyethyl starch solution is warranted given that there are effects on coagulation and renal function (Cittanova et al., 1996; Kozek-Langenecker, 2005; Blasco et al., 2008). Albumin solution (5%) can be administered for volume expansion immediately after hepatectomy, but there is no known benefit to its use in this population (Chhibber et al., 2007).

### Transfusion

Transfusion requirements for liver donation have gradually reduced with experience and advances in perioperative patient care (Shah et al., 2005; Middleton et al., 2006; Kim et al., 2012). Intraoperative blood loss is generally low, ranging from 72–2,000 mL with a median of 588 mL (Middleton et al., 2005), resulting in a transfusion rate of 1–5% (Jawan et al., 2005; Middleton et al., 2005; Patel et al., 2007). As a result, autologous blood transfusion is now rarely considered. Similarly, the intraoperative use of cell salvage may have limited benefit. However, its use offers few disadvantages and may be a reasonable choice in certain situations. Furthermore, having a cell salvage device readily available for unanticipated blood loss would seem prudent. The lack of effectiveness of acute normovolaemic haemodilution with reduced blood loss has led to the abandonment of this blood conservation modality in most centres (Adachi, 2003). Careful patient selection and consideration of current transfusion practice is the best guide for blood conservation efforts (Chan et al., 1998). Attempts to predict the need for blood transfusion in liver donor surgery will be exceptionally difficult as prediction rules for transfusion risk in liver resection surgery, where the risk of transfusion is 5–10 times higher, have been only modestly successful (Sima et al., 2009).

## Postoperative management

Patients are managed in the ICU or step-down units for the first 36–48 hours after surgery and then transferred to a regular surgical ward where daily assessment by the medical, surgical, and acute pain service continues until discharge. Patients are given parenteral magnesium and phosphate infusions until tolerating diet and then are transitioned to oral supplementation as required (Tan et al., 2003; Martin et al., 2005). Subcutaneous vitamin K (10 mg) is administered for the first 2–3 days after surgery depending on whether intraoperative intravenous vitamin K is given. The effects of vitamin K supplementation on postoperative coagulopathy are not known.

Platelet count reaches its nadir on postoperative day 2–3, while PT, INR, and aPTT reach their peaks on postoperative days 1–2 (Shah et al., 2005; Wang et al., 2006; Choi et al., 2007b). Other authors using thromboelastography have discovered a period of hypercoagulability following donor hepatectomy (Cerutti et al., 2004). Although only a small percentage of the overall population suffers from severe coagulation derangement, the use of epidural analgesia has been a subject of active debate because of the associated risk of epidural haematoma (Choi et al., 2007b). Thus intravenous patient-controlled analgesia and/or intrathecal morphine (Ko et al., 2009) and abdominal wall catheters infusing local anaesthetics (Hebbard, 2008; Niraj et al., 2009) have become alternatives for immediate postoperative pain control in live liver donors (Ko et al., 2009).

Pain management after liver resection is an important clinical consideration, particularly given that the incidence of inadequate postoperative pain control is reported to be as high as 81% (Wakata et al., 2011). Due to concerns with changes in postoperative coagulation profile the use of epidural analgesia is limited in many centres and patient-controlled intravenous analgesia is used more commonly. Using a numerical rating scale to assess postoperative discomfort, pain is rated as 4–6 out of 10, indicating moderate to severe postoperative pain (Clarke et al., 2011; Lee et al., 2012). However, opioid metabolism is slowed following liver resections, placing donors at risk of respiratory depression and oversedation (Beebe et al., 2011). Plasma morphine concentrations correlate with volume of liver removed, and given that up to 70% of a liver may be resected for donation this is particularly important (Rudin et al., 2007).

The use of non-steroidal analgesics is controversial as these agents have been implicated in postoperative bleeding. In many centres the use of these adjuncts is limited until the 2nd or 3rd postoperative day. However, the use of intravenous ketorolac when pain is adequately managed with intravenous morphine is of minimal benefit both in terms of the total dose of morphine required and the patient-reported pain score (Kao et al., 2012).

The oblique subcostal variant of the transversus abdominis plane (TAP) block has been described as a simple method to provide reliable analgesia for supra-umbilical incisions (Hebbard, 2008). Ultrasound-guided TAP blocks have been used with success in liver recipients (Milan et al., 2011) to reduce opiate consumption and allow early extubation. Placing catheters between the transversus abdominis and internal oblique plane, either by ultrasound (Niraj et al., 2009) or directly, affords the ability to prolong analgesia. The dangers of accidental liver perforation from catheter needles must be emphasized and will be limited by training and taking the appropriate precautions (Milan et al., 2011). Alternatively, abdominal catheters can be placed under direct vision as part of the surgical wound closure. Preliminary data from Toronto indicate that these abdominal wall catheters and the infusion of local anaesthetics can reduce intravenous narcotic requirements by as much as 40% (Hance Clarke, personal communication, presented at the ILTS Meeting 2012).

The use of acetaminophen, membrane-stabilizing agents (e.g. gabapentin), and alpha-2 agonists (e.g. clonidine and dexmedetomidine) should be agreed upon by anaesthesia and the attending surgical and medical teams. To date there is no published information that these agents are effective in management of postoperative pain in this population.

Liver regeneration occurs very rapidly in the donor, as assessed by volumetric magnetic resonance imagery (Marcos et al., 2000). Despite the regeneration of liver mass, the regeneration of functional liver, as assessed by indocyanine green pharmacokinetics, is somewhat slower (Niemann et al., 2002). The implications of the slower function recovery of the liver are unclear but should be kept in mind when prescribing medication dependent on liver metabolism for elimination.

There is significant impact on the liver donor even in the event-free case. Both physical and psychological measures and quality of life are negatively impacted for at least 3 months after surgery (Holtzman et al., 2009). Despite this impact on the donor's quality of life, the vast majority of donors would donate a second time if it were possible (Middleton et al., 2005; Chan et al., 2006; Holtzman et al., 2009). The issues of postoperative pain management and the incidence of chronic pain syndromes limiting return to baseline function need to be more thoroughly addressed.

## Donor morbidity and mortality

By far the most commonly used graft in adult-to-adult live donor liver transplant is the right lobe. This procedure can involve the removal of up to 70% of the donor liver. The use of the right lobe rather than the left reduces the risk of small-for-size graft syndrome in the recipient but imposes a potentially higher perioperative risk for the donor that must be appreciated and accounted for in the process of surgical consent (Salvalaggio et al., 2004; Middleton et al., 2005; Hwang et al., 2006). The use of the left lobe for adult-to-adult liver transplantation is still being considered in particular situations, but earlier experience with left lobe donation has not been favourable in adult-to-adult transplantation (Ben-Haim et al., 2001; Kanoh et al., 2002). When right lobe donation is not possible surgically, a Korean group has reported on the use of dual left lobe grafts from two living donors to work around the issue of small-for-size graft and secure the safety of the donor (Lee et al., 2001; Lee, 2010).

The incidence of postoperative morbidity and mortality is one of the first considerations for a potential liver donor. The second issue is the severity of the postoperative outcomes, and more recent publications have adopted the Clavien or modified Clavien grading system to allow for some objective assessment of the severity of postoperative complications (Clavien et al., 1994) (see Table 24.1). There is evidence that through optimization of donor selection and diligent patient care outcome is improving (Kim et al., 2012). However, it is sobering to keep in mind that deaths have been reported in the donor population with an incidence of 0.2–0.5% (Middleton et al., 2005; Trotter et al., 2006). Estimating the risk of mortality and morbidity from the literature is made more difficult by duplicate and underreporting of complications (i.e. reporting bias) (Table 24.1). The Adult to Adult Living Donor

Liver Transplantation Cohort Study (A2ALL) group reports the risk of complications at 40%, while the risk of death, liver failure, or residual disability is 1% (Abecassis et al., 2012). Biliary anastomotic leak and infection are the most common causes of morbidity (Wakata et al., 2011).

At least one intraoperative adverse event is reported in 50% of donors. The most common are hypothermia (39%), hypotension (26%), and blood product transfusion (17%) (Araz et al., 2012). These events are associated with increasing age, larger graft weight, low pH, and right hepatectomy.

There is an association between donor transfusion requirements and the development of the hypothermia. Donors who experienced intraoperative hypotension have a 48% higher risk of adverse events (Abecassis et al., 2012). Longer duration of surgery, younger age, lower body surface area, and urgent surgery are predictors of postoperative complications (Wakata et al., 2011). Diagnosed donor comorbidities appear to have no bearing on outcome. This is presumably because any such comorbidity is mild (Wakata et al., 2011).

Ninety-five percent of all complications resolve within 3 months; however, donors require 3–6 months to return to normal daily activity and 6–12 months for the liver volume and physical and mental quality of life to resume normal capacity (Wakata et al., 2011; Abecassis et al., 2012; Jin et al., 2012). Social function is better in donors more than 40 years of age, in a full-time occupation, and 2 years following surgery and is directly associated with the health of the recipient (Jin et al., 2012).

## Future areas of investigation

Regardless of live or cadaveric donor liver transplantation, ischemic reperfusion injury (I/R) is inevitable and is one of the main causes of postoperative hepatic dysfunction. Protective strategies against I/R vary from pharmacological to surgical techniques. Studies using ischaemic preconditioning by an inflow occlusion technique, i.e. the Pringle manoeuvre, have shown a protective role against I/R in deceased donor liver transplantation (Koneru et al., 2005, 2007). Although live donor liver transplantation has many advantages in regard to warm/cold ischaemic time, prevention of I/R can be a challenging issue, particularly in marginal grafts (i.e. older age donor and/or fatty liver) even in live donors, and needs to be further investigated in the future.

The use of live donors in the case of acute liver failure poses an additional challenge but has been conducted safely with good outcomes (Viana et al., 2008). A process has to be put in place to expedite preoperative evaluation, and the effectiveness of this process for both donor and recipient needs to be evaluated.

Surgical alternatives to conventional techniques are emerging. Upper midline incisions have been used (Lee et al., 2011). Hand-assisted laparoscopies, including methods with relatively small midline incisions, are now safer as experience improves (Berloco et al., 2011; Soyama et al., 2012). Single port laparoscopic-assisted right hepatectomy has been demonstrated to be associated with early discharge and better postoperative liver function tests (Choi et al., 2012). This presumably translates into better graft survival. There is a growing pressure to limit donor mortality and morbidity by using left lobe donation as frequently as possible. Small-for-size syndromes can be reduced by portal flow modulations and concomitant splenectomy in the recipient (Soejima et al., 2012).

Postoperative pain management in this valuable patient population should remain a priority consideration for clinical research. Not only is this research essential if we are to optimize clinical care, but also it offers a unique perspective on the relationship between acute and persistent postoperative pain. Similarly, live liver donors can serve as an excellent study population to establish whether surgical technique may attenuate postoperative pain. There is evidence that the type of surgical incision, i.e. upper midline compared to subcostal, can modify postoperative pain, but the comparative safety and efficacy of both needs to be further evaluated (Kim et al., 2009).

## Conclusion

We would like to echo the call of others for a worldwide outcome database for live liver donors so that changes in management can be guided by evidence and potential donor candidates given accurate risk assessments (Middleton et al., 2006; Mulligan, 2006; Trotter et al., 2006). As the number of cases of live donor liver transplantation increases worldwide, donor safety remains a critical concern.

## References

Abbas SM, Hill AG (2008) Systematic review of the literature for the use of oesophageal Doppler monitor for fluid replacement in major abdominal surgery. *Anaesthesia*, **63**(1):44–51.

Abdullah MH, Soliman HD, Morad WS (2011) External jugular venous pressure as an alternative to conventional central venous pressure in right lobe donor hepatectomies. *Exp Clin Transplant*, **9**(6):393–398.

Abecassis MM, Fisher RA, Olthoff KM, et al. (2012) Complications of living donor hepatic lobectomy—a comprehensive report. *Am J Transplant*, **12**(5):1208–1217.

Adachi T (2003) Anesthetic principles in living-donor liver transplantation at Kyoto University Hospital: experiences of 760 cases. *J Anesth*, **17**(2):116–124.

Araz C, Pirat A, Unlukaplan A, et al. (2012) Incidence and risk factors of intraoperative adverse events during donor lobectomy for living-donor liver transplantation: a retrospective analysis. *Exp Clin Transplant*, **10**(2):125–131.

Barr ML, Belghiti J, Villamil FG, et al. (2006) A report of the Vancouver Forum on the care of the live organ donor: lung, liver, pancreas, and intestine data and medical guidelines. *Transplantation*, **81**(10):1373–1385.

Beck-Schimmer B, Breitenstein S, Urech S, et al. (2008) A randomized controlled trial on pharmacological preconditioning in liver surgery using a volatile anesthetic. *Ann Surg*, **248**(6):909–918.

Beebe D, Singh H, Jochman J, et al. (2011) Anesthetic complications including two cases of postoperative respiratory depression in living liver donor surgery. *J Anaesthesiol Clin Pharmacol*, **27**(3):362–366.

Ben-Haim M, Emre S, Fishbein TM, et al. (2001) Critical graft size in adult-to-adult living donor liver transplantation: impact of the recipient's disease. *Liver Transplant*, **7**(11):948–953.

Berloco PB, Lai Q, Levi Sandri GB, et al. (2011) Laparoscopy in solid organ transplantation: a comprehensive review of the literature. *G Chir*, **32**(6-7):293–306.

Blasco V, Leone M, Antonini F, Geissler A, Albanese J, Martin C (2008) Comparison of the novel hydroxyethylstarch 130/0.4 and hydroxyethylstarch 200/0.6 in brain-dead donor resuscitation on renal function after transplantation. *Br J Anaesth*, **100**(4):504–508.

Bustelos R, Ayala R, Martinez J, et al. (2009) Living donor liver transplantation: usefulness of hemostatic and prothrombotic screening in potential donors. *Transplant Proc*, **41**(9):3791–3795.

Cerutti E, Stratta C, Romagnoli R, et al. (2004) Thromboelastogram monitoring in the perioperative period of hepatectomy for adult living liver donation. *Liver Transplant*, **10**(2):289–294.

Chan AC, Blumgart LH, Wuest DL, Melendez JA, Fong Y (1998) Use of preoperative autologous blood donation in liver resections for colorectal metastases. *Am J Surg*, **175**(6):461–465.

Chan SC, Liu CL, Lo CM, Lam BK, Lee EW, Fan ST (2006) Donor quality of life before and after adult-to-adult right liver live donor liver transplantation. *Liver Transplant*, **12**(10):1529–1536.

Chen CL, Chen YS, de Villa VH, et al. (2000) Minimal blood loss living donor hepatectomy. *Transplantation*, **69**(12):2580–2586.

Chhibber A, Dziak J, Kolano J, Norton JR, Lustik S (2007) Anesthesia care for adult live donor hepatectomy: our experiences with 100 cases. *Liver Transplant*, **13**(4):537–542.

Choi HJ, You YK, Na GH, Hong TH, Shetty GS, Kim DG (2012) Single-port laparoscopy-assisted donor right hepatectomy in living donor liver transplantation: sensible approach or unnecessary hindrance? *Transplant Proc*, **44**(2):347–352.

Choi SJ, Gwak MS, Ko JS (2007a) Can peripheral venous pressure be an alternative to central venous pressure during right hepatectomy in living donors? *Liver Transplant*, **13**(10):1414–1421.

Choi SJ, Gwak MS, Ko JS, et al. (2007b) The changes in coagulation profile and epidural catheter safety for living liver donors: a report on 6 years of our experience. *Liver Transplant*, **13**(1):62–70.

Cittanova ML, Leblanc I, Legendre C, Mouquet C, Riou B, Coriat P (1996) Effect of hydroxyethylstarch in brain-dead kidney donors on renal function in kidney-transplant recipients. *Lancet*, **348**(9042):1620–1622.

Clarke H, Chandy T, Srinivas C, et al. (2011) Epidural analgesia provides better pain management after live liver donation: a retrospective study. *Liver Transplant*, **17**(3):315–323.

Clavien PA, Camargo CA Jr, Croxford R, Langer B, Levy GA, Greig PD (1994) Definition and classification of negative outcomes in solid organ transplantation. Application in liver transplantation. *Annal Surg*, **220**(2):109–120.

Cole BT, Penrod KE, Hall FG (1953) The hematocrit and hemoglobin response of blood donors. *J Aviation Med*, **24**:227–229.

Dimartini A, Cruz RJ Jr, Dew MA, et al. (2012) Motives and decision making of potential living liver donors: comparisons between gender, relationships and ambivalence. *Am J Transplant*, **12**(1):136–151.

Ghobrial RM, Freise CE, Trotter JF, et al. (2008) Donor morbidity after living donation for liver transplantation. *Gastroenterology*, **135**(2):468–476.

Gordon EJ, Daud A, Caicedo JC, et al. (2011) Informed consent and decision-making about adult-to-adult living donor liver transplantation: a systematic review of empirical research. *Transplant*, **92**(12):1285–1296.

Gordon EJ, Bergeron A, McNatt G, Friedewald J, Abecassis MM, Wolf MS (2012) Are informed consent forms for organ transplantation and donation too difficult to read? *Clin Transplant*, **26**(2):275–283.

Gruttadauria S, Marsh JW, Vizzini GB, et al. (2008) Analysis of surgical and perioperative complications in seventy-five right hepatectomies for living donor liver transplantation. *World J Gastroenterol*, **14**(20):3159–3164.

Hebbard P (2008) Subcostal transversus abdominis plane block under ultrasound guidance. *Anesth Analg*, **106**(2):674–675.

Holtzman S, Adcock L, Dubay DA, et al. (2009) Financial, vocational, and interpersonal impact of living liver donation. *Liver Transplant*, **15**(11):1435–1442.

Hwang S, Lee SG, Lee YJ, et al. (2006) Lessons learned from 1,000 living donor liver transplantations in a single center: how to make living donations safe. *Liver Transplant*, **12**(6):920–927.

Hwang S, Lee SG, Moon DB, et al. (2010) Exchange living donor liver transplantation to overcome ABO incompatibility in adult patients. *Liver Transplant*, **16**(4):482–490.

Ikegami T, Taketomi A, Soejima Y, et al. (2009) Rituximab, IVIG, and plasma exchange without graft local infusion treatment: a new protocol in ABO incompatible living donor liver transplantation. *Transplantation*, **88**(3):303–307.

Jawan B, Cheng YF, Tseng CC, et al. (2005) Effect of autologous blood donation on the central venous pressure, blood loss and blood transfusion during living donor left hepatectomy. *World J Gastroenterol*, **1**(27):4233–4236.

Jin SG, Xiang B, Yan LN, et al. (2012) Quality of life and psychological outcome of donors after living donor liver transplantation. *World J Gastroenterol*, **18**(2):182–187.

Johnson M, Mannar R, Wu AV (1998) Correlation between blood loss and inferior vena caval pressure during liver resection. *Br J Surg*, **85**(2):188–190.

Jones RM, Moulton CE, Hardy KJ (1998) Central venous pressure and its effect on blood loss during liver resection. *Br J Surg*, **85**(8):1058–1060.

Kaneko J, Sugawara Y, Tamura S, et al. (2005) Coagulation and fibrinolytic profiles and appropriate use of heparin after living-donor liver transplantation. *Clin Transplant*, **19**(6):804–809.

Kanoh K, Nomoto K, Shimura T, Shimada M, Sugimachi K, Kuwano H (2002) A comparison of right-lobe and left-lobe graft for living-donor liver transplantation. *Hepatogastroenterology*, **49**(43):222–224.

Kao CW, Wu SC, Lin KC, et al. (2012) Pain management of living liver donors with morphine with or without ketorolac. *Transplant Proc*, **44**(2):360–362.

Kim SH, Cho SY, Lee KW, Park SJ, Han SS (2009) Upper midline incision for living donor right hepatectomy. *Liver Transplant*, **15**(2):193–198.

Kim SJ, Na GH, Choi HJ, Yoo YK, Kim DG (2012) Surgical outcome of right liver donors in living donor liver transplantation: single-center experience with 500 cases. *J Gastrointest Surg*, **16**(6):1160–1170.

Kim YK, Chin JH, Kang SJ, et al. (2009) Association between central venous pressure and blood loss during hepatic resection in 984 living donors. *Acta Anaesthesiol Scand*, **53**(5):601–606.

Kim YK, Shin WJ, Song JG, Jun IG, Hwang GS (2011) Does stroke volume variation predict intraoperative blood loss in living right donor hepatectomy? *Transplant Proc*, **43**(5):1407–1411.

Ko JS, Gwak MS, Choi SJ, et al. (2008) The effects of desflurane and propofol-remifentanil on postoperative hepatic and renal functions after right hepatectomy in liver donors. *Liver Transplant*, **14**(8):1150–1158.

Ko JS, Choi SJ, Gwak MS, et al. (2009) Intrathecal morphine combined with intravenous patient-controlled analgesia is an effective and safe method for immediate postoperative pain control in live liver donors. *Liver Transplant*, **15**(4):381–389.

Ko JS, Gwak MS, Choi SJ, et al. (2010) The effects of desflurane and sevoflurane on hepatic and renal functions after right hepatectomy in living donors. *Transplant Int*, **23**(7):736–744.

Ko JS, Kim G, Shin YH, et al. (2012) The effects of desflurane and isoflurane on hepatic and renal functions after right hepatectomy in living donors. *Transplant Proc*, **44**(2):442–444.

Koneru B, Fisher A, He Y, et al. (2005) Ischemic preconditioning in deceased donor liver transplantation: a prospective randomized clinical trial of safety and efficacy. *Liver Transplant*, **11**(2):196–202.

Koneru B, Shareef A, Dikdan G, et al. (2007) The ischemic preconditioning paradox in deceased donor liver transplantation-evidence from a prospective randomized single blind clinical trial. *Am J Transplant*, **7**(12):2788–2796.

Kozek-Langenecker SA (2005) Effects of hydroxyethyl starch solutions on hemostasis. *Anesthesiology*, **103**(3):654–660.

Lee KW, Kim SH, Han SS, et al. (2011) Use of an upper midline incision for living donor partial hepatectomy: a series of 143 consecutive cases. *Liver Transplant*, **17**(8):969–975.

Lee SG (2010) Living-donor liver transplantation in adults. *Br Med Bull*, **94**:33–48.

Lee SG, Hwang S, Park KM, et al. (2001) Seventeen adult-to-adult living donor liver transplantations using dual grafts. *Transplant Proc*, **33**(7-8):3461–3463.

Lee SH, Lim KC, Jeon MK, et al. (2012) Postoperative pain and influencing factors among living liver donors. *Transplant Proc*, **44**(2):363–365.

Lo CM, Fan ST, Liu CL, et al. (2004) Lessons learned from one hundred right lobe living donor liver transplants. *Ann Surg*, **240**(1):151–158.

Marcos A, Fisher RA, Ham JM, et al. (2000) Liver regeneration and function in donor and recipient after right lobe adult to adult living donor liver transplantation. *Transplant*, **69**(7):1375–1379.

Marsh JW, Gray E, Ness R, Starzl TE (2009) Complications of right lobe living donor liver transplantation. *J Hepatol*, **51**(4):715–724.

Martin GS, Moss M, Wheeler AP, Mealer M, Morris JA, Bernard GR (2005) A randomized, controlled trial of furosemide with or without albumin in hypoproteinemic patients with acute lung injury. *Crit Care Med*, **33**(8):1681–1687.

Melendez JA, Arslan V, Fischer ME, et al. (1998) Perioperative outcomes of major hepatic resections under low central venous pressure anesthesia: blood loss, blood transfusion, and the risk of postoperative renal dysfunction. *J Am Coll Surg*, **187**(6):620–625.

Middleton PF, Duffield M, Lynch SV, et al. (2006) Living donor liver transplantation—adult donor outcomes: a systematic review. *Liver Transplant*, **12**(1):24–30.

Milan ZB, Duncan B, Rewari V, Kocarev M, Collin R (2011) Subcostal transversus abdominis plane block for postoperative analgesia in liver transplant recipients. *Transplant Proc*, **43**(7):2687–2690.

Miller C, Florman S, Kim-Schluger L, et al. (2004) Fulminant and fatal gas gangrene of the stomach in a healthy live liver donor. *Liver Transplant*, **10**(10):1315–1319.

Mulligan DC (2006) A worldwide database for living donor liver transplantation is long overdue. *Liver Transplant*, **12**(10):1443–1444.

Nadalin S, Malago M, Valentin-Gamazo C, et al. (2005) Preoperative donor liver biopsy for adult living donor liver transplantation: risks and benefits. *Liver Transplant*, **11**(8):980–986.

Niemann CU, Roberts JP, Ascher NL, Yost CS (2002) Intraoperative hemodynamics and liver function in adult-to-adult living liver donors. *Liver Transplant*, **8**(12):1126–1132.

Niemann CU, Feiner J, Behrends M, Eilers H, Ascher NL, Roberts JP (2007) Central venous pressure monitoring during living right donor hepatectomy. *Liver Transplant*, **13**(2):266–271.

Niraj G, Kelkar A, Fox AJ (2009) Oblique sub-costal transversus abdominis plane (TAP) catheters: an alternative to epidural analgesia after upper abdominal surgery. *Anaesthesia*, **64**(10):1137–1140.

Ozkardesler S, Ozzeybek D, Alaygut E, et al. (2008) Anesthesia-related complications in living liver donors: the experience from one center and the reporting of one death. *Am J Transplant*, **8**(10):2106–2110.

Patel S, Orloff M, Tsoulfas G, et al. (2007) Living-donor liver transplantation in the United States: identifying donors at risk for perioperative complications. *Am J Transplant*, **7**(10):2344–2349.

Rudin A, Lundberg JF, Hammarlund-Udenaes M, Flisberg P, Werner MU (2007) Morphine metabolism after major liver surgery. *Anesth Analg*, **104**(6):1409–1414.

Salah T, Sultan AM, Fathy OM, et al. (2012) Outcome of right hepatectomy for living liver donors: a single Egyptian center experience. *J Gastrointest Surg*, **16**(6):1181–1188.

Salvalaggio PR, Baker TB, Koffron AJ, et al. (2004) Comparative analysis of live liver donation risk using a comprehensive grading system for severity. *Transplant*, **77**(11):1765–1767.

Scheingraber S, Rehm M, Sehmisch C, Finsterer U (1999) Rapid saline infusion produces hyperchloremic acidosis in patients undergoing gynecologic surgery. *Anesthesiology*, **90**(5):1265–1270.

Shah SA, Grant DR, Greig PD, et al. (2005) Analysis and outcomes of right lobe hepatectomy in 101 consecutive living donors. *Am J Transplant*, **5**(11):2764–2769.

Shah SA, Levy GA, Adcock LD, Gallagher G, Grant DR (2006) Adult-to-adult living donor liver transplantation. *Can J Gastroenterol*, **20**(5):339–343.

Shin WJ, Kim YK, Bang JY, Cho SK, Han SM, Hwang GS (2011) Lactate and liver function tests after living donor right hepatectomy: a comparison of solutions with and without lactate. *Acta Anaesthesiol Scand*, **55**(5):558–564.

Sima CS, Jarnagin WR, Fong Y, et al. (2009) Predicting the risk of perioperative transfusion for patients undergoing elective hepatectomy. *Ann Surg*, **250**(6):914–921.

Simpson MA, Pomfret EA (2012) Searching for the optimal living liver donor psychosocial evaluation. *Am J Transplant*, **12**(1):7–8.

Simpson MA, Kendrick J, Verbesey JE, et al. (2011) Ambivalence in living liver donors. *Liver Transplant*, **17**(10):1226–1233.

Smyrniotis V, Kostopanagiotou G, Theodoraki K, Tsantoulas D, Contis JC (2004) The role of central venous pressure and type of vascular control in blood loss during major liver resections. *Am J Surg*, **187**(3):398–402.

Soejima Y, Shirabe K, Taketomi A, et al. (2012) Left lobe living donor liver transplantation in adults. *Am J Transplant*, **12**(7):1877–1885.

Solus-Biguenet H, Fleyfel M, Tavernier B, et al. (2006) Non-invasive prediction of fluid responsiveness during major hepatic surgery. *Br J Anaesth*, **97**(6):808–816.

Soyama A, Takatsuki M, Hidaka M, et al. (2012) Standardized less invasive living donor hemihepatectomy using the hybrid method through a short upper midline incision. *Transplant Proc*, **44**(2):353–355.

Spiess BD, Royston D, Levy JH, et al. (2004) Platelet transfusions during coronary artery bypass graft surgery are associated with serious adverse outcomes. *Transfusion*, **44**(8):1143–1148.

Tan HP, Madeb R, Kovach SJ, et al. (2003) Hypophosphatemia after 95 right-lobe living-donor hepatectomies for liver transplantation is not a significant source of morbidity. *Transplant*, **76**(7):1085–1088.

Trotter JF (2005) Living donor liver transplantation: is the hype over? *J Hepatol*, **42**(1):20–25.

Trotter JF, Adam R, Lo CM, Kenison J (2006) Documented deaths of hepatic lobe donors for living donor liver transplantation. *Liver Transplant*, **12**(10):1485–1488.

Uehara M, Hayashi A, Murai T, Noma S (2011) Psychological factors influencing donors' decision-making pattern in living-donor liver transplantation. *Transplantation*, **92**(8):936–942.

Viana CF, Rocha TD, Cavalcante FP, Valenca JT Jr, Coelho GR, Garcia JH (2008) Liver transplantation for acute liver failure: a 5 years' experience. *Arq Gastroenterol*, **45**(3):192–194.

Wakata Y, Nakashima N, Taketomi A, Shirabe K, Maehara Y, Hagihara A (2011) Factors associated with the postoperative status of donor patients for living donor liver transplantation. *Liver Transplant*, **17**(12):1412–1419.

Wang WD, Liang LJ, Huang XQ, Yin XY (2006) Low central venous pressure reduces blood loss in hepatectomy. *World J Gastroenterol*, **12**(6):935–939.

Waters JH, Yazer M, Chen YF, Kloke J (2012) Blood salvage and cancer surgery: a meta-analysis of available studies. *Transfusion*, **52**(10):2167–2173.

Weng LC, Huang HL, Wang YW, Chang CL, Tsai CH, Lee WC (2012) The coping experience of Taiwanese male donors in living donor liver transplantation. *Nurs Res*, **61**(2):141–147.

Williams EL, Hildebrand KL, McCormick SA, Bedel MJ (1999) The effect of intravenous lactated Ringer's solution versus 0.9% sodium chloride solution on serum osmolality in human volunteers. *Anesth Analg*, **88**(5):999–1003.

# CHAPTER 25

# Paediatric liver transplantation: assessment and intraoperative care

James Bennett and Peter Bromley

## Introduction

About 8% of all liver grafts are performed in children. One-year survival after transplantation for most indications is more than 90% and long-term quality of life is good (McKiernan, 2011). Although results are comparable to those in adults, there are substantial differences between paediatric and adult practice: the causes and manifestations of both acute and chronic liver failure are distinct; size-matched donor organs are few, so techniques such as reduced and split-liver grafting and living-related liver transplantation are used much more often; technical problems related to small size and congenital anomalies are common; while physiological responses and post-transplant complications vary widely with age and indication. Moreover, the ethical and psychosocial issues encountered in children are often unique. Liver transplantation in children is a distinct subspecialty and requires the full range of specialist services available in a dedicated paediatric unit.

## Indications for liver transplantation in children

Indications for liver transplantation in children are shown in Table 25.1. Neonatal haemochromatosis presents in the first days of life and is the commonest cause of ALF in the newborn. Biliary atresia presents in the first few weeks of life, progresses slowly into a chronic condition of infancy, and is the commonest indication for liver transplantation in children less than 2 years of age. Alpha-1-antitrypsin deficiency may present in infancy but is more likely to affect older children or adults, who develop the symptoms of chronic liver disease. Wilson's disease is an autosomal recessive metabolic condition caused by a deficiency of ceruloplasmin and consequent deposition of copper in the liver and other tissues. It is usually a chronic condition affecting children of school age but may present acutely. Autoimmune hepatitis and cystic fibrosis are the most common conditions presenting in adolescence.

## Clinical manifestations of liver disease

Biliary atresia merits further discussion as it demonstrates the pattern of progressive liver disease in children. It is a rare congenital condition affecting 1:14,000 live births but accounts for around 50% of paediatric liver transplants worldwide and is the commonest indication in children under 2 years of age (data from the European Liver Transplant Registry). It typically presents in the first few weeks of life with jaundice and pale stools. Prompt assessment may allow timely surgery to establish bile flow by Kasai portoenterostomy. However, progressive liver disease often develops, with cholestasis, cirrhosis, and portal hypertension. These children are malnourished, icteric, and have abdominal distension from hepatosplenomegaly. Hospital admission is often necessary to treat variceal haemorrhage, spontaneous bacterial peritonitis, or recurrent cholangitis. Malabsorption and poor nutrition lead to failure to thrive and metabolic bone disease. The skin is often thin and bruises easily, with scratch marks from chronic itching.

## Extrahepatic manifestations of liver disease

Progressive liver disease can have profound effects on cardiorespiratory and renal function, with implications for anaesthesia and critical care.

### Cardiovascular function

Some liver conditions are associated with congenital cardiac malformations: Alagille syndrome is associated with distal pulmonary artery stenosis, and biliary atresia with atrial septal defects, anomalous pulmonary venous drainage, and ventricular septal defects, amongst others.

The commonest finding in ESLD is increased cardiac output secondary to reduced systemic vascular resistance, possibly associated with reduced clearance of vasoactive compounds, particularly nitric oxide. Cardiomyopathy is occasionally seen in children undergoing retransplantation, secondary to immunosuppression with tacrolimus, or in transplantation for unresectable hepatoblastoma after doxorubicin chemotherapy (Atkinson et al., 1995). Systemic hypertension also occurs in retransplant candidates and often requires treatment. Chest X-ray, ECG, and transthoracic echocardiogram must be carefully reviewed in all candidates before listing.

Portopulmonary hypertension is very rare in children and almost always is associated with Alagille syndrome, an autosomal dominant condition characterized by bile duct paucity, cholestasis, and cardiac, facial, and skeletal abnormalities. The cardiac anomaly is typically

**Table 25.1** Indications for liver transplantation in children: diagnostic categories

- Chronic liver disease:
  - Biliary atresia
  - Alagille syndrome
  - Autoimmune hepatitis
  - Caroli's syndrome
  - Cryptogenic cirrhosis
- Genetic conditions leading to chronic liver disease:
  - Alpha-1-antitrypsin deficiency
  - Progressive familial intrahepatic cholestasis
  - Cystic fibrosis
  - Wilson's disease
  - Glycogen storage disease types 3 and 4
- Metabolic conditions (enzyme defect in the liver with extrahepatic manifestations):
  - Urea cycle defects
  - Propionic acidaemia
  - Methylmalonic acidaemia
  - Primary hyperoxaluria type 1
  - Maple syrup urine disease
- Liver tumours:
  - Unresectable hepatoblastoma
- Acute liver failure
- Retransplantation

distal pulmonary artery stenosis, but there may be a spectrum of right heart abnormalities, and cardiology review is essential. Some units use stress echocardiography to assess the effect of increased cardiac output on pulmonary artery pressures; occasionally interventional cardiology techniques are necessary to treat complex lesions. Outcome from liver transplantation is acceptable, but mortality from cardiac causes is increased. The decision to list the child can be difficult, as the indication for transplant is often severe pruritus rather than decompensated liver disease (Kamath et al., 2010).

Occasionally routine echocardiography identifies coincidental cardiac anomalies, which may be a potential route for paradoxical embolization during liver transplantation, especially at reperfusion. The decision to close such defects must balance embolic risks against those of cardiac intervention in the presence of liver disease. If the lesions are not closed it is important to avoid any source of air entrainment during the procedure.

## Respiratory function

Respiratory compromise and hypoxaemia are common in advanced liver disease and are most often the result of reduced diaphragmatic splinting from ascites and hepatosplenomegaly. Improvement may be seen following treatment of ascites with diuretics or drainage. Pleural effusions are also common but rarely drained, as they tend to recur even following transplantation.

Cystic fibrosis is an autosomal recessive condition with an incidence of 1:3,000 live births, affecting the lungs, liver, pancreas, and sweat glands. Around a third of affected individuals develop liver disease, usually as teenagers, and this is the commonest non-respiratory cause of death. Liver disease with portal hypertension is an indication for liver transplantation, but potential candidates must be carefully assessed as respiratory failure, sepsis, and distal intestinal obstruction are common complications.

HPS is a condition comprising arterial hypoxaemia, liver disease, and pulmonary vascular dilatation (Rodríguez-Roisin and Krowka, 2008). It is most common in children with biliary atresia. Diagnosis is important because hypoxaemia from this cause may be out of proportion to the severity of liver disease and is an indication for early liver transplantation. The underlying pathology is generalized pulmonary vasodilatation with right to left shunting, although arteriovenous malformations may contribute in some cases (Schranz and Michel-Benke, 2004; Noli et al., 2008). The diagnosis is based on the presence of low oxygen saturation on pulse oximetry, dyspnoea, and clubbing, as long as chest imaging excludes other causes. Intrapulmonary shunting is confirmed by a positive contrast-enhanced echocardiogram or a Technetium-99-radiolabelled macro-aggregated albumin (99TcMAA) perfusion scan. Contrast appearing in the left atrium after three cardiac cycles, in the absence of an interatrial connection, is considered diagnostic in contrast-enhanced echocardiography. The 99mTcMAA scan is a more quantitative and invasive investigation, comparing the absorption of radiolabelled macro-aggregated albumin in the lungs against that in systemic tissues. A ratio less than 93% is abnormal and may indicate transplant. Transplantation leads to the resolution of hypoxia, sometimes slowly, but is associated with an increased morbidity and mortality compared with other indications (Al-Hussaini et al., 2010).

## Renal system

In most children with chronic liver disease, renal function is well preserved. There may be pre-existing renal disease associated with conditions such as polycystic liver and kidney disease and primary hyperoxaluria. Children with these conditions are often on dialysis at the time of transplant and require combined liver–kidney transplantation.

Renal dysfunction is often seen in children assessed for retransplantation of the liver. Indeed, renal failure remains a common complication of paediatric liver transplantation and its causes include early graft dysfunction, nephrotoxic drugs, and CNIs (MacDiarmid, 1996). Assessment should include serum urea and creatinine, but serum creatinine measurements may be misleading in liver disease because of reduced muscle mass and impaired hepatic synthesis. Creatinine clearance is a superior indicator of renal dysfunction.

HRS is a form of prerenal failure induced by renal vasoconstriction accompanying splanchnic vasodilatation. It is an uncommon complication of ESLD in children. In adults the vasopressin analogue terlipressin has been shown to improve renal function by inducing splanchnic vasoconstriction and there is some evidence of its efficacy in affected children (Yousef et al., 2010).

## Growth and development

Poor nutrition is common in children with ESLD and may profoundly affect growth and development. Causes include poor appetite due to abdominal distention and encephalopathy, fat malabsorption associated with cholestasis, reduced hepatic protein synthesis, and a catabolic state resulting from sepsis. Regular nutritional assessment is important and oral or tube feeding should be optimized before transplant as nutritional status has a major impact on outcome (MacDiarmid, 2001).

### Neurological function

Hepatic encephalopathy is an ominous and occasionally unrecognized sign in children with ESLD and may progress rapidly in ALF (see the section 'Acute liver failure'). There are a number of putative causes including hyperammonaemia, accumulation of false neurotransmitters, and alterations in cerebral blood flow and metabolism. Common causes such as hypoglycaemia and accumulation of sedative medication should be excluded.

## Investigation of paediatric liver disease

The investigation of liver disease is of great importance in affected children. Full blood count, clotting studies, serum urea, creatinine, electrolytes, and liver function tests are the minimum requirement, noting that normal ranges may be different in children. Anaemia is common, resulting from gastrointestinal bleeding or the marrow depression of chronic disease, as is thrombocytopaenia caused by portal hypertension and splenomegaly. White cell count may be reduced by depressed bone marrow function or increased in cholangitis and sepsis.

Serum sodium typically decreases in ESLD, sometimes aggravated by treatment with spironolactone, and values lower than 130 mEq/L are associated with increased mortality (Carey et al., 2010). PT and serum albumin reflect liver synthetic function. Although the liver is the only source of albumin, serum levels may also be reduced in malnutrition and the nephrotic syndrome. Compared to clotting factors, serum albumin concentration changes slowly due to its longer half-life.

Bilirubin is a breakdown product of the haem constituent of haemoglobin and is conjugated with glucuronide by hepatocytes to make it water-soluble. This conjugated form is measured as direct bilirubin. A raised level suggests biliary obstruction. Raised total bilirubin with a normal direct bilirubin assay suggests increased haem production, caused by haemolysis or failure of glucuronidation from hepatocyte loss. The transaminases ALT and AST are both released by hepatocytes when damaged, as in viral or drug-induced hepatitis. AST is a less specific test for liver disease because it is also released from erythrocytes and muscle. Alkaline phosphatase is found in the biliary ducts and bone and levels may be increased in cholestasis. Serum glutamyl transferase (γGT) is similarly raised with biliary obstruction but is a particularly sensitive marker because it is only found in the liver.

Specialized investigations identify specific aetiologies, e.g. alpha-1-antitrypsin (α1AT) assay for α1AT deficiency and alpha-fetoprotein (αFP) for hepatocellular cancer. Imaging studies such as ultrasound, CT, and MRI are routinely done to assess liver anatomy, vasculature, and blood flow.

A pretransplant review of immunization status is required. Routine childhood vaccines, supplemented by those against pneumococcus, hepatitis A and B, and influenza, should be given if needed. Live vaccines should be administered at least 2 weeks before transplantation (*Varicella zoster* and measles, mumps, and rubella (MMR) vaccines if over 6 months of age). Suspension from the transplant list during this period is advisable.

## Management on the transplant waiting list

The interval between listing and liver transplantation may be associated with disease progression and mortality, so severity-based prioritization on the waiting list is needed. This has been aided by scoring systems such as the PELD model for children less than 12 years of age with chronic liver disease. PELD is comprised of points for each of the following: bilirubin, INR, serum albumin, growth failure, and age < 1 year. The sum predicts risk of death and allows objective comparison between patients. Survival data appear to support the PELD model such that children with higher scores suffer worse outcomes (Bourdeaux et al., 2005; Barshes et al., 2006).

Diverse aetiologies and the wide variation in progression of paediatric liver disease may account for the observation that PELD appears less successful than MELD at predicting outcome (Olthoff et al., 2004). It is used less in Europe than in the US. Concerns include lack of scoring for the extrahepatic manifestations of liver disease, such as hepatopulmonary syndrome, and the competition between children and adult candidates for donor livers on the basis of different scoring systems. Potential liver transplant recipients with ALF and certain other indications, such as hepatoblastoma, are excluded from this model and need to be prioritized according to local or national criteria.

## Acute liver failure

The management of paediatric ALF is discussed in Chapter 26. This section will outline key issues in ALF as background for the description of intraoperative management of liver transplantation in this setting.

ALF is a syndrome of hepatic necrosis causing severe impairment of liver function in the absence of chronic liver disease. Paediatric ALF has a high mortality and its causes and evolution may differ distinctly from those seen in adults. Most notably, encephalopathy may be absent, particularly in smaller children. ALF accounts for around 10–15% of all paediatric liver transplants.

The aetiology varies with the age of the child. Neonatal haemochromatosis occurs in the newborn, with metabolic and infectious causes predominating in infancy and early childhood, and paracetamol toxicity and Wilson's disease occurring in older children. However, the cause remains obscure in around 50% of cases. The diagnosis of paracetamol overdose is particularly important because treatment with N-acetylcysteine is effective if administered early.

The presentation of ALF varies, but the condition may progress rapidly, so urgent referral to a specialist liver unit with intensive care and transplant facilities is essential. ALF is a multisystem disorder and requires a team approach, with the child closely monitored in a high-dependency or intensive care area. The aims are simultaneous diagnosis, treatment, and organ support to allow potential regeneration of the liver; however, liver transplantation remains the only effective treatment for severe hepatic necrosis.

Death from cardiovascular collapse and intracranial hypertension is common. Profound vasodilatation may cause cardiovascular instability requiring fluid and inotropic support. Respiratory function may be compromised by aspiration, infection, or acute lung injury. Acute renal failure is common and often necessitates renal replacement therapy.

Neurological symptoms can be subtle in the early phases and vary from mild behavioural changes, irritability, and confusion to coma and intracranial hypertension. The aetiology of hepatic encephalopathy in ALF remains unknown. Hyperammonaemia and the effects of false neurotransmitters are hypotheses. Ammonia is produced from gut flora and converted to urea by the liver. It is water soluble, and when metabolism is impaired it crosses the blood–brain barrier and causes astrocyte swelling, although the severity of hepatic encephalopathy does not always correlate with serum ammonia levels (see Table 25.2).

**Table 25.2** Grading of hepatic encephalopathy. (Data from Trey C and Davidson CS, 'The management of fulminant hepatic failure', *Progress in liver diseases*, 1970, 3, pp. 282–298)

| | |
|---|---|
| Grade 0 | Normal |
| Grade I | Slowness of mentation |
| Grade II | Drowsiness, disorientation, and confusion |
| Grade III | Sleepy but arousable, unresponsive to verbal commands |
| Grade IV | Unconscious and unresponsive to painful stimuli |

Early intubation and ventilation are recommended to ensure airway protection. Surges in intracranial pressure cause pupillary dilation and are treated with additional sedation, ventilation to normocapnia, and bolus doses of 0.5 g/kg of 20% mannitol to treat the associated hypo-osmolar state. The administration of 3% hypertonic saline has been shown to delay progression of encephalopathy in adults (Murphy, 2004). Therapeutic hypothermia shows promise, but there is little evidence to support its use at present and it may aggravate coagulopathy (Jalan et al., 2004).

Measurement of intracranial pressure has been advocated to guide therapy and ensure adequate cerebral perfusion pressure; however, it remains controversial due to the risk of intracranial haemorrhage in children with coagulopathy. Various extracorporeal liver support systems have been developed, aiming to replace the function of the damaged liver and stabilize the child until either sufficient hepatocyte regeneration occurs or liver transplantation becomes available. MARS™ uses a selective membrane and albumin adsorption to remove water-soluble and albumin-bound substances from the circulation, including bilirubin, ammonia, and bile acids. Small series in children have suggested improvements in hepatic encephalopathy and cardiovascular parameters. Other data suggest that plasma exchange with hemodialysis is superior to MARS™ in paediatric ALF (Schaefer et al., 2011). Human hepatocyte infusion into the peritoneum or portal vein may have potential in the treatment of selected patients with ALF and metabolic disorders in the future.

Liver transplantation remains the best treatment for children unlikely to regain hepatic function, although mortality still exceeds that for chronic indications. In part this may result from the inability to obtain a suitable donor organ quickly enough, which has led to the use of urgent living-related transplantation by some groups.

## Anaesthesia and intraoperative management

Liver transplantation is a major procedure and presents the operating room team with a formidable challenge. This section will describe common and predictable perioperative events and their empirical management, focusing on the physiological principles that are important to outcome. Much is based on the subtleties of experience, since published evidence is often lacking.

### Immediate preoperative assessment, induction, and monitoring

The patient must be assessed for any change in his or her condition since the time of listing, which may have been many months previously. Patients on the waiting list will be regularly reviewed in clinic, so significant deterioration will likely have been noted and communicated to the anaesthetic and surgical teams. However, an acute intercurrent illness, in particular infection, may present on the day of a planned transplant. The presence of untreated infection and incipient sepsis, marked by pyrexia, leucocytosis, metabolic acidosis, and raised C-reactive protein, may justify cancellation, but a consensus on the balance of risks should be sought between senior members of the hepatology, surgery, anaesthesia, and infectious diseases teams.

Hyponatraemia is common but usually mild. Values below 130 mmol/L prompt concern, since large and unavoidable intraoperative increases in serum sodium may cause disequilibrium myelinolysis and long-term neurological disability. Measures aimed at gradual, partial preoperative correction, including administration of hypertonic saline or haemofiltration, have been advocated, but evidence of benefit is lacking. In any case, there is usually too little time for these interventions and the balance of risks favours proceeding. However, very low values (< 124 mmol/L), when substantial blood product use is likely, might justify cancellation. A high preoperative potassium level, on the other hand, increases the risk of life-threatening arrhythmias perioperatively, especially at graft reperfusion, and may warrant preoperative or intraoperative haemofiltration.

Premedication is not routine, but benzodiazepines may be used for extreme anxiety. Parental presence at induction is to be encouraged and monitoring is placed as tolerated. An intravenous or inhalational technique is used. A rapid sequence induction is not usually needed.

Atracurium or cis-atracurium is the obvious choice for muscle relaxation. Intubation by the oral route is preferred; nasal intubation can be used but is rarely needed, since most patients can be extubated within 24–48 hours and coagulopathy may increase the risk of nasal bleeding.

A gastric tube is used for continuous passive drainage of the stomach. Central and peripheral temperature monitors are placed. An arterial line is used for continuous arterial pressure monitoring and intermittent blood gas analysis. The radial artery is preferred but the brachial is an acceptable alternative. Lower limb catheters may be used but pressure traces are lost during periods of aortic clamping, which may be necessary to create arterial inflow to the liver. Ultrasound visualization may assist with difficult placements.

### Venous access

Central venous catheterization above the diaphragm is essential, most commonly using the right internal jugular route, since the inferior vena cava is clamped during the procedure. A multilumen catheter is used for vasoactive drugs and monitoring and a separate large-bore cannula for rapid infusion. A 4F introducer sheath serves very well for volume administration in an infant, increasing to 8F in an adult-size patient. A large-bore peripheral cannula may be adequate for resuscitation fluids, and smaller cannulae can be used for maintenance crystalloids, opioids, and muscle relaxants.

Vasopressors, calcium, and sodium bicarbonate can cause tissue necrosis if extravasation occurs and should only be given by the central venous route. Strict asepsis must be maintained during insertion of central venous catheters (Centers for Disease Control and Prevention, 2011) and use of ultrasound is recommended.

## Temperature control

Normothermia should be maintained, using a forced-air warmer and/or warming mattress and fluid warming. A marked fall in temperature is noted on reperfusion of the graft, which is preserved at 4°C. Care should be taken not to exceed 37.5°C once core temperature is restored after reperfusion.

## Anaesthesia maintenance and fluids

Anaesthesia is maintained with desflurane or isoflurane in an air/oxygen mix. A continuous infusion of atracurium and an opioid is usual; the rate is titrated against clinical effect. Calcium chloride (or gluconate) and noradrenaline are infused through a central venous line. A calcium infusion is adjusted to have the blood-ionized calcium at 1.2–1.3 mmol/L at the time of reperfusion. The amount required is variable and depends on blood product use, but some calcium is usually needed even if there is no transfusion (Jawan et al., 2003). Noradrenaline is usually not required at high rates from the outset, except in some cases of ALF. However, we administer it at a low rate from the start, mainly to ensure that the response to an increased infusion rate is immediate.

Maintenance crystalloids are usually given, 0.9% sodium chloride or a balanced electrolyte solution (Hartmann's or Ringer's lactate). Glucose may be needed, especially in ALF. Any crystalloid regime has potential disadvantages, but electrolytes, glucose, blood gases, and lactate are measured frequently and should be kept within normal limits as far as possible. Red blood cells, FFP or a pooled plasma preparation, and platelets are ordered according to the recipient's body weight and anticipated blood loss (Hellstern and Solheim, 2011). Cryoprecipitate and factor concentrates are rarely needed and not routinely ordered.

## Red cell salvage

Cell salvage reduces dependence on and risks from donated blood. Device improvements in recent years have reduced the salvage volume required to produce reinfusable cells, increasing their use in paediatrics and lowering bank blood use by one-third to one-half. Although reliable, cell salvage machines require the presence of a trained technician. Use in tumour patients is controversial if not contraindicated, given evidence that tumour cells may be reinfused despite filtering (Esper and Waters, 2011).

## Monitoring

Routine cardiovascular monitoring includes central venous and invasive arterial pressures. The presence of a variable degree of pre-existing coagulopathy and the inevitable total loss of hepatic function intraoperatively make close monitoring of coagulation necessary. Long processing times for laboratory samples often make them impractical, and point-of-care measurement of PT/INR and aPTT is widely used, together with thromboelastography (TEG or ROTEM). These monitors allow a targeted administration of procoagulant blood products and drugs.

In adult liver transplantation cardiac function is monitored by either pulmonary artery catheterization with thermodilution or TEE using Simpson's method (Burtenshaw and Isaac, 2006), the latter gaining popularity in recent years. However, in children below 25 kg, PA catheters are difficult and risky to use. TEE is possible at much smaller sizes, but the presence of oesophageal varices and coagulopathy present unquantifiable risks. The PiCCO system measures cardiac output by arterial waveform analysis (Pulsion GmBH, Germany), requiring an arterial thermistor and calibration by thermodilution. However, an arterial catheter of at least 4F is required, restricting its use to older children. Techniques using lithium dilution, oesophageal Doppler, and transthoracic bio-impedance have also been described (Della Rocca et al., 2009; Funk et al., 2009). However, we no longer use cardiac output monitoring in sub-adult size patients, arguing that the benefits of advanced measurement methods do not justify the risks and that changes in cardiac output can be inferred from other data.

## Surgical technique and intraoperative care

In the first part of the procedure, the dissection phase, the surgical team will skeletonize the liver, isolating its vessels and adjacent vena cava in preparation for its removal (see Table 25.3). In the patient with chronic liver disease and portal hypertension, surgical division of extensive portosystemic collaterals and inflammatory adhesions around the vena cava may cause heavy bleeding. The anaesthetic tasks are to maintain optimum preload (a mainstay of the entire procedure) and to preserve physiological normality as far as possible. The choice of fluids for volume replacement depends on the starting point and the volume lost, but blood and clotting factor administration should allow the haematocrit to decline to about 25%, while a PT of 20 s (INR ≈ 2.0) is an acceptable target. Platelets are not normally given unless the count was very low to start with. Clotting and blood gas analysis is typically done hourly, but more often if major bleeding occurs. Glucose replacement and calcium infusion rates often edge upwards at this time. The length of the dissection phase depends on the degree of surgical difficulty; 2–4 hours is typical.

The anhepatic phase begins when the circulation to the native liver is interrupted and the organ is explanted. In all but the larger children this will entail completely occluding the inferior vena cava above and below the liver, which will result in a fall in venous return of 40% in most cases. This causes a corresponding fall in cardiac output and often a degree of arterial hypotension. This can be treated with judicious fluid administration, perhaps with

**Table 25.3** Key points in the intraoperative management of paediatric liver transplantation

| |
|---|
| ◆ Use invasive pressure monitoring |
| ◆ Place cannulae for rapid infusion |
| ◆ Ensure generous intravascular filling |
| ◆ Add vasopressors if needed to maintain perfusion pressure |
| ◆ Aim for moderate haemodilution (haematocrit ≈ 25%) and moderately prolonged coagulation parameters (INR ≈ 1.5–2.0) |
| ◆ Anticipate surgical events: caval clamping, reperfusion, cut surface bleeding |
| ◆ Ensure adequate reserves of blood products |

a low-dose vasopressor support. Too much fluid may aggravate venous stasis in the gut and kidneys and cause fluid overload when the vena cava is unclamped. Depending on surgical preference, the haemodynamic effects of portal clamping can be attenuated by creation of a portocaval shunt, in which the portal vein is temporarily anastomosed to the upper cava.

In this phase, glucose and calcium requirements may escalate markedly. Increasing metabolic acidosis and a rising serum lactate are consistent features. The acidosis is not normally treated with bicarbonate unless severe and clearly interfering with other vital functions. Modest hyperventilation may be helpful.

When caval and portal venous anastomoses are nearly complete, the graft is flushed to remove preservation fluid, air, heparin, and inflammatory mediators before restoring portal blood flow. The solution used varies between centres. After this, the portal and caval anastomoses are completed and unclamping of the vena cava and portal vein reperfuses the liver. The surgical team keeps the anhepatic phase as short as possible to minimize both warm ischaemia of the graft and the effects of venous stasis on the gut.

Reperfusion is almost always via the portal vein. The liver should immediately blush and fill with blood. A systemic effect is usually obvious within a few seconds. The classic reperfusion syndrome comprises a fall in heart rate, a rise in pulmonary artery pressure, and a fall of at least 30% in systemic arterial pressure (Aggarwal et al., 1993). The syndrome is now less often seen in its florid form, but some fall in systemic pressure is inevitable. Dysrhythmias may occur as potassium-rich preservation fluid enters the central circulation. Marked vasodilation occurs, often accompanied by myocardial depression. Both are treated with small boluses of adrenaline. Hypotension may be aggravated by anastomotic bleeding and by partial or complete reclamping of the vena cava to repair the leak. When filling is maintained, usually with boluses of colloid, persistent hypotension is usually attributed to systemic vasodilatation and treated with noradrenaline infusion. This is later tapered as the graft begins to function.

The majority of smaller children receive split cadaveric grafts, usually the left lobe or two segments from an adult liver. It is difficult for the surgeon to detect and seal all the significant vessels on the cut surface during preparation of the lobar graft, so split grafts can bleed heavily when reperfused. The ability to replace blood loss rapidly may be critical at this stage. If bleeding is severe, the surgical team may be asked to restrict portal vein flow into the graft intermittently for a few 10-s intervals. This is an extreme measure and potentially harmful to the graft but may be life-saving.

The hypotension following reperfusion tends to resolve in less than 30 minutes, and it is usually possible to reduce the rate of vasopressor infusion, even when as much as 0.5 mcg/kg/min noradrenaline has been needed. If hypotension is severe and persistent despite good filling pressures (CVP 10–12 mmHg), addition of a vasopressin infusion may be preferable to high doses of noradrenaline, since the latter may cause pulmonary hypertension, right heart failure, or splanchnic ischaemia. When the graft works well, vasopressors are typically discontinued before the patient reaches the ICU.

Once anastomotic and cut-surface bleeding has been controlled, the priority is to restore arterial flow to the graft, which will not be viable without a dual blood supply. An arterial conduit may be needed, carrying blood from the aorta to the graft hepatic artery(s). A secondary reperfusion phenomenon may be seen when the arterial flow is restored, but this is unusual if the portal flow has been satisfactory. Once arterial flow is restored, a surgical break to allow the liver a period of undisturbed perfusion may be beneficial. This is followed by a biliary drainage procedure, either a duct-to-duct or a Roux-en-Y anastomosis.

After the initial reperfusion period, continuing major blood loss is unusual and care should be taken to avoid overfilling, since correction of a low haematocrit and administration of coagulation factors may be required. Partial correction of coagulopathy to a PT of 15–18 s (INR about 1.5) before reperfusion may be prudent to attenuate later deterioration. Careful attention should be paid to the thromboelastogram, and platelet or cryoprecipitate therapy may be indicated. Fibrinolysis may occur and can be treated with tranexamic acid. If bleeding continues despite full conventional therapy, recombinant factor VIIa can be given as a last resort. However, overzealous treatment of coagulopathy or too high a haematocrit can predispose to vascular thrombosis or pulmonary embolism (Warnaar et al., 2008).

Glucose and calcium are not usually required after reperfusion unless graft function is poor. Insulin may be given if the glucose level is very high (≥ 15 mmol/L, but insulin resistance is typical until graft function is established. Thus infusion of insulin at high doses may risk hypoglycaemia, and bolus dosing or no treatment may be safer (De Wolf et al., 1987; Shangraw and Hexem, 1996).

Once biliary drainage is completed, drains are placed and the abdomen is closed. If full closure cannot be achieved without causing high intra-abdominal pressure, partial closure with a silastic patch may be the best option. The wound edges are then brought together in stages over several days.

Graft vessels may be examined with Doppler ultrasound at the end of surgery to ensure satisfactory flow, and this is repeated at 12- to 24-hour intervals on the ICU. When flow is poor or difficult to demonstrate, timely intervention can prevent hepatic infarction. When graft function is poor despite patent vessels, infusion of N-acetylcysteine may be considered (Lee et al., 2009). If deterioration continues, urgent retransplantation may be necessary.

## Intraoperative management in ALF

Ten to fifteen percent of primary liver transplants are carried out for ALF. Some important pathophysiological differences between acute and chronic liver failure in children are shown in Table 25.4.

In ALF the patient will be already intubated and ventilated in the ICU. Prophylactic administration of clotting factors is usual and glucose infusion is needed until soon after reperfusion, when hyperglycaemia occurs. Because there are no varices the dissection phase and explant are not usually associated with haemodynamic instability, but caval clamping may be less well tolerated because of the absence of portosystemic collaterals. Occasionally, devascularization of the necrotic liver is in itself associated with significant haemodynamic improvement, but in all cases a functioning graft allows a rapid reduction of vasopressor dose.

Intraoperative renal support is rarely required but may be useful in ALF, urgent retransplantation, or combined liver–kidney transplant. It is indicated to control severe acidosis and hyperkalaemia, but the following caveats apply. Vigorous preoperative dialysis should be avoided in patients on chronic intermittent dialysis because of the acute fluid shifts and electrolyte fluctuations it may cause. Intraoperative renal support will require an ICU or dialysis unit nurse and may be difficult to organize at short notice. Because

**Table 25.4** Differences between acute and chronic liver failure in children

| Acute | Chronic |
|---|---|
| Marked coagulopathy | Moderate coagulopathy or normal coagulation (especially with biliary cirrhosis) |
| High glucose requirement | Glucose requirement unusual |
| Encephalopathy, potentially with raised intracranial pressure | Encephalopathy unusual |
| Pronounced systemic vasodilatation, sometimes requiring vasopressor; high cardiac output | Low systemic vascular resistance and hyperdynamic circulation, but vasopressor need suggests sepsis |
| No significant varices or portosystemic collateral vessels | Portal hypertension usual, with varices, ascites, and hypersplenism |
| Acute renal failure common | Severe renal impairment unusual |

the machine cannot be positioned close to the patient, long outflow and return lines may cause significant cooling despite warming of the haemofilter; it may help to run the return limb back through a coaxial fluid warmer, such as the Hot-line™.

Urine output should be measured routinely, but caution is warranted in responding to low urine flows. Periods of renal hypoperfusion are unavoidable during liver transplantation, since caval clamping acutely raises renal venous pressure and is often associated with arterial hypotension. However, with adequate attention to intravascular filling and modest use of vasopressors, kidney function is surprisingly robust. Persistent severe oliguria otherwise suggests poor graft function.

## Retransplantation

Retransplantation is needed in 10–15% of paediatric liver grafts. Primary graft non-function or early infarction rapidly induces multi-organ failure and is managed perioperatively much as ALF. However, early retransplants and those performed within the first few weeks are surgically relatively easy, since all the dissection and vessel preparation have already been done. Late retransplantation, on the other hand, is complicated by dense adhesions and much higher blood loss. Retransplant associated with portal vein thrombosis may be uniquely challenging. Portal venous pressure is acutely raised and collateral vessels are large, numerous, and may bleed torrentially. Achieving adequate blood flow to the replacement liver may also be difficult and perioperative risk in these patients is very high. Despite these hazards, outcomes from retransplantation in paediatric recipients are often better than seen in the adult population.

## Conclusion

Paediatric liver transplantation is associated with excellent outcomes; in most cases the recipients exhibit excellent growth and normal development, with many attaining adulthood in good health. The diversity of indications, variation in size, and associated conditions present immense challenges to the anaesthetist. A thorough understanding of paediatric liver disease as well as the pathophysiological changes during liver transplantation is essential for success. Although there are many features common to both paediatric and adult liver disease, the extrapolation of adult techniques to children is not ideal. Future developments and techniques promise much for children with liver disease but are likely to present new medical and ethical challenges to all working with these patients.

## References


Aggarwal S, Kang Y, Freeman JA, et al. (1993) Postreperfusion syndrome: hypotension after reperfusion of the transplanted liver. *J Crit Care*, **8**(3):154–160.

Al-Hussaini A, Taylor RM, Samyn M, et al. (2010) Long-term outcome and management of hepatopulmonary syndrome in children. *Pediatr Transplant* 2010, **14**(2),276–282.

Atkinson P, Joubert G, Barron A, et al. (1995) Hypertrophic cardiomyopathy associated with tacrolimus in paediatric transplant patients. *Lancet*, **345**:894–896.

Barshes N, Lee T, Udell I, et al. (2006) The pediatric end-stage liver disease model (PELD) as a predictor of survival benefit and posttransplant survival in pediatric liver transplant recipients. *Liver Transplant*, **12**(3):475–480.

Bourdeaux C, Tri T, Gras J, et al. (2005) PELD score and posttransplant outcome in pediatric liver transplantation: a retrospective study of 100 recipients. *Transplantation*, **9**:1273–1276.

Burtenshaw AL, Isaac JL (2006) The role of transoesophageal echocardiography for perioperative cardiovascular monitoring during orthotopic liver transplantation. *Liver Transplant*, **12**(11):1577–1583.

Carey R, Bucuvalas J, Baliesteri W, et al. (2010) Hyponatraemia increases mortality in pediatric patients listed for liver transplantation. *Pediatric Transplant*, **14**:115–1120.

Centers for Disease Control and Prevention (2011) *Guidelines for the prevention of catheter-related blood stream infections.* CDC and Healthcare Infection Control Practices Advisory Committee (HICPAC). <www.cdc.gov/hicpac/pdf/guidelines/bsi-guidelines-2011.pdf>.

Della Rocca G, Brondani A, Costa MG (2009) Intraoperative hemodynamic monitoring during during organ transplantation: what is new? *Curr Opin Organ Transplant*, **14**(3):291–296.

De Wolf AM, Kang YG, Todo S, et al. (1987) Glucose metabolism during liver transplantation in dogs. *Anesth Analg*, **66**(1):76–80.

Esper SA, Waters JH (2011) Intra-operative cell salvage: a fresh look at the indications and contraindications. *Blood Transfusion*, **9**(2):139–147.

Funk DJ, Morretti EW, Gan TJ (2009) Minimally invasive cardiac output monitoring in the perioperative setting. *Anesth Analg*, **108**(3):887–897.

Hellstern P, Solheim BG (2011) The use of solvent/detergent treatment in pathogen reduction of plasma. *Transfus Med Hemother*, **38**(1):65–70.

Jalan R, Olde Damink SW, Deutz NE, Hayes PC, Lee A (2004) Moderate hypothermia in patients with acute liver failure and uncontrolled intracranial hypertension. *Gastroenterology*, **127**:1338–1346.

Jawan B, De Villa V, Luk H-N, et al. (2003) Ionized calcium changes during living-donor liver transplantation in patients with and without administration of blood-bank products. *Transplant Int*, **16**(7):510–514.

Kamath BM, Schwarz KB, Hadžić N (2010) Alagille syndrome and liver transplantation. *J Pedi Gastroenterol Nutr*, **50**(1):11–15.

Lee WM, Hynan LS, Rossaro L, et al. (2009) Intravenous N-acetylcysteine improves transplant-free survival in early stage non-acetaminophen acute liver failure. *Gastroenterol*, **137**(3):856–864.

MacDiarmid S (1996) Renal function in pediatric liver transplant patients. *Kid Intl Supp*, **53**:S77–84.

MacDiarmid SV (2001) Management of the pediatric liver transplant patient. *Liver Transplant*, **7**(Suppl):77–86.

McKiernan P (2011) Long-term care following paediatric liver transplantation. *Arch Dis Child Educ Pract Edn*, **96**:82–86.

Murphy N, Auzinger G, Bernal W, Wendon J (2004) The effect of hypertonic sodium chloride on intracranial pressure in patients with acute liver failure. *Hepatology*, **39**:464–470.

Noli K, Solomon M, Golding F, Charron M, Ling S (2008) Prevalence of hepatopulmonary syndrome in children. *Pediatrics*, **121**(3):522–527.

Olthoff K, Brown R, Delmonico F, et al. (2004) Summary report of a national conference: evolving concepts in liver allocation in the MELD and PELD era. *Liver Transplant*, **10**(Suppl):A6–A22.

Rodríguez-Roisin R, Krowka MJ (2008) Hepatopulmonary syndrome—a liver-induced lung vascular disorder. *N Engl J Med*, **358**:2378–2387.

Schaefer B, Schaefer F, Engelman G, et al. (2011) Comparison of Molecular Adsorbents Recirculating System (MARS) dialysis in children with acute liver failure. *Nephrol Dial Transplant*, **26**(11):3633–3639.

Schranz D, Michel-Behnke I (2004) Arteriovenous malformations and hepatopulmonary syndrome. *Lancet*, **364**(9428):26–27.

Shangraw RE, Hexem JG (1996) Glucose and potassium metabolic responses to insulin during liver transplantation. *Liver Transplant Surg*, **2**(6):443–54.

Warnaar N, Molenaar IQ, Colquhoun SD, et al. (2008) Intraoperative pulmonary embolism and intracardiac thrombus complicating liver transplantation: a systematic review. *J Thromb Haemost*, **6**(2):297–302.

Yousef N, Habes D Ackerman O, Durand P, Bernard O, Jacquemin E (2010) Hepatorenal syndrome: diagnosis and effect of terlipressin therapy in 4 paediatric patients. *J Paed Gastroenterol Nutr*, **51**:100–102.

## Further reading

European Liver Transplant Registry: <www.eltr.org>.

# CHAPTER 26

# Paediatric liver transplantation: critical care

Richard Neal and Oliver Bagshaw

## Introduction (supportive measures)

Respiratory support is indicated in patients with grade 3 or 4 encephalopathy in order to protect the airway, optimize care delivery (including placement of venous and arterial access lines), and prevent fluctuations in ICP (Riordan and Williams, 1997). Hepatic-specific considerations are as follows.

Hypoglycaemia, caused by impaired glycogen storage and gluconeogenesis, should be treated with IV glucose infusions as required to maintain blood glucose concentration > 4 mmol/L.

Coagulopathy can be treated with FFP, cryoprecipitate, and, if extreme, recombinant factor VII. However, since PT is routinely used to monitor the severity of the condition, products are usually given only for active bleeding, as prophylaxis for invasive procedures, or when very severe coagulopathy carries a high risk of spontaneous haemorrhage.

Hypotension is caused by systolic and diastolic myocardial dysfunction and vasoplegia, often associated with sepsis and relative adrenal suppression (Harry et al., 2002). Titrated volume administration, inotropic support with adrenaline, vasopressors including noradrenaline and vasopressin, and steroid administration are common treatment modalities. Echocardiographic assessment of cardiac function may be useful, especially when the response to these measures is inadequate.

## Pretransplant

All children listed for liver transplantation should have a thorough pretransplant assessment, which should target growth parameters, underlying diagnosis, and associated comorbidities. It also allows investigation to assess suitability and optimization of the patient.

A small number of patients awaiting transplantation will already be on the ICU; most of these will be cases of ALF.

## Acute liver failure

The aetiology of this condition has been reviewed in Chapter 25. ALF is a potentially fatal condition with a high mortality in those not receiving a transplant. Poor prognosis without transplantation is associated with age < 10 years, infantile metabolic liver disease, and familial erythrophagocytosis, seronegative hepatitis, severe coagulopathy (PT > 55 s), severe encephalopathy (grade 3–4), prolonged duration of illness before onset of hepatic encephalopathy, and coexisting renal failure.

The patient with ALF may be critically ill and require rapid assessment and stabilization prior to transfer to the paediatric intensive care unit (PICU) for ongoing care. ALF progressively leads to multi-organ system failure and intracranial hypertension. The management of ALF is directed towards hepatic support, the prevention and treatment of complications, and early consideration for liver transplantation.

Respiratory support is indicated in patients with severe ALF, particularly those with evidence of grade 3 or 4 encephalopathy, in order to protect the airway, optimize care delivery (including placement of venous and arterial access lines), and prevent fluctuations in ICP (Riordan and Williams, 1997). Specific considerations are now discussed.

## Hypoglycaemia

Loss of functional hepatocytes results in both impaired glycogen storage and gluconeogenesis. Hypoglycaemia should be identified and treated with IV dextrose infusions (10–50%) as required to maintain blood glucose level > 4 mmol/L.

## Coagulation abnormalities

Coagulation abnormalities are an effect of impaired hepatocyte production of clotting factors. They can usually be partially treated with vitamin K, FFP, cryoprecipitate, or even recombinant factor VII; but since PT is frequently used to monitor the progression of the condition, transfusion of clotting factors is reserved for cases of active bleeding or where the coagulopathy is so severe that there is a risk of spontaneous haemorrhage.

## Hypotension

Cardiac systolic and diastolic dysfunction, vasoplegic shock, sepsis, and relative adrenal suppression can all lead to profound hypotension. Echocardiographic assessment of cardiac function may be useful in addition to volume administration, inotropic support (adrenaline), vasopressor (noradrenaline and vasopressin), and steroid administration. Adrenal dysfunction is common in adult ALF and may contribute to metabolic and haemodynamic instability (Fede et al., 2012).

## Immune system dysfunction

The complement, neutrophil, and gut immune function are all impaired in ALF. Fever and white cell responses to infection are blunted. Infective complications are seen in a significant proportion of children; however, distinguishing sepsis from the multi-organ dysfunction seen in ALF can be difficult (Godbole et al., 2011). Pneumonia, urosepsis, and spontaneous bacterial peritonitis are all common foci of infection. Fungal infections are also seen in one-third of patients. Treatment with broad-spectrum antibiotics, oral selective bowel decontamination, antivirals, and antifungal agents is recommended.

## Hepatic encephalopathy

Hepatic encephalopathy is a consequence of synergistic metabolic neurotoxins which when present in sufficient concentrations interfere with the intercellular communication of the brain (predominantly due to effects in astrocytes), which lead to the clinical signs of impaired consciousness and altered behavior (Lizardi-Cervera et al., 2003). Acetylcysteine and epoprostenol infusions may improve cerebral oxygenation and reduce the brain's metabolic demand. EEG monitoring may assist in grading encephalopathy and with the detection of subclinical seizures. Treatments to minimize hepatic encephalopathy include minimizing enteral protein load, the addition of oral lactulose, and antibiotic therapy to decrease gut flora and consequently reduce ammonia production.

MARS® has been shown to remove water-soluble and albumin-bound toxins and provide renal support in cases of renal failure (Betrosian et al., 2007). MARS® therapy in adult ALF has been shown to improve both haemodynamic parameters and hepatic encephalopathy (Stange et al., 2002). Paediatric case series are limited. Evidence suggests that alternating the use of haemodialysis and plasma exchange may be superior in terms of ammonia and bilirubin clearance and reduction in INR (Schaefer et al., 2011).

## Cerebral oedema

Intracranial hypertension and cerebral oedema may be loosely correlated with the degree of hyperammonaemia. Astrocyte oedema (secondary to the conversion of ammonia to the organic osmol glutamine) and cerebral vasodilatation with loss of vascular autoregulation lead to raised ICP. CT of the brain is insensitive in identifying oedema; however, it may be useful to exclude intracranial bleeding. Management of intracranial hypertension may be achieved by targeting cerebral perfusion and MAP by volume expansion and vasopressor use. Strategies to improve cerebral perfusion may include head elevation (20–30°), midline positioning, osmotic therapy (hypertonic saline and mannitol), controlled hyperventilation, controlled hypothermia, and sedation (barbiturate coma). There are risks associated with hyperventilation (cerebral vasoconstriction and worsening of cerebral ischaemia) and with hypothermia (immune paresis). ICP monitoring is controversial due to the potential risks of bleeding, infection, and misinterpretation of the measured values. Whilst there is some case series evidence of benefit (Kamat et al., 2012), invasive ICP monitoring is not recommended in the routine care of the child with ALF.

## Renal failure

The incidence of acute renal failure is between 10 and 15% in paediatric ALF. The presence of renal failure is associated with reduced patient survival after OLT (McDiarmid, 1996). Renal support with CVVH or haemodialysis and filtration (CVVHDF) allows preoperative optimization of fluid balance, electrolytes, and acid-base status.

CVVH allows both fluid and solute removal; addition of the substitution fluid can be done in the predilution or postdilution setting. Predilution has the added benefit of giving a continuous flush to the haemofilter membrane, in effect diluting the blood flowing through it, which may decrease the incidence of clotting in the filter but also reduces solute clearance.

CVVHDF will usually be used when adequate management of acid-base balance is not being achieved in CVVH mode. If substitution fluid volumes of 150 ml/kg/hour have been used unsuccessfully in excess of 6 hours then CVVHDF should be considered. The volume of substitution will be the same as for other continuous renal replacement therapy modes, i.e. up to a maximum of 150–200 ml/kg/hour. The proportion of the substitution fluid infused as dialysate and post dilution will vary. A suggested starting point will be to infuse 50% as dialysate into the filter and 50% post dilution.

Therapeutic plasma exchange (TPE) with albumin/FFP solution can be used to clear toxins, plasma proteins, and autoantibody mediators. This process allows the removal of very large plasma proteins up to approximately 2 million Da.

A double volume plasma exchange can be calculated as requiring:

Double plasma volume = 2 × (Estimated blood volume (ml/kg) × weight (kg) × (1 − Haematocrit). For a 10-kg child, 80 ml/kg blood volume, haematocrit of 0.3.

Double plasma volume = 2 × (80 × 10) × (1 − 0.3) = 2 × 560 ml = 1120 ml

Substitution fluid rate 1,120/6 hours = 186 mL/hour.

In plasma exchange, unlike haemofiltration, replacement fluid is given post filter. Patients will likely require cryoprecipitate or platelets in addition to FFP for restoration of platelet and fibrinogen levels at the end of the plasma exchange.

## Palliative care decisions

There are a number of children with ALF who will not survive to liver transplantation or in whom performing the transplant is impossible. It may be necessary to discuss end-of-life management with families in these situations.

The decision to limit intensive care support or to provide palliative care rather than aggressive medical management is important and should be made with the agreement of the medical and nursing team and after consultation with the patient and their parents. The best interests of a patient must be the primary consideration in determining the care plan and are central to decision-making.

It recognizes the following three scenarios:

- Brain stem death, as determined by agreed professional criteria appropriately applied
- Imminent death, where physiological deterioration is occurring irrespective of treatment
- Inevitable death, where death is not immediately imminent but will follow and where prolongation of life by LST confers no overall benefit.

As can be seen from the RCPCH guidance statements, the underlying principle on determining the suitability of withdrawal of life-sustaining treatments should be based around the child's best interests. This decision will require an assessment of potential future or active suffering with ongoing treatments and the potential for future cure and quality of life.

Decisions relating to paediatric care are made for the most part between the doctor and the parent(s). Prognosis, risk to life, and perceived future potential 'quality of life' should be discussed and where possible the child's point of view should be considered.

The medical information guiding the decision to limit care or withhold life-sustaining intensive care is complicated, and although it is known that children who reach grade 4 encephalopathy have a poor prognosis (20% survival) and may develop cerebral oedema in the post-transplant period, this information in itself does not warrant withdrawal. In the pretransplant period, cerebral oedema, GI bleeding, and overwhelming sepsis are the most common causes of death.

Many children with severe organ dysfunction and ALF are supported and listed for transplant. In this situation it is reasonable to discuss do not attempt CPR (DNACPR) orders (Resuscitation Council (UK), 2014). A DNACPR order may be issued after consent is gained from the parent provided that a patient's condition is such that resuscitation is unlikely to succeed or if successful resuscitation would not be in the patient's best interest. If a cardiac arrest does not occur and an organ becomes available, it is then the role of the transplant anaesthesiologist and surgeon to determine whether the child is suitable for the team to proceed. Utilizing a precious donor organ and putting a child through an operation with no chance of recovery is unethical from both the 'patient's best interests' and utilitarian perspectives.

## Postoperative intensive care

### General principles

On admission of the post-transplant patient to the PICU it is essential to receive a comprehensive handover from the operative care team, including preoperative factors, anaesthetic management, surgical factors, and any complications or potential concerns. The ICU stabilization and initial management of the patient requires a carefully coordinated combined medical and nursing strategy. Routine ICU observations, such as continuous ECG, pulse oximetry, and continuous CVP and arterial pressure monitoring, are taken as a presumed baseline.

Patients require regular blood gas analyses (initially every 2–4 hours) and complete haematology, coagulation, and clinical chemistry blood panels (every 4–6 hours). The first set of blood test results will reflect the transitional physiology from reperfusion of the implanted liver, the residual metabolic derangements from the anhepatic period, and fluid resuscitation. A significant hyperchloraemic acidosis is frequently identified. This can be passively observed provided appropriate levels of respiratory support are in place and the cardiac output is deemed adequate, through surrogate markers such as blood pressure, central perfusion, urine output, mixed venous oxygen saturations, and serum lactate.

The position of the anaesthetic support lines and tubes should be assessed on an admission chest X-ray. The nasogastric tube, biliary drain, and urinary catheter should remain on free drainage and the surgical drains may require low-pressure suction.

Unit policy regarding postoperative fluid management varies and no single specific regime can be universally recommended. Provided the fluid volume, electrolyte composition, and glucose delivery are adjusted according to monitored levels, the patient is unlikely to come to any harm. A replacement solution for drain and nasogastric tube losses should be provided; a combination of human albumin (5%) and crystalloid is commonly used.

The graft will be assessed for function and signs of complications by both clinical examination and reviewing blood results; ominous signs are worsening coagulopathy, increased serum acidosis and lactate, climbing base deficit, and rising serum transaminases. A Doppler ultrasound scan of the graft vessels should take place at the end of surgery, again within the first 12–24 hours, and at any time if there is acute deterioration.

## Transplant medications

Transplant medications are all administered intravenously unless otherwise stated.

### Antibiotics

Broad-spectrum antibacterial agents are usually administered at induction of anaesthesia for the liver transplant procedure and continued in the post-transplant period, with review at 48 hours. Antiviral and antifungal agents are added postoperatively. An example of a current protocol includes piperacillin/tazobactam (ciprofloxacin if penicillin-allergic) and metronidazole at induction, followed by cotrimoxazole (po), aciclovir (dependent on EBV and CMV status of donor and recipient), nystatin (po), and ambisome in the early postoperative period.

### Immunosuppression

Immunosuppressive medication is initiated during the transplant operation and continued as per specific transplant protocol. A current regime comprises basiliximab day 0 and day 4; mycophenolate (po) from day 15; and tacrolimus (po) from day 0. Hydrocortisone (IV) is given in some selective cases, e.g. combined liver and renal transplantation, autoimmune liver disease, some retransplants, and where underlying condition requires long-term corticosteroids.

### Anti-acid medication

Anti-acid agents are used to prevent gastritis and ulceration and aim to maintain gastric pH > 5. A current regime starts with ranitidine, changing to sucralfate (po) or omeprazole (IV or po) if gastric pH remains < 5.

### Antiplatelet agents

Antiplatelet agents are prescribed to protect the graft from thrombotic complications; dipyridamole (po) is given if the platelet count is $> 50 \times 10^9$/L, adding aspirin (po) if $> 75 \times 10^9$/L. These are reviewed at 6 months post-transplant.

## Systems approach to postoperative care

### Respiratory system

In infants and small children undergoing liver transplantation, a relatively large graft may make abdominal closure difficult. It is therefore common practice to delay full closure, using a synthetic patch or leaving the abdomen open with a superficial occlusive dressing. Although this minimizes compression while the graft establishes function and oedema resolves, it necessitates 1–5 days of sedation and respiratory support in the ICU. When surgical closure is completed, abdominal pressure may still be high, and moderate levels of PEEP of 8–10 cm $H_2O$ may be required to maintain FRC and oxygenation. On extubation, these patients may need non-invasive ventilator support with CPAP or BiPAP for the same reason. The use of high-flow nasal cannula oxygen therapy may also be considered in these patients. Surgical wound pain and ascites may contribute to difficulties in weaning from mechanical ventilation, as may diaphragmatic weakness and dysfunction, especially in patients with pretransplant malnutrition. Pleural effusions are common and may require drainage.

In older children there is usually a window of opportunity in the first 12–24 hours to wean from ventilator support and extubate. The decision to wean and the weaning process will be guided by the PICU routine, considerations including graft status, other organ failure, inspired oxygen requirement, arterial blood gas measurements, and clinical assessment of the adequacy of spontaneous breathing. Fluid resuscitation, blood products, and hypoalbuminaemia can contribute to both interstitial pulmonary oedema and the development of TRALI mimicking ARDS. Pneumonia, atelectasis, haemothorax, or pneumothorax can also develop and delay ventilator weaning.

Additional respiratory complications associated with liver failure include HPS. HPS is associated with increased post-transplant mortality and these patients may require prolonged respiratory support, including inhaled nitric oxide and high-frequency oscillatory ventilation to improve lung recruitment and ventilation–perfusion matching.

### Cardiovascular system

Hypotension is usually a marker of intravascular volume depletion. In the immediate postoperative period (< 12–24 hours), hypotension, tachycardia, and falling haemoglobin (Hb) indicate bleeding. Haemorrhagic peritoneal drain fluid may be seen. The surgical team should be notified as soon as bleeding is suspected and blood transfused to a target Hb of 7–8.5 g/dL. After consultation with the surgical team, coagulopathy should also be corrected. Re-exploration may be required.

Inotrope and vasopressor infusions can usually be weaned as the effects of anaesthetic agents wear off and the graft establishes function. In patients with a persistent requirement for vasopressor therapy, bleeding, primary graft non-function, sepsis, and cardiac dysfunction should be suspected and managed appropriately.

Monitoring of CVP and arterial blood pressure is essential in the immediate postoperative period. CVP should be maintained at a high–normal level (6-10 cm $H_2O$) to provide optimal end-diastolic filling and cardiac output. It is important that hypovolaemia is avoided in the postoperative period as it may compromise hepatic artery flow and risk thrombosis.

Arrhythmias may be related to an underlying cardiac condition or acute electrolyte abnormalities. Bradycardia may be associated with steroid administration, but raised intracranial pressure from cerebral oedema or intracranial bleeding should also be considered. Tachyarrhythmias are more commonly associated with electrolyte disturbances such as hyperkalaemia, hypokalaemia, hypocalcaemia, and hypomagnesaemia. Close attention to fluid and blood product administration is essential to avoid iatrogenic causes.

### Sedation and analgesia

A number of factors will determine when postoperative sedation should be reduced or discontinued. These include age, graft size, pre-existing morbidity, intraoperative complications, cardiovascular stability, and need for further surgery. All patients require analgesia for a painful abdominal wound. Morphine is a suitable choice and is usually administered by continuous infusion at a dose of 20–60 μg/kg/hour.

Patients requiring a period of postoperative ventilation are usually commenced on an infusion of midazolam at a rate of 1–3 μg/kg/min, particularly if muscle relaxation is required. Midazolam should be avoided, or the dose greatly reduced, in children aged < 3 months and in those with hepatic or renal impairment. If midazolam alone provides inadequate sedation, then an $\alpha_2$-receptor agonist such as clonidine or dexmedetomidine may be added. Propofol is avoided because it is unlicensed in this setting and may trigger propofol infusion syndrome in susceptible patients.

Once the patient is extubated and ready to return to the ward the morphine infusion can be converted to nurse or patient-controlled analgesia. Paracetamol is given to supplement opiate analgesia, intravenously, rectally, or orally. Dosing is reduced in liver transplant patients.

Once enteral feeds have been re-established it may be possible to replace or supplement midazolam with an oral sedative such as chloral hydrate or clonidine. It is important to monitor the effects of all sedative drugs to avoid under- or overdosing. A useful system for this is the COMFORT score, a composite of behavioural and physiological dimensions each scored between 1 and 5, with lower values indicating greater sedation (Ista et al., 2005). This is undertaken on an hourly basis, with sedation titrated to maintain a score of 17–26. The score cannot be applied to patients who are receiving muscle relaxant agents.

### Fluid management

A strategy for fluid management should be agreed locally. It is important to consider total fluid balance in terms of all losses (urine output, insensible, drain, and GI tract) and fluid replacements. Volume, electrolyte composition (particularly sodium content), acid-base status, and albumin levels should all be considered. Regular monitoring of serum electrolytes, liver function tests, and blood gases should inform fluid selection.

Renal dysfunction commonly accompanies liver impairment following transplantation. The risk factors for renal dysfunction include pre-existing renal failure, intraoperative hypotension, prolonged surgery, nephrotoxic medication, and postoperative hypotension. In the postoperative period it is desirable to maintain a urine output of 1–2 mL/kg/hour. If urine output is reduced to < 0.5 mL/kg/hour for two consecutive hours it is important to review intravascular volume and cardiac output parameters and to exclude urinary retention and abdominal compartment syndrome. A fluid challenge should be considered. Occasionally a good diuresis following a diuretic challenge (e.g. furosemide 0.5–1.0 mg/kg IV) may provide reassurance, but the use of furosemide should be limited due to concerns it will lead to hypovolaemia and increase the risk of graft vessel thrombosis.

Investigations to help define the cause of a reduced urine output include a check for catheter patency, serum and urine osmolality, ultrasound scan of the bladder and kidneys, immunosuppressant levels, and measurement of intra-abdominal pressure. In the absence of immediately treatable causes, haemofiltration or dialysis may be required, particularly in the context of fluid overload, renal dysfunction, acidosis, or severe electrolyte disturbance, especially hyperkalaemia.

## Blood products

Blood product administration may be ongoing at the time the patient returns to the PICU. Administration of bank blood is guided by haemoglobin concentration, but in the presence of continued bleeding, platelet count, fibrinogen concentration, and whole blood viscoelastic testing (thromboelastography or thromboelastometry) are also important. The haemoglobin concentration should be kept between 7 and 8.5 g/dL to optimize blood flow to the graft, which may necessitate small volume transfusions if blood loss continues or if blood tests are numerous. A platelet count of above 50 – $10^9$/L is usually satisfactory in the absence of active bleeding. FFP and cryoprecipitate may be administered as required. An ongoing requirement for these products in the immediate postoperative period should raise concerns about graft function. Occasionally overtransfusion occurs, necessitating venesection to reduce the risk of hepatic arterial thrombosis.

## Abdominal compartment syndrome

Primary closure of the abdominal wall after liver transplantation is frequently not possible in infants and children due to the size of the graft. Attempted closure may lead to abdominal compartment syndrome.

Abdominal compartment syndrome is defined as an intra-abdominal pressure (IAP) > 12 mmHg (1 mmHg = 1.36 $cmH_2O$) with associated organ dysfunction (Malbrain et al., 2006; Cheatham et al., 2007). A grading system defines severity as follows: grade I (12–15 mmHg), grade II (16–20 mmHg), grade III (21–25 mmHg), and grade IV (> 25 mmHg). IAP measurement is usually obtained through an intravesical catheter (Bailey and Shapiro, 2000) and bladder instillation of up to 1 mL/kg volume (maximum 25 mL) is recommended in children to facilitate measurement. Perfusion of the abdominal organs is determined by the difference between MAP and IAP. IAP can be falsely elevated by muscle contractions, forced expiration, and poor pain control.

A raised IAP may lead to reduced cardiac output due to a reduction in venous return, increased systemic vascular resistance, and myocardial strain. This can lead to impaired global tissue oxygen delivery, revealed by increased venous extraction of oxygen, a rise in serum lactate, and evidence of end-organ hypoxia (confusion, agitation, poor urine output, gut ileus). Elevation of IAP causes multi-organ impairment and is independently associated with increased intensive care mortality (Malbrain et al., 2005). The effects include:

- Intestinal venous congestion, ischaemia, and a systemic inflammatory response secondary to bacterial translocation.
- Poor hepatic graft function from reduced hepatic arterial and portal venous inflow.
- Renal dysfunction with decreased glomerular filtration rate and acute tubular necrosis.
- Respiratory compromise from diaphragmatic splinting, hypoventilation, and ventilation–perfusion mismatch.
- Cerebral impairment due to increased venous pressure, reduced oxygen delivery, and poor hepatic neurotoxin clearance.

Elevated IAP should be actively identified and treated. Prevention strategies include staged abdominal wall closure with interval use of a prosthetic patch, reduction of graft size, and avoiding constrictive dressings (Thomas et al., 2010).

Treatment of elevated IAP requires the evacuation of the intestinal contents using nasogastric drainage, prokinetics, bowel enemas, and nil-by-mouth orders, as well as ascitic fluid drainage, analgesic control, neuromuscular blockade, and judicious diuresis. In the context of deteriorating organ function, vasoactive medications can be titrated to maintain an abdominal perfusion pressure of > 60 mmHg. If these measures are unsuccessful in reducing the IAP and reversing organ dysfunction then surgical abdominal decompression should be considered.

## Neurological system

Seizures may complicate the post-transplant period and have many causes. These include intracranial bleeding, electrolyte disturbances (hyponatraemia, hypomagnesaemia, hypocalcaemia), hypoglycaemia, hypoxia, and sepsis. However, the commonest cause remains immunosuppressant-related neurotoxicity. A full blood panel including glucose, extended electrolytes, immunosuppressant levels, full blood count, coagulation profile, liver and renal profiles, and arterial blood gas analysis should be performed urgently. The priority is to maintain cardiorespiratory function while pursuing a treatable cause. Brain CT and EEG may be indicated.

## Infection control

Immunosuppression in the post-transplant patient increases the risk of all types of infection, including primary bacterial, viral, and fungal infections, and reactivation of viruses and atypical micro-organisms. Bacterial infections predominate and are most common in the early post-transplant period, while viral infections, pneumocystis, and fungal infections appear later, sometimes requiring respiratory support in intensive care. Prophylaxis is of proven benefit. A typical protocol is given in the following sections. (Note: dosing is given as a guide and the responsibility for individual prescriptions remains with the prescriber. The authors cannot take responsibility for mistakes or misprints.)

### Antimicrobials

- Piperacillin/tazobactam: 90 mg/kg/dose 8 hourly for 48 hours, then review (if penicillin allergic: ciprofloxacin 5 mg/kg/dose 12 hourly)
- Metronidazole: 8 mg/kg/dose (maximum 500 mg) 8 hourly for 48 hours, then review

- Cotrimoxazole: up to 5 years 240 mg orally on alternate days; over 5 years 480 mg orally on alternate days

### Antivirals

Until the donor status for EBV and CMV is known all transplanted children are started on antiviral prophylaxis. Acyclovir IV 500 mg/m$^2$ 8 hourly, then orally at 200 mg qds if < 2 years or 400 mg qds if > 2 years of age. If the donor is EBV positive or CMV positive or the status is unknown, then acyclovir should be continued for 3 months post-transplant.

### Antifungals

Nystatin 100,000 units orally qds if > 10 kg or 50,000 units orally 6 hourly if < 10 kg. Systemic antifungals, e.g. liposomal amphotericin B (AmBisome®) 3 mg/kg IV for 7–10 days, should be used for prophylaxis only in selected high-risk groups of patients: ALF, prolonged ventilation, CVVH, retransplant, relaparotomy, biliary leak, and those with vascular complications. Patients already on fluconazole should be changed to amphotericin.

## Nutrition

Clear fluids (e.g. Dioralyte™) are introduced in small volumes when bowel sounds are heard and the child has passed stools. Full enteral fluids are started after consultation with the surgical team, once it is confirmed that clear fluids are tolerated.

Postoperative patients often become catabolic due to increased metabolic demands and inadequate calorie delivery. Pretransplant malnutrition may also be present. Every effort should be made to satisfy the patient's nutritional requirements at the earliest opportunity, using the enteral or parenteral routes or a combination of both.

### Enteral feeding

Enteral feeding is the preferred option in most patients. It is technically easier, has fewer side effects, and is cheaper than parenteral nutrition and less likely to damage the liver graft. Various preparations are available; their use depends on the age and calorie requirements of the patient, and on the availability of breast milk. Specialist dietetic advice should be sought to identify the best regime for the patient. Most feeds are delivered continuously, which allows superior absorption and is better tolerated by patients with respiratory compromise. It also permits assessment of absorption without the risk of large gastric aspirates and the potential for regurgitation or vomiting.

Tolerance of feeds should be confirmed by regular aspiration of the nasogastric tube. It is common to aspirate some feed, which can be replaced if the volume is small (< 5 mL/kg). Evidence of feed intolerance includes persistent large nasogastric aspirates, vomiting, abdominal pain, and diarrhoea.

Feed intolerance is common and often multifactorial. It can be overcome by reducing feed volumes, adding prokinetic drugs, or feeding via nasojejunal tube. In certain situations special feeds are indicated, including thickened feeds for gastric reflux, medium chain triglycerides (MCT) for chylothorax, and feeds that are lactose-free, predigested, or calorie-loaded, when volumes are limited or growth poor. As respiratory function improves, problems such as hunger and hypoglycaemia may be addressed by the introduction of bolus feeds. These are initially small volumes given 2 hourly, progressing to larger feeds 3–4 hourly as tolerated.

If enteral feeding is contraindicated, or if it is not established by 5–7 days after surgery, parenteral nutrition (PN) should be considered. However, PN should be replaced with enteral nutrition at the earliest opportunity.

## Other complications

### Graft dysfunction/thrombosis

Acute graft dysfunction presents a picture similar to ALF, with rising bilirubin, transaminases, lactate, and PT, accompanied by hypotension, hypoglycaemia, acidosis, and signs of neurological dysfunction. Urgent Doppler ultrasound assessment of hepatic artery blood flow should be undertaken. If no flow is seen, conventional or CTA should be done to confirm the diagnosis. This is a surgical emergency requiring immediate abdominal exploration.

If dysfunction is related to a poor quality graft, intraoperative complications, or compromised cardiac output in the postoperative period, liver function may be supported by the infusion of N-acetylcysteine by infusion (150 mg/kg/day). It may be necessary to relist for urgent retransplantation and intensive organ system support will be required.

Patients should undergo daily abdominal ultrasound examination in the postoperative period to assess vessel blood flow. If vascular anastamoses are considered to be at risk, a prophylactic heparin infusion may be administered. This can be stopped once feeding has been commenced and the patient established on aspirin and dipyridamole. It is typically stopped 7 days after transplant in any case.

### Rejection

Acute rejection tends to occur at 5–10 days post-transplant and presents as a derangement in liver enzymes and hyperbilirubinaemia. It is usually confirmed by liver biopsy and treated with either increased doses of existing immunosuppressive agents or high-dose steroid therapy. Ongoing assessment includes regular measurement of liver enzymes and repeat liver biopsy.

### Acute gastrointestinal bleeding

Bleeding from the GI tract is a relatively common problem following liver transplantation. It is most often related to acute ulceration and/or complications from pre-existing portal hypertension. Most bleeds can be managed conservatively by blood transfusion, correction of coagulopathy, and optimizing gastric protection therapy (ranitidine, omeprazole, and sucralfate).

### Failure to wean from the ventilator

There are many reasons why a child fails to wean from ventilation following liver transplantation, as outlined in Table 26.1.

Every effort should be made to address these complications and optimize the child's condition before attempting extubation. When difficulty is likely, planned use of non-invasive ventilatory support is prudent, using CPAP or BiPAP by facemask or nasal catheter, reducing support gradually over a number of days as the child's condition improves.

When it is clear that the child will not cope off the ventilator, early reintubation is recommended. This may prevent atelectasis, aspiration, acidosis, hypotension, and arrhythmias. It also allows the respiratory tract to be cultured for pathogens and aids

**Table 26.1** Failure to wean following liver transplantation

| Cause | Reason |
|---|---|
| Respiratory failure | Infection |
| | Fluid overload |
| | Pleural effusion |
| | Diaphragmatic paresis |
| | Diaphragmatic splinting |
| | Abdominal patch |
| | Muscle weakness |
| Cardiovascular failure | Hypovolaemia |
| | Impaired cardiac function |
| | Vasoplegia |
| Hepatic failure | Encephalopathy |
| | Impaired drug metabolism |
| | Hyperammonaemia |
| Renal failure | Fluid overload |
| | Electrolyte disturbances |
| | Uraemia |
| | Drug accumulation |
| Neurological failure | Encephalopathy |
| | Cerebral oedema |
| | Intracranial bleed |
| | PICU polyneuropathy |
| Sepsis | Pyrexia |
| | Failure of organ systems |
| | Respiratory infection |
| Pain | Poor secretion clearance |
| | Inadequate ventilatory effort |
| | Increased anxiety |
| | Increased oxygen consumption |
| Nutrition | Inadequate calorie intake |
| | Muscle wasting |
| | Excessive carbohydrate |
| Pharmacology | Residual drug effects |
| | Drug withdrawal |
| | Inadequate analgesia/sedation |

interventions such as drainage of pleural effusions and changing of central venous catheters.

## Conclusion

Paediatric liver transplant recipients may need no more than a few hours' postoperative ventilation or may suffer a complicated postoperative course involving the full range of organ support modalities. To achieve good outcomes the paediatric intensivist must combine sound knowledge of the underlying disease state and potential post-transplant complications with vigilance and timely intervention. Excellent communication with other specialist teams is also vital. Exemplary care is well rewarded, however, as long-term outcomes continue to improve and as skills refined in the management of these complex patients ultimately benefit a much wider group of critically ill children.

## References


Bailey J, Shapiro M (2000) Abdominal compartment syndrome. *Crit Care*, **4**(1):23–29.

Betrosian AP, Agarwal B, Douzinas EE (2007) Acute renal dysfunction in liver diseases. *World J Gastroenterol*, **13**(42):5552–5559.

Cheatham ML, Malbrain ML, Kirkpatrick A, et al. (2007) Results from the International Conference of Experts on Intra-abdominal Hypertension and Abdominal Compartment Syndrome. II. Recommendations. *Intensive Care Med*, **33**(6):951–962.

Fede G, Spadaro L, Tomaselli T, et al. (2012) Adrenocortical dysfunction in liver disease: a systematic review. *Hepatology*, **55**(4):1282–1291.

Godbole G, Shanmugam N, Dhawan A, et al. (2011) Infectious complications in pediatric acute liver failure. *J Pediatr Gastroenterol Nutr*, **53**(3):320–325.

Harry R, Auzinger G, Wendon J (2002) The clinical importance of adrenal insufficiency in acute hepatic dysfunction. *Hepatology*, **36**:395–402

Ista E, van Dijk M, Tibboel D, et al. (2005) Assessment of sedation levels in pediatric intensive care patients can be improved by using the COMFORT 'behavior' scale. *Pediatr Crit Care Med*, **6**(1):58–63.

Kamat P, Kunde S, Vos M, et al. (2012) Invasive intracranial pressure monitoring is a useful adjunct in the management of severe hepatic encephalopathy associated with pediatric acute liver failure. *Pediatr Crit Care Med*, **13**(1):e33–e38.

Larcher V, Craig F, Bhogal K, Wilkinson D, Brierley J, on behalf of the Royal College of Paediatrics and Child Health (2015) Making decisions to limit treatment in life-limiting and life-threatening conditions in children: a framework for practice. *Arch Dis Child*, 100:s1–s23.

Lizard-Cervera J, Almeda P, Guevera L, et al. (2003) Hepatic encephalopathy: a review. *Annal Hepatol*, **2**(3):122–130.

Malbrain ML, Chiumello D, Pelosi P, et al. (2005) Incidence and prognosis of intraabdominal hypertension in a mixed population of critically ill patients: a multiple-center epidemiological study. *Crit Care Med*, **33**(2):315–322.

Malbrain ML, Cheatham ML, Kirkpatrick A, et al. (2006) Results from the International Conference of Experts on Intra-abdominal Hypertension and Abdominal Compartment Syndrome. I. Definitions. *Intensive Care Med*, **32**(11):1722–1732.

McDiarmid SV (1996) Renal function in pediatric liver transplant patients. *Kidney Int Suppl*, **53**:S77–S84.

Resuscitation Council (UK) (2014) Decisions Relating to Cardiopulmonary Resuscitation, 3rd edn. <https://www.resus.org.uk/pages/decisionsrelatingtocpr.pdf.>

Riordan SM, Williams R (1997) Treatment of hepatic encephalopathy. *N Engl J Med*, **337**:473–479.

Schaefer B, Schaefer F, Engelman G, et al. (2011) Comparison of Molecular Adsorbents Recirculating System (MARS) dialysis in children with acute liver failure. *Nephrol Dial Transplant*, **26**(11):3633–3639.

Stange J, Hassanein TI, Mehta R, et al. (2002) The molecular adsorbents recycling system as a liver support system based on albumin dialysis: a summary of preclinical investigations, prospective, randomized, controlled clinical trial, and clinical experience from 19 centers. *Artif Organs*, **26**(2):103–110.

Thomas N, Thomas G, Verran D, et al. (2010) Liver transplantation in children with hyper-reduced grafts—a single-center experience. *Pediatr Transplant*, **14**(3):426–430.


## Further reading


European Liver Transplant Registry: <www.eltr.org>.

Suchy FJ, Sokol RJ, Balistreri WF (eds) (2007) *Liver Disease in Children*, 3rd edn. Cambridge University Press, Cambridge.

Cauli O, Rodrigo R, Llansola M, et al. (2009) Glutamatergic and GABAergic neurotransmission and neuronal circuits in hepatic encephalopathy. *Metab Brain Dis*, **24**:69.

Chu CJ, Wang SS, Lee FY, et al. (2001) Detrimental effects of nitric oxide inhibition on hepatic encephalopathy in rats with thioacetamide-induced fulminant hepatic failure. *Eur J Clin Invest*, **31**:156.

SECTION 7

# Intestinal and multivisceral

# CHAPTER 27

# Anaesthetic management of adult intestinal and multivisceral transplantation

Kyota Fukazawa, Ernesto A. Pretto, Jr., and Seigo Nishida

## Introduction

According to the US OPTN and Scientific Registry for Transplant Recipients, more than 29,000 cadaveric transplants were performed in the US in 2014. Of these, 139 were intestinal transplants (ITx), which include intestine and intestine with other organ (multivisceral) (OPTN, 2014). The majority of organs originated from deceased brain (DBD) or deceased cardiac donors (DCD), with only a few cases of living donor ITx. According to the Intestinal Transplant Registry, 2,887 intestinal transplants on 2,669 recipients were performed between April 1985 and March 2014 at 82 transplant centres worldwide (Grant et al., 2015). Therefore clinical experience in ITx is concentrated in only a few centres, most of which are located in the US. Nevertheless, numbers have been growing ever since the Center for Medicare and Medicaid Services (CMS, 2006) approved insurance coverage for intestinal, combined intestine and liver, or multivisceral transplantation in April 2001 (Abu-Elmagd et al., 2002). Current actuarial survival rates for ITx are 76%, 56%, and 43% at 1, 5, and 10 years, respectively (Grant et al., 2015). In 2013, 44.8% of intestine with liver and 19.6% of intestine transplants were in children aged 18 years old or less (Smith et al., 2015).

During the early experimental phase of ITx/MVTx, outcome was associated with a high incidence of graft rejection due to strong host expression of histocompatibility antigens, high number of resident lymphocytes, and colonization of micro-organisms (Grant et al., 2005). Graft survival has markedly improved since the early 1990s (Kaufman et al., 2001). This is attributable to multiple factors, among these: improvement of surgical techniques, perioperative anaesthetic management, new diagnostic tools for the early identification of acute rejection (e.g. introduction of zoom video endoscope in 1988), the introduction of new classes of immunosuppressive agents (e.g. calcineurin inhibitors (CNIs) and IL-2 suppressing agents), and standardized protocols for CMV prophylaxis. Today more than 76% of cases that survive more than 6 months after transplant no longer require Total parenteral nutrition (TPN), leading to marked improvement of quality of life. Over 90% of those recipients are able to lead normal social lives, comparable to that of healthy people. There are many recipients who have survived more than 16 years (Intestinal Transplant Association, 2005). However, the number of ITx/MVTx cases is 30 times less than liver transplants, and 5-year survival is only 56% compared to 72% for liver transplant recipients (Intestinal Transplant Association, 2005).

## Definitions

### Short bowel syndrome

Short bowel syndrome (SBS) occurs when the length of functional intestine is less than 200 cm. Intestinal absorption is proportional to the amount of residual intestine. According to guidelines from the American Gastroenterological Association (2003), patients at greatest nutritional risk generally have a duodenostomy or a jejuno-ileal anastomosis with < 35 cm of residual small intestine, jejunocolic or ileocolic anastomosis with < 60 cm of residual small intestine, or an end-jejunostomy with < 115 cm of residual small intestine. In patients with SBS the colon becomes an important digestive organ; therefore patients can be further subdivided into those with colon-in-continuity and those without colon-in-continuity.

### Intestinal transplantation

ITx refers to the transplant of the intestine only (including some part of the colon), also called isolated intestine transplant. Combined liver and intestine transplants are often performed and usually categorized as ITx or MVTx.

### Multivisceral transplantation

MVTx has not been clearly categorized and defined but usually refers to the transplantation of more than three intra-abdominal organs as a composite graft. Organs often transplanted as part of an MVTx procedure include liver, pancreas, spleen, stomach, duodenum, small intestine, portion of the colon, and kidney. Therefore MVTx is a separate category to the liver–intestine transplant procedure. In these cases, perioperative management will depend on the type of organs involved. For the purposes of this chapter we will consider anaesthetic and perioperative management in the following procedures: (1) isolated ITx or intestine plus one other organ (two organs) or MVTx (three or more organs); and (2) combined liver–intestine and/or involvement of other organs, such as kidney and pancreas.

# Indications

## Intestinal transplantation

ITx is indicated in patients with intestinal failure, which is defined as irreversible inability of the intestinal tract to fulfil the body's nutritional, fluid, and electrolytic requirements (see Figure 27.1) (Molmenti et al., 2009). Recipients typically develop 'short gut syndrome' after multiple resections of the small intestine, in some cases for the treatment of ulcerative colitis/Crohn's disease or after resection of ischaemic bowel due to mesenteric thrombosis. In short gut syndrome intestinal absorption of nutrients is often inadequate and TPN via central venous access is required to provide supplemental nutrients necessary to maintain life. However, indwelling central venous catheters (CVCs) can lead to bacterial infection or sepsis, as well as hypercoagulability with venous thrombosis. Frequent bacterial infections and lack of central venous access for TPN are common indications for ITx. TPN-induced irreversible hepatic dysfunction is also an indication for combined liver–intestine or multivisceral transplant.

The reported incidence of short gut syndrome is 1.8–2.0 per 1,000,000 population (Lennard-Jones, 1990; Moreno et al., 2005). In the US the Centers for Medicare and Medicaid Services (CMS) has classified indications for ITx into three categories: (1) inability to continue TPN at home; (2) high risk of death due to the underlying disease; and (3) intolerance to TPN due to frequent complications (see Table 27.1; Centers for Medicare and Medicaid Services, 2006). Heretofore, ITx has been contraindicated in recipients who simply want to improve their quality of life. This is because of the immediate risks of the procedure. As long-term survival increases with improvement of transplant outcomes, quality of life may become an indication (Grant et al., 2005).

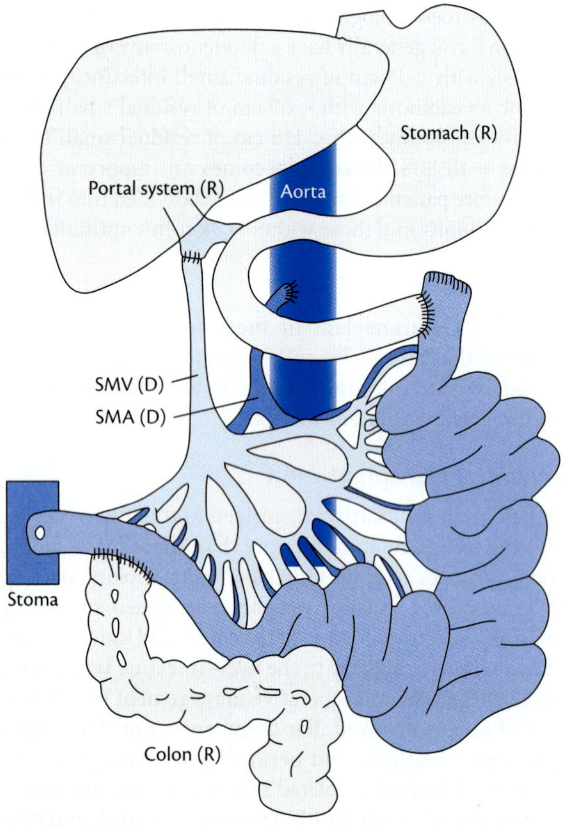


**Fig. 27.1** Intestinal transplantation. D, Donor; R, recipient; SMA, superior mesenteric artery; SMV, superior mesenteric vein.

## Combined liver–intestine transplantation

Combined liver–intestine transplantation is indicated in patients with intestinal failure and concomitant liver failure. Outcomes are worse than for ITX (Smith et al., 2015).Therefore it is important to undergo ITx before the onset of liver failure. It has been reported that liver dysfunction is reversible if successful ITx is performed prior to the development of liver failure. UNOS reports a high death rate among patients on ITx waiting lists compared to patients on other organ transplant waiting lists. On wait-lists the highest death rates are primarily among young children awaiting combined liver–intestine transplantation (Fecteau et al., 2001; Fryer et al., 2003). Modification of the organ allocation system as well as alternative surgical options (reduced size graft from an adult donor) have been proposed to minimize waiting-list death rates (Reyes et al., 1998; de Ville de Goyet et al., 2000).

## Multivisceral transplantation

MVTx is indicated in patients with irreversible multiple abdominal organ failure and abdominal tumours involving multiple organs, as well as in patients with short gut syndrome with TPN-induced liver failure (Figure 27.2). In addition, extensive vascular thrombosis involving the superior mesenteric venous system and/or portal venous system due to congenital coagulation disorders (e.g. protein C deficiency) may be an indication for MVTx. If concomitant kidney failure exists, the kidney is also included in the MVTx procedure. It is not uncommon that the surgical plan will change due to unforeseen anatomical and technical problems encountered intraoperatively.

Common pathological conditions associated with ITx are summarized in Table 27.2. In paediatric cases these include neonatal necrotizing colitis, obstruction of the small intestine, mid-gut volvulus, obstruction of the colon, gastroschisis, and motility disorders (see Chapter 28).

## Contraindications

Contraindications for ITx/MVTx include the presence of active infection, progressive malignant tumour, multi-organ failure, all conditions affecting the central nervous system (CNS), and psychiatric disease. These conditions need to be thoroughly assessed during the pretransplant screening process. See Table 27.2.

## Pretransplant assessment of recipients for ITx/MVTx

Before listing candidates for ITx/MVTx it is necessary to assess their medical, surgical, and mental health. The evaluation process is interdisciplinary, comprising gastroenterologists, transplant surgeons, transplant anaesthesiologists, cardiologists, psychiatrists, social workers, and dieticians.

High-risk patients include those with: (1) venous thrombosis of more than 50% of central venous access sites who therefore cannot receive TPN; (2) recurrent severe infections or sepsis due to indwelling intravenous catheters; (3) progressive liver dysfunction; (4) impaired renal function due to massive GI fluid losses; and (5) locally aggressive, non-metastasizing desmoid tumours

**Table 27.1** Indications for ITx. (Reprinted from *Gastroenterolgy*, 135, 1, Pironi L et al., 'Survival of Patients Identified as Candidates for Intestinal Transplantation: A 3-Year Prospective Follow-Up', pp. 61–71, Copyright 2008, with permission from Elsevier and the AGA Institute.)

| 1. Failure of TPN |
|---|
| 1a. Impending (total bilirubin $^{3}$ 3–6 mg/dL, progressive thrombocytopaenia, and progressive splenomegaly) or liver failure (portal hypertension, hepatosplenomegaly, hepatic fibrosis, or cirrhosis) because of parenteral nutrition liver injury |
| 1b. CVC-related thrombosis of $^{3}$ 2 central veins |
| 1c. Frequent central line sepsis: $^{3}$ 2 episodes/year of systemic sepsis secondary to line infections requiring hospitalization; a single episode of line-related fungaemia; septic shock or ARDS |
| 1d. Frequent episodes of severe dehydration despite intravenous fluid in addition to TPN |
| 2. High risk of death attributable to the underlying disease |
| 2a. Desmoid tumours associated with familial adenomatous polyposis |
| 2b. Congenital mucosal disorders (e.g. microvillus atrophy, intestinal epithelial dysplasia) |
| 2c. Ultra-SBS (gastrostomy, duodenostomy, residual small bowel £ 10 cm in infants and £ 20 cm in adults) |
| 3. Intestinal failure with high morbidity or low acceptance of TPN |
| 3a. Intestinal failure with high morbidity (frequent hospitalization, narcotic dependency) or inability to function (e.g. pseudo-obstruction, high-output stoma) |
| 3b. Patient's unwillingness to accept long-term TPN (e.g. young patients) |

Criteria were taken from those approved by the US Center for Medicine and Medicaid Services and from the paper of the American Society of Transplantation regarding paediatric ITx candidate. ARDS, acute respiratory distress syndrome; CVC, central venous catheter; SBS, short bowel syndrome; TPN, total parenteral nutrition.

that can only be removed by massive evisceration (Kaufman et al., 2001; Grant et al., 2005). These patients require careful pretransplant assessment and complex interdisciplinary decision-making.

Relatively low-risk patients include: (1) patients on TPN without problems; (2) infants and adults with an ultra-short intestine (less than 20–30 cm of small intestine); and (3) infants with total intestinal aganglionosis or microvillus inclusion disease, because these patients have very poor survival with TPN.

Pretransplant screening includes assessment of the underlying disease process, intestinal and liver function tests, screening studies for virus infection (EBV, CMV), blood and HLA typing, determination of panel reactive antibody (PRA) status, and coagulation studies (especially for patients with a history of vascular thrombosis). Citrullin level can be used to monitor the condition of the intestine. Patients with dysmotility syndrome may require manometry of the oesophagus and rectum. These results are also useful for transplant anaesthesiologists to plan intraoperative management. Information regarding whether to transplant the liver or not is most important because it changes the surgical approach and intraoperative anaesthetic management. The preoperative anaesthesia assessment of MVTx candidates includes an understanding of the underlying GI pathology, the patient's general condition, cardiovascular risk assessment, and assessment of vascular access.

## Cardiovascular risk assessment

Intraoperative haemodynamic fluctuations and significant tachycardia are common during ITx/MVTx. This is mainly due to hypovolaemia from massive fluid shifts and third space loss during surgery, as well as inflammatory reactions (e.g. ischaemia–reperfusion). Therefore cardiovascular risk assessment is particularly important. A complete history and physical examination before transplant will provide a gross estimate of cardiac reserve of the recipient and will determine the need for further cardiac testing. Recipients who are young (< 40 years old) with no cardiovascular risk factors and good exercise tolerance of > 4 MET require only a 12-lead ECG and transthoracic echocardiogram (TTE). Elderly patients and patients with higher cardiovascular risks require stress testing or coronary angiogram to ensure that cardiac reserve is sufficient to overcome cardiovascular stress during surgery. The decision whether to carry out advanced cardiovascular testing is determined based on American Heart Association (AHA) guidelines (Fleisher et al., 2007). ITx recipients with concomitant liver failure must be screened for pulmonary hypertension. The same screening criteria used for liver transplant recipients with portopulmonary hypertension are applicable to intestinal and multivisceral patients (Rodriguez-Roisin et al., 2004; Fukazawa et al., 2010). In liver transplant recipients there is an association between cardiopulmonary death and portopulmonary hypertension (Krowka et al., 2000). TTE is used for cardiovascular screening of pulmonary hypertension. Signs of elevated right ventricular systolic pressure (RVSP) require direct measurement of pulmonary artery pressure by right heart catheterization.

## Assessment of vascular access

In patients with thrombosis, establishing adequate vascular access can be a challenging undertaking for the transplant anaesthesiologist. Almost all patients have very limited vascular access due to thrombosis caused by hypercoagulability resulting from indwelling central venous cannulation for TPN. Therefore pretransplant evaluation should include venous Doppler studies or venograms to determine central vascular access (e.g. internal jugular vein, subclavian vein, external jugular vein, and brachial veins). If occluded, a plan for alternative venous access may be required (e.g. collateral veins, inferior vena cava (IVC) access from lumber approach, interosseous infusions, or intra-arterial). In those cases, early consultation with an interventional radiologist may be required to perform fluoroscopy-guided vascular cannulation. Intraoperative access to the azygos vein or the renal vein may be another option if all other options fail (see Figure 27.3). In those cases, the transplant procedure can be started with peripheral intravenous lines or femoral vein access, then switched to alternative sites by the surgeon intraoperatively. Communication between the transplant surgeon, anaesthesiologist, and interventional radiologists before transplant is particularly important in these situations and a detailed plan (including a backup plan) for vascular access needs to be well sorted out beforehand.

## Intraoperative monitoring

Major considerations for intraoperative monitoring are similar to those of major cardiac surgery or liver transplantation because of the risk of marked haemodynamic fluctuations associated with

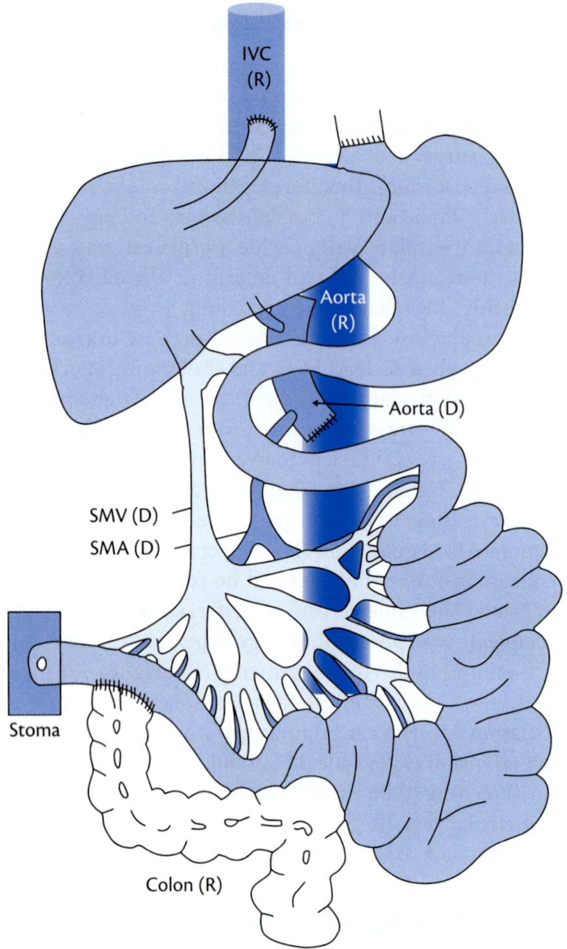


**Fig. 27.2** Multivisceral transplantation. D, Donor; R, recipient; IVC, inferior vena cava; SMA, superior mesenteric artery; SMV, superior mesenteric vein.

**Table 27.2** Contraindications for ITx. (Reprinted from Gastroenterolgy, 135, 1, Pironi L et al., 'Survival of Patients Identified as Candidates for Intestinal Transplantation: A 3-Year Prospective Follow-Up', pp. 61–71, Copyright 2008, with permission from Elsevier and the AGA Institute.)

| a. Absolute |
|---|
| a1. Non-resectable malignancy (local or metastatic) |
| a2. Severe congenital or acquired immunological deficiencies |
| a3. Advanced cardiopulmonary disease |
| a4. Advanced neurological dysfunction |
| a5. Sepsis with multisystem organ failure |
| a6. Major psychiatric illness |
| a7. Demonstrated patient non-compliance with medical recommendations |
| a8. Insufficient vascular patency for central venous access for ³ 6 months after ITx |
| b. Relative |
| b1. Age > 65 years (depending on associated vascular, cardiac, and respiratory disease) |
| b2. History of cancer in the past 5 years (depending on judgement of oncologist) |
| b3. Physical debilitation (risk of poor survival after ITx) |
| b4. Lack of family support (risk of low compliance after ITx) |

Criteria were taken from those approved by the US Center for Medicine and Medicaid Services and from the paper of the American Society of Transplantation regarding paediatric ITx candidate.

manipulation of major vessels and inflammatory reactions encountered during the procedure. When considering invasive monitoring it is important to take into account (1) the risk of postoperative infection and sepsis, because recipients require potent immunosuppressive medication intraoperatively and postoperatively, and (2) the risk of thrombosis, because the majority of candidates for ITx are hypercoagulable. Invasive arterial pressure monitoring is required in addition to standard anaesthetic monitoring (electrocardiogram, peripheral oxygen saturation, and non-invasive blood pressure). To avoid interruption of invasive arterial blood pressure monitoring during blood draws, we recommend the use of two arterial lines. A pulmonary artery catheter provides hands-free monitoring of central venous pressure (CVP) and pulmonary artery pressure (PAP), as well as continuous cardiac output and mixed venous oxygen saturation ($SvO_2$), which enables more precise fluid and haemodynamic management. Therefore if vascular access for pulmonary arterial catheter is possible, pulmonary arterial catheter is used, especially if transplantation of the liver is planned. Trans esophageal echocardiography (TOE) is useful to monitor cardiac function, volume status, and air/thromboembolism. TOE is relatively non-invasive with minimal risk for infection; thus its use in high-risk cases is highly recommended. However, the presence of oesophageal varices or a recent history of upper GI bleeding are relative contraindications to its use.

Serial arterial blood gas assessment is required to monitor the status of pulmonary gas exchange, acid-base status, electrolytes, glucose, and haematocrit. Coagulation monitoring is facilitated by the use of intraoperative Thromboelastogram (TEG). Coagulation monitoring includes platelet count/function, PT, aPTT, and

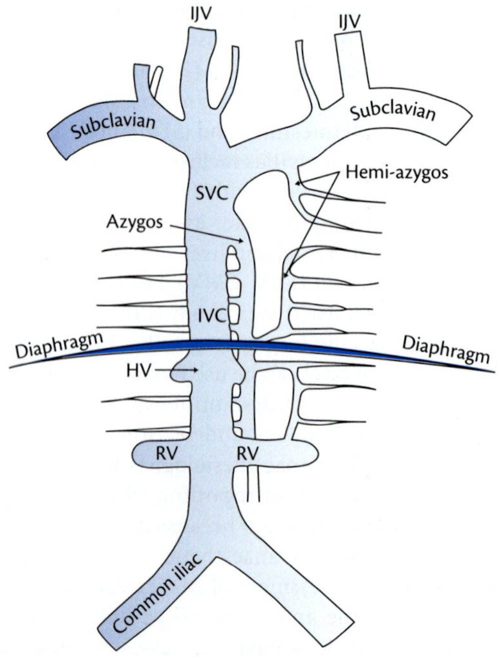


**Fig. 27.3** The venous system. HV, Hepatic vein; IJV, internal jugular vein; IVC, inferior vena cava ; SVC, superior vena cava; RV, renal vein.

fibrinogen. TEG enables quick, point-of-care assessment of coagulation status and provides a method for the early detection of hypercoagulation. In our institution, blood and blood component therapy is managed based solely on TEG results. Baseline TEG in ITx and MVTx recipients often shows hypercoagulability. Patients with concomitant liver failure may present with more complex combined coagulation abnormalities.

Generally, transplant recipients have a prior history of multiple open abdominal surgeries. Since blood loss from dissection of adhesions can occur, we recommend placement of two large-bore multilumen central venous lines. One of those lines can be used for the placement of a pulmonary artery catheter, if indicated. The other line can be used for intraoperative continuous venovenous hemodialysis (CVVHD) if required. Use of the femoral vein should be avoided because of the following considerations: (1) high risk of infection; and (2) the IVC might be occluded by thrombus or tumour, or clamped during transplant. Doppler ultrasound is very useful to localize and assess the patency of veins.

Before taking patients into the operating room, blood products (packed red blood cells (PRBCs), fresh frozen plasma (FFP), platelets) should be available and ideally in the room (at least 5–10 units each) prior to start. Based on the potential for surgical bleeding, severity of coagulopathy, and preoperative haematocrit, additional products should be ordered early, especially for recipients who have red blood cell antibodies. In case of massive blood loss, recipients with rare blood type, and recipients with red blood cell antibodies, direct communication with the blood bank or transfusion service is very important. Also usage of cell saver or a rapid infusion system should be anticipated.

## Intraoperative management

Transplant surgery is usually performed on an emergency basis whenever a donor organ becomes available, so as to minimize ischaemia time. In this case, patients are considered full stomach. ITx recipients often have multiple abdominal surgeries and gastric resections, resulting in delayed gastric emptying and abnormal anatomy of the stomach. Therefore rapid sequence induction of anaesthesia is recommended in liver and multivisceral transplant recipients. Placement of nasogastric tubes to evacuate the stomach before anaesthesia induction may help decrease the incidence of aspiration. Anaesthesia can be maintained with volatile anaesthetics, muscle relaxant, and opioid. Nitrous oxide is not recommended because it may cause distension of the GI tract, which may make anastomosis and abdominal closure difficult or increase the risk of air embolism during vascular anastomosis. Recipients with a history of multiple abdominal surgeries may have a higher requirement for opioids due to chronic use to control pain. Cisatracurium and doxacurium do not depend on liver metabolism or renal excretion and are ideal muscle relaxants for management of paralysis during ITx. The BIS monitor should be used to estimate depth of anaesthesia to avoid risk of awareness during surgery.

## Operative procedures

The transplant operation unfolds over three distinct phases: (1) dissection, (2) vascular anastomosis, and (3) GI tract reconstruction. During the dissection phase, bleeding is a major concern. For ITx the recipient's infrarenal aorta, infrarenal IVC, and portal vein need to be exposed for vascular anastomosis (see Figure 27.2). If the transplant includes a liver graft (liver–intestine or multivisceral transplant), the infrarenal aorta, supraceliac aorta, superior mesenteric artery (SMA), and suprahepatic vena cava need to be exposed. Dissection of multiple adhesions due to prior abdominal surgeries, venous collaterals from thrombosis or portal hypertension, and coagulopathy due to cirrhosis increase the risk of massive haemorrhage.

During the vascular anastomosis phase, anastomosis of the SMA or infrarenal aorta of the recipient with SMA of the donor is performed. If the donor arterial graft is not adequate, the donor mesenteric or carotid arteries can be used as interposition grafts. Venous anastomoses include: the donor portal venous system with the recipient portal venous system (e.g. portal vein of the donor to portal vein of the recipient); the donor portal vein to the recipient superior mesenteric vein (SMV); and the confluence of SMV to the recipient splenic vein. If the anastomosis to the recipient portal system is not possible, the donor portal vein can be anastomosed to the recipient inferior cava. As of now, there is no difference in post-transplant outcomes between portal–portal and IVC anastomoses (Shaffer et al., 1988, 1989; Hashimoto and Ohyanagi, 2003).

During MVTx, the donor SMA or aorta is anastomosed to the recipient aorta and the donor suprahepatic IVC is anastomosed to the recipient hepatic veins (Figure 27.2). In the majority of cases, the IVC at the confluence of the hepatic veins is partially cross-clamped, which is called the 'piggyback technique'. However, if complete cross-clamping of the IVC is needed, venovenous bypass (VVB) may be required to avoid haemodynamic collapse and intestinal congestion during the organ implantation phase.

Revascularization with reperfusion of the organs is often associated with major haemodynamic fluctuations, especially transplants that include the liver graft. The main reasons for this haemodynamic instability are: (1) a large volume of recipient blood sequestered in the donor graft immediately after reperfusion; (2) suppression of atrial (sinoatrial (SA) node) activity by cold, acidic preservation solution emanating from the liver/intestine graft; and (3) liberation of vasoactive inflammatory factors. Optimization of fluid status, correction of acid-base and electrolyte disturbances, and maintenance of body temperature, in addition to pretreatment with small bolus doses of vasopressor may be required before reperfusion. Also volume resuscitation, vasopressors, calcium chloride, or sodium bicarbonate may be necessary to treat reperfusion-related haemodynamic fluctuations.

Once haemostasis is achieved after reperfusion, reconstruction of the GI tract begins. For ITx the proximal jejunum of the donor graft is anastomosed to the recipient small intestine and a stoma is created at the distal end of the donor small intestine to avoid dilation of the small intestine. Postoperatively, acute rejection is monitored through this stoma using magnified fibreoptic endoscopy, starting in the immediate post-transplant period. In MVTx the donor stomach (partial or total) is anastomosed to the recipient oesophagus or stomach. After the anastomosis is completed, a feeding tube is advanced from the nose through to the jejunum. This feeding tube is carefully secured because it crosses the internal line of the anastomosis. If the feeding tube comes out inadvertently, fluorescent-guided replacement may be required.

The last step is closure of the abdominal wall, which is often challenging due to multiple defects of the abdominal wall from previous surgeries as well as intestinal or abdominal wall oedema. Prolonged exposure of the abdominal visceral organs during surgery results in significant third spacing of fluid, requiring close monitoring and careful titration of fluids to maintain intravascular volume. In our institution, crystalloid/colloid (albumin) 60%/40% fluid resuscitation is the preferred approach. As a consequence of the need for large or massive volume resuscitation, intestinal and abdominal wall oedema may preclude closure of the abdomen at the end of surgery, especially in paediatric recipients. This may require leaving the abdominal wall open to prevent abdominal compartment syndrome. If the closure is difficult, the abdominal wall is left open until bowel oedema subsides, after which stepwise closure of the abdomen is considered. Additionally, during the procedure partial resections of the donor small intestine, liver graft, or removal of the native spleen may be necessary to create space for transplanted organs. In some patients, multiple previous abdominal surgeries may also create an abdominal wall defect, which may require repair with a skin or muscle flap, mesh, or transplantation of a portion of the donor abdominal wall to facilitate abdominal closure without tension.

Once closure of the abdomen starts, increases in airway pressure (from compression of the diaphragm), decrease in blood pressure, and/or decrease in urine output may be observed and need to be carefully monitored and corrected promptly to avoid impaired perfusion of the grafts. Generally, intraoperative haemodynamic fluctuations in multivisceral graft recipients are similar to those observed in recipients of liver transplants and are due to low peripheral vascular resistance and compensatory increased cardiac output. After reperfusion, vascular resistance is further decreased.

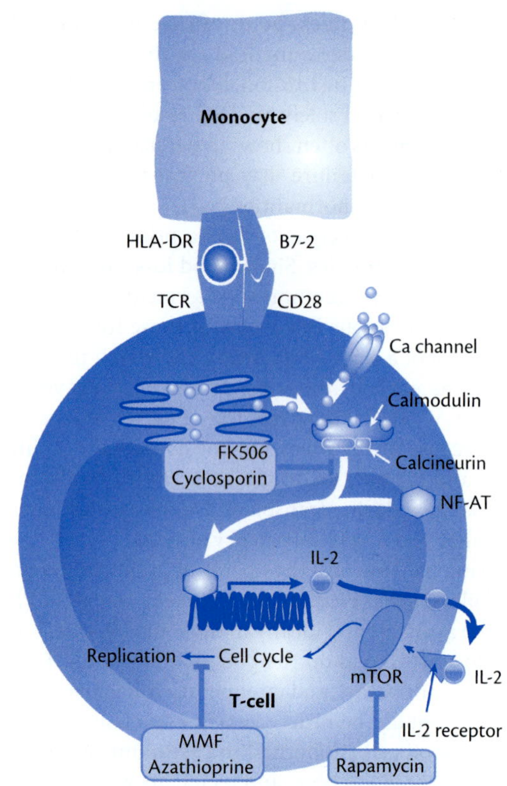


**Fig. 27.4** Site of action of immunosuppressive agents. HLA, Human leucocyte antigen; IL-2, interleukin 2; MMF, mycophenolate mofetil; mTOR, mammalian target of rapamycin; NF-AT, nuclear factor of activated T-cells; TCR, T-cell receptor.

## Immunosuppression and antibiotics

A description of the management of immunosuppressive therapy is beyond the scope of this chapter (see Chapter 11). However, we will briefly describe some important aspects of immune-suppressive agents and antibiotic therapy.

The most commonly used immunosuppression regimens during and post-transplant include: (1) calcineurin inhibitors (CNIs) (tacrolimus: Prograf); (2) macrolide antibiotics (rapamycin: Rapamune); (3) anti-IL-2 antibodies (daclizumub: Zenapax); (4) anti-CD52 antibody (alemtuzumab: Campath); (5) antithymocyte antibody (thymoglobulin); and (6) steroids See Figure 27.4. Tacrolimus, sirolimus, and steroids are mainly used for maintenance immunosuppression, while daclizumab, alemtuzumab, and antithymocyte globulin, as well as methylprednisolone are often used for induction of immunosuppression or treatment for acute rejection.

### Tacrolimus

Tacrolimus is a CNI that inhibits transcription in T-cells with decreases in the production of IL-2 and other cytokines, leading to inhibition of T-cell activation. To obtain therapeutic plasma concentration of tacrolimus early post-transplant, it is often administered during transplant or immediately following transplantation. It is often administrated as an infusion in order to establish a stable plasma concentration. Enteric administration is not used during the early postoperative period because drug absorption via the small intestine is dependent on the function of the recovering graft. Tacrolimus infusions should be used with caution because anaphylactic reactions have been reported (Takamatsu et al., 2001). Other possible side effects include renal and neuronal toxicity (seizure, headache), hyperglycaemia, and hypertension. Adjustment of plasma concentration is based on kidney and liver function to minimize side effects, and plasma concentration is often measured daily in the ICU.

### Rapamycin

Rapamycin is a macrolide antibiotic and relatively new immunosuppressive agent. It binds to tacrolimus-binding protein-12 and inhibits T-cell division. Rapamycin has low renal toxicity compared to tacrolimus and can be used in patients with renal dysfunction. Also it is often used with tacrolimus to decrease nephrotoxicity from tacrolimus. As with tacrolimus, the plasma concentration needs to be monitored, but it is often difficult to adjust the drug concentration even with daily monitoring.

### Antithymocyte antibody

Antithymocyte antibody is a polyclonal rabbit-derived antibody for human T-cell that attaches to the T-cell surface antigen and destroys T-cells. Also daclizumab (anti-IL-2 receptor antibody) and alemtuzumab (anti-CD52 antibody) are monoclonal antibodies and both are often used for induction of immunosuppression or treatment for rejection solely or in combination with tacrolimus or steroids. Anaphylaxis, fever, and shivering are known side effects of both medications. Premedication with steroids, acetaminophen, and antihistamine is required.

## Post-transplant management

After MVTx, recipients should remain intubated and transported to the intensive care unit. Intravascular volume continues to shift to third space at least for 2 days post-transplant and fluid replacement is a mainstay of post-transplant care. Other medical management includes sedation, ventilator management, acid-base electrolyte and metabolic control, prophylaxis for deep venous thrombosis, blood component therapy in case of surgical bleeding or coagulopathy, and antibiotic prophylaxis for infection. Tube feeding via a gastrojejunostomy (GJ) tube may start at 4–6 days after transplant. The primary reason to start tube feeding early post-transplant is to prevent loss of integrity of intestinal mucus membrane or loss of barrier function of the intestine. The transplanted intestine initiates peristalsis immediately after reperfusion, but it is less coordinated because of denervation of the graft. Absorption of carbohydrates, amino acids, and lipid absorption are all impaired and recovery takes several months. Supplements of medium-chain triglycerides and lipid-soluble vitamins (A, D, E, and K) are necessary for the first few months after transplant.

## Conclusion

ITx/MVTx has gained recognition as a viable treatment option for patients who are suffering from SBS and associated medical conditions. Before the era of ITx/MVTx, those patients received only supportive measures like nutritional support from indwelling central venous catheter. ITx/MVTx provides a life-saving, active treatment option for those patients. With improving recipient survival, the number of cases has been steadily rising and anaesthesiologists will have more opportunity to be involved in those cases.

ITx/MVTx is still in the stage of technical development. In the near future, further transplant research will uncover key pathways of intestinal ischaemic injury, which will allow researchers to develop novel therapies to attenuate ischaemia–reperfusion and preservation injury, as well as methods to non-invasively monitor levels of intestinal damage after transplantation due to rejection. Technical advances on the horizon include improved perioperative management of the intestinal and multivisceral transplant recipient; newer modalities for organ preservation, such as perfusion-preservation of abdominal organs, and the introduction of more effective and less toxic immunosuppressive treatment protocols, combined will improve the outcome of ITx/MVTx.

## References


Abu-elmagd K, Bond G, Reyes J, Fung J (2002) Intestinal transplantation: a coming of age. *Adv Surg*, **36**:65–101.

American Gastroenterological Association (2003) American Gastroenterological Association medical position statement: short bowel syndrome and intestinal transplantation. *Gastroenterology*, **124**:1105–1110.

Centers for Medicare and Medicaid Services (2006) *National Coverage Determination (NCD) for Intestinal and Multi-Visceral Transplantation (260.5)*. <http://www.cms.gov/medicare-coverage-database/details/ncd-details.aspx?ncdid=280&ncdver=2&searchtype=advanced&coverageselection=both&ncselection=ncd&policytype=final&s=all&keyword=intestinal&keywordlookup=title&keywordsearchtype=exact&kq=true&bc=iaaaabaaaaaa&>.

de Ville de Goyet J, Mitchell A, Mayer, et al. (2000) En block combined reduced-liver and small bowel transplants: from large donors to small children. *Transplantation*, **69**:555–559.

Fecteau A, Atkinson P, Grant D (2001) Early referral is essential for successful pediatric small bowel transplantation: the Canadian experience. *J Pediatr Surg*, **36**:681–684.

Fleisher LA, Beckman JA, Brown KA, et al. (2007) ACC/AHA 2007 Guidelines on perioperative cardiovascular evaluation and care for noncardiac surgery: executive summary: a report of the American College of Cardiology/American Heart Association Task Force on Practice Guidelines (Writing Committee to Revise the 2002 Guidelines on Perioperative Cardiovascular Evaluation for Noncardiac Surgery) developed in collaboration with the American Society of Echocardiography, American Society of Nuclear Cardiology, Heart Rhythm Society, Society of Cardiovascular Anesthesiologists, Society for Cardiovascular Angiography and Interventions, Society for Vascular Medicine and Biology, and Society for Vascular Surgery. *J Am Coll Cardiol*, **50**:1707–1732.

Fryer J, Pellar S, Ormond D, Koffron A, Abecassis M (2003) Mortality in candidates waiting for combined liver–intestine transplants exceeds that for other candidates waiting for liver transplants. *Liver Transplant*, **9**:748–753.

Fukazawa K, Poliac LC, Pretto EA (2010) Rapid assessment and safe management of severe pulmonary hypertension with milrinone during orthotopic liver transplantation. *Clin Transplant*, **24**:515–519.

Grant D, Abu-Elmagd K, Reyes J, et al. (2005) 2003 report of the Intestine Transplant Registry: a new era has dawned. *Ann Surg*, **241**:607–613.

Grant D, Abu-Elmagd K, Mazariegos J, et al. (2015) Intestinal Transplant Registry report: global activity and trends. *Am J Transplant*, **15**(1):210–219.

Hashimoto N, Ohyanagi H (2003) Metabolic effects of systemic venous drainage in small bowel transplantation. *Transplant Proc*, **35**:1567–1568.

Intestinal Transplant Association (2005) *Intestine Transplant Registry*. <http://www.transplantation-soc.org/section.php>.

Kaufman SS, Atkinson JB, Bianchi A, et al. (2001) Indications for pediatric intestinal transplantation: a position paper of the American Society of Transplantation. *Pediatr Transplant*, **5**:80–87.

Krowka MJ, Plevak DJ, Findlay JY, Rosen CB, Wiesner RH, Krom R (2000) Pulmonary hemodynamics and perioperative cardiopulmonary-related mortality in patients with portopulmonary hypertension undergoing liver transplantation. *Liver Transplant*, **6**:443–450.

Lennard-Jones JE (1990) Indications and need for long-term parenteral nutrition: implications for intestinal transplantation. *Transplant Proc*, **22**:2427–2429.

Molmenti E, Pyrsopoulos N, Tzakis A (2009) *Intestinal and Multivisceral Transplantation*. Paschalidis Medical Publications, London.

Moreno JM, Planas M, Lecha M, et al. (2005). The year 2002 national register on home-based parenteral nutrition. *Nutr Hosp*, **20**:249–253.

Reyes J, Fishbein T, Bueno J, Mazariegos G, Abu-Elmagd K (1998) Reduced-size orthotopic composite liver–intestinal allograft. *Transplantation*, **66**:489–492.

Rodriguez-Roisin R, Krowka MJ, Herve P, Fallon MB, Committee ERSTFP-HVDS (2004) Pulmonary–hepatic vascular disorders (PHD). *Eur Respir J*, **24**:861–880.

Shaffer D, Diflo T, Love W, Clowes GH, Maki T, Monaco AP (1988) Immunologic and metabolic effects of caval versus portal venous drainage in small-bowel transplantation. *Surgery*, **104**:518–524.

Shaffer D, Diflo T, Love W, Clowes GH, Maki T, Monaco AP (1989) Metabolic effects of systemic versus portal venous drainage of orthotopic small bowel isografts. *Transplant Proc*, **21**:2872–2874.

Smith JM, Skeans MA, Horslen SP (2015). OPTN/SRTR 2013 Annual Data Report: Intestinge. Am J Transplant 15(S2): 1–16

Takamatsu Y, Ishizu M, Ichinose I, et al. (2001) Intravenous cyclosporine and tacrolimus caused anaphylaxis but oral cyclosporine capsules were tolerated in an allogeneic bone marrow transplant recipient. *Bone Marrow Transplant*, **28**:421–423.


## Further reading


OPTN: <http://optn.transplant.hrsa.gov/data>.

# CHAPTER 28

# Paediatric intestinal and multivisceral transplantation: indications, selection, and perioperative management

Lydia M. Jorge and Obi Ekwenna

## Introduction

Solid organ transplantation is now considered a feasible treatment for children with end-stage organ dysfunction who otherwise would have a poor prognosis and dismal long-term survival. Advances in this field have provided the potential for markedly improved lifestyles. Three key factors over a period of decades emanating from several medical centres made transplantation of GI organs a possibility:

- Advances in vascular anatomy and surgical technique
- Discovery of and research into the immunological process of rejection
- Research in immunosuppressive medications, with progressive improvements in survival among transplant recipients

ITx and MVTx have evolved into an accepted therapeutic option for management of adults and children with life-threatening complications of intestinal failure (Reyes et al., 2002). Advances in surgical technique, medical management, immunosuppression, monitoring and treatment of rejection, and CMV prophylaxis for MVTx/ITx have improved outcomes in patients and graft survival rates. MVTx/ITx is performed in patients with SBS which is due to extensive intestinal resections for multiple pathologies that ultimately lead to malabsorption of nutrients. Long-term hyperalimentation with TPN is instituted for SBS but usually results in liver failure, along with other complications such as hypercoagulation, line sepsis, and venous thrombosis.

The incidence of SBS is not well known; however, it is estimated that 3 to–5 out of 100,000 babies born will develop SBS (Wallander et al., 1992; Weih et al., 2012). The aetiology of SBS often is a result of extensive surgical intervention in these patients, the consequence of which is a dramatic loss of intestinal mucosal surface area required for absorption of nutrients essential for normal physiological processes. This results in inadequate caloric intake, malabsorption of vitamins and electrolytes, severe malnutrition, and neurological complications.

The number of patients on the MVTx/ITx waiting list has increased steadily since the mid-1990s primarily among children. Children under the age of 6 represent 50% of all candidates with a median time to transplant of over 300 days (Magee et al., 2004). Because of the high mortality of patients on the waiting list, MVTx/ITx provides a modality of treatment that confers an improved quality of life and a survival advantage (Fryer et al., 2003).

## Special considerations for donor assessment and selection

Prior to MVTx/ITx careful assessment of the recipient is done by the transplant surgeon(s) to ensure proper size matching in each recipient. At the time of donor surgery, the donor undergoes selective intestinal decontamination with neomycin, erythromycin, and amphotericin B in addition to a third-generation cephalosporin (Abu-Elmagd et al., 2000). The organ donor procurement operation is similar to procurement for liver. An incision from the suprasternal notch to the pubic symphysis transversing the midline is carried out, exposing the abdominal contents and chest cavity. Various techniques with modification of the University of Pittsburgh protocol have been described in the procurement of the multivisceral graft (Starlz et al., 1984, 1991; Abu-Elmagd et al., 2000; Bueno et al., 2000). The key aspects of procurement are careful examination of intestines and other organs, with particular attention paid to evidence of trauma, mesenteric haematoma, or retroperitoneal haematoma and assessment of organ perfusion. Meticulous, precise, and decisive exposure of key structures is important to ensure organ procurement in a rapid fashion in case of unanticipated donor instability. The anatomical dissection and exposure of the inferior mesenteric vein (IMV), dissection of the infrarenal aorta, and exposure of the abdominal aorta below the take-off of the inferior mesenteric artery (IMA) ensure that heparin administration, aortic cannulation, cross-clamp, and organ cold perfusion can be completed quickly. Once the aorta and IMV are cannulated, an infusion of precooled organ preservation solution is administered.

After completion of the infrarenal aortic dissection, an essential element of multivisceral/intestine with/without liver allograft procurement is maintenance of the SMA–portal vein axis. The stomach, pancreas, and colonic dissections are then completed based on recipient needs assessment. After cold perfusion, the organs are harvested en bloc; the integrity of the mesentery is verified before wrapping the intestinal allograft in a surgical towel for careful transportation, ex-vivo preservation, and implantation (Yersiz et al., 2003).

Although DCD can yield transplantable organs for paediatric liver and kidney transplants, this is not an option at most transplant centres for paediatric MVTx/ITx (de Vries et al., 2010; Gozzini et al., 2010). Due to prolonged exposure to ischaemia, organs obtained from DCD donors have the least chance of being transplantable and produce less favourable outcomes compared to DBD (Reich et al., 2009). Intestines are exquisitely sensitive to ischaemia and the risk of dysfunction can be decreased or averted by selecting DBD donors. Thus SCD or heart-beating donors who have been declared dead by neurological criteria are exclusively used for paediatric MVTx/ITx.

Proper size matching is essential in donor selection since recipients usually have less abdominal mass from multiple procedures, stunted growth, or surgical conditions that affect abdominal closure post-transplantation (Reyes et al., 1998; Delriviere et al., 2000). Donors are usually 50–80% of recipient weight; however, some centres have demonstrated success with donors > 20% of recipient weight (Delriviere et al., 2000). By accepting larger donors, centres are able to improve organ allocation and decrease the morbidity and mortality associated with intestinal failure.

A controversial yet emerging area is living-donor intestinal transplantation. Benedetti et al. (2006) described the experience with 11 patients with overall 1- and 3-year patient survival at 82% with graft survival of 75%, and Ghafari et al. (2011) described an experience with six patients, of whom five were alive at long-term follow-up. Overall experience with living donation is limited to anecdotal results, but it presents an alternative to increasing the donor pool, reducing waiting time for patients with life-threatening intestinal disease.

## Indications

MVTx/ITx is performed for the following causes of SBS:

- Necrotizing enterocolitis
- Gastroschisis
- Intestinal atresia
- Volvulus
- Dysmotility syndromes (Hirshsprung's disease, megacystis microcolon, pseudo-obstruction)
- Microvolvulus inclusion disease
- Trauma
- Desmoid tumours
- Crohn's disease
- Gardner's syndrome
- Radiation-induced bowel injury
- High risk of death
- Severe SBS
    - Residual bowel < 10 cm paediatric
    - Residual bowel < 20 cm adult
    - Duodenostomy
    - Gastrostomy
- Failure to thrive
- Inability to continue TPN
- Catheter-associated central vein thrombosis
- TPN-associated liver cholestasis or dysfunction
- Multiple episodes of sepsis (two or more) with hospitalization

The dismal fate of patients with intestinal failure has dramatically changed since the 1960s. Much of the improved survival observed was initially due to the availability of TPN, which required continuous hospitalization; however, now most patients do well with convenient home-based infusions. After many years of evolution, ITx is now offered to patients who succumb to the inevitable complications of TPN in the form of infection, catheter-associated thrombosis, hepatic disease, renal disease, persistent GI dysfunction, and metabolic derangement. Paediatric intestinal failure remains a devastating condition, with MVTx/ITx providing an alternative for patients with life-threatening complications of TPN. The AST and CMS recommend MVTx/ITx for the following indications (Kaufman et al., 2001; Buchman et al., 2003):

## Contraindications

There are absolute and relative contraindications for MVTx/ITx (Table 28.1). The presence of the following conditions constitutes absolute or relative contraindications (Mangus et al., 2012):

Absolute:

- Severe respiratory failure/high-frequency
    - Active untreated systemic infections/sepsis (fungal, viral, bacterial)
- Extrahepatic infections
- HIV
- Advanced cardiopulmonary disease
- Cerebral oedema
- Dependence on mechanical ventilation or severe pulmonary hypertension
- Complete loss of vascular access or insufficient central venous access
- Extrahepatic malignancy or metastatic disease
- Large non-resectable tumours (large hepatoma, desmoid tumours)

**Table 28.1** Absolute contraindications for MVTx/ITx donation (Data from Abu-Elmagd, K., et al. (2000). Logistics and technique for procurement of intestinal, pancreatic, and hepatic grafts from the same donor. Annals of surgery. 232 (5), 680-687; and Reyes, J., et al. (2002). Pediatric intestinal transplantation: historical notes, principles and controversies. Pediatric transplantation. , 6 (3), 193-207.)

| |
|---|
| Hypoxia |
| End-organ dysfunction (renal, hepatic) |
| Prolonged cardiac arrest with cardiopulmonary resuscitation |
| Malignancy |
| Untreated sepsis |
| GI trauma |
| Prior GI surgery |
| Intestinal haemorrhage |
| Intra-abdominal contamination |
| Acquired immunodeficiency syndrome |
| Active viral hepatitis B or C, CMV |
| Active West Nile virus or rabies |
| Tuberculosis |
| Cold ischaemia time > 12 hours |
| *Obesity > 150% of ideal body weight or BMI 30 lb/m$^2$ |
| *High-risk sexual behaviour |
| *Recent history of intravenous drug abuse |

* Relative contraindication

- Severe neurological disorders
- Severe uncorrectable congenital abnormalities
- Significant psychiatric illness that may prevent adequate treatment post-transplant

Relative:

- Extremes of patient age
- Patient weight (< 10 kg)
- Anatomical elements (cavity size, vascular flow)
- Vascular thrombosis of portal vein and SMV
- Previous organ transplantation
- Renal failure
- Evidence of consistent non-compliance with medications and treatments
- Complete lack of family and social support
- Patients who are currently stable on TPN without signs of liver failure or other complications

In addition, patients who are unable to comply with immunosuppressive therapy and the recommended follow-up are at risk of graft loss and increased mortality. Therefore 'non-compliance' during pre-evaluation work-up and assessment is considered a relative contraindication at most centres.

## Surgical technique

The recipient operation is started when the donor organs are procured and confirmed to be satisfactory. Careful and meticulous laparotomy is performed, with particular attention to the presence of and in anticipation of stomas. The anatomical variations of grafts (Figure 28.1) used for MVTx/ITx are classified as multivisceral, modified multivisceral, composite liver–intestine-pancreas, non-composite liver–intestine, composite liver–intestine, and isolated intestine. The decision as to

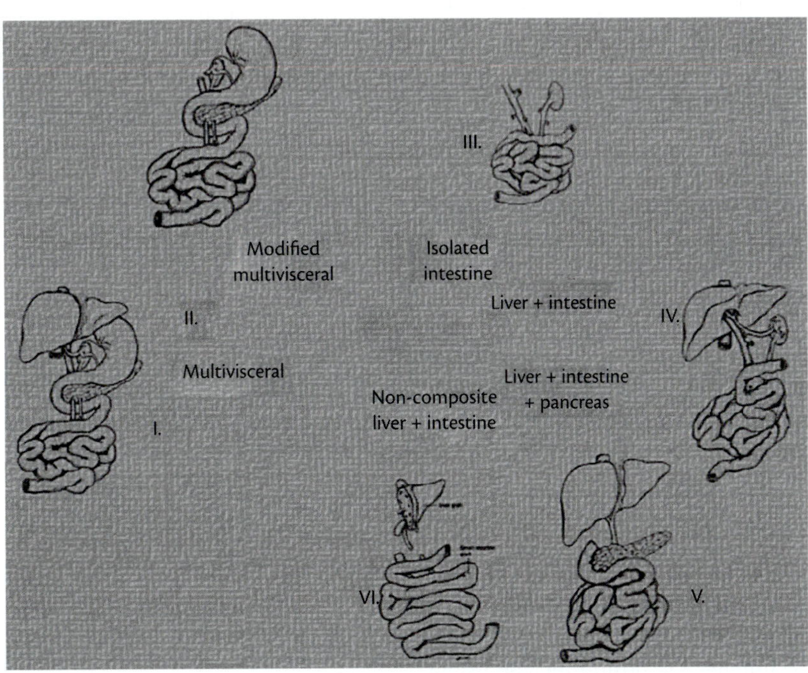


**Fig. 28.1** Anatomical variations of grafts used for MVTx/ITx. (Adapted from Kato T et al., *Annals of surgery*, 'Intestinal and multivisceral transplantation in children', 243, 6, pp. 756–764, copyright 2006, with permission from Wolters Kluwer.)

which type of graft is used is based on the recipient's underlying disease process, with slight variation based on transplant centre experience.

The multivisceral graft includes the stomach, duodenum, pancreas, small intestine, and liver for en-bloc transplantation. MVTx is reserved for patients with liver and intestinal failure and severe dysmotility or dysfunctional pancreas. The need for liver transplantation is 75% in patients with intestinal failure. The kidney may be included in patients with ESRD; additionally the spleen is included in some to help reduce the incidence of post-transplant lymphoproliferative disorder (Kato et al., 2006). The modified MVTx procedure involves all the GI organs except the liver; it is used in patients with preserved liver function.

The composite liver–intestine-pancreas is used mainly in the paediatric population to avoid back-table injury to the hepatic hilar structure while dissecting the pancreas off the composite graft and to avoid biliary reconstruction. A non-composite graft is used to accommodate any major size discrepancies encountered between the recipient and donor; this permits abdominal closure (Kato and Tzakis, 2004; Kato et al., 2006). Isolated intestinal transplantation is performed in patients who have no associated ESLD with intestinal failure.

Vascular anastomoses in the isolated intestinal graft are between the donor SMA and the recipient's SMA, or native aorta. The outflow or venous drainage is usually from the portal venous system of the graft to the IVC or portal system of the recipient. In a multivisceral or modified multivisceral graft or varied combined liver–intestine transplants, the donor and recipient aortas are anastomosed in an end-to-side fashion with an interposition aortic graft. The vena cava is anastomosed also in an end-to-side fashion with the hepatic veins for venous outflow using the piggyback technique (Nishida et al., 2006). Of note, when the recipient native stomach, pancreas, spleen, and duodenum are retained, oesophagogastric varices from venous obstruction can result. To prevent this, portocaval or splenorenal shunt procedure is performed to provide adequate venous drainage (Loinaz et al., 2005; Kato et al., 2007).

The bowel anastomosis in isolated intestinal and combined liver–intestinal transplantation is performed in a side-to-side fashion to the distal end of the native recipient intestine. The continuity of the bowel is established proximally and distally using standard general surgical technique with two-layer visceral anastomosis. Routine terminal ileostomy is created to allow for surveillance of the bowel after transplantation in case of rejection. Use of the donor colon was initially thought to increase the risk of graft loss; however, others have shown that inclusion of the donor colon is well tolerated (Todo et al., 1995; Kato et al., 2008). When the colon is used it is placed in an orthotopic position, anastomosed to the recipient colon, and usually an end colostomy is performed to allow for decompression.

Abdominal closure after MVTx/ITx can be challenging and exceptionally difficult. This is due to prior surgical operations in the recipients, leading to loss of abdominal domain from recurrent infections, scar formation, and contracted abdominal cavity. Thus abdominal closure may require temporary use of Gore-Tex or mesh to enclose the abdomen until resolution of intestinal oedema and inflammation. Other techniques for closure include use of abdominal wall transplantation and plastic surgery (Alexandrides et al., 2000; Levi et al., 2003).

## Anaesthetic management of the MVTx/ITx recipient

### Preoperative evaluation

With the continued refining of surgical technique and improvement of immunosuppression protocols, MVTx/ITx recipients have experienced increased survival and intestinal function over the years (OPTN, 2010). See Figure 28.2.

It has been shown that in patients with irreversible intestinal dysfunction, long-term survival is better achieved with ITx versus chronic TPN (Howard et al., 1991; Abu-Elmagd et al., 2009). However, the timing of referral to a transplant centre for initial evaluation of the candidate for MVTx/ITx has not yet been well established. Due to the shortage of available donors and the length of time once on the waiting list, it has been recommended that patients who potentially may need transplantation be referred for early evaluation (OPTN, 2010). A multidisciplinary team of transplant physicians and healthcare providers will examine the patient, review medical history and all previous surgical records, perform diagnostic studies, and obtain all necessary laboratory data in order to convene a panel that will thoroughly discuss eligibility for transplantation and decide on how to proceed for each individual patient's needs (Table 28.2). This team of specialists is comprised of transplant surgeons, transplant coordinators, paediatric gastroenterologist, the paediatric critical care physician, infectious disease specialist, paediatric anaesthesiologist, nutritionist, psychiatrist, social services, and child life specialists. Often other specialists may be consulted to further evaluate these patients, particularly if extensive cardiac, respiratory, or renal disease is present.

MVTx candidates must undergo a myriad of procedures and laboratory and diagnostic testing to obtain accurate information and data on their current state of health, as well as to determine the complexity of the surgical technique. Previous surgical interventions and the use of chronic TPN and venous access warrant a complete evaluation of the patient's GI and vascular anatomy. Diagnostic studies such as CT scans of the abdomen, oesophagogastroduodenoscopy (OGD), and colonoscopies with biopsies, barium studies, and motility studies will elucidate further the extent of GI dysfunction. The presence or absence of significant liver dysfunction/failure must be established. Synthetic function

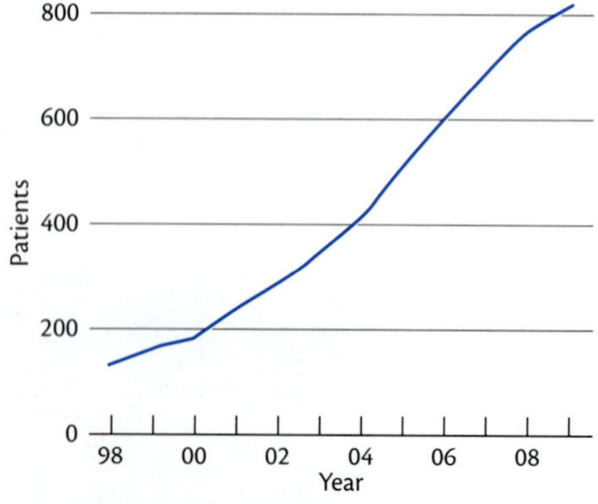


**Fig. 28.2** Number of ITx recipients alive with a functioning transplant. (SRTR 2012 Annual Data Report. Scientific Registry of Transplant Recipients. http://srtr.transplant.hrsa.gov/annual_reports/2012/Default.aspx. Accessed 22/12/14.)

**Table 28.2** Recommended preoperative studies in MVTx/ITx

| Systemic evaluation | Diagnostic images and laboratories |
|---|---|
| Neurological | CT brain with or without contrast, EEG |
| Cardiovascular | ECG, 2DECHO, cardiac catheterization to evaluate pulmonary HTN if present or hepatopulmonary HTN |
| Respiratory | CXR, CT chest, PFTs if pulmonary pathology present |
| GI | OGD, colonoscopy, barium swallow, gastric emptying study, D-xylose absorption study |
| Liver | US, biopsy, AST, ALT, alkaline phosphatase, bilirubin, ammonia, CT-abdomen |
| Renal | CMP, creatinine, renal US, ABG for acidosis |
| Vasculature | Intra-abdominal US of aorta, mesenteric artery, portal vein, SMV, upper and lower extremities, angiography may be needed for selected patients |
| Haematopoietic | ABO, CBC, PT, PTT, INR, HLA typing |
| Infectious disease | Blood cultures, urine cultures, pan culture for sources of infection, CMV, viral hepatitis A, B, C, HIV, TB, EBV |

2DECHO, Two-dimensional echocardiogram; PFTs, pulmonary function tests; OGD, oesophagogastroduodenoscopy; US, ultrasound; CMP, comprehensive metabolic panel; CBC, complete blood count.

of the liver is considerably decreased in patients with liver fibrosis. The presence of derangements in liver function tests (LFTs) such as ALT and AST, hyperbilirubinaemia, hypocholesterolaemia, hypoalbuminaemia, and coagulopathy are suggestive of hepatocyte destruction. The patient must be evaluated for signs of portal HTN manifested by oesophageal and GI varices, ascites, splenomegaly, and subsequent thrombocytopaenia. These tests along with the results of a liver biopsy will determine the level of necrosis and the need for MVTx versus modified MVTx. Extremely young patients with developmental delay or signs of encephalopathy should undergo a complete neurological evaluation including a CT scan of the brain to exclude any organic brain abnormalities including cerebral oedema. Doppler ultrasonography of vascular access from the upper and lower extremities and intra-abdominal vasculature flow may show occlusion of vessels. MRI may prove the extent of the occlusion. A summary of studies and laboratories is shown in Table 28.2 (Reyes et al., 1993; Stayer et al., 2012).

MELD and PELD are mathematical formulas designed as scoring systems for stratification of candidates at highest risk of death from not receiving a transplant. They are used in conjunction with all other evaluation tools in order to ascertain the urgency for liver transplantation. The MELD score is used in patients > 12 years of age and PELD is for patients < 11 years old. The MELD score is based on three laboratory values: serum creatinine (mg/dL), bilirubin (mg/dL), and INR. The formula is as follows (UNOS, 2009):

$$\text{MELD score} = 0.957 \times \text{Log}_e(\text{creatinine}) + 0.378 \times \text{Log}_e(\text{bilirubin}) + 1.120 \times \text{Log}_e(\text{INR}) + 0.643.$$

Maximum value of creatinine in the MELD score is 4.0. If the patient is on dialysis the creatinine value is 4.0.

The PELD score is calculated from five factors: bilirubin (mg/dL), INR, albumin (g/dL), growth failure, and age of listing. The formula is as follows:

$$\text{PELD score} = 0.480 \times \text{Log}_e(\text{bilirubin}) + 1.857 \times \text{Log}_e(\text{INR}) - 0.687 \times \text{Log}_e(\text{albumin}) + 0.436 + 0.667 \text{ (for patients with growth failure)}$$

Each calculated MELD or PELD score is then multiplied by 10 and rounded to the nearest whole number. Laboratory values less than 1 will be designated a value of 1.0. These score values range from 6–40 in ascending level of illness. These scores change according to the changing health status of the patient.

Once the transplant candidates have been thoroughly evaluated and discussed by the transplant committee, the decision is made by both the transplant team and patient's family whether or not to proceed. The status of the candidate is then determined. Status 1A indicates a patient whose life expectancy is less than a few days or hours if not immediately transplanted. Status 1B is given to the paediatric patient with limited life expectancy who is chronically and severely ill. The patient is then registered to the waiting list and all required information is provided to the match system via UNet—a web-based electronic program utilized by UNOS/OPTN to secure accurate data collection, security, and management. ABO verification must be collected and sent from two separate samples to ensure accuracy. The match system then evaluates each candidate on their waiting list and determines those recipients who are eligible or not due to ABO or size incompatibility. It also prioritizes each candidate according to his or her predetermined level of urgency and status (UNOS, undated).Since 2005 there has been a steady rise in the number of patients placed on the wait-list for ITx (with or without other organs) (Figure 28.3). Of these patients, over 71% were less than 17 years of age. In 2009, among

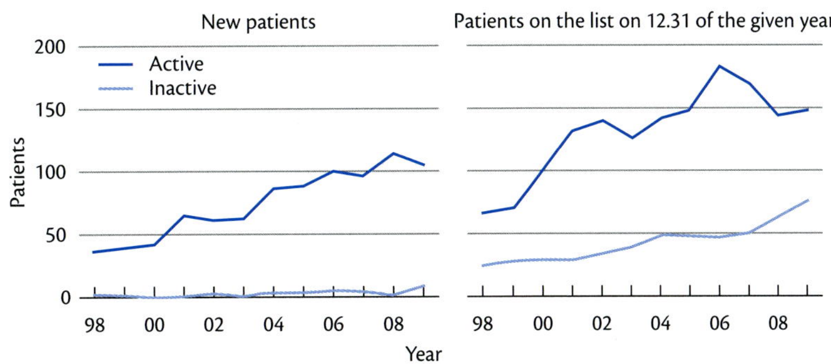


**Fig. 28.3** Patients on the wait-list for ITx as of 2008. (SRTR 2012 Annual Data Report. Scientific Registry of Transplant Recipients. http://srtr.transplant.hrsa.gov/annual_reports/2012/Default.aspx. Accessed 22/12/14.)

the patients on the waiting list for ITx, over 50% were actively listed for over 1 year, and among those transplanted, 52% were under the age of 17 (based on OPTN data from 1 October 2012).

Once a donor is identified, the recipient, his or her family, and transplant team members are notified several hours ahead of time in order to orchestrate the transport of the recipient and organs to the transplant centre. Many times the recipient is admitted from home. Once in the hospital, a preoperative evaluation including a concise history and physical examination is again obtained to assess for changes from the initial evaluation. NPO status is verified and requested. Current labs are obtained and the blood bank is notified to ensure that adequate blood products are available for the transplant surgery. Due to the high potential for massive blood loss and haemorrhage from patient coagulopathy, factor depletion, and platelet dysfunction often associated with liver disease, as well as the vascular nature of MVTx surgeries, it is imperative that the appropriate amount of blood products is ordered and immediately available in the operating room for transfusion. The amount of each blood product ordered varies and is institution dependent. In adults it is often recommended to have at least 10 units of PRBCs and 10 units of FFP in the operating room, along with 10 units of platelets as well as cryoprecipitate on standby. In the paediatric population this is equivalent to approximately 30–50 mL/kg of PRBCs and FFP and approximately 10–20 mL/kg of platelets and 1 unit of cryoprecipitate for every 5–10 kg (10–20 mL/kg) (Raife and Di Paola, 2004). PRBCs should be washed, irradiated, and leucocyte reduced to decrease the possibility of allergic reactions, decrease potassium load in older units, prevent transfusion-related graft-versus-host disease, and reduce the risk of transmission of CMV respectively.

## Intraoperative management of the MVTx/ITx recipient

Paediatric MVTx, in general, is a lengthy surgery taking over 12–14 hours. This complex organ transplant requires multiple procedures, high vigilance, rapid response to haemodynamic changes, and fluctuating stability of the recipient. The presence of two anaesthesia providers is often necessary and recommended. The anaesthesia team typically consists of a paediatric anaesthesiologist attending along with a fellow in paediatric anaesthesia and/or a mid-level anaesthesia provider, an anaesthesia technician, and a perfusion technician.

## Operating room preparation and equipment

Preparing the operating room and having the appropriate equipment available will ensure that the patient can have the best care possible. Along with the standard anaesthesia machine and basic physiological monitors, devices for more specialized haemodynamic monitoring, rapid transfusion of IV fluids and blood products, immediate analysis of intraoperative patient blood samples, and patient temperature control are necessary.

All patients, particularly paediatric patients, are prone to hypothermia in the operating room, with the majority of body temperature loss occurring through radiation (heat loss occurring between two objects in the environment). Hypothermia is associated with worsening coagulopathy, metabolic disturbances, arrhythmias, renal dysfunction, and interference with drug metabolism as well as immune responses. In an operating room environment at 22°C (72°F) radiant heat loss can account for almost 80% of the total patient heat loss (Flick, 2012). Maintaining the operating room environment warm during its preparation can decrease radiant heat loss. Convection heat loss (loss of heat to an environmental mass in motion such as air current or water current) accounts for 34% of body temperature decrease in a neutral environment. Proper use of air-warming blankets and IV fluid warmers can minimize this form of heat loss.

Standard anaesthesia ASA monitors should be placed prior to induction. Along with monitoring electrocardiography, blood pressure, and oxygen saturation through pulse oximetry, more invasive monitors are required in order to accurately and promptly diagnose and treat any haemodynamic changes which often occur during this complex surgery. Strict sterile techniques must always be used when placing invasive monitors, particularly in these immune-compromised patients. If the patient does not already have a central line placed preoperatively, it should be placed after induction, preferably in the IJ veins or subclavian veins due to the clamping of the IVC during MVTx. Central venous access is important for not only obtaining vascular access for fluid resuscitation and also for infusion of medications, but also the ability to monitor CVP and waveforms. Changes in this tracing from baseline can provide useful information about the patient's haemodynamic status and cardiac rhythm. Table 28.3 provides recommended sizes for central venous catheters according to weight in paediatric patients.

Proper placement of the central venous catheter must be ensured prior to its use. Ultrasound-guided placement of invasive lines has optimized direct visualization and access of vascular structures and improved the success rate of central line placements, with minimal risks. In order to minimize catheter-related complications such as perforations and arrhythmias the catheter tip should reside within the superior vena cava (SVC) just above the SVC–right atrium (RA) junction. This can be verified through chest radiograph, or if a TEE probe is being used you may see the tip of the catheter at the SVC–RA junction. A simple formula can also be used to estimate the allowable length of the catheter placed in the right IJ or subclavian veins. This formula can safely predict the location of the catheter to be approximately 1 cm above the SVC–RA junction (Andropoulos, 2012):

Patient height < 100 cm:

(Height ÷ 10) – 1 cm = length of catheter insertion

**Table 28.3** Central line catheter sizes and lengths in paediatrics (Reproduced with kind permission from Jorge, L et al., 2012, 'Central Venous Access in the Pediatric Patient', *Anesthesia Unplugged*, Second Edition, pp. 29–41. Copyright McGrawHill; Data from Andropoulos DB, 'Vascular access and monitoring'. In Andropoulos DB, Anaesthesia for congenital heart disease, Hoboken NJ: Blackwell; 2010, pp. 99–107)

| Patient weight (kg) | Internal jugular vein/ subclavian vein | Femoral vein |
|---|---|---|
| < 10 kg | 4F, 2 lumen, 8 cm | 4F, 2 lumen, 12 cm |
| 10–30 kg | 4F, 2 or 3 lumen, 12 cm | 4F, 2 or 3 lumen, 12—15 cm |
| 30–50 kg | 5F, 2 or 3 lumen, 12–15 cm | 5F, 2 or 3 lumen, 15 cm |
| 50–70 kg | 7F, 3 lumen, 15 cm | 7F, 3 lumen, 20 cm |
| > 70 kg | 8F, 2 or more lumen, 16 cm | 8F, 2 or more lumen, 20 cm |

F, French.

Patient height > 100 cm:

(Height ÷ 10) – 2 cm = length of catheter insertion

It is not uncommon that these patients typically will have very poor vascular access and central line placements may be very difficult. It may be necessary to have these catheters placed by an interventional radiologist under fluoroscopic guidance. If so, arrangements must be made ahead of time so that the patient may have this procedure done prior to organ transplantation, if at all possible. Percutaneous intravenous catheters (PICC lines) have been used for CVP monitoring and as infusion lines successfully. If the MVTx is also associated with kidney transplant or if the patient has renal failure requiring intraoperative haemodialysis, the dialysis catheter may further interfere with vascular access. Of note, catheters are not often placed below the diaphragm due to the partial or complete cross-clamping of the IVC and aorta during liver/MVTx. Typically two radial arterial lines are placed to continuously monitor blood pressure and for multiple arterial blood sampling. This is as a precaution in case one of the arterial lines renders itself non-functional during surgical transplant. Recently, SVV, determined by continuous monitoring of the arterial pressure waveform, has been shown to be effective as a preload and fluid-responsive parameter in adult patients undergoing liver transplantation. One study from Kasagi et al. (2012) in Tokyo, Japan, compared the use of SVV with CVP monitoring alone in 40 paediatric patients who underwent living donor liver transplantation. They determined that haemodynamic changes were less when SVV was used as the parameter for circulating blood volume. Further studies in children are needed to validate these findings. Pulmonary artery catheters are rarely used in paediatric patients. If a history of congenital cardiac disease or cardiomyopathy exists, the ability to place and interpret information provided by a TEE may be necessary. Caution to avoid bleeding with placement of this monitor must be taken. A Foley catheter and nasogastric tube is also placed in preparation to monitor urine output and decompress abdominal organs. An intraoperative CXR is obtained after all invasive lines and tubes are in place to ensure accurate placement and verify the presence of any abnormalities or complications (pneumothorax, haemothorax, inappropriate endotracheal tube positioning) which may need immediate intervention prior to the start of the surgery.

Massive haemorrhage can often occur with MVTx. Multiple larger bore peripheral IV access must be placed preferably in the upper extremities for rapid fluid resuscitation and blood transfusions. A blood salvage device as well as a rapid infusing system may be used in larger patients (above 30 kg). Blood products must be immediately available in the operating room (OR). If possible, the blood bank can be requested to wash the PRBCs to decrease their potassium load. If not, this may be accomplished with the use of the cell salvage system in the OR.

## Anaesthesia induction

Depending on the patient's level of consciousness, they may or may not require premedication with sedatives prior to entering the OR and this is given at the discretion of the experienced anaesthesia provider. Older children undergoing MVTx/ITx have been in and out of the hospital environment most of their lives, having experienced numerous procedures and surgeries. Their level of anxiety, as well as for their parents, may be extreme. Midazolam can be given orally (0.5–1 mg/kg, not to exceed 20 mg) or IV (0.03–0.1 mg/kg) for safe sedation.

Once in the OR, monitors are placed and the patient is preoxygenated with 100% oxygen. Dependent on the patient's IV access and NPO status, the anaesthesiologist may proceed with an inhalation induction or an IV induction. Keeping in mind that most patients have a degree of bowel dysfunction and delayed gastric emptying or may not be appropriately NPO due to the urgency of this procedure and time constraints, an IV rapid sequence induction with application of cricoid pressure may be warranted. The choice of IV induction agent may be dictated by the recipient's underlying physiological status and the preference of the anaesthesiologist. The use of succinylcholine or high-dose rocuronium has also been used for rapid muscle relaxation as long as no contraindications are present. The airway is immediately secured via direct laryngoscopy with an oral endotracheal tube. In paediatrics, the use of low-pressure cuffed endotracheal tubes is now proven to be safe, even in infants and children, as long as the appropriate size tube is used (Schmitz et al., 2006; Weiss et al., 2009). Cuffed endotracheal tubes have the advantage of minimizing aspiration from gastric contents, improving ventilation by creating a seal, and minimizing leaks around the endotracheal tube, and they avoid the need for multiple laryngoscopies due to inappropriate endotracheal tube size placement. Once the airway is secured and the patient is placed on mechanical ventilation maintaining oxygenation and applying appropriate PEEP to avoid atelectasis, the anaesthesia team proceeds to the placement of invasive monitors. Ensuring proper patient positioning to avoid potential nerve damage and decubitus ulcers from such a prolonged surgical procedure is extremely important. These patients are malnourished and prone to ulceration. All extremities must be padded and free of pressure. Specialized OR tables and foam mattresses are used to minimize pressure sores.

## Anaesthetic maintenance

A balanced general anaesthetic technique with oxygen, air, volatile agent, neuromuscular blocking medication for muscle relaxation, and the use of opioids for pain control is common practice. No study has shown one anaesthesia maintenance regimen to be far more superior than another for liver transplants, MVTx, modified MVTx, or ITx. This is left to the discretion and experience of the anaesthesiologist. Of note, nitrous oxide is typically avoided to prevent worsening of bowel distension. Some providers have used narcotic-based anaesthetic regimen with supplemental volatile agent as a primary anaesthetic drug with no significant sequela (Uejima, 2004). The presence of liver dysfunction may affect the volume of distribution, metabolism, and clearance of induction agents, opioids, and neuromuscular blocking medications, which can potentially prolong their effects and duration of action. Cisatracurium is often used for continued muscle relaxation due to its enzymatic degradation process; however, rocuronium, vecuronium, and pancuronium have also been used with minimal clinical complications. The use of a neuromuscular monitoring device is imperative to assess muscle relaxation throughout the surgery. Ultimately, once a functioning liver graft is transplanted and normal function resumes, so does drug metabolism and recovery from anaesthetic medications.

## Intraoperative concerns

In MVTx, dissection of the multiple organs, including the liver, can prove to be very difficult and time consuming and is associated with large fluid shifts. The presence of adhesions from previous surgeries and potential vascular abnormalities can be associated with significant bleeding. Vascular clamping and prolonged ischaemic times can lead to haemodynamic changes and potential end-organ dysfunction.

MVTx can be discussed in two stages. Stage 1 includes the resection of the native organs, known as abdominal exenteration where vessels are clamped and divided above their take-off from the aorta and the organs are dearterialized. Stage 2 involves the implantation, anastomosis, and reperfusion of the graft. Each stage can be associated with haemodynamic instability, blood loss, coagulopathy, hypothermia, and electrolyte abnormalities with varying degrees of severity.

### Hypotension

In stage 1, the liver can be carefully dissected from the IVC (piggyback technique), removed en bloc (total hepatectomy), or preserved as in modified MVTx. Hypotension is a common occurrence during this stage of the transplant. Common causes of hypotension to be considered are continuous bleeding, massive haemorrhage, and/or decrease in preload due to cross-clamping of major vessels such as the IVC and portal vein. Dampening of arterial waveform and respiratory variations along with a decrease in CVP, tachycardia, and developing metabolic acidosis are all potential signs of hypovolaemia. Typically, paediatric patients respond well to fluid boluses (10–20 mL/kg) to treat hypotension. Maintaining a CVP of 8–10 mm Hg during the transplant correlates with adequate perfusion pressures. Crystalloids should be delivered to compensate for the significant amount of insensible losses throughout the transplant at 10–50 mL/kg/hour. Colloids such as blood products and albumin are commonly given for fluid replacement. Colloids when compared to crystalloid administration have been thought to decrease the severity of bowel oedema that can impair intestinal motility, and abdominal wall closure. Transfusion of PRBCs is necessary to maintain a haematocrit around 30–35%. PRBCs are often washed to decrease allergic reactions by foreign plasma proteins and reduce potassium ($K^+$) load from older units. Formulas have been developed to estimate the volume of PRBCs needed to increase a patient's haemoglobin or haematocrit to a certain level. Typically, transfusing 10 mL/kg of PRBCs can raise the haemoglobin by 3 g/dL and the haematocrit by 10%:

Volume of PRBCs to be transfused (mL)

= 4.8 × weight (kg) × desired rise of haemoglobin (g/dL)

or

= 1.6 × weight (kg) × desired rise of haematocrit (%)

Use of this formula can predict a rise in haemoglobin of 0.95 (Miller and Hendrickson, 2012).

Excessive fluid hydration can impair hepatic venous drainage postperfusion as well as worsen bowel oedema and impair abdominal closure. Patients with persistent hypotension may require the use of vasoactive medications such as dopamine, dobutamine, or epinephrine. Hypocalcaemia, hyperkalaemia, hypokalaemia, and metabolic acidosis can commonly occur throughout the course of this surgery and can potentiate hypotension (Table 28.4).

With reperfusion of the graft in stage 2, hypotension can be commonly observed despite adequate hydration. Right ventricular dysfunction may occur due to increased pulmonary vasoconstriction along with bradycardia and dysrhythmias as a result of increased blood return, perfusion with high potassium load, acidic, cold fluids, and blood products. Correction of acidosis and hypocalcaemia to normal or slightly higher levels is recommended prior to reperfusion of the graft.

**Table 28.4** Intraoperative indices during MVTx/ITx

| Threshold of stability | Goal | Comments |
|---|---|---|
| MAP | > 60 mmHg | Fluid administration. Beware of pulmonary oedema and intestinal oedema. Monitor wedge pressure and CVP to avoid fluid overload |
| Vasoactive-drug requirement | < 10 µg/kg/min | Start with dopamine. With persistent hypotension add vasopressin, norepinephrine, epinephrine, or phenylephrine. Initiate hormone therapy for refractory hypotension |
| Urinary output | > 1.0 mL/kg/hour | Beware of diabetes insipidus |
| Left ventricular ejection fraction | > 45% | |
| Systolic blood pressure | > 90 mmHg | |
| CVP | 8–10 mmHg | Consider PA catheter to monitor wedge pressure |
| Blood sugar concentration | 60–150 mg/dL | Administer insulin |
| Temperature | > 35°C (36–37.5°C) | |
| Hb, INR, platelets | Hb > 7 g/dL<br>INR < 2.0<br>Platelets > 80,000 | No transfusion required if Hb is between 7 and 10 g/dL if patient is haemodynamically stable.<br>Transfuse if Hb < 10 g/dL and patient is haemodynamically unstable. Preferably use leukopoor and CMV seronegative blood products. |

### Management of hyper-/hypokalaemia

Hyperkalaemia can potentiate haemodynamic instability in MVTx similar to the effects seen in liver transplants and must be corrected prior to reperfusion. ECG changes typical for moderate to severe hyperkalaemia are peaked T-waves, wide QRS complex, and ST depression that can lead to significant bradycardia, ventricular fibrillation, and asystole if not corrected immediately. Potassium should be maintained below 3.5 mEq/L prior to reperfusion and can increase often > 1.5 mEq/L on graft perfusion. Treatments for hyperkalaemia consist of calcium administration to stabilize cardiac membrane. Promote intracellular shift of potassium by correcting acidosis with sodium bicarbonate, administration of glucose and insulin, and hyperventilation. Increasing diuresis with furosemide, a potassium-eliminating diuretic, can also decrease potassium levels. Ultimately, haemodialysis may be

**Table 28.5** Treatment for hyperkalaemia.

| | | |
|---|---|---|
| Stabilizes cardiac cell membranes | Calcium chloride | 10–20 mg/kg |
| | Calcium gluconate | 30–60 mg/kg |
| Shifts $K^+$ to intracellular | Sodium bicarbonate | 1–2 mEq/kg |
| | Tromethamine (THAM) 0.3 M solution | 3–6 mL/kg |
| | Glucose and regular insulin | 1–2 g/kg of glucose with 1 unit of insulin per 4 g of glucose IV |
| | Increase minute ventilation | |
| | Beta-agonist | Albuterol |
| $K^+$ removal | Furosemide | 0.5–1 mg/kg IV |
| | Kayexalate | 1 g/kg orally or rectally every 6 hours |
| | Haemodialysis | Immediate removal |

necessary if hyperkalaemia increases to dangerous levels, particularly in patients with ESRD or HRS and it may be required intraoperatively (Table 28.5).

Hypokalaemia can often be seen postperfusion. This may be due to several factors: iatrogenic treatment of hyperkalaemia, urinary losses, and uptake by liver and muscle cells. After stabilization of the patient and maintenance of urine output, replacement of potassium may be indicated.

### Glycaemic control

MVTx recipients experience a number of metabolic dysfunctions, one of which is maintaining blood glucose control. Hypoglycaemia is often a consequence of depleted glycogen stores and impaired gluconeogenesis. Their glucose is closely monitored intraoperatively and replaced with a glucose-containing solution and/or TPN as a maintenance infusion.

Hyperglycaemia after MVTx graft reperfusion is common and its cause is multifactorial. Release of glucose from ischaemic hepatocytes, blood product transfusions, steroid use for immunosuppression, hypothermia, and the surgical stress response can all increase glucose levels after reperfusion. Hyperglycaemia is associated with impaired wound healing and increased morbidity and mortality (McCowen et al., 2001; Van den Berghe et al., 2003; Kitabchi et al., 2009). It is important to maintain normoglycaemia by frequent laboratory analysis intraoperatively and insulin administration to sustain glucose levels of 80–150 mg/dL.

### Coagulopathy

Transplant recipients often are coagulopathic, particularly if significant liver dysfunction is present. This may worsen during the course of the MVTx. Continued visualization of the surgical field along with laboratory analysis of platelets, PT, PTT, and fibrinogen can be used to guide the treatment of the coagulopathy. TEG is a test used to analyze clot formation, strength, and fibrinolysis in real-time. It has been used in developing transfusion parameters in coagulopathic trauma and surgical patients. Maintaining normothermia can minimize the risk of clotting abnormalities. The goal for the MVTx recipient is to achieve a stable haemoglobin (8–10 mg/dL) and haematocrit (25–35%) with decreased bleeding due to coagulopathy and avoiding a hypercoagulable state that can cause vascular occlusion of the transplanted graft and hepatic artery. Cryoprecipitate may be indicated if fibrinogen levels fall below 100 mg/dL and is associated with continued bleeding. Platelet counts less than 100,000 are commonly observed after reperfusion and do not require platelet transfusion in the absence of significant bleeding. Finally, antifibrinolytics are not commonly used in paediatric patients due to the increased risk of vascular graft occlusion in such small recipients and vessel caliber.

## Conclusion

ITx and MVTx have advanced, from an experimental treatment to an accepted therapeutic option for the management of short gut syndrome and associated complications due to failure of TPN. The anatomical variations of grafts include: multivisceral, modified multivisceral, composite liver–intestine-pancreas, non-composite liver–intestine, composite liver–intestine, and isolated intestine. The decision to use which type of graft is based on the recipient's pathology and transplant centre experience. The multivisceral graft includes the stomach, duodenum, pancreas, small intestine, and liver for en-bloc transplantation. MVTx is reserved for patients with liver, intestinal failure, and severe dysmotility and/or a dysfunctional pancreas. In 75% of patients with SGS and chronic parenteral nutrition a liver transplant is also needed. The kidney may be included in patients with ESRD; additionally the spleen is included in some to help reduce the incidence of post-transplant lymphoproliferative disorder. Along with surgical advances and immunosuppression, patient outcomes and graft survival have improved dramatically. In some cases, long-term hyperalimentation with TPN results in liver failure, along with other complications such as hypercoagulation, line sepsis, or venous thrombosis, and may require concomitant liver transplantation.

The success of ITx and MVTx has resulted in a steady increase in the number of patients on the transplant wait-list, particularly young children. Children under the age of 6 represent 50% of all candidates with a median time to transplant of over 300 days. Unfortunately the scarcity of suitable organs has increased the mortality of patients on the waiting list. Finally, long-term survival after ITx and MVTx will continue to improve as experience with this complicated surgical procedure grows and as new sources or organs and enhanced preservation techniques become available.

## References

Abu-Elmagd K, Fung J, Bueno J, et al. (2000) Logistics and technique for procurement of intestinal, pancreatic, and hepatic grafts from the same donor. *Annal Surg*, **232**(5):680–687.

Abu-Elmagd K, Costa G, Bond G, et al. (2009) Five hundred intestinal and multivisceral transplantations at a single center: major advances with new challenges. *Annal Surg*, **250**:567–581.

Alexandrides I, Liu P, Marshall D, Nery J, Tzakis A, Thaller S (2000) Abdominal wall closure after intestinal transplantation. *Plastic Reconstructive Surg*, **106**(4):805–812.

Andropoulos D (2012) Monitoring and vascular access. In: Gregory G, Andropoulos D (eds) *Gregory's Pediatric Anesthesia*, 5th edn, pp. 381–418. Wiley-Blackwell, Oxford.

Benedetti E, Holterman M, Asolati M, Di Domenico S, Oberholzer J, Sankary H (2006) Living related segmental bowel transplantation: from experimental to standardized procedure. *Annal Surg*, **244**(5):694–699.

Buchman A, Scolapio J, Fryer J (2003) AGA technical review on short bowel syndrome and intestinal transplantation. *Gastroenterology*, **124**(4):1111–1134.

Bueno J, Abu-Elmagd K, Mazariegos G, Madariaga J, Fung J, Reyes J (2000) Composite liver–small bowel allografts with preservation of donor duodenum and hepatic biliary system in children. *J Pediatric Surg*, **35**(2): 291–295.

de Vries E, Snoeijs M, van Heurn E (2010) Kidney donation from children after cardiac death. *Crit Care Med*, **38**(1):249–253.

Delriviere L, Muiesan P, Marshall M, et al. (2000) Size reduction of small bowels from adult cadaveric donors to alleviate the scarcity of pediatric size-matched organs: an anatomical and feasibility study. *Transplantation*, **69**(7):1392–1396.

Evens A (2010) Multicenter analysis of 80 solid organ transplantation recipients with post-transplantation lymphoproliferative disease: outcome and prognostic factors in the modern era. *J Clin Oncol*, **28**(6):1038–1046.

Flick R (2012) Clinical complications in pediatric anesthesia. In: Gregory G, Andropoulos D (eds) *Gregory's Pediatric Anesthesia*, 5th edn, pp. 1152–1182. Wiley-Blackwell, Oxford.

Fryer J, Pellar S, Ormond D, et al. (2003) Mortality in candidates waiting for combined liver–intestine transplants exceeds that for other candidates waiting for liver transplants. *Liver Transplant*, **9**(7):748–753.

Fuster V, Ryden L, Cannom D, et al. (2011a) 2011 ACCF/AHA/HRS focused updates incorporated into the ACC/AHA/ESC 2006 guidelines for the management of patients with atrial fibrillation: a report of the American College of Cardiology Foundation/American Heart Association Task Force on practice guidelines. *Circulation*, **123**(10):e269–e367.

Fuster V, Ryden L, Cannom D, et al. (2011b) 2011 ACCF/AHA/HRS focused updates incorporated into the ACC/AHA/ESC 2006 Guidelines for the management of patients with atrial fibrillation: a report of the American College of Cardiology Foundation/ American Heart Association Task Force on Practice Guidelines developed in partnership with the European Society of Cardiology and in collaboration with the European Heart Rhythm Association and the Heart Rhythm Society. *J Am Coll Cardio*, **57**(11):e101–e198.

Ghafari J, Bhati C, John E, Tzvetanov I, Testa G, Jeon H (2011) Long-term follow-up in adult living donors for combined liver/bowel transplant in pediatric recipients: a single center experience. *Pediatr Transplant*, **15**(4):425–429.

Gozzini S, Perera M, Mayer D, Mirza D, Kelly D, Muiesan P (2010) Liver transplantation in children using non-heart-beating donors (NHBD). *Pediatr Transplant*, **14**(4):554–557.

Howard L, Heaphey L, Fleming C, Lininger L, Steiger E (1991) Four years of North American registry home parenteral nutrition outcome data and their implications for patient management. *J Parenter Enteral Nutr*, **15**:384–393.

Jorge L, Saab A, Elf R (2012) Central venous access in the pediatric patient. In Gallagher C, Ginsberg S, Lewis M, Park C, Schwengel D (eds) *Anesthesia Unplugged*, 2nd edn, pp. 29–41. McGraw-Hill, New York.

Kasagi Y, Hashimoto M, Kasuya S, et al. (2012) Usefulness of monitoring stroke volume variations for fluid management during pediatric living donor liver transplantation. *Open J Anesthesiol*, **2**:146–149.

Kato T, Tzakis A (2004) Noncomposite simultaneous liver and intestinal transplantation. *Transplantation*, **78**(3):485.

Kato T, Kleiner G, David A, et al. (2006a) Inclusion of spleen in pediatric multivisceral transplantation. *Transplant Proc*, **38**(6):1709–1710.

Kato T, Tzakis A, Selvaggi G, et al. (2006b) Intestinal and multivisceral transplantation in children. *Annal Surg*, **243**(6):756–764.

Kato T, Tzakis A, Selvaggi G, et al. (2007) Transplantation of the spleen: effect of splenic allograft in human multivisceral transplantation. *Annal Surg*, **246**(3):436–444.

Kato T, Selvaggi G, Gaynor J, et al. (2008) Inclusion of donor colon and ileocecal valve in intestinal transplantation. *Transplantation*, **86**(2):293–297.

Kaufman S, Atkinson J, Bianchi A, et al. (2001) Indications for pediatric intestinal transplantation: a position paper of the American Society of Transplantation. *Pediatr Transplant*, **5**(2):80–87.

Kitabchi A, Umpierrez G, Miles J, Fisher J (2009) Hyperglycemic crisis in adult patients with diabetes. *Diabetes Care*, **32**(7):1335.

Levi D, Tzakis A, Kato T, et al. (2003) Transplantation of the abdominal wall. *Lancet*, **361**(9376):2173–2176.

Lillehei R, Goot B, Miller F (1959a) Homografts of the small bowel. *Surg Forum*, **10**:197.

Lillehei R, Goot B, Miller F (1959b) The physiologic response of the small bowel of the dog to ischemia including prolonged in vitro preservation of the bowel with successful replacement and survivial. *Ann Surg*, **150**:543–560.

Loinaz C, Rodriguez M, Kato T, et al. (2005) Intestinal and multivisceral transplantation in children with severe gastrointestinal dysmotility. *J Pediatr Surg*, **40**(10):1598–1604.

Magee J, Bucuvalas J, Farmer D, et al. (2004) Pediatric transplantation. *Am J Transplant*, **4**:54–71.

Mangus R, Tector A, Kubal C, Fridell J, Vianna R (2012) Multivisceral transplantation: expanding indications and improving outcomes. *J Gastrointest Surg*, **17**(1):179–186.

McCowen K, Malhotra A, Bistrian B (2001) Stress induced hyperglycemia. *Crit Care Clin*, **17**:107.

Miller BE, Hendrickson JE (2012) Coagulation, bleeding, and blood transfusion. In Gregory GA, Andropoulos DB (eds) *Pediatric Anesthesia*, 5th edn, pp. 224–254. Wiley-Blackwell, Oxford.

Nishida S, Nakamura N, Vaidya A, et al. (2006) Piggyback technique in adult orthotopic liver transplantation: an analysis of 1067 liver transplants at a single center. *HPB (Oxford)*, **8**(3):182–188.

OPTN (2010) Annual Data Report of the US Organ Procurement and Transplantation Network and the Scientific Registry of Transplant Recipients 1998–2009. *Transplant Data*.

Raife T, Di Paola J (2004) Transfusion of the pediatric surgery, trauma, and intensive care unit patient. In Strauss R, Luban N, Hillyer C (eds) Handbook *Pediatric Transfusion* Medicine, pp. 137–148. Academic Press, Burlington, Massachusetts.

Reich D, Mulligan D, Abt P, Pruett T, Abecassis M, D'Alessandro A (2009) ASTS recommended practice guidelines for controlled donation after cardiac death organ procurement and transplantation. *Am J Transplant*, **9**:2004–2011.

Reyes J, Tzakis A, Todo S, Nour B, Starlz T (1993) Small bowel and liver/small bowel transplatation in children. *Semin Pediatr Surg*, **2**(4):289–300.

Reyes J, Fishbein T, Bueno J, Mazariegos G, Abu-Elmagd K (1998) Reduced-size orthotopic composite liver–intestinal allograft. *Transplantation,*, **66**(4):489–492.

Reyes J, Mazariegos G, Bond G, et al. (2002) Pediatric intestinal transplantation: historical notes, principles and controversies. *Pediatr Transplant*, **6**(3):193–207.

Rosendale J, Kauffman H, McBride M, et al. (2003a) Aggressive pharmacologic donor management results in more transplanted organs. *Transplantation*, **75**(4):482–487.

Rosendale J, Kauffman H, McBride M, et al. (2003b) Hormonal resuscitation yields more transplanted hearts, with improved early function. *Transplantation*, **75**(8):1336–1341.

Schmitz S, Henze G, Stutz K, et al. (2006) Evaluation of a new recommendation for improved cuffed tracheal tube size selection in infants and small children. *Acta Anaesthesiol Scand*, **50**:557–561.

Starlz T (1993) Cell migration and chimerism after whole organ transplantation: the basis for graft acceptance. *Hepatology*, **17**:1127–1152.

Starlz T, Hakala T, Shaw B, et al. (1984) A flexible procedure for multiple cadaveric organ procurement. *Surg Gynecol Obstetr*, **158**(3):223–230.

Starlz T, Todo S, Tzakis A, et al. (1991) The many faces of multivisceral transplantation. *Surg Gynecol Obstetr*, **172**(5):335–344.

Stayer S, Williams G, Andropolous D (2012) Anesthesia for transplantation. In: Gregory G, Andropoulos D (eds) *Gregory's Pediatric Anesthesia*, 5th edn, pp. 682–685. Wiley-Blackwell, Oxford.

Todo S, Tzakis A, Reyes J, et al. (1995) Intestinal transplantation: 4-year experience. *Transplant Proc*, **27**(1):1355–1356.

Uejima T (2004) Anesthetic management of the pediatric patient undergoing solid organ transplantation. *Anesthesiol Clin N Am*, **22**:809–826.

UNOS (undated) *Organ Allocation*. <http://www.unos.org/donation/index.php?topic=organ allocation>.

UNOS (2009) *MELD and PELD Calculator Documentation*. <http://www.unos.org/docs/meld peld calculator documentation>.

Van den Berghe G, Wouters P, Boullion R, et al. (2003) Outcome benefit of intensive insulin therapy in the critically ill: Insulin dose versus glycemic control. *Crit Care Med*, **31**:359.

Wallander J, Ewald U, Lackgren G, Tufveson G, Wahlberg J, Meurling S (1992) Extreme short bowel syndrome in neonates: an indication for small bowel transplantation? *Transplant Proc*, **24**(3):1230–1235.

Weih S, Kessler M, Fonouni H , et al. (2012) Current practice and future perspectives in the treatment of short bowel syndrome in children—a systematic review. *Langenbeck Arch Surg/Dtsch Gesellschaft Chirurg*, **397**(7):1043–1051.

Weiss M, Dullenkopf A, Fischer J, Keller C, Gerber A (2009) European Paediatric Endotracheal Intubation Study Group: prospective randomized controlled multi-centre trial of cuffed or uncuffed endotracheal tubes in small children. *Br J Anaesth*, **103**:867–873.

Yersiz H, Renz J, Hisatake G, et al. (2003) Multivisceral and isolated intestinal procurement techniques. *Liver Transplant*, **9**(8):881–886.

# CHAPTER 29

# Critical care of the intestinal and multivisceral transplant recipient

Lydia M. Jorge and Haran Fisher

## Postoperative care and nutritional support

At the conclusion of ITx and MVTx surgery, the surgeons will determine whether complete abdominal wound closure is feasible or if it should be performed as a series of staged closures. Due to the complexity of this surgery, respiratory function for most patients is maintained by mechanical ventilation and sedation and patients are transported to the ICU for further management. Close monitoring for haemodynamic changes, bleeding, metabolic and electrolyte disturbances, and organ dysfunction is continued. A careful balance of fluid hydration and vasoactive medications must be maintained to allow for appropriate organ perfusion and to avoid organ ischaemia, overhydration, and bowel oedema (which usually progresses within the first 24–48 hours after surgery). In severe cases the patient can develop abdominal compartment syndrome, as evidenced by increased abdominal distention, worsening respiratory function or failure, and decreased urine output with increased bladder pressures; this often requires immediate surgical intervention.

### Management of multivisceral graft and organ perfusion

Multivisceral and intestinal graft perfusion and viability must be maintained in the immediate postoperative period. Increasing oxygen delivery and tissue perfusion to the newly transplanted organs is most important. This can be accomplished in several key ways:

- Oxygen delivery:
  - Maintain cardiac output and function in the normal to high range
  - Maintain oxygen-carrying capacity with a haematocrit of 25–30%
  - Ensure oxygen saturation is > 95%
- Tissue perfusion:
  - Maintain preload with crystalloids, colloids, and blood products
  - Decrease blood viscosity
  - Maintain a relative hypocoagulable state

Hypotension is frequently encountered in the immediate postoperative period. It is usually a result of hypovolaemia, fluid shifts, and peritoneal fluid loss. IV fluid resuscitation and administration of albumin can resolve this. Vasoconstriction, particularly with alpha-adrenergic agents, should be avoided to minimize hypoperfusion to the graft. Hypertension can often result from aggressive fluid administration and volume overload, steroid use, nephrotoxicity, or poor pain control. If persistent, short-acting antihypertensive agents such as calcium channel blockers or beta-blockers can be administered. Table 29.1 provides a list of monitors and laboratory tests frequently evaluated in the postoperative period for MVTx and ITx recipients.

### Respiratory function

Early extubation is still the goal in order to avoid ventilatory acquired pneumonias in transplant recipients. However, pre-existing respiratory dysfunction remains a major deterrent. Other causes of prolonged intubation are volume overload, large graft size, and increased intra-abdominal pressures, pleural effusions, and ascites. Transient diaphragmatic dysfunction is typically a reversible process and can be diagnosed via ultrasonography or fluoroscopy. Extubation can be achieved within 48 hours after a transplant but may be delayed, particularly if closure of the abdominal wall is staged due to a large multivisceral graft.

### Renal function

Renal function is monitored closely throughout the perioperative period. Approximately 25% of transplant recipients have some form of renal dysfunction (Hauser et al., 2008). This can be related to an ongoing pre-existing renal dysfunction, acute renal insufficiency, or iatrogenic causes due to nephrotoxic medications or hypoperfusion. Many transplant recipients who present with relative decreases in GFR can progress to renal failure after transplantation. High-dose tacrolimus therapy prior to transplantation has been found to be a predictor of poor renal function. Tacrolimus toxicity has also been associated with a higher incidence of acute renal injury in part due to its unpredictable absorption and metabolism by the intestinal enterocytes. Tacrolimus toxicity is associated with high serum levels, elevated BUN and creatinine, and oliguria unresponsive to diuretic therapy and has been described as a predictor in decreases of GFR in both paediatric and adult populations after transplant (Hopfner et al., 2012). Haemodialysis or CVVHD may be required in patients with progressively worsening renal function unresponsive to medical management.

**Table 29.1** Continued postoperative monitoring of MVTx/ITx recipients in the ICU. (Reproduced from *Intensive Care Medicine*, 34, 9, 2008, 'Pediatric intestinal and multivisceral transplantation: a new challenge for the pediatric intensivist', pp. 1570-1579, Hauser et al., with kind permission from Springer Science and Business Media.)

| | |
|---|---|
| *Cardiac:* | *Respiratory function:* |
| Maintain adequate graft and organ perfusion | Maintain adequate ventilation/oxygenation |
| Optimize CVP | Arterial blood gas analysis |
| Optimize blood pressure | Lung-protective mechanical ventilation |
| ◆ Avoid vasoconstrictors if possible | ◆ Frequent respiratory rate, lower tidal volumes and peak pressures |
| ◆ Avoid hypotension | |
| Optimize oxygen delivery | Diaphragmatic dysfunction |
| ◆ Arterial saturation of $O_2$ > 95% | ◆ Difficulty with weaning ventilation |
| ◆ Haematocrit 27–30%, lower blood viscosity | |
| Bedside Doppler examination of stoma for perfusion | *Haematological:* |
| | Maintain a relative hypocoagulable state |
| | Check PT, PTT, INR, fibrinogen, platelet count |
| *Renal function:* | |
| Frequent analysis of electrolytes/CMP | |
| Correct any electrolyte and acid-base abnormalities | *Infections:* |
| Correct hyperglycaemia | Obtain frequent/daily blood cultures, drain cultures. |
| BUN/creatinine | |
| ◆ High levels of tacrolimus levels can correlate with renal dysfunction | Bronchoalveolar lavage if suspect pneumonia |
| Avoid hypermagnesaemia | |
| ◆ May potentiate tacrolimus neurotoxicity | |
| *GI function and nutrition:* | |
| Frequent liver function analysis (LFTs), bilirubin | |
| Amylase and lipase | |
| Evaluate nutrition status | |
| ◆ Check protein levels, albumin; monitor caloric intake, fat, glucose, electrolytes daily | |
| Monitor signs of rejection: | |
| ◆ Abdominal pain, obstruction, fevers | |
| ◆ Ostomy output, colour | |
| ◆ Frequent ileoscopies and biopsies twice a week post-operative | |

## Haematologic system

MVTx and ITx recipients commonly have neutropaenia, anaemia, and thrombocytopaenia postoperatively. This can persist for prolonged periods due to the use of myelosuppressive medications post-transplant. In the acute postsurgical period, transfusions should be limited to cases of severe anaemia associated with clinical signs and bleeding episodes. It is common to see haematocrit levels in the mid 20s and platelet counts below 100. Other causes include infectious aetiologies, immunomodulators, antibiotics, antiviral medications, and drug toxicity. A rare but deadly complication associated with transplant recipients is thrombotic microangiopathy (TMA). It causes tissue ischaemia and organ dysfunction from microvascular occlusion and thrombosis. TMA is associated with the use of tacrolimus and cyclosporine. It can manifest as multi-organ system deterioration, tissue ischaemia, and stroke. Plasmapheresis has been shown to aid in the treatment, along with discontinuation of the medication.

## Nutrition

The goal of MVTx is to achieve nutritional autonomy. This is a gradual process. Each centre differs on when to resume enteral feeds and this can vary from 3 days to several weeks post-op. Bedside evaluation of the intestinal stoma can provide useful information about bowel ischaemia, rejection, and function. Serum lactate levels gradually drop to normal after 24 hours postoperatively. Elevated lactic acid levels may be a sign of ongoing tissue ischaemia and may prompt surgical exploration. Gastroparesis is a common occurrence after surgery, particularly since the transplanted bowels' innervation is intrinsically mediated via Aurbach's and Meissner's plexi. Intestinal peristalsis starts slowly after reperfusion and it can take several days to weeks before optimal bowel function resumes. Oral administration of prokinetic medications can improve bowel motility. However, absorption of nutrients is delayed and affected by the mucosal damage sustained during tissue ischaemia and bowel denervation during organ procurement and preservation (Silver and Castellanos, 2000). Reperfusion injury of the transplanted graft has been shown to cause cell membrane damage by oxidative free radicals (Schroeder, 1994).

Nutrition is slowly introduced once the patient is stable and no signs of rejection are observed. Initially the patient is placed on TPN and enteral feeds are started. These formulas are designed by dieticians to meet each patient's nutritional energy, protein, vitamins, and mineral requirements. Feeds are gradually advanced to optimize nutrition to at least 50% of the patient's total energy needs. If the patient tolerates these formulas (including lipids, triglycerides, and fibre) he/she is weaned off the TPN, which may take several months. It may be necessary for some paediatric patients to require physical therapy in order to relearn oral feeding habits and decrease food aversion.

Vigilance for infection, rejection, and malignancy is important since these patients are at high risk for these complications. Broad-spectrum antibiotics and immunosuppressive agents are continued throughout the postoperative course. These topics are discussed in more detail in the sections on 'Infection', 'Rejection surveillance and effects', and 'Post-transplant lymphoproliferative disorder'.

## Infection

Sepsis continues to be the number-one cause of death in immunosuppressed MVTx recipients. Rejection of the transplanted organs can lead to abdominal infections that are difficult to treat in an already immunocompromised patient. The need for antirejection medications, which further weaken the patient's ability to prevent and fight infections, makes this a vicious cycle.

Almost all transplant recipients experience an episode of infection within the first 3 months post-transplant. Early on, the causes of infection can be derived from the donor or the recipient. Preoperative screening of both donor and recipient for possible sources of infection is important to form a plan for perioperative antibiotic, antiviral, and/or antifungal prophylactic treatment. Many microbes can appear as latent infections in the organ recipient, such as *Herpes simplex, Varicella zoster* virus, hepatitis B or C, tuberculosis, and toxoplasmosis. Chronic infections in these patients, such as indwelling central venous catheter infections, have increased the risk of antibiotic-resistant microbes to vancomycin, fluconazole, and other agents, further complicating treatment and morbidity.

In one study, bacteraemia and respiratory infections were the primary causes of infections in MVTx recipients, significantly increasing their mortality, particularly in the younger population < 1 year old (Kato et al., 2006b). Other sources of infection include central lines, abdominal drains, peritoneal fluid collections, surgical wounds, and urinary tract infections. The transplanted organs can also be a source of infection. Bacterial translocation from compromised bowel may require bowel decontamination regimens with multiple antifungal and antibiotic agents, principally in the setting of rejection. Later on, more opportunistic infections can cause serious complications in the immunosuppressed recipient, requiring prophylaxis, such as *Pneumocystis jirovecii* (known as *Pneumocystis carinii*), toxoplasmosis, leishmaniasis, histoplasmosis, *Coccidioides*, and *Cryptococcus*.

Viruses are also implicated in certain diseases and are copathogens in some opportunistic infections (Van den Berg et al., 1996; Fishman, 2007). CMV has been known to cause fever, neutropaenia, gastritis, oesophagitis, colitis, adrenal insufficiency, and encephalitis. Patients are placed on prophylaxis or treated with antiviral medications such as gancyclovir. Other viruses have been known to cause certain cancers. EBV is known to predispose these patients to lymphomas such as PTLD and HCV, causing hepatocellular carcinoma. Infections and complications with such microbes can result in graft failure and loss.

## Rejection surveillance and effects

Acute rejection is the most common complication from intestinal transplants. Some studies have shown that MVTx (which includes the liver) offers some protection from rejection (Abu-Elmagd et al., 1998, 2001; Tzakis et al., 2005). Patients are closely monitored for rejection postoperatively. The diagnosis of rejection is determined by a combination of clinical signs and histological tissue findings, which is the gold standard for diagnosis. Clinical signs often seen with rejection are fevers, abdominal pain, bleeding, diarrhoea, and changes in stoma output. Endoscopy is used for visualizing the transplanted bowel and obtaining multiple biopsies for tissue analysis. The stoma opening is used to facilitate the endoscopic procedure with direct visualization of the transplanted graft. Surveillance protocols have been developed and recommend frequent postoperative endoscopies performed 1–2 times a week for the first 2 weeks post-transplant, then once a week for the following 2 months, then once a month until stoma closure (Kato et al., 2006b).

A graded system of acute rejection has been determined depending on pathological findings, varying in degree of inflammation, mucosal injury, and apoptosis (Ruiz et al., 2004).

| | |
|---|---|
| Grade 0: | No rejection |
| Grade (IND): | Indeterminate (likely no rejection) |
| Grade 1: | Mild rejection |
| Grade 2: | Moderate rejection |
| Grade 3: | Severe rejection |

Depending on the severity of the rejection, treatment consists of steroid administration, adjustments of immunosuppression levels, and addition or modification of antilymphocyte medications. Ultimately, if the patient experiences severe rejection that is resistant to treatment, he/she may require a retransplant.

## Post-transplant lymphoproliferative disorder

PTLD is a malignancy associated with immune suppression and EBV infection. It is a type of lymphoma, usually B-cell lymphoma, but it can be non-B-cell type as well (T/NK cell). Some antirejection medications have also been associated with an increased incidence of PTLD such as muromonab-CD3 (OKT3) and tacrolimus (Kato et al., 2006b). Treatment for PTLD consists of antiviral medications, reduction of immunosuppression, and chemotherapeutic agents such as rituximab. Early tapering from immunosuppressive agents and antiviral prophylaxis may decrease the incidence of PTLD.

## Graft versus host disease

GVHD has been documented in all organ transplants. Antibodies from the transplanted organ/graft recognize and attack the host (recipient) as a foreign body. Intestines have a large amount of lymphoid tissue, which may increase the incidence of GVHD in ITx/MVTx recipients. It can be described as acute or chronic GVHD depending on the time of onset post-transplant (< 100 days or > 100 days, respectively).

Clinical manifestations of GVHD can involve the skin, liver, GI tract, and haematopoetic system. A maculopapular rash of the neck, shoulders, hands, and feet is the most common presentation. In severe cases, liver involvement can present without the skin rash. Non-specific liver dysfunction such as increased bilirubin and cholestasis may be seen in GVHD. Upper and lower GI involvement include nausea, vomiting, severe abdominal pain, and diarrhoea. Haematopoetic involvement can present as subtle but persistent thrombocytopaenia and decreased immunoglobulin levels (Shono et al., 2010). Skin and GI tract biopsies can be easily obtained to confirm diagnosis of GVHD. Liver biopsy may cause significant bleeding. Non-specific immunosuppressive drugs such as corticosteroids, cyclosporine, and tacrolimus are used as prophylaxis and treatment. Once again, the presence of this disorder and its treatment can further predispose these transplant patients to organ dysfunctions and infections.

## Immunosuppressive therapy following MVTx

The possibility of intestinal transplantation was first entertained at the beginning of the twentieth century (Carrel, 1905). Nonetheless, immunological manipulation proved to be challenging. The intestine is richly supplied with lymphoid tissue as well as a large mucosal surface area expressing class 2 MHC antigen. This creates an ideal situation for mutual rejection between the graft and host. Furthermore, the intestine is a hollow organ replete with multiple potentially infectious micro-organisms. It was once labelled as the 'largest undrained abscess' in the body. The thin mucosal monolayer can allow translocation of micro-organisms, thus allowing direct access to the systemic circulation (Middleton, 2005). Hence, early attempts at transplantation were a resounding failure due to a combination of acute graft rejection and sepsis and subsequent multiple-organ failure.

### The first era

Following the introduction of cyclosporine by Calne and colleagues, a renewed enthusiasm occurred in the field of ITx (Calne, 1978). Grant and colleagues reported in 1990 a successful case of intestine and liver transplantation in a patient with SBS and liver failure with underlying antithrombin-3 deficiency (Grant, 1990). Concomitant publications were based on two paediatric patients with SBS and liver failure who underwent composite allograft consisting of liver, stomach, duodenum, jejunum, and ileum (Williams, 1989; Starlz, 1989). In these two publications, cyclosporine was the backbone of the immunosuppressive regimen. The introduction of cyclosporine allowed for acceptable medium-term survival, although long-term rejection remained a significant challenge.

### The second era

In 1989 the development of the new immunosuppressant tacrolimus (FK-506), a CNI, allowed for transplantation to become more of a reality. As noted by Todo (1995), infection rather than acute rejection became the primary cause of mortality. This pointed to a need to fine-tune the degree of immunosuppression. Further, this powerful immune-modulating effect led to a resurgence of chronic rejection, possibly brought about by the near-complete loss of progressive tolerance that allowed during the earlier days of transplantation the use of minimal, if any, immunosuppression (McGeown, 1998). A possible explanation of the observation of high incidence of acute rejection as compared to a more acceptable level of chronic rejection may lie in the report by Starlz (1992) on the development of chimerism between the host and the recipient leucocytes. Thus the development of powerful immunosuppressive drugs, although very beneficial in the short term in combating acute rejection, may predispose to ablation of the beneficial effects brought about by engagement of host and donor leucocytes.

As noted by Cortesini (2004), the significant reduction in the T-helper and cytotoxic population in association with the expansion of antigen-specific suppressor and regulatory T-cells in the recipient brought about by the newer immunosuppressive drugs (campath 1H) allows a medium in which the graft is well tolerated under the gentle 'umbrella' of immunosuppression.

### The third era

The next significant advance in the field of immunosuppression occurred with the introduction of campath 1H (Cambridge Pathology). Being a monoclonal antibody directed against CD54 antibodies, it resulted in significant immunosuppression when combined with tacrolimus. However, these high degrees of immunosuppression led to episodes of severe infections. Initially this high degree of immunosuppression was attributed to the use of composite grafting. However, with the advancement of immunology and the creation of a single international registry it became apparent that stable chimerism, between the graft and the host, is essential for a successful outcome. This may well be achieved by engaging the host with the graft with concomitant judicious, small doses of immunosuppression which may lead to the development of mutual tolerance. This has become the goal of modern transplantation immunosuppression (Starlz, 1993).

Thus, based on the current literature and a 2008 review from the University of Pittsburgh which included 500 patients with ITx and MVTx in a single centre, it has been suggested that an initial induction regimen that involves either alemtuzumab (campath) or rabbit antithymocyte globulin (thymoglobulin) administered within 3 hours of reperfusion, with underlying immunosuppression provided with either tacrolimus and/or MMF, and the use of steroids for episodes of acute cellular rejection provides the best protocol for long-term survival (Abu-Elmagd, 2009).

In recent years the importance of donor-specific antibodies (DSA) has come to the forefront. While acute rejection could be managed successfully under most circumstances with steroids administration, long-term chronic rejection usually initiated by antibodies was largely resistant and impervious to steroid therapy. The detection of high-titre DSA both coincided with episodes of rejection and decreased long-term prognosis. Hence, if DSA could be neutralized, or at the least detected early, then measures could be instituted to improve outcome. To this end, single antigen fluorescent (Luminex) bead assays have been developed, which were not apparent with older established detection methods such as enzyme-linked immunoabsorbent assays. Once detected, for example in the pretransplant stage, strategies to neutralize their deleterious effect may include plasmapheresis and/or administration of immunoglobulin.

In the post-transplant stage, strategies to counterbalance chronic rejection brought about by DSA include routine administration of MMF with rescue rapamycin.

More novel techniques include complement-blocking drugs such as C1 (esterase) inhibitors, since this is the first step in the antibodies' activation of the complement cascade system. Further strategies include the administration of rituximab, which binds to CD20 on precursor and mature B-cells and induces their destruction, thus decreasing antibody production.

Since plasma B-cells play a significant role in the presentation of antigens to T-cells and subsequent T-helper and T-cytotoxic activation, rituximab may tame down this pathway as well. Nonetheless, rituximab has no effect on terminally differentiated B-cells as they lack CD20. It is this very population that yields the bulk of circulating antibodies. Bertezomib is a highly selective inhibitor of the 26S proteasome, which is currently used as standard therapy for multiple myeloma. Its indirect effects include suppression of NF-κB and induction of apoptosis. As such, it has been used following administration of tacrolimus and/or MMF in order to suppress DSA production (Berger, 2012).

Practically, MVTx/ITx recipients are monitored for clinical signs of rejection via endoscopic surveillance of loop or standard ileostomy. Initially during the 6 weeks following transplantation this is done two times a week, subsequently weekly for the next 6 weeks, and then monthly for the next 6 months, if there are no signs of rejection, that is high output through the ileostomy, bleeding, ileus, diarrhoea, abdominal pain, or fever (Lomax, 2011).

Recently the measurement of high-serum citrulline as a non-invasive surveillance and diagnostic tool for the development of acute rejection has been described. Hibi and colleagues prospectively collected over a period of 16 years (1995–2011) a total of 13,499 samples of citrulline from 111 consecutive paediatric MVTx/ITx (Hibi et al., 2012). Serum citrulline levels were found to be related to the degree of acute rejection. Based on their findings the authors recommend performing biopsy in an otherwise well patient after 3 months following transplantation, if citrulline levels are < 15 μmol/L or a 25% reduction from baseline.

## Quality of life

The definition of quality of life is drawn from the social sciences where it is defined as the physical, psychological, and social domains of health that are influenced by a person's experience, beliefs, expectations, and perception. Quality of life is more than just mere absence of dysfunction and stress; it is a composite score given to a subjective and fluid endpoint and it includes a sense of well-being and satisfaction. Since ITx and MVTx in paediatric patients are fairly recent surgical procedures, some of the insight regarding the quality of life has to be drawn from adults who underwent a similar procedure.

Home parenteral nutrition is at present the method of choice in providing nutrition to patients with irreversible intestinal failure. However, there is evidence that quality of life tends to decrease over time. Cameron and colleagues at Addenbrooke's Hospital in Cambridge, UK, assessed three groups of patients with intestinal failure (Cameron, 2002). Group 1 consisted of adult patients of mean age 36 years who were transplanted, group 2 of patients mean age 42 years on stable home parenteral nutrition, and group 3 of patients with complicated intestinal failures who were deemed inappropriate to transplant. Their results suggest that the first two groups had a similar quality of life as judged by the Nottingham Health Profile and SF-36 Short Form, whereby increasing score represented a decreasing quality of life. The authors noted that their sample size was small and thus not powered to detect significant differences.

Rovera in 1998 essentially found very similar results when he compared ten adult recipients of ITx with ten home TPN patients (Rovera, 1998). Essentially a similar quality of life was experienced in both groups, with the ITx group experiencing decreasing anxiety with the passage of time and increased adjustment in the post-transplant period.

The group of DiMartine from Pittsburgh published a more favourable result. Using the quality of life index (QOLI) which contains 26 domains that cover most of the adult daily living activities, this questionnaire includes 130 questions and takes about 30–45 minutes to complete (DiMartini, 1998). Two population groups were investigated: patients that had small bowel transplantation and patients that were on home TPN. The transplanted patients were further subdivided into three groups: TPN compared to pre-TPN, post-ITx compared to TPN, and post-ITx compared to pre-TPN. Although it could be argued that this stratification increased unnecessarily the complexity and created numerous subgroups, rendering statistical analysis prone to errors, nonetheless in the majority of domains examined a significant improvement in subjective feeling was experienced in the transplanted population. Specifically, patients who underwent small bowel transplantation were more likely to be compliant on medical treatment as well as exhibiting less signs of depression, e.g. alcohol consumption.

A more recent article by O'Keefe from Pittsburgh describes a population of 46 adult patients that underwent small bowel transplantation between June 2003 and July 2004. This group was assessed in comparison to 13 patients who were on home TPN and were either reluctant to undergo transplantation or deemed inappropriate for the procedure. Using the quality of life index, the transplanted group fared significantly better than the home TPN group (O'Keefe, 2007). Specifically, significant improvement was observed in mood parameters, namely anxiety, depression, cognitive emotion, appearance, stress experience, and parenting, as well as digestive and urinary function. Based on these largely favourable results, the author of this article recommended extending the criteria of suitability for small bowel transplantation from 'TPN failure' to a larger group of patients, viz 'at risk of developing TPN failure'.

A recent article by Pironi from Bologna compared 22 ITx recipients and 33 home parenteral nutrition patients for benign intestinal failure (Pironi, 2012). This was a cross-sectional study using a validated tool for assessment. The quality of life questionnaire consists of 48 items that pertain to the emotional, physical, and symptomatic issues. It is divided into seven multi-item functional scales encompassing: general health, ability to vacation, coping mechanism, physical status, nutritional assessment, employment, sexual function, and emotional function. Essentially their experience points to improvement in patient quality of life following ITx in respect of a decrease in GI symptoms, fatigue, enhancement of a sense of well-being associated with ability to eat, and freedom of movement without the hassle of TPN. The authors are quick to point out that although their results are generally favourable, they are by no means conclusive. They do support the role of rehabilitation following ITx for irreversible gut failure; however, the results do not indicate that a patient with poor quality of life on home parenteral nutrition is an indication for ITx. Nonetheless, it is prudent to conclude that most centres support the assertion that quality of life is superior in adult patients who have undergone ITx as opposed to patients on home parenteral nutrition.

Regarding the paediatric population, Ngo published his results using the Health-Related Quality of Life (HRQOL) and the Pediatric Quality of Life Inventory 4.0 (PedsQL4.0) in 24 patients with a median age of 6 years who underwent ITx (Ngo, 2011). Of note, the majority of patients were Latino males (58%) who underwent liver-inclusive transplants. The findings point towards a significant difference in social functioning as well as physical health between their group and a healthy group. A possible explanation for the relatively modest outcome may be the fact that both parents and children use their pretransplant experience as a reference point when answering the questionnaire. Further, the answers may represent a 'desire' to be healthy, rather than the actual current circumstances.

A more favourable report was published by Sudan in 2004. The Child Health Questionnaire was administered to both children and parents. The group consisted of 29 children who underwent ITx 1 year previously and had a functioning graft. Essentially the findings indicate that transplanted patient quality of life fared worse than normal children but was comparable to children with a chronic ailment, i.e. renal failure and haemodialysis (Sudan, 2004).

Based on the current relative paucity of information regarding paediatric patients' quality of life following ITx it would seem prudent to undergo this procedure in a well-selected population of patients in a tertiary centre well versed with the myriad of services required to support such challenging children.

## Future directions

PTLD is a serious although relatively uncommon complication following solid organ transplantation, occurring at a rate between 1 and 20% (Courthey, 2010). Typically it presents in the first year of life and is usually associated with EBV infection. The second peak occurs in the subsequent year and is usually not related to EBV infection. The pathological feature resembles non-Hodgkin lymphoma (NHL). Nonetheless, the prognosis is less favourable than in de-novo NHL. Predisposing factors include the degree of immunosuppression, with increased rates following administration of tacrolimus and OKT3. Cyclosporine, on the other hand, with close attention to therapeutic levels, does not appear to predispose to PTLD.

The mechanism of development appears to be related to B-cell chronic stimulation following an increase in foreign viral antigen load brought about by immunosuppression. Therapeutic strategies usually involve the administration of combination chemotherapy and immunotherapy with monoclonal antibodies (such as anti-CD20, anti-CD21, and anti-CD22). Rituximab, a monoclonal antibody directed against CD20, appears to offer the greatest beneficial impact. An article by Orjuela reported six paediatric patients with PTLD following solid organ transplantation who were treated with cyclophosphamide, rituximab, and prednisone (Orjuela, 2003). Five of the six patients had complete response. The sixth patient had a partial response at a median follow-up of 12.5 months. More guarded reports by Gross in a paediatric population, although still pointing toward a high response rate, nonetheless indicate a 58% event-free survival at 2 years (defined as absence of relapse, disease progression, drug toxicity, and death) (Gross, 2005). Although significant progress has been made in the treatment of PTLD, it is hoped that the newer agents that are currently being used as novel strategies for NHL, viz bertezomib, yttrium Y 90 ibritumomab tiuxetan and sirolimus, may be beneficial in treating PTLD as well (Gonzalez-Barca, 2007; Evens, 2010).

## Chronic rejection

A relatively new approach to immunosuppression minimization in children aims to take advantage of the newer immunosuppressive agents, while at the same time minimizing and possibly eliminating altogether the older agents, particularly the CNIs (cyclosporine A and tacrolimus) and corticosteroids due to their myriad adverse effects (Sarwal, 2008). Other agents that may be phased out sometime in the future include sirolimus and everolimus, due to their hyperlipidaemic effects and impaired wound healing, and MMF, due to its GI and bone marrow depression. Their minimization will usher in greater usage of the newer induction agents such as humanized interleukin-2 receptor (IL-2R) blockers (daclizumab and basiliximab), thymoglobulin, and campath.

A further future approach would involve tailoring the immunotherapy to the patient-specific genetic profile, e.g. inosine 5-monophosphate dehydrogenase 1 (IMPDH1) genetic polymorphism and MMF therapy. Short nucleotide polymorphism in the cytochrome P450 was associated with increased biopsy-proven rejection in the first year after renal transplantation. In addition, IMPDH2 isoform has been correlated with a higher incidence of MMF haematological and GI side effects. Progress in this field is likely to be slow due to the multiple genes governing the metabolism of a single drug. However, it is plausible that in the future both donor and recipient will undergo genotype testing (Wavamunno, 2008).

## Conclusion

The critical care of patients following ITx or MVTx poses a great challenge to the expertise of the ICU medical and nursing staff. The delivery of care requires good communication and cooperation among several disciplines including transplant medicine, surgery, infectious diseases, anaesthesiology, and nursing, with the support of ancillary services such as infection control, pharmacy, nutrition, and psychology, among others. In large-volume transplant programmes ICUs are staffed by medical and nursing staff specifically trained in the care of these complicated patients. Clinical care is guided by evidenced-based procedures and treatment protocols. In order to maximize care, specific physiological targets need to be set up in order to maximize preservation and full recovery of GI function. Further, validated protocols need to be in place so as to streamline care and avoid variability in quality of care. In this chapter we have reviewed selected topics particularly relevant to critical care of the adult and paediatric ITx and MVTx recipient, such as post-transplant infection, rejection, GVHD, lymphoproliferative disease, the evolution of immunosuppression therapy, and quality of life.

## References

Abu-Elmagd K, Reyes J, Todo S, et al. (1998) Clinical intestinal transplantation: new perspectives and immunologic considerations. *J Am Coll Surg*, **185**:512.

Abu-Elmagd K, Reyes J, Bond G, et al. (2001) Clinical intestinal transplantation: a decade of experience at a single center. *Annal Surg*, **234**(3):404–417.

Abu-Elmagd K, Costa G, Bond G, et al. (2009) Five hundred intestinal and multivisceral transplantations at a single center: major advances with new challenges. *Annal Surg*, **250**:567–581.

Berger M (2012) Immunologic challenges in small bowel transplantation. *Am J Transplant*, **12**:S2–S8.

Calne R (1978) Cyclosporin A in patients receiving renal allografts from cadaver donors. *Lancet*, **2**:1323–1327.

Cameron E (2002) Quality of life in adults following small bowel transplantation. *Transplant Proc*, **34**:965–966.

Carrel A (1905) The transplantation of organs. A preliminary communication. *JAMA*, **45**:1645.

Cortesini R (2004) The concept of 'partial' clinical tolerance. *Transplant Immunol*, **13**:101–104.

Courthey D (2010) Treatment advances in posttransplant lymphoproliferative disease. *Curr Opin Hematol*, **17**:1065.

Dujardin K, McCully R, Wijdicks E, et al. (2001) Myocardial dysfunction associated with brain death: clinical, echocardiographic, and pathologic features. *J Heart Lung Transplant*, **20**(3):350–357.

Evens A (2010) Multicenter analysis of 80 solid organ transplantation recipients with post-transplantation lymphoproliferative disease: outcome and prognostic factors in the modern era. *J Clin Oncol*, **28**(6):1038–1046.

Fishman J (2007) Infection in solid-organ transplant recipients. *N Engl J Med*, **357**(25):2601.

Flick R (2012) Clinical complications in pediatric anesthesia. In: Gregory G, Andropoulos D (eds) *Gregory's Pediatric Anesthesia*, 5th edn, pp. 1152–1182. Wiley-Blackwell, Oxford.

Fuster V, Ryden L, Cannom D, et al. (2011a) 2011 ACCF/AHA/HRS focused updates incorporated into the ACC/AHA/ESC 2006 guidelines for the management of patients with atrial fibrillation: a report of the American College of Cardiology Foundation/American Heart Association Task Force on practice guidelines. *Circulation*, **123**(10):e269–e367.

Fuster V, Ryden L, Cannom D, et al. (2011b) 2011 ACCF/AHA/HRS focused updates incorporated into the ACC/AHA/ESC 2006 Guidelines for the management of patients with atrial fibrillation: a report of the American College of Cardiology Foundation/American Heart Association Task Force on Practice Guidelines developed in partnership with the European Society of Cardiology and in collaboration with the European Heart Rhythm Association and the Heart Rhythm Society. *J Am Coll Cardiol*, **57**(11):e101–e198.

Gonzalez-Barca E (2007) Prospective phase 2 of extended treatment with rituximab in patients with B cell post transplant lymphoproliferative disease. *Haematologica*, **92**:1484–1494.

Grant D (1990) Successful small bowel/liver transplantation. *Lancet*, **335**:181–184.

Gross T (2005) Low dose chemotherapy for Epstein–Barr virus positive post transplant lymphoproliferative disease in children after solid organ transplantation. *J Clin Oncol*, **23**(27):6481–6488.

Hauser GJ, Kaufman SS, Matsumoto CS, Fishbein TS (2008) Pediatric intestinal and multivisceral transplantation: a new challenge for the pediatric intensivist. *Intens Care Med*, **34**(9):1570–1579.

Hibi T, Nishida S, Garcia J, et al. (2012) Citrulline level is a potent indicator of acute rejection in the long term following pediatric intestinal/multivisceral transplantation. *Am J Transplant*, **12**:S27–S32.

Hopfner R, Tran TT, Island ER, McLaughlin GE (2012) Nonsurgical Care of Intestinal and Multivisceral Transplant Recipients: a review for the intensivist. *J Inten Care Med*, **28**(4):215–229.

Kato T, Kleiner G, David A, et al. (2006a) Inclusion of spleen in pediatric multivisceral transplantation. *Transplant Proc*, **38**(6):1709–1710.

Kato T, Tzakis A, Selvaggi G, et al. (2006b) Intestinal and multivisceral transplantation in children. *Annal Surg*, **243**(6):756–764.

Lillehei R, Goot B, Miller F (1959a) Homografts of the small bowel. *Surg Forum*, **10**:197.

Lillehei R, Goot B, Miller F (1959b) The physiologic response of the small bowel of the dog to ischemia including prolonged in vitro preservation of the bowel with successful replacement and survivial. *Ann Surg*, **150**:543–560.

Lomax S (2011) Anaesthesia for intestinal transplantation. *Cont Educ Anaesth*, **2**:1–4.

Mangus R, Tector A, Kubal C, Fridell J, Vianna R (2012) Multivisceral transplantation: expanding indications and improving outcomes. *J Gastrointest Surg*, **17**(1):179–186

McGeown M (1998) Ten year results of renal transplantation with azathioprine and prednisolone as the only immunosuppression. *Lancet*, **1**:983–985.

Middleton S (2005) The current status of small bowel transplantation in the UK and internationally. *Gut*, **54**:1650–1657.

Miller BE, Hendrickson JE (2012) Coagulation, bleeding, and blood transfusion. In Gregory GA, Andropoulos DB (eds) *Pediatric Anesthesia*, 5th edn, pp. 224–254. Wiley-Blackwell, Oxford.

Ngo K (2011) Pediatric health related quality of life after intestinal transplantation. *Pediatr Transplant*, **15**:849–855.

O'Keefe S J D (2007) Nutrtion and quality of life following intestinal transplantation. *Am J Gastroenterol*, **102**(5):1093–1110.

OPTN (2010) Annual Data Report of the US Organ Procurement and Transplantation Network and the Scientific Registry of Transplant Recipients 1998–2009. *Transplant Data*

Orjuela M (2003) A pilot study of chemoimmunotherapy (cyclophosphamide, prednisone, and rituximab) in patients with post-transplant lymphoproliferative disorder following solid organ transplantation. *Clin Canc Res*, **9**:3945S–3952S.

Raife T, Di Paola J (2004) Transfusion of the pediatric surgery, trauma, and intensive care unit patient. In Strauss R, Luban N, Hillyer C (eds) *Handbook Pediatric Transfusion* Medicine, pp. 137–148. Academic Press, Burlington, Massachusetts.

Rosendale J, Kauffman H, McBride M, et al. (2003a) Aggressive pharmacologic donor management results in more transplanted organs. *Transplantation*, **75**(4):482–487.

Rosendale J, Kauffman H, McBride M, et al. (2003b) Hormonal resuscitation yields more transplanted hearts, with improved early function. *Transplantation*, **75**(8):1336–1341.

Rovera G (1998) Quality of life after intestinal transplantation. *Transplantation*, **66**(9):1141–1145.

Ruiz P, Bagni A, Brown R, et al. (2004) Histological criteria for the identification of acute cellular rejection in human small bowel allografts: results of the pathology workshop at the VIII International Small Bowel Transplant Symposium. *Transplant Proc*, **36**:335–337.

Sarwal M (2008) Out with the old, in with the new: immunosuppression minimization in children. *Curr Opin Organ Transplant*, **13**:513–521.

Shono Y, Ueha S, Wang Y, et al. (2010) Bone marrow graft-versus-host disease:early destruction of hematopoited nich after MHC mismatched hematopoitec stem cell transplantation. *Blood*, **115**(26):5401.

Silver H, Castellanos V (2000) Nutritional complications and management of intestinal transplant. *J Am Dietitic Assoc*, **100**(6):680–689.

Starlz T (1989) Transplantation of multiple abdominal viscera. *JAMA*, **261**:1449–1457.

Starlz T (1992) Cell migration, chimerism and graft acceptance. *Lancet*, **339**:1579–1582.

Starlz T (1993) Cell migration and chimerism after whole organ transplantation: the basis for graft acceptance. *Hepatology*, **17**:1127–1152.

Stayer S, Williams G, Andropolous D (2012) Anesthesia for transplantation. In: Gregory G, Andropoulos D (eds) *Gregory's Pediatric Anesthesia*, 5th edn, pp. 682–685. Wiley-Blackwell, Oxford.

Sudan D (2004) Quality of life after intestinal transplantation. *Am J Transplant*, **4**:407–413.

Todo S (1995) Outcome analysis of 71 clinical intestinal transplantation. *Annal Surg*, **220**:270.

Tzakis A, Kato T, Levi D, et al. (2005) 100 Multivisceral transplants at a single center. *Annal Surg*, **242**(2):480–491.

UNOS (undated) *Organ Allocation*. <http://www.unos.org/donation/index.php?topic=organ allocation>.

UNOS (2009) *MELD and PELD Calculator Documentation*. <http://www.unos.org/docs/meld peld calculator documentation>.

Van den Berg A, Klompmaker I, Haagsma E, et al. (1996) Evidence for an increased rate of bacterial infection in liver transplant patients with cytomegalovirus infection. *Clin Transplant*, **10**(2):224.

Wavamunno M (2008) Individualization of immunosuppression: concepts and rationale. *Curr Opin Organ Transplant*, **13**:604–608.

Williams J (1989) Splanchnic transplantation an approach to the infant dependent on parenteral nutrition who develops irreversible liver damage. *JAMA*, **261**:1458–1462.

SECTION 8

# Heart, lung, and heart–lung

# CHAPTER 30

# Perioperative management of the heart transplant recipient

Alan Ashworth and Andrew Roscoe

## Introduction

Heart transplantation (HTx) is the treatment of choice for certain patients with end-stage heart failure and cardiac disease (Stehlik, 2011). The first reported successful human-to-human HTx was performed at Groote Schuur Hospital, South Africa, in December 1967 (Barnard, 1967). The patient survived 18 days before succumbing to overwhelming lung infection. After the introduction of cyclosporin, the number of HTx increased dramatically from the early 1980s to peak during the mid-1990s (see Figure 30.1). Median survival for adult HTx is approximately 10 years (see Figure 30.2). The development of newer generation mechanical ventricular assist devices (VADs) may lead to the decline in the number of HTx surgeries over the next decade (Lietz and Miller, 2005).

## Donor organ management

Guidelines for the management of the potential organ donor are well recognized (Shemie, 2006; Mascia, 2009). The yield of transplantable hearts from potential donors is only 40%, mainly due to left ventricular dysfunction (Zaroff et al., 2003a, 2003b). Brainstem death produces a surge in the release of circulating catecholamines. This 'catecholamine storm' causes an increase in myocardial oxygen demand with the concomitant risk of myocardial ischaemia and potential myofibre death. Following this period there is typically a loss of sympathetic tone with resultant vasodilatation and hypotension. Reduced coronary perfusion during this time contributes further to myocardial injury (Costanzo, 2010). Traditional assessment of donor heart function involves invasive monitoring with central venous and PA catheters, in addition to direct surgical inspection. The routine use of donor echocardiography may increase the umber of hearts for successful transplantation (Venkateswaran, 2005). The yield of donor organs can be improved by the use of 'hormonal' therapy, which includes the administration of methylprednisolone, thyroxine, and vasopressin (Rosendale, 2003).

## Recipient candidates

The most common indications for HTx are dilated cardiomyopathy and end-stage heart failure secondary to coronary artery disease (see Figure 30.3). Ambulatory patients with end-stage heart failure should initially undergo cardiopulmonary exercise (CPX) testing to determine candidacy for HTx. A maximum CPX test is defined as one with a respiratory exchange ratio > 1.05 and achievement of an anaerobic threshold. In patients taking $^{2}$-blocking therapy, a cutoff for peak oxygen consumption ($VO_{2)}$ < 12 mL/kg/min is used to guide listing. In the absence of a beta-blocker, the cutoff for peak $VO_2$ < 14 mL/kg/min guides listing. In patients with submaximal CPX testing or ambiguity of testing, a heart failure survival score may be considered (Table 30.1) (Mehra, 2006).

Right heart catheterization should be performed as part of the routine work-up for transplant listing. Pulmonary hypertension (PHT) is one of the leading causes of right ventricular failure and early mortality after transplantation. When there is evidence of PHT (Table 30.2) a vasodilator challenge is given. Failure to show reversibility to an acute challenge should prompt hospitalization for active medical therapy in an attempt to reduce PVR. If medical therapy fails, mechanical support should be considered (Stobierska-Dzierzek, 2001). Patients presenting in cardiogenic shock may also be considered for transplant listing and are assessed on an individual basis. Vasoactive therapy and mechanical support may be required to bridge the critically ill patient to transplantation (Shanewise, 2004). Relative contraindications to HTx are listed in Table 30.3. Patients on the waiting list must be evaluated at 3- to 6-monthly intervals to assess response to therapy or detect the development of possible contraindications (Mehra, 2006).

## Anaesthetic management

### Preoperative assessment

Due to the urgency of HTx the time available to the anaesthetist for preoperative assessment is short (Shanewise, 2004; Ramakrishna, 2009). In some institutions patients who are candidates for HTx are evaluated at the preoperative clinic by an anaesthesiologist in order to identify risks, such as anticipated difficult intubation. Some may be in-patients on the urgent waiting list, which allows the anaesthesiologist more time for assessment. These patients are usually on a coronary care unit or ICU on infusions of inotropes and diuretics, and they may also be receiving renal replacement therapy. They may be supported by mechanical therapies such as left and/or right VADs or intra-aortic balloon pumps (IABPs). In 2009, 32% of patients were bridged to HTx with VADs (19% LVAD, 3% RVAD, and 5% left and right VAD) (Stehlik, 2011).

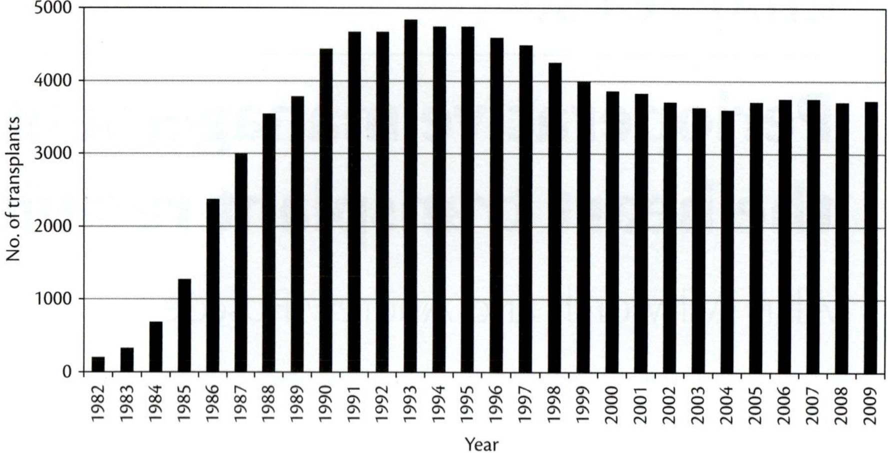


**Fig. 30.1** Number of heart transplants performed by year.

Preoperative assessment should cover all routine aspects for any patient coming to the operating theatre for an urgent procedure, with particular attention paid to fasting status, current level of cardiovascular support, the presence of implanted devices, medication, and recent hospital admissions. In addition, anaesthesiologists should aim to take note of any recent changes in symptoms and current medications, especially anticoagulants and antiplatelet therapy. Patients who are warfarinized should have an INR corrected to ≤ 1.5. A higher INR is likely to result in excessive bleeding (Hirsh, 1998). This can be achieved by vitamin K, FFP, or prothrombin complex concentrates (Costanzo, 2010). A history of previous cardiac surgery is important as it increases the time needed by the surgeons to prepare the recipient for transplantation and increases the risk of bleeding. These patients will need external defibrillator pads to be applied and blood immediately available prior to sternotomy. If the patient has an automatic implantable cardioverter-defibrillator (AICD), external defibrillator pads should be applied and it should be deactivated immediately prior to induction of anaesthesia.

Timing is crucial to minimize the donor heart ischaemic time and cardiopulmonary bypass (CPB) time for the recipient, so close communication is required between the team harvesting the donor heart and the team managing the recipient (Shanewise, 2004). Any anticipated anaesthetic or surgical difficulties should be highlighted so that extra time can be allowed. There is an association between longer ischaemic times and primary graft dysfunction (Costanzo, 2010).

Physical examination should focus on assessment of the airway and the patient's volume status. Investigations should aim to identify the presence of cardiac decompensation and end-organ damage. Many patients have renal and hepatic impairment secondary to low cardiac outputs and venous congestion (Banner, 2011). This results in altered drug pharmacokinetics due to decreased volume of distribution and drug clearance, leading to higher than expected drug plasma concentrations (Shammas and Dickstein, 1988). Hepatic impairment may also result in a coagulopathy. Investigations are limited due to the short time available but should include ECG, chest X-ray, and blood tests, including full blood count, electrolytes, renal function, liver function tests, coagulation, and blood cross-match. Many institutions also offer point-of-care testing of coagulation and platelet mapping, which is useful in patients on anticoagulant/antiplatelet therapy or in hepatic impairment. Thromboelastography has been demonstrated to reduce perioperative blood transfusion rates in patients undergoing complex cardiac surgery (Shore-Lesserson, 1999).

HTx recipients will have had an echocardiogram, pulmonary function tests, and left and right heart catheterizations as part of the transplant assessment. Right heart catheterization is very important to assess for the presence of PHT and the transpulmonary gradient (TPG). TPG is defined as the pressure drop between

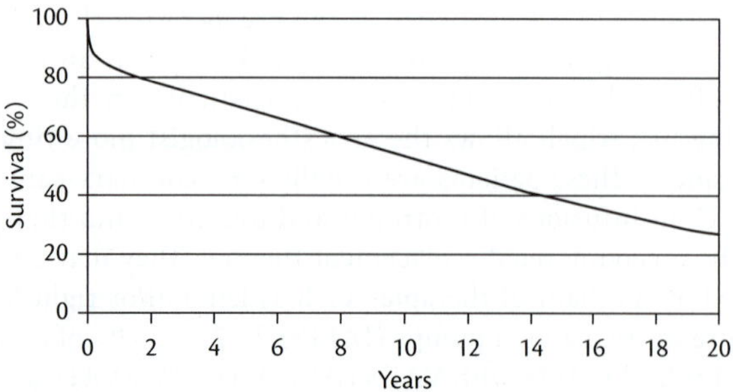


**Fig. 30.2** Survival for adult HTx.

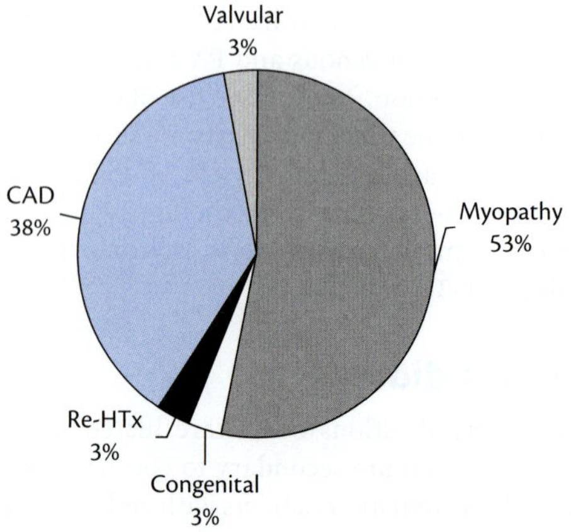


**Fig. 30.3** Indications for adult HTx. CAD, Coronary artery disease.

**Table 30.1** Criteria used in the calculation of Heart Failure Survival Score

| |
|---|
| Ischaemic cardiomyopathy |
| Resting heart rate |
| Left ventricular ejection fraction |
| Mean arterial blood pressure |
| Intraventricular conduction delay |
| Peak $VO_2$ |
| Serum sodium |

the pulmonary arterial system and the pulmonary veins and it is calculated as the mean PA pressure minus the pulmonary capillary wedge pressure (Mets, 2000). An elevated TPG indicates raised pulmonary vascular resistance and increases the risk of right ventricular failure on separation from CPB (Dickstein, 1998). A recent retrospective review of 120 patients with severe pulmonary hypertension found that if there is no significant reduction in PVR and TPG after 3–4 days of pharmacological therapy then mechanical circulatory support is the only option to bridge end-stage heart failure patients to transplantation (Mikus, 2011). Another review of 109 patients who had undergone orthotopic HTx found that a TPG ≥ 12 mmHg was associated with a five-fold increase in mortality at 6 months and the 1-year mortality was seven times higher compared to those who had a TPG < 12 mmHg (Erickson, 1990).

## Premedication

Premedication for HTx includes induction immunosuppressants (dependent on the institution's immunosuppressant protocol), antacids, and gastric prokinetics in patients who are not fasted. Sedatives should be used with caution due to the presence of end-organ damage and altered drug pharmacokinetics. Oversedation will lead to hypoxia and hypercarbia resulting in increased pulmonary vascular resistance and may precipitate right ventricular decompensation.

## Monitoring

Standard routine monitoring, including pulse oximetry, non-invasive blood pressure monitor, electrocardiograph, gas analysis (oxygen, carbon dioxide, and volatile anaesthetic agent), and airway pressure, is established prior to induction of anaesthesia (Birks, 2007). Patients undergoing HTx require additional monitoring: invasive arterial blood pressure, five-lead electrocardiograph, central venous pressure, PA pressure, cardiac output monitor, core temperature, urinary output, and TOE (Quinlan, 2006). Flotation of a PA catheter may be difficult due to cardiac chamber dilatation and severe tricuspid regurgitation. It is very important to remember to withdraw the PA catheter into the SVC prior to venous cannulation for CPB (Shanewise, 2004). BIS monitoring can be used but is not mandatory. High-risk cardiac surgery (ejection fraction < 30%, cardiac index < 2.1 L/min/m$^2$, and pulmonary hypertension) is a risk factor for intraoperative awareness (Myles, 2004); therefore all patients undergoing HTx are at increased risk of awareness. A prospective observational study found the incidence of awareness following cardiac surgery involving cardiopulmonary bypass to be 1.14% (Phillips, 1993), compared to 0.2% in studies investigating the incidence of awareness in patients undergoing non-cardiac surgery (Liu, 1991). Cerebral oximetry monitoring has been shown to reduce the incidence of major organ dysfunction and intensive care length of stay, and improve outcomes in major cardiac surgery (Murkin, 2007).

**Table 30.2** Definition of pulmonary hypertension in HTx assessment

| |
|---|
| Pulmonary artery systolic pressure > 50 mmHg |
| Transpulmonary gradient > 15 mmHg |
| Pulmonary vascular resistance > 3 Wood units |

**Table 30.3** Relative contraindications to listing for HTx

| | |
|---|---|
| Irreversible pulmonary artery hypertension | PVR > 5 Wood units |
| | TPG > 16 mmHg |
| Age > 70 years | |
| Body mass index > 30 kg/m$^2$ | |
| Active malignancy | |
| Diabetes mellitus | With evidence of end-organ damage |
| | Poor control with $HbA_{1C}$ > 7.5 |
| Irreversible renal dysfunction (eGFR < 40 mL/min) | |
| Severe symptomatic cerebrovascular or peripheral vascular disease | |
| Active tobacco smoking | |
| Active substance abuse | |
| Poor compliance with drug therapy | |

eGFR, Estimated glomerular filtration rate; $HbA_{1C}$, glycosylated haemoglobin; PVR, pulmonary vascular resistance; TPG, transpulmonary gradient.

### Transoesophageal echocardiography

The use of TOE during HTx is a class IIb indication—the current evidence suggests that it may be beneficial to patient outcome (Cheitlin, 2003). TOE should be used in all cases unless there are any contraindications (Hilberath, 2010). TOE is used intraoperatively to assess the presence of intracardiac thrombus (see Figure 30.4), pleural effusions, volume status, myocardial contractility, and aortic atherosclerosis. TOE is also used to aid separation from CPB by allowing direct visualization of left and right ventricular function and filling. It is important in the assessment of the surgical anastamoses (see Figure 30.5) and valvular function of the donor heart.

## Induction of anaesthesia

Timing of induction of anaesthesia is crucial to minimize the donor heart ischaemic time, which should be ideally less than 4 hours (Stehlik, 2011). Prolongation of the ischaemic time results in reduced function of the donor heart intraoperatively and postoperatively and increases the risk of primary graft dysfunction. The maximum ischaemic time is not known, but longer ischaemic

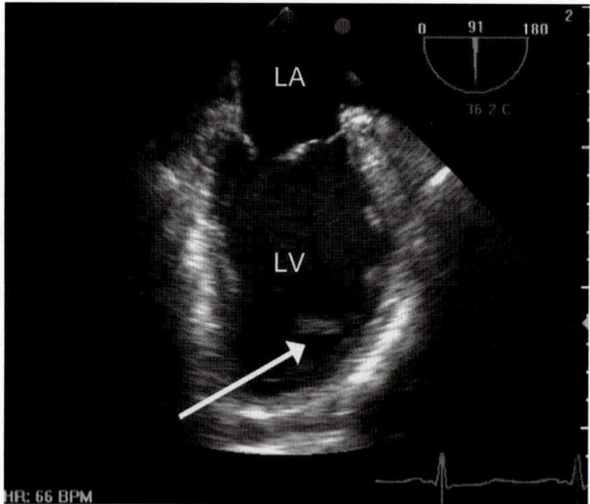

**Fig. 30.4** TOE mid-oesophageal two-chamber view, showing a thrombus (arrow) on the anterior wall of the left ventricle (LV). LA, Left atrium.

times can be accepted if there are no other risk factors for primary graft dysfunction. These risk factors include increased donor age, donor inotrope requirements, and donor cardiac dysfunction (Young, 1994; Costanzo, 2010). The timing of induction of anaesthesia involves close liaison between the anaesthetist, surgeon, and transplant coordinator.

The main goals of anaesthetic management for HTx are to avoid acute decompensation prior to CPB and the management of right heart failure and coagulopathy post-CPB. Patients with end-stage cardiac failure typically have an ejection fraction (EF) less than 20%, with a 'fixed' stroke volume. It is important to maintain adequate preload, but increasing the preload will not increase the stroke volume because of the patients' position on the Frank–Starling curve. These patients are also sensitive to an increase in afterload, which results in a reduction in stroke volume and cardiac output. Cardiac output becomes dependent on heart rate, so bradycardia will significantly reduce cardiac output. Patients with end-stage heart failure have high levels of circulating catecholamines, which maintain vasoconstriction.

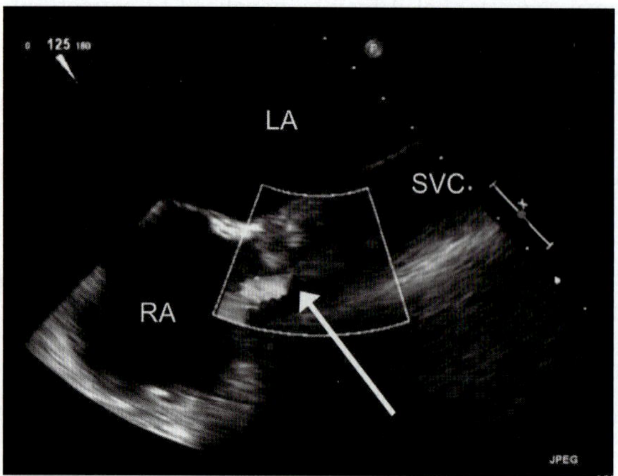

**Fig. 30.5** TOE mid-oesophageal modified bicaval view, showing superior vena cava (SVC) anastomotic stenosis, as demonstrated by colour flow Doppler (arrow). LA, Left atrium; RA, right atrium.

Cardiovascular decompensation can occur during induction of anaesthesia due to the reduction in sympathetic stimulation resulting in hypotension and reduced diastolic myocardial perfusion. If inotropes or mechanical support are running preoperatively they should be continued intraoperatively. It is important to remember that patients with end-stage heart failure have down-regulation of the β–receptors, so higher doses of β-agonist may need to be used (Shanewise, 2004).

The induction of anaesthesia is a particularly hazardous time for the HTx recipient due to the risk of cardiovascular decompensation, so the surgeons and perfusionists should be present to facilitate the rapid institution of CPB should the patient decompensate. Large-bore intravenous access, arterial line, central venous catheter, and PA catheter should be placed under local anaesthesia prior to induction of anaesthesia to allow rapid identification of a deterioration and rapid treatment (Dickstein, 1998). Particular attention should be paid to strict asepsis because the patient will be immunosuppressed in the postoperative period. External defibrillator pads should be applied if the patient has an AICD or had previous cardiac surgery. A modified rapid sequence induction may need to be performed if the patient is not adequately fasted.

The physiological goals of induction are to avoid reductions in preload, increases in afterload, myocardial depression, and bradycardia. Induction agents usually include high-dose opiates, a hypnotic, and a muscle relaxant. It is more important how the drug is used than which induction agent in chosen (Dickstein, 1998).

## Maintenance of anaesthesia

Anaesthesia can be maintained by either volatile or intravenous agents. There is more predictable pharmacology with volatile agents in the presence of renal or hepatic dysfunction (Shammas, 1988). Nitrous oxide may increase pulmonary vascular resistance and expands any air emboli and should be avoided (Schulte-Sasse, 1982). BIS monitoring can assist balancing the myocardial depression associated with anaesthetic agents and maintaining adequate depth of anaesthesia. High-dose steroids, usually methylprednisolone, are administered prior to release of the aortic cross-clamp and myocardial reperfusion (Aliabadi, 2011).

During myocardial reperfusion infusions of inotropes and vasopressors are usually started to aid separation from CPB. The donor heart is denervated, so indirect sympathomimetics will have no effect. Therefore it is important to use direct sympathomimetics such as isoprenolol, noradrenaline, adrenaline, or dopamine. Milrinone, a type three phosphodiesterase inhibitor, is an inotrope and vascular smooth muscle relaxant resulting in increased myocardial contractility and a reduction in pulmonary and systemic vascular resistance (Stobierska-Dzierzek, 2001). When combined with adrenaline it has synergistic effects on the patient's haemodynamic parameters (Bush, 1989). Levosimedan, a calcium sensitizer, is an inotrope and vasodilator which has successfully been used in patients with right ventricular dysfunction following HTx (Petaja, 2006; Perez Vela, 2008). Vasoactive drugs may also be needed to maintain an adequate MAP for adequate coronary perfusion.

## Antifibrinolytics

Antifibrinolytics such as tranexamic acid and aprotinin have been administered since at least 1995 in patients undergoing cardiac surgery to reduce postoperative chest drain losses and red blood cell transfusion (Del Rossi, 1989; Horrow, 1990, 1991; Isetta, 1991). A study of 70 patients who had undergone HTx investigated the haemostatic benefits of aprotinin. They found that there were no significant differences in blood loss between the aprotinin and control groups. They did, however, find that aprotinin reduced the need for blood transfusions in patients undergoing a re-do sternotomy (Prendergast, 1996). A retrospective review of 225 patients who had undergone HTx compared postoperative blood loss between patients who had received aprotinin and those who had been given tranexamic acid. They found that the blood loss postoperatively was the same in the two groups (Shuhaiber, 2008). Some institutions still use aprotinin for HTx, especially if the patient had previously undergone cardiac surgery.

### Separation from cardiopulmonary bypass

Prior to separation from CPB it is important to ensure that the usual conditions for separation are met: temperature, heart rate and rhythm, haematocrit, ventilation, arterial blood gases, acid-base and electrolytes, and activated clotting time (Mora-Mangano, 2006). TOE is used to ensure that all the air is evacuated from the heart, as any residual air is at risk of passing down the right coronary artery, compromising right ventricular function (Cheitlin, 2003). TOE is also used to assess ventricular filling, right and left ventricular function, and the surgical anastomotic sites.

Generally, the longer the ischaemic time, the poorer the initial function of the donor heart (Shanewise, 2004). The most common reason for failure to separate from CPB is right ventricular failure (Stobierska-Dzierzek, 2001). TOE is very useful for the diagnosis and management of right ventricular failure. Tricuspid regurgitation may also be present due to dilatation of the tricuspid annulus.

## Postoperative management

Continuous monitoring is continued during transfer and in the ICU. Inotropes and vasopressors should be continued into the postoperative period to maintain cardiovascular stability. There is, however, no evidence that the use of inotropes improves outcomes (Chen, 1998). Vasopressors, such as noradrenaline, should be used to maintain an adequate MAP, but vasopressin (Morales, 2003) or methylene blue (Leyh, 2003) may need to be added for patients in vasodilatory shock. Factors that affect the need for haemodynamic support include the preoperative status of the recipient and the myocardial protection of the donor heart, as well as the previously discussed risk factors for primary graft dysfunction. Recipient factors associated with prolonged haemodynamic support include reduced systemic vascular resistance, pulmonary hypertension, other end-organ damage, coagulopathy, and postoperative bleeding (Costanzo, 2010).

### Early complications

Pulmonary hypertension and right ventricular failure can complicate HTx recipients, requiring the use of pulmonary vasodilators such as inhaled nitric oxide (iNO) or glycerine trinitrite (Beck, 1992; Wagner, 1997; Argenziano, 1998). iNO results in selective pulmonary vasodilatation due to smooth muscle relaxation, which results in a reduction in PVR, increased pulmonary blood flow, and reduced right ventricular afterload. Because its action results in direct vasodilatation it does not exacerbate ventilation–perfusion mismatching. In a review of patients with right ventricular failure following LVAD insertion, TOE demonstrated that the right ventricular EF increased from 24% to 44% after 48 hours of iNO administration (Wagner, 1997). Although iNO has been used to reduce right ventricle afterload there is no level one evidence to support its use or to demonstrate a reduction in mortality (Griffiths and Evans, 2005). Sildenafil is a type five phosphodiesterase inhibitor which has been used for the management of PHT following HTx to aid the weaning of iNO (Costanzo, 2010). Prostanoids induce smooth muscle relaxation and can be administered intravenously or by inhalation. Prostaglandin $E_1$ ($PGE_1$) needs to be administered by infusion because of its short half-life. It undergoes first-pass metabolism in the pulmonary circulation, dramatically reducing but not eliminating the systemic side effects. Prostacyclin ($PGI_2$) can be administered by intravenous infusion or inhalation. If medical therapy fails then mechanical support, including IABP, ECMO, or VAD, can be used to support the circulation (Arafa, 2000; Kavarana, 2003; Ibrahim, 2007).

Postoperative bleeding can complicate any cardiac surgical procedure. Bleeding can be divided into surgical and non-surgical bleeding. Non-surgical bleeding is due to preoperative anticoagulation, platelet dysfunction, fibrinolysis or the development of a coagulopathy secondary to haemodilution, long duration of CPB, hypothermia, and inadequate reversal of heparin. Point-of-care testing of coagulation and platelet function is useful to allow the appropriate blood products to be administered (Costanzo, 2010).

Dysrrhythmias are common in the immediate postoperative period. Most patients following HTx will be in a sinus tachycardia due to the loss of vagal tone and up to 60% will be in right bundle branch block (Stecker, 2005). The incidence of bradyarrhythmias ranges from 8–64% (Miyamoto, 1990). This sinus node dysfunction is secondary to SA node ischaemia, surgical trauma, pharmacological treatment, age of donor, and ischaemic time. The incidence of sinus node dysfunction and the need for a permanent pacemaker has decreased with the introduction of bicaval and total heart techniques (Meyer, 2005). Temporary pacing is needed in 18–27% of patients and 4–7% require a permanent pacemaker (Montero, 1992). Atrial tachyarrhythmias complicate the postoperative period in 7–25% cases (Scott, 1992; Pavri, 1995; Cui, 2001). The postoperative incidence of atrial fibrillation (AF) increases with increasing donor and recipient age. The incidence of AF is not affected by surgical technique, but the reduction in size of the left atrium with the bicaval and total heart techniques reduces the incidence of atrial flutter (El Gamel, 1995; Cui, 2001). The onset of AF is significant if it occurs more than 2 weeks postoperatively as it may be associated with rejection and increased mortality (Dasari, 2009). Ventricular ectopics are very common postoperatively. Non-sustained ventricular tachycardia (VT) occurs in 2% of patients and is associated with longer ischaemic times and increased sensitivity to catecholamines (Stecker, 2005). Treatment of the tachyarrhythmias can be difficult due to the heart being denervated. Digoxin is ineffective, but beta-blockers, amiodarone, and calcium channel blockers can be effective due to their direct actions.

Antimicrobial prophylaxis is routine following HTx and should adhere to local guidelines. Bacterial infections are the most common infective complication, especially in the first postoperative week (Miller, 1994). Meticulous asepsis should be employed at all times. Isolation has not been shown to reduce the incidence of postoperative infections (Gamberg, 1987; Walsh, 1989).

Surgical complications include bleeding, anastomotic obstruction due to narrowing of the superior or inferior vena cava, the pulmonary veins or the PA, or kinking of the PA after the chest is closed if it is left too long, presenting as right ventricular failure (Dreyfus, 1990). Very large pericardial collections accumulate in up to 30% patients due to the implantation of a smaller heart into a large pericardial sac. A pericardial drain can be left in prophylactically if there are concerns (Al-Dadah, 2007).

Acute rejection can occur after reperfusion and usually presents as a gradual decline over the first 12 hours postoperatively. This is due to a combination of ischaemia, reperfusion, and myocardial oedema resulting in systolic and diastolic dysfunction. These patients may need haemodynamic support with the use of vasoactive and inotropic drugs, IABP, or VADs.

### Immunosuppression

Induction immunosuppression is an intense course of therapy aimed to reduce the pretransplant antigenic load, reduce the incidence of acute rejection, and prolong the graft survival, but the evidence base is poor. The use of induction immunosuppression is not universal in patients undergoing orthotopic HTx. In the first 6 months of 2010, 52% patients worldwide and 76% patients in Europe received induction immunosuppression (Hertz, 2011). A variety of agents can be used for induction immunosuppression: IL-2R antagonist, polyclonal ALG/ATG, OKT3, and alentuzumab. A review concluded that induction immunosuppression improved survival in patients at high risk of fatal rejection—those on pretransplant VAD support, of African-American race, age < 40, with four or more HLA mismatches, or highly sensitized (panel reactive antibody > 40%) (Ensor, 2009).

Maintenance of immunosuppression can be via monotherapy or combinations of agents. Commonly used agents include tacrolimus (a CNI), cyclosporine, mTOR, inhibitors sirolimus/everolimus, MMF/mycophenolic acid (MPA), azathioprine, and prednisolone (Ensor, 2009).

### Late complications

Long-term complications following HTx are frequently related to immunosuppressant therapy. Arterial hypertension is the most common morbidity, present in over 90% of HTx recipients at 5 years. Hyperlipidaemia is also very common and requires early aggressive therapy. Diabetes mellitus and renal dysfunction occur in one-third of recipients at 5 years (Hertz, 2011). Cardiac allograft vasculopathy is an accelerated form of coronary artery intimal hyperplasia, caused by both immunological and non-immunological factors. At 10 years 50% of recipients suffer from this life-threatening complication and it is often not amenable to revascularization due to the diffuse nature of the disease process (Wang, 2008). Malignancy affects 14% of survivors at 5 years, with skin cancers accounting for 40% of all neoplasms. Infection, rejection, and graft failure further contribute to late morbidity and mortality (Roussel, 2008; Hertz, 2011).

## Conclusion

In this chapter we have reviewed the perioperative management of HTx recipients, as well as the major challenges in their care. HTx has a median survival of approximately 10 years. The induction of anaesthesia is a particularly hazardous time for the HTx recipient due to the risk of cardiovascular decompensation. Physiological goals of induction are to avoid reductions in preload, increases in afterload, myocardial depression, and bradycardia. The most common reason for failure to separate from CPB is right ventricular failure. Finally, postoperative complications include pulmonary hypertension and right ventricular failure, bleeding, dysrhythmias, infection, and acute rejection.

## References


Al-Dadah AS, Guthrie TJ, Pasque MK, et al. (2007) Clinical course and predictors of pericardial effusion following cardiac transplantation. *Transplant Proc*, **39**:1589–1592.

Aliabadi A, Grommer M, Zuchermann A (2011) Is induction therapy still needed in heart transplantation. *Curr Opin Organ Transplant*, **16**:536–542.

Arafa OE, Geiran OR, Andersen K, et al. (2000) Intraaortic balloon pumping for predominantly right ventricular failure after heart transplantation. *Ann Thorac Surg*, **70**:1587–1593.

Argenziano M, Choudhri AF, Moazami N, et al. (1998) Randomized, double-blind trial of nitric oxide in LVAD recipients with pulmonary hypertension. *Ann Thorac Surg*, **65**:340–345.

Banner NR, Bonser RS, Clark AL, et al. (2011) UK guidelines for referral and assessment of adults for heart transplantation. *Heart*, **97**:1520–1527.

Barnard CN (1967) A human cardiac transplant: an interim report of a successful operation performed at Groote Schuur Hospital, Cape Town. *S Afr Med J*, **41**:1271–1274.

Beck JR, Mongero LB, Kroslowitz RM, et al. (1992) Inhaled nitric oxide improves hemodynamics in patients with acute pulmonary hypertension after high-risk cardiac surgery. *Perfusion*, **14**:37–42.

Birks RJS, Gemmell LW, O'Sullivan EP, et al. (2007) *Association of Anaesthetists of Great Britain and Ireland (AAGBI) guidelines—recommendations for standards of monitoring during anaesthesia and recovery*, 4th edn. AAGBI, London.

Bush A, Busst CM, Clarke B, et al. (1989) Effect of infused adenosine on cardiac output and systemic resistance in normal subjects. *Br J Clin Pharmacol*, **27**:165–171.

Cheitlin MD, Armstrong WF, Aurigemma GP, et al. (2003) ACC/AHA/ASE 2003 Guideline update for the clinical application of echocardiography: summary article. A report of the American College of Cardiology/American Heart Association Task Force on Practice Guidelines. *Circulation*, **108**:1146–1162.

Chen EP, Bittner HB, Davis RD, et al. (1998) Hemodynamic and inotropic effects of milrinone after heart transplantation in the setting of recipient pulmonary hypertension. *J Heart Lung Transplant*, **17**:669–678.

Costanzo MR, Dipchand A, Starling R, et al. (2010) The International Society of Heart and Lung Transplantation guidelines for the care of heart transplant recipients. Task Force 1: Peri-operative Care of the Heart Transplant Recipient. *J Heart Lung Transplant*, **29**:914–956.

Cui G, Tung T, Kobashigawa J, et al. (2001) Increased incidence of atrial flutter associated with the rejection of heart transplantation. *Am J Cardiol*, **88**:280–284.

Dasari TW (2009) Atrial fibrillation and atrial flutter in heart transplant patients: incidence, risk factors, and clinical outcomes. *J Heart Lung Transplant*, **28**:S167.

Del Rossi AJ, Ceraianu AC, Botros S, et al. (1989) Prophylactic treatment of postperfusion bleeding using EACA. *Chest*, **96**:27–30.

Dickstein ML (1998) Anesthesia for heart transplantation. *Semin Cardio-Thorac Vasc Anesth*, **2**:131–139.

Dreyfus G, Jebara VA, Couetil JP, et al. (1990) Kinking of the pulmonary artery: a treatable cause of acute right ventricular failure after heart transplantation. *J Heart Transplant*, **9**:575–576.

El Gamel A, Yonan NA, Grant S, et al. (1995) Orthotopic cardiac transplantation: a comparison of standard and bicaval Wythenshawe techniques. *J Thorac Cardiovasc Surg*, **109**:721–729.

Ensor CR, Cahoon WD, Hess ML, et al. (2009) Induction immunosuppression for orthotopic heart transplantation: a review. *Prog Transplant*, **19**:333–342.

Erickson KW, Costanzo-Nordin MR, O'Sullivan EJ, et al. (1990) Influence of preoperative transpulmonary gradient on late mortality after orthotopic heart transplantation. *J Heart Lung Transplant*, **9**:526–537.

Gamberg P, Miller JL, Lough ME (1987) Impact of protection isolation on the incidence of infection after heart transplantation. *J Heart Transplant*, **6**:147–149.

Griffiths MJ, Evans TW (2005) Inhaled nitric oxide therapy in adults. *N Engl J Med*, **353**:2683–2695.

Hertz MI, Aurora P, Benden C, et al. (2011) Scientific registry of the international society for heart and lung transplantation: introduction to the 2011 annual reports. *J Heart Lung Transplant*, **30**:1071–1077.

Hilberath JN, Oakes DA, Shernan SK, et al. (2010) Safety of transesophageal echocardiography. *J Am Soc Echocardiogr*, **23**:1115–1127.

Hirsh J (1998) Reversal of the anticoagulant effects of warfarin by vitamin K1. *Chest*, **114**:1505–1508.

Horrow JC, Hlavacek M Strong MD, et al. (1990) Prophylactic tranexamic acid decreases bleeding after cardiac operations. *J Thorac Cardiovasc Surg*, **99**:70–74.

Horrow JC, Van Riper DF, Strong MD, et al. (1991) The hemostatic effects of tranexamic acid and desmopressin during cardiac surgery. *Circulation*, **84**:2063–2070.

Ibrahim M, Hendry P, Masters R, et al. (2007) Management of acute severe perioperative failure of cardiac allografts: a single-centre experience with a review of the literature. *Can J Cardiol*, **23**:363–367.

Isetta C, Samat C, Kotaiche M, et al. (1991) Low-dose aprotinin or tranexamic acid treatment in cardiac surgery. *Anesthesiology*, **75**:A80.

Kavarana MN, Sinha P, Naka Y, et al. (2003) Mechanical support for the failing cardiac allograft: a single-centre experience. *J Heart Lung Transplant*, **22**:542–547.

Leyh RG, Kofidis T, Struber M, et al. (2003) Methylene blue: the drug of choice for catecholamine-refractory vasoplegia after cardiopulmonary bypass? *J Thorac Cardiovasc Surg*, **125**:1426–1431.

Lietz K, Miller LW (2005) Will left-ventricular assist device therapy replace heart transplantation in the foreseeable future? *Curr Opin Cardiol*, **20**:132–137.

Liu WHD, Thorp TAS, Graham SG, et al. (1991) Incidence of awareness with recall during general anaesthesia. *Anaesthesia*, **46**:435–437.

Mascia L, Mastromauro I, Viberti S, et al. (2009) Management to optimize organ procurement in brain dead donors. *Minerva Anestesiol*, **75**:125–133.

Mehra MR, Kobashigawa J, Starling R, et al. (2006) Listing criteria for heart transplantation: International Society for Heart and Lung Transplantation guidelines for the care of cardiac transplant candidates. *J Heart Lung Transplant*, **25**:1024–1042.

Mets B (2000) Anesthesia for left ventricular assist device placement. *J Cardio-Thorac Vasc Anesth*, **14**:316–326.

Meyer SR, Modry DL, Bainey K, et al. (2005) Declining need for permanent pacemaker insertion with the bicaval technique of orthotopic heart transplantation. *Can J Cardiol*, **21**:159–163.

Mikus E, Stepanenko A, Krabatsch T, et al. (2011) Left ventricular assist device or heart transplantation: impact of transpulmonary gradient and pulmonary vascular resistance on decision making. *Eur J Cardio-Thorac Surg*, **39**:310–316.

Miller LW, Naftel DC, Bourge RC, et al. (1994) Infection after heart transplantation: a multi-institutional study. Cardiac Transplant Research Database Group. *J Heart Lung Transplant*, **13**:381–392.

Miyamoto Y, Curtiss EI, Kormos RL, et al. (1990) Bradyarrhythmia after heart transplantation. Incidence, time course, and outcome. *Circulation*, **82**:313–317.

Montero JA, Anguita M, Concha M, et al. (1992) Pacing requirements after orthotopic heart transplantation: incidence and related factors. *J Heart Lung Transplant*, **11**:799–802.

Morales DL, Garrido MJ, Madigan JD, et al. (2003) A double-blind randomized trial: prophylactic vasopressin reduces hypotension after cardiopulmonary bypass. *Ann Thorac Surg*, **75**:926–930.

Mora-Mangano CT, Chow JL, Kanevsky M (2006) Cardiopulmonary bypass and the anesthesiologist. In: Kaplan JA, Reich DL, Lake CL, Konstadt SN (eds) *Cardiac Anesthesia*, 5th edn, pp. 893–935. WB Saunders, Philadelphia.

Murkin JM, Adams SJ, Novick RJ, et al. (2007) Monitoring brain oxygen saturation during coronary bypass surgery: a randomized, prospective study. *Anesth Analg*, **104**:51–58.

Myles PS, Leslie K, McNeil J, et al. (2004) Bispectral index monitoring to prevent awareness during anaesthesia: the B-aware randomised controlled trial. *Lancet*, **363**:1757–1763.

Pavri BB, O'Nunain SS, Newell JB, et al. (1995) Prevalence and prognostic significance of atrial arrhythmias after orthotopic cardiac transplantation. *J Am Coll Cardiol*, **25**:1673–1680.

Perez Vela JL, Corres Peiretti MA, Rubio Regidor M, et al. (2008) Levosimendan for postoperative ventricular dysfunction following heart transplantation. *Rev Esp Cardiol*, **61**:534–539.

Petaja LM, Sipponen JT, Hammainen PJ, et al. (2006) Levosimendan reversing low output syndrome after heart transplantation. *Ann Thorac Surg*, **82**:1529–1531.

Phillips AA, McLean RF, Devitt JH, et al. (1993) Recall of intraoperative events after general anaesthesia and cardiopulmonary bypass. *Can J Anaesth*, **40**:922–926.

Prendergast TW, Furukawa S, Beyer AJ 3rd, et al. (1996) Defining the role of aprotinin in heart transplantation. *Ann Thorac Surg*, **62**:670–674.

Quinlan JJ, Firestone S, Firestone LL (2006) Anesthesia for heart, lung and heart–lung transplantation. In: Kaplan JA, Reich DL, Lake CL, Konstadt SN (eds) *Cardiac Anesthesia*, 5th edn, pp. 845–865. WB Saunders, Philadelphia.

Ramakrishna H, Jaroszewski DE, Arabia FA (2009) Adult cardiac transplantation: a review of perioperative management Part I. *Ann Card Anaesth*, **12**:71–78.

Rosendale JD, Kauffman HM, McBride MA, et al. (2003) Hormonal resuscitation yields more transplanted hearts, with improved early function. *Transplantation*, **75**:1336–1341.

Roussel JC, Baron O, Perigaud C, et al. (2008) Outcome of heart transplants 15 to 20 years ago: graft survival, post-transplant morbidity and risk factors for mortality. *J Heart Lung Transplant*, **27**:486–493.

Schulte-Sasse U, Hess W, Tarnow J (1982) Pulmonary vascular responses to nitrous oxide in patients with normal and high pulmonary vascular resistance. *Anesthesiology*, **57**:9–13.

Scott CD, Dark JH, McComb JM (1992) Arrhythmia after cardiac transplantation. *Am J Cardiol*, **70**:1061–1063.

Shammas F, Dickstein K (1988) Clinical pharmacokinetics in heart failure: an updated review. *Clin Pharmacokinet*, **15**:94–113.

Shanewise J (2004) Cardiac transplantation. *Anesthesiol Clin N Am*, **22**:753–765.

Shemie SD, Ross H, Pagliarello J, et al. (2006) Organ donor management in Canada: recommendations of the forum on medical management to optimize donor organ potential. *CMAJ*, **174**:S13–32.

Shore-Lesserson L, Manspeizer HE, DePerio M, et al. (1999) Thromboelastography-guided transfusion algorithm reduces transfusions in complex cardiac surgery. *Anesth Analg*, **88**:312–319.

Shuhaiber JH, Goldsmith K, Large SR, et al. (2008) Does perioperative use of aprotinin reduce the rejection rate in heart transplant recipients? *Eur J Cardio Thorac Surg*, **33**:849–855.

Stecker EC, Strelich KR, Chugh SS, et al. (2005) Arrhythmias after orthotopic heart transplantation. *J Card Fail*, **11**:464–472.

Stehlik J, Edwards LB, Kucheryavaya AY, et al. (2011) The registry of the International Society for Heart and Lung Transplantation: twenty-eighth adult heart transplant report. *J Heart Lung Transplant*, **30**:1078–1094.

Stobierska-Dzierzek B, Awad H, Michler RE (2001) The evolving management of acute right-sided heart failure in cardiac transplant recipients. *J Am Coll Cardiol*, **38**:923–931.

Venkateswaran RV, Bonser RS, Steeds RP (2005) The echocardiographic assessment of donor heart function prior to cardiac transplantation. *Eur J Echocardiography*, **6**:260–263.

Wagner F, Dandel M, Gunther G, et al. (1997) Nitric oxide inhalation in treatment of right ventricular dysfunction following left ventricular assist device implantation. *Circulation*, **96**:291–296.

Walsh TR, Guttendorf J, Dummer S, et al. (1989) The value of protective isolation procedures in cardiac allograft recipients. *Ann Thorac Surg*, **47**:539–544.

Wang SS (2008) Treatment and prophylaxis of cardiac allograft vasculopathy. *Transplant Proc*, **40**:2609–2610.

Young JB, Naftel DC, Bourge RC, et al. (1994) Matching the heart donor and heart transplant recipient. Clues for successful expansion of the donor pool: a multivariable, multi-institutional report. The Cardiac Transplant Research Database Group. *J Heart Lung Transplant*, **13**:353–364.

Zaroff JG, Babcock WD, Shiboski SC (2003a) The impact of left ventricular dysfunction on cardiac donor transplant rates. *J Heart Lung Transplant*, **22**:334–337.

Zaroff JG, Babcock WD, Shiboski SC, et al. (2003b) Temporal changes in left ventricular systolic function in heart donors: results of serial echocardiography. *J Heart Lung Transplant*, **22**:383–386.

# CHAPTER 31

# Anaesthesia for heart–lung transplantation

Marcin Wąsowicz

## Introduction

Combined heart–lung transplantation is a highly complicated, rarely performed procedure. The number of heart–lung transplantations performed worldwide has been stable over the last few years and ranges from 75–114 annually (Christie et al., 2011). Most of the centres performing this type of transplantation are carrying out two to three operations per year. Indications for combined heart–lung transplantation have been narrowed and many patients who in the past would have received heart–lung transplantation would not receive it now. Instead it is now recommended to perform a double-lung transplantation accompanied by repair of the structural heart defect. The most common indications for heart–lung transplantation are congenital heart disease complicated by Eisenmenger syndrome, primary arterial pulmonary hypertension, and cystic fibrosis.

In the US the majority of heart–lung transplantations are performed in adult congenital heart patients who developed fixed pulmonary hypertension secondary to an intracardiac shunt. In Europe a large percentage of patients undergoing heart–lung transplantation are suffering from cystic fibrosis.

Anaesthesia and optimal perioperative management for this complex, high-risk surgical intervention requires expertise in both cardiac and thoracic anaesthesia. This includes an extensive knowledge of cardiac and pulmonary physiology and pathophysiology, lung isolation techniques, treatment of hypoxaemia, and the multi-organ impact of CPB and treatment of its implications. Additionally, anaesthesiologists providing perioperative care to patients undergoing heart–lung transplantation must be familiar with more advanced diagnostic and monitoring techniques (e.g. TEE and bronchoscopy). Heart–lung transplantation is a long procedure, quite often it is not the first surgery within the thoracic cavity of the patient and it is always performed with the use of CPB. For those reasons it is always complicated by severe coagulopathy and the subsequent complications of massive transfusion.

Since heart–lung transplantation is performed in very few centres the available literature is very limited and the optimal management of these procedures remains poorly described (Roselli and Smedira, 2004; Christie et al., 2011). The following section briefly describes the anaesthetic management for combined heart–lung transplantation based on experience acquired in the author's institution.

## Surgical considerations

A cardiac or thoracic surgeon usually performs combined heart–lung transplantation. In our institution it is usually a combined team from both specialties. In some institutions thoracic surgeons are routinely performing lung transplantation procedures and therefore are familiar with the techniques of extracorporeal circulation. From the experience of our hospital it seems that cooperation between thoracic and cardiac surgeons provides an optimal surgical approach for this type of transplantation. There have been no major changes in surgical technique for combined heart–lung transplantation since 1995 except for two technical aspects: replacement of tracheal anastomosis with separate bilateral bronchial anastomoses and placement of the lungs anterior to the phrenic nerves (Icenogle and Copeland, 1995; Griffith, 1999). These two modifications reduced the incidence of airway dehiscence, bleeding into the posterior mediastinum and improved exposure to the posterior structures in case chest reopening is necessary to control postoperative bleeding.

## Anaesthetic management for combined heart–lung transplantation

The literature describing the anaesthetic management of the patient undergoing combined heart–lung transplantation is very scarce and includes mainly reports from the International Society of Heart and Lung Transplantation (Christie et al. 2011). Subsequent paragraphs will summarize the current state of knowledge described as individual cases (Rose et al., 2011) and the experience of the institution where the author practices cardiac and thoracic anaesthesia. As mentioned before, the anaesthesiologist who is looking after the patient who is scheduled to undergo combined heart–lung transplantation should possess expertise in both cardiac and thoracic anaesthesia. Quite often these procedures are complex and require management by two anaesthesia consultants. They will need to manage haemodynamic derangements, hypoxaemia and ventilatory problems, and coagulopathy, and perform and interpret bronchoscopy and TEE.

### Preoperative assessment

Apart from standard preoperative evaluations before surgery, the anaesthesiologist preparing the patient for a combined cardiac and thoracic procedure must perform a detailed assessment of the respiratory and cardiovascular systems.

One of the most important parts of the assessment is thoughtful evaluation of the anatomy of the cardiovascular and respiratory system. Many patients scheduled to undergo combined heart–lung transplantation were born with congenital heart defects and subsequently developed pulmonary hypertension leading to Eisenmenger syndrome. Proper understanding of anatomy is also crucial for pre-anaesthetic planning of airway management, cannulation of arteries and central veins, and induction of general anaesthesia. Most of the patients considered as potential candidates for heart–lung transplantation already have an extensive description of their abnormal anatomy provided by cardiologists specializing in adult congenital heart disease patients. Additionally, existing pathology is usually documented by echocardiographic imaging and MRI. Careful review of the existing documentation will allow a full understanding of their abnormal anatomy and will allow for planning of their anaesthetic management prior to the CPB phase of the procedure.

Quite often, as a result of previous surgery or abnormal anatomy, we need to search for alternative approaches for induction of general anaesthesia and cannulation. For example, a patient may have undergone a Blalock–Taussig shunt operation in the past and the cannulation of his radial artery on the same side will result in underestimation of blood pressure. Other examples include a left-sided SVC draining directly into the coronary sinus and the presence of a Fontan circulation, meaning that we are dealing with single ventricle physiology and the pressure recorded from the central line will reflect mean pulmonary artery pressure. Presence of a Fontan shunt in a patient undergoing heart–lung transplantation implies that the function of the conduit is failing and induction of general anaesthesia with positive pressure ventilation might result in haemodynamic disaster due to rapid increase of afterload from positive pressure ventilation, with a circulation that is dependent on passive pulmonary blood flow. Quite often significant scarring and adherence of the RV to the sternum will dictate the need for awake femoral cannulation for the initiation of CPB prior to induction of anaesthesia or sternotomy.

In a patient suffering from cystic fibrosis, the usual presentation is a very fragile young patient with end-stage lung disease caused by chronic infections. Quite often the disease also affects the digestive system and the patient suffers from liver and pancreatic dysfunction.

An extensive description of the respiratory system evaluation is provided elsewhere (Slinger, 2011). Briefly, the anaesthesiologist who is assessing pulmonary function should concentrate on lung mechanics, pulmonary parenchymal function, and cardiorespiratory reserve. In a patient considered for combined heart–lung transplantation, assessment of the function of the respiratory system serves as a final confirmation of the decision to list the patient for transplantation. In most of the patients undergoing heart–lung transplantation, the dominating pathology is associated with irreversible pulmonary hypertension and loss of functional units of gas exchange or end-stage damage of pulmonary parenchyma caused by chronic inflammation (cystic fibrosis). A brief summary of the most important points for respiratory assessment are as follows:

- Evaluation of lung mechanics is assessed by spirometry. The value most commonly used by anaesthesiologists is FEV1.
- Maximal oxygen consumption is used to assess cardiopulmonary reserve.
- Diffusing capacity of carbon monoxide is measured to estimate the gas exchange function of lung parenchyma.

Any patient being prepared for combined heart–lung transplantation requires a very careful airway evaluation. Previous intrathoracic interventions often result in airway involvement, causing deviation or extensive scarring around large airways. Moreover, previous scars or anatomical abnormalities can affect or compress large vascular structures. Congenital malformations within the cardiovascular system and its significance for pre-bypass management were discussed previously. Apart from clinical symptoms the anaesthesiologist must examine the results of CT and MRI scans, which show precisely the extent of the disease and possible vascular involvement. A preoperative echocardiogram will be complementary to the radiological examination and should be routinely performed before combined heart–lung transplantation

The 'next leg' of preoperative evaluation focuses on the status of the other systems. The mortality and morbidity of patients undergoing heart–lung transplantation is strongly influenced by their preoperative severity of illness. Certainly mortality will be increased by the presence of renal and liver dysfunction. Unfortunately it is a frequent clinical scenario in this group of patients. Failure of the RV (due to fixed pulmonary hypertension) with coexisting tricuspid regurgitation causes chronic congestion of the liver, which can progress to cirrhosis. In the case of patients with cystic fibrosis, the primary disease commonly affects the liver. If diagnosis of liver cirrhosis is confirmed by liver biopsy the patient may be ineligible for surgery; however, many cardiologists believe that liver dysfunction might be reversed by transplantation and restoration of normal circulation and oxygenation. There are several perioperative implications of pre-existing liver dysfunction. Deficiency of coagulation factors, thrombocytopaenia, low albumin levels, and immunosuppression are among the most important ones.

The second common coexisting comorbidity for these patients is renal dysfunction caused by chronic hypoxia and congestion of splanchnic organs. As mentioned previously, heart–lung transplantation is a long procedure requiring a long bypass time, which is usually complicated by coagulopathy and commonly haemodynamic instability requiring the use of high doses of inotropic support. All those factors may contribute to deterioration of kidney function. If there is pre-existing severe renal dysfunction prior to transplantation, the postoperative period might be complicated by complete renal failure requiring renal replacement therapy.

## Anaesthetic management

The anaesthesiologist providing care during combined heart–lung transplantation faces multiple challenges. Therefore in many centres there are two anaesthesia consultants or one consultant and one experienced trainee (i.e. fellow) assigned for these cases. As mentioned previously, extensive experience and expertise in both cardiac and thoracic anaesthesia is mandatory. Quite often the anaesthesia team must simultaneously manage haemodynamic instability, hypoxaemia, problems with ventilation, and excessive bleeding. It is beyond the scope of this chapter to fully discuss all of the challenges of re-do intrathoracic surgery and anaesthesia, so they will be summarized briefly.

### Induction of anaesthesia

Induction of anaesthesia is one of the most crucial moments for perioperative management. Induction of general anaesthesia in patients with severe pulmonary hypertension might result in immediate haemodynamic collapse requiring urgent initiation of CPB. Factors contributing to haemodynamic instability are increased intrathoracic pressure precipitated by positive pressure ventilation, increased afterload for the RV, and decreased preload induced by the vasodilatory properties of induction agents. Patients who underwent the Fontan procedure prior to heart–lung transplantation will present the most classical example of this scenario. To secure a safe and controlled induction of general anaesthesia in a patient with pulmonary hypertension we usually recommend insertion of the arterial line, central line, and PA catheter prior to induction. It will allow rapid identification of the problem and allow for initiation of infusion of vasoactive drugs to support a potentially failing RV, decreasing pressures within the pulmonary circulation, and close monitoring of pressures within the pulmonary circulation.

Even though it is believed that in a patient with Eisenmenger syndrome pulmonary hypertension is fixed, we frequently observe variation of pulmonary pressure in these patients. These fluctuations can be caused by common physiological disturbances such as hypoxaemia, hypercarbia, and acidosis. Prompt correction of these abnormalities plus optimization of pre-afterload, chronotropy, or contractility usually allows smooth induction and maintenance of anaesthesia until CPB can be initiated. In a patient with cystic fibrosis with lungs filled with thick, copious secretions, frequent suctioning might be necessary to enable ventilation.

On the other hand, if heart–lung transplantation is not the first surgery within the thoracic cavity, rapid commencement of CPB ('crashing on pump') might not be possible due to difficulties establishing cannulation caused by adhesions and difficult surgical exposure of structures. Thus in some cases the anaesthesiologist and surgeon might decide on an alternative approach to rapidly establish CPB. The surgeon can cannulate femoral vessels prior to induction with use of local analgesia. Once vascular access is established and the patient is fully heparinized, induction of anaesthesia is initiated. In the case of any haemodynamic collapse during anaesthesia induction, the perfusionist can initiate CPB and the surgeon can then immediately proceed with a thoracotomy with a heart that will be decompressed and therefore less at risk of injury. Of course, this approach will extend the total CPB time, with all its negative consequences.

Following induction of anaesthesia, intubation will be achieved with either a single or double lumen tube. Even though the surgical procedure is performed with the use of CPB, some anaesthesiologists and surgeons find it useful to have the option to isolate the lungs (sequential bronchial anastomoses). One-lung ventilation can be useful when the surgeon completes the bronchial anastomosis or to prevent spillage between lungs in the case of haemoptysis. One-lung ventilation may also be used during dissection of the diseased lungs. Dissection can be challenging and is frequently accompanied by injury to lung parenchyma followed by a significant air-leak. To minimize the effects of this problem it might be decided to use one-lung ventilation. An alternative to the use of a double lumen tube is the bronchial blocker. Regardless of the technique of lung isolation, the position of the tube or device must be confirmed with use of bronchoscopy. Bronchoscopic assessment of the airway and bronchial anastomoses will be performed multiple times during the procedure and therefore proficiency of its use is another mandatory skill required for the anaesthesiologist responsible for the perioperative management of heart–lung transplantation recipients. After induction of anaesthesia, intubation, and stabilization of the haemodynamic status of the patient, the anaesthesiologist might decide to secure additional venous access primarily dedicated for rapid transfusion of blood products. Additional arterial access (usually the femoral artery) may also be useful. After initial stabilization the patient should receive prophylactic antibiotics and a first dose of immunosuppression (usually solumedrol).

TEE is another important diagnostic and monitoring tool routinely used during combined heart–lung transplantation. Use of TEE is one of the key components of intraoperative haemodynamic and anaesthetic management of patients undergoing these procedures. The important information obtained from intraoperative TEE during combined heart–lung transplantation includes assessment of left and RV function (diagnosis of new wall-motion abnormalities (often due to air entering the right coronary artery during reperfusion) and evaluation of the vascular anastomoses. It is a rare situation when there is a technical problem with the aortic anastomosis, but the IVC and SVC anastomoses might be more challenging and potentially be complicated by stenosis during suturing.

### Maintenance of anaesthesia

Maintenance of general anaesthesia can be achieved with the use of a volatile or intravenous anaesthetic technique or a combination of both (balanced anaesthesia) and is usually dictated by local practice. Preferentially, dissection of the diseased lungs to remove them is performed before initiation of CPB in order to reduce the total CPB time to minimize the complications of a prolonged pump run. This part of the procedure might require one-lung ventilation. Also, during this period we usually start an infusion of antifibrinolytics to minimize post-CPB blood loss. If the recipient of the heart–lung transplantation has an intracardiac shunt the anaesthesiologist is challenged to find a fine balance between pulmonary and systemic resistance. Excessive pulmonary vasodilation might result in increased left to right shunting and decreased oxygen delivery to the peripheral tissues. In contrast, excessive systemic vasodilation will result in increased right to left shunting and inadequate oxygen uptake. Since the time from induction to initiation of CPB might be long (re-do intrathoracic surgery), maintaining adequate oxygen uptake and delivery is crucial for preservation of other organ function.

## Cardiopulmonary bypass

CPB has three main functions during cardiac procedures: (1) replacing the function of the heart (circulation of the blood), (2) replacing the function of the lungs (oxygenation and $CO_2$ removal), and (3) diversion of the blood from the operating field to create optimal surgical conditions. To achieve these goals the SVC and IVC are cannulated and blood is passively drained into the CPB venous reservoir. The blood is then oxygenated and returned to the patient via an aortic cannula usually placed in the distal part of the ascending aorta. Since the primary function of CPB is to oxygenate blood and perfuse the vital organs, an important question for the anaesthesiologist is what perfusion/oxygenation is optimal? Even though it has been over 50 years since the first human use of extracorporeal circulation, there is no definite answer. Blood is exposed multiple times to the foreign surface of the extracorporeal circuit, causing a SIRS and microembolization, which can affect every organ of the human body. Apart from lung injury, CPB can contribute to cognitive dysfunction, renal injury or failure, pancreatitis, and, in the worst-case scenario, multi-organ dysfunction. It is the anaesthesiologist's role to prevent or minimize these complications. This part of the procedure is finished when dissection of the diseased lungs and heart is complete and new grafts are anastomosed. Depending on surgical preference the following anastomoses must be completed:

- Aortic
- Bicaval (SVC and IVC anastomosis)
- Tracheal or two bronchial anastomoses

During CPB the anaesthesiologist can prepare for several potential challenges he or she is going to face after discontinuation of CPB—coagulopathy, RV dysfunction or failure, hypoxaemia, and primary graft dysfunction. During this stage of the procedure the anaesthesiologist should secure the necessary blood products, prepare equipment that may be required for separation from bypass (for example, nitric oxide or rapid infusion system), and have an assistant available to help with all the necessary post-CPB activities aiming to stabilize the patient. We might also perform a thromboelastographic examination to detect more specifically which component of the coagulation system is affected (platelets, coagulation factors, or fibrinogen) in order to have the most appropriate blood products available for transfusion to reverse coagulopathy (Wąsowicz et al., 2010).

## Termination of CPB and reperfusion of new heart and lung grafts

This stage of the procedure usually presents several challenges for the anaesthesiologist responsible for the case. Before termination of CPB it is obligatory to complete a classical checklist, which includes bronchoscopic inspection of the tracheobronchial tree in order to confirm proper position of the endotracheal tube, assessment of the quality of anastomoses, and suction of any remaining secretions or pulmonoplegia that may contribute to hypoxaemia. Additionally, we need to confirm that the patient is normothermic, the haemoglobin level is ≥ 80g/L, the potassium and glucose levels are within normal limits, the ventilator is restarted, and the pacing wires are working. To decrease potential injury to the newly transplanted lung it is recommended to use the lowest possible $FiO_2$, reduce peak airway pressures, and use low tidal volumes. At the same time as a prevention of atelectasis we suggest the use of low to moderate PEEP. In case of hypoxaemia, a quick 'rule out' process must be performed. This checklist includes rapid bronchoscopy to confirm proper position of the endotracheal tube, which can always migrate too deeply, and suctioning of any residual secretions. At the same time a modified TEE examination should be performed to rule out any intracardiac shunting or LV dysfunction, which could result in pulmonary oedema.

If the findings of these examinations are negative, the most likely cause for hypoxaemia is primary graft dysfunction (PGD). Treatment of PGD usually includes a gradual increase in $FiO_2$ and PEEP, recruitment manoeuvres, and then initiation of therapy with selective pulmonary vasodilators (nitric oxide or prostacyclin). If all of the aforementioned therapies fail, ECMO should be initiated. In the case of normal heart function it might be a venovenous mode; however, if there is concomitant heart failure an arteriovenous mode should be utilized.

The second common problem occurring after termination of CPB is RV or biventricular failure. The anaesthesiologist looking after these patients must be familiar with all forms of circulatory support to provide haemodynamic stability during and after the surgery. Cardiac stability can be achieved by optimization of pre- and afterload, maintaining or improving contractility, and preservation of a stable sinus rhythm. One of the most worrisome haemodynamic problems complicating combined heart–lung transplantation procedures is RV dysfunction/failure. It is commonly caused by a rapid increase in the afterload (pressure) for the right side of the heart (PGD of the lung graft) or early rejection of the heart graft. The warning symptoms include RV distension visualized directly by the surgeon and the anaesthesiologist, a low cardiac output state, a CVP higher than the pulmonary artery diastolic pressure (PAD), and TEE features of RV failure. The treatment includes:

- Reduction of RV preload (e.g. promotion of diuresis with furosemide)
- Manoeuvres to decrease the pressure in the pulmonary circulation—hyperventilation, hyperoxia, and pharmacological support. Intravenous agents, which decrease afterload for the RV and improve its contractility, include dobutamine and milrinone. Inhalational pulmonary vasodilators (nitric oxide or prostacyclin) are used when a lack of response to intravenous agents occurs
- Preservation of good perfusion pressure to the RV and supporting ventricular interdependence—norepinephrine or vasopressin, and/or the use of an IABP
- Since stroke volume is usually fixed in RV failure, to increase the cardiac output it is recommended to increase the heart rate (e.g. A-V pacing)

If the haemodynamic situation deteriorates further, the only remaining option is to use an RVAD or venoarterial ECMO.

Most cases of combined heart–lung transplantation require a long CPB time. Duration of CPB directly correlates with the magnitude of coagulopathy. There are multiple mechanisms of excessive, non-surgical bleeding caused by extracorporeal circulation; among the most important are the dilutional effect, SIRS, platelet consumption, depleted amount of clotting factors, secondary fibrinolysis, and low haemoglobin. Pre-existing liver or kidney dysfunction can further aggravate non-surgical bleeding. On the other hand, when heart–lung transplantation is not the first intrathoracic surgery there is usually a significant surgical component of post-CPB bleeding, which makes management even more difficult. Treatment is based on the results of laboratory tests (INR, aPTT, fibrinogen level, and platelet count). Many centres use point-of-care devices, which deliver a quick assessment of the coagulation status based on results obtained from a whole-blood sample. Among the most popular ones are thromboelastography (Wąsowicz et al., 2010), sonoclot, and PFA-100.

Unfortunately, in most cases the magnitude of bleeding is so major that there is no time to wait for laboratory results and in many cases we use an empirical approach. This approach includes replacing all blood components, using high-dose antifibrinolytics, maintaining normothermia, and hoping that this strategy will work and bleeding will diminish. In the worst cases of non-surgical coagulopathy one might consider using activated recombinant factor VIIa (Puentes et al., 2015). Massive transfusion is associated with many complications, detailed discussion of which is beyond the scope of this chapter. There are two specific complications of transfusion that can start a vicious cycle of compounding complications. The first of these is transfusion-related lung injury, which on the operating table cannot be differentiated from PGD. The second is RV volume overload, which can further deteriorate RV dysfunction.

In our institution, for most heart–lung transplantation cases we secure at least two large-bore venous catheters to be able to transfuse large volumes of blood products in a relatively short period of time.

## Postoperative management.

Patients who are undergoing heart–lung transplantation are routinely transferred to an ICU. Detailed ICU care of heart–lung transplantation is beyond the scope of this chapter. Therefore we will discuss only the key components of early postoperative therapy. The best description of the clinical condition of a patient who is the recipient of a heart–lung transplantation being admitted to the ICU is 'controlled shock'. During the next couple of hours, and sometimes days, the ICU team will continue to stabilize the patient's haemodynamic status, ventilation, oxygenation, and coagulopathy. Further tasks will include prevention and treatment of potential infection and continuation of immunosuppression. The most common causes of unfavourable outcome of heart–lung transplantation during the early postoperative course are failure of the lung or heart grafts and postoperative infection.

## Conclusion

In this chapter we have briefly reviewed the perioperative management of combined heart–lung transplantation. This procedure is complex and should be performed only for selected cases in specialized centres which possess expertise in both cardiac and thoracic anaesthesia and surgery. In the majority of these centres a total of two to three transplantations are performed annually; therefore the available literature is very limited. We have described the important perioperative features and challenges encountered by the surgical team. In the preparation of the material for this chapter we have relied primarily on the experiences and clinical practice developed at the University of Toronto and Toronto General Hospital. Finally, anaesthesiologists responsible for the perioperative care of these patients must have extensive expertise in both cardiovascular and thoracic anaesthesia. Proficiency in TEE and bronchoscopy is mandatory.

## References

Christie JD, Edwards LB, Kucheryavaya AY, et al. (2010) The registry of the International Society of Heart and Lung Transplantation: twenty seventh official adult lung and heart–lung transplantation report. *J Heart Lung Transplant*, **30**:1104–1118.

Griffith BP, Magliato KE (1999) Heart–lung transplantation. *Op Tech Thor CV Surg*, **4**:124–141

Icenogle TB, Copeland JG (1995) A technique to simplify and improve exposure in heart–lung transplantation. *J Thorac Cardiovasc Surg*, **110**:1590–1593.

Puentes W, Roscoe A, Cypel M, et al. (2015) Succesful use of recombinant activated coagulation factor VII in a patient with veno-venous ECMO after lung transplantation. *Anaesthesiol Intensive Ther*, **47**(2):188–9. doi: 10.5603/AIT.a2014.0069. Epub 2014 Nov 23.

Rose J, Zimmerman H, Coelho-Anderson R, Copeland JG (2011) Twenty five year survival after heart–lung transplantation: a milestone. *J Heart Lung Transplant*, **30**:385–388.

Roselli EE, Smedira NG (2004) Surgical advances in heart and lung transplantation. *Anesth Clin N Am*, **22**:789–808.

Slinger P (2011) *Principles and Practice of Anesthesia for Thoracic Surgery*. Springer, Heidelberg.

Wąsowicz M, McCluskey SA, Wijeysundera DN, Yau TM, Meineri M, Karkouti K (2010) The incremental value of thromboelastography for prediction of excessive blood loss after cardiac surgery: an observational study. *Anesth Analg*, **111**:331–338.

# CHAPTER 32

# Lung transplantation

Derek Rosen, Marcelo Cypel, and Peter D. Slinger

## Introduction

Lung transplantation (LTx) is the definitive treatment for certain patients with end-stage lung disease. The term 'lung transplantation' includes lobar transplant, single-lung transplant (SLTx), and double-lung transplant (DLTx), most commonly performed as bilateral sequential lung transplant (BSLTx). SLTx and BSLTx are by far the most common operations and will be discussed in this chapter. The number of transplants has increased steadily since 1985, with over 3,200 transplants performed worldwide in 2009 (Christie et al., 2011). This increase is due primarily to a growth in the number of BSLTxs (see Figure 32.1). Median survival for adult LTx is 5.5 years, with 79% survival at 1 year, 53% at 5 years, and 30% at 10 years (Christie et al., 2011). Advantages of DLTx include less ventilation–perfusion mismatch and less risk of reperfusion pulmonary oedema (Baez and Castillo, 2008). Recipients of SLTx have lower survival rates after 1 year (Cai, 2007); however, this may reflect clinical factors which influenced the choice of procedure such as recipient diagnosis, age, and comorbidities (Christie et al., 2011) (see Figure 32.2).

## End-stage lung disease

The underlying disease processes in recipients of LTxs can be broadly categorized into obstructive, restrictive, suppurative, and pulmonary vascular. Figure 32.3 shows indications for LTx by diagnosis. COPD remains the most common indication, but transplants for idiopathic pulmonary fibrosis have increased considerably since 2005 (Christie et al., 2011).

### Obstructive diseases

This group of chronic lung diseases includes patients with COPD, $\alpha_1$-antitrypsin (AAT) deficiency, and bronchiolitis obliterans syndrome presenting for retransplantation. COPD (exclusive of AAT deficiency emphysema) is the fourth leading cause of death in the world and is the most common indication for LTx. Tobacco smoking is the main cause of COPD, which usually develops in middle-aged patients and predisposes them to comorbidities such as ischaemic heart disease, hypertension, and osteoporosis (Global Initiative for Chronic Obstructive Pulmonary Disease, 2010). Chronic inflammation in the lungs from noxious gases or particles causes airflow limitation due to a varying combination of small airways disease and parenchymal damage via an excess of proteases. The latter is characterized by destruction of elastin fibres in the alveoli and small airways, resulting in loss of elastic recoil, reduced number of functional alveolar units, and a reduced surface area for gas exchange. A loss of outward traction on the small airways causes airway collapse on expiration, gas trapping, and hyperinflation, known as intrinsic PEEP. This reduces inspiratory capacity and increases functional residual capacity especially on exercise, resulting in exertional dyspnoea (Global Initiative for Chronic Obstructive Pulmonary Disease, 2010). The disease is generally progressive, especially with continued exposure to noxious agents such as cigarette smoke.

A congenital deficiency of AAT, an antiprotease important in protecting the lung parenchyma from neutrophil elastases, results in development of severe emphysema at a young age.

Spirometry is used to diagnose COPD, classify severity, and monitor disease progression. A postbronchodilator ratio of FEV1 to forced vital capacity (FVC) below 0.7 is often used as a cutoff for the diagnosis of COPD. FEV1 less than 50% predicted for age and height in conjunction with this ratio is consistent with severe disease and FEV1 $< 30\%$ signifies very severe disease (Global Initiative for Chronic Obstructive Pulmonary Disease, 2010). Patients in this group may survive several years, making timing of transplantation complicated, with the question of transplantation for quality-of-life purposes arising. However, hospitalizations for acute exacerbations associated with $PaCO_2 \geq 50$ mmHg carry a poor prognosis with a 2-year mortality of 49% (Connors et al., 1996; Orens et al., 2006). To better guide timing of referral for LTx assessment the body mass, airflow obstruction, dyspnoea, and exercise capacity (BODE) index is used (Celliet al., 2004). It scores COPD patients from 0 to 10 and predicts their risk of death using BMI, degree of airway obstruction (percentage predicted FEV1), degree of dyspnoea (score on Modified Medical Research Council (MMRC) dyspnoea scale), and exercise capacity (distance walked in 6 minutes) (see Table 32.1). Patients with a BODE score $> 5$ should be referred for assessment and at scores of 7–10 have a median survival of 3 years, which is less than would be expected after transplantation.

The ISHLT guidelines for LTx in COPD are summarized in Table 32.2.

### Restrictive diseases

Idiopathic pulmonary fibrosis (IPF), also called usual interstitial pneumonia (UIP), is a form of chronic, progressive, fibrosing interstitial pneumonia of unknown cause occurring primarily in older adults, limited to the lungs, and associated with a typical histopathological and/or radiological pattern (Raghu et al., 2011). It is the most common form of idiopathic restrictive lung disease and the second most common indication for LTx (Orens et al., 2006). It carries a median survival of 3 years from the time of diagnosis (Nathan, 2005). It is more common in males than females, with

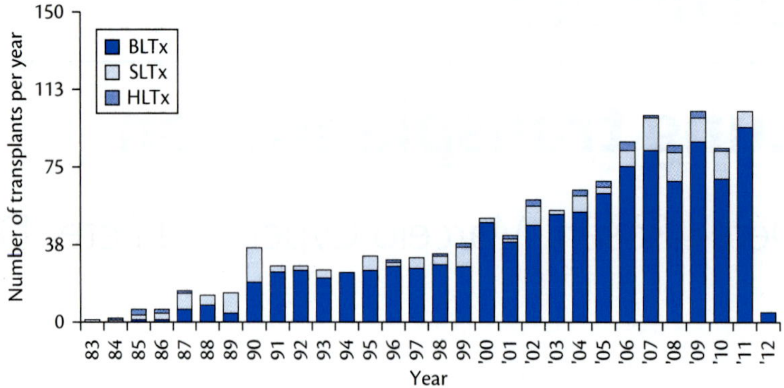


**Fig. 32.1** Number of LTx and HLTx procedures reported by year for the period 1983–2012 for Toronto General Hospital (BLTx = BSLTx) (HLTx =heart/lung transplant).

prevalence estimates ranging from 2 to 29 per 100,000 in the general population due to inconsistencies in its definition, which have been addressed in recent guidelines (Coultas et al., 1994; Raghu et al., 2006, 2011).

In IPF there is chronic inflammation and fibrosis of the alveolar walls, increasing the elastic recoil of the lungs and making them less distensible, with concomitant reduction in tidal volumes and functional residual capacity. Histology shows fibrotic areas consisting of dense collagen and proliferating fibroblasts and areas of honeycomb change, consisting of cystic fibrotic air spaces, alternating with normal parenchyma (DePaseo and Winterbauer, 1991; Raghu et al., 2011). This uneven distribution of disease through the lung causes ventilation–perfusion mismatch and resultant hypoxaemia (Ma and Slinger, 2011). Fibrosis of the alveolar capillary membrane impairs gas exchange, further adding to this hypoxaemia (Ma and Slinger, 2011).

IPF typically presents in the sixth and seventh decades of life with exertional dyspnoea, a dry cough, bibasilar fine inspiratory crackles, and finger clubbing (Raghu et al., 2011). It is a diagnosis of exclusion after other causes of interstitial lung disease have been ruled out and an UIP pattern is seen on a high-resolution computed tomography (HRCT) scan. Some patients also require surgical lung biopsy (Raghu et al., 2011). Disease progression is usually gradual over years but can occur rapidly, and IPF patients have the highest attrition rate of those awaiting transplant with a mortality rate of > 30% (Shorr, 2002). Patients frequently have comorbidities such as obstructive sleep apnoea, pulmonary hypertension, and connective tissue (Raghu et al., 2011).

Spirometry has been studied as a prognostic marker in IPF with varying results. FVC is typically reduced with a proportionate reduction in FEV1 and a normal or elevated FEV1/FVC ratio. Although some studies have shown that a 10% decrement in FVC over 6 months predicts reduced survival (Collard et al., 2003; Flaherty et al., 2003), the positive predictive value of such a decline is low (Orens et al., 2006). The most useful pulmonary function test appears to be the diffusing capacity of the lungs for carbon monoxide (DLCO), with < 39% predicted being associated with death within 2 years (Egan et al., 2005; Hamada et al., 2007). The 6-minute walk test (6-MWT), extent of HRCT changes, and histology are also prognostic and the ISHLT guidelines for transplantation are summarized in Table 32.3.

## Suppurative diseases

CF is the most common cause of bronchiectasis seen in LTx recipients and the third most common indication for transplant overall (Orens et al., 2006). It is an autosomal recessive disorder

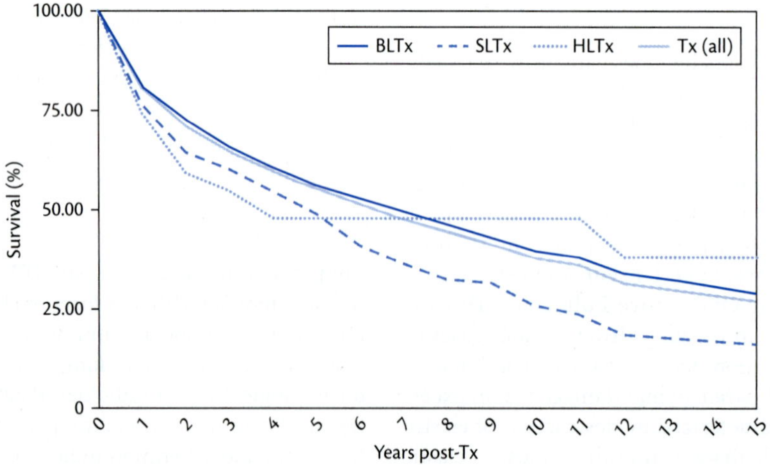


**Fig. 32.2** Percentage survival of patients in years following transplantation for the period 1983–2012 for Toronto General Hospital. TX (all), Combined lung and heart–lung transplant recipients.

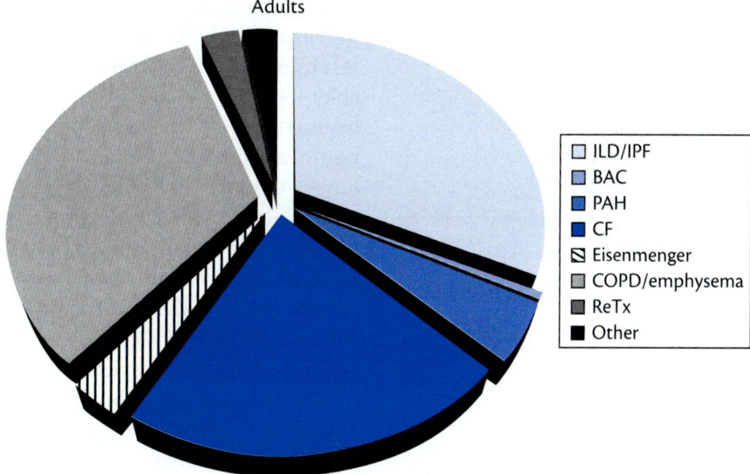


**Fig. 32.3** Proportion of lung and heart–lung transplantations according to recipient diagnosis for the period 1983–2102 at Toronto General Hospital. ILD/IPF, Interstitial lung disease/idiopathic pulmonary fibrosis; BAC, bronchoalveolar carcinoma; PAH, pulmonary artery hypertension; CF, cystic fibrosis; COPD, chronic obstructive pulmonary disease; ReTx, repeat transplantation.

most frequently seen in Caucasians but also affecting other racial groups. It is caused by a mutation in the cystic fibrosis transmembrane conductance regulator gene (CFTR) which codes for a chloride ion channel important in water and electrolyte transport across epithelial cells (Davies et al., 2007). This chloride channel defect results in abnormally viscous secretions, which cause obstruction in the respiratory tract, pancreas, biliary system, intestines, and sweat glands (Ma and Slinger, 2011). In the lungs this impairs mucociliary clearance, preventing CF patients from removing inhaled bacteria. There is also an excessive inflammatory response to pathogens, and the end result is chronic infection and inflammation with destruction of airway supporting tissue, bronchiectasis, haemoptysis, gas trapping, and eventual respiratory failure, the primary cause for the early mortality in these patients (Davies et al., 2007; Ma and Slinger, 2011).

Despite chronic colonization and infection with multiresistant organisms in the upper respiratory tract and sinuses which persist after transplantation, and the comorbidities inherent in the disease process, post-transplant survival of CF patients compares favourably with the survival of patients with other conditions (Egan et al., 2002; Bech et al., 2004; Orens et al., 2006). Infection with *Burkholderia cepacia* is associated with a poorer survival post-transplant and some centres will not transplant this subpopulation (De Soyza et al., 2001; Egan et al., 2002; Levine, 2004).

CF is characterized primarily by airflow obstruction, although varying degrees of restriction can occur. Early in the course of the disease the thickened mucus in the airways limits expiratory flow, and with disease progression damage to the airways results in collapse during exhalation and worsened obstruction (Ma and Slinger, 2011). Due to the heterogeneous multisystem nature of the disease, a consistent combination of predictors for survival has not been identified. Consideration for referral should occur when the FEV1 decreases to 30% of predicted or when there is a rapid decline in FEV1, an ICU admission, recurrent pneumothorax, or haemoptysis not controlled by embolization (Orens et al., 2006). The ISHLT guidelines for LTx in CF and other causes of bronchiectasis include oxygen-dependent respiratory failure, hypercapnia, and pulmonary hypertension.

**Table 32.1** Variables and point values used for computation of BMI, degree of airflow obstruction and dyspnoea, and exercise capacity (BODE) index. (Adapted from *The New England Journal of Medicine*, Celli BR et al., 'The Body-Mass Index, Airflow Obstruction, Dyspnea, and Exercise Capacity Index in Chronic Obstructive Pulmonary Disease', 350, 10, pp. 1005–1012, Copyright © 2004 Massachusetts Medical Society. Reprinted with permission from Massachusetts Medical Society.)

| Variable | Points on BODE index | | | |
|---|---|---|---|---|
| | 0 | 1 | 2 | 3 |
| FEV1 (% of predicted) | ≥ 65 | 50–64 | 36–49 | ≤ 35 |
| Distance walked in 6 minutes (m) | > 350 | 250–349 | 150–249 | ≤ 149 |
| MMRC dyspnoea scale | 0–1 | 2 | 3 | 4 |
| Body mass index (kg/m²) | > 21 | ≤ 21 | | |

## Pulmonary vascular diseases

Pulmonary artery hypertension (PAH) is defined as persistent elevation of mPAP> 25 mm Hg with pulmonary capillary wedge pressure < 15 mm Hg or elevation of exercise mPAP > 35 mm Hg (Subramaniam and Yared, 2007). In patients with PAH presenting for LTx, aetiologies include idiopathic or connective

**Table 32.2** ISHLT guidelines for LTx in COPD (Reprinted from *The Journal of Heart and Lung Transplantation*, 25, 7, Orens JB et al., 'International Guidelines for the Selection of Lung Transplant Candidates: 2006 Update—A Consensus Report From the Pulmonary Scientific Council of the International Society for Heart and Lung Transplantation', pp. 745–755, Copyright 2006, with permission from Elsevier and International Society for Heart and Lung Transplantation)

| BODE index 7–10 or at least one of the following: |
|---|
| Hospitalization for exacerbation with hypercapnia ($PaCO_2$ > 50 mmHg) |
| Pulmonary hypertension or cor pulmonale despite $O_2$ therapy |
| FEV1 < 20% predicted |

**Table 32.3** ISHLT guidelines for LTx in IPF. (Reprinted from *The Journal of Heart and Lung Transplantation*, 25, 7, Orens JB et al., 'International Guidelines for the Selection of Lung Transplant Candidates: 2006 Update—A Consensus Report From the Pulmonary Scientific Council of the International Society for Heart and Lung Transplantation', pp. 745–755, Copyright 2006, with permission from Elsevier and International Society for Heart and Lung Transplantation)

| |
|---|
| DLCO < 39% predicted |
| Decrement in FVC of > 10% over 6 months |
| Desaturation below 88% during 6-MWT |
| Honeycombing on HRCT (fibrosis score > 2) |

tissue disease-associated primary pulmonary hypertension (PPH), chronic hypoxaemic lung disease (COPD, IPF), and congenital heart disease with Eisenmenger syndrome (Ip and Slinger, 2011). They account for 4–6% of DLTxs currently performed (Christie et al., 2011; Azad, 2012). PPH is rare and is characterized by increased pulmonary vascular resistance due to vasoconstriction, smooth muscle proliferation (causing medial hypertrophy), and thrombosis-in-situ (Rubin, 1997).

Chronic pulmonary hypertension causes RV hypertrophy and dilatation. This dilatation causes shifting of the interventricular septum (IVS) towards the LV during systole, reducing the LV chamber size and impairing LV filling in diastole and LV contractile function (Subramaniam and Yared, 2007). The hypertrophied RV is dependent on MAP for flow through the right coronary artery and myocardial perfusion. RV ischaemia can develop rapidly during periods of systemic hypotension. This further compromises LV filling and cardiac output and can precipitate haemodynamic collapse (Subramaniam and Yared, 2007).

Patients with PPH tend to present with non-specific symptoms such as fatigue, exertional dyspnoea, angina, and syncope (Subramaniam and Yared, 2007). Abnormalities in lung function are usually mild and arterial hypoxaemia is usually always present. The 6-MWT correlates well with the severity of disease and can be used along with symptoms and haemodynamics to monitor progression and response to therapy (Rubin, 1997). Untreated the prognosis is poor with a median survival of 2.8 years (D'Alonzo et al., 1991); however, improvements in medical therapy with prostaglandins and endothelin antagonists have led to improved symptom control, quality of life, and survival (McLaughlin, 2006). ISHLT guidelines for LTx in PAH include persistent New York Heart Association (NYHA) class III or IV on maximal medical therapy, 6-MWT < 350 m, cardiac index < 2 L/min/m$^2$, and right atrial pressure > 15 mmHg (Orens et al., 2006).

## Donor selection

A major limitation to the number of transplants performed is a lack of acceptable donor organs. The largest source of donor organs is from DNDDs. Unfortunately, because of injuries acquired during the process of brain death, the average organ procurement rate remains disappointing. UNOS data reveal that only 2,489 individual lungs were transplanted from 8,089 deceased donors in 2007. As a comparison, 11,752 individual kidneys were transplanted from that same pool of organ donors.

A common strategy to maximize use of DNDD lungs has been to transplant ECD organs (i.e. those organs that fall outside of ISHLT standard criteria but are still believed to be transplantable) (Schiavon et al., 2012). Some transplant programmes have begun to explore the use of circulation-arrested donors, so-called non-heart-beating donors (NHBDs) as alternative sources for lungs (Wigfield and Love, 2011). Because most patients succumb as a result of cardiac arrest, the use of NHBDs could open a new pool of donor organs of such magnitude that ultimately the entire demand could be met. Two major problems with the use of ECD organs and NHBDs are the difficulty in assessing which lungs can be used safely (Wigfield and Love, 2011) and the time-critical nature of lung procurement due to ischaemia after death.

After declaration of brain death, consent for donation is discussed with relatives and, when available, donor registries can be checked. Ventilatory settings are altered to protect the potential donor lungs. This includes the use of small tidal volumes (6–8 mL/kg), in conjunction with pressure-controlled ventilation, with appropriate PEEP and recruitment manoeuvres (Angel et al., 2006; Kutsogiannis et al., 2006). Blood samples are obtained to check the blood group and to minimize the risk of donor-transmitted diseases. A chest radiograph is taken to exclude gross parenchymal or pleural abnormalities. A CT scan of the lungs may be available. A bronchoscopy should be performed to exclude gross infection, anatomical abnormalities, and pulmonary toilette. Finally, gas exchange capacity of the donor lungs can be assessed with an oxygen challenge (100% oxygen is delivered and the arterial oxygen partial pressure measured). A retrieval surgeon performs a direct evaluation by macroscopic observation and palpation to assess lung compliance and oedema. Palpation also is used to exclude intrinsic lung disease, areas of contusion, pneumonic infiltrates, or nodules before finally accepting the lungs. Observation of the ventilated lungs during deflation is important to assess acceptable elastic recoil, especially if donors have a smoking history. Donor lung assessment in controlled (Maastricht category III (Shemie et al., 2006)) NHBDs can be performed in the hours before planned termination of life support identical to the situation in DNDD donors.

The ISHLT criteria outlining ideal donors are strict and generally based on clinical impressions formed during the development of LTx rather than on medical evidence (de Perrot et al., 2005). These criteria are assessed during organ retrieval and are based on donor history, ABG, chest radiography, bronchoscopy, and physical examination of the lung. This clinical evaluation is imprecise and approximately 11–57% of lungs go on to PGD of varying severity, some of which may be the result of unrecognized donor injury. As a consequence, transplant clinicians remain conservative when choosing lungs for fear of potential PGD. It is estimated that 40% of rejected donor lungs could be used safely if more detailed and accurate evaluation were available to identify these lungs. The use of biomarkers to assess donor lung quality has been recently studied with very promising results. One of the studies demonstrated that the ratio of IL-6/IL-10 in the donor lung tissue was indeed more predictive of graft performance than clinical assessment (Kaneda et al., 2006; Anraku et al., 2008).

## Donor organ management

Donor lung preservation refers to the process of maintaining and protecting a donor lung from the time of lung procurement up until implantation into the recipient. Many factors such as temperature, perfusion volume and pressure, oxygenation, and degree of inflation may impact the likelihood of lung injury during storage or at the time of reperfusion. Much of the experimental work in LTx since 2005 has focused on optimizing methods of lung preservation to reduce the impact of ischaemia–reperfusion injury on post-transplant lung function (de Perrot et al., 2003b).

Preservation of the procured lungs is initiated with a hypothermic pulmonary artery flush of 50–60 mL/kg of a preservative solution, coupled with the topical administration of a cold solution (Hopkinson et al., 1998; Fischer et al., 2001). Flushing uniformly cools the lung tissue and removes blood from the pulmonary vascular bed, thereby preventing thrombosis and endothelial injury from retained neutrophils (de Perrot et al., 2003a). Anterograde and retrograde flushing appears to achieve better lung function than either alone and thus most centres do both (Venuta et al., 1999; Wittwer et al., 2005). Thereafter the lungs are transported at 4–8°C in a partially inflated state.

## Preservation solutions

The current preservation solution of choice used in most LTx centres is low potassium dextran (LPD) (Perfadex®). The key components of this solution are dextran and a low-potassium concentration. Dextran-40 in the LPD solution functions as an oncotic agent, tending to keep water in the intravascular compartment and thereby decreasing interstitial oedema formation. Dextran-40 also reduces the aggregation of erythrocytes and circulating thrombocytes, which may improve the microcirculation and reduce cellular activation (Keshavjee et al., 1992). The low-potassium concentration maintains normal PAPs during infusion. A further development is the dextran–glucose-based extracellular solution. The addition of glucose is designed to support aerobic metabolism and maintain cell integrity during prolonged ischaemia. This takes advantage of the unique aspect of lung physiology in transplantation; the inflated lung has the ability to supply oxygen to its parenchyma even during storage.

Several studies have found better early post-transplant outcomes (frequency of primary graft dysfunction, duration of ventilator dependence, and 30-day mortality) with LPD compared to other solutions. One of the largest studies retrospectively examined the likelihood of primary lung graft dysfunction among 157 consecutive patients whose donor lungs were preserved with one of three lung preservation solutions (Perfadex, Euro-Collins, and Papworth) (Oto et al., 2006). Perfadex was superior in preventing moderate to severe grades of primary graft dysfunction, and a trend towards superiority in other early post-transplant outcomes was also noted (Okada and Kondo, 2006; Minambres et al., 2007; Muhlfeld et al., 2007).

## Pharmacological additives

Two pharmacological agents, prostaglandins and glucocorticoids, have been used for lung preservation. These drugs have been given as pretreatment of the donor before flushing, as part of the flush perfusate itself, and as a treatment for the recipient during and after reperfusion. Prostaglandins $E_1$ ($PGE_1$, alprostadil) and $I_2$ ($PGI_2$, prostacyclin, and its synthetic analogue Iloprost) were originally chosen for lung preservation because their vasodilator activity offset the cold-induced vasoconstriction of the preservation solution and allowed a more even distribution of perfusate (Ueno et al., 1991; Mayer et al., 1992). Subsequent studies have found that prostaglandins have additional beneficial properties, including downregulation of proinflammatory cytokines and improvement of surfactant function, ameliorating ischaemia–reperfusion injury (de Perrot et al., 2001; Gohrbandt et al., 2005). Many centres routinely inject $PGE_1$ into the pulmonary artery just before flushing with preservation solution, although scientific data in humans are lacking.

High-dose methylprednisolone has become an empirical adjunct to most clinical protocols because of its anti-inflammatory actions (Venkateswaran et al., 2009). Methylprednisolone 15 mg/kg is typically administered intravenously to the donor before procurement and to the recipient usually immediately before reperfusion of the transplanted lung.

## Volume and pressure of preservation solution infusion

Scientific data are limited regarding the ideal volume of preservation solution; however, typically 60 mL/kg is infused over 15–20 minutes after lung extraction, as this is adequate to flush and cool the lungs (Fischer et al., 2001). The need for complete clearance of the vascular bed has to be balanced against the risk of injury to the low-pressure pulmonary vasculature. We typically use a perfusion pressure in the lower range (10–15 mmHg) and avoid exceeding a maximum perfusion pressure of 22 mmHg (30 cm $H_2O$) (Sasaki et al., 1996). Once the vascular bed has been flushed, perfusion is discontinued during storage.

## Lung inflation

Inflation of the lungs with an oxygen mixture during the ischaemic period protects the lung. Lung inflation is generally limited to 50% of the total lung capacity or to an airway pressure of 20 $cmH_2O$ to avoid overdistention (DeCampos et al., 1998; Kayano et al., 1999). Usually an inspired oxygen tension ($FiO_2$) ranging from 30–50% is used. Once the lungs have been inflated, the trachea is clamped for storage.

## Storage temperature

The ideal temperature for donor lung storage remains unclear. Hypothermia (4–8°C) reduces metabolic activity such that cell viability can be maintained in the face of ischaemia (5% of the metabolic rate at 37°C). Some experimental work has suggested that lungs preserved at 10°C instead of 4°C had superior lung function after transplantation (Wang et al., 1989; Ueno et al., 1991). However, the most common temperature for lung storage continues to be 4°C, as the logistics of transportation may prolong ischaemic time and necessitate the margin of safety provided by the lower temperature.

## Ischaemic time

The optimal and acceptable ischaemic times are not known, although the longer the ischaemic time, the greater the risk of severe reperfusion injury. Ischaemic times up to 8 hours are generally considered acceptable. The risks of PGD and 30-day mortality increase with more than 8 hours of ischaemia; however, ischaemic times of up to 10–12 hours have been successfully reported (Novick et al., 1999; Thabut et al., 2005). Therefore the decision to accept lungs with longer ischaemic times is made with the consideration of the constellation of other predictive risk factors in the

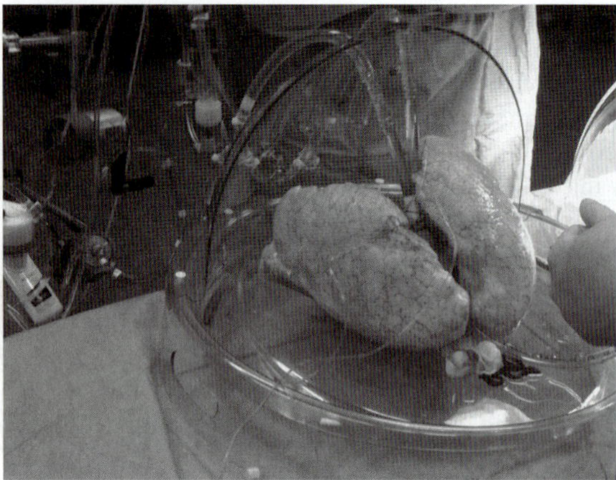

**Fig. 32.4** Ex-vivo donor lung perfusion. Inflow and outflow cannulae for perfusate, placed in the pulmonary artery and veins, can be seen entering at top of picture. An endotracheal tube can be seen at 4 o'clock in the trachea for ventilation.

lung donor (age, clinical variables, smoking history, etc.) and also consideration of the status or condition of the recipient.

### Ex-vivo lung perfusion

The increasing use of suboptimal donor lungs to increase the availability of donor organs and difficulties assessing lung function in NHBDs have made it necessary to explore alternative preservation techniques. Ex-vivo lung perfusion (EVLP) is a new preservation method that aims to recondition unacceptable donor lungs to optimize them for transplant. It has shown promising results (Rega et al., 2003; Steen et al., 2003; Cypel et al., 2008, 2009a; Ingemansson et al., 2009). During EVLP the donor lung is maintained under dynamic and physiological conditions so that real-time functional assessment and treatment of injured organs are possible (Cypel et al., 2009b) (see Figure 32.4). Using a lung-protective acellular perfusate, EVLP can maintain donor lungs for at least 12 hours at body temperature (37°C) without inducing injury (Cypel et al., 2008, 2009). During this acellular perfusion, evaluation of lung function ex vivo is also possible by pulmonary venous gas sampling, guiding decisions about the organs' suitability for transplant.

## Recipient selection

According to the international guidelines for the selection of LTx candidates, first published in 1998 (Maurer et al., 1998) and revised in 2006 (Orens et al., 2006), 'Lung transplantation is indicated for patients with chronic, end-stage lung disease who are failing maximal medical therapy, or for whom no effective medical therapy exists'. Listing for transplantation should occur when life expectancy after transplantation exceeds life expectancy without the procedure. In general this is when patients have less than 50% 2- to 3-year predicted survival, or NYHA class III or IV level of function, or both (Orens et al., 2006). Patients need to be free from major comorbidities and demonstrate high motivation, rehabilitation potential, acceptable nutritional status, a satisfactory psychological profile, and an adequate social support structure. Absolute and relative contraindications are listed in Table 32.4.

**Table 32.4** Absolute and relative contraindications to LTx. (Reprinted from *The Journal of Heart and Lung Transplantation*, 25, 7, Orens JB et al., 'International Guidelines for the Selection of Lung Transplant Candidates: 2006 Update—A Consensus Report From the Pulmonary Scientific Council of the International Society for Heart and Lung Transplantation', pp. 745–755, Copyright 2006, with permission from Elsevier and International Society for Heart and Lung Transplantation)

| Absolute contraindications | Relative contraindications |
|---|---|
| Malignancy in the last 2 years, with the exception of cutaneous squamous and basal cell tumours | Age > 65 years |
| Untreatable advanced dysfunction of another major organ system (e.g. heart, liver, or kidney) | Critical or unstable clinical condition (e.g. shock, mechanical ventilation, extracorporeal membrane oxygenation) |
| Chronic extrapulmonary infection including hepatitis B, C, HIV | Severely limited functional status with poor rehabilitation potential |
| Significant chest wall or spinal deformity | Colonization with highly resistant or highly virulent bacteria, fungi, or mycobacteria (including *P. cepacia*) |
| Documented non-compliance with medical therapy or follow-up | Obesity as defined by a BMI > 30 kg/m$^2$ |
| Untreatable psychiatric conditions impairing ability to comply with therapy | Severe or symptomatic osteoporosis |
| Substance addiction within previous 6 months | Other medical conditions that have not resulted in end-stage organ damage (e.g. diabetes mellitus, systemic hypertension) should be optimally treated before transplantation |
| Inadequate social support | |

Biological age is more important than chronological age; however, older recipients have a higher mortality (Yusen et al., 2010; Christie et al., 2011).

Donors and recipients are matched according to size and blood group and these are among the factors that affect waiting times. Smaller patients tend to wait longer than taller patients and women wait longer than men. Because the number of LTx recipients far exceeds the number of suitable donors, approximately 5–10% of recipients die each year while awaiting transplantation. Patients with IPF, CF, or PPH experience lower survival rates while awaiting LTx compared with patients who have emphysema or Eisenmenger syndrome (De Meester et al., 2001). In December 2011 in the US there were 1,700 patients awaiting LTx, with the median waiting time 136 days for listings in 2009. The implementation of the LAS system in the US in 2005, which uses medical urgency and expected outcome to prioritize donor lung allocation, dramatically reduced the number of active (eligible) waiting-list patients and median waiting times (Yusen et al., 2010). Prior to this, time on the transplant waiting list was primarily used to prioritize recipients. This led to very early listing resulting in average waiting times of around 2 years (Yusen et al., 2010). At Toronto General Hospital (TGH) the median wait time was 123 days for patients transplanted in 2011, with a mean of 193 days.

## Bridge to lung transplantation

Patients who are otherwise excellent candidates for LTx often die on the waiting list because they are too sick to survive until an organ becomes available. Currently, many of these patients are supported by maximal mechanical ventilation in the ICU, but this further aggravates the lung injury (Slutsky and Imai, 2003) and often leads to remote organ dysfunction with subsequent high mortality prior to or after LTx (Imai et al., 2003). For most of these patients, refractory hypercapnia and/or hypoxia will develop despite maximal ventilatory support and therefore ECMO is their only chance to survive until a compatible donor lung becomes available. Initial attempts at utilizing ECMO as a bridge to LTx were hindered by a high rate of complications and poor outcomes (Jurmann et al., 1991). Many centres came to view ECMO and mechanical ventilation as contraindications to LTx as it was believed that both compromised bronchial healing—the Achilles' heel of transplantation in the early days (Jurmann et al., 1991). In addition, the use of adult ECMO for acute respiratory failure (ARF) significantly declined after a negative National Institute of Health randomized trial in which survival after venoarterial ECMO was only 10% in patients with severe ARF (Zapol et al., 1979).

This combination of factors resulted in the concept of using ECMO as a bridge to LTx being largely discouraged. However, since 2005, improvements in LTx outcomes and patient selection, a better understanding of ventilator-associated lung injury, and significant improvements in artificial lung device technologies have made it possible to bridge these very sick patients to successful LTx (Fischer et al., 2006; Aigner et al., 2007; Strueber et al., 2009; Cypel et al., 2010; Olsson et al., 2010). In addition, recent studies have shown more promising results using ECMO for adults with ARF, with survival rates ranging from 50–80%. This includes the experience from Michigan with 100 patients (Kolla et al., 1997), the conventional ventilatory support versus extracorporeal membrane oxygenation for severe adult respiratory failure (CESAR) trial (Peek et al., 2009), and influenza A (H1N1)/ARDS reports (Davies et al., 2009; Freed et al., 2010). These improved survival rates for patients on ECMO are paralleled in the cohort of patients who are bridged to LTx with ECMO. A recent review from the UNOS experience totalling 51 such patients between 1987 and 2008 showed a 1-, 6-, 12-, and 24-month survival of 72%, 53%, 50%, and 45%, respectively, compared to 93%, 85%, 79%, and 70% for unsupported patients, respectively (Mason et al., 2010).

The most common complications during ECMO include haemorrhage, complications at the cannulation site, renal failure, neurological complications, and sepsis (Fischer et al., 2007).

## Anaesthesia for lung transplantation

### Preoperative assessment

Due to the emergent nature of LTx surgery, the anaesthesiologist usually has limited time for patient preoperative assessment. In many centres patients are seen by an anaesthesiologist in a preoperative assessment clinic prior to or soon after listing for transplantation in order to highlight anaesthetic considerations such as potentially difficult airways or distorted bronchial anatomy that may make double lumen tube placement difficult. At this visit invasive monitoring, postoperative intubation, analgesia, and blood transfusion are all discussed with the patient. A variety of baseline investigations are performed as part of the preoperative cardiorespiratory work-up both to assess suitability for transplantation and guide intraoperative management. Those performed at TGH are listed in Table 32.5. Patients should undergo intensive chest physiotherapy and be optimized by a respiratory therapist while on the waiting list.

**Table 32.5** Baseline investigations performed at Toronto General Hospital

| | |
|---|---|
| **Respiratory work-up** | Blood group and antibody screen |
| | Arterial blood gas on room air |
| | Pulmonary function testing (FEV1, FVC, DLCO, 6-MWT) |
| | CXR, CT scan Chest, ventilation/perfusion scan |
| **Cardiac work-up** | ECG, echocardiogram, radionuclide angiography (multigated acquisition scan) |
| Patients > 40 years | Cardiology consultation, nuclear cardiac stress testing |
| Men > 45 years, women > 50 years | Coronary angiography and right heart catheterization for PAP |
| **Infectious disease work-up** | Viral serology including HIV, hepatitis B, C, CMV, EBV; tuberculin skin test; sputum cultures |
| **Hepatic and renal function** | |
| **Osteoporosis work-up** | Bone mineral densitometry |

RV dysfunction and latent coronary artery disease are not uncommon in end-stage lung disease patients (Leibowitz et al., 1994; Vizza et al., 1998); however, the presence of non-critical coronary artery stenoses does not appear to influence morbidity and mortality after LTx (Choong et al., 2006). TEE has been shown to provide additional information in the pulmonary hypertensive population undetected by right and left heart catheterization and TTE (Singh and Bossard, 1997).

Aside from a routine anaesthetic assessment, important information to be gleaned from the preoperative evaluation includes:

- Underlying diagnosis: obstructive, restrictive, suppurative, pulmonary vascular disease. This will assist with planning the induction and ventilator settings for the patient
- ABG: this provides a baseline $PaCO_2$ on which to base intraoperative and postoperative levels
- PAP and RV function as assessed by echocardiography and right heart catheterization studies: these are two of the main determinants as to whether or not the procedure can be performed without CPB. Preoperative or intraoperative selective pulmonary vasodilator therapy may be indicated for severe pulmonary hypertension (Singh and Bossard, 1997)
- Antibiotic prophylaxis regimen: broad-spectrum antibiotics are given soon after induction. Piperacillin/tazobactam is the regimen of choice at Toronto General Hospital, with the exception of CF patients who are treated according to individual bacterial cultures

## Preoperative management

Recipients should abstain from solids for 6 hours and liquids for 2 hours and are advised to remain nil by mouth once called into hospital. Standard premedication usually involves immunosuppressants and antibiotics. Therapy for the underlying condition (oxygen, bronchodilators) should be continued until surgery. Routine preoperative sedation prior to entry into the operating room is not recommended as hypoventilation and hypercarbia can increase pulmonary vascular resistance and exacerbate pulmonary hypertension (Singh and Bossard, 1997).

## Intraoperative setup and monitoring

The patient is called to the operating room 2 hours before the donor lungs are expected to arrive (Boasquevisque et al., 2009). In addition to routine anaesthetic monitoring, invasive blood pressure is monitored, CVP is measured, and PACs are inserted. The latter provides valuable information in the setting of pulmonary hypertension, particularly during one-lung ventilation and PA clamping, when severe cardiopulmonary instability may be encountered (Singh and Bossard, 1997). It can also be used to measure cardiac output, which may be of benefit after separation from bypass.

Newer monitors may be adopted as familiarity with their use increases. Minimally invasive cardiac output monitors such as pulse contour analysis devices have been used during cardiac surgery and one-lung ventilation (OLV) and appear to correlate well with intermittent PA thermodilution measurements and may have a place in the future as familiarity increases (Button et al., 2007; Ishikawa et al., 2010). Reduced cerebral oxygen saturation is associated with a higher complication rate following thoracic surgery (Kazan et al., 2009) and cerebral oximetry has been shown to improve outcomes in major cardiac surgery (Murkin et al., 2007); however, its benefit in LTx has not been studied. Depth of anaesthesia monitors such as BIS reduce awareness in high-risk patient groups (Myles et al., 2004) and may be of benefit during LTx, particularly when the primary mode of anaesthesia is intravenous. The standard anaesthesia setup used at TGH is shown in Table 32.6.

At TGH a radial or brachial arterial line is inserted under local anaesthesia prior to induction, and if major blood loss or CPB is anticipated, a femoral arterial line is inserted when the patient is asleep. Central venous access is essential and along with the PAC is usually inserted once the patient is asleep, unless the patient is likely to decompensate on induction.

**Table 32.6** Toronto General Hospital operating room setup

| | |
|---|---|
| Monitoring | ECG (5 lead), NIBP, $SaO_2$, capnography, end-tidal $O_2$ monitoring, temperature, invasive BP, central venous pressure, PAP, urine output |
| IV access | Large-bore peripheral IV, internal jugular 8.5 FG swan sheath |
| Invasive lines | Arterial line, Swan–Ganz PAC, subclavian triple lumen central line |
| Infusions | Propofol, norepinephrine, and/or vasopressin, magnesium sulphate, insulin, and epinephrine as required |
| Emergency drugs | Phenylephrine, ephedrine, epinephrine, heparin (400 units/kg) |
| Airway | Double lumen tube, single lumen tube, flexible bronchoscope, spirometry, self-inflating bag, PEEP valve |

NIBP, Non-invasive blood pressure; FG, French Gauge.

A perfusionist and CPB machine should be present in the room for the entire case ('pump standby'), as emergency transition onto bypass may be needed at any time during the procedure.

Spirometry assists with protective ventilation of the transplanted lung by ensuring tidal volumes are kept at 5–7 mL/kg. Due to the large incisional surface area and insertion of cooled donor lungs, the patient is at high risk of hypothermia. Temperature monitoring and warming devices such as fluid warmers and forced-air heating blankets to maintain euthermia are essential. Intraoperative hypothermia can cause arrhythmias and coagulopathy.

## Induction of anaesthesia

LTx patients have minimal cardiorespiratory reserve and induction may precipitate cardiopulmonary collapse, so awareness of the pathophysiological processes at work is important (Myles et al., 1997; Banner et al., 2007). The sudden reduction in SVR and negative inotropic effects of intravenous and inhaled anaesthetic agents combined with the reduced venous return during positive pressure ventilation can compromise an already strained RV. Preoxygenation is recommended, but since ventilation–perfusion mismatch slows alveolar denitrogenation, it takes longer and can be monitored by end-tidal oxygraphy (Myles, 1998).

The preferred technique at TGH is to use a benzodiazepine (midazolam) and opioid- (fentanyl 5–10 mcg/kg or sufentanil 0.5–1 mcg/kg) based induction with a steroid intermediate (rocuronium) or long-acting (pancuronium) muscle relaxant. Ketamine (0.5–1 mg/kg) may be used to supplement this in patients with pulmonary hypertension to maintain SVR. Early assistance with ventilation as the patient begins to lose consciousness is important to prevent desaturation, which can be rapid in some patients, and hypercapnia, which is poorly tolerated in patients with pulmonary hypertension.

Patients with obstructive lung disease are at risk of dynamic hyperinflation (gas trapping) with positive pressure ventilation. Overdistention of the lungs causes elevated intrathoracic pressure, direct cardiac compression, impaired venous return, reduced RV filling, and reduced cardiac output with subsequent profound hypotension (Singh and Bossard, 1997; Boasquevisque et al., 2009). Sometimes ventilation needs to be paused and the endotracheal tube disconnected from the breathing circuit to allow adequate time for exhalation and restoration of venous return (Myles and Weeks, 1992; Quinlan and Buffington, 1993). Avoiding extrinsic PEEP and ventilating with a low respiratory rate and long expiratory time (inspiratory:expiratory ratio 1:3–5) to permit lung deflation may prevent this; however, marked acidaemia can become a limiting factor as $CO_2$ accumulates (Singh and Bossard, 1997). These patients are also at risk of bullous rupture causing a tension pneumothorax (Banner et al., 2007). The large alveolar dead space in these patients results in the end-tidal $CO_2$ underestimating the arterial $CO_2$ by unpredictable amounts and frequent blood gas sampling is necessary.

Patients with restrictive lung disease often require higher ventilation pressures (above 40 $cmH_2O$) and rates to deliver adequate minute ventilation and to benefit from increased levels of PEEP (Myles, 1998; Roscoe, 2011). If BSLTx is planned then the high ventilatory pressures required during OLV on the native lung to minimize hypercapnia can be tolerated since the damaged lungs will be removed.

In patients with suppurative lung diseases (most commonly CF) a single-lumen tube is often placed first to allow flexible bronchoscopy with a large suction port, lavage for microbiological culture, and pulmonary toilette before a double-lumen tube is placed (Boasquevisque et al., 2009). This may reduce sputum plugging and atelectasis, allowing better gas exchange. These recipients have mixed obstructive and restrictive defects, so ventilation strategies need to be suited to the individual but, in general, high inspiratory pressures are needed to deliver adequate tidal volumes. Hypercapnia is often a problem during OLV and frequent recruitment and repeated toilette of the airway may be required during the operation as lung manipulation can cause purulent secretions that obstruct the large airways (Ip and Slinger, 2011).

In patients with pulmonary vascular disease, induction of anaesthesia is a critical time and prior surgical femoral cannulation under local anaesthesia to prepare for urgent CPB may be considered in very high-risk patients (Myles, 1998). The goals on induction are to maintain systemic blood pressure and prevent rises in PVR. This is achieved by maintaining inotropic and chronotropic functions of the heart, optimizing preload, and preventing myocardial depression, hypoxaemia, and hypercapnia, which can increase PVR and cause acute right heart failure. The concomitant reduction in LV filling and systemic cardiac output results in profound hypotension, a further reduction in RV perfusion, and cardiovascular collapse (Feltracco et al., 2007).

Central venous access and PACs are generally inserted prior to induction. In severe cases, pulmonary vasodilators such as iNO or $PGI_2$ can be commenced before induction along with vasoactive agents to maintain systemic blood pressure. Norepinephrine appears to be better than phenylephrine for increasing SVR more than PVR (Subramaniam and Yared, 2007), and vasopressin is promising in this setting with some evidence that it increases SVR without affecting PVR (Dunser et al., 2001; Braun et al., 2004). Low-dose epinephrine, dopamine, dobutamine, and milrinone in conjunction with a vasopressor have all been used to provide inotropy if needed (Singh and Bossard, 1997; Myles, 1998; Subramaniam and Yared, 2007). Large opioid doses blunt the reflex increase in PVR in response to intubation and reduce the dose of intravenous anaesthetic agents required. Ketamine is considered the best induction agent due to favourable effects on pulmonary vasculature during controlled ventilation (Wiedemann and Diestelhorst, 1995). Table 32.7 summarizes disease-specific intraoperative complications.

**Table 32.7** Disease-specific intraoperative anaesthetic complications. (Reproduced from *Principles and practice of anesthesia for thoracic surgery*, 2011, 'Lung Transplantation', pp. 523–535, A. Roscoe, with kind permission from Springer Science and Business Media.)

| | |
|---|---|
| COPD/emphysema | Gas trapping with positive pressure ventilation leading to profound hypotension |
| | Pneumothorax |
| | Coronary artery disease often present |
| Pulmonary fibrosis | High ventilatory pressures associated with reduced venous return |
| | Secondary pulmonary hypertension |
| | Associated underlying pathologies, e.g. scleroderma |
| | Lung dissection can be prolonged due to scarring |
| Cystic fibrosis | Copious secretions impairing gas exchange |
| | Difficult to maintain normocapnia |
| | May require frequent pulmonary toilette |
| | Small patients (BMI < 20) and multiple lung adhesions leading to prolonged dissection and increased bleeding |
| | Often diabetic |
| Pulmonary hypertension | Poorly functioning RV |
| | Cardiovascular collapse on induction of anaesthesia |
| | CPB/ECMO required |

In general, a disposable polyvinylchloride left-sided double lumen tube is used for the airway, although for elective bypass cases a single lumen tube can be used (Banner et al., 2007). The practice at TGH is to do as much dissection as possible prior to heparinization and initiation of bypass to minimize bypass time and blood loss. A double lumen tube allows selective collapse of the lung being dissected and selective ventilation of the first transplanted lung while still on bypass. Positioning of the tube is confirmed with fibreoptic bronchoscopy and bronchoscopic washings are collected from all patients to assist in determining postoperative antimicrobial regimens if infection occurs. Occasionally the tube needs to be withdrawn slightly for the left main bronchial anastomosis. Bronchial blocker use has been described in a non-bypass case (Scheller et al., 1992); however, it needs repositioning in BSLTx and access to check the bronchial anastomosis and aspirate blood and secretions is limited (Horan et al., 1996).

## Transoesophageal echocardiography

The use of intraoperative TEE in LTx is listed as a IIb indication by the American College of Cardiology guidelines (Chetlin et al., 2003), suggesting that it may be beneficial to patient outcome. Our practice at TGH is to routinely perform intraoperative TEE during LTx if there is no contraindication such as oesophageal dysmotility in scleroderma patients.

Primarily, TEE is used as a monitor for fluid volume status since in the context of potential large-volume blood loss, LV and/or RV dysfunction, and vasoplegia following CPB it is very difficult to optimize preload based on CVP or PAC data (Della Rocca et al., 2009). TEE can also diagnose deteriorating RV function, which may occur secondary to increased pulmonary vascular resistance from hypercarbia or one-lung ventilation.

TEE is useful to diagnose a patent foramen oval (PFO), since this is often missed on a preoperative TTE and can result in an unexplained shunt and desaturation when PEEP is used or in cases of increased pulmonary vascular resistance (see Figure 32.5). If the transplantation is to be performed with CPB, the surgeon may choose to close a PFO during CPB.

TEE is useful to examine the vascular anastomoses to rule out stenosis after transplantation. It is usually possible to see the right PA anastomosis with TEE; however, the left PA anastomosis is commonly obscured by the left main stem bronchus. Both left and right pulmonary venous (PV)–left atrial (LA) anastomoses are normally easy to visualize with TEE. The left pulmonary venous anastomosis is often technically more difficult for the surgeon and thus more prone to stenosis (see Figure 32.6).

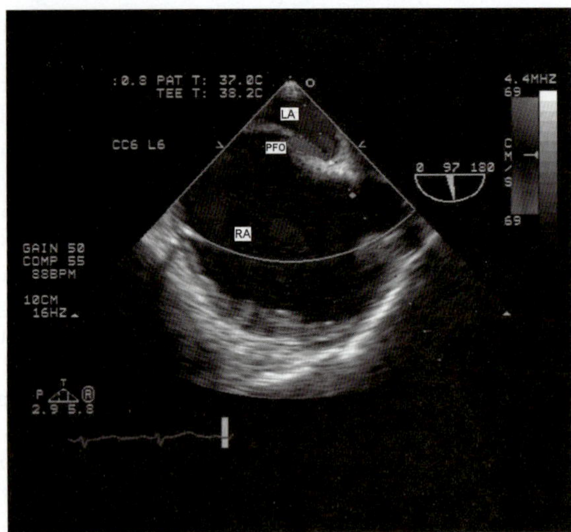


**Fig. 32.5** Mid-oesophageal TEE view of interatrial septum with flow Doppler demonstration of a patent foramen ovale (PFO) showing left to right shunt flow. This flow direction can be reversed in cases of increased pulmonary vascular resistance resulting in desaturation due to intracardiac shunt. RA, Right atrium; LA, left atrium.

It is a difficult team decision to decide whether to attempt to repair a PV–LA stenosis seen on TEE. It is possible that attempting to repair the stenosis may only make it worse. As a rough guide, if the diameter of the anastomotic orifice seems to be adequate (> 6 mm) we will usually not attempt a repair. Rarely, a thrombus may be seen at the orifice after a PV–LA anastomosis (see Figure 32.7).

During reperfusion of the lungs it is common to get systemic air microbubble emboli from the donor lungs. TEE gives an early warning of this problem, which may progress to right coronary artery air emboli and to acute right heart ischaemia and RV dysfunction. This is usually a transient complication and treatable with inotropes and vasopressors.

An uncommon intra-/postoperative haemodynamic complication in LTx is development of RV outflow tract obstruction. This leads to decreased cardiac output and hypotension most commonly in patients with RV hypertrophy following CPB and has been termed the 'suicide right ventricle'. This particular clinical scenario of tachycardia and hypotension, refractory to inotropes, can be very difficult to diagnose without TEE (see Figure 32.8).

Once the diagnosis is made the RVOT obstruction will usually respond to increased RV preload, decreased inotropy, and decreased heart rate. In rare cases an RV myomectomy has been required (Chen et al., 2009). Rarely, LV outflow tract obstruction has also been reported following LTx (Murtha and Guenther, 2002).

## Patient positioning and maintenance of anaesthesia

For BSLTx the patient is positioned supine with both arms out and at TGH a clamshell incision with sternal transection is the incision of choice; however, median sternotomy or anterolateral thoracotomies can be used. For SLTx the patient may be positioned in the lateral decubitus or supine positions, with lateral or anterolateral thoracotomy incisions respectively, the latter being useful if CPB is anticipated (Boasquevisque et al., 2009). Thromboembolic deterrent (TED) stockings and intermittent calf compressors are used for deep vein thrombosis prophylaxis and 5,000 units of subcutaneous heparin is given.

Maintenance of anaesthesia may be with low-dose potent inhaled anaesthetics (isoflurane or sevoflurane) (Singh and Bossard, 1997) or intravenous agents. Due to uncertain gas exchange in the native lungs and the potential for haemodynamic instability, our practice at TGH is to commence a propofol infusion early at 50 mcg/kg/min to ensure amnesia. Nitrous oxide may exacerbate pulmonary hypertension (Schulte-Sasse et al., 1982) and expand intravascular air emboli from the allograft, so it is avoided (McRae, 2006). Supplemental doses of fentanyl and muscle relaxant are administered or a sufentanil infusion can be used. All of our patients receive at least 4 g of magnesium sulphate to reduce the likelihood of perioperative arrhythmias.

In BSLTx the lung with the lowest perfusion is replaced first. Initiation of OLV will result in shunting of deoxygenated blood through the collapsed lung and this can cause significant

(a)

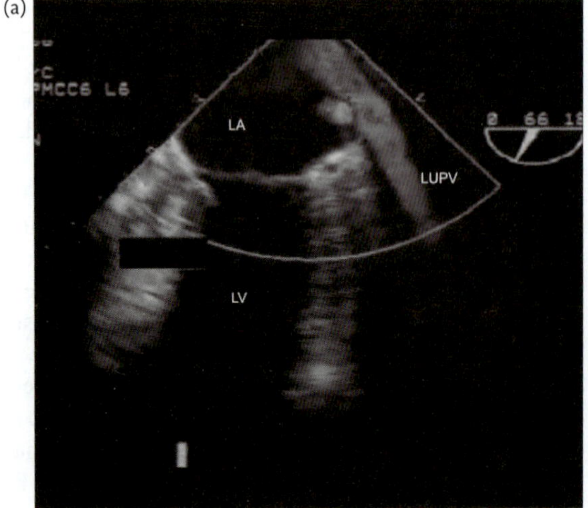


(b)

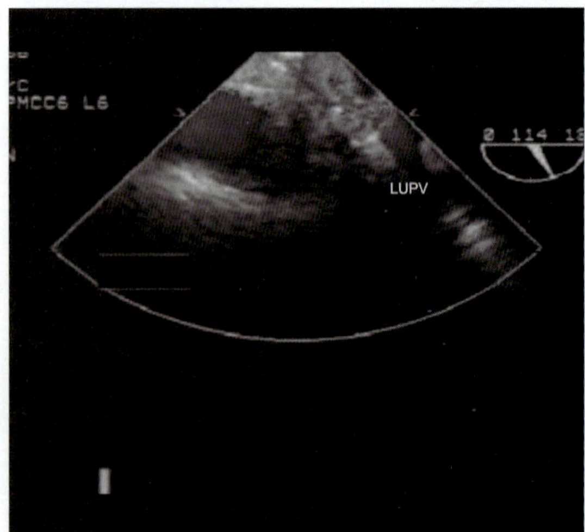


**Fig. 32.6** (**A**) Pretransplant mid-oesophageal TEE showing normal laminar left upper pulmonary vein (LUPV) flow pattern emptying into the left atrium (LA). LV, Left ventricle. (**B**) Post-transplant TEE view of LUPV shows stenosis at the anastomosis with the LA and a mosaic flow pattern into the LA. After discussion with the surgeon, the LUPV stenosis in this patient was not repaired and the patient recovered without complication.

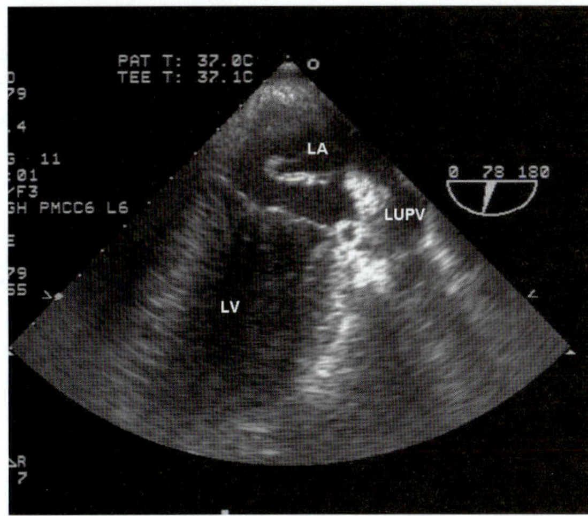


**Fig. 32.7** A linear thrombus is seen as extending from the orifice of the left upper pulmonary vein (LUPV) into the left atrium (LA) after LUPV anastomosis. This thrombus was removed by a suction passed through a left atriotomy by the surgeon without CPB. LV, Left ventricle.

hypoxaemia until the PA on that side is ligated. Elimination of $CO_2$ can be difficult during OLV and the aim is to achieve arterial blood gases similar to the patient's preoperative values (Myles, 1998). Permissive hypercapnia—allowing supraphysiological arterial $CO_2$ levels—is usually safe in the absence of pulmonary hypertension and avoids some of the problems with high airway pressures required during mechanical ventilation, such as reduced venous return while the chest is closed and lung hyperinflation (Myles, 1998). Pressure-controlled ventilation may be preferable to volume-controlled ventilation during OLV as it reduces peak airway pressures (Tugrul et al., 1997). Patients unable to tolerate OLV due to progressive hypercarbia will require CPB (Boasquevisque et al., 2009). During the dissection phase, serial blood gas sampling is undertaken to assess the adequacy of ventilation and

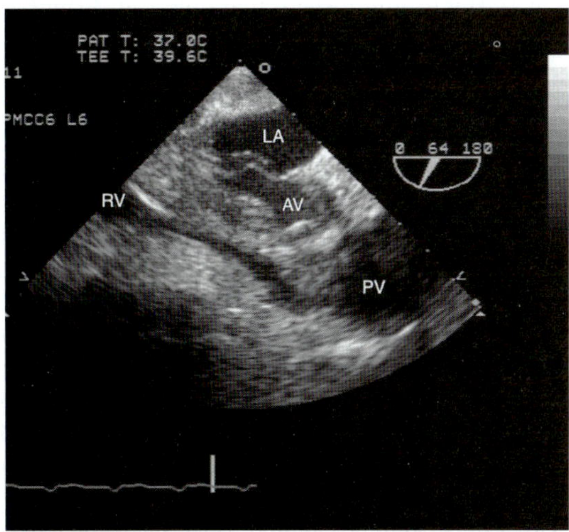


**Fig. 32.8** Dynamic obstruction of the RV outflow tract, which developed between the right ventricle (RV) and pulmonary artery (PA) in a patient with primary pulmonary hypertension following CPB for BLTx. LA, Left atrium; AV, aortic valve.

surgical blood loss is noted, as it can be considerable in pulmonary and cystic fibrotic patients and patients undergoing repeat transplantation. Mechanical manipulation of the heart during hilar dissection and allograft implantation can cause considerable haemodynamic instability, and judicious administration of fluid, vasopressors, and frequent communication with the surgeon are important during this stage.

## Management of RV dysfunction

Although surgical clamping of the PA during OLV will reduce shunt and improve oxygenation, it also causes an increase in PA pressure, which can precipitate RV failure in high-risk patients. The dilated RV causes bulging of the interventricular septum (IVS) into the LV, impairing LV filling and contractility, reducing cardiac output, and causing RV ischaemia and worsening RV function leading to cardiac arrest (Myles, 1998). In patients with pre-existing severe pulmonary hypertension, PA clamping will not be tolerated and elective CPB is employed. In patients with mild–moderately elevated pressures, temporary clamping can be employed and the effects on the PA pressure and RV monitored (Myles, 1998; Feltracco et al., 2007). TEE is very useful in these cases to promptly diagnose RV dysfunction (Pedoto and Amar, 2009).

Management of RV dysfunction is aimed at reducing PVR and RV afterload, increasing RV contractility, and increasing systemic blood pressure to improve right coronary artery blood flow and shift the IVS back toward the RV, improving LV output (Forrest, 2009). Non-pharmacological methods to reduce PVR such as increasing the $FiO_2$ to 1.0 and reducing $CO_2$ and acidosis may be of limited benefit during OLV. iNO at 20–40 parts per million (ppm) reduces PVR, improves oxygenation by redistributing blood flow to better ventilated areas of the lung, and can reverse RV failure (Fierobe et al., 1995; Myles, 1998; Krasuski et al., 2000; Rocca et al., 2001). Inhaled prostacyclin (epoprostenol, iloprost) therapy is a comparable alternative to iNO for reducing RV afterload and is cheaper (Haraldsson et al., 1998; Sablotzki et al., 2002; Baez and Castillo, 2008). Epinephrine (0.02–0.2 mcg/kg/min) can be used to improve RV function but at higher doses can cause pulmonary vasoconstriction (Myles, 1998; Subramaniam and Yared, 2007). Phosphodiesterase inhibitors such as milrinone also increase RV contractility and reduce PVR but cause systemic vasodilatation, necessitating co-administration of a vasoconstrictor such as norepinephrine or vasopressin to maintain coronary perfusion (Subramaniam and Yared, 2007; Forrest, 2009). Likewise, levosimendan, a newer inotrope, restores RV–PA coupling by increasing RV contractility and reducing PVR (Kerbaul et al., 2006) but also reduces SVR. It may be of future benefit. Norepinephrine has been shown to exert favourable effects on RV function in the setting of pressure overload (Martin et al., 1994; Forrest, 2009) and is the vasopressor of choice at TGH for these cases. It can be supplemented by vasopressin where necessary.

## Use of cardiopulmonary bypass and extracorporeal membrane oxygenation

There is variation amongst institutions in the frequency of elective CPB use. Approximately one-third of LTxs done at TGH utilize CPB (32/102 in 2011) (Azad, 2012). $PaCO_2$ is targeted around the patient's preoperative value. The heart is kept warm and beating and no aortic cross-clamp is used, unless the patient is undergoing concurrent coronary bypass or cardiac repair. After implantation of the first allograft, the heart is allowed to eject some blood and the allograft lung is gently ventilated.

The most common reason to use CPB electively is the presence of pulmonary hypertension (systolic PAP > 60 mmHg). These patients have RV dysfunction and a high risk of RV failure on clamping of one of the pulmonary arteries, necessitating bypass to unload the right heart. If the systolic PAP is < 50 mmHg the case is attempted off pump at TGH unless the patient has comorbidities such as advanced age (> 65) and ischaemic heart disease, when they are less likely to tolerate OLV and the cardiac manipulation required during the bronchial and vascular anastomoses around the hilum. Patients requiring intraoperative plasmapheresis to remove panel reactive antibodies form the third group done on CPB, since this is most conveniently performed during CPB.

The decision to initiate emergency CPB is based on the development of haemodynamic instability unable to be controlled by vasoactive agents, or severe gas exchange abnormalities, usually during one-lung ventilation. The main disadvantages of CPB include crystalloid loading increasing the risk of pulmonary oedema, the potential for massive bleeding associated with the anticoagulation required, and subsequent need for large amounts of blood products and coagulopathy (Quinlan and Buffington, 1993). The increase in pro-inflammatory cytokines from CPB is also well documented (Hall et al., 1997) and may be attenuated by the administration of high-dose steroids, more so if administered prior to initiation of CPB (Wan et al., 1996). For this reason we administer 500 mg of methylprednisolone on induction of anaesthesia rather than immediately prior to graft reperfusion (McRae, 2000). Whether or not CPB has a deleterious effect on early graft function or clinical outcome is still unclear. Some retrospective reviews have shown no adverse effects when CPB is used (Triantafillou et al., 1994; Szeto et al., 2002) while in others CPB has been associated with greater morbidity (longer period of mechanical ventilation, more pulmonary oedema) and short-term (1 month and 1 year) mortality (Aeba et al., 1994; Dalibon et al., 2006). The latter studies may, however, reflect the underlying pathology that led to the use of bypass rather than bypass itself. No prospective randomized controlled trials have been performed and the available evidence suggests that CPB should continue to be used where clinically indicated (Nagendran et al., 2011).

ECMO can provide an alternative to CPB if gas exchange is the major problem (Ko et al., 2001; Xu et al., 2010). Although it was associated with poorer outcomes in one previous retrospective review (Bittner et al., 2007), ECMO has largely replaced CPB for LTx in many centres. It is possible to continue ECMO into the ICU period if needed for lung support and less anticoagulation is required than with CPB.

## Plasmapheresis

Approximately 10–15% of LTx recipients are sensitized to HLA antigens (Appel et al., 2005). The development of anti-HLA antibodies is associated with hyperacute, acute, and chronic rejection in renal and cardiac transplants (Weil et al., 1981; Suciu-Foca et al., 1991) and it is possible that they have a similar role in LTx (Bittner et al., 2001; Appel et al., 2005). The detection of sensitized patients awaiting transplantation has increased with emergence of sensitive and specific HLA typing and antibody detection methods. HLA antigens can be identified and avoided at the time of transplant with the use of virtual cross-matching. This correlates well with prospective cross-matching (Stuckey et al., 2012). The rationale for peritransplant plasmapheresis is that by depleting anti-HLA antibodies with IVIG and/or plasma exchange with albumin and plasma, antibody-mediated (hyperacute) rejection is reduced in sensitized patients. It may also reduce the incidence of bronchiolitis obliterans (Appel et al., 2005).

## Fluid management

Optimizing preload is essential in managing intraoperative haemodynamics, especially during surgical manipulation of the heart, when periods of hypotension can be prolonged in the hypovolaemic patient. However, the lung allograft is prone to low-pressure pulmonary oedema thought to be due to re-expansion injury, ischaemia–reperfusion microvascular leak, oxygen free radicals, and loss of lymphatic drainage (Singh and Bossard, 1997; Baez and Castillo, 2008). A restrictive fluid administration regimen therefore seems prudent, similar to that for a pneumonectomy (Slinger, 1995), particularly when CPB is used, since these patients generally have a larger positive fluid balance (Myles, 1998). This may result in intraoperative hypotension, and judicious use of a vasopressor is required. A retrospective study by McIlroy et al. (2009) found that there was an inverse relationship between the volume of intraoperative colloid administered and the $PaO_2/FiO_2$ ratio at 12 hours, suggesting excessive colloid-impaired allograft function and delayed extubation (McIlroy et al., 2009). Blood products are transfused as clinically indicated. Whilst restrictive transfusion strategies in critically ill patients seem to be associated with better outcomes (Hebert et al., 1999; Vincent et al., 2002), transfusion-related immunomodulation may confer some benefit (Cicciarelli, 1990) and reduce the incidence of acute cellular rejection post-transplantation(Schneider, 2011).

Blood conservation techniques include the use of a cell saver and antifibrinolytics such as aprotinin and tranexamic acid. Aprotinin has been shown to reduce blood loss and transfusion requirements in patients undergoing LTx with (Kesten et al., 1995) and without (Balsara et al., 2009) CPB; however, retrospective studies have yielded conflicting results regarding its effects on acute graft function (Bittner et al., 2006; Marasco et al., 2010). Our practice at TGH is to administer tranexamic acid (30 mg/kg at the start of CPB and 16 mg/kg/hour infusion to a maximum dose of 100 mg/kg) only when CPB is used.

## Allograft reperfusion

The allograft is kept on a cooling jacket in the pleural cavity as it is implanted. The hilar anastomoses proceed from posterior to anterior, with the bronchial anastomosis being completed first, followed by the PA and the pulmonary veins via a left atrial cuff (Boasquevisque et al., 2009). Bronchoscopy is performed after the bronchial anastomosis to ensure its patency and to remove any blood and fluid from the large airways. The newly implanted lung is gently reinflated and ventilated, initially with air, limited peak airway pressures (< 25 $cmH_2O$), and PEEP of 5–10 $cmH_2O$ (McRae, 2000), keeping tidal volumes at 5–6 mL/kg to reduce mechanical stress (de Perrot et al., 2002). The PA is then unclamped over 10 minutes to promote gradual vascular recruitment and reduce lung injury caused by high flow reperfusion (Halldorsson et al., 1998; Pierre et al., 1998).

In BSLTx the native lung can be hand-ventilated with a high $FiO_2$ to maintain arterial oxygenation while the new allograft is reperfusing and ventilated at the above settings (Roscoe, 2011). Although some bleeding through the atrial patch is allowed prior to release of the atrial clamp to de-air the lung, hypotension on reperfusion is still common due to a combination of systemic release of stored pneumoplegia solution containing prostaglandins, inflammatory mediators from the ischaemic lung, and air embolism into the (usually right) coronary arteries (Myles, 1998; Baez and Castillo, 2008). ST segment changes are commonly seen in the inferior ECG leads and they usually resolve when the hypotension is treated with vasopressors such as phenylephrine and/or norepinephrine (Myles, 1998; Feltracco et al., 2007). Sometimes epinephrine (5- to 50-mcg boluses) is needed. The acute increase in the cross-sectional area of the pulmonary vasculature on reperfusion of the allograft may contribute to the hypotension and necessitate judicious fluid administration (Feltracco et al., 2007).

After the initial period of reperfusion, the $FiO_2$ to the allograft is increased to $FiO_2$ 0.5 and two-lung ventilation is resumed and $FiO_2$ adjusted as needed. A period of risk for hypoxaemia ensues as the ventilation goes to the compliant allograft, whilst the perfusion may predominantly go to the native lung since the vasculature in the allograft initially is relatively constricted. Rapid clamping of the native PA will improve this ventilation–perfusion mismatch; however, the entire cardiac output is now forced through the allograft, which can worsen pulmonary oedema if reperfusion injury has occurred (McRae, 2000). Refractory hypoxaemia or high PA pressures at this stage may necessitate the use of CPB for implantation of the second lung. In practice there does not seem to be a difference in lung injury between the first and second implanted lungs, suggesting this increased flow is of less consequence than might be anticipated (Sheridan et al., 1998). Once the second allograft is implanted and reperfused, haemostasis is obtained and the chest closed. A recruitment manoeuvre is undertaken after chest closure and PAPs are noted if they have been troublesome.

Ischaemia–reperfusion injury, also called PGD, is caused by oxygen free radicals formed when the ischaemic lung tissue is reoxygenated and results in pulmonary endothelial cell injury, the recruitment and activation of neutrophils, and complement activation leading to increased vascular permeability (McRae, 2000). Clinically this manifests as hypoxaemia despite increasing $FiO_2$, reduced lung compliance, rising pulmonary pressures, and in severe cases frank pulmonary oedema. It is the most common early complication of LTx, occurring within the first 72 hours and affecting 10–30% of recipients depending on how it is defined (Table 32.8) (Prekker et al., 2006). It is associated with increased mortality which persists beyond the first year, and management includes the use of low tidal volume ventilation, PEEP, and iNO or prostaglandins (McRae, 2000; Christie et al., 2005b). iNO improves oxygenation in cases of PGD by improving V/Q matching and reducing pulmonary vascular resistance, but its routine use to prevent PGD does not seem to be of benefit (de Perrot et al., 2003; Meade et al., 2003; Botha et al., 2007). Prostaglandin $E_1$ infusion has been shown to improve lung function in animal models of PGD and is used in some centres (de Perrot et al., 2003). ECMO has been used to treat severe PGD with some success (Oto et al., 2004; Hsu et al., 2008).

**Table 32.8** Modified ISHLT recommendations for grading of PGD severity, based solely on measured $PaO_2/FiO_2$ ratio (Adapted from *The Journal of Heart and Lung Transplantation*, 24, 10, Christie et al, 'Report of the ISHLT Working Group on Primary Lung Graft Dysfunction part II: definition. A consensus statement of the International Society for Heart and Lung Transplantation', pp. 1454–1459, Copyright 2005, with permission from Elsevier and the International Society for Heart and Lung Transplantation.)

| Grade | $PaO_2/FiO_2$ | Radiographic infiltrates consistent with pulmonary oedema |
|---|---|---|
| 0 | > 300 | Absent |
| 1 | > 300 | Present |
| 2 | 200–300 | Present |
| 3 | < 200 | Present |

$PaO_2/FiO_2$ ratio is calculated as the ratio of partial pressure of oxygen in arterial blood (mm Hg) to fractional inspired oxygen concentration (≤1.0).

## Analgesia

Good postoperative analgesia is imperative to allow the patient to cooperate with chest physiotherapy, and to prevent muscle deconditioning, pulmonary complications, and the development of chronic pain (Feltracco et al., 2010). Intraoperative analgesia at TGH is with high-dose fentanyl or sufentanil, since the patients are not extubated at the end of the case. Postoperative analgesic options are similar to those for an elective thoracotomy, with thoracic epidural anaesthesia (TEA) and parenteral opioid-based techniques being the most commonly employed. Adjunctive analgesics include acetaminophen and NSAIDs, although the latter should be used with caution due to the increased risk of renal impairment when used with cyclosporin (Altman et al., 1992). TEA has traditionally been considered the analgesic gold standard for thoracotomy, reducing complications such as atelectasis and pneumonia and the surgical stress response (Groben, 2006). Specific to LTx, a review of retrospective studies by Pottecher et al. (2011) found that TEA reduced the length of ICU stay and the number of respiratory complications.

However, the benefits of epidural analgesia need to be weighed against the risk of epidural haematoma, as some patients undergo emergency intraoperative bypass, which requires systemic heparinization. The risk is difficult to quantify and has been estimated with 95% confidence to be from 1 in 1,500 (maximum risk) to 1 in 150,000 (minimum risk) patients given thoracic epidurals, then heparinized for CPB (Ho, 2000). There have been no reports to date of major neurological damage related to perimedullary bleeding due to epidural catheterization in LTx (Feltracco et al., 2010); however, neuraxial haematoma following instrumentation has occurred in other anticoagulated patients (Ho, 2000). Our practice at TGH is to give all patients parenteral opioid via patient-controlled analgesia (PCA) once awake, with epidurals being inserted postoperatively only in those patients with severe ongoing pain despite PCA after coagulopathy has been excluded.

An alternative regional anaesthesia technique utilizes extrapleural (paravertebral) catheters, which have been shown to provide equivalent analgesia to TEA with less hypotension when used for thoracotomy (Joshi et al., 2008), with presumably low risk of epidural haematoma if inserted by the surgeons under direct vision.

## Postoperative care

Although most patients are transferred to the ICU intubated, early extubation in the operating room is feasible, particularly after SLTx, with appropriate patient selection and good analgesia (Hansen et al., 2003; Rocca et al., 2003). Avoidance of prolonged mechanical ventilation reduces the risk of barotrauma and the need for ongoing sedation and has been associated with improved oxygenation, reduced extravascular lung water, lower PA pressures, and reduced requirement for vasoactive drug (norepinephrine) support (Rocca et al., 2003). For patients remaining intubated, the endotracheal tube is changed to a single lumen tube and the patient is kept sedated with propofol for transfer to the ICU. A nasogastric tube is passed to facilitate early administration of enteral immunosuppression and patients are maintained on a protective ventilation strategy (2000).

## Conclusion

The anaesthetic management must be adapted to the underlying diagnosis of the recipient. The lung is the most sensitive of all the major transplant organs to ischaemic injury and the time from retrieval to reperfusion is critical. Recent advances such as ex-vivo donor graft perfusion have increased the number of available donor lungs for transplantation. The use of cardiopulmonary bypass during LTx varies widely between centres and is being replaced by ECMO in many centres. Intraoperative TEE gives valuable information about cardiac function, filling volumes, and vascular anastomoses during LTx.

## References


Aeba R, Griffith BP, Kormos RL, et al. (1994) Effect of cardiopulmonary bypass on early graft dysfunction in clinical lung transplantation. *Ann Thorac Surg*, **57**:715–722.

Aigner C, Wisser W, Taghavi S, et al. (2007) Institutional experience with extracorporeal membrane oxygenation in lung transplantation. *Eur J Cardiothorac Surg*, **31**:468–473, discussion 473–474.

Altman RD, Perez GO, Sfakianakis GN (1992) Interaction of cyclosporine A and nonsteroidal anti-inflammatory drugs on renal function in patients with rheumatoid arthritis. *Am J Med*, **93**:396–402.

Angel LF, Levine DJ, Restrepo MI, et al. (2006) Impact of a lung transplantation donor-management protocol on lung donation and recipient outcomes. *Am J Resp Crit Care Med*, **174**:710–716.

Anraku M Cameron MJ, Waddell TK, et al. (2008) Impact of human donor lung gene expression profiles on survival after lung transplantation: a case-control study. *Am J Transplant*, **8**(10):2140–2148.

Appel JZ, Hartwig MG, Davis RD, Reinsmoen NL (2005) Utility of peritransplant and rescue intravenous immunoglobulin and extracorporeal immunoadsorption in lung transplant recipients sensitized to HLA antigens. *Hum Immunol*, **66**:378–386.

ARDSNet (2000) Ventilation with lower tidal volumes as compared with traditional tidal volumes for acute lung injury and the acute respiratory distress syndrome. The Acute Respiratory Distress Syndrome Network. *N Engl J Med*, **342**:1301–1308.

Azad S (2012) *Re: Toronto General Hospital lung transplant registry.*

Baez B, Castillo M (2008) Anesthetic considerations for lung transplantation. *Semin Cardio-Thorac Vasc Anesth*, **12**:122–127.

Balsara KR, Morozowich ST, Lin SS (2009) Aprotinin's effect on blood product transfusion in off-pump bilateral lung transplantation. *Interactive Cardiovasc Thorac Surg*, **8**:45–48.

Banner N, Polak J, Yacoub M (2007) *Lung Transplant*. Cambridge University Press, Cambridge.

Bech B, Pressler T, Iversen M, et al. (2004) Long-term outcome of lung transplantation for cystic fibrosis—Danish results. *Eur J Cardio-Thorac Surg*, **26**:1180–1186.

Bittner HB, Dunitz J, Hertz M, Bolman MR, Park SJ (2001) Hyperacute rejection in single lung transplantation—case report of successful management by means of plasmapheresis and antithymocyte globulin treatment. *Transplantation*, **71**:649–651.

Bittner HB, Richter M, Kuntze T (2006) Aprotinin decreases reperfusion injury and allograft dysfunction in clinical lung transplantation. *Eur J Cardio-Thorac Surg*, **29**:210–215.

Bittner HB, Binner C, Lehmann S, Kuntze T, Rastan A, Mohr FW (2007) Replacing cardiopulmonary bypass with extracorporeal membrane oxygenation in lung transplantation operations. *Eur J Cardio-Thorac Surg*, **31**:462–467, discussion 467.

Boasquevisque CH, Yildirim E, Waddel TK, Keshavjee S (2009) Surgical techniques: lung transplant and lung volume reduction. *Proc Am Thorac Soc*, **6**:66–78.

Botha P, Jeyakanthan M, Rao JN, et al. (2007) Inhaled nitric oxide for modulation of ischemia-reperfusion injury in lung transplantation. *J Heart Lung Transplant*, **26**:1199–1205.

Braun EB, Palin CA, Hogue CW (2004) Vasopressin during spinal anesthesia in a patient with primary pulmonary hypertension treated with intravenous epoprostenol. *Anesth Analg*, **99**:36–37.

Button D, Weibel L, Reuthebuch O, Genoni M, Zollinger A, Hofer CK (2007) Clinical evaluation of the FloTrac/Vigileo system and two established continuous cardiac output monitoring devices in patients undergoing cardiac surgery. *Br J Anaesth*, **99**:329–336.

Cai J (2007) Double- and single-lung transplantation: an analysis of twenty years of OPTN/UNOS registry data. *Clin Transplant*, **2007**:1–8.

Celli BR, Marin JM, Casanova C, et al. (2004) The body-mass index, airflow obstruction, dyspnea, and exercise capacity index in chronic obstructive pulmonary disease. *N Engl J Med*, **350**:1005–1012.

Chetlin MD, Armstrong WF, Aurigemma GP, et al. (2003) ACC/AHA/ASE 2003 Guideline Update for the Clinical Application of Echocardiography: summary article. A report of the American College of Cardiology/American Heart Association Task Force on Practice Guidelines (ACC/AHA/ASE Committee to Update the 1997 Guidelines for the Clinical Application of Echocardiography). J Am Soc Echocardiogr, 16: 1091–1110

Chen F, Hanaoka N, Hasegawa S, et al. (2009) Right ventricular outflow tract obstruction after bilateral lung transplantation. *Thorac Cardiovasc Surg*, **57**:48–50.

Choong CK, Meyers BF, Guthrie TJ, Trulock EP, Patterson GA, Moazami N (2006) Does the presence of preoperative mild or moderate coronary artery disease affect the outcomes of lung transplantation? *Ann Thorac Surg*, **82**:1038–1042.

Christie JD, Carby M, Bag R, Corris P, Hertz M, Weill D (2005a) Report of the ISHLT working group on primary lung graft dysfunction. Part II: definition. A consensus statement of the International Society for Heart and Lung Transplantation. *J Heart Lung Transplant*, **24**:1454–1459.

Christie JD, Kotloff RM, Ahya VN, et al. (2005b) The effect of primary graft dysfunction on survival after lung transplantation. *Am J Respir Crit Care Med*, **171**:1312–1316.

Christie JD, Edwards LB, Kucheryavaya AY, et al. (2011) The Registry of the International Society for Heart and Lung Transplantation: twenty-eighth adult lung and heart-lung transplant report (2011) *J Heart Lung Transplant*, **30**:1104–1122.

Cicciarelli J (1990) UNOS Registry data: effect of transfusions. *Clin Transplant*, **1990**:407–416.

Collard HR, King TE, JR, et al. (2003) Changes in clinical and physiologic variables predict survival in idiopathic pulmonary fibrosis. *Am J Respir Crit Care Med*, **168**:538–542.

Connors AF, Thomas C, Harrell F, et al. (1996) Outcomes following acute exacerbation of severe chronic obstructive lung disease. *Am J Respir Crit Care Med*, **154**:959–967.

Coultas DB, Zumwalt RE, Black WC, Sobonya RE (1994) The epidemiology of interstitial lung diseases. *Am J Respir Crit Care Med*, **150**:967–972.

Cypel M, Yeung JC, Hirayama S, et al. (2008) Technique for prolonged normothermic ex vivo lung perfusion. *J Heart Lung Transplant*, **27**;1319–1325.

Cypel M, Rubacha M, Yeung J, et al. (2009a) Normothermic ex vivo perfusion prevents lung injury compared to extended cold preservation for transplantation. *Am J Transplant*, **9**:2262–2269.

Cypel M, Liu M, Rubacha M, et al. (2009b) Functional repair of human donor lungs by IL-10 gene therapy. *Sci Transl Med*, **1**:1–9.

Cypel M, Waddell TK, de Perrot M, et al. (2010) Safety and efficacy of the novalung interventional lung assist (iLA) device as a bridge to lung transplantation. *J Heart Lung Transplant*, **29**(2):S88.

D'Alonzo GE, Barst RJ, Ayres SM, et al. (1991) Survival in patients with primary pulmonary hypertension. Results from a national prospective registry. *Annal Intern Med*, **115**:343–349.

Dalibon N, Geffroy A, Moutafis M, et al. (2006) Use of cardiopulmonary bypass for lung transplantation: a 10-year experience. *J Cardio-Thorac Vasc Anesth*, **20**:668–672.

Davies A, Jones D, Bailey M, et al. (2009) Extracorporeal membrane oxygenation for 2009 influenza A (H1N1). *JAMA*, **302**:1888–1895.

Davies JC, Alton EW, Bush A (2007) Cystic fibrosis. *BMJ*, **335**:1255–1259.

Della Rocca G, Brondani A, Costa MG (2009) Intraoperative hemodynamic monitoring during organ transplantation: what is new? *Curr Opin Organ Transplant*, **14**: 291–296.

de Meester JMAS, Persijn G, Haverich A (2001) Listing for lung transplantation: life expectancy and transplant effect, stratified by type of end-stage lung disease, the Eurotransplant experience. *J Heart Lung Transplant*, **20**:518–524.

de Perrot M, Fischer S, Liu M, et al. (2001) Prostaglandin E1 protects lung transplants from ischemia–reperfusion injury: a shift from pro- to anti-inflammatory cytokines. *Transplantation*, **72**:1505–1512.

de Perrot M, Imai Y, Volgyesi GA, et al. (2002) Effect of ventilator-induced lung injury on the development of reperfusion injury in a rat lung transplant model. *J Thorac Cardiovasc Surg*, **124**:1137–1144.

de Perrot M, Liu M, Waddell T, Keshavjee S (2003a) Ischemia–reperfusion-induced lung injury. *Am J Respir Cell Mol Biol*, **28**:616–625.

de Perrot M, Liu M, Waddell TK, Keshavjee S (2003b) Ischemia–reperfusion-induced lung injury. *Am J Resp Crit Care Med*, **167**:490–511.

de Perrot M, Bonser RS, Dark J, et al. (2005) Report of the ISHLT Working Group on primary lung graft dysfunction. Part III: donor-related risk factors and markers. *J Heart Lung Transplant*, **24**:1460–1467.

DeCampos KN, Keshavjee S, Liu M, Slutsky AS (1998) Optimal inflation volume for hypothermic preservation of rat lungs. *J Heart Lung Transplant*, **17**:599–607.

Depaseo WJ, Winterbauer RH (1991) Intersitial lung disease. *Disease-a-Month*, **37**:67–133.

de Soyza A, Mcdowell A, Archer L, (2001) *Burkholderia cepacia* complex genomovars and pulmonary transplantation outcomes in patients with cystic fibrosis. *Lancet*, **358**:1780–1781.

Dunser MW, Mayr AJ, Ulmer H, et al. (2001) The effects of vasopressin on systemic hemodynamics in catecholamine-resistant septic and post-cardiotomy shock: a retrospective analysis. *Anesth Analg*, **93**:7–13.

Egan JJ, Martinez FJ, Wells AU, Williams T (2005) Lung function estimates in idiopathic pulmonary fibrosis: the potential for a simple classification. *Thorax*, **60**:270–273.

Egan TM, Detterbeck FC, Mill MR, et al. (2002) Long term results of lung transplantation for cystic fibrosis. *Eur J Cardio-Thoracic Surg*, **22**:602–609.

Feltracco P, Serra E, Barbieri S, et al. (2007) Anesthetic concerns in lung transplantation for severe pulmonary hypertension. *Transplant Proc*, **39**:1976–1980.

Feltracco P, Barbieri S, Milevoj M, et al. (2010) Thoracic epidural analgesia in lung transplantation. *Transplant Proc*, **42**:1265–1269.

Fierobe L, Brunet F, Dhainaut JF, et al. (1995) Effect of inhaled nitric oxide on right ventricular function in adult respiratory distress syndrome. *Am J Respir Crit Care Med*, **151**:1414–1419.

Fischer S, Matte-Martyn A, de Perrot M, et al. (2001) Low-potassium dextran preservation solution improves lung function after human lung transplantation. *J Thorac Cardiovasc Surg*, **121**:594–596.

Fischer S, Simon AR, Welte T, et al. (2006) Bridge to lung transplantation with the novel pumpless interventional lung assist device NovaLung. *J Thorac Cardiovasc Surg*, **131**:719–723.

Fischer S, Bohn D, Rycus P, et al. (2007) Extracorporeal membrane oxygenation for primary graft dysfunction after lung transplantation: analysis of the Extracorporeal Life Support Organization (ELSO) registry. *J Heart Lung Transplant*, **26**:472–477.

Flaherty KR, Mumford JA, Murray S, et al. (2003) Prognostic implications of physiologic and radiographic changes in idiopathic interstitial pneumonia. *Am J Resp Crit Care Med*, **168**:543–548.

Forrest P (2009) Anaesthesia and right ventricular failure. *Anaesth Inten Care*, **37**:370–385.

Freed DH, Henzler D, White CW, et al. (2010) Extracorporeal lung support for patients who had severe respiratory failure secondary to influenza A (H1N1) 2009 infection in Canada. *Can J Anaesth*, **57**:240–247.

Global Initiative for Chronic Obstructive Pulmonary Disease (2010) *Global Stategy for the Diagnosis, Management and Prevention of Chronic Obstructive Pulmonary Disease*. <http://www.goldcopd.org/uploads/users/files/goldreport_april112011.pdf>.

Gohrbandt B, Sommer SP, Fischer S, et al. (2005) Iloprost to improve surfactant function in porcine pulmonary grafts stored for twenty-four hours in low-potassium dextran solution. *J Thorac Cardiovasc Surg*, **129**:80–86.

Groben H (2006) Epidural anesthesia and pulmonary function. *J Anesth*, **20**:290.

Hall RI, Smith MS, Rocker G (1997) The systemic inflammatory response to cardiopulmonary bypass: pathophysiological, therapeutic, and pharmacological considerations. *Anesth Analg*, **85**:766–782.

Halldorsson A, Kronon M, Allen BS, et al. (1998) Controlled reperfusion after lung ischemia: implications for improved function after lung transplantation. *J Thorac Cardiovasc Surg*, **115**:415–424, discussion 424–425.

Hamada K, Nagai S, Tanaka S, et al. (2007) Significance of pulmonary arterial pressure and diffusion capacity of the lung as prognosticator in patients with idiopathic pulmonary fibrosis. *Chest*, **131**:650–656.

Hansen LN, Ravn JB, Yndgaard S (2003) Early extubation after single-lung transplantation: analysis of the first 106 cases. *J Cardio-Thorac Vasc Anesth*, **17**:36–39.

Haraldsson A, Kieler-Jensen N, Nathorst-Westfelt U, et al. (1998) Comparison of inhaled nitric oxide and inhaled aerosolized prostacyclin in the evaluation of heart transplant candidates with elevated pulmonary vascular resistance. *Chest*, **114**:780–786.

Hebert PC, Wells G, Blajchman MA, et al. (1999) A multicenter, randomized, controlled clinical trial of transfusion requirements in critical care. Transfusion requirements in critical care investigators, Canadian Critical Care Trials Group. *N Engl J Med*, **340**:409–417.

Ho AMH (2000) Neuraxial blockade and hematoma in cardiac surgery: estimating the risk of a rare adverse event that has not (yet) occurred. *Chest*, **117**:551–555.

Hopkinson DN, Bhabra MS, Hooper TL (1998) Pulmonary graft preservation: a worldwide survey of current clinical practi. *J Heart Lung Transplant*, **17**:525–531.

Horan BF, Cutfield GR, Davies IM, et al. (1996) Problems in the management of the airway during anesthesia for bilateral sequential lung transplantation performed without cardiopulmonary bypass. *J Cardio-Thorac Vasc Anesth*, **10**:387–390.

Hsu HH, Ko WJ, Chen JS, et al. (2008) Extracorporeal membrane oxygenation in pulmonary crisis and primary graft dysfunction. *J Heart Lung Transplant*, **27**:233–237.

Imai Y, Parodo J, Kajikawa O, et al. (2003) Injurious mechanical ventilation and end-organ epithelial cell apoptosis and organ dysfunction in an experimental model of acute respiratory distress syndrome. *JAMA*, **289**:2104–2112.

Ingemansson R, Eyjolfsson A, Mared L, et al. (2009) Clinical transplantation of initially rejected donor lungs after reconditioning ex vivo. *Ann Thorac Surg*, **87**:255–260.

Ip D, Slinger P (2011) Lung: management during surgery. In: Andrew A, Klein CJL, Joren C, Madsen (eds) *Organ Trasplantation: A Clinical Guide*. Cambridge University Press, Cambridge.

Ishikawa S, Shirasawa M, Fujisawa M, Kawano T, Makita K (2010) Compressing the non-dependent lung during one-lung ventilation improves arterial oxygenation, but impairs systemic oxygen delivery by decreasing cardiac output. *J Anesth*, **24**:,17–23.

Joshi GP, Bonnet F, Shah R, Wilkinson, et al. (2008) A systematic review of randomized trials evaluating regional techniques for postthoracotomy analgesia. *Anesth Analg*, **107**:1026–1040.

Jurmann M J, Haverich A, Demertzis S, Schaefers HJ, Wagner TO, Borst HG (1991) Extracorporeal membrane oxygenation as a bridge to lung transplantation. *Eur J Cardiothorac Surg*, **5**:94–97; discussion 98.

Kaneda H, Waddell TK, de Perrot M, et al. (2006) Pre-implantation multiple cytokine mRNA expression analysis of donor lung grafts predicts survival after lung transplantation in humans. *Am J Transplant*, **6**:544–551.

Kayano K, Toda K, Naka Y, Pinsky DJ (1999) Identification of optimal conditions for lung graft storage with Euro-Collins solution by use of a rat orthotopic lung transplant model. *Circulation*, **100**:II257–II261.

Kazan R, Bracco D, Hemmerling TM (2009) Reduced cerebral oxygen saturation measured by absolute cerebral oximetry during thoracic surgery correlates with postoperative complications. *Br J Anaesth*, **103**:811–816.

Kerbaul F, Rondelet B, Demester JP, et al. (2006) Effects of levosimendan versus dobutamine on pressure load-induced right ventricular failure. *Crit Care Med*, **34**:2814–2819.

Keshavjee SH, Yamazaki F, Yokomise H, et al. (1992) The role of dextran 40 and potassium in extended hypothermic lung preservation for transplantation. *J Thorac Cardiovasc Surg*, **103**:314–325.

Kesten S, de Hoyas A, Chaparro C, Westney G, Winton T, Maurer JR (1995) Aprotinin reduces blood loss in lung transplant recipients. *Ann Thorac Surg*, **59**:877–879.

Ko WJ, Chen YS, Lee YC (2001) Replacing cardiopulmonary bypass with extracorporeal membrane oxygenation in lung transplantation operations. *Artif Organs*, **25**:607–612.

Kolla S, Awad SS, Rich PB, Schreiner RJ, Hirschl RB, Bartlett RH (1997) Extracorporeal life support for 100 adult patients with severe respiratory failure. *Ann Surg*, **226**:544–564; discussion 565–566.

Krasuski RA, Warner JJ, Wang A, Harrison JK, Tapson VF, Bashore TM (2000) Inhaled nitric oxide selectively dilates pulmonary vasculature in adult patients with pulmonary hypertension, irrespective of etiology. *J Am Coll Cardiol*, **36**:2204–2211.

Kutsogiannis DJ, Pagliarello G, Doig C, Ross H, Shemie SD (2006) Medical management to optimize donor organ potential: review of the literature. *Can J Anaesth*, **53**:820–830.

Leibowitz DW, Caputo AL, Shapiro GC, et al. (1994) Coronary angiography in smokers undergoing evaluation for lung transplantation: is routine use justified? *J Heart Lung Transplant*, **13**:701–703.

Levine SM (2004) A survey of clinical practice of lung transplantation in North America. *Chest*, **125**:1224–1238.

Ma M, Slinger P (2011) Anesthesia for patients with end-stage lung disease. In: Slinger P (ed) *Principles and Practice of Anesthesia for Thoracic Surgery*. Springer, New York.

Marasco SF, Pilcher D, Oto T, et al. (2010) Aprotinin in lung transplantation is associated with an increased incidence of primary graft dysfunction. *Eur J Cardio-Thorac Surg*, **37**:420–425.

Martin C, Perrin G, Saux P, Papazian L, Gouin F (1994) Effects of norepinephrine on right ventricular function in septic shock patients. *Inten Care Med*, **20**:444–447.

Mason DP, Thuita L, Nowicki ER, Murthy SC, Pettersson GB, Blackstone EH (2010). Should lung transplantation be performed for patients on mechanical respiratory support? The US experience. *J Thorac Cardiovasc Surg*, **139**:765–773.

Maurer R, Estenne M, Higenbottam T, Glanville AR (1998) International guidelines for the selection of lung transplant candidates. *Heart Lung: J Acute Crit Care*, **27**:223–229.

Mayer E, Puskas JD, Cardoso PF, Shi S, Slutsky AS, Patterson GA (1992) Reliable eighteen-hour lung preservation at 4 degrees and 10 degrees C by pulmonary artery flush after high-dose prostaglandin E1 administration. *J Thorac Cardiovasc Surg*, **103**:1136–1142.

Mclroy DR, Pilcher DV, Snell GI (2009) Does anaesthetic management affect early outcomes after lung transplant? An exploratory analysis. *Br J Anaesth*, **102**:506–514.

McLaughlin VV (2006). Survival in patients with pulmonary arterial hypertension treated with first-line bosentan. *Eur J Clin Invest*, **36**(Suppl 3):10–15.

McRae K (2006) Anesthesia for intrathoracic transplantation. In: Cheng D, David T (eds) *Perioperative Care in Cardiac Anesthesia and Surgery*. Lippincott, Williams & Wilkins, Philadelphia.

McRae KM (2000) Pulmonary transplantation. *Curr Opin Anaesthesiol*, **13**:53–59.

Meade MO, Granton JT, Matte-Martyn A, et al. (2003) A randomized trial of inhaled nitric oxide to prevent ischemia–reperfusion injury after lung transplantation. *Am J Respir Crit Care Med*, **167**:1483–1489.

Minambres E, Gonzalez-Castro A, Rabanal JM, et al. (2007) Comparative study of two preservation solutions in the initial function after bilateral human lung transplantation. *Med Intens*, **31**:1–5.

Muhlfeld C, Muller K, Pallesen LP, et al. (2007) Impact of preservation solution on the extent of blood-air barrier damage and edema formation in experimental lung transplantation. *Anat Rec (Hoboken)*, **290**:491–500.

Murkin JM, Adams SJ, Novick RJ, et al. (2007) Monitoring brain oxygen saturation during coronary bypass surgery: a randomized, prospective study. *Anesth Analg*, **104**:51–58.

Murtha W, Guenther C (2002) Dynamic left ventricular outflow tract obstruction complicating bilateral lung transplantation. *Anesth Analg*, **94**:558–559.

Myles PS (1998) Aspects of anesthesia for lung transplantation. *Semin Cardio-Thorac Vasc Anesth*, **2**:140–154.

Myles PS, Weeks AM (1992) Alpha 1-antitrypsin deficiency: circulatory arrest following induction of anaesthesia. *Anaesth Intens Care*, **20**:358–362.

Myles PS, Weeks AM, Buckland MR, Silvers A, Bujor M, Langley M (1997) Anesthesia for bilateral sequential lung transplantation: experience of 64 cases. *J Cardio-Thorac Vasc Anesth*, **11**:177–183.

Myles PS, Leslie K, McNeil J, Forbes A, Chan MTV (2004) Bispectral index monitoring to prevent awareness during anaesthesia: the B-Aware randomised controlled trial. *Lancet*, **363**:1757–1763.

Nagendran M, Maruthappu M, Sugand K (2011) Should double lung transplant be performed with or without cardiopulmonary bypass? *Interactive Cardiovasc Thorac Surg*, **12**:799–804.

Nathan SD (2005) Lung transplantation: disease-specific considerations for referral. *Chest*, **127**:1006–10016.

Novick RJ, Bennett LE, Meyer DM, Hosenpud JD (1999) Influence of graft ischemic time and donor age on survival after lung transplantation. *J Heart Lung Transplant*, **18**:425–431.

Okada Y, Kondo T (2006) Impact of lung preservation solutions, Euro-Collins vs. low-potassium dextran, on early graft function: a review of five clinical studies. *Annal Thorac Cardiovasc Surg*, **12**:10–14.

Olsson KM, Simon A, Strueber M, et al. (2010) Extracorporeal membrane oxygenation in nonintubated patients as bridge to lung transplantation. *Am J Transplant*, **10**(9):2173–2178.

Orens JB, Estenne M, Arcasoy S, et al. (2006) International guidelines for the selection of lung transplant candidates: 2006 update—a consensus report from the Pulmonary Scientific Council of the International Society for Heart and Lung Transplantation. *J Heart Lung Transplant*, **25**:745–755.

Oto T, Rosenfeldt F, Rowland M, et al. (2004) Extracorporeal membrane oxygenation after lung transplantation: evolving technique improves outcomes. *Ann Thorac Surg*, **78**:1230–1235.

Oto T, Griffiths AP, Rosenfeldt F, et al. (2006) Early outcomes comparing Perfadex, Euro-Collins, and Papworth solutions in lung transplantation. *Ann Thorac Surg*, **82**:1842–1848.

Pedoto A, Amar D (2009) Right heart function in thoracic surgery: role of echocardiography. *Curr Opin Anaesthiol*, **22**:44–49.

Peek GJ, Mugford M, Tiruvoipati R, et al. (2009) Efficacy and economic assessment of conventional ventilatory support versus extracorporeal membrane oxygenation for severe adult respiratory failure (CESAR): a multicentre randomised controlled trial. *Lancet*, **374**:1351–1363.

Pierre AF, Decampos KN, Liu M, et al. (1998) Rapid reperfusion causes stress failure in ischemic rat lungs. *J Thorac Cardiovasc Surg*, **116**:932–942.

Pottecher J, Falcoz PE, Massard G, Dupeyron JP (2011) Does thoracic epidural analgesia improve outcome after lung transplantation? *Interactive CardiovascThorac Surg*, **12**:51–53.

Prekker ME, Nath DS, Walker AR, et al. (2006) Validation of the proposed International Society for Heart and Lung Transplantation grading system for primary graft dysfunction after lung transplantation. *J Heart Lung Transplant*, **25**:371–378.

Quinlan JJ, Buffington CW (1993) Deliberate hypoventilation in a patient with air trapping during lung transplantation. *Anesthesiology*, **78**:1177–1181.

Raghu G, Weycker D, Edelsberg J, Bradford WZ, Oster G (2006) Incidence and prevalence of idiopathic pulmonary fibrosis. *Am J Respir Crit Care Med*, **174**:810–816.

Raghu G, Collard HR, Egan JJ, et al. (2011) An official ATS/ERS/JRS/ALAT statement: idiopathic pulmonary fibrosis: evidence-based guidelines for diagnosis and management. *Am J Respir Crit Care Med*, **183**:788–824.

Rega FR, Jannis NC, Verleden GM, Lerut TE, van Raemdonck DE (2003) Long-term preservation with interim evaluation of lungs from a non-heart-beating donor after a warm ischemic interval of 90 minutes. *Annal Surg*, **238**:782–792.

Rocca GD, Passariello M, Coccia C, et al. (2001) Inhaled nitric oxide administration during one-lung ventilation in patients undergoing thoracic surgery. *J Cardio-Thorac Vasc Anesth*, **15**:218–223.

Rocca GD, Coccia C, Costa GM, et al. (2003) Is very early extubation after lung transplantation feasible? *J Cardio-Thorac Vasc Anesth*, **17**:29–35.

Roscoe A (2011) Lung transplantation. In: Slinger P (ed) *Principles and Practice of Anesthesia for Thoracic* Surgery. Springer, New York.

Rubin L (1997). Primary pulmonary hypertension. *N Engl J Med*, **336**:111–117.

Sablotzki A, Hentschel T, Gruenig E, et al. (2002) Hemodynamic effects of inhaled aerosolized iloprost and inhaled nitric oxide in heart transplant candidates with elevated pulmonary vascular resistance. *Eur J Cardio-Thorac Surg*, **22**:746–752.

Sasaki M, Muraoka R, Chiba Y, Hiramatu Y (1996) Influence of pulmonary arterial pressure during flushing on lung preservation. *Transplantation*, **61**:22–27.

Scheller MS, Kriett JM, Smith CM, Jamieson SW (1992) Airway management during anesthesia for double-lung transplantation using a single-lumen endotracheal tube with an enclosed bronchial blocker. *J Cardio-Thorac Vasc Anesth*, **6**:204–207.

Schiavon M, Falcoz PE, Santelmo N, Massard G (2012) Does the use of extended criteria donors influence early and long-term results of lung transplantation? *Interact Cardiovasc Thorac Surg*, **14**:183–187.

Schneider F (2011) Effect of blood transfusion on lung transplant rejection. *Am J Respir Crit Care Med*, **183**:A1132.

Schulte-Sasse U, Hess W, Tarnow J (1982) Pulmonary vascular responses to nitrous oxide in patients with normal and high pulmonary vascular resistance. *Anesthesiology*, **57**:9–13.

Shemie SD, Ross H, Pagliarello J, et al. (2006) Organ donor management in Canada: recommendations of the forum on medical management to optimize donor organ potential. *CMAJ*, **174**:S13–S32.

Sheridan BC, Hodges TN, Zamora MR, et al. (1998) Acute and chronic effects of bilateral lung transplantation without cardiopulmonary bypass on the first transplanted lung. *Ann Thorac Surg*, **66**:1755–1758.

Shorr AF (2002) Outcomes for patients with sarcoidosis awaiting lung transplantation. *Chest*, **122**:233–238.

Singh H, Bossard RF (1997) Periopcrativc anaesthetic considerations for patients undergoing lung transplantation. *Can J Anesth*, **44**:284–299.

Slinger PD (1995) Perioperative fluid management for thoracic surgery: the puzzle of postpneumonectomy pulmonary edema. *J Cardio-Thorac Vasc Anesth*, **9**:442–451.

Slutsky AS, Imai Y (2003). Ventilator-induced lung injury, cytokines, PEEP, and mortality: implications for practice and for clinical trials. *Intens Care Med*, **29**:1218–1221.

Steen S Liao Q, Wierup PN, et al. (2003) Transplantation of lungs from non-heart-beating donors after functional assessment ex vivo. *Ann Thorac Surg*, **76**:244–252.

Strueber M, Hoeper MM, Fischer S, et al. (2009) Bridge to thoracic organ transplantation in patients with pulmonary arterial hypertension using a pumpless lung assist device. *Am J Transplant*, **9**:853–857.

Stuckey LJ, Kamoun M, Chan KM (2012) Lung transplantation across donor-specific anti-human leukocyte antigen antibodies: utility of bortezomib therapy in early graft dysfunction. *Annal Pharmacother*, **46**:e2.

Subramaniam K, Yared JP (2007) Management of pulmonary hypertension in the operating room. *Semin Cardio-Thorac Vasc Anesth*, **11**:119–136.

Suciu-Foca N, Ho E, King DW, et al. (1991) Soluble HLA and anti-idiotypic antibodies in transplantation: modulation of anti-HLA antibodies by soluble HLA antigens from the graft and anti-idiotypic antibodies in renal and cardiac allograft recipients. *Transplant Proc*, **231**:295.

Szeto WY, Kreisel D, Karakousis GC, et al. (2002) Cardiopulmonary bypass for bilateral sequential lung transplantation in patients with chronic obstructive pulmonary disease without adverse effect on lung function or clinical outcome. *J Thorac Cardiovasc Surg*, **124**:241–249.

Thabut G, Mal H, Cerrina J, et al. (2005) Graft ischemic time and outcome of lung transplantation: a multicenter analysis. *Am J Respir Crit Care Med*, **171**:786–791.

Triantafillou AN, Pasque MK, Huddleston CB, et al. (1994) Predictors, frequency, and indications for cardiopulmonary bypass during lung transplantation in adults. *Ann Thorac Surg*, **57**:1248–1251.

Tugrul M, Camci E, Karadeniz H, Senturk M, Pembeci K, Akpir K (1997) Comparison of volume controlled with pressure controlled ventilation during one-lung anaesthesia. *Br J Anaesth*, **79**:306–310.

Ueno T, Yokomise H, Oka T, et al. (1991) The effect of PGE1 and temperature on lung function following preservation. *Transplantation*, **52**:626–630.

Venkateswaran RV, Dronavalli V, Lambert PA, et al. (2009) The proinflammatory environment in potential heart and lung donors: prevalence and impact of donor management and hormonal therapy. *Transplantation*, **88**:582–588.

Venuta F, Rendina EA, Bufi M, et al. (1999) Preimplantation retrograde pneumoplegia in clinical lung transplantation. *J Thorac Cardiovasc Surg*, **118**:107–114.

Vincent JL, Baron JF, Reinhart K, et al. (2002) Anemia and blood transfusion in critically ill patients. *JAMA*, **288**:1499–1507.

Vizza CD, Lynch JP, Ochoa LL, Richardson G, Trulock EP (1998) Right and left ventricular dysfunction in patients with severe pulmonary disease. *Chest*, **113**:576–583.

Wan S, Desmet JM, Antoine M, Goldman M, Vincent JL, Leclerc JL (1996) Steroid administration in heart and heart–lung transplantation: is the timing adequate? *Ann Thorac Surg*, **61**:674–678.

Wang LS, Yoshikawa K, Miyoshi S, et al. (1989) The effect of ischemic time and temperature on lung preservation in a simple ex vivo rabbit model used for functional assessment. *J Thorac Cardiovasc Surg*, **98**:333–342.

Weil R, Clarke D, Iwaki Y, et al. (1981) Hyperacute rejection of a transplanted human heart. *Transplantation*, **32**(1):71–72.

Wiedemann K, Diestelhorst C (1995) The effect of sedation on pulmonary function. *Anaesthesist*, **44**(Suppl 3):S588–S593.

Wigfield CH, Love RB (2011) Donation after cardiac death lung transplantation outcomes. *Curr Opin Organ Transplant*, **16**:462–468.

Wittwer T, Franke UF, Fehrenbach A, et al. (2005) Experimental lung transplantation: impact of preservation solution and route of delivery. *J Heart Lung Transplant*, **24**:1081–1090.

Xu LF, Li X, Guo Z, et al. (2010) Extracorporeal membrane oxygenation during double-lung transplantation: single center experience. *Chin Med J (Engl)*, **123**:269–273.

Yusen RD, Shearon TH, Qian Y, et al. (2010) Lung transplantation in the United States, 1999–2008. *Am J Transplant*, **10**:1047–1068.

Zapol WM, Snider MT, Hill JD, et al. (1979) Extracorporeal membrane oxygenation in severe acute respiratory failure. A randomized prospective study. *JAMA*, **242**:2193–2196.

# CHAPTER 33

# Intensive care management of heart, lung, and heart–lung transplant recipients

Andrew C. Steel

## Introduction to heart transplantation

Heart transplantation has made remarkable progress since the early pioneering work of Norman Shumway (Shumway et al., 1966) and Christian Barnard's ground-breaking successful procedure (Barnard, 1968). The year 2011 saw the hundred-thousandth heart transplant recipient. Unlike the 1980s, when only 20% of transplanted patients were alive at 1 year, it is an established treatment modality for selected patients with end-stage heart failure who are not responding to any other maximal medical or surgical therapy. Recipients in 2011 should expect more than 90% of their cohort to be alive at 12 months, and for patients surviving to 1 year after transplant the median survival has reached 14 years (Stehlik et al., 2011). This advance has resulted from concurrent progress in all aspects of care: not only surgical techniques, but also appropriate patient selection, adequate donor management, organ procurement, and the prevention of perioperative complications through excellent intraoperative anaesthetic management and postoperative intensive care.

### Transition from the operating theatre to the ICU

The process of weaning from CPB is often challenging and can predict the nature of the first 48 hours of postoperative care. After the period of coronary reperfusion, allowing the myocardium to recover, the performance of the graft becomes apparent. The preservation of the myocardium, at the time of procurement, the recipient PAP, and the length of the ischaemic time are probably the most critical determinants of RV and LV function. Additional influences (see Table 33.1) include surgical technique (biatrial vs bicaval vs orthotopic vs heterotopic) and donor–recipient size matching which also affect postoperative management strategies. Inevitably there is a period of time during which the patient requires active haemodynamic support.

Patient transfer to the ICU and the initial period of intensive care management are critical to the success of this long-anticipated period of the recipient's life. The quality of the communication between team members at this point is crucial to the seamless transfer of care. There are several key pieces of information from the patient's medical history that must be reviewed, e.g. medications, allergies, cardiac assist devices, pulmonary hypertension, and renal function. In terms of the intraoperative period there are equally important details that should be directly communicated to the ICU team including: separation from bypass, TEE findings, risk of ongoing haemorrhage, transfusions given, vasoactive medications, immunosuppression induction therapy, and antibiotic prophylaxis given. To ensure that important details of the patient's history are not missed, and the therapeutic goals are established, many transplant programmes have adopted intraoperative (Weiser et al., 2010) and postoperative checklists and developed preprinted order sheets for postoperative care.

### Postoperative monitoring

The intraoperative monitoring of the cardiac transplantation patient typically includes: (1) continuous 5-lead ECG monitoring; (2) invasive arterial pressure monitoring; (3) direct measurement of right atrial pressure (RAP) or central venous pressure (CVP); (4) measurement of left atrial or pulmonary artery wedge pressure (PAWP); (5) intermittent or continuous thermodilution measurement of CO; (6) continuous measurement of arterial oxygen saturation; (7) intraoperative TEE; and (8) continuous assessment of urinary output.

On arrival, a chest radiograph is performed to determine the position of the PAC and central venous catheter and, importantly, to establish the validity of subsequent trends in pressure and oximetry measurements. In the postoperative period it would be advantageous to then add daily chest radiograph and 12-lead ECG, performed additionally pro re nata (PRN, as required). In our institution we use continuous mixed venous ($SvO_2$) oximetric catheters in our cardiac transplants and find this a useful index of cardiac output.

Baseline blood values to be measured on arrival are listed in Table 33.2.

## Immediate postoperative management

The early intensive care management of the newly transplanted heart allograft is relatively similar in approach to that for routine open-heart surgery. Care is centred on the maintenance of haemodynamic stability as the allograft adopts normal function following separation from CPB.

**Table 33.1** Factors determining initial allograft function. (Data from Costanzo, M.R., et al. 2010. The International Society of Heart and Lung Transplantation Guidelines for the care of heart transplant recipients. J.Heart Lung Transplant., 29, (8) 914-956 available from: PM:20643330.)

| Donor factors | Recipient factors |
|---|---|
| Older age donor | Preoperative condition |
| Infection preprocurement procedure | Vasomotor tone (especially significant if lowered by ACE inhibitors or amiodarone (Chin et al., 1999)) |
| Drug toxicities, e.g. cocaine, alcohol | Severity and reversibility of pulmonary hypertension |
| Prolonged ischaemic time > 4 hours | Pulmonary function |
| Anatomical abnormalities, e.g. coronary artery disease, valvular abnormality, ventricular hypertrophy, atresia of the coronary sinus ostium | Renal function and volume status |
| Donor–recipient size mismatch | Haemorrhage |
| Preservation of donor heart | Immunological compatibility |

## Heart rate and rhythm

Cardiac transplantation patients typically need chronotropic and inotropic support for a few days in the ICU, after which time the infusions can be weaned as tolerated. Bradycardia is relatively common in the postoperative period, commonly due to sinus bradycardia or slow junctional rhythms (Scott et al., 1994), and less frequently heart block. Where biatrial technique has been employed it may be difficult to discern whether atrioventricular dissociation is truly present because there will be a donor and recipient P wave on the ECG. There will be a degree of diastolic dysfunction in the extended period following reperfusion of the graft and therefore bradycardia is poorly tolerated. Optimally a heart rate of 90–110 beats per minute should be achieved, with atrial or atrioventricular pacing, or with infusion of isoproterenol in the event of sinus bradycardia.

**Table 33.2** Admission assessment of the heart transplant patient

| Investigation | Time/frequency |
|---|---|
| Complete blood count (CBC) | Admission, 12-hourly |
| Creatinine, blood urea nitrogen (BUN) | Admission, 12-hourly |
| Electrolytes (K, Na, Cl, Mg, Ca) | Admission, 6-hourly |
| Lactate | Admission, 6-hourly |
| Troponin I (TnI) | Admission, 12-hourly |
| Creatine kinase (CK) | Admission, 12-hourly |
| Glucose | Admission, with ABG |
| 12-lead ECG | Admission, daily, PRN |
| Chest radiograph | Admission, daily, PRN |
| Arterial blood gas (ABG) | Admission, PRN |
| Mixed venous blood gas (MVBG) | Admission, 4-hourly, PRN |

Older series published in the literature describe the incidence of postoperative pacing, beyond the second week, up to 25% following transplantations (Montero et al., 1992). However, more recent studies suggest that with modern surgical techniques 20–38% of patients require temporary pacing with bicaval and biatrial anastomosis, respectively (Weiss et al., 2008) and less than 5% of patients may require permanent pacemaker implantation after transplantation. Where necessary the implantation of a dual-chamber, rate-responsive device would seem the most appropriate choice.

Dysrrhythmias, particularly atrial flutter or fibrillation, are common after transplantation. Although there is some association between these arrhythmias and acute rejection, most episodes are not related to rejection (Pavri et al., 1995). The therapeutic strategy for the management of such dysrrhythmias is similar in approach to non-transplanted patients, with some important exceptions. These are the fundamental, physiological response of the denervated heart (see the section 'Physiology and pharmacology of the transplanted heart'), e.g. the transplanted heart is exquisitely sensitive to adenosine, and digoxin is less effective, and the interactions of agents (e.g. diltiazem) with the CNIs such as cyclosporine.

## Preload and afterload

Although hypovolaemia is poorly tolerated by the transplanted heart, preload should be carefully controlled (see Table 33.3). CVP or RAP and PCWP in isolation are neither exact *measurements* of volume status nor excellent surrogates (Michard et al., 2000). However, a rising trend is an indication of a graft under strain. Therefore targeting an RAP or PCWP of 8–10 mmHg remains a consistent goal in the immediate postoperative period. This is routinely achieved with strict control of fluid input and either infusion or repeated boluses of diuretics such as furosemide and metolazone.

# Physiology and pharmacology of the transplanted heart

## Physiology

The allograft should be performing significantly better than the explanted heart and therefore patients should be afforded significant clinical improvement. However, the new heart will not

**Table 33.3** Indicators of adequacy and goals for cardiac output

| Upstream indicators | Downstream indicators |
|---|---|
| Assess flow and pressure in the heart and great vessel. The traditional variables used to assess the haemodynamic status of the critically ill and at-risk patient | Account for alterations in the microvasculature as oxygen and metabolic needs vary Such variables estimate adequacy of cardiac output and perfusion pressure |
| Systemic blood pressure | Urine output |
| Heart rate | Serum lactate |
| CVP | Base deficit |
| PCWP | $SvO_2$ and $ScvO_2$ |
| Cardiac output | $SvCO_2$ and tissue $CO_2$ levels |

be without some physiological derangement. Where the biatrial technique is used there will be an anastomosis between donor and recipient atria—which will not be synchronous. Because the native P wave cannot traverse the suture line it has no influence on the chronotropic activity of the transplanted heart. Therefore many heart transplant recipients will lose up to 15% of the atrial systolic contribution to stroke volume. This is not the case with a bicaval technique and atrial contraction is more forceful in those patients (Freimark et al., 1995).

The haemodynamic characteristics of the transplanted heart are somewhat restrictive over the first few days to weeks, even in the absence of rejection. This will become less clinically apparent over time, but in 10–15% of patients a fluid challenge will reveal a persistent impairment of ventricular filling (Glazier et al., 1994). During long-term follow-up, ejection fraction, fractional shortening, and intracardiac pressures are largely normal.

Explanting of the recipient's heart will sever both afferent and efferent pathways, i.e. the transplanted heart has no sympathetic, parasympathetic, or sensory innervation. Sympathetic reinnervation, mainly of the anteroseptal wall, may occur after heart transplantation. This significantly improves the performance of the graft, but which patients will experience this is unpredictable (Bengel et al., 2001). The interruption of the afferent pathway results in impairment of the RAAS response to rising filling pressures. It will also render the patient at risk of silent ischaemia or infarction without experiencing classical angina pectoris.

The efferent innervation contains sympathetic and parasympathetic pathways. The loss of CNS control of the heart rate will cause the resting heart rate to be higher and less responsive to volume changes and vasomotor tone. The transplanted heart relies upon circulating catecholamines for enhancement of performance.

## Pharmacology

Intrinsic mechanisms and coronary autoregulation remain intact after heart transplantation. Carotid sinus massage and the Valsalva manoeuvre have no effect on the heart rate (Gelb, 1987). Other effects associated with heart denervation include loss of cardiac baroreflexes and loss of sympathetic response to laryngoscopy and tracheal intubation (Spann and Van, 1998). The denervated heart may have a more blunted heart rate response to inadequate anaesthetic depth or analgesia (Gelb, 1987).

Because heart denervation has important implications for the pharmacology of many drugs often used in the perioperative period, the therapeutic plan must take these differences into account. In the denervated heart the catecholamine response is different from that in the normal heart because intact sympathetic nerves are required for the normal uptake and metabolism of catecholamines. Receptor density is unchanged and the transplanted heart will respond to direct-acting drugs (e.g. sympathomimetics). Epinephrine and norepinephrine may exhibit an augmented inotropic effect in the recipient and both tend to have higher inotropic to vasoconstrictor predominance. Dopamine acting predominantly through release of norepinephrine is a less effective inotrope in the management of the transplant patient, having primarily dopaminergic and α effect (Bristow, 1990). The inotropic effects of isoproterenol and dobutamine are preserved and are both effective in the denervated heart.

Vagolytic drugs, such as atropine and glycopyrrolate, will be ineffective in increasing heart rate. Therefore when immediate chronotropy is required, drugs such as ephedrine and isoproterenol must be used. A summary of the changes associated with common drugs and their effect on the transplanted heart is given in Table 33.4.

## Right heart function

The leading causes of mortality in the first 30 days after heart transplantation are: graft failure, MOF, infection (non-CMV), acute rejection, cardiac allograft vasculopathy (CAV), and renal failure (see Figure 33.1) (Stehlik et al., 2011).

Failure to wean a heart transplant patient from CPB is most commonly the result of right heart failure. Echocardiography shows a dilated, poorly contracting RV and (usually) an underfilled, vigorously contracting LV. Severe tricuspid regurgitation as a consequence of dilatation of the annulus is also often seen. Chronically elevated left heart pressures cause high PVR in the recipient's lungs and are an important factor contributing to acute RV failure post-transplantation. The donor RV is unaccustomed to the high afterload and acutely fails. The RV may also be more susceptible than the LV to ischaemic injury between procurement and reperfusion.

**Table 33.4** The pharmacological responses of the transplanted heart

| Agent | Action | Effect on transplanted organ |
|---|---|---|
| Epinephrine | Direct agonism of β1, β2, α1 ADR | Augmented inotropic effect (β vs α agonism) following denervation |
| Norepinephrine | Direct agonism of β1, α1 ADR | Augmented inotropic effect (β vs α agonism) following denervation |
| Dobutamine | Direct agonism of β1 ADR | Normal action |
| Isoproterenol | Direct agonism of β1 ADR | Normal action |
| Ephedrine | Indirect agonism of α1 and β1 ADR | Reduced effect |
| Phenylephrine | Direct agonism of α1 ADR | Normal action |
| Dopamine | Reduced action via NE release, DA and α1 ADR agonism preserved | Reduced inotropic effect |
| β-blockers | Direct antagonism of β ADR | Increased sensitivity |
| Atropine | Vagolytic | No effect on heart rate |
| Pancuronium | Norepinephrine release | No tachycardia, normal systemic effect |
| Succinylcholine | Increased vagal tone | No bradycardia with repeated dosing |
| Neostigmine | Denervation | No bradycardia |
| Digoxin | Direct myocardial effect, denervation | Normal increase in contractility, minimal AV node effect |
| Adenosine | AV nodal blockade | Increased or prolonged blockade |
| Nitroglycerin | Baroreflex, no longer intact | No reflex tachycardia |

ADR, Adrenoreceptor; NE, norepinephrine; DA, dopaminergic; AV, atrioventricular.

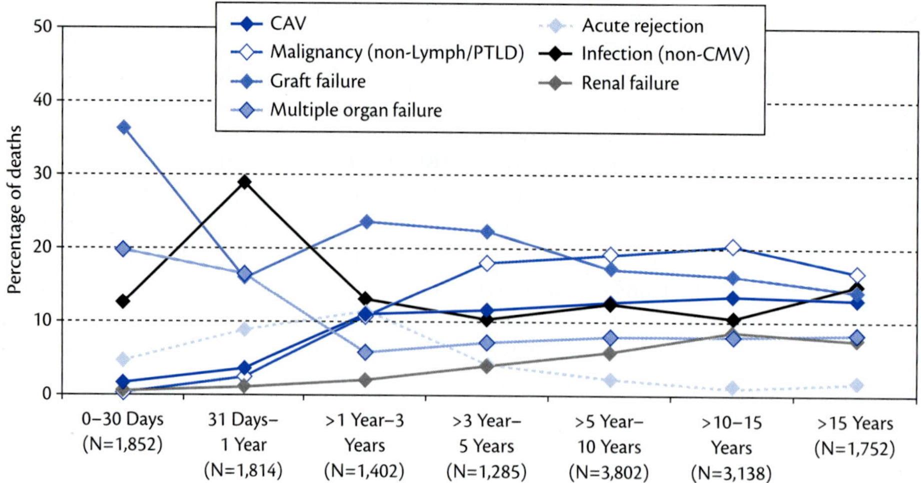


**Fig. 33.1** Relative incidences of the leading causes of post-transplant death in adult heart allograft recipients January 2000– June 2010. CAV, Cardiac allograft vasculopathy; CMV, cytomegalovirus; PTLD, post-transplant lymphoproliferative disorder. (Reprinted from *The Journal of Heart and Lung Transplantation*, 30, 10, Stehlik et al., 'The Registry of the International Society for Heart and Lung Transplantation: Twenty-eighth Adult Heart Transplant Report—2011', pp. 1078–1094, Copyright 2001, with permission from Elsevier and the International Society for Heart and Lung Transplantation.)

Treatment of right heart failure during heart transplantation has three major components: decreasing the afterload (PVR) and increasing myocardial contractility whilst maintaining an adequate systemic blood pressure to ensure sufficient RV perfusion. Adequate oxygenation and ventilation must be conserved to avoid pulmonary vasoconstriction from hypoxia and hypercarbia. Vasodilators such as nitroglycerine, sodium nitroprusside, $PGE_1$, and prostacyclin may be infused to reduce PVR but may affect SVR and cause hypotension. The phosphodiesterase inhibitor milrinone will increase contractility and decrease PVR but often requires simultaneous infusion of a vasoconstrictor to maintain SVR. The vasoconstrictors used to increase arterial blood pressure will also increase PVR, and achieving the proper balance of pulmonary and systemic vascular tone can be difficult.

Inhaled agents provide more selective pulmonary vasodilatation. NO is a potent vasodilator with a selective effect on the pulmonary vasculature because of its rapid breakdown in the lung. Administration has been shown to reduce PVR and improve RV function after CPB, and it may decrease the incidence of postoperative RV dysfunction (Rajek et al., 2000). $PGI_2$ (iloprost) can be nebulized and may be more effective than NO in decreasing PVR without decreasing systemic blood pressure in patients immediately after cardiac surgery, including heart transplantation (Sablotzki et al., 2002, 2003).

## Mechanical support

When cardiac failure after heart transplantation is severe and refractory to medical intervention, a mechanical assist device may be required. Although it is usually employed as an LV assist, IABP may be helpful in acute RV failure by improving perfusion and may provide the necessary support until function improves. In circumstances of extreme ventricular dysfunction following transplantation, right, left, or biventricular assist devices may be needed. The rationale of VAD insertion in this setting is that there may be a relatively quick recovery of ventricular function. One large centre (Kavarana et al., 2003) has found that almost half of the patients requiring VAD support after heart transplantation can be weaned but usually within 4 days, after which time the prognosis is very poor. Where there is both cardiac and pulmonary dysfunction many centres will opt for venoarterial extracorporeal membrane oxygenation (VA-ECMO) support instead of VAD insertion.

## Immunosuppression

*A fine balance exists between the risk of life-threatening rejection and the risk of life-threatening infection.* The finer points of immunosuppression will vary from centre to centre, 'all of which are certain that their particular immunosuppression cocktail is clearly the best' (Hosenpud, 2005) and all of which are to the same goal. The general principles are consistently the same (see Table 33.5): high dose induction immediately prior to surgery, followed by permanent combination therapy for maintenance. The intensity and combination is then adjusted according to side effects, e.g. neurotoxicity, organ dysfunction, especially kidney, and suspected or biopsy-proven episodes of rejection.

## Infection

All solid organ transplantation recipients are at risk for opportunistic infections as a result of their general health status, technical complications of surgery, use of parenteral nutrition, and immunosuppression. Complications resulting from infection are a major cause of death within the first year following heart transplant and the highest cause in the 30-day to 12-month period (Figure 33.1) (Stehlik et al., 2011). In addition to infection with common organisms such as *Pseudomonas aeruginosa* and *Staphylococcus aureus*, the immunocompromised heart transplant recipient is susceptible to organisms not ordinarily pathogenic to humans. All successful transplant programmes therefore must have policies and guidelines for both the prophylaxis and treatment of infection. The adopted strategy should be evidence-based, in context with local data (e.g. antibiograms), and supported by key individuals

**Table 33.5** Immunosuppression for heart transplant patients

| Agent | Mechanism of action |
|---|---|
| Methylprednisolone | Regulation of gene suppression leading to systemic suppression of inflammation and immune response |
| Antithymocyte globulin | T-cell depleting agent, modulation of integrins and cell adhesion molecules that facilitate leucocyte adhesion to the endothelium |
| Prednisolone | Regulation of gene suppression leading to systemic suppression of inflammation and immune response |
| Cyclosporine, tacrolimus | CNI preventing IL-2 production and full activation of T-cells |
| Azathioprine | Purine analogue incorporated into replicating DNA, blocking de-novo pathway of purine synthesis |
| Mycophenylate mofetil | Inhibition of purine synthesis necessary for T-cell activation |
| Sirolimus, everolimus | Target of rapamycin (TOR) inhibition |

including those with expertise in infectious diseases and antibiotic stewardship.

Infections in the early postoperative period can result from graft-transmitted pathogens from the donor. Therefore rapid communication between transplant centres and OPOs is needed in order for transplant teams to modify antibacterial regimens to target known pathogens in the donor. The larger source of early postoperative infections is nosocomial infections, i.e. those developing more than 48 hours after admission (Husain et al., 2011), such as catheter-related bloodstream infection (CRBSI), and ventilator-associated pneumonia. The presentation and natural course of these diseases will often be atypical, as the intense immunosuppression used during this period will retard the development of the inflammatory response.

Catheters remain the leading cause of early bloodstream infections in heart transplant patients. Like most patient populations, the cause of CRBSI is largely Gram-positive micro-organisms such as *Staphylococcus epidermidis*, although frequently the origin of a bloodstream infection in a heart transplant patient with multiple catheters is not determined. Prevention measures are fundamental in any critical care unit and must include education and training for all staff (Berenholtz et al., 2004), maximal sterile barrier precautions during catheter insertion, a 2% chlorhexidine/70% alcohol preparation for skin antisepsis (Maki et al., 1991), and avoiding the routine replacement of catheters (Cook et al., 1997). Management without catheter removal may be undertaken when indicated, although practice in our institution would be to remove even tunnelled lines in the event of confirmed CRBSI. Empiric therapy should cover Gram-positive, multidrug-resistant and Gram-negative bacteria, along with *Candida*. Prolonged antibiotic treatment exceeding 14 days is still recommended and should be continued up to 4–6 weeks in the case of *Staphylococcus aureus* (Mermel et al., 2009).

Although unlikely to manifest in the early postoperative ICU period, CMV is the most frequent opportunistic infection post-transplant. The ideal regimen for prophylaxis is much debated but not the necessity (Kotton et al., 2010). Prophylaxis against CMV should be initiated within 24–48 hours after surgery (Costanzo et al., 2010). In our institution it would be routine to administer ganciclovir (IV) or valganciclovir (po) for CMV prophylaxis in all heart transplants unless both recipient *and* donor are identified as CMV negative.

Generally, standard surgical antibacterial prophylaxis is recommended in transplant recipients, targeted to prevent surgical site infections. However, this regimen needs modification in circumstances in which there is a high risk of donor-derived bacterial infection. Surgical wound complications are more frequent in patients undergoing heart transplantation than in other heart surgery patients. Again this is probably attributable to the presence of additional risk factors in these patients, such as immunosuppression and mechanical assist devices. If a chronically infected device such as a VAD or a pacemaker is present, then perioperative antibiotics should be selected based upon microbiological sensitivities.

All solid organ transplantation recipients are at risk for invasive fungal infections as a result of their general health status, technical complications of surgery, use of parenteral nutrition, and immunosuppression. *Candida* and *Aspergillus* species have been reported as the most common fungal pathogens associated with invasive disease, although differences in the distribution of infections exist based on the organ transplanted. In lung and heart transplant recipients the reported annual incidence of invasive fungal infections lies between 15% and 35% (Dhar et al., 2012), with almost half of cases in heart transplant recipients occurring during the first 100 days post-transplant (Neofytos et al., 2010).

## Acute rejection

Approximately one-quarter of patients will be hospitalized for an episode of rejection during the first 12 months following transplantation (Lehmkuhl et al., 2009). If they survive the episode it will have a lasting detrimental long-term effect on their prognosis. The fundamental management of early rejection begins with early diagnosis, before the development of myocardial injury and endothelial cell proliferation. With adequate and aggressive immunosuppression regimes rejection remains uncommon in the first 14 days. However, because it is not uncommon for patients to remain longer on the ICU for the management of postoperative complications, an understanding of the mechanisms and appearance is important for the intensivist.

Allograft rejection traditionally has been classified into four classes: hyperacute rejection, acute cellular rejection, acute humoral rejection, and chronic rejection (see Table 33.6). The clinical presentation of rejection in cardiac transplant recipients can be variable and signs and symptoms fall into three groups: constitutional upset, myocardial irritability, and pump dysfunction or failure (Kirklin, 2005). Constitutional upset is vague and insidious in onset and includes symptoms such as malaise, fever, and discomfort. It is difficult to distinguish such symptoms from those experienced in a convalescent period following major surgery and critical illness, yet they may represent significant rejection.

Detection of anti-HLA antibodies that cause hyperacute and acute humoral rejection can be performed with pretransplant screening. A sample of the recipient's serum is combined with a 'panel' of known HLA antigens expressed on cells or materials from individuals felt to be representative of the potential donor

**Table 33.6** Classification of allograft rejection (Reproduced from Libby P et al., 'Macrophages and atherosclerotic plaque stability', *Current Opinion in Lipidology*, 7, 5, pp. 330–335, copyright 1996 with permission from Wolters Kluwer Health, Inc.)

| Classification | Mechanism |
|---|---|
| Hyperacute | Typically secondary to preformed, donor-specific Ab, e.g. ABO incompatibility |
| Acute cellular | $T_{helper}$-cell mediated |
| Acute humoral | Acquired or pre-existing anti-HLA Ab, e.g. expressed Ag on cell membranes of T-cells and B-cells |
| Chronic | Multifactorial insult and endothelial injury from both immune and non-immune mediators, e.g. overexpression of endothelial adhesion molecules (Libby et al., 1996) |

Ab, Antibody; Ag, antigen; HLA, human leucocyte antigen.

pool. This PRA test determines the percentage of possible donor HLA antigens targeted by the recipient's preformed circulating antibodies and is equivalent to the probability a recipient will reject a donor organ. In most centres a PRA ≥ 10% is the threshold above which virtual or real-time prospective cross-match should be done and antibody burden reduction performed, e.g. plasmapheresis.

Determining the presence of early rejection is difficult not least because correlation between clinical evidence, or presentation, and histology is poor. The gold standard for surveillance and investigation of acute cellular rejection since 1975 has been endomyocardial biopsy (EMB). This would be performed via the internal jugular approach or femoral vein for right heart biopsy and via femoral artery for left heart biopsy. The diagnosis of acute cellular rejection is based on the finding of lymphocytic infiltration and graded according to defined standards—the ISHLT EMB grading system, which is beyond the scope of this chapter. The risks of performing EMB depend on the clinical state of the patient and the experience of the operator. In a prospective analysis the incidence of complications arising from the biopsy procedure was found to be 3.3%, including two deaths (Deckers et al., 1992).

## Cardiac allograft vasculopathy

Chronic graft rejection is known as CAV, transplant vasculopathy, or transplant-associated coronary artery disease. It is a late complication and together with malignancy it represents the principal cause of death among long-term survivors of heart transplantation. Chronic allograft rejection usually presents as accelerated coronary artery disease. Because of the anatomical denervation, heart transplant recipients may have significant myocardial ischaemia without any clinical symptoms of pain.

Although milder forms of CAV do not compromise cardiac contractility, severe disease can lead to significant systolic and diastolic dysfunction (Uretsky et al., 1992). The clinical picture usually includes fatigue, ventricular dysrhythmias, congestive heart failure, and silent myocardial infarction on the ECG, and it can even present as sudden death.

The lesions of CAV can be treated by percutaneous coronary intervention (PCI) or grafted. However, because CAV compromises the entire vasculature, once it develops, any procedure to reopen epicardial arteries will be relatively ineffective, because current procedures cannot open small *intramyocardial* arteries. Disease progression has been somewhat attenuated by the introduction of target of rapamycin (TOR) inhibitors, sirolimus (Keogh et al., 2004), and everolimus (Eisen et al., 2003); however, for some patients cardiac retransplantation may be the only definitive, effective treatment option (Radovancevic et al., 2003).

## Malignancy

That which causes immunosuppression will elevate risk for the development of malignancy, and malignancies represent the leading cause of death among recipients at 5, 10, and 15 years post-transplant (Stehlik et al., 2011). The most important malignancies are PTLD and skin cancer. For heart transplant recipients, high-risk characteristics for PTLD include EBV seronegative patients (increased further by a seropositive donor), aggressive maintenance immunosuppression (including OKT3 induction) (Everly et al., 2007), and younger age (Ippoliti et al., 2011).

## Introduction to lung transplantation

The first human lung transplantation was performed as a combined heart and lung transplant in 1963 (Hardy et al., 1963). The patient survived almost 3 weeks before dying with renal failure. Following the important introduction of cyclosporine, the first isolated and successful lung transplant was performed in Toronto in 1983 (Toronto Lung Transplant Group, 1986). Since then the procedure has become an accepted, almost routine treatment option for patients with severe life-threatening respiratory diseases that are refractory to conventional therapies. The bilateral sequential lung transplant, with separate hilar anastomoses, was introduced in 1992 (Patterson, 1992) and is now the standard procedure for the majority of patients (Kaiser et al., 1991).

In 2005, 2,169 lung transplantations were performed, and that year bilateral sequential lung transplantation (DLTx) surpassed single lung transplants (SLTx) (Trulock et al., 2007). Overall survival after lung transplantation has now greatly improved. This is largely because of advances in surgical technique, improvements in immunosuppressive therapy, and earlier recognition and management of complications. In the immediate postoperative phase haemorrhage and mechanical complications are major concerns. In the perioperative phase, ischemia–reperfusion injury remains the gravest concern. With time, the consequences of multisystem organ failure, acute rejection, and infectious complications predominate.

### Immediate postoperative management

Attentive perioperative management of the lung transplant patient is of utmost importance to early and long-term outcomes. Since the operative procedure has been widely standardized, results of lung transplantation are much more dependent on the non-operative treatment strategies applied during this critical period. Patient care is delivered by a team of physicians and nurses who are supported by physiotherapists, psychologists, and other disciplines. The critical factor for success is the optimal coordination of these efforts through the preoperative and postoperative periods. This chapter intends to address the most important aspects of these cooperational efforts.

All lung transplant recipients are admitted to the ICU directly following their surgery. Immediate postoperative care can be defined by the various management issues, some of which are unique to this group of patients.

## Ventilator management and weaning

The patient's airway will be exchanged from a double lumen tube to a single lumen suction above the cuff endotracheal tube in the OR at the end of the procedure. Ventilation strategy from the time of bronchial anastomosis onwards should be protective—low tidal volumes (4–6 mL/kg ideal body weight) and low airway pressures. In the OR, initially pressure control is used with inspiratory pressures ($P_{insp}$) of 15–18 $cmH_2O$ and PEEP between 5 and 10 $cmH_2O$. $FiO_2$ is minimized to maintain saturations > 92% and reduce the contribution of oxygen and its potential to form oxidative free radicals, to avoid causing graft injury.

Ventilation management in the immediate postoperative period depends upon allograft function and the patient's overall condition. No clinical studies to date have proven benefit of any particular mode of ventilation in early lung transplantation. In our ICU facility it is practice to manage lung transplant recipients initially with PCV and assist-control (A/C) ventilation. On arrival in the ICU ABG analysis is performed on 100% oxygen and the same ventilation settings from the OR. At this stage, patients with an arterial partial pressure of oxygen ($PaO_2$) > 500 are considered to have an optimally functioning graft. To put this into context, a normal 40-year-old male with the same settings, and assuming a normal $PaCO_2$ of 40 mmHg, should have a $PaO_2$ of approximately 650 mmHg.

Partial pressure of arterial oxygen divided by the calculated partial pressure of oxygen in the alveolus ($PaO_2/P_AO_2$) may better reflect gas exchange over a broader range of $FiO_2$, but because of the simplicity of calculation, the ($PaO_2$:$FiO_2$) is used clinically. A–a gradient is not commonly used to assess graft function as it has such a wide variance with $FiO_2$. In one series the A–a gradient, when breathing 100% oxygen, varied from 8 to 82 mmHg in patients < 40 years of age and from 3 to 120 mmHg in patients > 40 years of age (Kanber et al., 1968).

After settling the patient, a chest radiograph is performed and then ventilator settings are weaned. Our ventilation strategy would be similar to that of the ARDS Network protocol—conservative, protective tidal volume range of 5–7 mL/kg, plateau pressures < 32 cm $H_2O$, and goals of $SpO_2$ > 92% and pH > 7.3 (Acute Respiratory Distress Syndrome Network, 2000). Patients are nursed in semirecumbent position (Drakulovic et al., 1999) and continually assessed by intensive care physicians, nurses, and respiratory therapists. Particularly we are vigilant of changes in oxygenation or deterioration in lung compliance—both indicators of early graft dysfunction.

SLTx performed for emphysema can pose different challenges. Native and donor lungs will have very different mechanical properties, e.g. the native emphysematous lung has higher compliance than donor lung. In these patients lower PEEP is often used, but if the transplanted lung becomes dysfunctional and requires higher inspiratory pressure and PEEP, the native, compliant lung can become overinflated. This can compress pulmonary vessels in the native lung and shunt pulmonary blood flow to the transplant lung. Mediastinal shift towards the transplant lung can lead to significant compromise of cardiac output. Isolated lung ventilation with double-lumen, endotracheal tube with each lung ventilated independently may be employed—although it is rarely necessary in our experience. Placing these patients with graft down and native lung up will increase gravitational flow of the blood to better ventilate the lung, improving V/Q mismatch and it may improve oxygenation.

For donor lungs that are too large for the recipient, downsizing by plication or by lobectomy has been performed. When severe hyperinflation develops, lung volume reduction surgery of the native lung is sometimes needed. Size differences of 10–25% between a donor lung and a recipient thoracic cage have been reported to be acceptable.

Recipients transplanted with severe, refractory pulmonary hypertension are not weaned immediately. Such patients often demonstrate labile pulmonary hypertension as well as frequent episodes of desaturation with minimal provocation. These patients are ventilated for at least 24–48 hours with assist-control ventilation along with sedation and neuromuscular blockade where required. Gradual weaning is continued after 24–48 hours or when frequent desaturation is no longer an issue.

## Fluid management and haemodynamics

Haemodynamic status can be somewhat volatile during the first few hours. Patients are routinely monitored with pulmonary artery flotation catheters (PAFCs), and $SvO_2$ and cardiac index (CI) are closely followed. Vasopressors and/or inotropes are added to support systemic perfusion and oxygen delivery when needed. Commonly used agents include norepinephrine, epinephrine, and milrinone. The addition of milrinone has the added benefit of greater lusitropy, synergistic action with epinephrine, and a degree of pulmonary artery dilatation (Colucci, 1991). Fluid therapy should be relatively restricted to reduce pulmonary capillary pressure and endothelial leak, whilst maintaining adequate urine output and systemic perfusion. Later in the postoperative stay diuretics are used to maintain urine output and help mobilize fluids. In most recipients there is a degree of pulmonary oedema due to capillary leak, severed lymphatics, 'third space' sequestration, and consequent to volume given during CPB.

Haematocrit is kept in the range of 25–30% , although no studies are available to support this. Clinical evidence of coagulopathy is corrected with the administration of FFP or specific coagulation factor replacement where required.

Postoperative hypotension can be due to any of several reasons including: hypovolaemia, systemic inflammatory response, haemorrhage, acute myocardial injury, epidural or medication effects, hyperinflation of a native lung in SLTx patients, pulmonary embolism, vascular obstruction, and anaphylaxis. As with open-heart procedures, pericardial tamponade can still occur from localized clot formation and despite breaching of the pericardium at the time of pulmonary vein anastomosis.

## Postoperative analgesia

Post-thoracotomy or clamshell incision pain has both nociceptive and neuropathic components. The acute phase of postoperative pain, which can last for several weeks, is aggravated by the presence of intercostal drains, and exacerbated by movement—especially coughing and deep inspiration. As a result of poor analgesia, early mobilization, essential to recovery, is delayed. There is also an established correlation between the severity of the acute phase and the development of postoperative complications, including chronic post-thoracotomy pain (Katz et al., 1996).

Early mobilization and rehabilitation following surgery requires a multilateral approach and fundamental to this process is immaculate postoperative analgesia. Intravenous opioids alone are inadequate without significant adverse events (Savage et al., 2002). Pain control can be achieved when a variety of routes of administration, agents, and interventions are employed—multimodal analgesia. Pain is targeted in a receptor-based approach using acetaminophen, opioids such as hydromorphone, and using 'opioid-sparing' analgesic properties of $\beta_2$ receptor agonism (dexmedetomidine, clonidine), NMDA receptor channel blockade (ketamine), and gabapentin. As discussed below, NSAIDs such as ketorolac and ibuprofen should be avoided at all cost because of their synergistic nephrotoxicity with CNIs.

Current evidence remains in favour of the use of TEA as part of a multimodal strategy for improving outcomes after lung transplant (Pottecher et al., 2011). Indeed, the benefit has been shown in terms of not only duration of mechanical ventilation but also reducing the ICU length of stay and the number of respiratory complications. Importantly, it has been shown in the literature that the risk of epidural haematoma is rare even where CPB is used. However, many clinicians, and patients, may feel that the devastating outcome of such a rare complication outweighs the benefit of TEA (Ronald et al., 2006).

### Early mobilization

Many patients listed for lung transplantation will experience severe deconditioning prior to their surgery. This is worsened and even accelerated if there are postoperative complications. Mobilization and physiotherapy of the patient after transplantation is critical and has substantial evidence supporting its benefit in the long-term outcome (Wickerson et al., 2010). In TGH, early mobilization is aggressively pursued and attempted on the first postoperative day, even if a patient is not extubated and is still requiring vasoactive medications. Frequent, early chest physiotherapy, including percussion and postural drainage, is used to help clear secretions and recruit atelectatic lung units. Theoretically, this activity stimulates 'ergoreceptors', enhancing the release of neurotransmitters and endorphins. This supports recovery through, for example, early weaning from mechanical ventilation, decreased delirium, and improved affect.

## Complications

In the immediate postoperative phase, worry regarding cardiovascular stability, haemorrhage, and other mechanical complications predominates. However, in the early period of the ICU stay the development of respiratory failure remains the gravest concern. The most common causes of respiratory failure are reperfusion injury (55%) and perioperative cardiovascular/haemorrhagic events (36%), and the mortality rate for patients who develop respiratory failure is approximately 45%. In the first postoperative week, reperfusion injury and infection are leading causes, whereas in the second week, rejection, infection, and airway problems become more prevalent.

### Primary graft dysfunction

PGD is synonymous with ischemia–reperfusion injury, post-transplant ALI, ARDS, and primary graft failure. Like ALI, it is a disease spectrum (see Table 33.7), of which severe PGD remains the primary cause of 30-day mortality, representing more than a quarter of deaths (27.1%) in the first month post-transplant (Christie et al., 2011). PGD is also associated with longer median hospital stay (47 vs 15 days) and longer duration of mechanical ventilation (15 vs 1 day) (Christie et al., 2005b). Amelioration would certainly improve both early and late transplantation outcomes; unfortunately neither improvements in procurement and implantation surgical techniques nor post-operative intensive care have resulted in a notable reduction of PGD after transplant (Kuntz et al., 2009).

**Table 33.7** ISHLT grading of primary graft dysfunction (Reproduced from Libby P et al., 'Macrophages and atherosclerotic plaque stability', *Current Opinion in Lipidology*, 7, 5, pp. 330–335, copyright 1996 with permission from Wolters Kluwer Health, Inc)

| Grade | $PaO_2/FiO_2$ | Radiographic infiltrates (consistent with pulmonary oedema) |
|---|---|---|
| 0 | > 300 | Absent |
| 1 | > 300 | Present |
| 2 | 200–300 | Present |
| 3 | < 200 | Present |

PGD typically occurs within the first 48 hours and up to 72 hours following implantation. The characteristics of the condition are: primarily impaired gas exchange with intrapulmonary shunt, diminishing lung compliance, pulmonary oedema, pulmonary infiltrates on chest radiograph, increased vascular resistance (PVR), and (if biopsy performed) diffuse alveolar damage (DAD). The underlying pathogenesis is not well understood, not beyond that of ARDS, and it represents a summation of acute injuries related to the donor lung, the transplantation process (retrieval, preservation, implantation, and reperfusion), and recipient risk factors.

Although many donor and recipient risk factors for post-transplantation PGD have been identified, few clinical studies have analyzed their relative impact. 'Traditional' inherent donor's risk factors are increased age, smoking history, and female gender, whereas acquired donor factors include the occurrence of brain death, prolonged ventilation, aspiration, pneumonia, trauma, and haemodynamic instability before organ retrieval. Recipient's risk factors include pulmonary fibrosis, pre-existing pulmonary hypertension, and the use of CPB.

### Treatment of severe primary graft dysfunction

Treatment remains primarily supportive for ARDS and most patients with PGD improve within the first 72 hours after transplantation. However, a small minority progress to develop a severe form of PGD and present an extremely challenging group to manage. Although ALI in this context is essentially reversible, it results in profound hypoxaemia, refractory acidosis, and eventually MOF.

It is very important to rule out other causes of respiratory failure at this stage of the clinical course, especially overhydration, infection, haemorrhage, and pulmonary venous obstruction. The latter can cause outflow obstruction and may present on chest X-ray as a more discrete, lobar opacification.

No firm consensus currently exists regarding the optimal postoperative care strategy and there have been no clinical studies that have systematically and specifically evaluated the effect of various modalities (mechanical ventilation, fluid management, circulatory support, etc.) on outcome. The general principles of treatment of patients with PGD are outlined in Table 33.8.

## Neurological complications

Neurological complications are common and occur in 25–31% of lung transplant recipients (Goldstein et al., 1998; Mateen et al., 2010). Severe complications necessitating hospital admission or evaluation are most commonly stroke or encephalopathy. Neurological complication of any severity, but particularly severe forms (hazard ratio 7.2), are associated with an increased risk of death (Mateen et al., 2010).

**Table 33.8** Treatment of severe primary graft dysfunction

| Therapeutic intervention | Strategy |
|---|---|
| Ventilation | ◆ Protective ventilation (VTe 4–6 mL/kg, Pplat < 32 cm$H_2O$, minimal $FiO_2$, higher PEEP<br>◆ Goals: $SpO_2$ > 92%, pH > 7.25 |
| Fluid management | ◆ Avoid excessive administration of fluids, including blood products, that raise capillary pressure<br>◆ Use of early renal replacement therapy for uraemia |
| Vasoactive medications | ◆ Use of inotropic agents to maintain adequate CI and systemic blood pressure<br>◆ Decreased augmentation of stroke volume with fluids |
| Nitric oxide | ◆ Exogenous NO and replenish cGMP levels<br>◆ Reduce PVR and improve V/Q matching<br>◆ Restore pulmonary capillary integrity<br>◆ Decrease leucocyte migration and platelet aggregation<br>◆ Decrease endothelin-1 production |
| Prostaglandins ($PGE_1$) | ◆ Mediate inflammation and regulation of blood flow<br>◆ Increase cAMP—reduces neutrophil adhesion, capillary permeability, and platelet aggregation<br>◆ Vasodilatation |
| Surfactant protein-A (SP-A) | ◆ Administration of nebulized exogenous SP-A-enriched surfactant—inactivated at a slower rate than endogenous<br>◆ Some improvement in oxygenation and compliance of allograft |
| Extracorporeal support | ◆ VV-ECMO or carbon dioxide removal ($ECCO_2r$) for haemodynamically stability<br>◆ Veno-arterial support (VA-ECMO) for those not stable<br>◆ Reserved ordinarily for the most severe PGD<br>◆ Early (< 24 hours) more successful and in specific populations, e.g. pulmonary hypertension<br>◆ Not advocated later than 7days post-transplant |

Pplat, Plateau pressure; VV-ECMO, venovenous extracorporeal membrane oxygenation; $ECCO_2r$, extracorporeal $CO_2$ elimination; VTe, exhaled tidal volume.

It is beyond the scope of this chapter to exhaustively describe all the neurological complications of solid organ transplant. However, the neurotoxicity of immunosuppressive agents deserves some discussion. This is not an infrequent complication and will occur in the context of new or established therapy and low, normal, or high plasma levels. The more likely causative agents are cyclosporine, tacrolimus, and corticosteroids. Frequent clinical presentations of neurotoxicity include seizures, encephalopathy, tremor, chorea, and even peripheral neuropathy. It has been suggested that concurrent hypomagnesaemia or hypocholesterolaemia are precipitating factors for neurotoxicity related to cyclosporine (de Groen et al., 1987). This is not consistently found, but low magnesium levels are certainly unfavourable—lowering seizure thresholds and increasing dysrrhythmias.

## Renal complications

Renal dysfunction (as defined by the Acute Kidney Injury Network) is common and seen in up to 23.9% of lung transplant recipients, but only 1.6% require long-term dialysis at the end of the first postoperative year and 2.5% at 5 years (Christie et al., 2011). Injury is often multifactorial including hypovolaemia and acute tubular necrosis, cyclosporine use, contrast-induced nephropathy, and other medications, e.g. amino glycosides. Renal dysfunction at 30 days is highly predictive of renal function at 5 years (Ishani et al., 2002).

In addition to the desired immunosuppressive effect, administration of CNIs is associated with the nearly universal consequence of nephrotoxicity. Acute nephrotoxicity is a result of intense vasoconstriction at the preglomerular (afferent) arterioles, leading to a decrease in renal blood flow and glomerular filtration rate. These effects are dose-related and can be reversible upon withdrawal of the agent. Table 33.9 lists the immunosuppressive agents commonly used in lung transplantation.

With this in mind, extremely high doses of CNIs should be avoided and patients with high creatinine levels are given basiliximab (anti-CD25 monoclonal antibody on IL-2 receptor) during the perioperative period instead. Furthermore, and even when postoperative analgesia is challenging, NSAIDs should be avoided at all cost and diuretics used on an as needed, not overzealous, basis.

## Acute rejection

Acute rejection is usually seen after the first week post-transplant but rarely within the first week. It presents as poor graft function and diffuse infiltrates. In these cases, rapid reassessment of donor–recipient cross-match is done. It is very important to try to exclude infection first as a cause of problem. Rejection is treated with high-dose steroids, antilymphocytic drugs, or plasmapheresis. The presence of preformed antibodies to donor organ-specific HLA or ABO antigens is thought to play a central role in hyperacute rejection, which is a fulminant, rapidly evolving, fatal clinical syndrome that may occur immediately after transplantation. Patients who have PRA levels > 25% receive plasmapheresis and intravenous immunoglobulin both prior to and following transplantation. The benefits of these interventions, however, remain to be proven.

## Infection and sepsis

Lung transplant recipients are at particularly high risk for developing pneumonia due to the unique susceptibility of

**Table 33.9** Immunosuppression regime for lung transplantation

| Preoperative | Intraoperative | Early ICU postoperative | Late ICU or HDU postoperative |
|---|---|---|---|
| Cyclosporine 5 mg/kg po (max 350 mg) | | Cyclosporine 5 mg/kg q 12-hourly po | |
| Tacrolimus 0.05 mg/kg po | | Tacrolimus 0.1 mg/kg q 12-hourly po | |
| | Methylprednisolone 500 mg IV on induction | Methylprednisolone (day 1–3) 0.5 mg/kg/day IV | |
| | | | Prednisolone (day 4) 0.5 mg/kg/ day po |
| | | Azathioprine | |
| | | Mycophenolate mofetil | |
| | | Basiliximab (day 0) 20 mg IVI or bolus | Basiliximab (day 4) 20 mg IVI or bolus |
| | | Thymoglobulin | |

HDU, High-dependency unit; IVI, intravenous infusion.

transplanted lung to bacterial and fungal infections. Lung allograft is denervated with decreased mucociliary clearance and cough reflex. In addition to generalized immunosuppression, lung is the only allograft continuously exposed to the environment and colonizing micro-organisms of the upper respiratory airways. Pneumonia is a significant contributor to poor outcome and mortality in lung transplant recipients, accounting for approximately 35% of deaths in the first year post-transplantation. *Pseudomonas aeruginosa* is the most frequent agent of respiratory infections, followed by *Staphylococcus aureus*. Therefore empiric antibiotic prophylaxis must consider these micro-organisms. In TGH the current standard is to use piperacillin/tazobactam as prophylaxis for non-CF patients. In the event that Gram-positive cocci are found in donor sputum, vancomycin is added until speciation and susceptibilities are known.

Recipients with CF or other suppurative lung disease, i.e. bronchiectasis, are at increased risk since there is association between pretransplant colonizing micro-organisms and early pneumonias in these patients. Their perioperative prophylaxis must depend upon their previous culture and sensitivity results and should be planned by infectious disease experts. In most cases, aggressive *Pseudomonas* infection cover will be the strategy for prophylaxis with a combination of ceftazidime, meropenem, and inhaled tobramycin. The role of selective decontamination of the digestive tract in lung transplantation has yet to be established.

Other factors promoting infection include the use of multiple invasive devices (endotracheal intubation, nasogastric tube, chest tubes, etc.) as well as immunosuppression. Orogastric tube should be preferred over the nasogastric route to reduce the incidence of sinus infections.

## Dysrrhythmia

Postoperative atrial dysrhythmia is seen in 20–39% of lung transplantation patients, with the peak incidence 2 days after transplant (Nielsen et al., 2004). This period corresponds to early sympathetic stimulation, peaks in pain, and fluid shift that occur immediately after surgery. There are also the additional confounding factors of hypoxia and graft dysfunction.

Careful attention should be paid to fluid balance to prevent atrial dilatation and activation of the RAAS, which has been implicated in the genesis of AF. Similarly, aggressive diuresis should be avoided, as it will produce hypotension, tachycardia, hypomagnesaemia, and hypokalaemia—all of which predispose patients to AF. Older patients and those with primary pulmonary hypertension are at further risk.

Ventricular rate control with metoloprolol, diltiazem, or digoxin is effective in up to one-quarter of such cases. The primary anti-arrhythmic used in the adult critical care population is amiodarone. Its early action on the β-adrenergic receptors offers excellent rate control, and its later potassium channel antagonism contributes to potential for cardioversion. However, amiodarone is not ideal in the short term in the ICU, nor preferred for long-term use due to its potential pulmonary toxicity (Donaldson et al., 1998).

Immediate correction of hypomagnesaemia and hypokalaemia is very important in the early ICU period. With aggressive treatment, sinus rhythm can be restored in almost all patients and anticoagulation largely avoided. Development of postoperative AF has been found to result in a longer ICU stay and may be associated with increased mortality (Nielsen et al., 2004; Isiadinso et al., 2011). It is our practice to anticoagulate patients with AF, persisting for more than 48 hours, with intravenous infusion of heparin.

## Gastrointestinal complications

Many patients have GI symptoms in the early postoperative period. Nausea and vomiting are common, and ileus is frequently due to the same factors, i.e. narcotics, immobility, and electrolyte disturbance. Gastroparesis can lead to vomiting and increase risk of aspiration, and chronic aspiration may contribute to long-term graft failure. Gastroparesis is perhaps caused by foregut parasympathetic dysfunction due to the surgery. Motility agents are prescribed immediately if high residuals (> 300 mL) are seen with enteral tube feeds.

Patients who have undergone lung transplantation should have bowel routine ordered when started on a regimen of PCA or an epidural in the ICU. This should include stool softener, stimulant laxatives, and if there has been no bowel movement after 72 hours, the use of a bisacodyl suppository.

Patients with CF are prone to distal intestinal obstruction syndrome (DIOS), in which ileocaecal obstruction is caused by viscid mucofaeculent material. This occurs in approximately 10% of CF patients undergoing lung transplantation (Morton et al., 2009). Therefore all lung transplant recipients with CF should have bowel routine and bowel preparation solution (a combination preparation of polyethylene glycol 3350 and electrolyte) as a preventive measure. It is initiated after the transplantation at 50–100 mL/hour until passage of stools. When non-operative therapy is unsuccessful, patients with DIOS require early aggressive management with timely laparotomy with enterotomy and possible stoma formation.

### Airway complications

Bronchial anastomosis used to be a common site of complications when end-to-end bronchial anastomosis combined with an omentopexy was performed. Advancements in surgical technique using telescoping anastomosis, with the cartilaginous portions of the donor and recipient bronchi intussuscepted and without use of omentum or other tissue wrap, have reduced focal necrosis to 1.4% of recipients with this method.

Bronchial stenosis has been reported to range from 1.6% to 24.4%. It is seen at the anastomotic site but rarely at the segmental non-anastomotic site. Several factors may impair airway healing after transplant which might contribute to this complication including ischaemia due to lack of blood flow to donor bronchus, inadequate organ preservation, rejection, immunosuppression, and infection. Balloon dilatation, laser therapy, and stenting in combination are effective in up to 90% of patients. If endoscopic therapies fail, surgical options are employed depending upon the extent and location of stenosis. Surgical options include reconstruction of bronchial anastomosis, sleeve resection with or without parenchymal sacrifice, and retransplantation.

## Heart–lung transplantation

Following Shumway's early pioneering work in heart transplantation, Reitz and colleagues (Reitz, 2011) performed the first successful heart–lung transplant in 1981 and the TGH group achieved successful SLTx a few years later.

Indications for combined heart–lung transplantation have become restricted because of the success of isolated lung transplantation and the limited availability of donors. Even in patients with severe pulmonary hypertension and RV dysfunction, lung transplantation is a very good option (Kramer et al., 1994). However, combined heart–lung transplantation procedure is necessary in patients with irreparable congenital cardiac lesions, such as ventricular septal defect (VSD) leading to Eisenmenger syndrome, and severe combined cardiopulmonary disease such as that seen with CF.

Unlike bilateral sequential lung transplant the operative procedure must be performed with CPB. The heart and lungs are removed, with care taken to preserve the phrenic nerves and to address the bronchial artery circulation—so as to reduce postoperative bleeding complications. Next, the donor heart and lungs are inserted en bloc and the tracheal anastomosis is performed. Following this the right atrial anastomosis is performed, followed by the aortic anastomosis. Care is taken to keep the donor trachea as short as possible because of the limited vascularity of the area. In recent years many institutions have favoured bilateral bronchial anastomosis instead of tracheal—reducing complications of surgery, especially haemorrhage.

The critical care management of heart–lung transplant recipients requires a combined understanding and experience of managing both the heart and the lung transplant recipient. Many of the key responsibilities of the intensivist and therapeutic protocols are central to the management of all cardiothoracic transplant patients. The haemodynamic goals and management outlined for heart transplant recipients and the ventilation strategy for both heart and lung transplant recipients are essential for patients undergoing combined transplantation.

The surgical procedure is unlikely to be the patient's first cardiothoracic operation. It will require extensive dissection during the process of explanation and always requires prolonged CPB. When combined with the associated comorbidities of congenital heart disease or CF, the result is that complications are more frequent and more significant. Haemorrhage may occur due to extensive dissection and systemic pulmonary collaterals in congenital heart disease, complicated by multifactorial coagulopathy. As with all cardiothoracic surgical patients, it must be treated aggressively and with far higher thresholds for transfusion than stable ICU patients (Hebert et al., 1999). Other early complications include tracheal anastomotic dehiscence, acute reperfusion injury due to long ischaemic times, and infection. Heart–lung recipients have three times as many infections as heart recipients and this contributes to their early mortality rate. Infection is the major cause of mortality in the first 6 months and rejection thereafter (Christie et al., 2011).

## Conclusion

In this chapter we have reviewed the intensive care management of recipients of heart, heart–lung, and lung transplants. These procedures are complex and should be performed at highly specialized and experienced transplant centres. Since 2005 we have gained substantial experience in the management of these cases. Clinical experience gained coupled with advances in immunosuppressive regimens have resulted in higher survival rates and better quality of life. Furthermore, as intraoperative procedures have become widely standardized, results of cardiothoracic transplantation are much more dependent on the non-operative treatment strategies applied during the immediate postoperative period. Therefore the quality of the communication and teamwork among the various interdisciplinary members of the transplant team are crucial elements in the delivery of care. We have also presented evidence to illustrate that the essential approach to the management of the transplanted heart includes careful control of cardiac indices, in particular preload. Another critical aspect is the fact that the transplanted heart is without sympathetic, parasympathetic, or sensory enervation. In the immediate postoperative period, ventilation management is dependent upon allograft function and the patient's overall condition. Finally, we have advocated for a protective ventilation strategy aimed at supporting the patient and not normalizing physiological parameters. It is important to note that the leading causes of morbidity and mortality in these patients in the first 30 days after transplantation are graft failure, MOF, infection, and renal failure.

## References

Acute Respiratory Distress Syndrome Network (2000) Ventilation with lower tidal volumes as compared with traditional tidal volumes for acute lung injury and the acute respiratory distress syndrome. *N Engl J Med*, **342**(18):1301–1308.

Barnard CN (1968) Human cardiac transplantation. An evaluation of the first two operations performed at the Groote Schuur Hospital, Cape Town. *Am J Cardiol*, **22**(4):584–596.

Bengel FM, Ueberfuhr P, Schiepel N, Nekolla SG, Reichart B, Schwaiger M (2001) Effect of sympathetic reinnervation on cardiac performance after heart transplantation. *N Engl J Med*, **345**(10):731–738.

Berenholtz SM, Pronovost PJ, Lipsett PA, et al. (2004) Eliminating catheter-related bloodstream infections in the intensive care unit. *Crit Care Med*, **32**(10)2014–2020.

Bristow MR (1990) The surgically denervated, transplanted human heart. *Circulation*, **82**(2):658–660.

Chin C, Feindel C, Cheng D (1999) Duration of preoperative amiodarone treatment may be associated with postoperative hospital mortality in patients undergoing heart transplantation. *J Cardio-Thorac Vasc Anesth*, **13**(5): 562–566.

Christie JD, Carby M, Bag R, Corris P, Hertz M, Weill D (2005a) Report of the ISHLT working group on primary lung graft dysfunction. Part II: definition. A consensus statement of the International Society for Heart and Lung Transplantation. *J Heart Lung Transplant*, **24**(10):1454–1459.

Christie JD, Sager JS, Kimmel SE, et al. (2005b) Impact of primary graft failure on outcomes following lung transplantation. *Chest*, **127**(1):161–165.

Christie JD, Edwards LB, Kucheryavaya AY, et al. (2011) The Registry of the International Society for Heart and Lung Transplantation: twenty-eighth adult lung and heart–lung transplant report—2011. *J Heart Lung Transplant*, **30**(10):1104–1122.

Colucci WS (1991) Cardiovascular effects of milrinone. *Am Heart J*, **121**(6 Pt 2):1945–1947.

Cook D, Randolph A, Kernerman P, et al. (1997) Central venous catheter replacement strategies: a systematic review of the literature. *Crit Care Med*, **25**(8):417–1424.

Costanzo MR, Dipchand A, Starling R, et al. (2010) The International Society of Heart and Lung Transplantation guidelines for the care of heart transplant recipients. *J Heart Lung Transplant*, **29**(8):914–956.

de Groen PC, Aksamit AJ, Rakela J, Forbes GS, Krom RA (1987) Central nervous system toxicity after liver transplantation. The role of cyclosporine and cholesterol. *N Engl J Med*, **317**(14):861–866.

Deckers JW, Hare JM, Baughman KL (1992) Complications of transvenous right ventricular endomyocardial biopsy in adult patients with cardiomyopathy: a seven-year survey of 546 consecutive diagnostic procedures in a tertiary referral center. *J Am Coll Cardiol*, **19**(1):43–47.

Dhar D, Dickson JL, Carby MR, Lyster HS, Hall AV, Banner NR (2012) Fungal infection in cardiothoracic transplant recipients: outcome without systemic amphotericin therapy. *Transpl Int*, **25**(7):758–764.

Donaldson L, Grant IS, Naysmith MR, Thomas JS (1998) Acute amiodarone-induced lung toxicity. *Inten Care Med*, **24**(6):626–630.

Drakulovic MB, Torres A, Bauer TT, Nicolas JM, Nogue S, Ferrer M (1999) Supine body position as a risk factor for nosocomial pneumonia in mechanically ventilated patients: a randomised trial. *Lancet*, **354**(9193):1851–1858.

Eisen HJ, Tuzcu EM, Dorent R, et al. (2003) Everolimus for the prevention of allograft rejection and vasculopathy in cardiac-transplant recipients. *N Engl J Med*, **349**(9):847–858.

Everly MJ, Bloom RD, Tsai DE, Trofe J (2007) Posttransplant lymphoproliferative disorder. *Ann Pharmacother*, **41**(11):1850–1858.

Freimark D, Czer LS, Aleksic I, et al. (1995) Improved left atrial transport and function with orthotopic heart transplantation by bicaval and pulmonary venous anastomoses. *Am Heart J*, **130**(1):121–126.

Gelb AW (1987) Anaesthesia for organ transplantation. *Can J Anaesth*, **34**(Suppl 1):S12–S15.

Glazier JJ, Mullen GM, Johnson MR, et al. (1994) Factors associated with the development of persistently depressed cardiac output during the first year after cardiac transplantation. *Clin Cardiol*, **17**(9):489–494.

Goldstein LS, Haug MT 3rd, Perl J, et al. (1998) Central nervous system complications after lung transplantation. *J Heart Lung Transplant*, **17**(2):185–191.

Hardy JD, Webb WR, Dalton ML Jr, Walker GR Jr (1963) Lung Homotransplantation in Man. *JAMA*, **186**:1065–1074.

Hebert PC, Wells G, Blajchman MA, et al. (1999) A multicenter, randomized, controlled clinical trial of transfusion requirements in critical care. Transfusion requirements in critical care investigators, Canadian Critical Care Trials Group. *N Engl J Med*, **340**(6):409–417.

Hosenpud JD (2005) Immunosuppression in cardiac transplantation. *N Engl J Med*, **352**(26):2749–2750.

Husain S, Mooney ML, Danziger-Isakov L, et al. (2011) A 2010 working formulation for the standardization of definitions of infections in cardiothoracic transplant recipients. *J Heart Lung Transplant*, **30**(4):361–374.

Ippoliti G, Pellegrini C, Nieswandt V (2011) Controversies about induction therapy. *Transplant Proc*, **43**(6)2450–2452.

Ishani A, Erturk S, Hertz MI, Matas AJ, Savik K, Rosenberg ME (2002) Predictors of renal function following lung or heart–lung transplantation. *Kidney Int*, **61**(6):2228–2234.

Isiadinso I, Meshkov AB, Gaughan J, et al. (2011) Atrial arrhythmias after lung and heart–lung transplant: effects on short-term mortality and the influence of amiodarone. *J.Heart Lung Transplant*, **30**(1):37–44.

Kaiser LR, Pasque MK, Trulock EP, Low DE, Dresler CM, Cooper JD (1991) Bilateral sequential lung transplantation: the procedure of choice for double-lung replacement. *Ann Thorac Surg*, **52**(3):438–445.

Kanber GJ, King FW, Eshchar YR, Sharp JT (1968) The alveolar-arterial oxygen gradient in young and elderly men during air and oxygen breathing. *Am Rev Respir Dis*, **97**(3)376–381.

Katz J, Jackson M, Kavanagh BP, Sandler AN (1996) Acute pain after thoracic surgery predicts long-term post-thoracotomy pain. *Clin J Pain*, **12**(1):50–55.

Kavarana MN, Sinha P, Naka Y, Oz MC, Edwards NM (2003) Mechanical support for the failing cardiac allograft: a single-center experience. *J Heart Lung Transplant*, **22**(5):542–547.

Keogh A, Richardson M, Ruygrok P, et al. (2004) Sirolimus in de novo heart transplant recipients reduces acute rejection and prevents coronary artery disease at 2 years: a randomized clinical trial. *Circ*, **110**(17):2694–2700.

Kirklin JK (2005) Is biopsy-proven cellular rejection an important clinical consideration in heart transplantation? *Curr Opin Cardiol*, **20**(2):127–131.

Kotton CN, Kumar D, Caliendo AM, et al. (2010) International consensus guidelines on the management of cytomegalovirus in solid organ transplantation. *Transplantation*, **89**(7):779–795.

Kramer MR, Valantine HA, Marshall SE, Starnes VA, Theodore J (1994) Recovery of the right ventricle after single-lung transplantation in pulmonary hypertension. *Am J Cardiol*, **73**(7):494–500.

Kuntz CL, Hadjiliadis D, Ahya VN, Kotloff RM, Pochettino A, Lewis J, Christie JD (2009) Risk factors for early primary graft dysfunction after lung transplantation: a registry study. *Clin Transplant*, **23**(6):819–830.

Lehmkuhl HB, Arizon J, Vigano M, et al. (2009) Everolimus with reduced cyclosporine versus MMF with standard cyclosporine in de novo heart transplant recipients. *Transplantation*, **88**(1):115–122.

Libby P, Geng YJ, Aikawa M, et al. (1996) Macrophages and atherosclerotic plaque stability. *Curr Opin Lipidol*, **7**(5):330–335.

Maki DG, Ringer M, Alvarado CJ (1991) Prospective randomised trial of povidone-iodine, alcohol, and chlorhexidine for prevention of infection associated with central venous and arterial catheters. *Lancet*, **338**(8763):339–343.

Mateen FJ, Dierkhising RA, Rabinstein AA, Van de Beek D, Wijdicks EF (2010) Neurological complications following adult lung transplantation. *Am J Transplant*, **10**(4):908–914.

Mermel LA, Allon M, Bouza E, et al. (2009) Clinical practice guidelines for the diagnosis and management of intravascular catheter-related infection: 2009 update by the Infectious Diseases Society of America. *Clin Infect Dis*, **49**(1):1–45.

Michard F, Boussat S, Chemla D, et al. (2000) Relation between respiratory changes in arterial pulse pressure and fluid responsiveness in septic patients with acute circulatory failure. *Am J Respir Crit Care Med*, **162**(1):134–138.

Montero JA, Anguita M, Concha M, et al. (1992) Pacing requirements after orthotopic heart transplantation: incidence and related factors. *J Heart Lung Transplant*, **11**(4 Pt 1):799–802.

Morton JR, Ansari N, Glanville AR, Meagher AP, Lord RV (2009) Distal intestinal obstruction syndrome (DIOS) in patients with cystic fibrosis after lung transplantation. *J Gastrointest Surg*, **13**(8):1448–1453.

Neofytos D, Fishman JA, Horn D, et al. (2010) Epidemiology and outcome of invasive fungal infections in solid organ transplant recipients. *Transpl Infect Dis*, **12**(3):220–229.

Nielsen TD, Bahnson T, Davis RD, Palmer SM (2004) Atrial fibrillation after pulmonary transplant. *Chest*, **126**(2):496–500.

Patterson GA (1992) Bilateral lung transplant: indications and technique. *Semin Thorac Cardiovasc Surg*, **4**(2):95–100.

Pavri BB, O'Nunain SS, Newell JB, Ruskin JN, William G (1995) Prevalence and prognostic significance of atrial arrhythmias after orthotopic cardiac transplantation. *J Am Coll Cardiol*, **25**(7):1673–1680.

Pottecher J, Falcoz PE, Massard G, Dupeyron JP (2011) Does thoracic epidural analgesia improve outcome after lung transplantation? *Interact Cardiovasc Thorac Surg*, **12**(1)51–53.

Radovancevic B, McGiffin DC, Kobashigawa JA, et al. (2003) Retransplantation in 7,290 primary transplant patients: a 10-year multi-institutional study. *J Heart Lung Transplant*, **22**(8):862–868.

Rajek A, Pernerstorfer T, Kastner J, et al. (2000) Inhaled nitric oxide reduces pulmonary vascular resistance more than prostaglandin E(1) during heart transplantation. *Anesth Analg*, **90**(3):523–530.

Reitz BA (2011) The first successful combined heart–lung transplantation. *J Thorac Cardiovasc Surg*, **141**(4):867–869.

Ronald A, Abdulaziz KA, Day TG, Scott M (2006) In patients undergoing cardiac surgery, thoracic epidural analgesia combined with general anaesthesia results in faster recovery and fewer complications but does not affect length of hospital stay. *Interact Cardiovasc Thorac Surg*, **5**(3):207–216.

Sablotzki A, Hentschel T, Gruenig E, et al. (2002) Hemodynamic effects of inhaled aerosolized iloprost and inhaled nitric oxide in heart transplant candidates with elevated pulmonary vascular resistance. *Eur J Cardio-Thorac Surg*, **22**(5):746–752.

Sablotzki A, Czeslick E, Gruenig E, et al. (2003) First experiences with the stable prostacyclin analog iloprost in the evaluation of heart transplant candidates with increased pulmonary vascular resistance. *J Thorac Cardiovasc Surg*, **125**(4):960–962.

Savage C, McQuitty C, Wang D, Zwischenberger JB (2002) Postthoracotomy pain management. *Chest Surg Clin N Am*, **12**(2):251–263.

Scott CD, Dark JH, McComb JM (1994) Sinus node function after cardiac transplantation. *J Am Coll Cardiol*, **24**(5):1334–1341.

Shumway NE, Lower RR, Stofer RC (1966) Transplantation of the heart. *Adv Surg*, **2**:265–284.

Spann JC, Van MC (1998) Cardiac transplantation. *Surg Clin N Am*, **78**(5):679–690.

Stehlik J, Edwards LB, Kucheryavaya AY, et al. (2011) The Registry of the International Society for Heart and Lung Transplantation: twenty-eighth adult heart transplant report—2011. *J Heart Lung Transplant*, **30**(10):1078–1094.

Toronto Lung Transplant Group (1986) Unilateral lung transplantation for pulmonary fibrosis. *N Engl J Med*, **314**(18):1140–1145.

Trulock EP, Christie JD, Edwards LB, et al. (2007) Registry of the International Society for Heart and Lung Transplantation: twenty-fourth official adult lung and heart–lung transplantation report 2007. *J Heart Lung Transplant*, **26**(8):782–795.

Uretsky BF, Kormos RL, Zerbe TR, et al. (1992) Cardiac events after heart transplantation: incidence and predictive value of coronary arteriography. *J Heart Lung Transplant*, 11(3 Pt 2):S45–S51.

Weiser TG, Haynes AB, Dziekan G, Berry WR, Lipsitz SR, Gawande AA (2010) Effect of a 19-item surgical safety checklist during urgent operations in a global patient population. *Ann Surg*, **251**(5):976–980.

Weiss ES, Nwakanma LU, Russell SB, Conte JV, Shah AS (2008) Outcomes in bicaval versus biatrial techniques in heart transplantation: an analysis of the UNOS database. *J Heart Lung Transplant*, **27**(2):178–183.

Wickerson L, Mathur S, Brooks D (2010) Exercise training after lung transplantation: a systematic review. *J Heart Lung Transplant*, **29**(5):497–503.

# CHAPTER 34

# Heart and lung transplantation in the paediatric and neonatal population: the current era

Mazen Faden and Elod Szabo

## Introduction to paediatric heart transplantation

The first paediatric heart transplantation was performed by a team led by Adrian Kantrowitz in 1967 (Kantrowitz et al., 1968; Bailey, 2009). The recipient was a 19-day-old infant with Ebstein's anomaly. Anencephalic donor heart, surface cooling, and no CPB was used. The infant initially appeared well but suffered an unexplained sudden cardiac arrest 6 hours after transplantation.

It was not until the 1980s when paediatric heart transplantation was embraced again (Mendeloff, 2002). Developments in recipient selection, donor management, surgical technique, and perfusion strategies, as well as improvements in immunosuppression and post-transplant management made paediatric heart transplantation a viable treatment option for certain congenital heart diseases (CHDs) and the standard therapy for end-stage heart failure related to cardiomyopathies (Canter et al., 2007; Huddleston, 2009; Conway and Dipchand, 2010). In many aspects paediatric heart transplantation is dissimilar to adult heart transplantation. The variety of aetiology, the small size of organs, the immature immune system, the effects of long-term immunosuppression, the unique psychosocial development of the child, and the intense involvement of the parents in the decision-making process all pose distinctive challenges, best managed by heart centres with a dedicated transplant team.

Since the early 1990s, nearly 10,000 paediatric transplantations have been performed worldwide in about 90 centres. The annual number of children transplanted has plateaued at 450–500 per annum during this time. The median survival in the current era is 18.4 years for patients who received a transplant during infancy and 12 years for those transplanted as an adolescent (Kirk et al., 2011). Data on paediatric transplantation are collected in the registries of the ISHLT and Pediatric Heart Transplant Study (PHTS). They both provide invaluable information in a field that is driven by consensus guidelines based on expert opinion (Dipchand et al., 2005; Canter et al., 2007). In this chapter we discuss the various indications for paediatric heart transplantation and the perioperative management of children undergoing heart transplantation or implantation of mechanical assist devices.

## Indications

The main diagnoses leading to heart transplantation in the paediatric population include cardiomyopathy of various aetiologies with end-stage heart failure and CHD not amenable to surgical palliation (Kirk et al., 2011; ISHLT). Re-transplantation and transplantation for previously palliated CHD are further groups of growing significance (Kirk et al., 2011; Huddleston, 2009).

### Cardiomyopathies

Cardiomyopathy (CMP) is a disease characterized by abnormal myocardial structure and function in the absence of coronary artery disease, hypertension, valvular disease, and CHD sufficient to cause the observed myocardial abnormality (Elliott et al., 2008). Here we adopt the clinically oriented classification of CMP by the European Society of Cardiology (Elliott et al., 2008) and discuss the major subtypes of CMP relevant for the current topic.

### Dilated cardiomyopathy

Dilated cardiomyopathy (DCM) is characterized by decreased contractility and dilatation of the LV. Mitral regurgitation secondary to ventricular dilatation may develop and atrial and ventricular arrhythmias are also common in patients with DCM. End-stage heart failure related to DCM can be complicated by pulmonary vascular disease and pulmonary hypertension (PHT).

DCM constitutes over half of all paediatric CMP (Lipshultz et al., 2003; Nugent et al., 2003) and is the most frequent diagnosis in children receiving heart transplantation (Conway and Dipchand, 2011; and according to the ISHLT), accounting for 76% of all listed CMP cases (Canter et al., 2007). Paediatric DCM is the consequence of a variety of aetiologies including viral, metabolic, toxic, and genetic causes (Towbin et al., 2006; Wilkinson et al., 2010). Approximately two-thirds of the cases are idiopathic. Major causes of acquired DCM include viral myocarditis (46% of non-idiopathic cases) (Towbin et al., 2006; Kühl and Schultheiss, 2010) and the late progressive complication of anthracycline chemotherapy (Singal and Iliskovic, 1998; Chatterjee et al., 2010; Rathe et al., 2010). Familial DCM, about 20% of cases, includes diseases with *multisystem involvement*, such as muscular dystrophies, mitochondrial diseases, and inborn errors of metabolism

(Hsu and Canter, 2010) and familial *isolated* DCM associated with over 30 genes, most of which have autosomal dominant inheritance (Kärkkäinen and Peuhkurinen, 2007; Jefferies and Towbin, 2010; Alvarez et al., 2011; Hershberger and Siegfried, 2011). The incidence of paediatric DCM is 0.57 cases per 100,000 children in the US (Towbin et al., 2006), corroborated by similar data in Australia (Daubeney et al., 2006).

Paediatric DCM has significant mortality: freedom from death and transplantation at 1 year after diagnosis is 72% and 69% and at 5 years 63% and 54%, respectively. Shift in medical therapy from digoxin and diuretics to angiotensin-converting enzyme inhibitors and β-adrenergic receptor blockers, mirroring adult DCM therapy, failed to improve the outcome of paediatric DCM (Kantor et al., 2010). Though wait-list mortality of paediatric DCM is relatively low, heart transplantation provides clear survival benefit compared to the natural history of the disease (Kirk et al., 2009b). DCM associated with *viral myocarditis*, on the other hand, has a relatively good prognosis: with 77% freedom from death and transplantation at 1 year and 70% at 5 years according to the Pediatric Cardiomyopathy Registry (PCMR) (Alvarez et al., 2011). Individual centres report even better transplant-free survival rates (Lee et al., 1999; Amabile et al., 2006) and emphasize the importance of mechanical circulatory support in bridging to recovery or transplant (Lee et al., 1999; Teele et al., 2011; Wilmot et al., 2011). A review of the Extracorporeal Life Support Organization registry confirms the role and power of ECMO in bridging myocarditis to recovery, demonstrating 73% decannulation due to adequate recovery and 61% final survival (Rajagopal et al., 2010).

## Anthracycline-induced cardiomyopathy

Anthracyclines are effective chemotherapeutic agents in several childhood malignancies (Weiss, 1992). Anthracyclines, independent of their antineoplastic action involving various mechanisms of DNA damage and topoisomerase II inhibition (Gewirtz, 1999; Takemura and Fujiwara, 2007), cause reactive oxygen species-induced mitochondrial toxicity (Wallace, 2007). This latter effect leads to dose-dependent, cumulative, irreversible cardiomyopathy. The incidence of chronic cardiotoxicity progressively increases over 500 mg/m$^2$ of cumulative doxorubicin (Hoff et al., 1979; Swain et al., 2003). However, there is great interindividual variability in susceptibility to anthracycline toxicity (Jamieson and Boddy, 2011), and life-long surveillance is recommended following low-dose therapy as well (Rathe et al., 2010). The established disease carries a very poor prognosis of 50% 1-year mortality (Hoff et al., 1979). The central issue of cardiac transplantation for anthracycline-induced CMP is the cancer recurrence rate, i.e. can a child be transplanted prior to reaching the 5-year disease-free period? To this end, successful transplantation has been reported in a child only 5 months into remission (Morgan and Pahl, 2002), and a multicentre, retrospective analysis by Ward et al. (2004) demonstrates acceptable transplantation outcomes and low risk of cancer recurrence in early transplant recipients. Such early transplantations remain controversial, however, and most centres observe 2 years of remission prior to considering listing for transplantation. Close collaboration with the oncologist is mandated in individual decision-making and has the potential of shortening the waiting period for listing.

## Hypertrophic cardiomyopathy

Hypertrophic cardiomyopathy (HCM) is the second most common paediatric CMP, representing 42% of Registry cases (Lipshultz et al., 2003; Nugent et al., 2003). HCM encompasses a morphologically similar but diverse group of disorders with varied aetiology and outcome (Colan et al., 2007). About 75% of paediatric HCM is idiopathic; the rest of the cases are equally distributed in the categories of inborn errors of metabolism, malformation syndromes, and neuromuscular disorders. Though 42 specific causes were identified in the PCMR, the majority of cases fell into three disease entities, Pompe's disease, Noonan's syndrome, and Friedreich ataxia, representing each of the above subsets of HCM.

The distinguishing feature of HCM is the presence of increased ventricular wall thickness in the absence of haemodynamic loading conditions sufficient to cause the hypertrophy. Systolic function is preserved or enhanced, there is associated diastolic dysfunction, and dynamic outflow tract obstruction frequently complicates haemodynamics (Maron et al., 2006; Hickey et al., 2012). Myocardial ischaemia is relatively common, and it is a consequence of increased wall thickness and altered small vessels and capillaries (Maron et al., 1986; Tanaka et al., 1987). In a cohort of children with HCM at a tertiary paediatric centre, 28% incidence of myocardial bridging with compression of an epicardial coronary artery, an additional substrate of ischaemia, was noted, with associated poor outcome (Yetman et al., 1998).

The clinical presentation of HCM varies from no symptoms to severely limiting obstructive symptoms of dyspnoea, angina, syncope, and sudden cardiac death (Maron et al., 1982; Ommen, 2011). HCM is a major cause of sudden cardiac death in children (Liberthson, 1996), the pathomechanism likely being ischaemia rather than malignant ventricular arrhythmias (McKenna and Deanfield, 1984; McKenna et al., 1988). Children presenting before 1 year of age have the poorest outcomes of all paediatric HCM, regardless of aetiology (Colan et al., 2007); 36% of these infants presented with congestive heart failure (CHF) in the Registry and nearly half of them died. In particular, infantile Pompe's disease is associated with severe HCM that is fatal by 2 years of age. Similarly, infantile Noonan's syndrome has a high risk of presenting with CHF and of having a poor outcome. However, children who survive infancy have an annual mortality rate of 1% (Colan et al., 2007). In the small subset of children who present with CHF, symptoms likely progress to an end-stage phase (Spirito et al., 1987; Biagini et al., 2005; Ommen, 2005), brought about by progressive dilatation of the hypertrophied LV or increasingly severe restrictive physiology (Canter and Kantor, 2007; Gajarski et al., 2009). These children comprise the majority of paediatric HCM listed for transplantation, 6% of all paediatric CMP listed (Dipchand et al., 2009). Other, infrequent, indications include failure of medical therapy and surgical septal myectomy (Coutu et al., 2004; Canter and Kantor, 2007; Gajarski et al., 2009). Risk factors for listing and poor outcome include presentation under 1 year of age, with lower LV shortening fraction and higher LV wall thickness (Colan et al., 2007; Dipchand et al., 2009; Gajarski et al., 2009).

## Restrictive cardiomyopathy (RCM)

RCM is a rare disease, with a prevalence of only 2-5% of all pediatric CMP in the US and Australia (Lipshultz et al. 2003; Nugent et al. 2003; Denfield and Weber 2010). However, it accounts for

11% of pediatric CMP listed for transplantation (Dipchand et al., 2009), attesting to the poor natural history of the illness. RCM is a progressive disease with 2-year survival of less than 50% (Chen et al., 2001; Russo and Webber, 2005; Zangwill et al., 2009). Familial occurrence is common, and a number of sarcomeric and cytoskeletal protein defects, reviewed in detail by Denfield and Weber (2010), have been identified with both autosomal dominant and recessive inheritance. However, the aetiology of the disease is usually unclear. The most common form of RCM is tropical, and in some populations endemic, endomyocardial fibrosis (Mocumbi et al., 2008). Currently, this disease bears no relevance to the topic and is not discussed further.

The hallmark of RCM is restrictive ventricular physiology in the presence of normal or reduced diastolic volumes and normal wall thickness (Elliott et al., 2008). Time of diagnosis can be late, with presenting symptoms of dyspnoea and exercise intolerance, as a consequence of limited cardiac output and progressive PHT (Weller et al., 2002; Russo and Webber, 2005; Denfield and Weber, 2010). Children without signs of heart failure may experience subclinical ischaemia and are at high risk of sudden cardiac death (Rivenes et al., 2000).

Medical therapy is limited to anticoagulation, careful diuresis if symptoms of CHF are present, and pre-emptive placement of implantable cardioverter-defibrillator—a high-risk procedure. Because of the poor survival and rapidly progressive nature of the disease (Chen et al., 2001; Weller et al., 2002; Russo and Webber, 2005; Zangwill et al., 2009) early transplant evaluation and listing is generally advocated (Dipchand et al., 2009; Zangwill et al. 2009; Denfield and Weber, 2010; Pahl et al., 2010). There is no consensus on pretransplant cardiac catheterization to determine the magnitude of PVR (Pahl et al., 2010), which is often quite high at the time of diagnosis (Weller et al., 2002; Russo and Webber, 2005). We do not advocate catheterization, as it is not possible to reliably evaluate the responsiveness of the pulmonary vasculature, a decisive factor in transplantation (discussed in the section 'Contraindications'), in RCM, and, in our institutional experience, we have not encountered irreversibly elevated PVR in this population (A. Dipchand, personal communication). A small percentage of symptomatic children may experience event-free survival (Chen et al., 2001; Weller et al., 2002; Russo and Webber, 2005). Due to the small cohorts, unfortunately, no consistent risk factors assisting in early listing could be identified (Russo and Webber, 2005; Denfield and Weber, 2010).

## Congenital heart disease

Historically, heart transplantation was the primary management option for hypoplastic left heart syndrome (HLHS) (Bailey et al., 1993; Bailey, 2009). During the period of 1988–1995, 84% of infant heart transplantation was performed for CHD, the majority of these being HLHS (Kirk et al., 2011). The combination of limited donor organ pool and improvement in surgical palliation of HLHS, however, shifted the indications of infant heart transplantation. In the current era, CHD represents 63% of infant heart transplantations. Generally, *primary transplantation for CHD* is reserved for infants afflicted by congenital heart malformations for which the outcome of surgical palliation is poor. These include (1) HLHS with poor RV function, severe tricuspid valve regurgitation, or pulmonary valve disease; (2) pulmonary atresia with intact ventricle septum and RV-dependent coronary circulation (Ashburn et al., 2004; Calder et al., 2007); (3) severe truncus arteriosus not amenable to primary repair; and (4) complex heterotaxy syndromes (Larsen et al., 2002; Lim et al., 2005).

Transplantation for *repaired CHD* is another group of CHD-related transplantations that needs mention. Certain repairs, such as the atrial switch operation of transposition of the great arteries (Roos-Hesselink et al., 2004) and the transannular patch repair of tetralogy of Fallot (Nollert et al., 1997), carry a significant long-term risk of cardiac death in the form of sudden cardiac death or CHF. These groups of patients are older, in their early and late adulthood, at the time of developing CHF, and therefore will not be discussed further.

Transplantation for *partially palliated CHD*, in essence, considers children with single ventricles who are not candidates for completion Fontan secondary to pulmonary vascular disease or significant AV valve regurgitation.

### Failed Fontan

Transplantation for *palliated CHD*, i.e. failed Fontan, is a category of growing significance. Palliation of single-ventricle lesions to Fontan circulation even under optimal conditions is plagued by a late phase of increasing risk of death (Fontan et al., 1990; Tweddell et al., 2009). The number of children with failed Fontan circulation is magnified by the increasing number of ever-complex single-ventricle lesions being palliated in recent years. Overall, this is the largest single group of children with CHD receiving heart transplant (Bernstein et al., 2006).

Children with failing Fontan circulation require heart transplantation as a consequence of progressive ventricular failure or failing Fontan physiology in the absence of focal correctable anatomical problems (Davies et al., 2009; Griffiths et al., 2009). Failing Fontan physiology is characterized by multiple morbidities in the face of preserved ventricular function. These debilitating, late complications of Fontan circulation include intractable arrhythmias, thromboembolic events, hepatic dysfunction, aortopulmonary collaterals, progressive cyanosis as a consequence of pulmonary arteriovenous malformations, persistent pleural effusions, protein-losing enteropathy (PLE), and plastic bronchitis. The enteric lymphatic disorder PLE is characterized by low serum albumin and immunoglobulins, coagulation abnormalities (Jahangiri et al., 1997), peripheral oedema, ascites, and chronic diarrhoea (Mertens et al., 1998). PLE and plastic bronchitis, likely the pulmonary analogue to PLE, are particularly worrisome complication and due to the absence of adequate medical treatment carry a 50% 5-year mortality (Mertens et al., 1998; Davies et al., 2009). Therefore these children are referred early to a transplant team for evaluation and timely listing.

Failed Fontan children are exceedingly high risk to transplant secondary to multiple prior surgeries, limited vascular access, immunocompromised and malnourished state, likelihood of HLA sensitization related to multiple exposures, the need for pulmonary artery reconstruction (Chen et al., 2004), the presence of aortopulmonary collaterals, and the possibility of elevated PVR (Khambadkone et al., 2003; Mitchell et al., 2004b). Survival of transplanted failed Fontan children is somewhat less than survival of children transplanted for other CHD or other diagnoses (Jayakumar et al., 2004; Bernstein et al., 2006; Davies et al., 2009). Children with preserved ventricular function and failing Fontan physiology have over three times risk of early death after transplantation compared to children with Fontan with failing ventricle (Griffiths et al., 2009; Simpson et al., 2012). Remarkably, however, the chronic complications of Fontan circulation necessitating heart transplantation, including PLE, resolve after transplantation (Jayakumar et al., 2004; Gamba et al., 2004; Mitchell et al., 2004a; Bernstein et al., 2006).

## Retransplantation

Retransplantation constitute a minor group of paediatric heart transplantations, representing 6% of transplantations annually (Kirk et al., 2011). Major aetiologies include post-transplant vasculopathy, graft failure due to acute rejection, and early primary graft failure. Outcomes of paediatric retransplantation for primary graft failure and rejection are inferior; 1-year survival of early retransplantation is 56% vs 85% for primary transplantation, as noted in the PHTS database (Chin et al., 2006). In fact, one of the significant risk factors for 1-year mortality is retransplantation (Kirk et al., 2011). Therefore such heart transplantations are relatively contraindicated (Chin et al., 2006). However, for those who survived more than a year after primary transplantation, especially with underlying allograft coronary vasculopathy, survival after retransplantation is comparable to primary transplantation (Chin et al., 2006; Kirk et al., 2011).

## Other indications

The following are rare conditions leading to heart failure and subsequent transplant listing.

Heart failure on an *ischaemic basis* is extremely rare in children. However, it can happen in the following circumstances: late diagnosis of anomalous origin of the left coronary artery from the pulmonary artery, not recovering after reimplantation; severe Kawasaki disease with distal stenoses (Checchia et al., 1997); and perioperative injury to the coronary arteries, as in arterial switch operation, resulting in irreversible LV dysfunction.

Further uncommon indications are intractable life-threatening tachyarrhythmias and unresectable primary cardiac tumours (Freedom et al., 2000; Conway and Dipchand, 2010).

## Contraindications

The purpose of pretransplant assessment is to identify factors that would complicate or contraindicate cardiac transplantation. The assessment includes full cardiac evaluation, including cardiac catheterization, as indicated, to determine anatomy, haemodynamic profile, and PVR. Other organ systems are evaluated and appropriate consultations called for to optimize therapy of affected end-organs and determine long-term outcome. Immunological assessment includes blood group and HLA typing and screening of PRAs. Thorough evaluation of the psychosocial functioning of the patient and the family is essential to identify behavioural aspects that would indicate future non-compliance, a major problem in the adolescent population (Ringewald et al., 2001). This multidisciplinary, comprehensive assessment of the transplant candidate is best performed by a transplant team led by a paediatric transplant cardiologist. Such a team should include physicians and other healthcare providers representing every aspect of the transplantation process (see Table 34.1).

**Table 34.1** Pretransplant assessment: tests and consultations. (Reprinted from *Pediatric Clinics*, 57, 2, Conway et al., 'Heart Transplantation in Children', pp. 353–373, Copyright 2010, with permission from Elsevier..)

| | |
|---|---|
| Cardiology | ECHO, ECG, CXR, exercise test, cardiac catheterization, MRI/MRA, CT angiography |
| Haematology/ immunology | Blood group, HLA typing, PRA, immunoglobulins |
| Serology | EBV, CMV, VZV, HSV, HIV, hepatitis B and C titres |
| Chemistries | Renal function, liver function, lipid profile |
| Transplant team consultations | Social work, psychiatry, adolescent medicine, physiotherapy, occupational health, dietician |
| Additional consultations | Anaesthesiology, genetics, metabolics, neurology, nephrology |

VZV, Varicella-zoster virus; HSV, herpes simplex virus.

Contraindications can be divided into two major categories: general, applicable to any organ transplant, and those specifically related to cardiovascular status. The number of absolute contraindications has decreased over the years (Dipchand et al., 2005; Canter et al., 2007; Conway and Dipchand, 2011); in particular, factors that are now considered relative contraindications and can be deemed as pushing the boundaries of cardiac transplantation include transplantation in children with PHT, HLA-sensitization, and ABO-incompatible (ABOi) transplantation. Definite contraindications are listed in Table 34.2 and selected ones are detailed below.

Severe end-organ dysfunction is a general contraindication and is relative in case of renal and hepatic dysfunction as long as the dysfunction is a consequence of heart failure and recovery is expected. However, being on dialysis is a significant risk factor for 1-year mortality (relative risk 2.01 compared to DCM alone) (Kirk et al., 2011) and serum creatinine constitutes a continuous risk factor for the same (according to the ISHLT).

Though some argue that there are no anatomical reasons precluding transplantation (Huddleston, 2009), severe hypoplasia of the branch pulmonary arteries and severe pulmonary vein stenosis are listed as contraindications in consensus guidelines (Dipchand

**Table 34.2** Definite contraindications to paediatric heart transplantation

| |
|---|
| Severe, irreversible end-organ damage (i.e. liver failure with cirrhosis) |
| Multisystem organ dysfunction |
| Active infection or malignancy |
| Severe progressive non-cardiac disease associated with limited survival (i.e. chromosomal, metabolic, neurological disorders) |
| Severe hypoplasia of the branch pulmonary arteries |
| Severe pulmonary vein stenosis |
| Severe irreversible pulmonary hypertension (?) |
| Prohibitive psychosocial circumstances |
| Retransplantation during an acute rejection episode |

et al., 2005; Canter et al., 2007). Additionally, it is worth noting that diagnosis of CHD is a risk factor for primary graft failure (Huang et al., 2004) and carries a relative risk of 1-year mortality of 1.97 compared to DCM (Kirk et al., 2011).

Long-standing heart failure is frequently complicated by *elevated* PVR. Elevated PVR is a graded risk factor for RV failure, primary graft rejection, and mortality after cardiac transplantation (Kirklin et al., 1988; Bando et al., 1993; Bourge et al., 1993; Murali et al., 1993; Gajarski et al., 1994; Huang et al., 2004; Hoskote et al., 2010). For this reason, an indexed PVR (PVRi) of 6 WU/m$^2$ or a transpulmonary gradient > 15 mmHg was considered a contraindication to transplantation (Addonizio et al., 1987; Murali et al., 1993; Costanzo et al., 1995; Canter et al., 2007). However, it is now clear that transplantation is feasible in patients with increased PVR if the pulmonary vasculature is responsive to vasodilators and the PVR index can be lowered below 6 WU/m$^2$ (Gajarski et al., 1994; Canter et al., 2007; Giglia and Humpl, 2010). A recent retrospective study of a large single-centre experience by Chiu et al. further clarifies the role elevated PVR plays in early transplant mortality (Chiu et al., 2012). In their analysis the authors found that in children with PVRi < 9 WU/m$^2$, of whom a significant portion were not responsive to vasodilator therapy, early mortality is minimal. PVRi > 9 WU/m$^2$ portended a 30-day mortality of 21%. Pulmonary vascular reactivity predicts lower PVRi after transplantation and an overall better outcome (Zales et al., 1993; Gajarski et al., 1994; Drakos et al., 2007). Still, even reversible PVR elevation carries a significant risk of post-transplant mortality (Butler et al., 2005; Hoskote et al., 2010).

Cardiac catheterization in combination with respiratory mass spectrometry determination of $O_2$ consumption (Davies et al., 1984) provides accurate measurement of PVR in most children. However, the direct Fick principle employed in this method is known to be inaccurate in the presence of high pulmonary blood flow (Cigarroa et al., 1989) and cannot be considered a 'gold standard'. MRI is emerging as a potentially more reliable method to assess PVR (Muthurangu et al., 2004; Kuehne, 2005). Nonetheless, evaluation of PVR and reactivity in complex CHD with variable sources of pulmonary blood flow, in failing Fontan circulation (Carey et al., 1998; Mitchell et al., 2004b), and in restrictive LV physiology remain challenging (Conway and Dipchand, 2010; Pahl et al., 2010).

Recently, the advent of bridging to transplantation has called into question the irreversibility of fixed PHT. A variety of VADs permitted mechanical unloading of the LV, decreased PVR, and allowed successful transplantation in adults (Zimpfer et al., 2007; Liden et al., 2009) and children (Gandhi et al., 2008) with previous diagnosis of non-reactive elevated PVR.

The presence of donor-specific anti-HLA antibodies defines recipient sensitization. Transplantation of *sensitized recipients* entails a significant risk of early graft failure and consequent increased mortality (Kobashigawa et al., 1996; Jacobs et al., 2004; Wright et al., 2007; Kirk et al., 2011). Pretransplant assessment involves the determination of sensitization by testing the serum of the recipient against a random panel of lymphocytes, known as the PRA screen. A PRA titre over 10% signifies sensitization (Betkowski et al., 2002; Haddad et al., 2009). The likelihood of high PRA titre is increased after multiple blood transfusions, repair of CHD with homograft material (Shaddy et al., 1996; Hooper et al., 2005), and VAD placement (Pagani et al., 2001; Itescu and John, 2003), factors predictably present in children with complicated pretransplant heart failure history. A negative cross-match for donor-specific HLA antibodies would rule out humoral rejection, but the necessary logistics involved would increase wait-list time and limit the donor pool to the local area (Conway and Dipchand, 2010). There are no consensus guidelines to transplanting children with high PRA levels. Treatment strategies include intravenous immunoglobulin G, intraoperative plasmapheresis, rituximab, and cyclophosphamide administration (Pisani et al., 1999; Wright et al., 2007; Haddad et al., 2009; Conway and Dipchand, 2010). Results of various centres are promising with the use of such aggressive immunosuppressive protocols, albeit at the price of frequent early rejections (Holt et al., 2007; Pollock-BarZiv et al., 2007). This approach, however, is encouraging as the frequency of rejection after 3–6 months decreases to the level seen in non-sensitized recipients.

## Mechanical circulatory support—bridge to transplantation

In recent years, mechanical circulatory support has emerged as an important measure to improve wait-list mortality (Blume et al., 2006; Hetzer et al., 2006; Morales et al., 2011; Fraser et al., 2012) and allocation of donor hearts (Goldman et al., 2003). In fact, use of VADs is now common, and transplantation occurred after bridging in 21% of patients (7.3% ECMO, 9.2% LVAD, 4.8% biventricular assist device (BiVAD)) according to the latest Registry (ISHLT). In the paediatric population, options for such a support were limited in the past. Older children can be successfully supported with adult-size VADs (Blume et al., 2006); however, until recently, the mainstay of mechanical support in smaller children has been the ECMO circuit.

The first successful long-term mechanical circulatory support in a child was achieved by the German Heart Institute (Warnecke et al., 1991). The device used, the Berlin Heart EXCOR® (BH), developed by the German Heart Institute (now Berlin Heart GmbH, Berlin, Germany), is a paracorporeal pneumatically driven pulsatile-flow circulatory support device. The BH is the only circulatory assist system able to support children from neonates (youngest being a 2-kg 3-day-old neonate) to adolescents, with available stroke volumes ranging from 10 mL to 80 mL (Hetzer et al., 2006). Accumulated evidence from Europe (Hetzer et al., 1999) and, lately, the US (Imamura et al., 2009; Jeewa et al., 2010; Fraser et al., 2012) establishes the BH as the preferred mode to bridge children to transplantation. Specific reasons include less mortality, longer time of support, less bleeding and infectious complications, and the ability to rehabilitate children after implantation. In particular, survival to transplantation, or recovery, on continued support was 57% vs 86% in a cohort of 21 children in each of an ECMO and BH group, respectively (Imamura et al., 2009). Wait-list mortality in a single-centre study was 38% and 13% for ECMO and BH patients, respectively (Jeewa et al., 2010), and a recent multicentre trial asserted a median survival time for historical control of children on ECMO of 13 days, whereas such an endpoint had not been reached in the prospective BH cohort at 174 days (Fraser et al., 2012).

Transplant survival after bridging is equivalent to survival of children transplanted without the need for VAD (Blume et al., 2006; Huebler et al., 2011). However, significant morbidity for BH bridging in the form of infection, bleeding, and stroke remains (Hetzer et al., 2006; Sharma et al., 2006; Imamura et al., 2009; Fraser et al., 2012). The greatest risk factor for early complications and mortality following BH implantation is history of CHD (Blume et al., 2006; Huebler et al., 2011). Some of this early mortality has been forestalled by elective early implantation (Blume et al., 2006; Hetzer et al., 2006). Specifically, in the largest single-centre experience (Hetzer et al., 2006), in infants and in postcardiotomy children, implantation of BH prior to the development of end-organ damage improved survival from 0% to 78% and 57%, respectively. Multivariate analysis of the initial multicentre US BH study identified BiVAD implantation in contrast to LVAD as a significant risk factor for mortality (35% vs 14%) (Morales et al., 2011). Advancing technology holds the promise to further improve the complication profile of VAD treatment of children: the third-generation continuous-flow device, HeartWare (HeartWare Inc, Miami Lakes, Florida), implantable in children over 30 kg, has a superior thromboembolic profile (no events in seven children) compared to BH (Miera et al., 2011).

BH implantation requires CPB. The anaesthetic considerations for this procedure must observe, in addition to the ones for a CPB, the degree of myocardial failure and end-organ damage, specificities of an (un)palliated CHD, and the necessity of supporting the RV in case of an LVAD-only implantation. LV unloading may not immediately decrease RV afterload; inotropic support for the RV and efforts to reduce PVR are often indicated.

Children with in-situ BH will inevitably require further invasive procedures, including heart transplantation. These children are stable, having recovered from secondary organ damage. They are anticoagulated according to the manufacturer's recommendation and institutional preference but retain significant risk for thromboembolic events. Their distinct haemodynamic profile is determined by the interaction of the pump and the native cardiovascular system devoid of regulatory feedback loop. The presence of a BH-trained perfusionist is required for any procedure that has the potential of upsetting this interaction. The fixed stroke volume of the BH translates into fixed cardiac output unless the pumping rate is changed. The BH is designed such that filling of the pumping chamber can easily be monitored, and the surgical field has to be set up to allow visual monitoring. Invasive monitoring should be considered for any major procedure. The inability of the BH to compensate for a drop in SVR leads to inadequate perfusion pressures. Similarly, an increase in venous capacitance or significant fluid shifts compromise the preload-sensitive pumping. Maintenance of adequate filling of the vascular system can be achieved with α-adrenergic agents and the judicious use of fluids. A comprehensive list of anaesthetic considerations for children with in-situ BH is shown in Table 34.3.

**Table 34.3** Anaesthetic considerations of in-situ Berlin Heart

| | Considerations | Recommendations |
|---|---|---|
| Preoperative | Time of implantation | Has child recovered from multi-organ failure? |
| | Aetiology of heart failure | Consider anaesthetic implications of multisystem disease |
| | Continuous risk of serious thromboembolic events | Note baseline neurological status, level, and mode of anticoagulation; examine BH chambers for presence of clot |
| | Logistics and timing of transport to OR | While not as involved as ECMO transportation, planning and communication are essential |
| Intraoperative | Monitoring | Invasive monitoring for major procedures; pump chambers covered with transparent drapes; presence of BH nurse |
| | RVAD generates negative pressure | Minimize risk of air embolism during central venous line placement |
| | Induction and maintenance | With the exception of ketamine, all agents decrease blood pressure secondary to decreased SVR and increased venous capacitance—titration to effect is important |
| Haemodynamics of BH | Fixed CO, preload dependence, no vascular feedback loop | Use α-agonists to augment both venous return and SVR; consider volume replacement if necessary; if in need of increased CO, adjust BH rate |
| | *LVAD only*—RV function is crucial | Consider implications and treatment of PHT (appropriate ventilation and analgesia, iNO) and RV failure (milrinone, epinephrine, and norepinephrine as second choice) |
| | Sudden deterioration of haemodynamics | Rule out mechanical problems: pneumatic hose kinking, tamponade, LV inflow cannula obstruction; in *LVAD-only*: PHT crisis, malignant arrhythmia |
| Redo thoracotomy | Prolonged surgical exposure and increased bleeding | Administer antifibrinolytics; ensure blood products available |
| Postoperative | Pain control and ICU care | As after heart transplantation; or ICU care and early extubation for major procedures and stepdown unit for minor procedures—continued presence of BH nurse |

## ABO-incompatible transplantation

The number of unallocated paediatric organs related to size discrepancy and ABOi is substantial. According to earlier estimates, less than half of available donor hearts are transplanted to suitable recipients (Boucek, 2001). To decrease the paediatric wait-list mortality and lessen the number of unallocated hearts the ABO barrier was intentionally crossed in the mid-1990s at the Hospital for Sick Children, Toronto (West et al., 2001). The immature immune system of the infant characterized by delayed development of responses to carbohydrate antigens, including delayed production of anti-A and anti-B isohaemagglutinins (Fong et al., 1974), made such a strategy successful compared to the lethal outcomes of inadvertent adult ABOi heart transplantations (Cooper, 1990). The maximum acceptable isohaemagglutinin titre, i.e. the upper age limit for successful ABOi transplantation, is not known. At our institute the upper ages include several children transplanted in their second year of life (A. Dipchand—personal communication), while the published oldest ABOi heart recipient was 5 years old at time of transplantation (Bućin et al., 2006).

When an ABOi heart transplantation is performed in the presence of low titres of isohaemagglutinins in the recipient's plasma, a plasma exchange is carried out upon initiation of CPB (West et al., 2001; Dipchand, 2011). Blood product management (see Table 34.4) is critically important during ABOi transplantation to safeguard against transfusion of isohaemagglutinins directed against the donor organ or the recipient (West et al., 2001; Conway and Dipchand, 2010; Dipchand, 2011). These transfusion guidelines must be followed indefinitely after an ABOi heart transplantation, and it is recommended that these children are cared for where there is an institutional level of understanding of their unique blood product requirements (Conway and Dipchand, 2010).

The practice of ABOi heart transplantation had a substantial impact on the outcomes of end-stage heart failure in infants. Wait-list mortality dramatically decreased without an adverse effect on survival after transplantation (West et al., 2001, 2006). No hyperacute antibody-mediated rejection was observed, and short-term and immediate-term results are comparable to ABOi transplantation (West et al., 2006; Roche et al., 2008; Dipchand et al., 2010). In particular, in analyzing the outcomes of the largest single-centre cohort of ABOi vs ABO-compatible heart recipients, 35 vs 45 infants (< 14 months old) respectively, Dipchand et al. demonstrated indistinguishable outcomes, including no difference in survival, rejection, renal dysfunction, allograft vasculopathy, or post-transplant lymphoproliferative disorder (Dipchand et al., 2010). As a result, these authors recommend that children under 2 years of age have their isohaemagglutinin titres checked prior to listing and be considered for ABOi transplantation (Conway and Dipchand, 2010; Dipchand et al., 2010).

Since the initial report, several paediatric heart centres embraced the practice and reported similarly good outcomes (Daebritz et al., 2007; Roche et al., 2008). Most ABOi heart recipient children develop selective donor-specific isohaemagglutinin deficiency, presumably as a result of exposure of the immature immune system to donor ABO antigens (Fan et al., 2004). Furthermore, a multicentre study demonstrated decreased de-novo synthesis of class II HLA antibodies after ABOi heart transplantation, suggesting a potentially protective effect of breaching the ABO barrier (Urschel et al., 2010).

**Table 34.4** Blood groups of the products to use in ABOi transplantation. (Adapted with kind permission from the Heart Transplantation Clinical Protocols, The Hospital for Sick Children, Dipchand, A., 2011, 'The Hospital for Sick Children Heart Transplant Program - Clinical Protocols', pp.1–141.)

| Patient's group | Donor's group | Red cells *plasma depleted* | FFP | Cryoprecipitate | Platelets |
|---|---|---|---|---|---|
| O | A | O | A | A | A or AB (2nd choice O or B concentrated)[a] |
| O | B | O | B | B | B or AB (2nd choice O or A concentrated)[a] |
| O | AB | O | AB | AB, A or B | AB (2nd choice A or B concentrated, 3rd choice O concentrated)[a] |
| A | B | A | AB | AB or B[a] | AB (2nd choice B concentrated, 3rd choice A or O concentrated)[a] |
| A | AB | A | AB | AB, A or B[a] | AB (2nd choice A or B concentrated, 3rd choice O concentrated)[a] |
| B | A | B | AB | AB or A[a] | AB (2nd choice A concentrated, 3rd choice B or O concentrated)[a] |
| B | AB | B | AB | AB, A or B[a] | AB (2nd choice A or B concentrated)[a] |

[a]If unavailable, consult with transplant physician, medical director, or haematopathologist on call about the possibility of switching ABO group.

## Donation after cardiac death

Prior to the development of criteria for brain death (Harvard Medical School, 1968), all transplantation relied on DCD organs. To improve the growing paediatric donor organ shortage, the practice of DCD has been reintroduced to paediatric transplantation (Boucek et al., 2008; Naim et al., 2008; Yoo et al., 2011). However, inherent controversies exist relating to the lack of precise definition of death and the fact that determination of death after cardiac arrest relies on indirect measurements of circulatory arrest. Accordingly, there is significant variability in policies across jurisdictions regarding the diagnostic procedures required to satisfy criteria for circulatory arrest and the length of time required before confirmation of death and initiation of organ procurement (Dhanani et al., 2011).

The time elapsed after cardiac arrest that ensures irreversibility of the physiological process of dying yet allows viability of donor organs is not known. The shortest time reported (75 s) (Boucek et al., 2008) ignited a heated debate (Bernat, 2008; Curfman et al., 2008; Truog and Miller, 2008; Veatch, 2008), highlighting the fundamental problem with DCD heart transplantation. That is to say, the fact that the donor heart is restarted in the recipient's body negates death by circulatory arrest and therefore violates the 'dead donor rule'. Despite these contentious issues, paediatric DCD transplantation has the potential to ameliorate the scarcity of paediatric donor organs and, with consistent, evidence-based guidelines and a shift from various definitions of death towards emphasizing valid informed consent (Truog and Miller, 2008, 2010), can satisfy ethical obligations and ensure public trust.

## Outcomes

### Survival

Survival after paediatric heart transplantation continues to improve (Kirk et al., 2011; and according to the ISHLT). Median survival of infant, children, and adolescent transplantation is 18.4, 16.4, and 12 years, respectively. The highest risk of death is incurred during the first 6 months after transplantation. Median conditional survival after this period is > 20, 19.3, and 16 years for the above age groups, respectively. Risk factors for early morbidity include diagnosis of CHD (vs CMP), retransplantation, degree of end-organ failure and pretransplantation support (mechanical assist, ventilatory support, dialysis), and a PRA over 10%. Centre volume is a risk factor for infant transplantation, with a clear survival advantage in centres performing more than ten transplantations a year (Davies et al., 2011; and according to the ISHLT).

### Transplant morbidity and surveillance

The purpose of post-transplantation surveillance is to detect transplant-related complications and initiate timely treatment in order to limit morbidity and mortality. As multiple organ systems are potentially affected, the surveillance is a comprehensive, detail-oriented process that should be done at the transplanting centre. Routine bloodwork includes haematology, renal and liver function tests, and therapeutic drug level monitoring. Cardiac follow-up includes ECG, echocardiography, exercise testing, cardiac catheterization, and endomyocardial biopsy. We briefly discuss major morbidities in the following five sections.

### Rejection

Rejection is a primary cause of mortality, responsible for 15% of deaths during the first year following transplantation (Kirk et al., 2011). Treated rejection during this period is associated with a 6% decrease in survival at 5 years according to the most recent ISHLT Registry report (Kirk et al., 2011). Rejection associated with haemodynamic compromise has an 18% mortality (Pahl et al., 2001; Chin et al., 2004). Risk factors for such an episode include non-white race and older age of recipient. Induction therapy and the type of antimetabolite bore no relevance to rejection episodes during the first year; however, children on tacrolimus experienced fewer episodes of rejection (27%) compared to children treated with cyclosporin (42%). The difference in the number of rejection episodes does not translate into a difference in conditional survival (Kirk et al., 2011). Episodes of rejection may occur without clinical symptoms, and therefore endomyocardial biopsy is the gold standard for screening and diagnosis of rejection (Conway and Dipchand, 2010).

### Infection

Infections are a cause of significant early mortality and remain a continuous threat in immunosuppressed children (Conway and Dipchand, 2010; Kirk et al., 2011). It is of utmost importance to observe aseptic technique when performing invasive procedures in transplanted children and to provide the appropriate antibiotics for specific surgical procedures. However, prophylaxis for infective endocarditis is not recommended unless valvulopathy is present (Wilson et al., 2007).

### Cardiac allograft vasculopathy

Cardiac allograft vasculopathy (CAV) is a serious transplant-related morbidity with a linear increase in prevalence with time from transplant (Kirk et al., 2011; and according to the ISHLT). Risk factors include a history of being highly sensitized and age at time of transplantation: 8 years after transplant, 78%, 75%, and 55% of infant, child, and adolescent patients were free of CAV, respectively. Rejection during the first year, induction therapy, and the specifics of immunosuppressive therapy were not part of the risk profile. Graft survival is severely influenced by CAV, being only 48% at 5 years after transplant when CAV is present.

### Renal dysfunction and hypertension

Renal dysfunction is a multifactorial comorbidity (Sachdeva et al., 2007; Kirk et al., 2011). Pretransplant low cardiac output state and diuretic use contribute to the aetiology. The presence of renal dysfunction declines after transplantation. However, there is a gradual increase in prevalence the longer the children were followed (Sachdeva et al., 2007). Eleven years after transplant 5% of children are dependent on renal replacement therapy (Kirk et al., 2011). Presence of renal insufficiency at 6 months after transplant is a strong predictor of chronic kidney disease at 5 years (Sachdeva et al., 2007). Other risk factors include African-American race, younger age at transplant, and a high level of CNIs. Once renal dysfunction is detected it is essential to avoid or minimize nephrotoxic medications, including CNIs, to decrease the likelihood of further deterioration (Conway and Dipchand, 2010).

Hypertension is common in children after transplantation; an earlier Registry report stated 69% at 8 years follow-up (Kirk et al., 2009a). Ongoing steroid therapy is clearly the major contributor to hypertension (according to the ISHLT). Treatment is obligatory to reduce long-term risk of coronary artery disease and renal dysfunction.

### Malignancy

Another significant and time-dependent morbidity, caused by the immunosuppressive therapy, is post-transplant malignancy, with a prevalence of 15% at 13 years after transplantation (Kirk et al., 2011). Unlike adults who develop skin, solid-organ, and lymphoid neoplastic disease, children almost exclusively are affected by PTLD (Kirk et al., 2011). The development of PTLD is linked to primary infection of EBV after transplantation (Webber et al., 2006). Treatment varies depending on the histology and stage of the disease and includes, among others, lowering immunosuppression and administering antiviral agents while monitoring rejection. Outcomes are satisfactory, with survival of 60% and event-free survival over 40% 5 years after PTLD diagnosis (Webber et al., 2006).

## Perioperative management

### Preanaesthetic assessment and considerations

Children on the waiting list for heart transplantation can be classified into four groups in terms of the acuity of their heart disease: (1) children at home, stable on heart failure medication, a minority in our current practice; (2) children on the cardiac floor with intravenous inotropic medication (i.e. milrinone) and CPAP ventilatory support; (3) children may be in the cardiac ICU on maximal medical therapy of various inotropes and mechanical ventilation; and (4) children may be in the ICU (or cardiac floor) following implantation of a mechanical circulatory assist device. Anaesthetic considerations of the first group are governed by the primary disease-related concerns. Namely, for this group of children the anaesthetic technique of induction and maintenance should take into consideration the need to observe the specific physiological goals for HCM, RCM, and palliated CHD, as reviewed in the literature (Rosenthal and Hammer, 2011; White, 2011; Ing et al., 2012). Perioperative care of children in groups (2) and (3) has to reflect the fact that they are in end-stage heart failure. Specifics of the BH in-situ group (4) have been discussed in the section 'Mechanical circulatory support' (and see Table 34.3).

Medical charts of listed children are quite comprehensive and must be reviewed by the anaesthesiologist. Particular attention, beyond the usual airway, anaesthetic history, allergy, and primary disease, has to be paid to the full cardiac work-up, including previous cardiac surgical history, ECHO and catheterization data, peripheral vessel imaging, blood group and PRA status, and end-organ involvement. Members of the transplant team need to communicate with each other not only to determine optimal OR time but also to emphasize specific concerns related to their own field, such as the need for plasmapheresis in case of high PRA titre, the potential for significant perioperative bleeding related to previous sternotomies in cyanotic CHD, the specific management goals of a mechanical assist device, or the cannulation site for rapid-access CPB. Logistics and timing of transportation need to be resolved as part of the preanaesthetic assessment.

Clinical examination should focus on airway, current haemodynamic and respiratory status, vascular access, and the need and possibility of preoperative sedation. In our experience, a significant portion of children in groups (2) and (3) do not tolerate sedation, while this is not the case for children arriving from home or who are rehabilitated by a VAD. These children are often very anxious and their careful sedation is of prime importance.

## Intra- and postoperative management

The level of monitoring in children coming for heart transplantation varies from non-invasive, minimal to 'fully lined', complete with arterial line and central venous cannula or PICC line in place. Induction of children with limited cardiovascular reserve is a particularly critical time of perioperative care. Induction has to be performed being mindful of sudden deterioration in haemodynamic or respiratory status. Therefore it is advantageous to have invasive monitoring in place to allow careful titration of induction medication. However, placement of such monitors in the awake or even the sedated child with limited reserve is counterproductive. We advocate slow, watchful titration of induction agents, observing vital signs, particularly mental status. In addition, adopting the pioneering work of Dr Hoffman and colleagues (Hoffman et al., 2005), prior to induction we place near-infrared spectroscopy (NIRS) probes on both the forehead and the T12–L2 flank region to allow monitoring of regional oxygen delivery as an indication of cardiac output.

The type of induction medications is of minor importance; combination of fentanyl, midazolam, propofol, ketamine, and sevoflurane as dictated by the underlying diagnosis and clinical state of the child and the preference of the anaesthesiologist is entirely acceptable. It is essential to have the ability to increase ongoing inotrope infusions, and resuscitating drugs have to be at hand during induction. Furthermore, access site for rapid cannulation has to be prepped and draped prior to induction, as the clinical situation, e.g. limited function and redo sternotomy, commands. Induction is followed by expeditious airway control and establishment of appropriate vascular access and full invasive monitoring.

Pre-bypass maintenance is a high narcotic, low inhalational agent technique, with ongoing inotrope support as needed. Surgical exposure can be lengthy in redo sternotomies and bleeding may be substantial as a consequence of both prior surgeries and coagulopathy related to end-organ damage and lingering anticoagulation. Volume replacement needs to observe the conservative blood product management of transplantation.

Issues faced after the donor heart is implanted include global myocardial dysfunction related to ischaemia time, RV dysfunction and PHT, physiology of the denervated heart, bleeding, and transfusion management. In preparation for separating from CPB support, metabolic derangements have to be addressed, normothermia needs to be achieved, and requisite lung compliance ensured. Our institutional preference is to administer 50–100 mcg/kg of milrinone bolus prior to coming off pump, and our inotrope management for separation includes infusion of isoproterenol to drive the denervated heart at a heart rate that provides sufficient cardiac output. Milrinone is continued at 0.66–0.99 mcg/kg/min and a modest drip of epinephrine is maintained to overcome any myocardial dysfunction. Post-CPB vasodilatory shock is rare in children, with; reported incidence of 3% in a 300-patient cohort (Killinger et al., 2009); however, the multivariate analysis of this study identified only heart transplantation and VAD placement as highly predictive of the condition (Killinger et al., 2009). Vasopressin and/or norepinephrine drips can be added to avert the shock state. Post-CPB vasodilatory shock is, usually, not a lasting condition, but it can complicate the management of post-transplant RV failure.

Post-CPB RV failure and PHT are pivotal matters in paediatric heart transplantation, requiring early and aggressive treatment by the anaesthesiologist. Acute RV failure following heart transplantation is common—25% incidence in a paediatric single-centre study (Hoskote et al., 2010)—and has major consequences in the form of increased early morbidity and mortality (Bourge et al., 1993; Hoskote et al., 2010; and according to the ISHLT) and, in earlier era, decreased long-term survival (Hosenpud et al., 2000). Both donor and recipient factors are implicated in the aetiology. Brain death initiates a sympathetic storm causing transient cardiac dysfunction (White et al., 1995; Novitzky, 1997), predominantly on the right side of the donor heart (Bittner et al., 1995; Stoica et al., 2006). Elevated PVR prior to transplantation and suboptimal right heart protection during prolonged ischaemia may be additional factors setting the stage for acute RV failure following coupling of the donor heart and the recipient pulmonary vasculature. However, in the largest study to date (Hoskote et al., 2010), multivariate analysis identified pretransplant elevated PVR and the primary diagnoses of RCM and CHD only, and no donor variables, as significant risk factors. It is important to note that the absence of these risk factors does not preclude RV failure. In fact, 72% of RV failure happened in children who had acceptable pretransplantation PVR in Hoskote's review (Hoskote et al., 2010).

Management of post-transplant RV failure revolves around pulmonary vasodilation, normalization of coronary perfusion, inotropic support, and timely decision to perform an atrial septostomy, or institute mechanical support of the RV. In anticipation of PHT, it is best to separate from the bypass circuit with slightly alkaline pH, compliant lungs, optimal PEEP, modest hyperventilation, and high $FiO_2$. An iNO delivery system has to be available in the OR in case such pulmonary vasodilatory measures failed. Any indication of PHT, as evidenced by inspection (struggling RV, RV distention), by TEE (decreased RV contractility and dilatation, increasing tricuspid regurgitation), or by other monitoring means (increasing RA pressure, decreasing NIRS reading), should prompt aggressive acceleration of pharmacological therapy: iNO for selective pulmonary vasodilation, increased epinephrine infusion for inotropic support of the RV, and a vasopressor infusion to ensure coronary perfusion. Increasing SVR will have the added benefit of improving LV output by supporting (stenting) the interventricular septum. Along these lines, it is critical to reduce preload to the ischaemic distended RV and not to try to improve haemodynamics with volume administration. If the above measures prove insufficient, the goal is to gain some degree of haemostasis and establish mechanical support for the RV in the form of ECMO or RVAD. RV function is expected to improve with unloading and maintained coronary perfusion. PVR and reactivity decrease as well (Gajarski et al., 1994). Children who were mechanically supported for RV failure had an acceptable outcome: 60% survival in Hoskote's cohort (Hoskote et al., 2010).

## Conclusion

Heart transplantation is a highly effective treatment for end-stage heart failure in children. Even though the paediatric transplant field was originally lagging behind adult heart transplantation, continuing advancement, such as ABOi transplantation, transplantation in sensitized children, and miniaturization of assist devices, forced by the scarcity of donor organs, places the field at the forefront of transplant medicine. The extreme end of physiological vulnerability, the complex pathologies present, the steadily advancing field, and the enormous impact make anaesthesia for these children challenging and immensely rewarding at the same time.

## Introduction to paediatric lung transplantation

In this section we generally refer to the chapter on adult lung transplantation (Chapter 32) and will only discuss pertinent differences in indications and management.

The first successful paediatric lung transplantation was performed in 1987 at the University of Toronto in a 16-year-old boy with familial pulmonary fibrosis (Mendeloff, 2002). The accomplishment was a direct consequence of the success of adult lung transplantation pioneered by the Toronto Lung Transplant Program. According to the ISHLT Registry, since then a total of over 1,700 paediatric lung transplantations have been performed, and the annual number of transplants has increased to 100–120 in recent years (Benden et al., 2011; and according to the ISHLT). The number of centres reporting lung transplantation in children increased to 49; however, there are only three centres performing more than ten transplantations a year, accounting for 28% of the procedures. The age distribution of recipients remained the same over the years: 70% are 12–17 years old, 18% are 6–11 years old. Transplantations in infants continues to be rare, with only a handful of transplants reported yearly. The main indication in children over 6 years of age is CF, accounting for 56% and 72% of transplants in the 6–11 and 12–17 years age groups, respectively. Diagnoses of recipients under 6 years of age are distributed in four major categories: idiopathic pulmonary arterial hypertension, idiopathic pulmonary fibrosis, CHD, and surfactant protein B deficiency. Under 1 year of age, CHD (including pulmonary venous stenosis) is the most common (24.4%) diagnosis, followed by surfactant protein B deficiency (17.4%) (according to the ISHLT).

### Indications, contraindications, and outcomes

Apart from the leading diagnosis, CF, a common indication in adults, there are a number of unique paediatric conditions that will cause end-stage respiratory failure, as a result of either progressive parenchymal disease or critical pulmonary vascular disease. General contraindications are similar to contraindications of heart and adult lung transplantation and include active malignancy, sepsis, and tuberculosis, severe neuromuscular disease, refractory non-adherence, multiple organ dysfunction, HIV infection, and hepatitis C infection with histological liver disease (Faro et al., 2007). Relative contraindications are centre-specific and include mechanical ventilation, poorly controlled diabetes mellitus, renal insufficiency, scoliosis, and chronic airway infection with multiresistant organisms. In particular, airway colonization of CF patients by *Burkholderia cepacia* complex constitutes an absolute contraindication at most transplant centres. However, the risk of poor transplant outcomes depends on the actual species and strain, with *Burkholderia cenocepacia* E12 colonization carrying a particularly high mortality risk with or without transplantation (Murray et al., 2008; Solomon et al., 2010). The Toronto Program by successfully employing a combination of strategies (antibiotic synergy testing, triple antibiotics, reduced immunosuppression) is pushing the limits of lung transplantation in this high-mortality population (Nash et al., 2010; Solomon et al., 2010).

Lung transplantation for CHD-related PHT is performed as repair of the cardiac lesion and concomitant lung transplantation. Lesions associated with irreversible PHT and subsequent need for lung transplantation include tetralogy of Fallot with pulmonary atresia (TOF/PA) and inadequate pulmonary vascular bed, pulmonary venous stenosis, VSD with PHT despite adequate repair, and late diagnosis of VSD. Despite the complexity of the surgical procedure and the related perioperative morbidity, outcomes are comparable to heart–lung transplantation in children with PHT and single ventricle anatomy or poor LV function (Choong et al., 2005), permitting better allocation of infant donor hearts. More recent analysis from one of the major paediatric lung transplant centres, however, points to the futility of transplanting the TOF/PA group (Grady et al., 2009). Whereas median survival of other CHD-related lung transplants (over 6 years) is favourable to survival of overall paediatric lung transplants (4.3 years), median survival of children transplanted for TOF/PA is only 47 days. The heterogeneous nature of the pulmonary blood supply in TOF/PA constitutes a high-risk pathology, resulting in a challenging surgical procedure and very high perioperative morbidity (Grady et al., 2009).

Children born with null-mutation in the surfactant protein B gene lack functional surfactant and develop irreversible respiratory failure in the neonatal period (Nogee et al., 1993). Until gene therapy becomes feasible, lung transplantation in the first few months of life is the only treatment option. Outcomes of transplantation for these children are comparable to outcomes of other infant transplantations (Hamvas et al., 1997).

## Surgical procedure and perioperative care

The surgical procedure and perioperative care for children are essentially the same as in adults. The cardinal difference is the near-universal use of CPB. CPB is used in children with PHT and haemodynamic instability. Additionally, stable, sequential lung isolation is technically not possible in small children, precluding the bilateral sequential lung transplant technique. In smaller children, haemodynamic instability arises easily as a consequence of the very restricted surgical field and the presence of extensive adhesions and/or vascularized scar tissue. In order to maintain haemodynamic stability under such circumstances, the anaesthetist is bound to abandon restrictive fluid administration, one of the tenets of lung transplantation (McIlroy et al., 2009) (see Chapter 32). Despite the disadvantages, such as heparinization, increased blood product use, and circuit-related inflammatory response, CPB is a favourable option to a prolonged, dubious struggle to maintain haemodynamics. As discussed in Chapter 32, the use of CPB may be an independent risk factor for primary graft dysfunction. However, the largest single centre comparison of adult and paediatric lung transplantation outcomes demonstrates no difference in primary graft dysfunction between the two groups, suggesting no influence of CPB (Meyers et al., 2005).

Owing to the relative frequency of PHT, we would like to emphasize that induction in this population is a critical moment: means to decrease PHT (iNO) and maintain RV function and haemodynamics (norepinephrine and epinephrine) have to be ready and the OR has to be prepared for urgent cannulation.

## Outcomes

Survival and other outcome measures are similar in children and adult lung transplant recipients (Meyers et al., 2005; Solomon et al., 2010; and according to the ISHLT). Five-year overall survival is 53% and 7-year survival is 45%, with significantly better survival in the 1–11 years recipient group (Benden et al., 2011). Survival improved over the years; however, the improvement is only an indication of better early survival; survival after the first transplant year has not changed since the early years of paediatric lung transplantation (Zafar et al., 2011). Bronchiolitis obliterans syndrome remains the leading cause of death beyond the first transplant year, while early deaths are dominated by infection and graft failure (Benden et al., 2011). Functional status of long-term survivals is excellent, i.e. there are no limitations in activity reported, in over 80% of these children (Görler et al., 2009; and according to the ISHLT).

# Conclusion

Lung transplantation remains a viable but challenging therapeutic option for end-stage lung disease in children, reflecting both the difficulties of lung transplantation in general and the challenges of the paediatric transplant population in particular.

# References


Addonizio LJ, et al. (1987) Elevated pulmonary vascular resistance and cardiac transplantation. *Circulation*, **76**(5 Pt 2):V52–55.

Alvarez JA, et al. (2011) Competing risks for death and cardiac transplantation in children with dilated cardiomyopathy: results from the pediatric cardiomyopathy registry. *Circulation*, **124**(7):814–823.

Amabile N, et al. (2006) Outcome of acute fulminant myocarditis in children. *Heart (Br Cardiac Soc)*, **92**(9):1269–1273.

Ashburn DA, et al. (2004) Determinants of mortality and type of repair in neonates with pulmonary atresia and intact ventricular septum. *J Thoracic Cardiovasc Surg*, **127**(4):1000–1007, discussion 1007–1008.

Bailey LL (2009) The evolution of infant heart transplantation. *J Heart Lung Transplant* **28**(12):1241–1245.

Bailey LL et al. (1993) Bless the babies: one hundred fifteen late survivors of heart transplantation during the first year of life. The Loma Linda University Pediatric Heart Transplant Group. *J Thorac Cardiovasc Surg*, **105**(5):805–14, discussion 814–5.

Bando K, et al. (1993) Improved survival following pediatric cardiac transplantation in high-risk patients. *Circulation*, **88**(5 Pt 2):II218–II223.

Benden C, et al. (2011) The Registry of the International Society for Heart and Lung Transplantation: fourteenth pediatric lung and heart-lung transplantation report—2011. *J Heart Lung Transplant*, **30**(10):1123–1132.

Bernat JL (2008) The boundaries of organ donation after circulatory death. *N Engl J Med*, **359**(7):669–671.

Bernstein D et al. (2006) Outcome of listing for cardiac transplantation for failed Fontan: a multi-institutional study. *Circulation*, **114**(4)273–280.

Betkowski AS et al. (2002) Panel-reactive antibody screening practices prior to heart transplantation. *J Heart Lung Transplant* **21**(6):644–650.

Biagini E et al. (2005) Dilated-hypokinetic evolution of hypertrophic cardiomyopathy: prevalence, incidence, risk factors, and prognostic implications in pediatric and adult patients. *J Am Coll Cardiology*, **46**(8):1543–1550.

Bittner HB, et al. (1995) Myocardial beta-adrenergic receptor function and high-energy phosphates in brain death—related cardiac dysfunction. *Circulation*, **92**(9 Suppl):II472–II478.

Blume ED, et al. (2006) Outcomes of children bridged to heart transplantation with ventricular assist devices: a multi-institutional study. *Circulation*, **113**(19):2313–2319.

Boucek MM (2001) Breaching the barrier of ABO incompatibility in heart transplantation for infants. *N Engl J Med*, **344**(11):843–844.

Boucek MM et al. (2008) Pediatric heart transplantation after declaration of cardiocirculatory death. *N Engl J Med*, **359**(7):709–714.

Bourge RC et al. (1993) Pretransplantation risk factors for death after heart transplantation: a multiinstitutional study. The Transplant Cardiologists Research Database Group. *J Heart Lung Transplant*, **12**(4):549–562.

Bućin D, Johansson S, Lindberg LO (2006). Heart transplantation across antibodies against human leukocyte antigen and ABO-post-transplant follow-up of donor reactive antibodies. *Xenotransplantation*, **13**(2):101–104.

Butler J, et al. (2005) Pre-transplant reversible pulmonary hypertension predicts higher risk for mortality after cardiac transplantation. *J Heart Lung Transplant*, **24**(2)170–177.

Calder AL, Peebles CR, Occleshaw CJ (2007) The prevalence of coronary arterial abnormalities in pulmonary atresia with intact ventricular septum and their influence on surgical results. *Cardiol Young*, **17**(4)387–396.

Canter CE, Kantor PF (2007) Heart transplant for pediatric cardiomyopathy. *Prog Pediatr Cardiol*, **23**(1):67–72.

Canter CE, et al. (2007) Indications for heart transplantation in pediatric heart disease: a scientific statement from the American Heart Association Council on Cardiovascular Disease in the Young; the Councils on Clinical Cardiology, Cardiovascular Nursing, and Cardiovascular Surgery and Anesthesia; and the Quality of Care and Outcomes Research Interdisciplinary Working Group. *Circulation*, **115**(5):658–676.

Carey JA, et al. (1998) Orthotopic cardiac transplantation for the failing Fontan circulation. *Eur J Cardio-Thorac Surg*, **14**(1):7–13, discussion 13–14.

Chatterjee K, et al. (2010) Doxorubicin cardiomyopathy. *Cardiology*, **115**(2):155–162.

Checchia PA, et al. (1997) Cardiac transplantation for Kawasaki disease. *Pediatrics*, **100**(4):695–699.

Chen JM, et al. (2004) Trends and outcomes in transplantation for complex congenital heart disease: 1984 to 2004. *Annal Thorac Surg*, **78**(4):1352–1361.

Chen SC, Balfour IC, Jureidini S (2001) Clinical spectrum of restrictive cardiomyopathy in children. *J Heart Lung Transplant*, **20**(1):90–92.

Chin C, et al. (2004) Risk factors for recurrent rejection in pediatric heart transplantation: a multicenter experience. *J Heart Lung Transplant*, **23**(2):178–185.

Chin C, et al. (2006) Cardiac re-transplantation in pediatrics: a multi-institutional study. *J Heart Lung Transplant*, **25**(12):1420–1424.

Chiu P, et al. (2012) What is high risk? Redefining elevated pulmonary vascular resistance index in pediatric heart transplantation. *J Heart Lung Transplant*, **31**(1):61–66.

Choong CK, et al. (2005) Repair of congenital heart lesions combined with lung transplantation for the treatment of severe pulmonary hypertension: a 13-year experience. *J Thorac Cardiovasc Surg*, **129**(3):661–669.

Cigarroa RG, Lange RA, Hillis LD (1989) Oximetric quantitation of intracardiac left-to-right shunting: limitations of the Qp/Qs ratio. *Am J Cardiol*, **64**(3):246–247.

Colan SD, et al. (2007) Epidemiology and cause-specific outcome of hypertrophic cardiomyopathy in children: findings from the Pediatric Cardiomyopathy Registry. *Circulation*, **115**(6):773–781.

Conway J, Dipchand AI (2010) Heart transplantation in children. *Pediatr Clinic N Am*, **57**(2):353–73, table of contents.

Conway J, Dipchand AI (2011) Transplantation and pediatric cardiomyopathies: Indications for listing and risk factors for death while waiting. *Prog Pediatr Cardiol*, **32**(1):51–54.

Cooper DK (1990) Clinical survey of heart transplantation between ABO blood group-incompatible recipients and donors. *J Heart Transplant*, **9**(4):376–381.

Costanzo MR, et al. (1995) Selection and treatment of candidates for heart transplantation. A statement for health professionals from the Committee on Heart Failure and Cardiac Transplantation of the Council on Clinical Cardiology, American Heart Association. *Circulation*, **92**(12):3593–3612.

Coutu M, et al. (2004) Cardiac transplantation for hypertrophic cardiomyopathy: a valid therapeutic option. *J Heart Lung Transplant*, **23**(4):413–417.

Curfman GD, Morrissey S, Drazen JM (2008) Cardiac transplantation in infants. *N Engl J Med*, **359**(7):749–750.

Daebritz SH, et al. (2007) Blood type incompatible cardiac transplantation in young infants. *Eur J Cardio-Thorac Surg*, **31**(3):339–43, discussion 343.

Daubeney PEF, et al. (2006) Clinical features and outcomes of childhood dilated cardiomyopathy: results from a national population-based study. *Circulation*, **114**(24):2671–2678.

Davies NJ, et al. (1984) Pulmonary vascular resistance in children with congenital heart disease. *Thorax*, **39**(12):895–900.

Davies R, et al. (2009) Transplantation for the 'failed' Fontan. *Progr Pediatr Cardiol*, **26**(1):21–29.

Davies RR, et al. (2011) Increased short- and long-term mortality at low-volume pediatric heart transplant centers: should minimum standards be set? Retrospective data analysis. *Annal Surg*, **253**(2):393–401.

Denfield SW, Weber SA (2010) Restrictive cardiomyopathy in childhood. *Heart Fail Clin*, **6**(4):445–452, viii.

Dhanani S, Hornby L, Ward R, Shemie S (2011) Variability in the determination of death after cardiac arrest: a review of guidelines and statements. *J Intensive Care Med*, 27(4):238–252.

Dipchand A (2011) The Hospital for Sick Children Heart Transplant Program. *Clin Protocols*, :1–141.

Dipchand A, Cecere R, Delgado D, et al. (2005) Canadian Consensus on cardiac transplantation in pediatric and adult congenital heart disease patients 2004: executive summary. *Can J Cardiol*, **21**(13):1145–1147.

Dipchand AI, et al. (2009) Outcomes of children with cardiomyopathy listed for transplant: a multi-institutional study. *J Heart Lung Transplant*, **28**(12):1312–1321.

Dipchand AI, et al. (2010) Equivalent outcomes for pediatric heart transplantation recipients: ABO-blood group incompatible versus ABO-compatible. *Am J Transplant*, **10**(2):389–397.

Drakos SG, et al. (2007) Effect of reversible pulmonary hypertension on outcomes after heart transplantation. *J Heart Lung Transplant*, **26**(4):319–323.

Elliott P, et al. (2008) Classification of the cardiomyopathies: a position statement from the European Society Of Cardiology Working Group on Myocardial and Pericardial Diseases. *Eur Heart J*, **29**(2):270–276.

Fan X, et al. (2004) Donor-specific B-cell tolerance after ABO-incompatible infant heart transplantation. *Nat Med*, **10**(11):1227–1233.

Faro A, Mallory GB, Visner GA, et al. (2007) American Society of Transplantation executive summary on pediatric lung transplantation. *Am J Transplant*, **7**(2):285–292.

Fong SW, Qaqundah BY, Taylor WF (1974) Developmental patterns of ABO isoagglutinins in normal children correlated with the effects of age, sex, and maternal isoagglutinins. *Transfusion*, **14**(6):551–559.

Fontan F, et al. (1990) Outcome after a 'perfect' Fontan operation. *Circulation*, **81**(5):1520–1536.

Fraser CD, et al. (2012) Prospective trial of a pediatric ventricular assist device. *N Engl J Med*, **367**(6):532–541.

Freedom RM, et al. (2000) Selected aspects of cardiac tumors in infancy and childhood. *Pediatr Cardiol*, **21**(4):299–316.

Gajarski RJ, et al. (1994) Intermediate follow-up of pediatric heart transplant recipients with elevated pulmonary vascular resistance index. *J Am Coll Cardiol*, **23**(7):1682–1687.

Gajarski R, et al. (2009) Outcomes of pediatric patients with hypertrophic cardiomyopathy listed for transplant. *J Heart Lung Transplant*, **28**(12):1329–1334.

Gamba A, et al. (2004) Heart transplantation in patients with previous Fontan operations. *J Thorac Cardiovasc Surg*, **127**(2):555–562.

Gandhi SK, et al. (2008) Beyond Berlin: heart transplantation in the 'untransplantable'. *J Thorac Cardiovasc Surg*, **136**(2):529–531.

Gewirtz DA, (1999) A critical evaluation of the mechanisms of action proposed for the antitumor effects of the anthracycline antibiotics adriamycin and daunorubicin. *Biochem Pharmacol*, **57**(7):727–741.

Giglia TM, Humpl T (2010) Preoperative pulmonary hemodynamics and assessment of operability: is there a pulmonary vascular resistance that precludes cardiac operation? *Pediatr Crit Care Med*, **11**(2 Suppl):S57–69.

Goldman AP, et al. (2003) The waiting game: bridging to paediatric heart transplantation. *Lancet*, **362**(9400):1967–1970.

Görler H, et al. (2009) Lung and heart-lung transplantation in children and adolescents: a long-term single-center experience. *J Heart Lung Transplant*, **28**(3):243–248.

Grady RM, et al. (2009) Dismal lung transplant outcomes in children with tetralogy of Fallot with pulmonary atresia compared to Eisenmenger syndrome or pulmonary vein stenosis. *J Heart Lung Transplant*, **28**(11):1221–1225.

Griffiths ER, et al. (2009) Evaluating failing Fontans for heart transplantation: predictors of death. *Annal Thorac Surg*, **88**(2):558–563, discussion 563–564.

Haddad H, Isaac D, Legare JF, et al. (2009) Canadian Cardiovascular Society Consensus Conference update on cardiac transplantation 2008: executive summary. *Can J Cardiol*, **25**(4):197–205.

Hamvas A, et al. (1997) Lung transplantation for treatment of infants with surfactant protein B deficiency. *J Pediatrics*, **130**(2):231–239.

Harvard Medical School (1968) A definition of irreversible coma. Report of the Ad Hoc Committee of the Harvard Medical School to examine the definition of brain death. *JAMA*, **205**(6):337–340.

Hershberger RE, Siegfried JD (2011) Update 2011: clinical and genetic issues in familial dilated cardiomyopathy. *J Am Coll Cardiol*, **57**(16):1641–1649.

Hetzer R, et al. (1999) Pulsatile pediatric ventricular assist devices: current results for bridge to transplantation. *Semin Thoracic Cardiovasc Surg Pediatr Card Surg Annu*, **2**:157–176.

Hetzer R, et al. (2006) Improvement in survival after mechanical circulatory support with pneumatic pulsatile ventricular assist devices in pediatric patients. *Annal Thorac Surg*, **82**(3):917–924, discussion 924–925.

Hickey EJ, et al. (2012) Hypertrophic cardiomyopathy in childhood: disease natural history, impact of obstruction, and its influence on survival. *Annal Thorac Surg*, **93**(3):840–848.

Hoff Von DD, et al. (1979) Risk factors for doxorubicin-induced congestive heart failure. *Annal Intern Med*, **91**(5):710–717.

Hoffman GM, Ghanayem NS, Tweddell JS (2005) Noninvasive assessment of cardiac output. *Semin Thorac Cardiovasc Surg Pediatr Card Surg Annu*, **2005**:12–21.

Holt DB, et al. (2007) Mortality and morbidity in pre-sensitized pediatric heart transplant recipients with a positive donor crossmatch utilizing peri-operative plasmapheresis and cytolytic therapy. *J Heart Lung Transplant*, **26**(9):876–882.

Hooper DK, et al. (2005) Panel-reactive antibodies late after allograft implantation in children. *Annal Thorac Surg*, **79**(2):641–644, discussion 645.

Hosenpud JD, et al. (2000) The Registry of the International Society for Heart and Lung Transplantation: seventeenth official report 2000. *J Heart Lung Transplant*, **19**(10):909–931.

Hoskote A, et al. (2010) Acute right ventricular failure after pediatric cardiac transplant: predictors and long-term outcome in current era of transplantation medicine. *J Thorac Cardiovasc Surg*, **139**(1):146–153.

Hsu DT, Canter CE (2010). Dilated cardiomyopathy and heart failure in children. *Heart Fail Clin*, **6**(4):415–32, vii.

Huang J, et al. (2004) Risk factors for primary graft failure after pediatric cardiac transplantation: importance of recipient and donor characteristics. *J Heart Lung Transplant*, **23**(6):716–722.

Huddleston C (2009) Indications for heart transplantation in children. *Progr Pediatr Cardiol*, **26**(1):3–9.

Huebler M, et al. (2011) Pediatric heart transplantation: 23-year single-center experience. *Eur J Cardio-Thorac Surg*, **39**(5):e83–e89.

Imamura M, et al. (2009) Bridge to cardiac transplant in children: Berlin Heart versus extracorporeal membrane oxygenation. *Annal Thorac Surg*, **87**(6):1894–1901, discussion 1901.

Ing RJ, Ames WA, Chambers NA (2012) Paediatric cardiomyopathy and anaesthesia. *Br J Anaesth*, **108**(1):4–12.

Itescu S, John R (2003) Interactions between the recipient immune system and the left ventricular assist device surface: immunological and clinical implications. *Annal Thorac Surg*, **75**(6 Suppl):S58–65.

Jacobs JP, et al. (2004) Pediatric cardiac transplantation in children with high panel reactive antibody. *Annal Thorac Surg*, **78**(5):1703–1709.

Jahangiri M, et al. (1997) Coagulation factor abnormalities after the Fontan procedure and its modifications. *J Thorac Cardiovasc Surg*, **113**(6):989–92, discussion 992–993.

Jamieson D, Boddy AV, (2011) Pharmacogenetics of genes across the doxorubicin pathway. *Expert Opin Drug Metab Toxicol*, **7**(10):1201–1210.

Jayakumar KA, et al. (2004) Cardiac transplantation after the Fontan or Glenn procedure. *J Am Coll Cardiol*, **44**(10):2065–2072.

Jeewa A, et al. (2010) Outcomes with ventricular assist device versus extracorporeal membrane oxygenation as a bridge to pediatric heart transplantation. *Artific Organ*, **34**(12):1087–1091.

Jefferies JL, Towbin JA (2010) Dilated cardiomyopathy. *Lancet*, **375**(9716):752–762.

Kantor PF, et al. (2010) The impact of changing medical therapy on transplantation-free survival in pediatric dilated cardiomyopathy. *J Am College Cardiol*, **55**(13):1377–1384.

Kantrowitz A, et al. (1968) Transplantation of the heart in an infant and an adult. *Am J Cardiol*, **22**(6):782–790.

Kärkkäinen S, Peuhkurinen K (2007) Genetics of dilated cardiomyopathy. *Annal Med*, **39**(2):91–107.

Khambadkone S, et al. (2003) Basal pulmonary vascular resistance and nitric oxide responsiveness late after Fontan-type operation. *Circulation*, **107**(25):3204–3208.

Killinger JS, et al. (2009) Children undergoing heart transplant are at increased risk for postoperative vasodilatory shock. *Pediatr Crit Care Med*, **10**(3):335–340.

Kirk R, Edwards LB, et al. (2009a) Registry of the International Society for Heart and Lung Transplantation: twelfth official pediatric heart transplantation report—2009. *J Heart Lung Transplant*, **28**(10):993–1006.

Kirk R, Naftel D, et al. (2009b) Outcome of pediatric patients with dilated cardiomyopathy listed for transplant: a multi-institutional study. *J Heart Lung Transplant*, **28**(12):1322–1328.

Kirk R, et al. (2011) The Registry of the International Society for Heart and Lung Transplantation: fourteenth pediatric heart transplantation report—2011. *J Heart Lung Transplant*, **30**(10):1095–1103.

Kirklin JK, et al. (1988) Pulmonary vascular resistance and the risk of heart transplantation. *J Heart Transplant*, **7**(5):331–336.

Kobashigawa JA, et al., 1996. Pretransplant panel reactive-antibody screens: are they truly a marker for poor outcome after cardiac transplantation? *Circulation*, **94**(9):294–297.

Kuehne T (2005). Magnetic resonance imaging guided catheterisation for assessment of pulmonary vascular resistance: in vivo validation and clinical application in patients with pulmonary hypertension. *Heart (Br Cardiac Soc)*, **91**(8):1064–1069.

Kühl U, Schultheiss H-P (2010) Myocarditis in children. *Heart Fail Clin*, **6**(4):483–496, viii–ix.

Larsen RL, et al. (2002) Usefulness of cardiac transplantation in children with visceral heterotaxy (asplenic and polysplenic syndromes and single right-sided spleen with levocardia) and comparison of results with cardiac transplantation in children with dilated cardiomyopathy. *Am J Cardiol*, **89**(11):1275–1279.

Lee KJ, et al. (1999) Clinical outcomes of acute myocarditis in childhood. *Heart (Br Cardiac Soc)*, **82**(2):226–233.

Liberthson R (1996) Sudden death from cardiac causes in children and young adults. *N Engl J Med*, **334**(16):1039–1044.

Liden H, et al. (2009) Does pretransplant left ventricular assist device therapy improve results after heart transplantation in patients with elevated pulmonary vascular resistance? *Eur J Cardio-Thorac Surg*, **35**(6):1029–1034, discussion 1034–1035.

Lim JSL, et al. (2005) Clinical features, management, and outcome of children with fetal and postnatal diagnoses of isomerism syndromes. *Circulation*, **112**(16):2454–2461.

Lipshultz SE, et al. (2003) The incidence of pediatric cardiomyopathy in two regions of the United States. *N Engl J Med*, **348**(17):1647–1655.

Maron BJ, et al. (1982) Hypertrophic cardiomyopathy in infants: clinical features and natural history. *Circulation*, **65**(1):7–17.

Maron BJ, et al. (1986) Intramural ('small vessel') coronary artery disease in hypertrophic cardiomyopathy. *J Am Coll Cardiol*, **8**(3):545–557.

Maron MS, et al. (2006) Hypertrophic cardiomyopathy is predominantly a disease of left ventricular outflow tract obstruction. *Circulation*, **114**(21):2232–2239.

McIlroy DR, Pilcher DV, Snell GI (2009). Does anaesthetic management affect early outcomes after lung transplant? An exploratory analysis. *Br J Anaesth*, **102**(4):506–514.

McKenna WJ, Deanfield JE (1984) Hypertrophic cardiomyopathy: an important cause of sudden death. *Arch Dis Childhood*, **59**(10):971–975.

McKenna WJ, et al. (1988) Arrhythmia and prognosis in infants, children and adolescents with hypertrophic cardiomyopathy. *J Am Coll Cardiol*, **11**(1):147–153.

Mendeloff EN (2002) The history of pediatric heart and lung transplantation. *Pediatr Transplant*, **6**(4):270–279.

Mertens L, et al. (1998) Protein-losing enteropathy after the Fontan operation: an international multicenter study. PLE study group. *J Thorac Cardiovasc Surg*, **115**(5):1063–1073.

Meyers BF, et al. (2005) Primary graft dysfunction and other selected complications of lung transplantation: a single-center experience of 983 patients. *J Thorac Cardiovasc Surg*, **129**(6):1421–1429.

Miera O, et al. (2011) First experiences with the HeartWare ventricular assist system in children. *Annal Thorac Surg*, **91**(4):1256–1260.

Mitchell MB, Campbell DN, Boucek MM (2004a) Heart transplantation for the failing Fontan circulation. *Semin Thorac Cardiovasc Surg*, 7:56–64.

Mitchell MB, Campbell DN, Ivy D, et al. (2004b) Evidence of pulmonary vascular disease after heart transplantation for Fontan circulation failure. *J Thorac Cardiovasc Surg*, **128**(5):693–702.

Mocumbi AO, et al. (2008) A population study of endomyocardial fibrosis in a rural area of Mozambique. *N Engl J Med*, **359**(1):43–49.

Morales DLS, et al. (2011) Bridging children of all sizes to cardiac transplantation: the initial multicenter North American experience with the Berlin Heart EXCOR ventricular assist device. *J Heart Lung Transplant*, **30**(1):1–8.

Morgan E, Pahl E (2002) Early heart transplant in a child with advanced lymphoma. *Pediatr Transplant*, **6**(6):509–512.

Murali S, et al. (1993) Preoperative pulmonary hemodynamics and early mortality after orthotopic cardiac transplantation: the Pittsburgh experience. *Am Heart J*, **126**(4):896–904.

Murray S, et al. (2008) Impact of burkholderia infection on lung transplantation cystic fibrosis. *Am J Resp Crit Care Med*, **178**(4):363–371.

Muthurangu V, et al. (2004) Novel method of quantifying pulmonary vascular resistance by use of simultaneous invasive pressure monitoring and phase-contrast magnetic resonance flow. *Circulation*, **110**(7):826–834.

Naim MY, et al. (2008) The Children's Hospital of Philadelphia's experience with donation after cardiac death. *Crit Care Med*, **36**(6):1729–1733.

Nash EF, et al. (2010) Survival of *Burkholderia cepacia* sepsis following lung transplantation in recipients with cystic fibrosis. *Transplant Inf Dis*, **12**(6):551–554.

Nogee LM, et al. (1993) Brief report: deficiency of pulmonary surfactant protein B in congenital alveolar proteinosis. *N Engl J Med*, **328**(6):406–410.

Nollert G, et al. (1997) Long-term survival in patients with repair of tetralogy of Fallot: 36-year follow-up of 490 survivors of the first year after surgical repair. *J Am Coll Cardiol*, **30**(5):1374–1383.

Novitzky D (1997) Detrimental effects of brain death on the potential organ donor. *Transplant Proc*, **29**(8):3770–3772.

Nugent AW, et al. (2003) The epidemiology of childhood cardiomyopathy in Australia. *N Engl J Med*, **348**(17):1639–1646.

Ommen SR (2005) There is much more to the recipe than just outflow obstruction. *J Am Coll Cardiol*, **46**(8):1551–1552.

Ommen SR (2011) Hypertrophic cardiomyopathy. *Curr Problem Cardiol*, **36**(11):409–453.

Pagani FD et al. (2001) Development of anti-major histocompatibility complex class I or II antibodies following left ventricular assist device implantation: effects on subsequent allograft rejection and survival. *J Heart Lung Transplant*, **20**(6):646–653.

Pahl E, et al. (2001) Death after rejection with severe hemodynamic compromise in pediatric heart transplant recipients: a multi-institutional study. *J Heart Lung Transplant*, **20**(3):279–287.

Pahl E, Dipchand AI, Burch M (2010) Heart transplantation for heart failure in children. *Heart Fail Clin*, **6**(4):575–89.

Pisani BA, et al. (1999) Plasmapheresis with intravenous immunoglobulin G is effective in patients with elevated panel reactive antibody prior to cardiac transplantation. *J Heart Lung Transplant*, **18**(7):701–706.

Pollock-BarZiv SM, et al. (2007) Pediatric heart transplantation in human leukocyte antigen sensitized patients: evolving management and assessment of intermediate-term outcomes in a high-risk population. *Circulation*, **116**(11 Suppl):I172–I178.

Rajagopal SK, et al. (2010) Extracorporeal membrane oxygenation for the support of infants, children, and young adults with acute myocarditis: a review of the Extracorporeal Life Support Organization registry. *Crit Care Med*, **38**(2):382–387.

Rathe M, et al. (2010) Long-term cardiac follow-up of children treated with anthracycline doses of 300 mg/m2 or less for acute lymphoblastic leukemia. *Pediatr Blood Cancer*, **54**(3):444–448.

Ringewald JM, et al. (2001) Nonadherence is associated with late rejection in pediatric heart transplant recipients. *J Pediatr*, **139**(1):75–78.

Rivenes SM, et al. (2000) Sudden death and cardiovascular collapse in children with restrictive cardiomyopathy. *Circulation*, **102**(8):876–882.

Roche SL, et al. (2008) Multicenter experience of ABO-incompatible pediatric cardiac transplantation. *Am J Transplant*, **8**(1):208–215.

Roos-Hesselink JW et al. (2004) Decline in ventricular function and clinical condition after Mustard repair for transposition of the great arteries (a prospective study of 22-29 years). *Eur Heart J*, **25**(14):1264–1270.

Rosenthal DN, Hammer GB (2011) Cardiomyopathy and heart failure in children: anesthetic implications. *Paediatr Anaesth*, **21**(5):577–584.

Russo LM, Webber SA (2005) Idiopathic restrictive cardiomyopathy in children. *Heart (Br Cardiac Soc)*, **91**(9):1199–1202.

Sachdeva R, et al. (2007) Determinants of renal function in pediatric heart transplant recipients: long-term follow-up study. *J Heart Lung Transplant*, **26**(2):108–113.

Shaddy RE, et al. (1996) Prospective analysis of HLA immunogenicity of cryopreserved valved allografts used in pediatric heart surgery. *Circulation*, **94**(5):1063–1067.

Sharma MS, et al. (2006) Ventricular assist device support in children and adolescents as a bridge to heart transplantation. *Annal Thorac Surg*, **82**(3):926–932.

Simpson KE, et al. (2012) Failed Fontan heart transplant candidates with preserved vs impaired ventricular ejection: 2 distinct patient populations. *J Heart Lung Transplant*, **31**(5):545–547.

Singal PK, Iliskovic N (1998) Doxorubicin-induced cardiomyopathy. *N Engl J Med*, **339**(13):900–905.

Solomon M, Grasemann H, Keshavjee S (2010) Pediatric lung transplantation. *Pediatr Clin North Am*, **57**(2):375–91, table of contents.

Spirito P, et al. (1987) Occurrence and significance of progressive left ventricular wall thinning and relative cavity dilatation in hypertrophic cardiomyopathy. *Am J Cardiol*, **60**(1):123–129.

Stoica SC, et al. (2006) Brain death leads to abnormal contractile properties of the human donor right ventricle. *J Thorac Cardiovasc Surg*, **132**(1):116–123.

Swain SM, Whaley FS, Ewer MS (2003) Congestive heart failure in patients treated with doxorubicin: a retrospective analysis of three trials. *Cancer*, **97**(11):2869–2879.

Takemura G, Fujiwara H (2007) Doxorubicin-induced cardiomyopathy from the cardiotoxic mechanisms to management. *Prog Cardiovasc Dis*, **49**(5):330–352.

Tanaka M, et al. (1987) Quantitative analysis of narrowings of intramyocardial small arteries in normal hearts, hypertensive hearts, and hearts with hypertrophic cardiomyopathy. *Circulation*, **75**(6):1130–1139.

Teele SA, et al. (2011) Management and outcomes in pediatric patients presenting with acute fulminant myocarditis. *J Pediatr*, **158**(4):638–643.

Towbin JA, et al. (2006) Incidence, causes, and outcomes of dilated cardiomyopathy in children. *JAMA*, **296**(15):1867–1876.

Truog RD, Miller FG (2008) The dead donor rule and organ transplantation. *N Engl J Med*, **359**(7):674–675.

Truog RD, Miller FG (2010) Counterpoint: are donors after circulatory death really dead, and does it matter? No and not really. *Chest*, **138**(1):16–8, discussion 18–19.

Tweddell JS, et al. (2009) Fontan palliation in the modern era: factors impacting mortality and morbidity. *Annal Thorac Surg*, **88**(4):1291–1299.

Urschel S, et al. (2010) Absence of donor-specific anti-HLA antibodies after ABO-incompatible heart transplantation in infancy: altered immunity or age? *Am J Transplant*, **10**(1):149–156.

Veatch RM (2008) Donating hearts after cardiac death—reversing the irreversible. *N Engl J Med*, **359**(7):672–673.

Wallace KB (2007) Adriamycin-induced interference with cardiac mitochondrial calcium homeostasis. *Cardiovasc Toxicol*, **7**(2):101–107.

Ward KM, et al. (2004) Pediatric heart transplantation for anthracycline cardiomyopathy: cancer recurrence is rare. *J Heart Lung Transplant*, **23**(9):1040–1045.

Warnecke H, et al. (1991) Mechanical left ventricular support as a bridge to cardiac transplantation in childhood. *Eur J Cardio-Thorac Surg*, **5**(6):330–333.

Webber SA, et al. (2006) Lymphoproliferative disorders after paediatric heart transplantation: a multi-institutional study. *Lancet*, **367**(9506):233–239.

Weiss RB (1992) The anthracyclines: will we ever find a better doxorubicin? *Semin Oncol*, **19**(6):670–686.

Weller RJ, et al. (2002) Outcome of idiopathic restrictive cardiomyopathy in children. *Am J Cardiol*, **90**(5):501–506.

West LJ, et al. (2001) ABO-incompatible heart transplantation in infants. *N Engl J Med*, **344**(11):793–800.

West LJ, et al. (2006) Impact on outcomes after listing and transplantation, of a strategy to accept ABO blood group-incompatible donor hearts for neonates and infants. *J Thorac Cardiovasc Surg*, **131**(2):455–461.

White M, et al. (1995) Cardiac beta-adrenergic neuroeffector systems in acute myocardial dysfunction related to brain injury. Evidence for catecholamine-mediated myocardial damage. *Circulation*, **92**(8):2183–2189.

White MC (2011) Approach to managing children with heart disease for noncardiac surgery. *Paediatr Anaesth*, **21**(5):522–529.

Wilkinson D, et al. (2010) The pediatric cardiomyopathy registry and heart failure: key results from the first 15 years. *Heart Fail Clinic*, **6**(4):401–413, vii.

Wilmot I, et al. (2011) Effectiveness of mechanical circulatory support in children with acute fulminant and persistent myocarditis. *J Cardiac Fail*, **17**(6):487–494.

Wilson W (2007) Prevention of infective endocarditis: guidelines from the American Heart Association: a guideline from the American Heart Association Rheumatic Fever, Endocarditis, and Kawasaki Disease Committee, Council on Cardiovascular Disease in the Young, and the Council on Clinical Cardiology, Council on Cardiovascular Surgery and Anesthesia, and the Quality of Care and Outcomes Research Interdisciplinary Working Group. *Circulation*, **116**(15):1736–1754.

Wright EJ, et al. (2007) Cardiac transplant outcomes in pediatric patients with pre-formed anti-human leukocyte antigen antibodies and/or positive retrospective crossmatch. *J Heart Lung Transplant*, **26**(11):1163–1169.

Yetman AT, et al. (1998) Myocardial bridging in children with hypertrophic cardiomyopathy—a risk factor for sudden death. *N Engl J Med*, **339**(17):1201–1209.

Yoo PS, Olthoff KM, Abt PL (2011) Donation after cardiac death in pediatric organ transplantation. *Curr Opin Organ Transplant*, **16**(5):483–488.

Zafar F, et al. (2011) Two decades of pediatric lung transplant in the United States: have we improved? *J Thorac Cardiovasc Surg*, **141**(3):828–832.

Zales VR, et al. (1993) Pharmacologic reduction of pretransplantation pulmonary vascular resistance predicts outcome after pediatric heart transplantation. *J Heart Lung Transplant*, **12**(6 Pt 1):965–972, discussion 972–973.

Zangwill SD, et al. (2009) Outcomes of children with restrictive cardiomyopathy listed for heart transplant: a multi-institutional study. *J Heart Lung Transplant*, **28**(12):1335–1340.

Zimpfer D, et al. (2007) Post-transplant survival after lowering fixed pulmonary hypertension using left ventricular assist devices. *Eur J Cardio-Thorac Surg*, **31**(4):698–702.

## Further reading

International Society for Heart and Lung Transplantation (ISHLT): <http://www.ishlt.org/registries>.

Pediatric Heart Transplant Study (PHTS): <www.uab.edu/phts>.

SECTION 9

# Special considerations

# CHAPTER 35

# Geriatric transplant anaesthesia

Fouad G. Souki and Michael C. Lewis

## Introduction

The elderly comprise a growing fraction of the population. In 2012, individuals older than 65 years in the US numbered 41.5 million (13.4%), with 5.7 million being older than 80. Estimates suggest that almost 20% of US citizens will be older than 65 by the year 2030. With the aging of the population, and associated increases in pathologies, it is only natural that the demand for medical and surgical services will expand. This increasing need will include organ transplantation.

Historically, elderly patients were seen as higher-risk recipients with shorter life expectancy. These aged patients have largely been excluded from transplantation. However, advances in surgical technique, perioperative care, and immunosuppressants have broadened the indications for organ transplantation to the benefit of the old (Adani et al., 2009). Age, by itself, is no longer considered a contraindication for organ transplantation. In the US, transplantation of patients older than 65 years has increased from 2.1% to 15.5% between 1988 and 2014, with some elderly having repeat transplants. As of 27 February 2015, 21% of candidates on the organ transplant list are older than 65. Of those, 84.5% are registered for a kidney, 12.3% for liver, 2.7% for heart, and 1.4% for lung transplantation. Only 9 elderly patients are registered for a kidney–pancreas transplant, 7 for pancreas, one for intestine, and one for heart–lung (OPTN, 2015).

Despite the increased acceptability of transplantation in the elderly, aged patients still pose greater challenges than younger adults when undergoing surgery. Decreased physiological reserve, frailty, and co-existing disease, such as cardiovascular, pulmonary, endocrine, and renal, increase perioperative morbidity and mortality related to transplant procedures (Herrero et al., 2003; Audet et al., 2010). The continuous scarcity of organ donors has led to ethical questions regarding transplantation in the elderly when outcome and life expectancy are considered. Transplantation success depends on careful evaluation and patient selection with optimal perioperative management (Frühauf et al., 2004). This chapter addresses the physiological changes in the elderly, outcome of organ transplantation, preoperative work-up, and anaesthetic management.

## Physiological changes in the elderly

The elderly represent a unique surgical population that challenges the practitioner by presenting variable physiological and pharmacological puzzles along with co-existing diseases. Aging is associated with the gradual decrease of physiological reserve by 1% per year after the age of 30 (Barash, 2009). By age 70, basal metabolic rate has decreased by 40% (Jones, 1989). Co-existing diseases are common in the elderly and further diminish organ reserve and function.

### Cardiovascular

Aged alterations occur in cardiac efficiency, blood vessels, autonomic control, cardiac conduction, and ischaemic preconditioning. Aging is associated with decreased contractility, LV wall thickening, hypertrophy, myocardial stiffening, impaired diastolic relaxation and filling, diastolic dysfunction, and decreased β-adrenergic sensitivity (Priebe, 2000). Diastolic dysfunction is common in the elderly and associated with increased mortality (Phillip et al., 2003; Rooke, 2003; Matyal et al., 2009). Vascular stiffness leads to systolic hypertension and contributes to the aforementioned heart changes. With aging, the decrease in the response to β-receptor stimulation (Rooke, 2003) and baroreflex control (Ebert et al., 1992) means less heart rate response to catecholamines (i.e. exercise). Sympathetic nervous system activity increases and parasympathetic activity decreases lead to greater intraoperative haemodynamic lability (Folkow and Svanborg, 1993). Due to a decrease in vagal tone, increased heart rate may be limited after administration of atropine or glycopyrrolate. In addition, loss of sinoatrial node cells may make these patients more prone to sick sinus syndrome. Lastly, aging appears to diminish the cardiac protective effects of ischaemic preconditioning (Rooke, 2003). Vascular disease involving the coronaries is prevalent in more than 50% of elderly people (Audet et al., 2010). These processes compromise the heart's ability to buffer changes in circulatory volume, resulting in a disposition to either CHF or hypotension (Robinson et al., 2011).

### Respiratory

As with the cardiovascular system, changes occur in both lung structure and function. Increasing age results in decreased respiratory response to hypoxaemia and hypercapnia, increased lung compliance, decreased chest wall compliance, decreased alveolar surface area, and increased airway resistance and closing volume. Moreover, respiratory muscle mass and strength also decrease with age (Zaugg and Lucchinetti, 2000). These changes lead to an increase in the work of breathing, residual volume, decreased vital capacity, and worsening ventilation–perfusion matching. Susceptibility to hypoxaemia is increased by the gradual age-related decrease in resting arterial oxygen tension. A higher risk for aspiration and pneumonia can be seen due to dysfunctional swallowing caused by decrease in laryngopharyngeal sensation and motor function (Aviv, 1997).

Age is a significant risk factor for postoperative pulmonary complications, mainly atelectasis, acute bronchitis, and pneumonia (Seymour and Vaz, 1989; Smetana et al., 2006; Smetana, 2009). The risk of a postoperative pulmonary complication doubles in patients aged 60–69 and triples in patients aged 70–79 compared to young patients (Qaseem, 2006; Sieber and Barnett, 2011). Postoperative pulmonary complications account for 40% of deaths in patients over the age of 65 (Zaugg and Lucchinetti, 2000). Anaesthesia, severe COPD, and high-risk procedures such as upper abdominal or intrathoracic surgery have also been associated with increased postoperative pulmonary complications (Sprung et al., 2006; Cook and Lisco, 2009). Residual anaesthetic drugs contribute to decreased pharyngeal muscle tone, impaired airway protection, aspiration, increased susceptibility to airway obstruction, and decreased arousal in response to hypoxia and hypercarbia in the PACU (Kaw et al., 2006).

### Neurological

Biochemical, anatomical, and functional changes have been described in the aging brain. Neurotransmitter functions change with aging (Mrak et al., 1997; Peters, 2002). However, coupling of cerebral electric activity, cerebral metabolic rate, and cerebral blood flow are unchanged (Ge et al., 2002). Brain mass decreases slowly, beginning at approximately age 50 such that at the age of 80 the brain has typically lost 10% of its weight (Drachman, 2006). Memory decline occurs in more than 40% of individuals older than age 60 (Small, 2001) and at 85 years of age nearly 50% have significant cognitive impairment. Decreases in brain reserve with aging are manifested by decreases in activity of daily living, increased sensitivity to anaesthetic medications, delayed emergence, increased risk of perioperative delirium, and postoperative cognitive dysfunction (Dyer et al., 1995). Alterations in neurotransmitter levels and neuronal circuits lead to pharmacodynamic changes and changes in sensitivity to anaesthetic agents (Eger, 2001; Matsuura et al., 2009). Increased brain sensitivity along with decreased drug clearance leads to an average dose requirement decrease of 50% for propofol and midazolam in the elderly (Bell et al., 1987; Schnider et al., 1999; Shafer, 2000). Likewise, the older brain appears to be more sensitive to opioids, which are approximately twice as potent in elderly patients (Shafer, 2000; Bowie and Slattum, 2007). Perhaps the best-known anaesthetic effect of brain aging is the 6% decrease in minimum alveolar concentration (MAC) per decade after the age of 40 (Mapleson, 1996). This decline further accelerates after 50 years of age (Nickalls and Mapleson, 2003; Das et al., 2010).

### Hepatic, metabolic, and renal

Aging involves a number of changes in morphology and function of the liver that can lead to a decrease in resistance to pathogenic noxae and an inferior regenerative capacity. As in most aging organs, the decline in function is gradual. No functional laboratory test can be directly related to an influence of aging on the liver (Dal Santo, 2011). Hepatic blood flow decreases with aging (Stell and Wall, 2003; Le Couteur et al., 2009), mostly associated with a 35% decrease in liver mass (Wynne et al., 1989; Wynne, 2005). The decrease in liver mass and hepatic blood flow may have a role in the decline in hepatic metabolism of drugs and anaesthetics (Schmucker, 2001; Wynne, 2005). The reduction in hepatic first-pass metabolism of highly extracted drugs (such as morphine) results in increased plasma drug concentration. While phase 1 reactions (oxidation, reduction, hydrolysis) seem to be most affected by aging, phase 2 reactions (glucuronidation, methylation, sulfation, acylation) are not (Schmucker, 2001; Mangoni and Jackson, 2004).

Altered pharmacological responses of elderly patients are further affected by changes in plasma protein binding, body composition, metabolism, and pharmacodynamics (Sadean and Glass, 2003; Vuyk, 2003; Bowie and Slattum, 2007). As one ages there is a decrease in lean body mass and total body water and an increase in body fat. Due to these changes, intravenous drug bolus administration will cause an increase in the serum concentration of drugs and a prolongation of effect (Shafer, 2000; Singh and Antognini, 2010).

The elderly usually have decreased plasma and total body water with decreased vascular capacitance and kidney function (Navaratnarajah and Jackson, 2013). The aging kidney is characterized by a decrease in renal blood flow, renal mass, GFR, creatinine clearance, tubular function, ability to handle acid load, and thirst response. Renal blood flow decreases by 10% per decade after the age of 50 (Weinstein and Anderson, 2010). Decrease in blood flow is accompanied by a reduction in renal mass, with a loss of 20–25% between the ages of 30 and 80 years. Age-related decline in GFR is often considered the most important pharmacokinetic change in old age. GFR, normally 125 mL/min in young adults, decreases to approximately 80 mL/min at 60 years of age and to about 60 mL/min at 80 years. Creatinine clearance decreases by approximately 1 mL/min/year after the age of 40. Thus drugs that depend on renal function for clearance may accumulate in the elderly. The aging kidney has limited ability to dilute and concentrate urine due to decreased tubular function (Esposito et al., 2010; Weinstein and Anderson, 2010). Impaired tubular activity in the elderly may also lead to decreased acid excretion and perioperative metabolic acidosis (Esposito and Dal Canton, 2010). With age the kidney is also less effective at retaining salt in response to renin–aldosterone plasma activity (Anderson, 1997; Esposito and Dal Canton, 2010). Decreased response to thirst, renin–aldosterone, and ADH systems affects water balance in the old (Hajjar, 1997; Kenney and Chiu, 2001).

Sick elderly patients will often have hyponatraemia due to inadequate electrolyte and water ingestion and regulatory mechanisms (O'Neill, 1996 ; Kenney and Chiu, 2001; Morgan et al., 2002; Hsieh and Power, 2009). Reductions in flow paired with a reduced response to vasodilatory stimuli render the elderly kidney susceptible to the harmful effects of reduced cardiac output, hypotension, hypovolaemia, and haemorrhage (Cook and Rooke, 2003).

## Liver transplantation in the elderly

### Aetiology

Many diseases causing liver failure are age specific and some are increasingly common in patients of advancing age. In the elderly the most common indications for liver transplantation are hepatocellular carcinoma, cirrhosis caused by hepatitis C virus, primary biliary cirrhosis, primary sclerosing cholangitis, and alcoholic cirrhosis (Bjøro et al., 2000; Collins et al., 2000; Bilbao et al., 2008; Floreani, 2009; Audet et al., 2010); in the general adult population, chronic hepatitis C and/or alcoholic liver disease are the most common aetiologies leading to transplantation. The peak incidence of primary biliary cirrhosis occurs in the elderly, with the median age of diagnosis just over 60 (Newton et al., 2000; Neuberger, 2003; Keswani et al., 2004; Lipshutz et al., 2007). During 1990–1998, primary biliary cirrhosis, primary sclerosing cholangitis, and acute hepatic failure were the most frequent diagnoses requiring transplantation in one report (Bjøro et al., 2000). In a survey carried out between 1996 and 2004, the main indication for liver transplantation in the elderly was post-necrotic cirrhosis (59%), followed by hepatocellular carcinoma (33%) over cirrhosis, with half of the patients having hepatitis C virus (Bilbao et al., 2008). For patients older than 70 years of age the most common cause of liver failure requiring liver transplantation was hepatitis C (48%), followed by cryptogenic cirrhosis (18%) (Lipshutz et al., 2007). In one study, 58.5% of cirrhotic patients aged above 80 had hepatitis C virus (Hoshida et al. 1999).

Alcoholic liver disease may be relatively common in seniors. Age of presentation in patients with alcoholic liver disease was > 60 years in 28% of patients and > 70 years in 6% (Potter and James, 1987; Keswani et al., 2004). Drugs may also be the cause of hepatocellular, cholestatic, or mixed damage, which reveals itself as an 'acute hepatitis' or overlap with a previous chronic hepatopathy, worsening the prognosis (Schiødt et al., 2009; Dal Santo, 2011).

## Outcome

Liver transplantation is the standard treatment for decompensated ESLD and clinical outcomes afterwards are excellent, with recent 1- and 5-year survival rates approximating 90% and 75% in young adults, respectively (Cross et al., 2007; Adani et al., 2009). There has been an important change in trend among liver transplant recipients. Increasing numbers of recipients are older. The percentage of recipients aged 65 years or older has gradually increased from 1.7% in 1988 to 15.5% (956/6,142) by November 2014. In February 2015, 3,181 elderly patients were candidates for liver transplantation, 20.7 % of all liver transplant candidates (OPTN, 2015). This change in trend has been due greatly to improvements in surgical, immunological, and perioperative care leading to acceptable graft and patient survival.

During the initial era of transplantation, theoretical shorter life expectancy of older adults led to the initial exclusion of patients aged 50 and older. Reports of good outcome after transplantation in older patients began emerging in the mid-1980s. Early reports of transplants performed in the 1980s showed the survival rates for elderly patients were 71.3% after 1 year and 65.5% after 3 years, comparable to young adults at the time (Stieber et al., 1991). As selection and techniques improved, later work revealed no important differences in survival, initial transplant hospitalization, or the incidence of infection and rejection between the young and elderly (Pirsch et al., 1991). Patient survival was 83% at 2 years for recipients 60 years of age and above compared to 76% patient survival in adult recipients who were under the age of 60 (Pirsch et al., 1991). Further work confirmed that the outcome of liver transplant in patients over 60 is comparable to that observed in patients under that age (Donovan et al., 1996; Kryzhanovski and Beller, 1997; De la Peña et al., 1998).

Eventually studies compared outcome in patients > 65, 70, and 75 years of age (Bjøro et al., 2000; Lipshutz et al., 2007; Taner et al., 2012). Other researchers compared patients aged > 65 years with those aged 60–65. Patient 1-year survival was 75% and 3-year survival 62%, which was not significantly lower than that of younger patients (Bjøro et al., 2000). Bilbao also showed that results in patients > 65 years old are comparable to those < 65 years if older candidates are carefully selected (Bilbao et al., 2008). Survival at 1, 3, 5, and 10 years was 82%, 75%, 72%, and 70% for the < 65 years group vs 77%, 66%, 55%, and 55% for the > 65 years group, respectively, with fewer infections and rejections occurring in the elderly postoperatively (Bilbao et al., 2008). Short-term studies of elderly liver transplant recipients have demonstrated that operative course, length of hospitalization, incidence of perioperative complications, and overall patient survival are comparable with their younger adult counterparts (Adani et al., 2009). With improvements in management, liver transplantation in the elderly became successful and less controversial. Three studies are especially noteworthy: all demonstrated 5-year survival rates greater than 70% and mortality rates comparable to those of younger populations (Donovan et al., 1996; Kryzhanovski and Beller, 1997; Taner et al., 2012).

Results in elderly liver transplants are comparable to younger recipients, yet the elderly have a lower survival rate. In 1998 a multicentre review of 735 liver transplant recipients analyzed by age revealed a lower patient survival for recipients over age 60 than for younger adults (81% vs 90%) (Zetterman et al., 1998). Another study in 1999 concluded that 3-year survival for patients over age 70 was comparable to those under age 60, though there was a trend for decreased patient survival (Rudich and Busuttil, 1999). In 2000, data published on 91 seniors who underwent transplantation at the University of Wisconsin showed poor long-term patient survival after liver transplantation (Collins et al., 2000). Five-year patient survival was 52% for patients over age 60 and 75% for patients under age 60; 10-year patient survival was 35% and 60% in seniors and young adults, respectively. Although seniors older than 65 years were found to have worse outcomes than those who were 60–65, the majority of seniors who survive liver transplantation have full or only minimally limited functional status (Keswani et al., 2004).

In 2009, 143 transplants were performed for patients who were 70 years old or more. The overall survival rate was significantly attenuated for the septuagenarians versus the younger cohort. After 5 years of follow-up this disparity exceeded 10–15%, depending on the populations being compared. The 5-year actuarial survival rates were 72.7% for patients who were younger than 70 years and 55.2% for patients who were 70 years or older (Schwartz et al., 2012). In 2008, Kemmer (Kemmer et al., 2008), using the UNOS database, showed that 5-year patient survival was 62% for patients aged 65 and over and 70.3% for patients aged 50–64. The 10-year patient and graft survival was 60% and 57% for < 65 years vs 42% and 40% for > 65 years, respectively (Kemmer et al., 2008). Recent data showed improved survival in elderly patients. Survival rates at 1, 3, and 5 years for recipients 60 years of age were 91.1%, 84.9%, and 79.2%, respectively (Taner et al., 2012). Patient survival rates at 1, 3, and 5 years for recipients between 60 and 74 years of age were 88.9%, 80.4%, and 73.2%, respectively (Taner et al., 2012). These and other studies mean that an increasing number of patients over 60 years old can be listed for liver transplantation and receive a liver allograft with satisfying results (Lipshutz et al., 2007; Adani et al., 2009; Ballarin et al., 2011; Taner et al., 2012). Age 70 years or more did not constitute a strong risk factor (Lipshutz et al., 2007).

Many of the studies advocated allocation of liver transplants to low-risk seniors (Schwartz et al., 2012). The data suggest that long-term mortality of low-risk patients would be similar to their younger counterparts (Schwartz et al., 2012). The findings of a comprehensive analysis of the UNOS database determined that recipients aged 60 and older who lacked three or more risk factors (from among mechanical ventilation, diabetes mellitus, hepatitis C, renal insufficiency, and combined donor and recipient age of 120 and older) had the same clinical outcomes as younger recipients (Aloia et al., 2010). In a prospective analysis of 208 consecutive liver transplant recipients, older adults consumed a similar amount of postoperative resources (days in hospital, days in intensive care, use of consultative services, reoperative rates, and 90-day readmission rates) as subjects younger than 60 and there were no differences in survival rates between the two groups (Shankar et al., 2011).

Although liver transplant is being performed in increasingly challenging circumstances (i.e. older recipients with more comorbidity undergoing transplant with high MELD scores and suboptimal donor organs), beneficial transplant outcomes in the US remain robust (OPTN, 2012).

### Risk factors

An empirical approach to the decision of whether to proceed with liver transplantation should take into account age, severity of illness, and comorbid conditions. Increased age at time of transplantation is a poor prognostic indicator (Herrero et al., 2003; Lipshutz et al., 2007; Zhang et al., 2011). Age is a component of the older recipient prognostic score, which is an aggregate score of five prognostic factors generated from univariate and multivariate modelling of UNOS/OPTN data. Among these factors, the summed total of donor and recipient ages has the highest predictive value in forecasting poor patient survival (Aloia et al., 2010). Cirrhosis is also the major risk factor affecting prognosis and survival in elderly with hepatic cancer undergoing transplantation (Hoshida et al., 1999).

The main causes of early mortality in patients over 65 years of age were recurrence of underlying disease and medical causes (infectious, cardiac, and neurological diseases) (Zetterman et al., 1998) (Bilbao et al., 2008). Cardiovascular complications were significantly more frequent in the elderly. Death due to sepsis or cardiovascular disease would explain half of the deaths in the first year (Lipshutz et al., 2007). Cardiovascular causes of mortality are increased in the elderly by 9% (Audet et al., 2010), and in the literature the mortality of patients with CAD who undergo liver transplantation may be as high as 50% (Plotkin et al., 1996, 1998). Other risk factors for death in patients over 65 are preliver transplant renal insufficiency (Bilbao et al., 2008), preoperative hospitalization, cold ischaemia time, and hepatitis C/ethanol (Lipshutz et al., 2007). The most common cause of late mortality in elderly liver recipients was malignancy (35.0%), whereas most of the young adult deaths were the result of infectious complications (24.2%) (Collins et al., 2000).

Despite an increase in cardiovascular risk (Carey et al., 1995; Plotkin et al., 1996; Keswani et al., 2004), osteoporotic fractures ( Leidig-Bruckner et al., 2001; Ninkovic et al., 2001; Keswani et al., 2004), and neoplasia (Sheiner et al., 2000; Haagsma et al., 2001; Xiol et al., 2001), it has been shown across the board that liver transplantation tremendously improves the quality of life of any recipient when compared with pretransplant status (Lipshutz et al., 2007). Elderly patients should undergo transplantation at an earlier time point in the spectrum of ESLD.

## Kidney transplantation in the elderly

As in the case of liver transplantation, the rate of kidney transplantation in the elderly has increased through the years, driven by an increase in longevity and ESRD. According to the United States Renal Data System, the prevalence of ESRD in the US is increasing disproportionately to its incidence, likely because patients are living longer with ESRD. Nearly half of all new patients are older than 65 and one-third of patients are older than 70 years (Collins et al., 2012; Knoll, 2012).

Access to transplantation decreases with advancing age (Huang et al., 2009). There is a 30% decrease in access to transplantation for each decade increase in age (Huang et al., 2009). While 21% of patients aged 18–39 and 16% of those 40–59 years were listed for kidney transplantation, only 3.4% of patients older than 70 and 0.5% of those 80 years and more were listed (Collins et al., 2012).

The AST evaluation guidelines state that 'there should be no absolute upper age limit for excluding patients whose overall health and life situation suggest that transplantation will be beneficial'(Kasiske et al., 2002). These guidelines also recommend that elderly patients with ESRD be screened more aggressively for cardiovascular disease and malignancy (Kasiske et al., 2002). Older transplant candidates should have a reasonable probability of surviving beyond current waiting times for transplantation (Knoll, 2012).

In 2014, 19.6% of kidney transplants were performed in recipients older than 65 compared to 2.4% in 1988. In February 2015, 21,839 elderly patients out of 101,586 candidates (equating to 21%) were awaiting a kidney transplant (OPTN, 2015).

### Outcome

Patients of all ages gained additional years of life with transplant compared to dialysis. Jassal et al. (2003) showed that in all age groups up to 85 years, life expectancy improved after transplantation, with decreases in mortality of 41–61% depending on the study (Wolfe et al., 1999; Rao et al., 2007). This survival advantage translated into a 4-year increase in life expectancy in one report (Wolfe et al., 1999). However, older transplant recipients have decreased patient and transplant survival compared with younger recipients. Five-year survival of deceased donor transplant recipients older than 65 years is 67% compared to 89% for those aged 30–49 (Knoll, 2012). For live donor transplant recipients, 5-year survival was 80% for the elderly and 94% for young adults (Knoll, 2012). Causes of first-year mortality among renal transplant recipients older than 60 in the US are: infection 38%, cardiovascular 35%, cerebrovascular 7%, malignancy 5%, and haemorrhage 2% (Kauffman et al., 2007).

Elderly recipients are more likely to have comorbid conditions at the time of transplant than younger patients. These conditions are associated with higher post-transplant mortality. In patients older than 60, a history of angina/CAD, COPD, or diabetes increases the odds of 1-year mortality anywhere from 30% to 121% compared with recipients older than 60 with no comorbidities (Kauffman et al., 2007). When patients older than 60 received an ECD kidney or experienced delayed graft function, the presence of any of the earlier-described comorbidities increased the odds of mortality in the first year in the order of 59% to 351% (Kauffman et al., 2007).

The risk of cardiovascular disease increases with the progression of kidney disease (Go et al., 2004). Likewise, advancing age increases the risk for cardiovascular death in ESRD patients. As per AST guidelines, elderly patients with ESRD should be screened more aggressively for cardiovascular disease and malignancy. Similar to the dialysis population, the most common cause of death in kidney transplant patients is cardiovascular disease (Ojo et al., 2000). However, the risk of cardiovascular death for all age groups is greater for wait-listed patients than for transplant patients (Meier-Kriesche et al., 2001b). Thus it can be inferred that transplantation is associated with a decreased risk of cardiovascular death compared with dialysis (Huang et al., 2009).

Older transplant recipients experience more infectious complications and less acute rejection, but the risk of transplant loss from rejection is increased compared with younger patients (Meier-Kriesche et al., 2000; Tullius and Milford, 2011).

In general, older patients are more susceptible to infectious death than younger patients (Meier-Kriesche et al., 2000). Infectious death represents the most common cause of first-year mortality in transplant patients older than 60, a period during which the relative degree of immunosuppression is the highest (Kauffman et al., 2007). These data show that the elderly are more vulnerable to the effects of immunosuppression, perhaps because of age-related immunosenescence. Nevertheless, despite the increased effect of age on infectious death with transplantation, transplantation is associated with a lower risk of infection-related mortality in all age groups compared with dialysis (Meier-Kriesche et al., 2001b).

The type of transplanted donor kidney affects survival in elderly recipients. Data suggest that living donor kidneys might be the best treatment option for the elderly, just as they are for younger individuals. Use of living donors, even older living donors, provides significantly better outcomes for elderly recipients compared with the use of deceased donors (Chang et al., 2012; Knoll, 2012). Four-year transplant survival was greatest in elderly patients who received a transplant from either a younger living donor (81%) or an older living donor (78%), and both were significantly better than either SCD (70%) or ECD (57%) transplants (Gill et al., 2008). (ECDs are defined as those aged 60 or older or those aged 50–59 with at least two of the following conditions: history of hypertension, creatinine level >1.5 mg/dL, or cerebrovascular cause of death (Knoll, 2012).) However, in the absence of a living donor, survival is improved significantly in the elderly by accepting an ECD organ rather than waiting for an SCD deceased donor (Chang et al., 2012). Rao et al. (2007) confirmed that even elderly patients 70 years and older have a survival advantage with an ECD kidney and a 25% survival benefit.

Researchers Schold and Meier-Kriesche (2006) found that patients 65 years and older had a slightly longer life expectancy if they accepted an ECD kidney within 2 years of starting dialysis therapy rather than waiting 4 years to receive either an SCD or a living donor kidney. Importantly, they also showed that as waiting time accumulated, the relative likelihood of receiving a transplant decreased significantly for those who were at least 65 years old.

ECD transplantation should be offered to all elderly candidates without a living donor who otherwise would have a prolonged wait for an SCD kidney, and all elderly diabetic candidates regardless of anticipated waiting time (Huang et al., 2009; Knoll, 2012). In the US and other regions, the use of ECD kidneys has become common practice in the elderly. In 2006, 34.3% of ECD kidneys were given to patients older than 65. The Eurotransplant International Foundation has chosen to preferentially allocate kidneys from deceased donors aged 65 years or older to recipients who also are at least 65 (this is known as the 'old for old' programme) (Knoll, 2012).

To sum up, although older transplant patients have a higher risk for mortality than their younger counterparts, elderly transplant patients have improved quality of life and a lower risk of mortality compared to dialysis. There is also survival benefit associated with ECD transplantation compared with dialysis; however, patient and graft outcomes are worse with ECD transplantation compared with living donor and SCD transplantation.

## Multivisceral transplantation in the elderly

MVTx includes the simultaneous transplantation of multiple abdominal viscera including the stomach, duodenum, pancreas, and small intestine, with liver (MVTx) or without liver (modified MVT (MMVTx)). Indications include intestinal failure alone, intestinal failure with cirrhosis, complete portal mesenteric thrombosis, slow-growing central abdominal tumours, intestinal pseudo-obstruction, and frozen abdomen. Patients who are candidates for this procedure generally have a terminal condition that is non-responsive to standard medical or surgical therapy (Harper and Jamieson, 2011). The development of cirrhosis associated with chronic parenteral nutrition is a catastrophic situation that leads to death in most patients who are not rescued by transplantation (Goulet et al., 2004), with 60–70% of the patients referred for intestinal transplantation already having some degree of irreversible liver failure (Fryer, 2007). The common element in all variants is transplantation of the small bowel. Inclusion of the colon, pancreas, spleen, kidney, and abdominal wall is performed as appropriate to the baseline pathology and centre preference (Levi et al., 2003; Tzakis et al., 2005). Early referral is still the best practice when considering intent to treat (Gupte et al., 2007; Vianna et al., 2008). In the US in 2011, 18 centres performed intestinal transplants. In 2007 policies regarding organ allocation in the US were changed, giving priority to paediatric patients waiting combined liver–pancreas–intestinal transplant.

Since 2006 the number of new intestinal transplant candidates listed each year has decreased, likely reflecting increased medical and surgical treatment for intestinal failure. Historically, the most common organ transplanted with the intestine was the liver; this practice decreased substantially from a peak of 52.9% in 2007 to 30% in 2012 (OPTN, 2014).

From 2001–2012 only 20 cases of intestinal transplants were performed in patients > 65 years of age out of 1,004 performed in adults >18 years old. 2001 is the first year an adult > 65 years of age underwent intestinal transplant (according to UNOS data), although this procedure has been performed since 1990. In 2012 only one intestinal transplant was performed in the elderly out of 50 transplanted in adults > 18 years of age; 20 of the 50 intestinal transplants in adults were in recipients > 50 years of age. As of 28 February 2015 only one elderly was registered for an intestinal transplant out of 84 adults on the OPTN database (OPTN, 2015).

### Outcome

Outcomes vary between centres, between the types of intestinal transplants, and among adult and paediatric patients. Graft survival has continued to improve. Graft failure in the first 90 days after transplant occurred in 15.7% of 2011–2012 intestinal transplant recipients, compared with 21% in 2001–2002 (OPTN, 2014). Rehospitalization is common, having occurred in 86.1% of 2007–20012 recipients by 6 months post-transplant and in almost all by 1 year (OPTN, 2014). Patient and graft survival at 1 year following intestinal and multivisceral transplantation has been reported to be 80% and 75%, respectively, approaching that of other solid-organ recipients (Hanto et al., 2005). Indeed, high-volume centres are reporting 1-year survival rates for isolated small bowel grafts in excess of 90% (Messing et al., 1999; Vianna et al., 2008). Longer-term results remain more modest, with a 5-year patient and graft survival of 48% and 45%, respectively, in MVTx performed in the 1990s (Chan et al., 1999). Since 2000, 5-year patient survival rate is near 60% for all adult and paediatric intestinal recipients. Unfortunately, patients with higher risk of death include very old and very young individuals (Ruiz et al., 2007).

Isolated intestinal transplants are more commonly performed in adults, while MVTx are most commonly performed in infants (Pironi et al., 2004). According to the UNOS database (1987–2009), out of 759 intestinal transplants in 687 patients, 463 (61%) were isolated and 296 (39%) were combined with liver. Patient survival for primary isolated intestinal transplant at 1, 3, and 5 years was 84%, 66.7%, and 54.2% and primary liver–intestine transplant was 67%, 53.3%, and 46%, respectively (Desai et al., 2012).

The complexity of the MVTx procedure, with its steep learning curve and high-risk patients, requires meticulous attention to all medical and surgical details and may still end in failure. In one report spanning 6 years, ten patients older than 60 years underwent MVTx; they had 50% graft and patient survival. When patients with renal failure at transplant were excluded, the overall patient survival at 3 years was 63% (Mangus et al., 2013). The presence of renal failure was an important marker for worse outcomes and these potential transplant recipients should be closely scrutinized. Factors found to be associated with improved patient survival in that report included younger recipient age. Moreover, many of the patients who experienced early death were severely debilitated at the time of transplant. Though all patients underwent standard pretransplant screening, debility and frailty are difficult to measure and may be more pronounced in these patients who have often accumulated months and years of poor nutrition and inactivity. Given the complexity of managing these patients, care must be taken in patient selection to optimize long-term outcomes (Mangus et al., 2013). Donor age >40 years had a very significant negative effect for outcome in combined liver–intestine graft recipients (Abu-Elmagd et al., 2001; Pironi et al., 2004).

As with other solid abdominal organ transplants, absolute contraindications to intestinal transplantation include severe cardiopulmonary disease, severe systemic infections with multiple organ failure, aggressive malignancy, and severe neurological impairment. HIV infection is currently considered a relative contraindication for solid organ transplantation (Vianna et al., 2008). The age of the patient is not a usual limitation; however, the overall health of the patient, including nutritional status, is of importance in the patient's ability to tolerate transplantation (Cameron et al., 2002; Pironi et al., 2004). Almost by definition, patients who have undergone intestinal transplant have a poor nutritional status, which directly impacts wound and anastomotic healing. Doppler ultrasonography of the neck veins and extremities provides a venous map for the anaesthesiologist who must place central venous lines for the transplant procedure. It is not uncommon for patients to have lost one or more of the six major routes of venous access during the course of their illness.

The transplant team must assess the patient's suitability for transplantation in great detail, including anatomical and technical considerations, physiological function and reserve, immunological factors, and psychological issues, in particular pain and drug dependence, which are common in this patient population (Harper and Jamieson, 2011). Optimization aims to improve fitness for major surgery and the complicated and prolonged postoperative period, particularly in regard to cardiorespiratory function and nutritional status. In addition, identification and effective treatment of ongoing sepsis is crucial and may require significant intervention, including repeated surgery.

Fluid management following intestinal transplantation is one of the most challenging parts of postoperative management. Monitoring and replacement of water and electrolytes must be meticulous, as losses from the transplanted bowel can be very variable and complicated by profound fluid shifts following major surgery and the transfer from long-standing parenteral to enteral nutrition. In particular, the risk of dehydration and acute renal failure persists for several months following transplantation.

The early postoperative course is very challenging for some patients, especially for recipients of combined liver–intestinal and multivisceral transplants (Abu-Elmagd et al., 2001). Post-transplant complications include rejection (50% MMVTx and 17% MVTx), infection (> 90% in the first year), GVHD (13%), and post-transplant lymphoproliferative disorder (5%) (Mangus et al., 2013). The most important early complications are acute rejection and sepsis, which frequently occur together. Sepsis remains the leading cause of death in bowel transplant patients in the perioperative and long-term periods (Vianna et al., 2008). The major complications like graft thrombosis, ischaemia, and technical failure have all reduced, especially since the 1990s (Abu-Elmagd et al., 2001).

## Pancreatic transplantation in the elderly

Pancreas transplant remains a viable option for β-cell replacement in insulin-dependent diabetes mellitus, mostly type 1. Although the number of pancreas transplants has been decreasing steadily since 2000, outcomes continue to improve for all groups of pancreas transplant: simultaneous pancreas–kidney transplant (SPKTx) and solitary pancreas transplant (pancreas after kidney transplant (PAKTx) and pancreas transplant alone (PTxA)). The improving outcomes are mainly due to improvements in immunosuppression, surgical technique, and donor–recipient selection. The decrease in the number of pancreas transplants is partly attributable to improved insulin delivery systems, concerns about outcomes after solitary PTxA, and potentially a renewed interest in islet transplant. Even though isolated reports suggest that 5-year islet transplant outcomes at a single centre have matched pancreas transplant outcomes, the current consensus seems to be that pancreas transplant is superior to islet transplant in efficiency and durability. This view may change in the future, resulting in more islet transplants being performed. Rates of post-transplant rehospitalization are high, most occurring in the first 6 months. Rejection rates are highest for PTxA recipients, who also experience higher incidence of post-transplant lymphoproliferative disorder.

Since 2000 the number of new candidates on the pancreas waiting list has steadily decreased, with a gradual increase in the proportion of older candidates (aged 50–64 years).

### Outcome

While pancreatic transplant in adults above 50 years of age comprises 20–25% of all pancreas transplants, pancreatic transplantation in the elderly is rare. As of 30 November 2014, only 28 lone pancreatic transplants have been performed in patients older than 65 years. In 2014 only 2 out of 227 pancreatic transplants were performed in an elderly recipient. For SPKTx, 0 out of 661 was performed in the elderly in 2014. As of 27 February 2015, only 7 elderly patients were awaiting a pancreatic transplant (OPTN, 2015).

## Immunosuppression

The aging process significantly affects the immune response. Although there is heterogeneity among individual patients, in general terms both innate and adaptive immunity show decreases with increased age (Martins et al., 2005; Huang et al., 2009). These changes are believed to contribute to the observation of decreased acute rejection in elderly transplant recipients and an increased susceptibility to infectious illness, decreased response to immunizations, and a higher incidence of neoplasia (Ershler, 1988; Weigle, 1989; Meier-Kriesche et al., 2001a). This seemingly undesirable immune senescence might paradoxically improve outcome in older transplant recipients by theoretically reducing the incidence and severity of allograft rejection and requirements for immunosuppressive drugs (Keswani et al., 2004; Audet et al., 2010).

Reduction in drug dosage used after transplantation to reduce side effects (cataracts, diabetes mellitus, infection, and osteopaenia) can often be achieved and is particularly beneficial to older patients. While some centres noted significantly fewer acute liver rejection episodes in the elderly compared to younger adults, with immunosuppression regimens containing cyclosporine (Shaw, 1992; Emre et al., 1993; Filipponi et al., 2001), others showed no difference (Stieber et al., 1991; Collins et al., 2000). An analysis involving more than 70,000 kidney transplant recipients (Meier-Kriesche et al., 2000) showed that the incidence of acute rejection decreased steadily with increased age. For patients aged 18–29 years, the 6-month acute rejection rate was 28% compared to only 19.7% for those older than 65 (Meier-Kriesche et al., 2000). Conversely, death due to infection increased dramatically with age from 0.8% in 18- to 29-year-olds to 4.8% in the oldest age group (Meier-Kriesche et al., 2000). Importantly, these differences in rejection and infection were independent of baseline immunosuppression. In a more recent analysis using the UNOS database, Tullius and Milford (2011) confirmed these findings and found a steady decrease in acute rejection with increasing recipient age. For patients 18 years of age the rejection rate was 28%, compared to only 14% for those aged 70 years (Tullius and Milford, 2011).

Consequences of acute rejection may be greater in the elderly. In an analysis of 48,821 transplant recipients the adjusted annual rate of transplant loss among those with rejection was significantly higher for elderly patients. A variety of cofactors including comorbidities, drug–drug interactions, diet, renal and hepatic function, and immune senescence may influence the overall effect of immunosuppressive medications (Huang et al., 2009). Side effects of commonly used immunosuppressive medications include weight gain, diabetes, hypercholesterolaemia, and hypertension, all of which may contribute significantly to cardiovascular risk (Huang et al., 2009).

## Ethical considerations of transplantation in the elderly

Today the donor organ shortage seems to be the major limiting factor for the application of transplantation. As the need for organ transplantation in the geriatric population increases and the geriatric population continues to age and grow, the gap between demand and supply will continue to widen. Therefore it is important that use of these scarce organs provides net benefits to the patient and society. The question that we are often faced with is 'What level of survival is good enough?' (Lipshutz et al., 2007). In an outcome-based approach, the practice of using grafts for older patients and concerns of potentially decreasing access to younger patients is a legitimate concern. A major consideration in the development of an equitable organ allocation scheme is the balance of utility, in which organs are offered to those candidates who would derive the greatest benefit from transplantation, versus justice, in which all age groups have equal access to donated organs (Huang et al., 2009).

To address the question of justice and utility properly, one should not exclude patients from transplant based only on age any more than one should transplant a younger patient with multiple comorbidities that would result in similar short- and long-term outcomes. The decision-making of accepting an organ often has to be blinded to the age of the recipient to avoid bias, and patient evaluation should be based on physiological rather than chronological age (Ballarin et al., 2011). For liver transplantation, the MELD score includes the variables that influence death the most. Although age was one highly significant variable to predict death from liver disease, it is excluded from the MELD formula so we would not discriminate against older recipients. Patients aged 75 years can receive a marginal-quality liver graft with good graft and patient survival (Taner et al., 2012). According to the Social Security Actuarial Publications, a man and woman aged 75 years are expected to live an additional 10.46 and 12.43 years, respectively. Fifty percent of liver transplants in the elderly can extend life by at least 5 years, which is half of their remaining life expectancy in an otherwise poor outcome due to ESLK and/or hepatocellular carcinoma (Taner et al., 2012).

## Anaesthetic management

### Preoperative

Geriatric patients are a heterogeneous population with wide disparity between physiological and chronological age. Advancing age is associated with a steady decline in organ function reserve and inability to compensate for physiological stress. Multiple acute and chronic comorbidities may co-exist. Patients can have complex medication regimens. All these attributes lead to increased surgical morbidity and mortality with age and end-stage organ disease (Leung and Dzankic, 2001; Monk et al., 2005; McNicol et al., 2007; Story, 2008).

The preoperative assessment of the patient is composed of four interrelated functions: risk stratification; history and physical examination, including functional assessment; preoperative testing; and preoperative optimization (Robinson et al., 2011). Elderly patients must have reasonable functional and health status before being considered for transplant. While certain elements of the pretransplant evaluation are routine for all patients, others are determined by comorbid conditions common to the elderly. Preoperative evaluation of older patients for transplantation is focused on the functional status of the cardiopulmonary system and requires careful screening to exclude malignancy, bone disease, and other diseases of the aged (Keswani et al., 2004). Advancing age is an independent risk factor for the development of CAD (Kannel and Vokonas, 1992), and the prevalence of CAD in patients with ESLD is similar to and may even exceed that of the general population. Carey et al. (1995) demonstrated a 27% prevalence of moderate to severe CAD in patients with liver disease and age greater than 50. Moreover, the mortality of patients with CAD who undergo liver transplantation may be as high as 50% (Plotkin et al., 1996; Keswani et al., 2004).

Elderly patients are more likely to require a functional cardiac study and carotid artery analysis before listing for transplantation compared to younger patients (Keswani et al., 2004). Stress testing combined with myocardial imaging should be undertaken. To that end, DSE has been shown to be efficacious as a screening test to detect CAD in patients undergoing liver transplantation (Plevak, 1998). In a study evaluating the utility of DSE in patients undergoing liver transplantation, Plotkin et al. (1998) showed that only patients with wall motion abnormalities on DSE had significant CAD. DSE had a 100% positive and negative predictive value for significant CAD. Donovan et al. (1996) reported that a negative stress echocardiogram is helpful in ruling out perioperative cardiac events in patients without typical angina symptoms or a history of CAD; however, a positive stress echocardiogram must be confirmed by a cardiac catheterization (Keswani et al., 2004).

A retrospective study of kidney–pancreas transplant recipients evaluated the predictive value of non-invasive cardiac testing (standard echocardiography, stress echocardiography, exercise tolerance testing, and nuclear myocardial perfusion) for postoperative cardiac events and concluded that these tests had a 97% negative predictive value 1 year post-testing and 1 year post-transplant with a 3% risk of missing coronary disease (Lin et al., 2001). Cardiac testing does not predict all cardiac events up to 1 year post-testing in this high-risk patient population with diabetes and renal failure (Lin et al., 2001). For stress echocardiography, 5 of the 43 patients (12%) with negative tests had a myocardial infarction post-transplant, including two intraoperative events. The negative predictive value was 93% for events within 1 year post-testing and 88% for events within 1 year post-transplant (Lin et al., 2001).

Patients who have a history of CAD or a positive stress test should undergo coronary angiography and angioplasty as indicated before transplantation. Cardiac catheterization remains the gold standard for identifying CAD; many centres proceed with cardiac catheterization as a first test for patients with a strong clinical history of CAD, diabetes, or symptoms of exertional angina (Keeffe et al., 2001). Diabetes mellitus may be the most important risk factor for the presence of CAD in patients with liver disease (Carey et al., 1995). Cardiac catheterization, regardless of stress test results, may be advisable in these patients. A positive cardiac stress test should also lead to cardiac catheterization for confirmation of CAD (Keswani et al., 2004).

Questions remain as to what degree of lesion requires intervention and what type of treatment is best. Most subcritical coronary stenosis in surgical patients can be medically managed. However, investigators report a perioperative death rate of more than 50% in transplant recipients with CAD who were managed medically (Plotkin et al., 1996). Further myocardial infarction during transplant surgery has occurred with as little as 30% vessel occlusion. Studies show that at least one critical coronary artery lesion occurs in 5–26% of all liver transplant candidates who are asymptomatic (Carey et al., 1995; Plotkin et al., 1996; Tiukinhoy-Laing et al., 2006). Patients requiring coronary artery bypass grafts do not do well in the long term; therefore this population is not considered as transplant candidates. However, if there is a defined small lesion that is stented in the absence of other complicating factors, such as hepatopulmonary syndrome in an older patient, the patient may be considered (Lipshutz et al., 2007). In contrast to ischaemic heart disease, most patients with advanced liver disease have myocardial defects that cause systolic and diastolic impairments that are not always evident at rest. There are also underlying electrophysiological defects that cause an uncoupling of mechanical and electrical activity. Cirrhotic cardiomyopathy can be subtle and some patients will develop frank heart failure when exposed to pharmacological or physiological stress such as liver transplantation (Mandell et al., 2008).

The results from three screening tests were used in one report to assess for transplant eligibility: DSE, pulmonary function test, and ECG interpretation (Taner et al., 2012). Similar to young adult transplant candidates, if an elderly patient is not physiologically fit, with major cardiac or pulmonary issues, he/she should not undergo transplantation. Pulmonary arterial hypertension carries a high mortality rate for patients undergoing liver transplantation (Krowka et al., 2000). If the echocardiogram interrogation of the pulmonary artery suggests elevated pulmonary arterial pressures, a right-heart catheterization should be performed.

Proper evaluation and management of the elderly individual can allow these patients to undergo this life-saving procedure. When considering reducing risk in the elderly patient, a few important factors are: the use of β-blockade and statins, the importance of blood pressure control perioperatively, and the utility of a preoperative ECG. In general, β-blockers should be continued around surgery and administered perioperatively to high-risk individuals undergoing intermediate- or high-risk surgery as outlined by the American College of Cardiology Foundation/AHA guidelines. Indiscriminate and widespread use of β-blockers is not recommended. Perioperatively, statin use should not be abruptly discontinued. Statins in the perioperative period are indicated in patients with high-risk indices undergoing intermediate- and high-risk surgery.

Older patients with ESRD who are assessing transplantation often have more complex issues to contemplate than their younger counterparts, including cognitive impairment, decreased functional status, and frailty (Brown and Johansson, 2010; Tamura and Yaffe, 2011). Mild cognitive impairment and dementia occur with greater frequency in older individuals and this increase is even greater in patients with ESRD. For example, only 10–30% of young and middle-aged dialysis patients have cognitive impairment compared with 30–55% of those older than 75 years (Tamura and Yaffe, 2011). Despite the high prevalence, practice guidelines do not recommend routine testing for cognitive impairment, even in high-risk elderly patients, prior to transplantation (Kasiske et al., 2002). Screening for cognitive impairment may be an important first step in the transplantation evaluation process for elderly patients with ESRD since it would identify patients who are at increased risk of functional decline, hospitalization, and death post-transplantation (Tamura and Yaffe, 2011).

Frailty describes a distinct syndrome that is becoming increasingly recognized as an important predictor of survival and prognosis. It appears to provide a marker of decreased physiological reserve and may be an important preoperative risk factor for older patients (Brown and Johansson, 2010; Makary et al., 2010; Garonzik-Wang et al., 2012 ; Partridge et al., 2012). Frailty is not defined as one single disease entity; the most comprehensive definition includes five features: unintentional weight loss, weakness (decreased grip strength), slow walking speed, low physical activity, and self-reported exhaustion (Makary et al., 2010). Frailty is associated with functional decline, loss of independence, and increased mortality. After elective general surgery, frail patients had a higher incidence of adverse events and length of discharge (Makary et al., 2010; Robinson et al., 2011).

Frailty is highly prevalent in dialysis patients and this prevalence increases with age. For example, Johansen et al. (2007) showed that 44% of dialysis patients younger than 40 years met the criteria for frailty compared with 78% of patients older than 70 years. Frailty is a significant predictor of both hospitalization and mortality in dialysis patients (Johansen et al., 2007). With regard to transplantation and major surgery, frailty also has emerged as an important risk factor. In an analysis involving 594 patients who were at least 65 years old and undergoing elective surgery, Makary et al. (2010) showed that frailty was associated independently with increased risk of perioperative complications, length of stay, and the likelihood of being discharged to an assisted-living facility if previously living at home. Frailty as defined previously was found in 25% of 183 patients presenting for kidney transplantation and was associated with increased risk of delayed transplant function (Garonzik-Wang et al., 2012). Frailty, like cognitive impairment, is highly prevalent and is emerging as an important predictor of outcomes in elderly patients with ESRD. Assessing frailty and cognitive impairment has the potential to better refine who among the many elderly transplant candidates should proceed with transplantation.

Based on the results of work-up, liver transplant teams need to assess the perioperative and long-term risks of each individual patient. Success of transplantation is all about selection of the recipient and selection of the donor (Lipshutz et al., 2007). Results in patients > 65 years old are comparable to those < 65 years if older liver transplant candidates are carefully selected (Bilbao et al., 2008). Donor graft quality is also of significant importance; the concept of the liver donor risk index (DRI) was introduced to evaluate the organ's quality (Feng et al., 2006) and to predict allograft survival (Avolio et al., 2008). Meticulous pretransplant assessment of the recipient is necessary to exclude patients with age-associated disease and confirm the capacity of the recipient to face the transplant operation and long-term immunosuppression (Lipshutz et al., 2007).

## Intraoperative

The major factors governing anaesthesia in the elderly are increased risk of adverse outcomes (Turrentine et al., 2006), loss of functional reserve, altered pharmacological responses, and increased sensitivity to anaesthetics. Older patients represent a heterogeneous group and each anaesthetic should be personally tailored. In general, 'start low, go slow' remains a valid axiom when taking care of elderly patients—and older patients require less anaesthesia compared to younger counterparts. The elderly CNS is more sensitive to anaesthetics and opioids and thus doses should be decreased; the MAC of inhalational agents predictably decreases by 6% every decade after age 40 and opioid doses can be reduced by 50% in older patients. Cirrhotic patients are prone to encephalopathy or present with it and thus require less anaesthetic doses.

Metabolic changes related to aging, organ failure, frailty, and decreased intravascular volume further affect drug action, so drugs with least dependence on renal and hepatic function are preferred (i.e. remifentanil, cisatracurium, esmolol). In the same way, isoflurane is better avoided due to its prolonged CNS effects (Motsch et al., 1998; Arar et al., 2005; Agoliati et al., 2010) and excessive cardiac depressant properties in the elderly (Peduto et al., 1998). Rapid sequence induction is recommended to protect the airway from aspiration due to gastro-oesophageal reflux. Preinduction insertion of invasive monitoring lines must be guided by the clinical presentation of the patient but is not usually performed. Portable ultrasound devices can reduce the number of failed attempts at central vein catheter or arterial line insertion (Hatfield and Bodenham, 1999).

Intraoperatively, the physician has to deal with the effects of the diseased transplanted organ along with the decreased reserves of the elderly. Liver failure has multisystem effects. Extrahepatic manifestations (cardiac, pulmonary, renal, neurological, metabolic) should be taken into consideration when treating a cirrhotic patient to optimize clinical outcomes. Apart from the regular monitors and access to the arterial line and central line, haemodynamic monitors that include continuous cardiac output and mixed-venous oxygen saturation are generally recommended. Cardiac function monitoring such as PAC and TEE are crucial in the elderly undergoing liver or multivisceral transplantation and help in assessment of preload and ventricular wall motion (Jacque, 2004). The use of TEE can facilitate estimation of the patient's volume status and detection of wall motion abnormalities or myocardial ischaemia, and serve as a sensitive indicator of air or thrombus in the right heart. At the University of Miami Jackson Memorial Hospital, a 'double stick' of the right internal jugular vein is routinely performed, into which a 9-F introducer and 12-F triple-lumen catheter are inserted. The right heart is catheterized using a PAC with continuous cardiac output monitoring capabilities. Two arterial catheters are inserted for monitoring and frequent blood sampling for ABGs, haematocrit, electrolytes, glucose, and thromboelastography (Jacque, 2004).

Age-related cardiac changes are amongst the most predictable and important physiological changes that impact anaesthesia administration. It is estimated that one-third of patients with normal preoperative LV function have diastolic dysfunction. These patients are very susceptible to fluid overload in the perioperative period. On the other hand, the impaired β-receptor responsiveness reduces an older patient's ability to respond to an increase in demand through increased heart rate alone and the elderly patient becomes very reliant on vascular tone and preload. The elderly vascular system may be less responsive to pressors when needed, thus requiring higher doses. Anaesthetics and alterations in autonomic function make it more difficult for older patients to maintain their body temperature, and because postoperative hypothermia increases the risk of adverse outcomes (Schmied et al., 1996; Lenhardt et al., 1997; Insler and Sessler, 2006), temperature control in elderly surgical patients requires more attention. Maintenance of a normal core body temperature is also essential to prevent worsening of the patient's coagulation status. Preoperative lung disease may affect ventilation and oxygenation. Moreover, decrease in chest wall compliance and decreased respiratory muscle strength due to advanced age may lead to hypoventilation and postoperative pulmonary complications, particularly with residual effects of neuromuscular blockade. Extubation of an elderly patient in the OR post-transplant may be challenging and requires that all criteria be completely met.

Technical issues during surgery and the risk factors that the patient brings to the OR will primarily determine how well the patient does (Leung and Dzankic, 2001; McNicol et al., 2007).

### Postoperative

Surgery in the very old patient carries a higher rate of morbidity and mortality (Finlayson and Birkmeyer, 2001; Leung and Dzankic, 2001; Monk et al., 2005; McNicol et al., 2007; Story, 2008). In addition to death, myocardial infarction, and CHF, older patients are unusually prone to postoperative delirium, cognitive dysfunction, aspiration, pneumonia, atelectasis, sepsis, adverse drug reactions, malnutrition, falls, and failure to return to ambulation or to home (Robinson et al., 2011). Postoperative care of the geriatric patient is complex. ICU and hospital stays may be more prolonged. Cardiovascular morbidities such as those related to CAD, CHF, and abdominal aortic aneurysm are more common with increasing age and their development perhaps is accelerated after liver transplant (Taner et al., 2012).

Pulmonary complications, including infections, are the most common complication of the elderly patient undergoing surgery (Seymour and Vaz, 1989). Postoperative pulmonary complications account for 40% of deaths in patients over the age of 65 (Zaugg and Lucchinetti, 2000). The risk of a postoperative pulmonary complication doubles in patients aged 60–69 years and triples in patients aged 70–79 compared to young patients (Qaseem, 2006; Sieber and Barnett, 2011). Pain, anaesthetics, neuromuscular blockers, atelectasis, fluid shifts, and other postoperative physiological changes accentuate age-related changes in respiratory mechanics and control. Similarly, age-related alterations in pharyngeal function and diminished cough are aggravated by anaesthetics, muscle relaxants, pharyngeal instrumentation, and upper abdominal or neck surgery. The latter predispose the elderly to aspiration, and precautions should be taken. TEE use increases risk of aspiration postoperatively (Hogue et al., 1995). Poor pain control may also be a contributing factor to the development of postoperative pulmonary complications.

Neurological changes, delirium, and postoperative cognitive dysfunction (POCD) are more common than in the young. After liver transplantation, 11.7% of recipients > 65 years old suffered minor neurological manifestation that resolved spontaneously (Audet et al., 2010). Delirium is an acute confusional state, usually appearing 1–3 days after surgery; it may persist for weeks to months in afflicted patients. The aetiology is multifactorial and includes acute medical conditions (sepsis, hypoxaemia, urinary tract infections, alcohol withdrawal, abnormal electrolytes, hypoxia), medications (meperidine, diphenhydramine, scopolamine, benzodiazepines), and pain. Patients with pre-existing dementia, baseline cognitive difficulties, and depression carry a higher risk of developing delirium postoperatively. Delirium is associated with an increase in morbidity and mortality as well as an increase in the length of stay and dependent living situations. Low-dose haloperidol (1.5 mg/day) has been shown to reduce the length and severity of delirium and may have some utility in high-risk patients. In contrast to delirium, POCD refers to a specific cognitive disorder generally recognized in the postoperative period and is ultimately diagnosed through neuropsychological testing. Studies have demonstrated that almost 10% of elderly patients receiving a general anaesthesia had some cognitive dysfunction 3 months after surgery.

Sepsis is another common cause of death in the postoperative period. Due to immune senescence, fewer immunosuppressive doses and lower levels may be needed (Lipshutz et al., 2007). Overimmunosuppression should be avoided in older candidates as its effects could worsen the pre-existing diseases common in elderly patients (Bilbao et al., 2008).

Although some extrahepatic sequelae of cirrhosis may be reversible after liver transplantation, some may not, or given clinical severity may compromise the feasibility of the transplant process. Morbidity like osteoporosis, gout, urinary retention, hypertension, new-onset diabetes, and non-melanomatous skin cancers are relatively common in the post-transplant period in all age groups. Perioperative renal dysfunction may occur due to anaesthetic and surgical stress, pain, sympathetic stimulation, and renal vasoconstrictive drugs. Preoperative comorbid disease was found to be a more significant source of postoperative complications than anaesthetic management or age (Leung and Dzankic, 2001; McNicol et al., 2007).

## Conclusion

Organ transplantation is one of the most costly and complex surgical procedures, but it has proven effectiveness in enhancing the quality and longevity of life in suitable individuals. Prudent allocation of this precious resource is required because of organ shortage. Advanced age alone should not exclude a patient from transplantation; however, it mandates thorough pretransplant evaluation and careful long-term follow-up (Keswani et al., 2004). Preoperative screening in the aged population should be detailed to exclude cardiovascular disease, bone disease, and malignancy, with attention to quality of life and functional status. Physiology, and not chronology, should ultimately guide decision-making in pretransplantation assessment (Adani et al., 2009).

Well-selected older adults fare just as well as younger recipients after transplant and do not consume excess postoperative resources. Similar to younger recipients, donor quality strongly impacts patient and transplant outcomes in the elderly, who should, when possible, undergo transplantation earlier in the spectrum of disease. There is no magic bullet for the elderly; instead vigilance, careful titration of medication, and a thorough understanding of physiological changes and commonly encountered comorbidities are needed. Comprehensive evidence-based geriatric perioperative care might have particular value in prevention of delirium and pneumonia, in pain management, and in improving functional status on discharge. Although outcome is eventually determined by the patient's initial functional status and surgery specifics, the anaesthesiologist has a unique role because he/she contributes significantly to preoperative assessment and intraoperative and postoperative management.

## References


Abu-Elmagd K, Reyes J, Bond G, et al. (2001) Clinical intestinal transplantation: a decade of experience at a single center. *Annal Surg*, **234**(3):404–417.

Adani GL, Baccarani U, Lorenzin D, et al. (2009) Elderly versus young liver transplant recipients: patient and graft survival. *Transplant Proc*, **41**(4):1293–1294.

Agoliati A, Dexter F, Lok J, et al. (2010) Meta-analysis of average and variability of time to extubation comparing isoflurane with desflurane or isoflurane with sevoflurane. *Anesth Analg*, **110**(5):1433–1439.

Aloia TA, Knight R, Gaber AO, Ghobrial RM, Goss JA (2010) Analysis of liver transplant outcomes for united network for organ sharing recipients 60 years old or older identifies multiple model for end-stage liver disease-independent prognostic factors. *Liver Transplant*, **16**(8):950–959.

Anderson S (1997) Ageing and the renin-angiotensin system. *Nephrol Dialysis Transplant*, **12**(6):1093–1094.

Arar C, Kaya G, Karamanlioglu B, Pamukcu Z, Turan N (2005) Effects of sevoflurane, isoflurane and propofol infusions on post-operative recovery criteria in geriatric patients. *J Int Med Res*, **33**(1):55–60.

Audet M, Piardi T, Panaro F, et al. (2010) Liver transplantation in recipients over 65 yr old: A single center experience. *Clin Transplant*, **24**(1):84–90.

Aviv JE (1997) Effects of aging on sensitivity of the pharyngeal and supraglottic areas. *Am J Med*, **103**(5A):74S–76S.

Avolio AW, Siciliano M, Barbarino R, et al. (2008) Donor risk index and organ patient index as predictors of graft survival after liver transplantation. *Transplant Proc*, **40**(6):1899–1902.

Ballarin R, Montalti R, Spaggiari M, et al. (2011) Liver transplantation in older adults: our point of view. *J Am Geriatr Soc*, **59**(7):1359–1361.

Barash PG (2009) *Clinical Anesthesia*, 6th edn, pp. 877–888. Wolters Kluwer/Lippincott Williams & Wilkins, Philadelphia.

Bell GD, Spickett GP, Reeve PA (1987) Intravenous midazole for upper gastrointestinal endoscopy: a study of 800 consecutive cases relating dose to age and sex of patient. *Br J Clin Pharmacol*, **23**(2):241–243.

Bilbao I, Dopazo C, Lazaro JL, et al. (2008) Our experience in liver transplantation in patients over 65 yr of age. *Clin Transplant*, **22**(1):82–88.

Bjøro K, Höckerstedt K, Ericzon BG, et al. (2000) Liver transplantation in patients over 60 years of age. *Transplant Int*, **13**(Suppl 1):S165–S170.

Bowie MW, Slattum PW (2007) Pharmacodynamics in older adults: a review. *Am J Geriatr Pharmacother*, **5**(3):263–303.

Brown EA, Johansson L (2010) Old age and frailty in the dialysis population. *J Nephrol*, **23**(5):502–507.

Cameron EAB, Binnie JAH, Jamieson NV, Pollard S, Middleton SJ (2002) Quality of life in adults following small bowel transplantation. *Transplant Proc*, **34**(3):965–966.

Carey WD, Dumot JA, Pimentel RR, et al. (1995) The prevalence of coronary artery disease in liver transplant candidates over age 50. *Transplant*, **59**(6):859–864.

Chan S, McCowen KC, Bistrian BR, et al. (1999) Incidence, prognosis, and etiology of end-stage liver disease in patients receiving home total parenteral nutrition. *Surgery*, **126**(1):28–34.

Chang P, Gill J, Dong J, et al. (2012) Living donor age and kidney allograft half-life: implications for living donor paired exchange programs. *Clin J Am Soc Nephrol*, **7**(5):835–841.

Collins AJ, Foley RN, Chavers B, et al. (2012) US renal data system 2011 annual data report. *Am J Kidney Dis*, **59**(1):e1–e27.

Collins BH, Pirsch JD, Becker YT, et al. (2000) Long-term results of liver transplantation in patients 60 years of age and older. *Transplantation*, **70**(5):780–783.

Cook DJ, Rooke GA (2003) Priorities in perioperative geriatrics. *Anesth Analg*, **96**(6):1823–1836.

Cook MW, Lisco SJ (2009) Prevention of postoperative pulmonary complications. *Int Anesthesiol Clin*, **47**(4):65–88.

Cross TJS, Antoniades CG, Muiesan P, et al. (2007) Liver transplantation in patients over 60 and 65 years: An evaluation of long-term outcomes and survival. *Liver Transplant*, **13**(10):1382–1388.

Dal Santo P (2011) Chronic liver diseases in the elderly. *Riv Ital Med Lab*, **7**(2):106–112.

Das S, Forrest K, Howell S (2010) General anaesthesia in elderly patients with cardiovascular disorders: choice of anaesthetic agent. *Drugs Aging*, **27**(4):265–282.

De la Peña A, Herrero JI, Sangro B, et al. (1998) Liver transplantation in cirrhotic patients over 60 years of age. *Rev Espan Enfermed Dig*, **90**(1):9–14.

Desai CS, Gruessner AC, Khan KM, et al. (2012) Isolated intestinal transplants vs. liver-intestinal transplants in adult patients in the united states: 22 yr of OPTN data. *Clin Transplant*, **26**(4):622–628.

Donovan CL, Marcovitz PA, Punch JD, et al. (1996) Two-dimensional and dobutamine stress echocardiography in the preoperative assessment of patients with end-stage liver disease prior to orthotopic liver transplantation. *Transplantation*, **61**(8):1180–1188.

Drachman DA (2006) Aging of the brain, entropy, and Alzheimer disease. *Neurology*, **67**(8):1340–1352.

Dyer CB, Ashton CM, Teasdale TA (1995) Postoperative delirium: a review of 80 primary data-collection studies. *Arch Intern Med*, **155**(5):461–465.

Ebert TJ, Morgan BJ, Barney JA, Denahan T, Smith JJ (1992) Effects of aging on baroreflex regulation of sympathetic activity in humans. *Am J Physiol*, **263**(3):Pt 2, H798–H803.

Eger EI 2nd (2001) Age, minimum alveolar anesthetic concentration, and minimum alveolar anesthetic concentration-awake. *Anesth Analg*, **93**(4):947–953.

Emre S, Mor E, Schwartz ME, et al. (1993) Liver transplantation in patients beyond age 60. *Transplant Proc*, **25**(1):1075–1076.

Ershler WB (1988) Biomarkers of aging: immunological events. *Exp Gerontol*, **23**(4–5):387–389.

Esposito C, Dal Canton A (2010) Functional changes in the aging kidney. *J Nephrol*, **23**(15):S41–S45.

Feng S, Goodrich NP, Bragg-Gresham JL, et al. (2006) Characteristics associated with liver graft failure: the concept of a donor risk index. *Am J Transplant*, **6**(4):783–790.

Filipponi F, Roncella M, Boggi U, et al. (2001) Liver transplantation in recipients over 60. *Transplant Proc*, **33**(1–2):1465–1466.

Finlayson EV, Birkmeyer JD (2001) Operative mortality with elective surgery in older adults. *Effective Clin Pract*, **4**(4):172–177.

Floreani A (2009) Liver disorders in the elderly. *Best Pract Res Clin Gastroenterol*, **23**(6):909–917.

Folkow B, Svanborg A (1993) Physiol cardiovascular aging. *Physiol Rev*, **73**(4):725–764.

Frühauf NR, Frilling A, Malagó M, Broelsch CE (2004) Liver transplantation in elderly patients. *Urol Ausgabe A*, **43**(8):942–946.

Fryer JP (2007) Intestinal transplantation: current status. *Gastroenterol Clin N Am*, **36**(1):145–159.

Garonzik-Wang JM, Govindan P, Grinnan JW, et al. (2012) Frailty and delayed graft function in kidney transplant recipients. *Arch Surg*, **147**(2):190–193.

Ge Y, Grossman RI, Babb JS, Rabin ML, Mannon LJ, Kolson DL (2002) Age-related total gray matter and white matter changes in normal adult brain. Part I: volumetric MR imaging analysis. *Am J Neuroradiol*, **23**(8):1327–1333.

Gill J, Bunnapradist S, Danovitch GM, Gjertson D, Gill JS, Cecka M (2008) Outcomes of kidney transplantation from older living donors to older recipients. *Am J Kidney Dis*, **52**(3):541–552.

Go AS, Chertow GM, Fan D, McCulloch CE, Hsu C (2004) Chronic kidney disease and the risks of death, cardiovascular events, and hospitalization. *N Engl J Med*, **351**(13):1296–1305, 1370.

Goulet O, Ruemmele F, Lacaille F, Colomb V (2004) Irreversible intestinal failure. *J Pediatr Gastroenterol Nutr*, **38**(3):250–269.

Gupte GL, Beath SV, Protheroe S, et al. (2007) Improved outcome of referrals for intestinal transplantation in the UK. *Arch Dis Childhood*, **92**(2):147–152.

Haagsma EB, Hagens VE, Schaapveld M, et al. (2001) Increased cancer risk after liver transplantation: a population-based study. *J Hepatol*, **34**(1):84–91.

Hajjar RR (1997) Age-related issues in volume overload and hyponatremia in the elderly. *J Nutr, Health Aging*, **1**(3):146–150.

Hanto DW, Fishbein TM, Pinson CW, et al. (2005) Liver and intestine transplantation: summary analysis, 1994–2003. *Am J Transplant*, **5**(4):II, 916–933.

Harper SJF, Jamieson NV (2011) Intestinal and multivisceral transplantation. *Surgery*, **29**(7):342–347.

Hatfield A, Bodenham A (1999) Portable ultrasound for difficult central venous access. *Br J Anaesth*, **82**(6):822–826.

Herrero JI, Lucena JF, Quiroga J, et al. (2003) Liver transplant recipients older than 60 years have lower survival and higher incidence of malignancy. *Am J Transplant*, **3**(11):1407–1412.

Hogue CW Jr, Lappas GD, Creswell LL, et al. (1995) Swallowing dysfunction after cardiac operations: associated adverse outcomes and risk factors including intraoperative transesophageal echocardiography. *J Thorac Cardiovasc Surg*, **110**(2):517–522.

Hoshida Y, Ikeda K, Kobayashi M, et al. (1999) Chronic liver disease in the extremely elderly of 80 years or more: clinical characteristics, prognosis and patient survival analysis. *J Hepatol*, **31**(5):860–866.

Hsieh M, Power DA (2009) Abnormal renal function and electrolyte disturbances in older people. *J Pharm Prac Res*, **39**(3):230–234.

Huang, E, Segev DL, Rabb H (2009) Kidney transplantation in the elderly. *Semin Nephrol*, **29**(6):621–635.

Insler SR, Sessler DI (2006) Perioperative thermoregulation and temperature monitoring. *Anesth Clin N Am*, **24**(4):823–837.

Jacque JJ (2004) Anesthetic considerations for multivisceral transplantation. *Anesth Clin N Am*, **22**(4):741–751.

Jassal SV, Krahn MD, Naglie G, et al. (2003) Kidney transplantation in the elderly: a decision analysis. *J Am Soc Nephrol*, **14**(1):187–196.

Johansen KL, Chertow GM, Jin C, Kutner NG (2007) Significance of frailty among dialysis patients. *J Am Soc Nephrol*, **18**(11):2960–2967.

Jones RM (1989) Anaesthesia in old age. *Anaesthesia*, **44**(5):377–378.

Kannel WB, Vokonas PS (1992) Demographics of the prevalence, incidence, and management of coronary heart disease in the elderly and in women. *Ann Epidemiol*, **2**(1–2):5–14.

Kasiske BL, Cangro CB, Hariharan S, et al. (2002) The evaluation of renal transplantation candidates: clinical practice guidelines. *Am J Transplant*, **1**(Suppl 2):1–95.

Kauffman HM, McBride MA, Cors CS, Roza AM, Wynn JJ (2007) Early mortality rates in older kidney recipients with comorbid risk factors. *Transplantation*, **83**(4):404–410.

Kaw R, Michota F, Jaffer A, Ghamande S, Auckley D, Golish J (2006) Unrecognized sleep apnea in the surgical patient: implications for the perioperative setting. *Chest*, **129**(1):198–205.

Keeffe BG, Valantine H, Keeffe EB (2001) Detection and treatment of coronary artery disease in liver transplant candidates. *Liver Transplant*, 7(9):755–761.

Kemmer N, Safdar K, Kaiser TE, Zacharias V, Neff GW (2008) Liver transplantation trends for older recipients: regional and ethnic variations. *Transplantation*, **86**(1):104–107.

Kenney WL, Chiu P (2001) Influence of age on thirst and fluid intake. *Med Sci Sports Exercise*, **33**(9):1524–1532.

Keswani RN, Ahmed A, Keeffe EB (2004) Older age and liver transplantation: a review. *Liver Transplant*, **10**(8):957–967.

Knoll GA (2012) Kidney transplantation in the older adult. *Am J Kidney Dis*, **61**:790–797.

Krowka MJ, Plevak DJ, Findlay JY, Rosen, CB, Wiesner RH, Krom RAF (2000) Pulmonary hemodynamics and perioperative cardiopulmonary-related mortality in patients with portopulmonary hypertension undergoing liver transplantation. *Liver Transplant*, **6**(4):443–450.

Kryzhanovski VA, Beller GA (1997) Usefulness of preoperative noninvasive radionuclide testing for detecting coronary artery disease in candidates for liver transplantation. *Am J Cardiol*, **79**(7):986–988.

Le Couteur DG, Everitt A, Lebel M (2009) The aging liver. *Geriatr Aging*, **12**(6):319–322.

Leidig-Bruckner G, Hosch S, Dodidou P, et al. (2001) Frequency and predictors of osteoporotic fractures after cardiac or liver transplantation: a follow-up study. *Lancet*, **357**(9253):342–347.

Lenhardt R, Marker E, Goll V, et al. (1997) Mild intraoperative hypothermia prolongs postanesthetic recovery. *Anesthesia*, **87**(6):1318–1323.

Leung JM, Dzankic S (2001) Relative importance of preoperative health status versus intraoperative factors in predicting postoperative adverse outcomes in geriatric surgical patients. *J Am Geriatr Soc*, **49**(8):1080–1085.

Levi DM, Tzakis AG, Kato T, et al. (2003) Transplantation of the abdominal wall. *Lancet*, **361**(9376):2173–2176.

Lin K, Stewart D, Cooper S, Davis CL (2001) Pre-transplant cardiac testing for kidney–pancreas transplant candidates and association with cardiac outcomes. *Clin Transplant*, **15**(4):269–275.

Lipshutz GS, Hiatt J, Ghobrial RM, et al. (2007) Outcome of liver transplantation in septuagenarians: a single-center experience. *Arch Surg*, **142**(8):775–781.

Makary MA, Segev DL, Pronovost PJ, et al. (2010) Frailty as a predictor of surgical outcomes in older patients. *J Am Coll Surg*, **210**(6):901–908.

Mandell MS, Lindenfeld JA, Tsou M, Zimmerman M (2008) Cardiac evaluation of liver transplant candidates. *World J Gastroenterol*, **14**(22):3445–3451.

Mangoni AA, Jackson SHD (2004) Age-related changes in pharmacokinetics and pharmacodynamics: basic principles and practical applications. *Br J Clin Pharmacol*, **57**(1):6–14.

Mangus RS, Tector AJ, Kubal CA, Fridell JA, Vianna RM (2013) Multivisceral transplantation: expanding indications and improving outcomes. *J Gastrointest Surg*, **17**(1):179–187.

Mapleson WW (1996) Effect of age on MAC in humans: a meta-analysis. *Br J Anaesth*, **76**(2):179–185.

Martins PNA, Pratschke J, Pascher A, et al. (2005) Age and immune response in organ transplantation. *Transplantation*, **79**(2):127–132.

Matsuura T, Oda Y, Tanaka K, Mori T, Nishikawa K, Asada A (2009) Advance of age decreases the minimum alveolar concentrations of isoflurane and sevoflurane for maintaining bispectral index below 50. *Br J Anaesth*, **102**(3):331–335.

Matyal R, Hess PE, Subramaniam B, et al. (2009) Perioperative diastolic dysfunction during vascular surgery and its association with postoperative outcome. *J Vasc Surg*, **50**(1):70–76.

McNicol L, Story DA, Leslie K, et al. (2007) Postoperative complications and mortality in older patients having non-cardiac surgery at three Melbourne teaching hospitals. *Med J Australia*, **186**(9):447–452.

Meier-Kriesche H, Ojo A, Hanson J, et al. (2000) Increased immunosuppressive vulnerability in elderly renal transplant recipients. *Transplantation*, **69**(5):885–889.

Meier-Kriesche H, Srinivas TR, Kaplan B (2001a) Interaction between acute rejection and recipient age on long-term renal allograft survival. *Transplant Proc*, **33**(7-8):3425–3426.

Meier-Kriesche H, Ojo AO, Hanson JA (2001b) Exponentially increased risk of infectious death in older renal transplant recipients. *Kidney* Int, **59**(4):1539–1543.

Messing B, Crenn P, Beau P, et al. (1999) Long-term survival and parenteral nutrition dependence in adult patients with the short bowel syndrome. *Gastroenterology*, **117**(5):1043–1050.

Monk TG, Saini V, Weldon BC, Sigl JC (2005) Anesthetic management and one-year mortality after noncardiac surgery. *Anesth Analg*, **100**(1):4–10.

Morgan AL, Sinning WE, Weldy DL (2002) Age effects on body fluid distribution during exercise in the heat. *Aviation Space Environ Med*, **73**(8):750–757.

Motsch J, Epple J, Fresenius M, Neff S, Schmidt W, Martin E (1998) Desflurane versus isoflurane in geriatric patients. A comparison of psychomotor recovery and postoperative well-being. *Anasth Intens Notfallmed Schmerzther*, **33**(5):313–320.

Mrak RE, Griffin WST, Graham DI (1997) Aging-associated changes in human brain. *J Neuropathol Exp Neurol*, **56**(12):1269–1275.

Navaratnarajah A, Jackson SHD (2013) The physiology of ageing. *Medicine (UK)*, **41**(1):5–8.

Neuberger J (2003) Liver transplantation for primary biliary cirrhosis. *Autoimmun Rev*, **2**(1):1–7.

Newton JL, Jones DE, Metcalf JV, et al. (2000) Presentation and mortality of primary biliary cirrhosis in older patients. *Age Ageing*, **29**(4):305–309.

Nickalls RW, Mapleson WW (2003) Age-related iso-MAC charts for isoflurane, sevoflurane and desflurane in man. *Br J Anaesth*, **91**(2):170–174.

Ninkovic M, Love SA, Tom B, Alexander GJM, Compston JE (2001) High prevalence of osteoporosis in patients with chronic liver disease prior to liver transplantation. *Calcified Tissue Int*, **69**(6):321–326.

Ojo AO, Hanson JA, Wolfe RA, Leichtman AB, Agodoa LY, Port FK (2000) Long-term survival in renal transplant recipients with graft function. *Kidney Int*, **57**(1):307–313.

O'Neill PA (1996) Aging and salt and water balance. *Rev Clin Gerontol*, **6**(4):305–313.

OPTN (2012) *OPTN/SRTR 2011 Annual Data Report*. Department of Health and Human Services, Health Resources and Services Administration, Healthcare Systems Bureau, Division of Transplantation, Rockville, Maryland.

OPTN (2014) *OPTN/SRTR 2012 Annual Data Report*. Department of Health and Human Services, Health Resources and Services Administration, Rockville, Maryland:

OPTN (2015) *National Data*. <http://optn.transplant.hrsa.gov/converge/latestdata/step2.asp?>.

Partridge JSL, Harari D, Dhesi JK (2012) Frailty in the older surgical patient: a review. *Age Ageing*, **41**(2):142–147.

Peduto VA, Peli S, Micucci G, et al. (1998) Maintenance of and recovery from anaesthesia in elderly patients. A clinical comparison between sevoflurane and isoflurane. *Minerva Anestesiolog*, **64**(9 Suppl 3):18–25.

Peters A (2002) Structural changes that occur during normal aging of primate cerebral hemispheres. *Neurosci Biobehav Rev*, **26**(7):733–741.

Phillip B, Pastor D, Bellows W, Leung JM (2003) The prevalence of preoperative diastolic filling abnormalities in geriatric surgical patients. *Anesth Analg*, **97**(5):1214–1221.

Pironi L, Spinucci G, Paganelli F, et al. (2004) Italian guidelines for intestinal transplantation: potential candidates among the adult patients managed by a medical referral center for chronic intestinal failure. *Transplant Proc*, **36**(3):659–661.

Pirsch JD, Kalayoglu M, D'Alessandro AM, et al. (1991) Orthotopic liver transplantation in patients 60 years of age and older. *Transplantation*, **51**(2):431–433.

Plevak DJ (1998) Stress echocardiography identifies coronary artery disease in liver transplant candidates. *Liver Transplant Surg*, **4**(4):337–339.

Plotkin JS, Scott VL, Pinna A, Dobsch BP, De Wolf AM, Kang Y (1996) Morbidity and mortality in patients with coronary artery disease undergoing orthotopic liver transplantation *Liver Transplant Surg*, **2**(6):426–430.

Plotkin JS, Benitez RM, Kuo PC, et al. (1998) Dobutamine stress echocardiography for preoperative cardiac risk stratification in patients undergoing orthotopic liver transplantation. *Liver Transplant Surg*, **4**(4):253–257.

Potter JF, James OFW (1987) Clinical features and prognosis of alcoholic liver disease in respect of advancing age. *Gerontology*, **33**(6):380–387.

Priebe HJ (2000) The aged cardiovascular risk patient. *Br J Anaesth*, **85**(5):763–778.

Qaseem T (2006) Risk assessment for and strategies to reduce perioperative pulmonary complications. *Annal Intern Med*, **145**(7):553.

Rao PS, Merion RM, Ashby VB, Port FK, Wolfe RA, Kayler LK (2007) Renal transplantation in elderly patients older than 70 years of age: results from the Scientific Registry of Transplant Recipients. *Transplantation*, **83**(8):1069–1074.

Robinson TN, Wu DS, Stiegmann GV, Moss M (2011) Frailty predicts increased hospital and six-month healthcare cost following colorectal surgery in older adults. *Am J Surg*, **202**(5):511–514.

Rooke GA (2003) Cardiovascular aging and anesthetic implications. *J Cardio-Thorac Vasc Anesth*, **17**(4):512–523.

Rudich S, Busuttil R (1999) Similar outcomes, morbidity, and mortality for orthotopic liver transplantation between the very elderly and the young. *Transplant Proc*, **31**(1–2):523–525.

Ruiz P, Kato T, Tzakis A (2007) Current status of transplantation of the small intestine. *Transplantation*, **83**(1):1–6.

Sadean MR, Glass PSA (2003) Pharmacokinetics in the elderly. *Best Practice Res Clin Anaesth*, **17**(2):191–205.

Schiødt FV, Chung RT, Schilsky ML, et al. (2009) Outcome of acute liver failure in the elderly. *Liver Transplant*, **15**(11):1481–1487.

Schmied H, Kurz A, Sessler DI, Kozek S, Reiter A (1996) Mild hypothermia increases blood loss and transfusion requirements during total hip arthroplasty. *Lancet*, **347**(8997):289–292.

Schmucker DL (2001) Liver function and phase I drug metabolism in the elderly: a paradox. *Drugs Aging*, **18**(11):837–851.

Schnider TW, Minto CF, Shafer SL, et al. (1999) The influence of age on propofol pharmacodynamics. *Anesthesia*, **90**(6):1502–1516.

Schold JD, Meier-Kriesche HU (2006) Which renal transplant candidates should accept marginal kidneys in exchange for a shorter waiting time on dialysis? *Clin J Am Soc Nephrol*, **1**(3):532–538.

Schwartz JJ, Pappas L, Thiesset HF, et al. (2012) Liver transplantation in septuagenarians receiving model for end-stage liver disease exception points for hepatocellular carcinoma: the national experience. *Liver Transplant*, **18**(4):423–433.

Seymour DG, Vaz FG (1989) A prospective study of elderly general surgical patients: II. Post-operative complications. *Age Ageing*, **18**(5):316–326.

Shafer SL (2000) The pharmacology of anesthetic drugs in elderly patients. *Anesth Clin N Am*, **18**(1):1–29.

Shankar N, Albasheer M, Marotta P, Wall W, McAlister V, Chandok N (2011) Do older patients utilize excess health care resources after liver transplantation? *Annal Hepatol*, **10**(4):477–481.

Shaw BW Jr (1992) Liver transplantation in patients over 60 years of age. *Liver Update Function Dis*, **5**:3–4.

Sheiner PA, Magliocca JF, Bodian CA, et al. (2000) Long-term medical complications in patients surviving ≥5 years after liver transplant. *Transplantation*, **69**(5):781–789.

Sieber FE, Barnett SR (2011) Preventing postoperative complications in the elderly. *Anesth Clin*, **29**(1):83–97.

Singh A, Antognini JF (2010) Perioperative pharmacology in elderly patients. *Curr Opin Anaesthesiol*, **23**(4):449–454.

Small SA (2001) Age-related memory decline: current concepts and future directions. *Arch Neurol*, **58**(3):360–364.

Smetana GW (2009) Postoperative pulmonary complications: an update on risk assessment and reduction. *Cleveland Clin J Med*, **76**(Suppl 4):S60–S65.

Smetana GW, Lawrence VA, Cornell JE, American College of Physicians (2006) Preoperative pulmonary risk stratification for noncardiothoracic surgery: systematic review for the American College of Physicians. *Annal Intern Med*, **144**(8):581–595.

Sprung J, Gajic O, Warner DO (2006) Review article: age related alterations in respiratory function—anesthetic considerations. *Can J Anaesth*, **53**(12):1244–1257.

Stell D, Wall WJ (2003) The impact of aging on the liver. *Geriatr Aging*, **6**(3):36–37.

Stieber AC, Gordon RD, Todo S, et al. (1991) Liver transplantation in patients over sixty years of age. *Transplantation*, **51**(1):271–273.

Story DA (2008) Postoperative complications in elderly patients and their significance for long-term prognosis. *Curr Opin Anaesthesiol*, **21**(3):375–379.

Tamura MK, Yaffe K (2011) Dementia and cognitive impairment in ESRD: diagnostic and therapeutic strategies. *Kidney Int*, **79**(1):14–22.

Taner CB, Ung RL, Rosser BG, Aranda-Michel J (2012) Age is not a contraindication for orthotopic liver transplantation: a single institution experience with recipients older than 75 years. *Hepatol Int*, **6**(1):403–407.

Tiukinhoy-Laing SD, Rossi JS, Bayram M, et al. (2006) Cardiac hemodynamic and coronary angiographic characteristics of patients being evaluated for liver transplantation. *Am J Cardiol*, **98**(2):178–181.

Tullius SG, Milford E (2011) Kidney allocation and the aging immune response. *N Engl J Med*, **364**(14):1369–1370.

Turrentine FE, Wang H, Simpson VB, Jones RS (2006) Surgical risk factors, morbidity, and mortality in elderly patients. *J Am Coll Surg*, **203**(6):865–877.

Tzakis AG, Kato T, Levi DM, et al. (2005) 100 Multivisceral transplants at a single center. *Annal Surg*, **242**(4):480–493.

Vianna RM, Mangus RS, Tector AJ (2008) Current status of small bowel and multivisceral transplantation. *Adv Surg*, **42**:129–150..

Vuyk J (2003) Pharmacodynamics in the elderly. *Best Practice Res Clin Anaesth*, **17**(2):207–218.

Weigle WO (1989) Effects of aging on the immune system. *Hospital Prac*, **24**(12):112–116, 118.

Weinstein JR, Anderson S (2010) The aging kidney: physiological changes. *Adv Chronic Kidney Dis*, **17**(4):302–307.

Wolfe RA, Ashby VB, Milford EL, et al. (1999) Comparison of mortality in all patients on dialysis, patients on dialysis awaiting transplantation, and recipients of a first cadaveric transplant. *N Engl J Med*, **341**(23):1725–1730.

Wynne H (2005) Drug metabolism and ageing. *J Br Menopause Soc*, **11**(2):51–56.

Wynne HA, Cope LH, Mutch E, Rawlins MD, Woodhouse KW, James OFW (1989) The effect of age upon liver volume and apparent liver blood flow in healthy men. *Hepatology*, **9**(2):297–301.

Xiol X, Guardiola J, Menendez S, et al. (2001) Risk factors for development of de novo neoplasia after liver transplantation. *Liver Transplant*, **7**(11):971–975.

Zaugg M, Lucchinetti E (2000) Respiratory function in the elderly. *Anesthesiol Clin N Am*, **18**(1):47–58, vi.

Zetterman RK, Belle SH, Hoofnagle JH, et al. (1998) Age and liver transplantation: a report of the liver transplantation database. *Transplantation*, **66**(4):500–506.

Zhang Y, Zhang Q, Li H, et al. (2011) Prognostic factors for late mortality after liver transplantation for benign end-stage liver disease. *Chinese Med J*, **124**(24):4229–4235.

# CHAPTER 36

# Transfusion medicine and organ transplantation

Richard Charlewood and Kerry Gunn

## Introduction

Rates of transfusion in organ transplantation have reduced since the 1990s. The mean number of red cells transfused to a liver recipient was 12 units in the late 1990s but is now as low as 0.5 units, with some centres reporting almost 80% of patients not requiring any blood transfusion (Triulzi, 2001; Massicotte et al., 2012). Transfusion rates in other organ transplant settings have shown a similar decreasing trend. Nevertheless, transfusion remains an essential part of the toolbox for transplantation.

## Issues with blood and blood components

### ABO compatibility for ABO-incompatible transplants

ABO antigens are oligosaccharides, attached not only to red cells but also to platelets, endothelial cells, and most epithelial cells. ABO antibodies directed against any ABO antigens not expressed by the host are typically formed in the first few months of life in response to naturally occurring food and bacterial antigens. The significance of these so-called naturally occurring antibodies is in providing compatible blood components for transfusion as well as organs for organ transplantation. Where the organ is ABO identical, these antibodies are only of significance for transfusions. Where the organ is not ABO-compatible, one of two situations arise—where the organ is compatible with the recipient, termed a minor incompatibility (e.g. O organ to an A recipient) or where the organ is incompatible, termed a major incompatibility (e.g. A organ to an O recipient). Where both the organ and recipient are mutually incompatible, this is termed a bidirectional incompatibility (e.g. A organ to a B recipient).

It is therefore essential to be sure of the donor blood group. In massive transfusion of group O red cells (e.g. following trauma) the donor's blood may reflect the transfused cells and appear to be O. Particular care must be taken when assigning a blood group to the donor if he/she is multiply transfused prior to the first blood group being taken.

ABOi-incompatible organ transplants have a higher rate of acute rejection. Measurement of the titre of ABO antibodies in the recipient may assist in predicting the likelihood of this occurring and the appropriateness of interventions to reduce it (Tobian et al., 2008). This can be performed manually, using tubes or gel cards, or by flow cytometry. The manual methods are simpler but less precise, whereas the latter is more costly and more difficult to set up but more reproducible (Ata et al., 2012).

ABOi transplantation is discussed elsewhere (see Chapter 11). However, in the ABOi live donor setting, plasma exchange and immunosuppression are commonly used in renal transplantation to reduce ABO titres (Tobian et al., 2008; Takahashi and Saito, 2013). The replacement fluid in plasma exchanges does not usually contain clotting factors because FFP is associated with a higher rate of adverse reactions than the alternatives (e.g. albumin, saline). This has the potential to create a dilutional coagulopathy. Although not usually clinically significant, this may need to be corrected prior to any surgical intervention. Prior to the transplant it is important that the last exchange uses plasma (e.g. FFP) to ensure that the recipient is able to clot normally at the time of surgery and that the patient's clotting profile is checked preoperatively. This does not apply for immunoadsorption where ABO antibodies are selectively removed by column adsorption extracorporeally. Although immunoadsorption is somewhat more efficient than plasma exchange and does not affect other plasma proteins, its cost and small number of indications mean its use is not widespread (Hur et al., 2011).

Once the transplant has taken place, selection of the ABO group for transfusion is complicated by the presence of ABO antigens on the endothelium of the transplanted organ and the recipient, as well as the circulating red cells. The significance of this is that a transfusion that is ABOi with the organ may lead to antibody binding to the transplanted organ's endothelium and a vasculitis. This in turn may lead to graft rejection.

Lastly, donor lymphocytes in the transplanted organ may produce ABO antibodies if a minor incompatibility exists, or they may produce other antibodies directed at the recipient's red cells. In this situation, haemolysis of the recipient's red cells may arise, typically abruptly 1–3 weeks after transplantation, with spontaneous resolution within 3 months. This phenomenon is termed passenger lymphocyte syndrome. It occurs particularly in organs with extensive lymphoid tissue such as liver and lungs. Haemolysis is most commonly due to ABO mismatch with an O organ, but other blood group systems have also been reported (Smith, 2010). The antibodies normally bind to the red cells or endothelium, but may occasionally also be free-floating and then can give rise to an ABO grouping anomaly in the blood bank. Good communication with the haematology laboratory and blood bank will ensure this is detected early.

There is no standardized approach to transfusion support in minor ABOi transplants. The various possibilities can be grouped into the following categories: transfusing only recipient group red cells (i.e. ignoring the minor ABOi incompatibility); transfusing donor group red cells from the time of surgery (i.e. reducing the level of donor-incompatible red cells in circulation); or waiting for serological evidence of antibody formation in either a positive direct antiglobulin test or an incompatible cross-match before switching to donor group red cells. Because the risk is lowest in renal transplants (red cell antibodies in 17%, haemolysis in 9%), a watch and wait approach is prudent. The risk is higher in liver transplants (antibodies in 40%, haemolysis in 29%) and highest in heart–lung transplants (antibodies in 70%, haemolysis in 70%), as liver and lung contain large number of antibody-producing leucocytes. For these organs the second two options should be considered. Plasma transfusions should be of the recipient group or of the universal plasma donor group, AB.

## Red cell alloimmunization

There are over 20 different red cell blood group systems and many different individual red cell antigens. While 'naturally occurring' ABO antibodies are formed in infancy, antibodies to other blood group antigens (e.g. Rh(D), Kell) are typically formed only following alloimmunization, due to transfusion, pregnancy, or transplantation. These antibodies may wane over time and potentially disappear altogether. However, in a phenomenon called the anamnestic response, the memory cells still present can, on re-exposure to the antigen, cause a rapid resurgence in the antibody to the point of causing clinically significant haemolysis.

In the pretransplant period, a restrictive transfusion policy will reduce the risk of alloantibody formation. Although largely out of the transplanter's hands, there is evidence that transfusion of donations collected from donors of the recipient's own ethnic background may also reduce the risk of alloimmunization (Olujohungbe et al., 2001). This observation is of relevance when considering transferring transplant-recipients away from their ethnic community.

Not all transfusion recipients will mount an immune response to allogeneic red cells, although the published rate varies widely, from 2% to 21% (Zalpuri et al., 2012). Factors such as immune suppression, the recipient's red cell phenotype, the number of units transfused, and other presumed to be inherited factors influence whether a recipient produces antibodies directed to the transfused red cells.

The risk of red cell alloimmunization can be reduced in two ways. First, matching the phenotype of the red cells for transfusion to the recipient's phenotype for clinically significant antigens greatly reduces the risk of antibody formation but inevitably increases costs. The Rh and Kell blood group systems accounted for 60% of red cell antibodies in a UK study of liver transplant recipients (Mushkbar et al., 2013). Providing prophylactically matched red cells for these two blood groups could be justifiable. Second, reducing the number of units transfused also significantly reduces the risk of alloimmunization, with a 3.6-fold higher risk of alloimmunization after 40 units transfused compared with only 5 units (Zalpuri et al., 2012).

Platelet transfusions are also a potential source of red cell alloimmunization as there is a small amount of donor red cells in each platelet component, sufficient to sensitize a recipient to Rh(D). Passive prophylaxis to the D antigen is readily available by providing a dose Rh D immunoglobulin if Rh(D)-incompatible platelets are transfused. This option is not available for red cell transfusions as it would lyse the transfused red cells and is not readily available for any other red cell antigens.

## Fresh vs old red cells

The impact of the age of red cell components at the time of transfusion has become topical in recent years. Concerns have been raised that the use of older red cell components is associated with increased morbidity and mortality in a range of clinical settings.

Storage lesions develop in refrigerated red cells and are well described (van de Watering, 2011b):

- Loss of 2,3-diphosphoglycerate (2,3DPG) with associated decrease in ability to release oxygen in the tissues due to an altered oxygen dissociation curve
- Altered red cell shape makes red cells less deformable and less able to traverse capillary beds and sinusoids
- Refrigeration-induced loss of function of the Na/K channel with a rise in extracellular potassium in the unit
- Haemolysis of red cells
- Release of cytokines, histamine, complement, lipids, proinflammatory CD40 ligand, and bioactive lipid peroxidases (especially in non-leucodepleted components)
- Binding of nitric oxide leading to vasoconstriction

Although these changes are well established in vitro, the clinical importance of the storage lesion is still a matter of some debate. Clinical consequences ascribed to the storage lesion include:

- Transfusion-related immunomodulation (TRIM) with secondary increase in the risk of infectious complications, spread of malignancy, and reduction in rejection of solid organ transplants (only the last has been convincingly demonstrated clinically)
- Increased hospital and ICU length of stay
- Organ failure
- Increased mortality in some studies

Contrary arguments to provision of fresh blood include:

- Increased risk of transfusion-associated graft versus host disease (TA-GVHD)
- Increased mortality in some studies

A number of studies, systematic reviews, and meta-analyses have attempted to address this question (Vamvakas, 2010; Wang et al., 2012; Lelubre and Vincent, 2013), but many have significant methodological flaws (van de Watering, 2011a; Flegel, 2012; Warkentin and Eikelboom, 2012). A number of large randomized control trials (ABLE, RECESS, and Transfuse) are in progress in an attempt to address this question.

## HLA immunization

Formation of HLA antibodies in potential organ recipients not only limits the availability of organs but also can cause graft rejection. Fresh non-frozen components carry leucocytes that express HLA antigens, and there is a correlation between the number of transfusions and the rate of sensitization (Scornik and Meier-Kriesche, 2011; Balasubramaniam et al., 2012). Ten to sixteen percent of renal transplant candidates who have received leucodepleted or non-leucodepleted transfusions with no other route of sensitization develop HLA antibodies. The presence of HLA antibodies is associated with longer wait times for transplantation and, when directed against (organ) DSA, with poorer outcomes. Leucodepleting components do not appear to reduce the risk of sensitization. As a result, while it may be necessary to transfuse patients, a restrictive transfusion policy and effective patient blood management should be adopted (Scornik and Meier-Kriesche, 2011; Balasubramaniam et al., 2012; Scornik et al., 2013).

## Cytomegalovirus

CMV is a member of the *Herpes* family of viruses, spread by a variety of body fluids as well as transfusion and transplantation. The virus typically establishes life-long latency in leucocytes. Although clinical illness is unusual and typically self-limiting in the immunocompetent host, acute infection or reactivation in the immunosuppressed patient may cause substantial morbidity and mortality. CMV infection is one of the commonest complications affecting organ transplant recipients, with significant direct morbidity, occasional mortality, as well as indirect effects impacting outcomes (Kotton et al., 2010). Thirty to ninety percent of people in developed countries have evidence of prior CMV infection (Staras et al., 2006; Crough and Khanna, 2009). Development of CMV infection in the transplant recipient may therefore arise due to (Kotton et al., 2010):

- Reactivation of the infection in the organ recipient
- Transmission from the transplanted organ
- Transmission by blood transfusion

If the recipient is either already infected pretransplant or exposed via an organ from a CMV-infected donor, there is little to be gained in trying to restrict transfusions to CMV-safer components. Symptomatic CMV infection is more likely to develop from the infected organ or by reactivation of the recipient's past infection.

CMV-safer transfusions are classically provided either as blood from donors that have tested negative for CMV antibodies or by leucodepleting the blood by filtration prior to transfusion, thereby removing the viral reservoir in the blood. Neither of these methods totally eliminates the risk. CMV antibody-negative donors may be in the viraemic early stages of the infection, the window period, and leucodepletion does not eliminate cell-free viral particles found in the period leading up to and soon after seroconversion to CMV positivity (Ziemann et al., 2007).

The difference between the two methods of prevention is, at most, small. In an early large study of 521 haemopoietic stem-cell transplant recipients receiving either CMV-negative components or bedside-filtered components, there was no statistically significant difference in CMV infection (0.8% vs 1.2%), disease (0% vs 1.2%), or survival (Bowden et al., 1995). A subsequent meta-analysis showed a slight difference favouring CMV-negative donations over leucodepletion (Vamvakas, 2005); however, the issue remains controversial and is not regarded as resolved (Bilgin et al., 2011). Whether there is additive benefit in leucodepleting CMV-negative donations has not been tested and is unlikely to be, as it would require many thousands of patients to demonstrate a clinical benefit (Laupacis et al., 2001).

An interesting alternative approach examined blood donors who had been CMV-positive for at least a year, showing these were less likely to have CMV DNA in their donation (Drew and Roback, 2007; Ziemann et al., 2007). This approach has yet to be confirmed or accepted into clinical practice.

Due to the immunosuppression associated with solid organ transplantation, CMV-safer transfusions are appropriate for transplants where both donor and recipient are CMV-negative. If universal prestorage leucodepletion is in place, the safety afforded by leucodepletion is probably sufficient for most types of transplant. Concern is sometimes raised about the impact CMV has on a newly transplanted lung in CMV-negative lung transplant donor–recipients pairs. However, reviews that considered this particular issue concluded there was no evidence to support leucodepleting CMV-negative donations, and that either CMV-negative or leucodepleted components were sufficient (Kotton et al., 2010; SaBTO, 2012).

## Leucodepletion

Leucodepletion offers many advantages to the transplant recipient. Reduction in platelet refractoriness has been well demonstrated (Slichter et al., 2005): up to 50% reduction in postoperative infection (Blumberg et al., 2007), a reduction in febrile non-haemolytic transfusion reactions (Brown and Navarrete, 2011), and a reduction in pathogen transmission: bacteria, intracellular viruses, and parasites.

Leucodepletion can be provided in two forms—filtration at the bedside for selected patients, or universal filtering of all units by the blood provider service, either pre or post storage. Although some of the gains to be had from leucodepletion can be achieved with selective bedside leucodepletion, universal prestorage leucodepletion offers better patient outcomes even for those patients that would warrant bedside filtration (Da Ponte et al., 2005). The cost of these benefits for all patients has been a source of much debate (van de Watering, 2004), but many countries have nevertheless implemented universal leucodepletion.

## Irradiation

GVHD is a well-recognized complication in organ transplantation whereby donor lymphocytes engraft in the recipient and mount an immune attack. Sources of these lymphocytes include the organ itself, concomitant haematopoietic stem-cell infusions from the organ donor, and transfusions (Triulzi and Nalesnik, 2001). TA-GVHD, although rare, is almost uniformly fatal (King and Ness, 2011). In the setting of organ transplantation, the situations where TA-GVHD is a risk are as follows (Treleaven et al., 2011; American Association of Blood Banks, 2014):

- Donations from blood relatives
- Matched platelet transfusions, typically given for platelet refractoriness
- The use of powerful immunosuppressive drugs such as alemtuzamab
- Granulocyte infusions

Irradiation prevents TA-GVHD by inducing breaks in lymphocyte DNA in the unit for transfusion, preventing multiplication of the lymphocyte. It is only required for components that do or may contain viable cells such as whole blood, red cells, platelets, and fresh plasma but not FFP.

Recent developments have contributed to both an increased and decreased risk of TA-GVHD. While irradiation is not currently routinely recommended for solid organ transplant recipients, new potent immunosuppressants may put patients at risk until a requirement to irradiate has been established (O'Brien et al., 2013). Conversely, in some blood services, the advent of pathogen reduction systems effectively prevents TA-GVHD without the problems of hyperkalaemia (Fast, 2012). These systems aim to prevent the transmission of unknown pathogens by modifying any nucleic acids in the donation, preventing the lymphocytes from proliferating in the recipient. Leucodepletion also appears to substantially reduce, but not entirely eliminate, the risk of TA-GVHD (Bolton-Maggs and Cohen, 2012).

Irradiating red cells causes the sodium–potassium pump to fail, leading to a rise in extracellular potassium. Although this is reabsorbed by the red cells after transfusion, there is a risk of hyperkalaemia in the patient if the red cells are administered too quickly. Apart from this, irradiated components are as safe to transfuse as non-irradiated units, provided their shortened shelf-life is observed.

### Preoperative anticoagulant reversal

Patients prior to transplantation, especially cardiac transplantation, may be taking warfarin or other anticoagulants. This represents a significant risk for surgical bleeding, but cessation of anticoagulants may cause unnecessary thromboembolic risk. A risk assessment of the relative importance of these two factors is needed prior to surgery.

Key anticoagulants to consider include vitamin K antagonists (e.g. warfarin/coumadin), thrombin and clotting factor inhibitors (e.g. dabigatran, rivaroxiban, apixaban), antiplatelet agents (e.g. aspirin, clopidogrel), and heparin (unfractionated or low molecular weight). Guidelines exist for reversal of these agents prior to surgery (Dunning et al., 2008; Bauer, 2012; Hartman and Teruya, 2012; Kaatz et al., 2012; Kruger et al., 2012). It is beyond the scope of this chapter to cover these in detail; suffice to say that broad principles include planning the anticoagulant/antiplatelet reversal well in advance of surgery, as timed withdrawal of medication is a key plank to controlled reversal. Where the patient is at high risk of thrombosis, bridging agents such as heparin may be required. Temporary or emergency reversal may be available, depending on the drug being used. Reversal agents include prothrombin complex concentrates for warfarin and rivaroxiban, platelets for antiplatelet agents, protamine for heparin and humanized antibody fragments such as idarucizumab, being trialled for dabigatran reversal.

## Issues with patients

### The red cell alloimmunized patient

Depending on the type of transplant, the alloimmunized patient can present a significant challenge to transplant co-ordination. Although renal transplants seldom require blood, liver transplants may on occasion consume large numbers of red cell units. Cross-matched units need to be available at all times once the potential organ recipient is close enough to the top of the list for transplantation. Because the availability of antigen-negative units may be limited, this requires close co-ordination with the local blood bank and blood provider. However, not all antibodies are clinically significant and this needs to be established with the blood bank at the outset. It should be borne in mind that there might be substantial delays in obtaining blood for transfusion once the prearranged stock is exhausted. If this should occur, there may be a role for giving incompatible units during brisk haemorrhage and reverting to compatible units towards the end of the transplant. In this case, close co-ordination with the blood bank is required (Ramsey et al., 1989). Careful preparation of the recipient can further reduce the risk of a shortage of cross-matched red cells. Important areas include addressing pre-existing anaemia and coagulation disturbances, as well as meticulous attention to haemostasis and tolerance of intraoperative anaemia.

### Cold agglutinins and cardiac surgery

Cold agglutinins are circulating antibodies, usually IgM, that are able to agglutinate the patient's own red cells, typically below body temperature. These can lead to symptoms such as haemolysis and peripheral ischaemia. In asymptomatic patients, the presence of cold agglutinins is generally regarded as a nuisance finding. However, in the context where patients may be deliberately subjected to hypothermia, the presence of cold agglutinins with a thermal amplitude that reaches the patient's hypothermic core temperature becomes more relevant. Concern has been expressed that, during hypothermia, agglutination may cause haemolysis or microvascular obstruction, both in the patient and in the bypass circuitry. The literature has been unclear on the relevance of these antibodies; suffice to say that, if detected, the type of surgery may be changed, possibly to a less effective or less safe operation. Alternatively, the cold agglutinins may be treated with rituximab, intravenous immunoglobulins, and plasmapheresis, leading to delayed surgery. A recent review and large retrospective study, however, has concluded that routine cold agglutinin screening improve neither patient care nor CPB outcomes. Instead, looking for the few at-risk patients with a preoperative history, intraoperative vigilance and in-the-field adjustment of CPB based on clinical suspicion are recommended. (Jain et al., 2013).

## Delivery

### Massive transfusion

In the critically bleeding patient, rapid delivery of blood components is essential. To aid this a protocol is needed that, once activated, allows the blood bank to prepare components ahead of time, facilitating their transfusion as soon as they are required. Much has been written on the importance of high plasma and platelet to red cell ratios (e.g. 1:1 FFP:red cells) (Borgman et al., 2007; Shaz et al., 2010; Thomas et al., 2010), but this remains controversial (Snyder et al., 2009; de Biasi et al., 2011; Dzik et al., 2011). Less explored but nevertheless of importance, and possibly the reason massive transfusion protocols achieve good patient outcomes, is the significance of a delivery system that operates promptly and efficiently (Riskin et al., 2009).

It goes without saying that achieving haemostasis is essential in reducing transfusion requirements. This is particularly important in cardiac and pulmonary surgery where the recipient is receiving cardiac bypass or ECMO. It is also true in liver transplantation where abnormal coagulation may be present in the dissection, anhepatic and postreperfusion phases of surgery. Haemostasis is discussed in detail in Chapter 37.

### Intraoperative transfusion

Since the 1990s there has been a consistent reduction in blood product usage during liver transplantation (Triulzi, 2001; Massicotte et al., 2012). Attempts to relate the degree of bleeding and transfusion to traditional coagulation tests preoperatively have shown poor correlation and, in fact, use of FFP to correct an elevated INR may increase red cell transfusion (DuPont et al., 1996; Caldwell et al., 2006). Pre-existing anaemia is a predictor of red cell transfusions in liver transplantation (Massicotte et al., 2012). The decision-making for which product is indicated is covered in other chapters, but significant advancement has recently been made in reducing unnecessary blood product transfusions by reduced CVP techniques, venesection, and not treating abnormal coagulation parameters in the absence of clinical bleeding (Massicotte et al., 2012). This is important, as numerous studies have highlighted the association of red cell transfusions and bleeding with negative outcomes after liver transplantation (Ramos et al., 2003). However, these studies typically suffer from confounding by indication (Middelburg et al., 2010), and clear evidence that poor outcomes are caused by the deleterious effect of blood products rather than more severe systemic disease or greater blood loss is lacking.

In a retrospective study, platelet transfusions were shown to be an independent risk factor for patient and graft survival after liver transplant (de Boer et al., 2008). It is suggested that platelet transfusion can worsen reperfusion injury by inducing endothelial cell apoptosis (Sindram et al., 2000). Apheresis-derived platelets have been shown to be associated with a lower incidence of alloimmunization and infectious complications (Ness and Campbell, 2001). In a smaller study from a group using leucodepleted whole blood derived and apheresis platelets, a negative correlation could not be found (Nixon et al., 2009).

The use of low CVP during anaesthesia, use of moderate vasopressor, and the lack of prophylactic FFP use can lead to a significant reduction in blood product use and a 79.6% incidence of transplantation without blood products (Massicotte et al., 2012). While there is no study that directly compares the outcome of patients receiving liberal vs restrictive blood transfusions for the same MELD score or bleeding, the suggested benefit or methods to reduce unnecessary blood transfusions are likely to improve outcome. FFP-free haemostatic management of liver transplantation is also possible using fractionated plasma products, i.e. fibrinogen concentrate, prothrombin complex concentrates, and factor VIII. Noval-Padillo et al. (2010) compared thromboelastometry-guided algorithms for administration of fibrinogen concentrate to maintain a normal fibrinogen-dependent graph (fib-tem®) and compared this to historical controls that received FFP. Fibrinogen concentrate was used in 45% of the patients and was associated with a 53% reduction in red cell use and a 63% reduction in FFP use. There are no randomized studies comparing 'traditional' and fractionated product use in liver transplantation, but numerous studies in cardiac surgery indicate a significant reduction in blood product use when using an algorithmic approach to product use with thromboelastography, either TEG® or ROTEM®.

### Fractionated products vs fresh components

Fractionated products (also called blood derivatives) are highly purified protein concentrates (Table 36.1) prepared by a large-scale fractionation process typically using thousands of units of donated plasma per batch of product. This is distinct from plasma (fresh, fresh frozen, thawed, or pooled) that is minimally processed donated plasma.

There are three main advantages of using fractionated products. First their purity and pharmaceutical-style batch production mean their contents and concentrations are known and consistent with few if any contaminating proteins. Second, modern fractionation processes typically include one or more viral inactivation steps such as heat, pH, nanofiltration, and solvents. This provides much greater confidence in the infectious safety of the products compared with fresh components. However, it should be borne in mind though that for developed nations, plasma components such as FFP typically have a viral infection risk of the order of only one in a million. The third advantage is the ease of delivery of the product. Fractionated products are usually stored refrigerated or at room temperature, making for faster dispensing than frozen plasma, and they have significantly smaller volumes than plasma so are quicker to administer. However, some are provided in powder form and reconstitution can take time if frothing is to be avoided.

There are two main disadvantages of fractionated products. The first is cost. Fractionation is an expensive process, with fractionated products costing two or more times that of plasma for the equivalent amount of the specific protein. The second disadvantage is that the purified products do not provide balanced coagulation support. Although a cocktail of a few prothrombotic and antithrombotic factors can be given to patients, a physiological product, as found in FFP, is not currently available. This generally results in a significantly prothrombotic state postinfusion, with implications for postinfusion thrombotic risk and thromboprophylaxis.

## Patient blood management

Increased emphasis is being placed on blood conservation following studies showing increased mortality associated with transfusion (Marik and Corwin, 2008) and convincing evidence that a

**Table 36.1** Examples of fractionated (plasma-derived) blood products

| Type of fractionated blood product | Examples of fractionated blood product |
|---|---|
| Albumin solutions | Hypertonic (also called 'salt-poor') or isotonic (4–5%) |
| Clotting factor concentrates | Factor VIII and vWF, Factor IX |
| | Anti-thrombin III, Protein C |
| | Prothrombin complex (factors II, IX, X ± VII) |
| | Fibrinogen |
| Immunoglobulin concentrates | Intravenous, intramuscular, and subcutaneous |
| | Hyperimmune immunoglobulins (e.g. Rh D immunoglobulin, Tetanus immunoglobulin) |
| Enzymes | C1-esterase inhibitor |

restrictive transfusion strategy is safe or possibly even advantageous in most groups of patients, including those with pre-existing cardiac disease (Carson et al., 2012b). Blood conservation rests on three pillars (Figure 36.1)—optimizing erythropoiesis, minimizing blood loss during surgery, and optimizing physiological reserves of anaemia (Spahn et al., 2008).

If surgery is anticipated, optimizing erythropoiesis, by first looking for anaemia, should be done at a time that allows for investigation and treatment of the anaemia. Even mild anaemia is associated with a significantly increased rate of transfusion (Beattie et al., 2009).

In certain circumstances, notably in renal failure and Jehovah's Witnesses, anaemia can be treated, either pre- or post-transplant, using erythropoietin. Care about patient selection and the target haemoglobin concentration needs to be taken, as erythropoietin is associated with thrombotic risks (Lippi et al., 2010).

Managing bleeding is more complicated in settings where transfusion is restricted due to the patient's physiology or where the patient refuses transfusion. Preoperative management includes identifying and managing any bleeding risk, minimizing iatrogenic blood loss (e.g. blood sampling in the paediatric population), together with planning and, if necessary, even rehearsing the surgical procedure. In highly selected cases, preoperative autologous blood collection may be warranted, but in general this is no longer recommended as it generally leads to increased donation-associated risks, worsening preoperative anaemia, and is of low clinical efficacy (Boulton and James, 2007).

Meticulous surgical haemostasis, blood-sparing surgical technique, maintaining normothermia, as well as using antifibrinolytic drugs such as tranexamic acid will assist in reducing surgical blood loss. In addition, cell salvage may recover up to half of the red cell requirement in liver transplantation. Intraoperative monitoring of coagulopathy/haemostasis, ideally using near-patient testing, will guide blood component management and reduce transfusion requirements (Luddington, 2005). Blood substitutes remain investigational.

When transfusion is required, a restrictive strategy should be employed (Carson et al., 2012a, 2012b). A transfusion can be withheld until the haemoglobin levels are 70 g/L or less in adult and paediatric ICU patients and 80 g/L in the postoperative surgical patient with good supporting evidence. Transfusion is also appropriate where patients are symptomatic (angina, orthostatic hypotension, tachycardia unresponsive to fluid resuscitation, or CHF), although this is usually not relevant in the intraoperative setting. Clear guidance is lacking in acute coronary syndromes, although tolerance of anaemia is reduced. While the transfusion trigger is one aspect, the target haemoglobin also needs to be considered. The original Transfusion Requirements in Critical Care (TRICC)

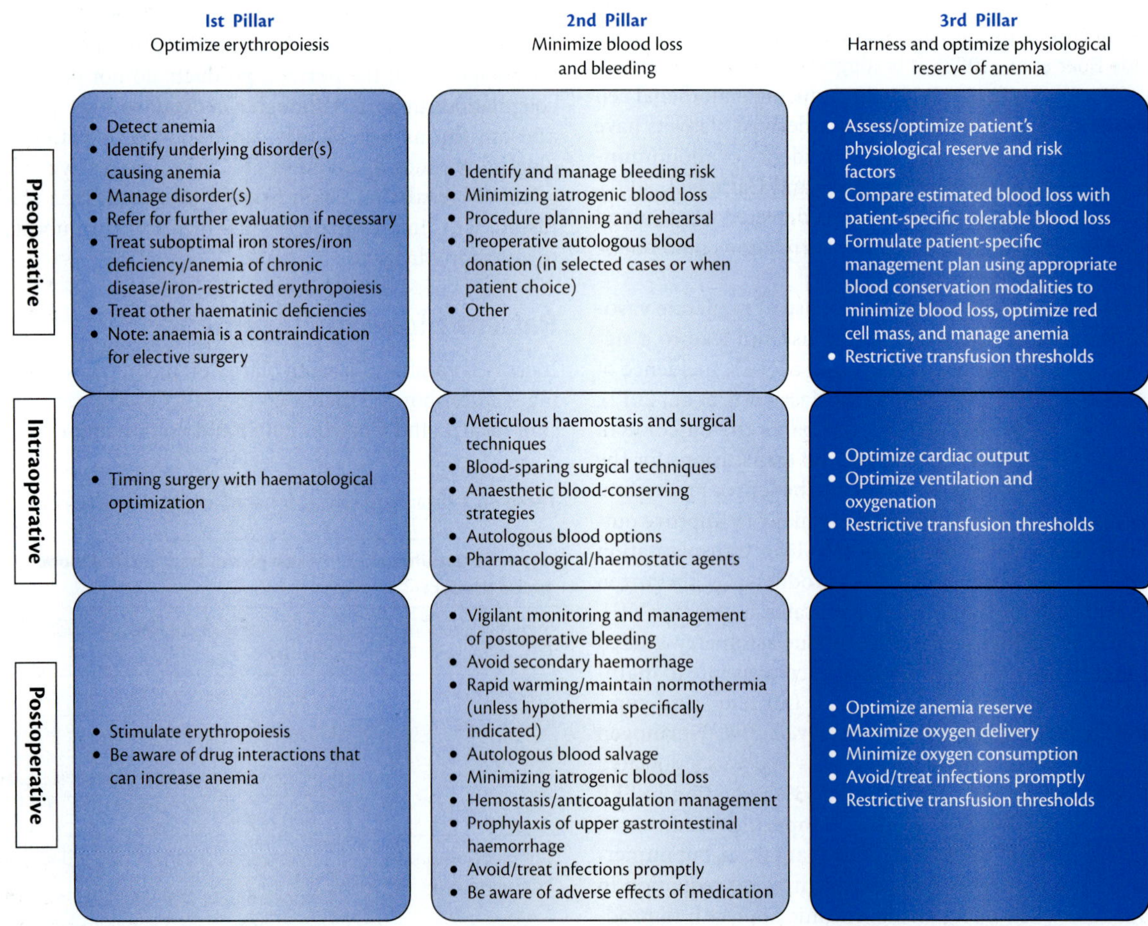


**Fig. 36.1** Patient blood management. (Republished with permission of AlphaMed Press, from *The Oncologist*, 'Five Drivers Shifting the Paradigm from Product-Focused Transfusion Practice to Patient Blood Management', Hoffman et al., 16, pp. 3–11, 2011; permission conveyed through Copyright Clearance Center, Inc.)

study targeted patients' post-transfusion haemoglobin levels to the 80–90 g/L range (Hébert et al., 1999), with little evidence available to contradict that position.

## Complications of transfusion

### Transfusion-related acute lung injury

TRALI—non-cardiogenic pulmonary oedema with an onset within 6 hours of transfusion—is one of the leading causes of death from transfusion, with a mortality rate in the range of 5–25% (Silliman et al., 2005). The commonest cause of this syndrome is infusion of donor-derived HLA antibodies directed coincidentally at the recipient's cognate HLA antigens. However, it is believed that the infusion of biologically active lipids, such as in the supernatant of older platelet components, may also be capable of triggering TRALI. Unusually, it is possible for donor-derived antigens in non-leucodepleted blood to be the cause of TRALI in an HLA-sensitized recipient. TRALI is frequently unrecognized and under-reported, with one prospective study in cardiac surgery finding possible TRALI in 16 of 668 patients and only one of the 16 reported to the blood bank (Vlaar et al., 2011). In unilateral lung transplantation TRALI may affect only the transplanted lung (Stoclin et al., 2013). Treatment for TRALI remains supportive.

Internationally, various countries have been putting measures in place to reduce the risk of TRALI (Wendel et al., 2007). These range from male-only plasma donations to reduce the risk of pregnancy-acquired HLA antibodies, to screening donors for HLA antibodies or pooling plasma to dilute specific antibodies. All of these measures appear to be successful in achieving their goal, with different impacts on the costs and logistics of the blood supply.

### Transfusion-associated circulatory overload

Transfusion-associated circulatory overload (TACO) is characterized by any four of the following: acute respiratory distress, tachycardia, increased blood pressure, acute or worsening pulmonary oedema on frontal chest radiograph, and evidence of positive fluid balance, occurring within 6 hours of completion of transfusion. Finding a raised brain natriuretic peptide (BNP) adds further support for a diagnosis of TACO (ISBT, 2011). Although often considered as an unfortunate consequence, TACO has an appreciable morbidity and mortality. Of 163 reports received by the UK Serious Hazards of Transfusion programme, 70 either died or suffered major morbidity due to or contributed by transfusion (Bolton-Maggs and Cohen, 2012). Management is diuresis and supportive care, but prevention is a better approach. The elderly and the very young are at increased risk of TACO, particularly those with comorbidities such as cardiac failure, renal impairment, hypoalbuminaemia, and fluid overload. Patients at risk should be identified before commencing the transfusion and appropriate measures taken, such as diuresis and slow transfusion, to prevent TACO. Transfusions in non-emergent situations should take place during the day and with close monitoring.

### Infectious risks

Although the risk of a transfusion-transmitted viral infection, especially HIV, remains one of recipients' biggest concerns (AuBuchon, 2004), the reality is that for most countries where solid organ transplantation is being conducted the risks of a transfusion-acquired HIV, hepatitis B, or hepatitis C infection are less than one in a million transfusions (Seed et al., 2005; Al Shaer et al., 2012; Bolton-Maggs and Cohen, 2012; S.F. O'Brien et al., 2012). Risks of other infections such as West Nile virus, malaria, *Babesia*, dengue, and variant CJD are more geographically localized but also remain rare events in the developed world. Steps to reduce infectious risk include careful donor screening, infectious testing including nucleic acid testing, and, in some countries, pathogen inactivation using a variety of means to disrupt viral, bacterial, and parasitic nucleic acids.

Bacterial risk from platelet transfusions is higher than viral risk, due to the storage of platelets at room temperature for up to 5–7 days, with bacteria found in 0.03–0.12% of platelet units (Larsen et al., 2005). The bacteria are typically skin commensals; however, in one study, 17% were Gram-negative organisms (Fang et al., 2005). Because the majority of organisms are relatively benign, septicaemia due to platelet transfusion is rare. Nevertheless, this is an area where many blood services are now aiming to further reduce risk. Bacterial contamination of red cell units is also rare: 1 in $10^5$–$10^7$ red cell units transfused. When it occurs, septicaemia and fatality in the recipient is most commonly due to *Yersinia enterocolitica* because of its ability to reproduce at red cells' storage temperature of 2–8°C (Guinet et al., 2011).

### Transfusion-related immunomodulation

As far back as 1973, TRIM was recognized with reduction of renal graft rejection following transfusion (Opelz et al., 1973). Much work has been done in this field, looking particularly at risks of postoperative infection, cancer growth and recurrence in non-leucodepleted transfusions. Unfortunately, despite over 150 clinical studies, a definite conclusion has yet to be drawn (Vamvakas and Blajchman, 2001). Nevertheless, it remains plausible that the effect does exist and it seems likely to be either HLA-mediated and/or via apoptotic cells affecting the innate immune system (Dzik, 2003). Leucodepletion may ameliorate at least some of the TRIM effect, as shown in reduced postoperative infections following leucodepletion (Blumberg et al., 2007) and in poorer outcomes for renal transplants (F.J. O'Brien et al., 2012).

### Haemolytic transfusion reactions

Haemolysis may be due to passenger lymphocyte syndrome (as described in the section 'ABO compatibility for ABO-incompatible transplants'. This may be seen in 9%, 29% and 70% of kidney, liver, and heart–lung minor incompatible transplants, respectively (Ramsey, 1991). Haemolytic reactions, acute and delayed, due to pregnancy and transfusion-induced antibodies are rare and ABO haemolytic transfusion reactions, typically as a result of error, are rarer still.

### Microchimerism

Detection of donor-derived leucocytes persisting in recipients' circulation was first reported in 1995 (Lee et al., 1995). Although much remains unanswered, of the factors established, the condition of the recipient and the viability of the leucocytes appear to be most prominent. Trauma seems to be an important predisposing factor to microchimerism, with leucocytes persisting for decades afterwards, presumably having engrafted in the recipient (Utter et al., 2008). Leucodepletion does not appear to reduce the likelihood of microchimerism. Initial concerns that microchimerism could lead on to a form of chronic GVHD do not appear to be supported in practice (Utter et al., 2006).

## Conclusion

Transfusion has been described as a minitransplant of viable cells into the recipient. As with solid organ transplantation, careful selection of the recipient as well as of the components is needed for an optimal outcome. Although safer than organ transplantation, transfusion is nevertheless associated with a variety of complications. Awareness of these is important for prompt recognition and management.

## References


Al Shaer L, Abdul Rahman M, John TJ, et al. (2012) Trends in prevalence, incidence, and residual risk of major transfusion-transmissible viral infections in United Arab Emirates blood donors: impact of individual-donation nucleic acid testing, 2004 through 2009. *Transfusion*, **52**(11):2300–2309.

American Association of Blood Banks (2014) *Standards for Blood Banks and Transfusion Services*, 29th edn. AABB, Bethesda, Maryland.

Ata P, Cetinkaya F, Ozgezer T, et al. (2012) Flow cytometric detection of anti-AB antibody titers in blood group O recipients of blood group A2 donor kidneys. *Transplant Proc*, **44**(6):1706–9.

AuBuchon JP (2004) Managing change to improve transfusion safety. *Transfusion*, **44**(Sept):1377–1383.

Balasubramaniam GS, Morris M, Gupta A, et al. (2012) Allosensitization rate of male patients awaiting first kidney grafts after leuko-depleted blood transfusion. *Transplantation*, **93**(4):418–422.

Bauer K (2012) Reversal of antithrombotic agents. *Am J Hematol*, **87**(Suppl 1— February):S119–S126.

Beattie WS, Karkouti K, Wijeysundera DN, et al. (2009) Risk associated with preoperative anemia in noncardiac surgery: a single-center cohort study. *Anesthesiology*, **110**(3):574–581.

Bilgin YM, van de Watering LMG, Brand A (2011) Clinical effects of leucoreduction of blood transfusions. *Neth J Med*, **69**, 441–450.

Blumberg N, Zhao H, Wang H, et al. (2007) The intention-to-treat principle in clinical trials and meta-analyses of leukoreduced blood transfusions in surgical patients. *Transfusion*, **47**(4):573–581.

Bolton-Maggs P, Cohen H (2012) *The 2011 Annual SHOT Report, Serious Hazards of Transfusion (SHOT) Steering Group*. SHOT, Manchester.

Borgman MA, Spinella PC, Perkins JG, et al. (2007) The ratio of blood products transfused affects mortality in patients receiving massive transfusions at a combat support hospital. *J Trauma*, **63**(4):805–813.

Boulton FE, James V (2007) Guidelines for policies on alternatives to allogeneic blood transfusion. 1. Predeposit autologous blood donation and transfusion. *Transfus Med*, **17**(5):354–365.

Bowden RA, Slichter SJ, Sayers M, et al. (1995) A comparison of filtered leukocyte-reduced and cytomegalovirus (CMV) seronegative blood products for the prevention of transfusion- associated CMV infection after marrow transplant. *Blood*, **86**:3598–3603.

Brown CJ, Navarrete CV (2011) Clinical relevance of the HLA system in blood transfusion. *Vox Sang*, **101**(2):93–105.

Caldwell SH, Hoffman M, Lisman T, et al. (2006) Coagulation disorders and hemostasis in liver disease: pathophysiology and critical assessment of current management. *Hepatology*, **44**(4):1039–1046.

Carson JL, Grossman BJ, Kleinman S, et al. (2012a) Red blood cell transfusion: a clinical practice guideline from the AABB. *Annal Intern Med*, **157**:49–58.

Carson JL, Carless PA, Hebert PC (2012b) Transfusion thresholds and other strategies for guiding allogeneic red blood cell transfusion. *Cochrane Database Syst Rev*, **4**(5):CD002042.

Crough T, Khanna R (2009) Immunobiology of human cytomegalovirus: from bench to bedside. *Clin Microbiol Rev*, **22**(1):76–98.

Da Ponte A, Bidoli E, Talamini R, et al. (2005) Pre-storage leucocyte depletion and transfusion reaction rates in cancer patients. *Transfus Med*, **15**:37–43.

De Biasi AR, Stansbury LG, Dutton RP, et al. (2011) Blood product use in trauma resuscitation: plasma deficit versus plasma ratio as predictors of mortality in trauma. *Transfusion*, **51**(Sept):1925–1932.

De Boer MT, Christensen MC, Asmussen M, et al. (2008) The impact of intraoperative transfusion of platelets and red blood cells on survival after liver transplantation. *Anesth Analg*, **106**(1):32–44.

Drew W, Roback J (2007) Prevention of transfusion-transmitted cytomegalovirus: reactivation of the debate? *Transfusion*, **47**:1955–1958.

Dunning J, Versteegh M, Fabbri A, et al. (2008) Guideline on anti-platelet and anticoagulation management in cardiac surgery. *Eur J Cardio-Thoracic Surg*, **34**(1):73–92.

DuPont J, Messiant F, Declerck N (1996) Liver transplantation without the use of fresh frozen plasma. *Anesth Analg*, **83**:681.

Dzik WH (2003) Apoptosis, TGF beta and transfusion-related immunosuppression: biologic versus clinical effects. *Transfus Apheresis Sci*, **29**(2):127–129.

Dzik WH, Blajchman MA, Fergusson D, et al. (2011) Clinical review: Canadian National Advisory Committee on Blood and Blood Products—massive transfusion consensus conference 2011: report of the panel. *Crit Care*, **15**(6):242.

Fang CT, Chambers LA, Kennedy J, et al. (2005) Detection of bacterial contamination in apheresis platelet products: American Red Cross experience, 2004. *Transfusion*, **45**(12):1845–1852.

Fast LD (2012) Developments in the prevention of transfusion-associated graft-versus-host disease. *Br J Haematol*, **158**(5):563–568.

Flegel W (2012) Fresh blood for transfusion: how old is too old for red blood cell units? *Blood Transfus*, **10**(3):247–251.

Guinet F, Carniel E, Leclercq A (2011) Transfusion-transmitted *Yersinia enterocolitica* sepsis. *Clin Infect Dis*, **53**(6):583–591.

Hartman SK, Teruya J (2012) Practice guidelines for reversal of new and old anticoagulants. *Disease-a-Month*, **58**(8):448–461.

Hébert PC, Wells G, Blajchman MA, et al. (1999) A multicenter, randomized, controlled clinical trial of transfusion requirements in critical care. Transfusion Requirements in Critical Care Investigators, Canadian Critical Care Trials Group. *N Engl J Med*, **340**(6):409–417.

Hofmann A, Farmer S, Shander A (2011) Five drivers shifting the paradigm from product-focused transfusion practice to patient blood management. *Oncologist*, **16**(Suppl 3):3–11.

Hur M, Moon HW, Kwon SW (2011) ABO-incompatible kidney transplantation. In: Ortiz J, Andre J (eds) *Understanding the Complexities of Kidney Transplantation*, pp. 332–348. InTech, Rijeka.

ISBT (2011) *ISBT Working Party on Haemovigilance*. International Haemovigilance Network, Manchester.

Jain MD, Cabrerizo-Sanchez R, Karkouti K, et al. (2013) Seek and you shall find-but then what do you do? cold agglutinins in cardiopulmonary bypass and a single-center experience with cold agglutinin screening before cardiac surgery. *Transfus Med Rev*, **27**(2):65–73.

Kaatz S, Kouides PA, Garcia DA, et al. (2012) Guidance on the emergent reversal of oral thrombin and factor Xa inhibitors. *Am J Hematol*, **87**(Suppl 1):S141–S145.

King KE, Ness PM (2011) How do we prevent transfusion-associated graft-versus-host disease in children? *Transfusion*, **51**(5):916–920.

Kotton CN, Kumar D, Caliendo, AM, et al. (2010). International consensus guidelines on the management of cytomegalovirus in solid organ transplantation. *Transplantation*, **89**(4), 779–795.

Kruger PC, Le Viellez AS, Herrmann RP (2012) Prothrombinex-VF use in warfarin reversal and other indications. *Med J Aus*, **196**(7):462–465.

Larsen CP, Ezligini F, Hermansen NO, et al. (2005) Six years' experience of using the BacT/ALERT system to screen all platelet concentrates, and additional testing of outdated platelet concentrates to estimate the frequency of false-negative results. *Vox Sang*, **88**(2):93–97.

Laupacis A, Brown J, Costello B, et al. (2001) Prevention of posttransfusion CMV in the era of universal WBC reduction: a consensus statement. *Transfusion*, **41**(April):560–569.

Lee TH, Donegan E, Slichter S, et al. (1995) Transient increase in circulating donor leukocytes after allogeneic transfusions in immunocompetent recipients compatible with donor cell proliferation. *Blood*, **85**(5):1207–1214.

Lelubre, C, Vincent, J-L (2013) Relationship between red cell storage duration and outcomes in adults receiving red cell transfusions: a systematic review. *Critical Care*, **17**(2):R66.

Lippi G, Franchini M, Favaloro EJ (2010) Thrombotic complications of erythropoiesis-stimulating agents. *Semin Thrombosis Hemostasis*, **36**(5):537–549.

Luddington RJ (2005) Thrombelastography/thromboelastometry. *Clin Lab Haematol*, **27**(2):81–90.

Marik PE, Corwin HL (2008) Efficacy of red blood cell transfusion in the critically ill: a systematic review of the literature. *Crit Care Med*, **36**(9):2667–2674.

Massicotte L, Lenis S, Thibeault L, et al. (2005) Reduction in blood transfusions during liver transplantation. *Can J Anaesth*, **52**:545–546.

Massicotte L, Denault AY, Beaulieu D, et al. (2012) Transfusion rate for 500 consecutive liver transplantations: experience of one liver transplantation center. *Transplantation*, **93**(12):1276–1281.

Middelburg RA, van de Watering LMG, van der Bom JG (2010) Blood transfusions: good or bad? Confounding by indication, an underestimated problem in clinical transfusion research. *Transfusion*, **50**:1181–1183.

Mushkbar M, Watkins E, Doughty H (2013) A UK single-centre survey of red cell antibodies in adult patients undergoing liver transplantation. *Vox Sang*, **105**(4):341–345.

Ness PM, Campbell SA (2001) Single donor versus pooled donor platelet concentrates. *Curr Opin Hematol*, **8**(6):392–396.

Nixon C, Gunn K, Main T, et al. (2009) Platelets and survival after liver transplantation. *Anesth Analg*, **108**:1354–1355.

Noval-Padillo JA, León-Justel A, Mellado-Miras P, et al. (2010) Introduction of fibrinogen in the treatment of hemostatic disorders during orthotopic liver transplantation: implications in the use of allogenic blood. *Transplant Proc*, **42**(8):2973–2974.

O'Brien FJ, Lineen J, Kennedy CM, et al. (2012) Effect of perioperative blood transfusions on long term graft outcomes in renal transplant patients. *Clin Nephrol*, *77*:432–437.

O'Brien KL, Pereira SE, Wagner J, et al. (2013) Transfusion-associated graft-versus-host disease in a liver transplant recipient: an unusual presentation and review of the literature. *Transfusion*, **53**(1):174–180.

O'Brien SF, Yi Q-L, Fan W, et al. (2012) Current incidence and residual risk of HIV, HBV and HCV at Canadian Blood Services. *Vox Sang*, **103**(1):83–86.

Olujohungbe A, Hambleton I, Stephens L, et al. (2001) Red cell antibodies in patients with homozygous sickle cell disease: a comparison of patients in Jamaica and the United Kingdom. *Br J Haematol*, **113**(3):661–665.

Opelz G, Sengar D, Mickey M, et al. (1973) Effect of blood transfusions on subsequent kidney transplants. *Transplant Proc*, **5**(1):253–259.

Opelz G, Graver B, Mickey MR, et al. (1981) Lymphocytotoxic antibody responses to transfusions in potential kidney transplant recipients. *Transplantation*, **32**(3):177–183.

Ramos E, Dalmau A, Sabate A, et al. (2003) Intraoperative red blood cell transfusion in liver transplantation: influence on patient outcome, prediction of requirements, and measures to reduce them. *Liver Transplant*, **9**(12):1320–1327.

Ramsey G (1991) Red cell antibodies arising from solid organ transplants. *Transfusion*, **31**(1):76–86.

Ramsey G, Cornell FW, Hahn LF, et al. (1989) Incompatible blood transfusions in liver transplant patients with significant red cell alloantibodies. *Transplant Proc*, **21**(3):3531.

Riskin DJ, Tsai TC, Riskin L, et al. (2009) Massive transfusion protocols: the role of aggressive resuscitation versus product ratio in mortality reduction. *J Am Coll Surg*, **209**(2):198–205.

SaBTO (2012) *Report of the Cytomegalovirus Steering Group*. <https://www.gov.uk/government/publications/sabto-report-of-the-cytomegalovirus-steering-group>.

Scornik, JC, Bromberg JS, Norman DJ, et al. (2013) An update on the impact of pre-transplant transfusions and allosensitization on time to renal transplant and on allograft survival. *BMC Nephrol*, **14**:217.

Scornik JC, Meier-Kriesche H-U (2011) Blood transfusions in organ transplant patients: mechanisms of sensitization and implications for prevention. *Am J Transplant*, **11**(9):1785–1791.

Seed CR, Kiely P, Keller AJ (2005) Residual risk of transfusion transmitted human immunodeficiency virus, hepatitis B virus, hepatitis C virus and human T lymphotrophic virus. *Intern Med J*, **35**(10):592–598.

Shaz BH, Dente CJ, Nicholas J, et al. (2010) Increased number of coagulation products in relationship to red blood cell products transfused improves mortality in trauma patients. *Transfusion*, **50**(2):493–500.

Silliman CC, Ambruso DR, Boshkov LK (2005) Review article transfusion-related acute lung injury. *Injury*, **105**(6):2266–2273.

Sindram D, Porte RJ, Hoffman MR, et al. (2000) Platelets induce sinusoidal endothelial cell apoptosis upon reperfusion of cold ischaemic rat liver. *Gastroenterology*, **118**(1):183–191.

Slichter SJ, Davis K, Enright H, et al. (2005) Factors affecting post-transfusion platelet increments, platelet refractoriness, and platelet transfusion intervals in thrombocytopenic patients. *Blood*, **105**(10):4106–4114.

Smith, EP (2010) Hematologic disorders after solid organ transplantation. *Hematology Am Soc Hematol Educ Program*, **2010**:281–286.

Snyder CW, Weinberg JA, McGwin G Jr, et al. (2009) The relationship of blood product ratio to mortality: survival benefit or survival bias? *J Trauma*, **66**(2):358–362.

Spahn DR, Moch H, Hofmann A, et al. (2008) Patient blood management. The pragmatic solution for the problems with blood transfusions. *Anesthesiology*, **109**(6):951–953.

Staras SAS, Dollard SC, Radford KW, et al. (2006) Seroprevalence of cytomegalovirus infection in the United States, 1988–1994. *Clin Inf Dis*, **43**(9):1143–1151.

Stoclin A, Delbos F, Dauriat G, et al. (2013) Transfusion-related acute lung injury after intravenous immunoglobulin treatment in a lung transplant recipient. *Vox Sang*, **104**(2):175–178.

Takahashi K, Saito K (2013) ABO-incompatible kidney transplantation. *Transplant Rev*, **27**(1):1–8.

Thomas D, Wee M, Clyburn P, et al. (2010) Blood transfusion and the anaesthetist: management of massive haemorrhage. *Anaesthesia*, **65**(11):1153–1161.

Tobian AAR, Shirey RS, Montgomery RA, et al. (2008) The critical role of plasmapheresis in ABO-incompatible renal transplantation. *Transfusion*, **48**(11):2453–2460.

Treleaven J, Gennery A, Marsh J, et al. (2011) Guidelines on the use of irradiated blood components prepared by the British Committee for Standards in Haematology blood transfusion task force. *Br J Haematol*, **152**(1):35–51.

Triulzi DJ (2001) Transfusion support in solid-organ transplantation. *Transfus Med Update*, **4**:1–4.

Triulzi DJ, Nalesnik MA (2001) Microchimerism, GVHD, and tolerance in solid organ transplantation. *Transfusion*, **41**(March):419–426.

Utter GH, Nathens AB, Lee T-H, et al. (2006) Leukoreduction of blood transfusions does not diminish transfusion-associated microchimerism in trauma patients. *Transfusion*, **46**(11):1863–1869.

Utter GH, Lee T, Rivers RM, et al. (2008) Microchimerism decades after transfusion among combat-injured US veterans from the Vietnam, Korean, and World War II conflicts. *Transfusion*, **48**(8):1609–1615.

Vamvakas EC (2005) Is white blood cell reduction equivalent to antibody screening in preventing transmission of cytomegalovirus by transfusion? A review of the literature and meta-analysis. *Transfus Med Rev*, **19**(3):181–199.

Vamvakas EC (2010) Meta-analysis of clinical studies of the purported deleterious effects of 'old' (versus 'fresh') red blood cells: are we at equipoise? *Transfusion*, **50**(3):600–610.

Vamvakas EC, Blajchman MA (2001) Deleterious clinical effects of transfusion-associated immunomodulation: fact or fiction? *Blood*, **97**(5):1180–1195.

Van de Watering L (2004) What has universal leucodepletion given us: evidence from clinical trials? *Vox Sang*, **87**(Suppl 2):139–142.

Van de Watering L (2011a) Pitfalls in the current published observational literature on the effects of red blood cell storage. *Transfusion*, **51**(8):1847–1854.

Van de Watering L (2011b) Red cell storage and prognosis. *Vox Sang*, **100**(1):36–45.

Vlaar APJ, Hofstra JJ, Determann RM, et al. (2011) The incidence, risk factors, and outcome of transfusion-related acute lung injury in a cohort of cardiac surgery patients: a prospective nested case-control study. *Blood*, **117**(16):4218–4225.

Wang D, Sun J, Solomon SB, et al. (2012) Transfusion of older stored blood and risk of death: a meta-analysis. *Transfusion*, **52**(6):1184–1195.

Warkentin TE, Eikelboom JW (2012) Old blood bad? Either the biggest issue in transfusion medicine or a nonevent. *Transfusion*, **52**(6):1165–1167.

Wendel S, Biagini S, Trigo F, et al. (2007) Measures to prevent TRALI. *Vox Sang*, **92**(3):258–277.

Zalpuri S, Zwaginga JJ, le Cessie S, et al. (2012) Red-blood-cell alloimmunization and number of red-blood-cell transfusions. *Vox Sang*, **102**(2):144–149.

Ziemann M, Krueger S, Maier AB, et al. (2007) High prevalence of cytomegalovirus DNA in plasma samples of blood donors in connection with seroconversion. *Transfusion*, **47**(11):1972–1983.

# CHAPTER 37

# Coagulation and haemodynamic monitoring

Mark Hayman and Andrew Watts

## Coagulation monitoring

Whole-blood coagulation testing provides information about the overall coagulation status of patients in surgical and non-surgical settings. Standard laboratory tests of coagulation (including aPTT, PT, INR, platelet counts, and fibrinogen levels) were designed to evaluate specific anticoagulant treatments and not specifically to provide information about the risk of bleeding or to guide management with either anticipated or established patient bleeding. Indeed, these laboratory tests correlate poorly with bleeding risk and transfusion requirements and provide only delayed information due to a lengthy turnaround time (Cammerer et al., 2003; Hardy et al., 2004). This prompted interest in the development of more immediate and relevant measures of haemostasis that can be used to reliably guide clinical coagulation management. Point-of-care (POC) measures of global haemostasis, particularly viscoelastic haemostatic assays (VHAs) (including TEG and thromboelastometry (ROTEM)), provide rapid information on clot formation including rate of clot formation, clot strength, and clot stability. They have been used increasingly, supplemented by standard laboratory tests, to assist in the management of haemostasis in OLT. Together with advancements in surgical technique and anaesthetic management, they have changed the approach to perioperative haemostasis management in OLT.

### Evidence supporting VHA use in liver transplant surgery

VHAs have been used to guide transfusion and correction of coagulopathy in liver transplantation surgery for many years (Kang et al., 1985; Kang, 1995; Harding et al., 1997). In 1985 Kang first demonstrated that TEG-directed therapy reduced transfusion of red cells and FFP as compared to standard laboratory-guided coagulation monitoring. A greater understanding of the complex changes in coagulation in ESLD and during transplantation has evolved with time. POC testing and in particular TEG/ROTEM is now widely used as one component of a multifactorial approach to haemostasis management. This approach includes restrictive fluid therapy (or low CVP anaesthesia), antifibrinolytic drugs, and improvements in surgical techniques. The result is a dramatic reduction in blood product use during OLT. However, most randomized clinical trial (RCT) evidence that supports the utility of VHAs to reduce bleeding is in cardiac surgery (Ashfari, Cochrane Database, 2011). In OLT there are limited prospective RCT data to suggest that the use of TEG can reduce plasma replacement (Wang et al., 2010). Increased use of VHAs has coincided with a reduction in transfusion and, while much of the evidence is anecdotal, their use is now considered a standard of care in many centres. A systematic Cochrane analysis concluded there is evidence that VHAs reduce the combined use of FFP and platelets but no evidence of a reduction in individual factor use or a reduction in mortality (Wikkelsoe et al., 2011).

Standard VHAs have provided numerous insights into the complex and dynamic changes in coagulation during OLT surgery. More recently, specific assays to extend the standard VHA measurements, including platelet function tests, have become available to add to the current understanding. The principles of operation of each of these techniques, the advantages and limitations of each test, the use of these tests in OLT, and evidence that support their use will be discussed.

## The standard VHAs: TEG and ROTEM

### Principles

VHAs are in-vitro whole-blood measures of overall haemostasis. They display changes in viscoelasticity as thrombin generation leads to fibrin polymerization and clot formation followed by clot dissolution. The VHA reflects the combined effects of red and white cells, platelets, fibrinogen, and anti- and procoagulant proteins as components in the complex cellular and non-cellular process of clot formation and clot dissolution (fibrinolysis). They are dynamic tests that provide real-time qualitative information on the rate of clot formation, clot strength or firmness, and fibrinolysis. This is in contrast to the traditional measures of coagulation, PT, and aPTT, which assay only enzymatic components of the coagulation system in plasma and provide only static quantitative information.

The principle of operation of these tests is simple. TEG® was originally developed in 1948 in Germany by Hartert and was first used in liver transplant surgery in Pennsylvania in the US in the 1970s. In the original test, 3.6 mL of whole blood was added to a cup which was oscillated through $4^0$ 45'. Today, kaolin or celite is added as an activator to promote clot formation. A transducer pin is then submerged into a cup which is oscillated back and forth slowly over 10 s to mimic slow venous flow (Figure 37.1). As clot forms, the shear strain on the pin increases and the pin begins to move as it becomes coupled by fibrin strands to the oscillating cup. In TEG the shear strain is converted into an electrical signal via an electrical–mechanical transducer.

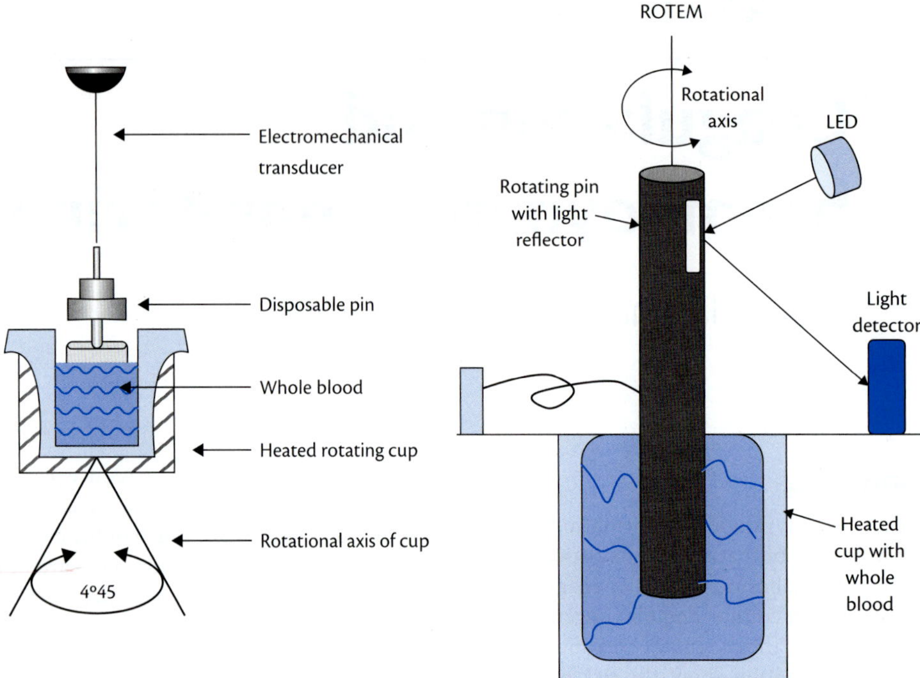


**Fig. 37.1** Principle of operation of TEG and ROTEM. Formation of fibrin strands in whole blood changes the shear elasticity, which is recorded by changes in rotation of the pin. (TEG® 5000 Hemostasis Analyzer Cup and Pin Image is used be permission of Haemonetics Corporation.)

This is displayed graphically as an evolving trace in real time on a computer display as a measure of clot strength (in shear elasticity units of dynes per second) over time (seconds) together with numerical results and normal ranges (Figure 37.2). New systems utilize digitized recordings of the changes in strain, employ single-use cups, and often include interpretive software that improves the ease of use and reproducibility of the tests.

The term thromboelastograph derives from the original systems that used a metal cup with a pin and a needle that burnt a trace directly onto thermosensitive paper. With repeated use these cups could develop scratches and dents that limited the accuracy and reproducibility of the assays. The traditional method of placing a torsion pin in an oscillating cup is also used in the ThromboElastoMeter-Automated (TEM-A) (Framar Hemologix, Rome, Italy). The ROTEM® (Tern International GmbH, Munich, Germany) uses a rotating pin in a fixed cup, but rather than a strain sensor it uses a light-emitting diode and an optical sensor to record the reflected light signal (Figure 37.1). Changes in this signal reflect changes in movement of the pin as clot forms. The evolving thromboelastometric trace displaying clot firmness against time is generated. The optical detection system within ROTEM is designed to make the system less prone to disruption by mechanical shocks. The

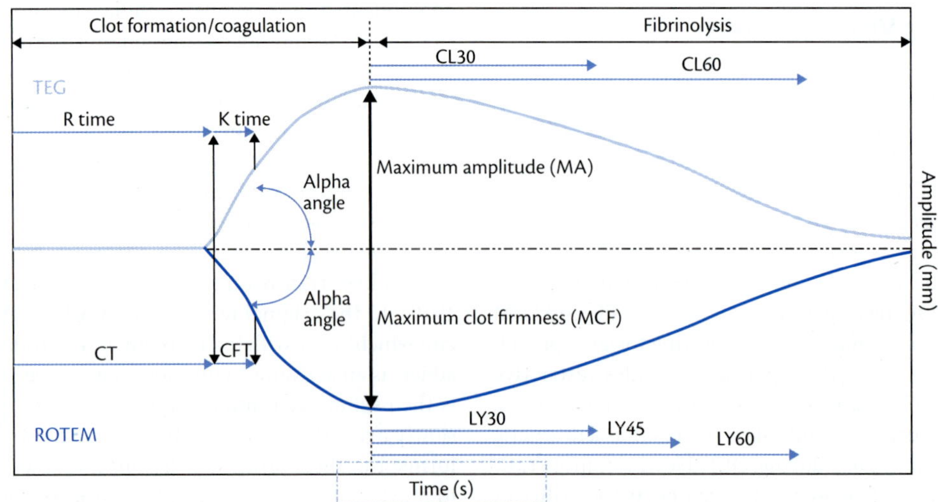


**Fig. 37.2** Typical TEG (top) and ROTEM (bottom) tracing. See Table 37.1 for details of the different reported parameters. (Reproduced with kind permission from Haemontics Corporation.)

conversion of the torsion into a digital signal or *metered* parameter has been used in the naming of the TEM-A and ROTEM systems, but the underlying principle of the test is the same in both thromboelastography and thromboelastometry systems.

TEG and ROTEM systems provide similar parameters of coagulation but are named differently by the respective companies (see Table 37.1). The results are not directly comparable partly due to the different activators used in the systems (the ROTEM system uses a proprietary INTEM activator solution which contains partial thromboplastin phospholipid). The tests provide information on the time to first clot formation (the reaction or 'r' time), rate of clot formation (alpha angle), the time to reach a certain clot strength (typically 20 mm, the 'kinetic' or 'K' time), the strength of clot formed or maximum amplitude (MA), and information about fibrinolysis as the test continues and lysis progresses. Representative normal and abnormal traces with interpretation are shown in Table 37.2.

## Extended viscoelastic haemostatic assays

In addition to the standard global assessment of haemostasis, a range of different specific assays can be used to delineate separate components of the coagulation system, enabling a more focused approach to replacement of blood factors or coagulation-modifying drugs (see Table 37.3). Both ROTEM and TEG systems allow for multiple tests to be run concurrently, facilitating a comparison between the different assays.

### Heparinase

Heparinase neutralizes exogenous and endogenous heparin and is useful particularly during the anhepatic and reperfusion phases of OLT.

### Fibrinolysis

Fibrinolysis is common in OLT. The potential response to antifibrinolytics is useful in OLT cases to guide antifibrinolytic therapy. ROTEM antifibrinolytic assay (APTEM) contains the antifibrinolytic plasmin inhibitor aprotinin. When combined with the EXTEM activator this assay gives information about the presence of mild fibrinolysis more rapidly than waiting for the tail of a normal TEG trace to evolve. This enables earlier use of specific antifibrinolytic drugs such as one of the lysine analogues (tranexamic acid or epsilon amino-caproic acid).

**Table 37.1** Standard TEG and ROTEM parameters

| Parameters | TEG | ROTEM |
|---|---|---|
| Reaction time (time from start to point when trace is 2 mm above baseline) | R time | Clot time (CT) |
| Rate of clot formation | Alpha angle | Alpha angle (angle of tangent at 2 mm amplitude) + maximum clot formation rate (CFR) |
| Time to form clot from 2–20 mm above baseline | K time | Clot formation time (CFT) |
| Clot strength | MA | Maximum clot firmness (MCF) + time to MCF |
| Amplitude (A) at set time (minutes) | A30, A60 | A5, A10,... |
| Clot lysis (CL/LY) at set times (minutes) | LY30, LY60 | LY30, LY45, LY60 |
| Time to lysis | Clot Lysis Time (CLT) from MA to 2mm | Clot lysis time (CLT) 10% reduction from MCF |

**Table 37.2** Normal and abnormal VHA traces. The normal trace is shown in light grey to highlight differences from normal of the various abnormal traces

| VHA trace | Key features | Graphical trace |
|---|---|---|
| Normal | Normal time to clot formation, rate of clot formation, maximum clot strength, minimal lysis 30min after MA. | 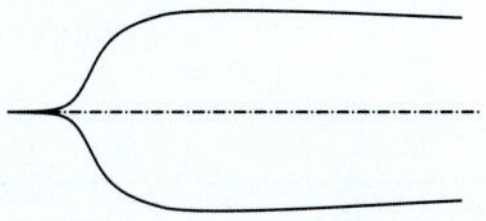 |
| Global hypocoagulable state | Prolonged R time, reduced rate of clot formation, reduced maximum clot strength | 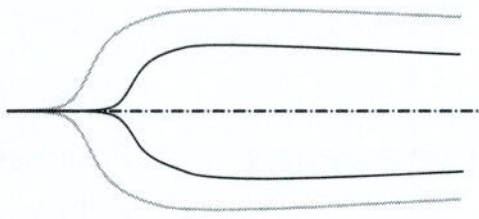 |
| Hypercoagulable state | Shortened R time, increased maximum amplitude | 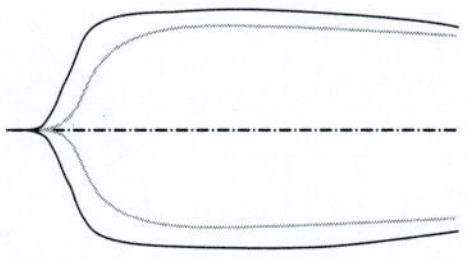 |
| Coagulation factor deficiency | Prolonged R time, reduced rate of clot formation, no change in maximum clot strength | 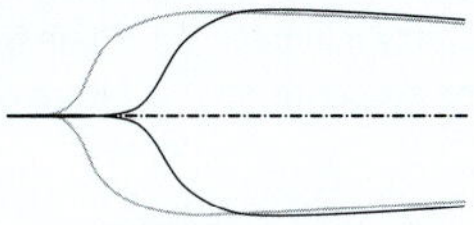 |
| Platelet or fibrinogen deficiency | Normal R time, reduced alpha angle, reduced maximum clot strength | 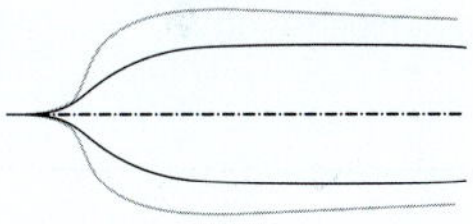 |
| Hyperfibrinolysis | Reduced clot lysis time with rapid tapering of trace from maximum amplitude and high LY30. | 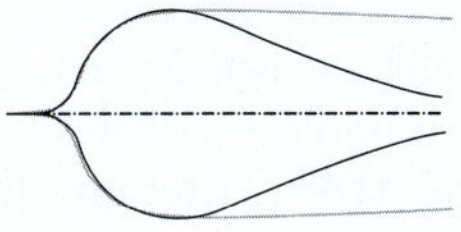 |

## Platelet function and fibrinogen contribution to clot

A major limitation of the standard TEG and ROTEM assays is the inability to reliably assess platelet function. In order to overcome this, the assessment of abnormal platelet function is provided using specific platelet activators, including ADP and arachidonic acid, to assess the inhibition of platelets by specific antiplatelet drugs. ROTEM FIBTEM assay provides inhibition of platelets, resulting in clot due to fibrin alone. The ROTEM EXTEM assay (tissue factor) can be combined with the FIBTEM assay to identify the contribution of platelets to clot formation by comparing the difference between these two assays. A low maximum clot firmness $(MCF)_{FIBTEM}$ suggests a deficiency of fibrinogen and a normal $MCF_{FIBTEM}$ in the presence of a low $MCF_{EXTEM}$ suggests a functional platelet deficiency. Thus comparison of the $MCF_{FIBTEM}$ and the $MCF_{EXTEM}$ allows for differentiation of a functional

**Table 37.3** Typical progression of a TEG/ROTEM trace during an OLT case

| Time in surgery | Key features of trace | Trace |
|---|---|---|
| Baseline | Combined factor and platelet deficiency | |
| Early anhepatic | Fibrinolysis developing | |
| Late anhepatic | Prolonged r time, reduced MA, lysis | |
| Early reperfusion | Flat-line trace with no clot formation | |
| Thirty minutes postreperfusion | Some spontaneous return of coagulation | |
| Ninety minutes postreperfusion | Return close to baseline | |

platelet deficiency and a fibrinogen deficiency. The TEG system also provides a PlateletMapping™ assay using arachidonic acid and ADP to determine the contribution of platelet dysfunction as a component of abnormal TEG traces.

Beyond TEG and ROTEM assays, a range of specialized POC platelet function analyzers have been developed. Interest has been generated by the need to assess response to and presence of antiplatelet drugs. As it is uncommon for patients presenting for OLT to be on antiplatelet medications these devices are not generally used in the OLT setting. Further, these monitors require the patients to have a constant haematocrit during testing. Their use has not been validated in the intraoperative setting (Table 37.4).

## Preanalytical and analytical considerations of use of VHAs

### Normal ranges

A feature of all the VHAs is that the normal ranges for the parameters measured are large. This may be a feature of any 'global' test of haemostasis (MacDonald and Luddington, 2010). The normal ranges differ for TEG and ROTEM systems, making comparative studies difficult. Further, activators used may differ and thus comparisons between systems and results may be meaningless. Consequently, VHAs provide a useful measure of change from a baseline reading in a particular individual over the course of an operation or clinical episode rather than being a reliable single-measure diagnostic tool. Indeed, that is how VHAs are used in OLT surgery where a baseline measurement is typically taken and then repeat measurements made intraoperatively, and

**Table 37.4** Extended VHAs and names used for each by TEG and ROTEM systems

| Assay | TEG | ROTEM |
|---|---|---|
| Global clot formation activator | Kaolin | INTEM (partial thromboplastin phospholipid) |
| Heparinase | Heparinase cuvettes can used with any activator | HEPTEM |
| Tissue factor activation | RapidTEG (also includes kaolin) | EXTEM |
| Platelet Function assay | PlateletMapping® ADP and AA assays | Comparison of difference between EXTEM and FIBTEM (this is not platelet function) |
| Antifibrinolytics assay | | APTEM (aprotinin added to assay) |
| Fibrin contribution to clot | Functional fibrinogen assay | FIBTEM |

sometimes beyond, into the postoperative period, to guide blood product, coagulation factor, and antifibrinolytic management.

Factors known to affect VHA traces include the haematocrit, heparin, pH, temperature, age, gender, and infection. These will be discussed as they relate to OLT (Table 37.3).

#### *Haematocrit*

Haematocrit affects clot strength and needs to be considered in the context of a VHA trace. For example, in the context of anaemia, ROTEM has been shown to display an inverse relationship between haematocrit and MCF without any change in thrombin generation (Spiezia et al., 2008). Typically an ABG analysis will be performed at the time of a VHA reading which will provide information on the haematocrit plus ionized calcium and extracellular pH, which all impact on coagulation. Interpretation of the VHA trace should be made in the context of these factors that may impact the trace as much as, if not more so, than any coagulation component deficiencies.

#### *Heparin effects*

Circulating heparin levels that will result in a flat TEG trace only slightly prolong the aPTT, highlighting the sensitivity of the TEG to heparin effects (MacDonald and Luddington, 2010). Fortunately heparin can be readily neutralized by the use of a heparinase assay. Endogenous circulating heparinoids (endogenous heparin-like glycosaminoglycans) are elevated in cirrhosis and liver failure and these also have a heparin effect on the TEG (Kettner et al., 1998). Heparin and heparinoid effects typically become substantial during the anhepatic phase, due to the absence of clearance, and upon reperfusion, due to release of heparin administered to the donor prior to liver harvesting. VHAs can thus help distinguish coagulopathy due to heparin from other factor deficiencies. Awareness of this heparin sensitivity is important when sampling from lines that may contain heparin. Typically, parallel heparinase and standard traces will be run on separate channels to allow quick identification of any heparin effects from baseline.

#### *pH and temperature considerations*

Hypothermia and acidosis impact the coagulation system and both can result in impaired VHA traces (MacDonald and

Luddington, 2010). Both TEG and ROTEM heat the blood sample to 37°C as a default to reflect normothermic conditions. Alternatively these systems can be set to heat the blood sample to match the current temperature of the patient. This produces a trace that reflects the haemostatic status of the patient but will not allow differentiation of temperature effects from any coagulation factor deficiency effects. Consequently it is recommended that these tests be conducted at normal body temperature unless the aim is to demonstrate the impact of hypothermia on coagulation.

#### *Sampling technique and time to test*

The process of blood aspiration can affect TEG results. This may relate to the shear forces during aspiration that can give erroneously shortened activation times and increased clot firmness (Frumento et al., 2002). Frumento demonstrated that samples from a CVC, associated with the highest shear forces, produced shorter R times and higher MAs than arterial or sheath introducer samples. Gentle aspiration of blood should be used to minimize activation of platelets and coagulation factors leading to erroneous VHA results (Chitlur and Lusher, 2010). The sample should be loaded into TEG/ROTEM immediately (< 6 minutes). Careful mixing of the activator with the blood sample in the TEG requires careful reaspiration using the pipette or by stirring, and in ROTEM this is achieved automatically using the electronic pipette. The same sampling site should be used throughout an OLT case to enable accurate comparisons between sequential traces. Whilst the use of fresh uncitrated blood is the preferred method of conducting a POC VHA test, if this is not available blood can be citrated, stored, and subsequently recalcified before analysis at least 1 hour and less than 8 hours later (Camenzind et al., 2000). Use of citrated blood yields a reduced clot onset time, a greater alpha angle, and a reduced maximum clot strength, indicating that citrate does not completely inhibit coagulation factor and platelet activation in stored blood.

#### *Infection*

Infection in cirrhotic patients has an effect on TEG due to a heparin effect. This has been demonstrated in cirrhotic patients in whom a heparin effect was seen only in the infected patients. The effect was reversed with resolution of infection (Papatheodoridis et al., 1999; Montalto et al., 2002).

#### *Age and gender*

Female gender and increasing age contribute to a more hypercoagulable baseline state. This is often not used when referring to normal ranges (MacDonald and Luddington, 2010). Age is weakly correlated with TEG variables (r time = 19.5 − 0.09 × age, maximum amplitude = 53.3 + 0.07 × age, alpha angle = 52.8 + 0.2 × age in years) (Ng, 2000).

#### *Intravenous fluid therapy*

Different intravenous fluids have been implicated in disturbances of the coagulation pathways, the most notable, historically, being high-molecular-weight starches. The newer medium-length starches, such as 6% HES, may also have a detrimental effect on coagulation in patients with ESLD. Dilution of blood with 6% HES results in a reduction in maximum amplitude and at higher levels of dilution all parameters of TEG are affected (Bang et al., 2011).

### Interpreting VHAs in the context of liver failure

The coagulation changes in acute and chronic liver failure patients presenting for liver transplant are complex. The typical haemostatic profile in chronic liver failure includes a reduction in coagulation factors and inhibitors, a decrease in fibrinolytic proteins, an increase in coagulation factors VIII and vWF, and a thrombocytopaenia possibly with platelet dysfunction (Lisman and Porte, 2010). It has long been observed that despite markedly prolonged INR measurements and thrombocytopaenia, chronic liver failure patients often do not present with spontaneous clinical bleeds. The bleeding related to portal hypertension may reflect venous pressure changes more than an underlying hypocoagulable state (Boks et al., 1986; Sharara and Rockey, 2001).

The concept of a fragile rebalanced haemostasis has been proposed, reflecting the fact that while procoagulant factors are diminished in liver failure, there is a concomitant reduction in anticoagulant factors that may *rebalance* the coagulation (Lisman and Porte, 2010). This rebalancing is, however, relatively unstable as both pro- and anticoagulant factors are reduced, thus diminishing the tolerance of the system to perturbations. This may explain the findings in a study of acute liver injury and ALF patients in whom, despite INRs of 3.4 ± 1.7, mean TEG parameters were normal (Stravitz et al., 2011). The mechanisms proposed in this study were an increase in clot strength with increasing severity of liver injury, increased factor VIII levels, and a matched decline in pro- and anticoagulant proteins. Anecdotally this not an uncommon observation and it highlights the utility and limitations of VHAs. This rebalancing may explain why patients with traditional measures of coagulation suggesting a hypocoagulable state are able to undergo OLT without the use of blood component replacement. It may also explain the occurrence of thrombotic complications including deep vein thrombosis, pulmonary embolus (PE), and portal vein thrombosis in patients with liver disease. To further illustrate this point, while an abnormal VHA trace may imply a coagulopathic state, it may also imply a hyperactivation of fibrinolysis activated by venous clot formation or a disseminated intravascular coagulation-like state. Indeed, in one series in which PE occurred in 4% of patients undergoing OLT, a flat-line TEG or TEG showing marked lysis was predictive of the development of a PE (Sakai et al., 2011).

## VHAs as part of a multifactorial approach to haemostasis

Whilst a baseline VHA may be relatively normal at the start of surgery, this can and often does change during the course of liver transplant surgery (Table 37.3). The changes in VHA, in conjunction with standard laboratory tests, clinical assessment of the type of bleeding, the fluid status of the patient, presence of hypothermia, the acid-base status, haematocrit, and ionized calcium levels, can provide valuable information to guide a more systematic approach to haemostasis management. This rational approach should utilize blood management protocols and algorithms, which have been shown to reduce blood product usage compared to clinical judgement (Kang et al., 1985; Avidan et al., 2004). These should ideally be developed and customized for each institution by a multidisciplinary team.

Presently there remains great variability between centres in the approach to haemostasis management and there are no universally agreed thresholds for transfusion of blood components in OLT (Dalmau et al., 2009). Future research may provide a guide to a more rational and evidence-based approach to the use of these assays to help minimize blood loss and exposure to homologous blood products. Comparison of standardized transfusion algorithms comparing ROTEM, TEG, and traditional coagulation tests in a prospective study would provide some valuable guidance towards this goal (Coakley et al., 2006) .

### Point-of-care prothombin time tests

New portable POC PT and INR measurement devices have recently become available, providing more rapid results than traditional laboratory-based methods. They can utilize capillary blood samples or blood sampled from indwelling vascular lines. They have been shown to correlate well in outpatient settings with standard laboratory-based measurements of PT (Colella et al., 2012; Peña et al., 2012). Systems currently available include the i-STAT (Abbott Point-of-Care, Princeton, New Jersey, US), Coagucheck (Roche, US), and the Hemochron® Whole Blood Coagulation System (ITC, New Jersey, US). Whilst their use in OLT is not yet reported, it seems likely that these will become incorporated into the POC assessment of haemostasis in the future.

### Further resources

An e-learning resource with access to recent lectures relating to perioperative coagulation management is provided at <www.perioperativebleeding.org>. The manufacturers of TEG and ROTEM systems provide information and applications to assist learning about their respective systems.

## Haemodynamic monitoring

The pathophysiology of liver failure is characterized by multiple haemodynamic changes that necessitate invasive real-time haemodynamic monitoring to guide anaesthetic management during OLT. Patients with ESLD may present with variable degrees of cardiac dysfunction, a reduction in SVR, and possibly PHT. A hyperdynamic circulation, characterized by a low SVR and a high or high–normal CO, is common. Liver reperfusion may be associated with marked haemodynamic changes, and detailed beat-to-beat haemodynamic monitoring is especially useful at this time to guide appropriate interventional therapy.

Routine haemodynamic monitoring in liver transplant surgery includes invasive arterial pressure, CVP, and often right heart and PAP monitoring. CO monitoring using intermittent thermodilution or continuous cardiac output (CCO) measurement is often employed, together with TOE assessment. Peripheral arterial waveform analysis, aortic pulse contour analysis, echocardiography, and oesophageal Doppler have all been used in the interest of providing more accurate and less invasive haemodynamic monitoring.

While invasive haemodynamic monitoring is used universally in liver transplant surgery to guide therapy, no correlation between haemodynamic variability and patient or graft survival has yet been demonstrated (Milan et al., 2011).This section outlines the particular features of the common and more recent monitoring techniques and highlights the relative advantages and disadvantages of each. Table 37.5 provides a summary of the different modalities employed.

**Table 37.5** Range of haemodynamic variables used in OLT

| Parameter | Common use in OLT | Limitations and risks |
|---|---|---|
| Arterial pressures | Beat-to-beat arterial pressure monitoring to guide vasoactive therapy | Radial pressure may underestimate central aortic pressures in vasodilatory states especially during reperfusion |
| Central venous pressures | Low CVP commonly used to limit blood loss during dissection and anhepatic phase | Little correlation between circulating blood volume and CVP |
| Pulmonary artery pressures | Used to confirm presence of PHT and response to vasodilator therapy | Risk of pulmonary artery rupture with distal balloon occlusion |
| Intermittent thermodilution cardiac output | Gold standard for intermittent CO measurement | Slow, requires repeat measurements, dependent on operator technique |
| Continuous cardiac output | Automated rolling average of CO measurements using heating filament and thermodilution technique | Similar to ITCO, less operator dependent |
| Central and mixed venous saturation | Measure of global venous oxygen saturation, used as a surrogate measure of total body oxygen supply | Mixed venous saturation often elevated in ESLD, target or normal range in OLT unknown, confounded during manipulation of liver, IVC clamping and release and during reperfusion of transplanted liver |
| Peripheral waveform analysis | Minimally invasive measure of CO and LV contractility | Not validated in OLT as an adequately accurate alternative to ITCO |
| Oesophageal Doppler | Non-invasive Doppler measure of CO | Requires accurate placement and prone to error with displacement. |
| Blood and fluid volumes | Echocardiography provides most immediate measure of cardiac volume status, thoracic and global end-diastolic volumes derived from aortic pulse contour analysis | Echocardiography provides most robust and reliable measures of cardiac volumes, pulse contour-derived measures have not been compared to echo-derived measurements in OLT |

### Arterial lines

Invasive arterial pressure monitoring is a standard monitor in OLT, and many centres place two lines to enable frequent arterial blood sampling and to provide redundancy in the event of a failure of one of the catheters. The technique and risks of this monitoring technique are well known and comprehensively described elsewhere. There are a few particular considerations in this patient population that need to be considered. There may be a clinically significant difference between femoral and radial systolic pressure readings (92 vs 76 mmHg during reperfusion, for example) but not between mean pressures (Arnal et al., 2005). This was most marked during reperfusion and is accentuated by the use of vasoconstrictor therapy. Attention to MAP rather than systolic readings is thus advocated, particularly during reperfusion, to guide fluid and vasopressor therapy, especially when using radial arterial catheters. Systolic pressure variation and pulse pressure variation, measures of the change in arterial systolic pressure between inspiration and expiration during controlled ventilation, are more reliable measures of fluid responsiveness than CVP (Marik et al., 2009) and thus may provide a more useful measure of volume status than CVP (Schroeder and Kuo, 2008).

## Central venous catheters

CVCs are routinely used in OLT to provide CVP and $ScvO_2$ measurements, in addition to providing vascular access for vasoactive drug administration.

### Central venous pressure

There is good evidence that low CVP anaesthesia reduces blood loss during liver resection (Jones et al., 1998; Chen et al., 2000; Wang et al., 2006). This strategy has been extended to OLT. The limited evidence in this context does suggest a reduction in blood loss (Schroeder et al., 2004; Massicotte et al., 2006; Feng et al., 2010) and may be mechanistically explained by a reduction in portal venous pressures with low CVP (Massicotte et al., 2010). Despite the relative paucity of high-quality evidence, this strategy is commonly utilized during the dissection phase of OLT. Massicotte demonstrated reduced blood transfusion requirements with low CVP targets and phlebotomy (Massicotte et al., 2006). More recently, a CVP of either < 5 mmHg or < 40% of baseline CVP was associated with a reduction in blood loss and transfusion volume without compromising renal function (Feng et al., 2010). It may be that avoiding an acutely elevated CVP, which was typical with pre-emptive fluid and coagulation factor loading in the past, is more important than a 'low' CVP target. CVP is an unreliable indicator of circulating blood volume and right heart filling and changes do not correlate well with cardiac filling or CO in OLT (Gelman, 2008; Massicotte et al., 2010). Consequently CVP, both absolute values and trends, whilst still commonly used to guide filling status, should be used cautiously, if at all. Alternative measures of volume status such as fluid responsiveness (a change in stroke volume in response to fluid loading) and echocardiographic measures of end-diastolic volumes should be considered.

### Central venous oxygen saturation

$ScvO_2$ is measured by intermittent blood sampling from the distal lumen of a CVC or monitored continuously using a CVC with an oximeter incorporated into the catheter (an example of such a catheter is the Edwards Presep CVC). $SvO_2$ and $ScvO_2$ have both been investigated as markers of the global balance between oxygen supply and demand. Interest in $SvO_2$ and $ScvO_2$ is long-standing and has been most extensively investigated in goal-directed therapy in the treatment of sepsis (Rivers et al., 2001). Central venous saturation measured in the right atrium using a CVC has been proposed as a surrogate measure for $SvO_2$. There is evidence in high-risk general surgery that an $ScvO_2$ < 72% is associated with increased postoperative complications (Collaborative Study Group on Perioperative $ScvO_2$ Monitoring, 2006). $ScvO_2$ has been studied in OLT and has been shown to correlate well with $SvO_2$ in the pre-anhepatic phase of surgery but does not correlate with $SvO_2$ or CO in the reperfusion phase. This possibly reflects inadequate mixing of blood returning from the splanchnic circulation and thus limits its value in liver transplantation (el-Masry et al., 2009; Dahmani et al., 2010).

### Complications of central venous catheters

Infection, vascular injury, and thrombosis are all well-recognized complications of CVCs. Diligent aseptic technique during insertion and management of central lines is especially important in these immunocompromised patients. Use of the subclavian vein is generally avoided because of coagulopathy and the risk of pneumothorax at the time of surgery.

## Pulmonary artery catheters

The PAC remains the gold standard for the measurement of CO and the measurement of PAP. Intermittent and/or continuous CO monitoring can be used. PACs can also be used for mixed venous saturation measurements (intermittent or continuous).

### Thermodilution cardiac output using pulmonary artery catheters

CO can change many-fold during the course of OLT. The traditional method of intermittent thermodilution cardiac output (ITCO) measurements requires a sequence of measurements, typically three or four, which can be averaged to provide a more accurate estimate of CO. This is time-consuming and limits its utility during episodes of marked change in CO such as liver manipulation, vascular clamping, and liver reperfusion. Continuous CO thermodilution catheters overcome some of these limitations and provide a regularly updated rolling trend of CO by incorporating a small filament that is heated rapidly and repeatedly and the temperature recorded at the distal thermistor. This system averages readings taken over several minutes, depending on the stability of the circulation, and does not provide instantaneous measurements.

### Limitations of cardiac output in OLT

During reperfusion of the liver and the variable washout temperature of the transplant effluent, thermodilution techniques of CO measurement, both intermittent and continuous, can be unreliable (Nissen et al., 2009b). Further, they do not provide beat-to-beat measurement of CO during periods of rapid changes in CO. For this reason other methods of CO measurement have been explored, including peripheral waveform analysis, echocardiography, and Doppler methods.

### Pulmonary artery pressures and role in portopulmonary hypertension

PPHTN is defined as PAH associated with portal hypertension with or without advanced hepatic disease. PACs remain the gold standard method for the diagnosis and quantification of this condition and can provide information about response to vasodilator therapy in these patients. TOE is useful in screening these patients and can also provide information on the degree of compensation of the RV and complements the data provided by the PAC. Occurring in 4–6% of patients undergoing liver transplant (Giusca et al., 2011), this alone justifies the use of pulmonary catheters in those patients with a confirmed or suspected diagnosis of PHT.

### Mixed venous oxygen saturation

$SvO_2$ provides information on the balance between oxygen consumption and delivery (CO and haematocrit). It is typically measured in the RV outflow tract or proximal PA using a PAC. Continuous measurement of $SvO_2$ is enabled with the newer PAC systems (such as the Edwards Vigilance II system). The threshold $SvO_2$ that should be targeted in OLT to ensure adequate oxygen delivery in ESLD is unknown. $SvO_2$ is typically elevated in ESLD but there is a redistribution of blood flow to different vascular beds, and hence an elevated $SvO_2$ may reflect increased arterio-venous shunting across some vascular beds rather than adequate oxygen delivery to all organs (el-Masry et al., 2009). Moreover, the correlation between $SvO_2$ and CO may be poor in OLT.

### Pulmonary artery occlusion pressures

The measurement of PAOP has been shown to have no consistent correlation with measures of preload such as stroke volume and CI (Costa et al., 2007). This, combined with the small risk of the devastating complication of PA rupture, means this is commonly not measured.

## Peripheral arterial waveform analysis

### Explanation of method

Quantitative peripheral arterial waveform analysis involves an analysis of the shape of the pressure waveform measured peripherally and a calculation of the beat-to-beat CO. The maximal slope of the pressure tracing is related to the LV contractility and the area under the curve is related to stroke volume. The relationships are not straightforward and are altered by changes and differences in haemodynamic variables including vascular compliance and SVR (Thiele and Durieux, 2011). CO is calculated using a complicated analysis of several waveform variables and relies on assumptions about vascular compliance, reflected pressure waves, and extrapolation back to central aortic pressures. These assumptions used to calculate CO may not be valid in rapidly changing haemodynamic states encountered during OLT. Indeed, these techniques have not yet reached a level of accuracy acceptable for clinical use in OLT. The benefits of this technique are that it is less invasive than the PAC, it provides rapid beat-to-beat analysis, and it is largely operator independent. With ongoing refinement of these monitors and their algorithms, accuracy and reliability as CO trending monitors may ultimately achieve a level of accuracy that makes them a useful tool in OLT.

### Clinical evidence

Most evidence relating to these devices is from the cardiac surgery literature and relates to comparisons with intermittent thermodilution methods of CO measurement. In this setting the accuracy of these devices has not been demonstrated to be acceptable for clinical use and changes in haemodynamic conditions result in changes that are not reliable even for trending of CO. The evidence from the liver transplant setting is more limited but instructive (Biancofiore et al., 2009, 2011; Krejci et al., 2010; Akiyoshi et al., 2011). In a series of 21 cirrhotic patients undergoing liver transplant, waveform analysis using the latest software version of the Vigileo/Flotrac system (Edwards, California, US) was compared with intermittent bolus thermodilution measurements of CO. This study showed a percentage error between the two techniques of 52% and only a moderate correlation ($r = 0.67$) between the two methods of measuring CI. These figures remain outside the generally accepted limits for acceptable agreement and trending (Critchley et al., 2010; Biancofiore et al., 2011).

### Aortic pulse contour analysis for cardiac output and volume measurement

A variation on the peripheral arterial waveform analysis technique is the use of a pulse contour of the aortic pressure waveform to derive a stroke volume and CO measurement (PCCO). This technique is used in the PiCCO system (Pulsion Medical System, Munich, Germany), which also uses the pulse contour to derive measures of intrathoracic, or global end-diastolic, volume indices. These systems use a customized femoral artery pressure catheter equipped with a distal thermistor. When combined with injection of a cold fluid bolus from a central line in the jugular or subclavian vein this enables the measurement of a transpulmonary CO and derivation of volume indices. These monitors are most extensively used in intensive care but have been shown to give intermittent and continuous CO measurements that correlate well with PAC CO measures during OLT (Della Rocca et al., 2002). The accuracy of this measure of CO has not been established during liver reperfusion and it may be subject to the same limitations as the transpulmonary thermodilution technique during this phase. The calculation of a measure of end-diastolic cardiac chamber volume index is a potentially useful guide to the volume status of a patient during OLT. Using this index it has been demonstrated that cirrhotic patients with hyperdynamic circulations may have a reduced circulating blood volume (Henriksen et al., 1989; Costa et al., 2007).

## Echocardiography

The use of TEE in OLT is presented elsewhere in the book (see Chapter 22). Echocardiography can provide valuable qualitative and quantitative information about cardiac structure and function and its use is now established in liver transplantation. TOE can provide quantitative pressure measurements, flow measurements (including CO), and valvular area and regurgitation quantification. It can also provide qualitative rapid visualization of global and regional ventricular contractility, ventricular filling, emboli (both air and thrombus), presence of patent foramen ovale or atrial septal defects, and the dilatation of acute LV or RV failure. It provides comprehensive and robust information that is dynamic and real time. When combined with other haemodynamic data it can provide an unparalleled understanding of the cardiovascular status. Concerns about the risk of tearing oesophageal varices during placement need to be considered, but this risk appears to be low.

## Oesophageal Doppler

Oesophageal Doppler has been investigated in many surgical settings as a relatively minimally invasive monitor of CO. The evidence in support of these monitors is limited and most comes from studies of elective abdominal surgery where the devices were used to guide fluid therapy to optimize CO. There is limited experience with their use in OLT. In a small series that demonstrated wide limits of agreement between oesophageal Doppler and the PAC in OLT it was concluded that this monitor is not interchangeable with the PAC (Perilli et al., 2009). Given the limited evidence in support of this monitor, plus the increasing use of TOE, it is rarely used in OLT.

## Cerebral monitoring

Maintenance of adequate cerebral oxygen delivery is an important consideration in OLT as patients may present with cerebral oedema and elevated ICP. Cerebral monitoring to optimize oxygen delivery and brain protection is available using a range of modalities, although none has been shown, in controlled trials, to change neurological outcomes. Non-invasive monitors include raw and processed EEG monitors, cerebral oximeters, and transcranial Doppler (TCD). Invasive monitors include ICP and jugular bulb venous saturation monitors ($SjvO_2$). Despite the limited evidence of outcome benefit, experience with their use provides some instructive insights. As part of a multimodal monitoring protocol they may provide information to guide intensive care and intraoperative management and ultimately may become more widely used in selected cases once evidence as to their utility increases.

### Near-infrared spectroscopy

NIRS measures the oxygen saturation of tissues and cerebral NIRS systems have been developed as non-invasive monitors to detect cerebral ischaemia and desaturation (Murkin and Arango, 2009). NIRS systems typically include two to four fibreoptic light sources and detectors that are placed bilaterally over the frontal cortex. They provide a measure of the oxygen saturation in the venous and arterial blood in the superficial cerebral tissue and display absolute saturation readings and trend data. Most experience with these monitors is from neonatal intensive care and cardiac surgery. In a small series of patients undergoing OLT, NIRS was shown to move in parallel with MAP in a few patients, whilst in the majority no change was identified over a wide range of blood pressure, suggesting that cerebral autoregulation was intact (Nissen et al., 2009a). Whilst no evidence of outcome benefit exists, this monitor may be useful in identifying patients in whom cerebral autoregulation is not intact or when ICP is elevated and in whom diligent management of systemic arterial blood pressure may be particularly important in order to maintain adequate cerebral blood flow and cerebral oxygenation.

### Transcranial Doppler

TCD utilizes a window in the temporal skull to measure the flow velocity in the middle cerebral arteries (MCAs) bilaterally. On the assumption that the large MCA diameter does not change, this velocity can be used as an indirect measure of blood flow. It provides flow velocity and pulsatility information and can (1) demonstrate if autoregulation is intact with changes in cerebral perfusion pressure; (2) show differences in flow between the two hemispheres; and (3) provide a visualization and quantification of embolic material to the brain (Fodale et al., 2007). The experience in OLT is limited. It has been used in patients with ALF and intracranial hypertension to guide therapy and judge when to proceed to liver transplant (Bindi et al., 2008). It has been used beyond the perioperative period into the intraoperative period to guide management, as demonstrated in a case report of a patient with ALF and cerebral oedema (Sidi and Mahla, 1995). In this case, TCD was shown to correlate well with an invasive ICP monitor and was considered useful in diagnosing elevated ICP and in guiding management (representative traces are illustrated in Figure 37.3). Limitations include the difficulty in applying and securing the transducer probes, the need for training and experience in interpreting the traces, and that in approximately one-quarter of patients reliable Doppler traces are not obtainable. For these reasons, despite its potential utility, it is not a widely used monitor in OLT.

### Raw and processed EEG

Raw EEG monitoring has been available since OLT was first performed. The expertise required to set up and interpret raw EEG has limited its uptake in intraoperative care and it is rarely used outside the ICU in these patients. The more recent processed EEG monitors, including the Bispectral Index Monitor (Covidien, US) and Entropy (GE, US), provide easy to use processed EEG information that has been designed to assess the adequacy of anaesthesia to prevent awareness. In addition to the processed indices (BIS, state entropy (SE)/response entropy (RE)), they also enable display

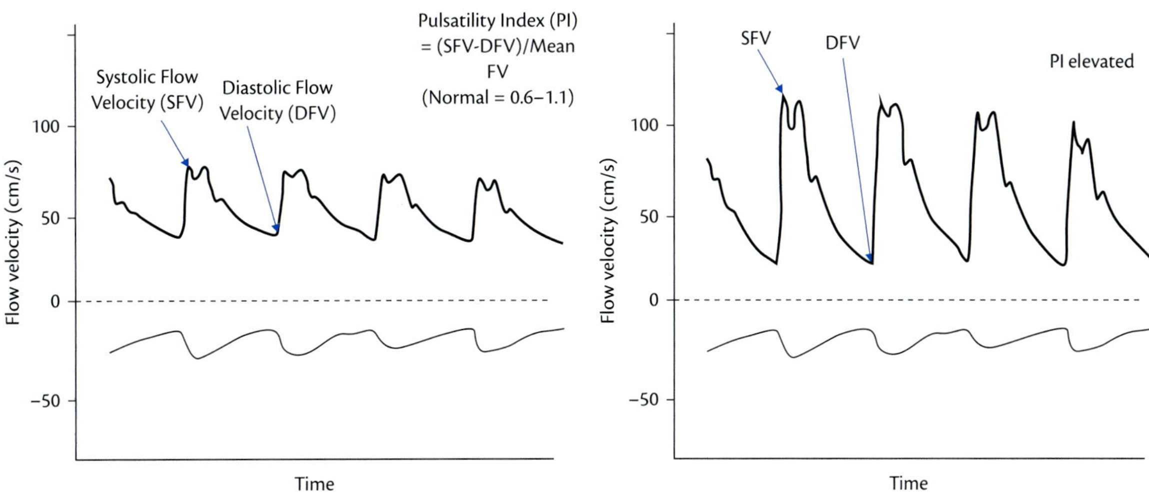


**Fig. 37.3** Left: typical normal TCD trace with mean flow velocity = 55 cm/s. Right: patient with elevated ICP demonstrating reduced diastolic flow velocity and elevated pulsatility index (PI).

of a raw EEG trace that can be interpreted with moderate training. They may provide useful information to guide the dose of anaesthesia, identify seizure activity, and determine return of cortical electrical activity in patients with an electrically silent EEG. BIS has been used to guide the titration of anaesthetic agents such as propofol (Tremelot et al., 2008) and isoflurane (Toprak et al., 2011) during the different phases of OLT when clearance may be altered significantly. BIS was used in a case of ALF to monitor cortical electrical activity. After reaching a state of electrical silence preceding and during transplant, BIS recovered to a value of 40 2 hours following surgery and the patient subsequently regained full consciousness (Okawa et al., 2011). This case highlights the potential utility of processed EEG monitoring in predicting emergence and success of graft function with resolution of the metabolic encephalopathy.

## Intracranial pressure monitors

ICP monitors are used to guide the intra- and perioperative management of patients for OLT with suspected or confirmed elevated ICP. They are invasive monitors and provide a direct measure of ICP and display a characteristic pressure waveform. Monitors can be placed intraparenchymally, into the extradural space, into the subarachnoid space using a bolt, or intraventricularly. The relative merits of each technique are outlined in Table 37.6 and typical normal and abnormal ICP waveforms are shown in Figure 37.4.

The risk of intracranial haemorrhage during the placement of intraparenchymal catheters in patients who are coagulopathic is a major concern. A recent audit of patients with ALF and severe encephalopathy identified an intracranial haemorrhage rate of 10.3% with ICP monitor placement, half of which were found incidentally on radiological imaging (Vaquero et al., 2005). In this series from multiple US centres, use of ICP monitors varied widely and they were used in 28% of these patients. There are no accepted guidelines for coagulation and factor replacement prior to ICP monitor placement (Davis et al., 2004), and practice consequently varies widely. Recombinant factor VIIa has been used prophylactically before placement of these catheters in a small series, with no haemorrhagic complications recorded (Le et al., 2010).

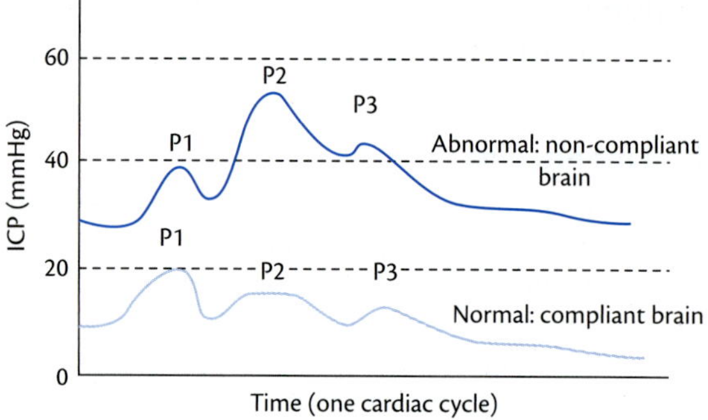


**Fig. 37.4** ICP trace—normal trace below, abnormal trace above. The ICP waveform originates from the arterial pressure wave and typically has three representative waves: P1 is the percussive wave which is the arterial pressure wave transmitted from the choroid plexus, P2 is the tidal wave and amplitude increases as compliance reduces, P3 represents the dicrotic notch of aortic valve closure.

**Table 37.6** ICP monitors—principles, advantages, and disadvantages

| Position | Principle | Advantage | Limitations |
|---|---|---|---|
| Intraventricular | Pressure transduced from within lateral ventricle | Accurate ICP measurement, allows CSF drainage | Invasive, difficult if ventricles compressed, risk of infection |
| Intraparenchymal | Fibreoptic-tipped catheter, can also be placed subdurally | Requires zeroing only on insertion, better quality waveforms than other techniques, no need to adjust transducer heights | No CSF access, fragile, cannot be recalibrated after placement |
| Subarachnoid bolt or screw | Subarachnoid placement of transducer | Less invasive, low rate of infection | Less accurate at elevated ICP, requires frequent recalibration, no access to CSF |
| Epidural or subdural | Use fluid column or fibreoptic system, least invasive technique | Least invasive technique, easily placed, low infection risk | No CSF access |

## Jugular venous oximetry ($SjvO_2$)

Measurement of the oxygen saturation in the jugular bulb gives an estimation of global cerebral oxygen consumption. Normal ranges, assuming normal arterial oxygenation, are 55–75%. This figure is lower than normal $SvO_2$ and reflects the higher oxygen extraction of the brain. $SjvO_2$ is a function of arterial oxygen content, cerebral blood flow, and cerebral metabolic rate for oxygen ($CMRO_2$) and consequently reflects changes in these parameters. It has been used to guide interventions such as cerebral perfusion pressure and arterial $CO_2$ tension management to improve and preserve adequate brain oxygenation. Most experience with this technique comes from the management of head-injured

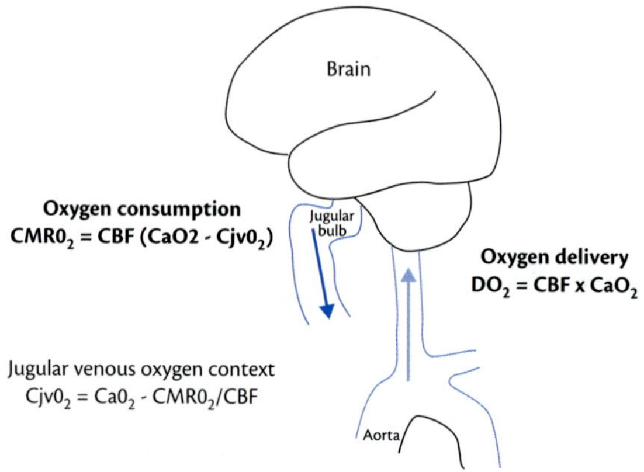


**Fig. 37.5** Determinants of $SjvO_2$ include arterial oxygen content ($CaO_2$), cerebral metabolic rate ($CMRO_2$), and cerebral blood flow (CBF). Changes in any of these will impact on $SjvO_2$.

**Table 37.7** Causes of high and low jugular venous oxygen saturation ($SjvO_2$)

| | |
|---|---|
| Low $SjvO_2$ < 55% | ◆ Increased cerebral oxygen extraction (arterial desaturation, elevated ICP, decreased CBF (such as with hypocapnia), low haematocrit)<br>◆ Increased $CMRO_2$ (fever, seizures) |
| High $SjvO_2$ > 75% | ◆ Elevated CBF (loss of autoregulation or hypercarbia)<br>◆ Elevated ICP, resulting in regional shunting, or, if very high, no cerebral blood flow at all<br>◆ Reduced CMRO2 due to hypothermia, drugs |

patients with elevated ICP (Figure 37.5). It is an invasive monitoring technique and is very sensitive to movement of the catheter tip from the jugular bulb. It does not provide information about oxygenation of the posterior fossa as venous outflow from there is not predominantly from the jugular veins. A continuous oximetry reading can now be provided using fibreoptic oximeters that provide a trend. This may be more useful in guiding management than relying on intermittent and sporadic saturation measurements. There is no literature published on the use of jugular venous oximetry in OLT, but it remains used in some ICUs to guide the management of refractory elevated ICP. Table 37.7 summarizes the common causes of low and high $SjvO_2$ readings.

## Conclusion

This chapter has attempted to cover a broad range of monitoring techniques used in the immediate perioperative period of liver transplantation. POC coagulation monitoring has contributed to the evolution and sophistication of blood management during and immediately after transplantation. Standard invasive haemodynamic monitoring is considered routine, but some of the more novel modes of cardiovascular and neurological monitoring require further research and investigation to clarify their role(s) in both the intraoperative and intensive care management of liver failure and transplantation.

## References


Akiyoshi K, Kandabashi T, Kaji J, et al. (2011) Accuracy of arterial pressure waveform analysis for cardiac output measurement in comparison with thermodilution methods in patients undergoing living donor liver transplantation. *J Anesth*, **25**:178–183.

Arnal D, Garutti I, Pérez-Peña J, Olmedilla L, Tzenkov IG (2005) Radial to femoral arterial blood pressure differences during liver transplantation. *Anaesthesia*, **60**:766–771.

Avidan MS, Alcock EL, Da Fonseca J, et al. (2004) Comparison of structured use of routine laboratory tests or near-patient assessment with clinical judgement in the management of bleeding after cardiac surgery. *Br J Anaesth*, **92**:178–186.

Bang SR, Kim YH, Kim GS (2011) The effects of in vitro hemodilution with 6% hydroxyethyl starch (HES) (130/0.4) solution on thrombelastograph analysis in patients undergoing liver transplantation. *Clin Transplant*, **25**:450–456.

Biancofiore G, Critchley LA, Lee A, et al. (2009) Evaluation of an uncalibrated arterial pulse contour cardiac output monitoring system in cirrhotic patients undergoing liver surgery. *Br J Anaesth*, **102**:47–54.

Biancofiore G, Critchley LAH, Lee A, et al. (2011) Evaluation of a new software version of the FloTrac/Vigileo (version 3.02) and a comparison with previous data in cirrhotic patients undergoing liver transplant surgery. *Anesth Analg*, **113**:515–522.

Bindi ML, Biancofiore G, Esposito M, et al. (2008) Transcranial doppler sonography is useful for the decision-making at the point of care in patients with acute hepatic failure: a single centre APOS experience. *J Clin Monitor Comput*, **22**:449–452.

Boks AL, Brommer EJ, Schalm SW, Van Vliet HH (1986) Hemostasis and fibrinolysis in severe liver failure and their relation to hemorrhage. *Hepatology*, 6:79–86.

Camenzind V, Bombeli T, Seifert B, et al. (2000) Citrate storage affects thrombelastograph analysis. *Anesthesiology*, **92**:1242–1249.

Cammerer U, Dietrich W, Rampf T, Braun SL, Richter JA (2003) The predictive value of modified computerized thromboelastography and platelet function analysis for postoperative blood loss in routine cardiac surgery. *Anesth Analg*, **96**:51–57, table of contents.

Chen H, Merchant NB, Didolkar MS (2000) Hepatic resection using intermittent vascular inflow occlusion and low central venous pressure anesthesia improves morbidity and mortality. *J Gastrointest Surg*, **4**:162–167.

Chitlur M, Lusher J (2010) Standardization of thromboelastography: values and challenges. *Semin Thromb Hemost*, **36**:707–711.

Coakley M, Reddy K, Mackie I, Mallett S (2006) Transfusion triggers in orthotopic liver transplantation: a comparison of the thromboelastometry analyzer, the thromboelastogram, and conventional coagulation tests. *J Cardiothorac Vasc Anesth*, **20**:548–553.

Colella MP, Fiusa MM, Orsi FL, De Paula EV, Annichino-Bizzacchi JM (2012) Performance of a point-of-care device in determining prothrombin time in an anticoagulation clinic. *Blood Coagul Fibrinolysis*, **23**:172–174.

Collaborative Study Group on Perioperative $ScvO_2$ Monitoring (2006) Multicentre Study on peri- and postoperative central venous oxygen saturation in high-risk surgical patients. *Crit Care*, **10**:R158.

Costa MG, Chiarandini P, Della Rocca G (2007) Hemodynamics during liver transplantation. *Transplant Proc*, **39**:1871–1873.

Critchley LA, Lee A, Ho AM (2010) A critical review of the ability of continuous cardiac output monitors to measure trends in cardiac output. *Anesth Analg*, **111**:1180–1192.

Dahmani S, Paugam-Burtz C, Gauss T, et al. (2010) Comparison of central and mixed venous saturation during liver transplantation in cirrhotic patients: a pilot study. *Eur J Anaesthesiol*, **27**:714–719.

Dalmau A, Sabaté A, Aparicio I (2009) Hemostasis and coagulation monitoring and management during liver transplantation. *Curr Opin Organ Transplant*, **14**:286–290.

Davis JW, Davis IC, Bennink LD, et al. (2004) Placement of intracranial pressure monitors: are 'normal' coagulation parameters necessary? *J Trauma*, **57**:1173–1177.

Della Rocca G, Costa MG, Pompei L, Coccia C, Pietropaoli P (2002) Continuous and intermittent cardiac output measurement: pulmonary artery catheter versus aortic transpulmonary technique. *Br J Anaesth*, **88**:350–356.

El-Masry A, Mukhtar AM, El-Sherbeny AM, Fathy M, El-Meteini M (2009) Comparison of central venous oxygen saturation and mixed venous oxygen saturation during liver transplantation. *Anaesthesia*, **64**:378–382.

Feng Z-Y, Xu X, Zhu S-M, Bein B, Zheng S-S (2010) Effects of low central venous pressure during preanhepatic phase on blood loss and liver and renal function in liver transplantation. *World J Surg*, **34**:1864–1873.

Fodale V, Schifilliti D, Conti A, Lucanto T, Pino G, Santamaria LB (2007) Transcranial Doppler and anesthetics. *Acta Anaesth Scand*, **51**:839–847.

Frumento RJ, Hirsh AL, Parides MK, Bennett-Guerrero E (2002) Differences in arterial and venous thromboelastography parameters: potential roles of shear stress and oxygen content. *J Cardiothorac Vasc Anesth*, **16**:551–554.

Gelman S (2008) Venous function and central venous pressure: a physiologic story. *Anesthesiology*, **108**:735–748.

Giusca S, Jinga M, Jurcut C, Jurcut R, Serban M, Ginghina C (2011) Portopulmonary hypertension: from diagnosis to treatment. *Eur J Intern Med*, **22**:441–447.

Harding SA, Mallett SV, Peachey TD, Cox DJ (1997) Use of heparinase modified thrombelastography in liver transplantation. *Br J Anaesth*, **78**:175–179.

Hardy JF, De Moerloose P, Samama M (2004) Massive transfusion and coagulopathy: pathophysiology and implications for clinical management. *Can J Anaesth*, **51**:293–310.

Henriksen JH, Bendtsen F, Sorensen TI, Stadeager C, Ring-Larsen H (1989) Reduced central blood volume in cirrhosis. *Gastroenterology*, **97**:1506–1513.

Jones RM, Moulton CE, Hardy KJ (1998) Central venous pressure and its effect on blood loss during liver resection. *Br J Surg*, **85**:1058–1060.

Kang Y (1995) Thromboelastography in liver transplantation. *Semin Thromb Hemost*, **21**(Suppl 4):34–44.

Kang YG, Martin DJ, Marquez J, et al. (1985) Intraoperative changes in blood coagulation and thrombelastographic monitoring in liver transplantation. *Anesth Analg*, **64**:888–896.

Kettner SC, Gonano C, Seebach F, et al. (1998) Endogenous heparin-like substances significantly impair coagulation in patients undergoing orthotopic liver transplantation. *Anesth Analg*, **86**:691–695.

Krejci V, Vannucci A, Abbas A, Chapman W, Kangrga IM (2010) Comparison of calibrated and uncalibrated arterial pressure-based cardiac output monitors during orthotopic liver transplantation. *Liver Transpl*, **16**:773–782.

Le TV, Rumbak MJ, Liu SS, Alsina AE, Van Loveren H, Agazzi S (2010) Insertion of intracranial pressure monitors in fulminant hepatic failure patients: early experience using recombinant factor VII. *Neurosurgery*, **66**:455–458, discussion 458.

Lisman T, Porte RJ (2010) Rebalanced hemostasis in patients with liver disease: evidence and clinical consequences. *Blood*, **116**:878–885.

Macdonald SG, Luddington RJ (2010) Critical factors contributing to the thromboelastography trace. *Semin Thromb Hemost*, **36**:712–722.

Marik PE, Cavallazzi R, Vasu T, Hirani A (2009) Dynamic changes in arterial waveform derived variables and fluid responsiveness in mechanically ventilated patients: a systematic review of the literature. *Crit Care Med*, **37**:2642–2647.

Massicotte L, Lenis S, Thibeault L, Sassine MP, Seal RF, Roy A (2006) Effect of low central venous pressure and phlebotomy on blood product transfusion requirements during liver transplantations. *Liver Transpl*, **12**:117–123.

Massicotte L, Perrault M-A, Denault AY, et al. (2010) Effects of phlebotomy and phenylephrine infusion on portal venous pressure and systemic hemodynamics during liver transplantation. *Transplantation*, **89**:920–927.

Milan Z, Taylor C, Duncan B, Kedilaya H, Sylvester D (2011) Statistical modeling of hemodynamic changes during orthotopic liver transplantation: predictive value for outcome and effect of marginal donors. *Transplant Proc*, **43**:1711–1715.

Montalto P, Vlachogiannakos J, Cox DJ, Pastacaldi S, Patch D, Burroughs AK (2002) Bacterial infection in cirrhosis impairs coagulation by a heparin effect: a prospective study. *J Hepatol*, **37**:463–470.

Murkin JM, Arango M (2009) Near-infrared spectroscopy as an index of brain and tissue oxygenation. *Br J Anaesth*, **103**(Suppl 1):i, 3–13.

Nissen P, Pacino H, Frederiksen HJ, Novovic S, Secher NH (2009a) Near-infrared spectroscopy for evaluation of cerebral autoregulation during orthotopic liver transplantation. *Neurocrit Care*, **11**:235–241.

Nissen P, Van Lieshout JJ, Novovic S, Bundgaard-Nielsen M, Secher NH (2009b) Techniques of cardiac output measurement during liver transplantation: arterial pulse wave versus thermodilution. *Liver Transpl*, **15**:287–291.

Okawa H, Ono T, Hashiba E, Tsubo T, Ishihara H, Hirota K (2011) Use of bispectral index monitoring for a patient with hepatic encephalopathy requiring living donor liver transplantation: a case report. *J Anesth*, **25**:117–119.

Papatheodoridis GV, Patch D, Webster GJ, Brooker J, Barnes E, Burroughs AK (1999) Infection and hemostasis in decompensated cirrhosis: a prospective study using thrombelastography. *Hepatology*, **29**:1085–1090.

Peña JR, Lewandrowski K, Lewandrowski EL, Gregory K, Baron JM, Van Cott EM (2012) Evaluation of the i-STAT point-of-care capillary whole blood prothrombin time and international normalized ratio: comparison to the Tcoag MDAII coagulation analyzer in the central laboratory. *Clin Chim Acta*, **413**(11–12):955–959.

Perilli V, Avolio AW, Sacco T, et al. (2009) Use of an esophageal echo-Doppler device during liver transplantation: preliminary report. *Transplant Proc*, **41**:198–200.

Rivers EP, Ander DS, Powell D (2001) Central venous oxygen saturation monitoring in the critically ill patient. *Curr Opin Crit Care*, **7**:204–211.

Sakai T, Matsusaki T, Dai F, et al. (2011) Pulmonary thromboembolism during adult liver transplantation: incidence, clinical presentation, outcome, risk factors, and diagnostic predictors. *Br J Anaesth*, 108(3):469–477.

Schroeder RA, Kuo PC (2008) Pro: low central venous pressure during liver transplantation—not too low. *J Cardio-Thorac Vasc Anesth*, **22**:311–314.

Schroeder RA, Collins BH, Tuttle-Newhall E, et al. (2004) Intraoperative fluid management during orthotopic liver transplantation. *J Cardiothorac Vasc Anesth*, **18**:438–441.

Sharara AI, Rockey DC (2001) Gastroesophageal variceal hemorrhage. *N Engl J Med*, **345**:669–681.

Sidi A, Mahla ME (1995) Noninvasive monitoring of cerebral perfusion by transcranial Doppler during fulminant hepatic failure and liver transplantation. *Anesth Analg*, **80**:194–200.

Spiezia L, Radu C, Marchioro P, et al. (2008) Peculiar whole blood rotation thromboelastometry (ROTEM) profile in 40 sideropenic anaemia patients. *Thromb Haemost*, **100**:1106–1110.

Stravitz RT, Lisman T, Luketic VA, et al. (2011) Minimal effects of acute liver injury/acute liver failure on hemostasis as assessed by thromboelastography. *J Hepatology*, 56(1):129–136.

Thiele RH, Durieux ME (2011) Arterial waveform analysis for the anesthesiologist: past, present, and future concepts. *Anesth Analg*, **113**:766–776.

Toprak HI, Sener A, Gedik E, et al. (2011) Bispectral index monitoring to guide end-tidal isoflurane concentration at three phases of operation in patients with end-stage liver disease undergoing orthotopic liver transplantation. *Transplant Proc*, **43**:892–895.

Tremelot L, Restoux A, Paugam-Burtz C, et al. (2008) Interest of BIS monitoring to guide propofol infusion during the anhepatic phase of orthotopic liver transplantation. *Ann Fr Anesth Reanim*, **27**:975–978.

Vaquero J, Fontana RJ, Larson AM, et al. (2005) Complications and use of intracranial pressure monitoring in patients with acute liver failure and severe encephalopathy. *Liver Transpl*, **11**:1581–1589.

Wang S-C, Shieh J-F, Chang K-Y, et al. (2010) Thromboelastography-guided transfusion decreases intraoperative blood transfusion during orthotopic liver transplantation: randomized clinical trial. *Transplant Proc*, **42**:2590–2593.

Wang WD, Liang LJ, Huang XQ, Yin XY (2006) Low central venous pressure reduces blood loss in hepatectomy. *World J Gastroenterol*, **12**:935–939.

Wikkelsoe AJ, Afshari A, Wetterslev J, Brok J, Moeller AM (2011) Monitoring patients at risk of massive transfusion with thrombelastography or thromboelastometry: a systematic review. *Acta Anaesth Scand*, **55**:1174–1189.

# CHAPTER 38

# Specialized equipment and procedures: blood salvage, rapid infusion systems, and renal replacement therapy

Andrew Watts and Kirstin Naguit

## Blood salvage

Intraoperative red blood cell salvage (ICS) and autologous blood transfusion are considered a routine part of the transplant anaesthesiologist's armamentarium during OLT, to reduce both exposure to allogeneic blood and demands placed on the finite resources of local blood banks. Early reports of ICS demonstrated that blood could be salvaged and returned to patients, yet its value and safety were questioned (Dzik and Jenkins, 1985, Van Voorst et al., 1985; Kang et al., 1991) More recently, literature demonstrating the value of ICS abounds in non-transplant circles (Ashworth and Klein, 2010), but there is still reticence to use ICS during liver transplantation, with doubts expressed about cost-effectiveness and risk of transmission of infection and malignancy (Kemper et al., 1997; Phillips et al., 2006). That said, its use is routine and value largely undisputed.

The initial impetus for ICS in OLT was driven by frequently encountered massive blood loss and transfusion requirements in the early experience of this surgery. Initial use of ICS demonstrated a reduction in allogeneic blood exposure by transfusion of salvaged blood (rather than an overall reduction in transfusion requirements). The potential complications associated with ICS in liver transplant surgery were recognized from early experience (Kang et al., 1991). From the mid-1990s awareness of the risks of transmission of blood-borne infections including viruses (hepatitis B, hepatitis C, HIV, CMV, EBV), bacteria, and prions in banked blood provided greater impetus for use of ICS. More recently, appreciation of other adverse effects of allogeneic blood transfusion such as TRIM, TRALI, and increased morbidity and mortality have provided further motivation for the use for ICS and return of salvaged blood (Massicotte et al., 2005; Shander et al., 2007; De Boer et al., 2008).

More recently, improvements in surgical technique, anaesthetic management of coagulopathy, use of antifibrinolytic drugs, and changes in anaesthetic fluid management philosophy (low CVP and in some institutions intraoperative phlebotomy (Massicotte et al., 2006) have combined to reduce blood loss and the need for transfusion in OLT. However, OLT can still be associated with both predictable and unpredictable major haemorrhage, massive transfusion, and the need for ICS. Factors that predict high transfusion requirements vary widely (Findlay et al., 2000). There appear to be institution and patient factors involved. Retransplantation or previous major abdominal surgery, low preoperative haemoglobin, use of VVB, placement of intraoperative portocaval shunt, and high MELD score may predict increased transfusion requirements (Findlay and Retke, 2000; Phillips et al., 2006; Mangus et al., 2007). Finally, OLT is now offered to Jehovah's Witnesses and ICS may be acceptable to these patients as a means to avoid blood transfusion.

### Technology

ICS involves the use of a device to collect the shed red cells from the surgical field (with an anticoagulant), which are then separated, washed, and then reinfused into the patient. The technology of cell salvage has evolved since its inception in the 1960s. Haemonetics developed the first system commercially available in the 1980s. There are now numerous commercial systems available—Haemonetics Cell Saver 5 and Cell Saver Elite (see Figure 38.1), Cobe BRAT 2 (Baylor Rapid Autotransfusion) Cell Saver, and Fresenius CATS (continuous autotransfusion system) device amongst others. The performance of commercial machines is similar and which one is purchased depends upon physician and institutional preference (Burman et al., 2002).

Blood is suctioned from the operative site via a double lumen tubing so that blood can be mixed with an anticoagulant—heparin or acid citrate dextrose solution A (ACDA) (see Figure 38.2). The flow of anticoagulant is manually controlled and adjusted for the rate of blood aspiration from the surgical field. Low-pressure suction (< 150 mmHg) is used to minimize haemolysis. Salvaged blood is passed via a filter (40–150 μm) to a reservoir (usually a cardiotomy reservoir) where it is held until there is sufficient blood for processing. At this point, the salvaged blood is pumped into a centrifuge bowl where it is concentrated and washed. The bowl size used varies (70–275 mL) depending on the size of the patient (paediatric vs adult) and anticipated blood loss. Sterile saline or plasmalyte

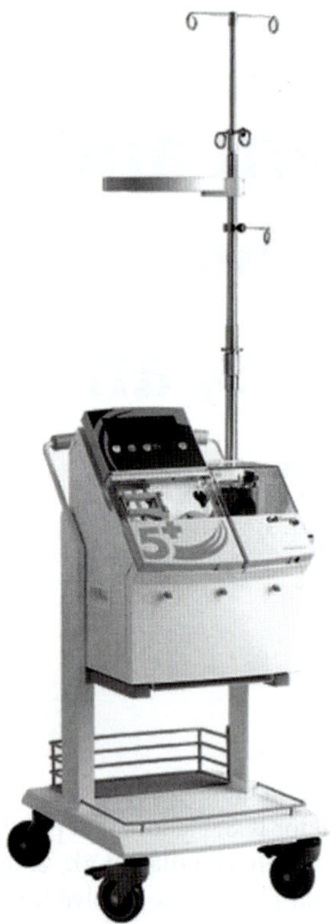

Fig. 38.1 Blood salvage device. (Reproduced with kind permission from Haemontics Corporation.)

solutions are used to wash the salvaged blood in the centrifuge bowl at 3,600–5,650 rpm depending upon the machine characteristics and wash cycle chosen (Burman et al., 2002; Naumenko et al., 2008). Manufacturers usually recommend using an automatic cycle but this may be overridden in some machines. The higher density red cells migrate to the outer wall of the spinning bowl. Waste from the centrifugation process (white cells, platelets, free haemoglobin, plasma, and heparin) is collected in a bag and disposed of. The processed red cells are suspended for retransfusion as required and can be stored for up to 4 hours at room temperature prior to reinfusion. The haematocrit of the salvaged blood is approximately 55–75%. In cases of major haemorrhage, two cell savers may be used to avoid wastage of spilled blood.

Potential complications associated with use of the cell saver include haemolysis, air embolism, coagulopathy, incomplete washing resulting in contamination with microaggregates causing microembolism, contamination with drugs, infection transmission, and the theoretical risk of transmission of cancer cells with recurrence (see the section 'Malignancy'). Transfusion of large volumes of salvaged red cells is that alone. The cell saver blood is devoid of platelets and plasma coagulation components, so large-volume infusion will result in a dilutional coagulopathy that will need to be monitored and corrected. There are very few absolute contraindications to cell salvage and those that are present a clear danger to the patient. This includes anything that would result in red cell lysis if administered with the salvaged red cells such as sterile water, hydrogen peroxide, alcohol, and any hypotonic solution (e.g. glycine) (Esper et al., 2011). Relative

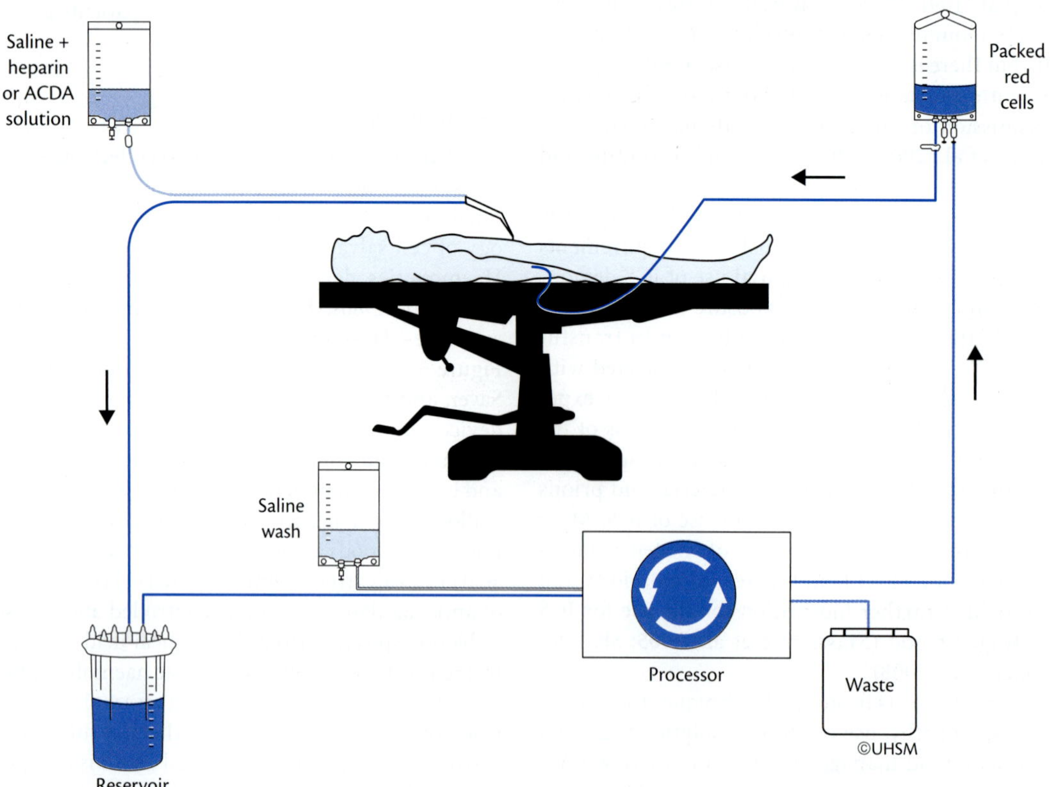


Fig. 38.2 Blood salvage circuit. (This figure is provided courtesy of the Department of Medical Illustration at University Hospital of South Manchester NHS Foundation Trust.)

contraindications to cell salvage include contaminants (urine, bowel contents, ascites, amniotic fluid, infection); malignancy; pharmacological agents (prothrombotic/clotting agents and anti-coagulants, methyl methacrylate (bone cement)); and haematological disorders.

Leucocyte depletion filters (LDFs) are frequently used in conjunction with ICS as they are felt to reduce side effects of salvaged blood and improve safety (Fergusson et al., 2004). Leucodepletion is achieved by a combination of mechanical sieving and direct adherence of cells to the fibres (Steneker et al., 1992). Removal of cancer cells and bacteria is felt to occur by a similar mechanism. In OLT the major limitations of LDFs are the slow flow rates associated with their use, it is recommended that they are not used in a pressurized system, and their filtering ability is limited to the equivalent of approximately 2 units of packed cells.

Operation of the cell saver requires training and is performed by an anaesthetic technician or perfusionist under supervision of the anaesthetist. A record of volumes processed, anticoagulation, and blood returned to the patient is essential. Regular audit and quality control of cell-salvaged blood should be undertaken.

## Cost savings

The volumes of blood returned to the patient vary considerably and, as noted before, predictors of blood loss are variable. Hence, the cost-effectiveness of ICS has been questioned (Duffy and Tolley, 1997; Kemper et al., 1997) and some have only shown it to be of benefit when transfusion requirements are in excess of the equivalent of 10 units of red cells (Dzik and Jenkins, 1985; Williamson et al., 1989; Kemper et al., 1997). These earlier studies may reflect the lower unit cost of red blood cells (RBCs) historically, early technology, and outsourcing of cell salvage management. Cost benefit has been shown more recently (Phillips et al., 2006). In 660 patients transplanted between 1997 and 2006 considerable cost savings (US $531,305) were demonstrated by using ICS. Moreover, the mean saving per patient increased from US $51 prior to leucodepletion to more than US $600 postleucodepletion. Most benefit was gained among patients having retransplantation. The study factored in disposable costs, equipment maintenance, and the clinical perfusionist's salary.

Cost-effectiveness has also been shown with small-volume transfusion figures (Massicotte et al., 2007). The centre studied uses low CVP targets, phlebotomy without volume replacement, vasopressors, and strict protocol-driven blood product transfusion. In this historical, observational study the authors were able to demonstrate that even by reducing allogeneic blood usage by 1.7 units of packed cells they could save approximately CAN $700 per case. The authors also factored in the cost of disposable equipment and the clinical perfusionist's cost. The breakeven point for cost-effectiveness in this study was 0.67 RBC units.

It should be noted that no studies examining cost-effectiveness of ICS attempt to factor in secondary costs implicated with blood transfusion. These are best recognized with allogeneic blood and include increased mortality, morbidity, length of ICU stay, and reduced patient and graft survival (Koch et al., 2006; De Boer et al., 2008).

## Malignancy

Use of ICS in patients with HCC is contentious. It is recognized that tumour cells are detected in peripheral blood in oncological surgery (Kudo et al., 2004; Stoffel et al., 2005; Catling et al., 2008; Liang et al., 2008) and in 1986 the American Medical Council stated that ICS was contraindicated in cases of malignancy (Council Scientific Affairs, 1986). In urological and gynaecological cancer surgery there is no evidence of increased recurrence rates of cancer either biochemically or clinically among patients when ICS is used, despite detection of tumour-specific proteins in peripheral blood (Nieder et al., 2005) and antibody-labelled cancer cells after processing and prior to reinfusion (Stoffel et al., 2005). Since 2008 the use of ICS for urological malignancies has been endorsed by the National Institute for Health and Clinical Excellence (NICE, 2008) and practiced widely. However, concern still exists in transplantation circles about the use of ICS and some consider known HCC an absolute contraindication to ICS (Phillips et al., 2006). This concern may be heightened because of the routine use of immunosuppression postoperatively and the potential increased risk of tumour recrudescence (Yokoyama et al., 1991; Foltys et al., 2009).

Fujinomoto et al. (1991) could not detect malignant cells after processing and filtration of red cells in patients undergoing hepatectomy, but this may just reflect dated technology. Contrary to this, others have reported circulating tumour cells in patients with advanced HCC (Kar and Carr, 1995) and release of AFP mRNA-expressing cells from the hepatic vein during liver resection (Jones et al., 1999). Liver transplantation differs from resection in that there is less tumour manipulation. The liver is not transected and is removed en bloc, so potential for tumour spillage may be reduced. The ability to reduce tumour load may be enhanced by the use of LDFs (Stoffel et al., 2005). LDF filters in conjunction with double washing of blood with a cell saver produced the greatest reduction in HCC cells but did not eliminate all cancer cells in an in-vitro model (Jones et al., 1999). Gwak et al. (2005) studied the ability of an LDF to filter HCC cells from a saline suspension. They used PCR technology to increase the sensitivity of their testing. They divided the test group into six varying tumour loads per 200 mL saline—10 cells up to $2 \times 10^7$ cells. The LDF was able to filter HCC cells in vitro but could not completely remove all tumour cells at high HCC loads. The authors recommended the use of two filters in series to improve safety when ICS is used in OLT.

For patients with HCC, application of and evidence for ICS with or without LDF in clinical transplantation is sparse. Liang et al. (2008) studied a small group of patients with HCC who had blood salvaged during OLT but not returned. The cell saver blood was collected, processed, and filtered through two LDFs. Samples of blood were taken after processing and then after passage through each LDF. The blood was then centrifuged to separate possible HCC cells. Detection of HCC cells was performed using reverse transcriptase—PCR technique to detect the AFP mRNA in the shed blood. In this study, 15 of 32 patients had HCC cells detected in processed cell saver blood, but only patients who had (1) tumours outside of both Milan and UCLA criteria and (2) tumour rupture during surgery had HCC cells detected after passage through the first (two patients) and second (one patient) LDF. Thus these filters may reduce tumour load but practicalities in OLT may restrict their use.

Blood may be returned to liver transplant patients with HCC with or without the use of an LDF (Muscari et al., 2005; Massicotte et al., 2007; Foltys et al., 2011). Two studies specifically examined HCC recurrence following OLT in patients when ICS was used and the salvaged blood reinfused (Muscari et al., 2005; Foltys et al., 2011). In the study by Muscari et al. (2005) patients were followed for a minimum of 12 months. This figure was chosen as 95% of HCC recurrences occur within this period. Recurrence rates were similar among patients who had ICS (6.4%) compared with those in whom ICS was not used (6.3%, $P$ = 0.9). The group in whom ICS was utilized had more macroscopic neoplastic vascular thrombosis (a recognized risk for cancer recurrence (Marsh et al., 1997; Margarit et al., 2002)) as well as fewer patients who received treatment for their cancer whilst on the waiting list.

More recently, Foltys et al. (2011) found that absence of recurrence of HCC at 5 years was similar in patients in whom ICS was used (86%) compared with patients in whom it was not used (69%, $P$ = 0.29). Further, 5-year survival was similar in each group. On multivariate analysis the only predictors of recurrence in these patients were microvascular invasion ($P$ = 0.015) and Up-to-Seven criteria ($P$ = 0.005) (Mazzaferro et al., 2009). In both studies (Muscari et al., 2005; Foltys et al., 2011) the tumour characteristics in both patient groups were similar and fewer patients in whom ICS was used had pretransplant treatment of their cancers. Current literature evidence would suggest that cancer should not be considered an absolute contraindication to ICS. Further, although use of LDFs does decrease the risk of exposure to reinfused cancer cells, it does not eliminate it completely.

### Infection

Microbiological contamination of cell saver blood occurs during most surgical procedures. The most common source of bacterial contamination is from the skin or environmental (Ezzedine et al., 1991; Kang et al., 1991). Patients undergoing OLT may have underlying infection preoperatively (spontaneous bacterial peritonitis, biliary sepsis), bile and bowel contents may be spilled intraoperatively, and immunosuppression postoperatively is routine. Bacterial contamination is considered by some to be an absolute contraindication to ICS in liver transplantation (Phillips et al., 2006). However, a causal relationship between contaminated cell salvaged blood and adverse clinical outcomes or an increase in postoperative infection has not been demonstrated (Jeng et al., 1998; Bowley et al., 2006; Feltracco et al., 2007).

Cell saver processing reduces bacterial contamination and this is further reduced after filtration through an LDF (Waters et al., 2003). The authors inoculated expired red cells with varying bacterial loads, processed the blood, and passed blood through an LDF with 300 mmHg of pressure. Cell saver washing and the use of an LDF significantly reduced bacterial load. However, at high bacterial load, the washing and filtration process is overwhelmed and significant bacterial contamination of the salvaged blood may occur. Bacterial contamination of salvaged blood occurs in more than 50% of liver transplant patients (Feltracco et al., 2007; Liang et al., 2010). Reinfusion of this salvaged blood does not predispose to postoperative infection (Liang et al., 2010). Factors that may predispose to bacteria being present in shed blood are the existence of SBP and longer duration of surgery. The finding that reinfusion of cell saver blood does not increase the risk of infection is consistent with other literature regarding 'dirty' cases such as penetrating abdominal trauma (Ozmen et al., 1992; Bowley et al., 2006).

The presence of SBP or enteric content contamination should not be considered an absolute contraindication to the use of cell salvage in transplantation. Rather, because cell saver processing and the use of LDF blood significantly reduce bacterial contamination and there is no evidence of increased risk of postoperative infection, its use should be considered even when preoperative sepsis is apparent. A separate suction apparatus should be used initially for ascites when present and during surgery on the bile ducts or when the bowel is opened (for jejunostomy) for added safety.

## Rapid infusion systems

Rapid infusion systems (RISs) enable infusion of large volumes of fluids at normothermia in surgery where blood loss may be large and at times unpredictable. These systems were developed partially in response to the advent of liver transplantation. In early descriptions of liver transplant surgery, more than 5% of patients required more than 100 units of red cells intraoperatively, and in response to these needs Sassano, in collaboration with Haemonetics Corporation, developed the RIS (see Figure 38.3). This was the first commercially available system and was marketed from 1986, although it was not used universally. Many transplant units developed their own in-house systems that were essentially modifications of a CPB system. These systems worked well and met the requirements of the time. They had a cardiotomy reservoir for storage of blood products and fluids, a water bath for heating, but required large prime volumes (the equivalent of 4 units of PRBCs or more) and so are of less value

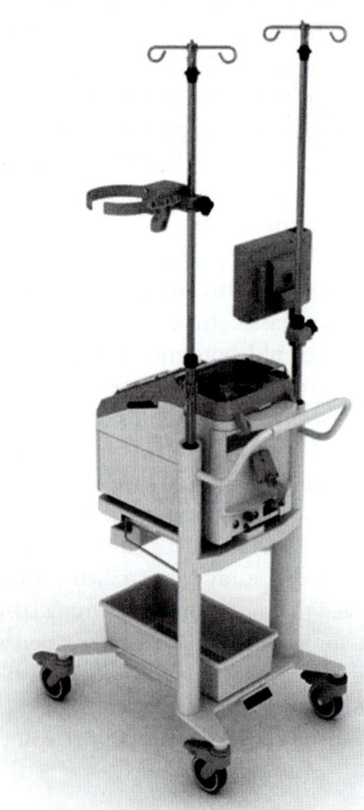

**Fig. 38.3** Initial rapid infusion system (RIS). (Reproduced with kind permission from Haemontics Corporation.)

in current transplantation practice as transfusion volumes have significantly diminished. Further, they occupy a large footprint in the operating room that has limited space. With time, commercial systems have become available and refined to meet today's demands.

An ideal RIS must be able to infuse large volumes of fluid rapidly (up to 1,500 mL/min) at normothermia. There must be accurate control of fluid infusion rates and temperature. Initial commercial systems used coiled tubing in water baths, heating plates, or a countercurrent exchange mechanism to heat the infusing fluid (Haemonetics RIS, Level 1). Some of these devices had limited capabilities to heat fluids at high flow rates and as a consequence infusate temperature could be substantially reduced (Kempen et al., 2000; Barcelona et al., 2003). Newer systems heat fluid by electromagnetic induction (FMS 2000, Belmont) or dry thermal technology (ThermaCor 1200) and have an improved capability to deliver warm fluids at high flows. In addition to providing rapid infusion, an RIS should be able to bolus fluid safely. Either a roller-pump or pressure infuser controls flow in contemporary systems. A semi-occlusive roller-pump enables more accurate determination of flow rates than automatic pressurized systems. Large-bore intravenous access facilitates rapid infusion and either central veins or access in veins that can be viewed and monitored is advised.

The system must be simple to set up, when speed may be of the essence and to minimize the risk of error. The operator and anaesthetist must be aware and alert to potential errors with the machine's use. In high-pressure systems, extravasation of fluid and tissue damage may occur. Inadvertent fluid recirculation rather than infusion into the patient has been reported with the Haemonetics machine (Kempen et al., 2000). This can only occur in systems that have a recirculation circuit. Inadvertent preferential filling of empty infusion bags can occur with other systems if lines are left unclamped, and exsanguination of the patient can occur when the RIS is disconnected from large-bore venous access if clamps and caps are not routinely applied.

Air embolism is well documented with RIS and fatal cases have been reported (Linden et al., 1997; Adhikary and Massey, 1998). The Level 1 and Ranger systems have gas-permeable membranes of 0.57 and 17.7 $cm^2$, respectively, that vent air. The Ranger system membrane's larger surface area enables more effective venting of air (Eaton and Dhillon, 2003), but if pressurized neither system can remove all air (Schoor et al., 2004; Zoremba et al., 2011). Since 2002 the manufacturers of the Level 1 have made available an ultrasonic air detector and automatic line clamp that is designed to prevent air embolism (TGA Australia). The FMS 2000 has two ultrasonic air detectors. The first is located after the fluid chamber, running from the fluid bags and prior to the roller-pump, and the second in-line air detector monitors air that may enter the patient line (Kempen et al., 2000). Fast simple de-airing of the machines will ensure fluid infusion is not interrupted for significant time periods.

Other safety features have been incorporated to help prevent patient harm. In addition to air detection and elimination, the system should monitor line pressure and reduce roller-pump speed and infusion rates at increasing pressure; have high-pressure alarms and stop infusing when the line pressure exceeds a given value; have temperature monitoring to prevent overheating of fluid; and have a simple mechanism to filter and remove debris.

The decision of what system to buy for a transplant unit will depend upon the physicians' requirements, initial cost outlay, and the cost of consumables as well as the functional and safety characteristics mentioned above.

## Renal replacement therapy

Renal replacement therapy (RRT) describes a range of treatments that are available for the management of patients with acute renal failure, fluid overload, and metabolic instability. Intermittent haemodialysis and CRRT are the most frequently used. CRRT affords more gradual metabolic control and fluid removal that may be advantageous in the unstable patient. RRT also facilitates in electrolyte management and nutritional support (Petroni and Cohen, 2002).

Renal insufficiency is a common finding (~ 25%) in patients with advanced liver disease and cirrhosis (Blackwell et al., 2003). The causes of renal dysfunction in liver disease include HRS, acute tubular necrosis (ATN), glomerular disease (e.g. associated with viral hepatitis, alcohol, amyloid, diabetes, and hypertension), tubulo-interstitial disease (e.g. associated with primary biliary cirrhosis), and renal impairment due to primary graft non-function after liver transplantation (Davenport, 2009a). The importance of renal disease and its negative impact on patients with advanced cirrhosis was highlighted with the introduction of the MELD score in 2002. The MELD scoring system applies a weighting for renal impairment (but not structural kidney disease) and has resulted in patients with renal impairment being prioritized for liver transplantation (Ginés and Schrier, 2009). Acute renal failure requiring CRRT in patients awaiting transplant is a predictor of mortality (65%) and also portends a worse clinical outcome following transplantation (Wong et al., 2005). Zand et al. (2011) demonstrated that postoperative haemodialysis is a risk factor for long-term mortality, with only 37% patient survival at 5 years after liver transplantation.

The indications for CRRT are well defined (see Table 38.1). Large-volume transfusion, haemodynamic instability, and metabolic derangement may worsen renal function among patients with pre-existing renal disease. CRRT can afford better control of acid-base status and electrolyte abnormalities and facilitate volume management in patients. However, there is a paucity of evidence for the introduction of CRRT intraoperatively in OLT. Townsend et al. (2009) demonstrated the feasibility of CRRT

**Table 38.1** Indications for continuous renal replacement therapy. These indications do not only pertain to liver transplant patients (Adapted from Petroni K and Cohen N, 'Continuous Renal Replacement Therapy: Anesthetic Implications', *Anesthesia & Analgesia*, 94, 5, pp. 1288–1297, copyright 2002, with permission from Wolters Kluwer Health, Inc. and International Anesthesia Research Society)

| Renal | Non-renal |
|---|---|
| Uraemia | Increased intracranial pressure |
| Hyperkalaemia | Congestive heart failure |
| Metabolic acidosis | Pulmonary oedema |
| Fluid overload | Adult respiratory distress syndrome |
| | Multiple organ dysfunction syndrome |
| | Sepsis |

intraoperatively in a small retrospective observational study, but the decision for dialysis was based on non-specific criteria. The patients who received CRRT had high MELD score (> 30), pre-existing renal dysfunction (AKI or established CRRT), high lactate, and other evidence of organ dysfunction (ventilator or inotrope dependence). The decision to continue CRRT in patients from the ICU with established renal failure is less contentious.

## Principles of continuous renal replacement therapy

There are three processes underlying RRT: ultrafiltration, convection, and diffusion. Ultrafiltration and convection are linked processes (see Figure 38.4). Ultrafiltration is the process by which water is transported across the semipermeable membrane by a transmembrane pressure gradient (the difference between hydrostatic pressure and plasma oncotic pressure). The water permeability and surface area of the membrane, as well as the transmembrane pressure gradient, influences the rate of filtration. In convection, fluid moving across the semipermeable membrane carries with it a solute. This process is known as 'solvent drag'. The size of the solute transported across is limited by membrane pore size. Increasing the ultrafiltration rate allows more fluid and thus more solute to be 'dragged' across the membrane (O'Reilly and Tolwani, 2005).

Diffusion and convection describe the movement of solute across a semipermeable membrane. In diffusion, solutes move from a high to a low concentration (see Figure 38.5). This electrochemical concentration gradient is generated by countercurrent flow of a dialysate (solution containing electrolytes) along the length of the membrane. Factors that influence the rate of solute diffusion include rate of blood flow, rate of dialysate flow, concentration gradient across the membrane, size of the solute, duration of treatment, membrane surface area, and pore size (Bellomo, 2009).

Table 38.2 describes the most commonly used modes of CRRT in critically ill patients and the intraoperative setting. CVVH results in the removal of large amounts of solute and water due to high ultrafiltration rate (UFR), leading to volume contraction that may lead to hypotension and loss of electrolytes. Replacement fluid is thus given to avoid hypovolaemia and to replenish desired solutes prior to blood return to the patient. In CVVHD, solutes can be either removed from or transferred to the patient, depending on their concentration in the dialysate (Figure 38.5). The blood flow rate is faster than the countercurrent dialysate flow, to avoid equilibration. Dialysate can be administered with or without fluid removal from the patient. CVVHDF is a combination of CVVH and CVVHD (see Figures 38.6 and 38.7). To date there are no convincing clinical data to support one mode of CRRT over another (Antoun and Palevsky, 2009).

Replacement fluids can be administered prefilter or postfilter. The advantage of prefilter replacement is decreased risk of filter clotting, but solute clearance is reduced due to dilution of solutes in the blood, which in turn reduces the concentration gradient. Postfilter replacement results in increased risk of filter clotting due to haemoconcentration within the filter (O'Reilly and Tolwani, 2005). Fluid removal rates are calculated independently of replacement fluid rates.

CRRT modalities commonly used are shown in Table 38.2. Those not routinely used in the setting of liver failure include peritoneal dialysis, slow continuous ultrafiltration (SCUF), continuous arteriovenous haemofiltration (CAVH), continuous arteriovenous haemodialysis (CAVHD) and continuous arteriovenous haemodiafiltration (CAVHDF).

## Requirements for continuous renal replacement therapy

### Vascular access

To undertake CRRT, a double-lumen haemodialysis catheter must be placed in a central vein (internal jugular, subclavian, or femoral). The catheters range between sizes 11 and 14 French, with the inflow and outflow lumens arranged in a coaxial manner or side by side. For intraoperative use it is preferable to have the catheter in an internal jugular vein. Attempted insertion into a subclavian vein may result in a pneumothorax or bleeding, particularly in the coagulopathic patient. Thrombocytopaenia or coagulopathy may need to be corrected prior to catheter insertion. Femoral catheters are difficult to access, cannot be visualized under surgical drapes, and are less desirable. Catheter malfunction can result in poor flows and high pressure that may lead to inadequate haemodialysis. Malfunction can be attributed to kinking, malposition, intraluminal thrombus, or a fibrin sheath around the catheter tip (Vijayan, 2009).

### Dialysis machine and fluids

The choice of dialysis machine is usually made at an institutional level. A variety of commercial machines are available (see Table 38.3). The unit consists of an extracorporeal circuit, a haemofilter, a blood pump, and a variety of other fluid pumps. With

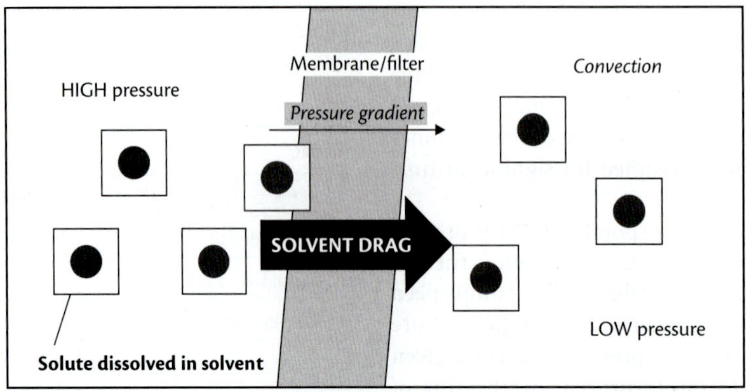


**Fig. 38.4** Ultrafiltration and convection during CRRT. (Courtesy of Patrick Neligan, Department of Intensive Care, University College Hospital, Galway, Ireland.)

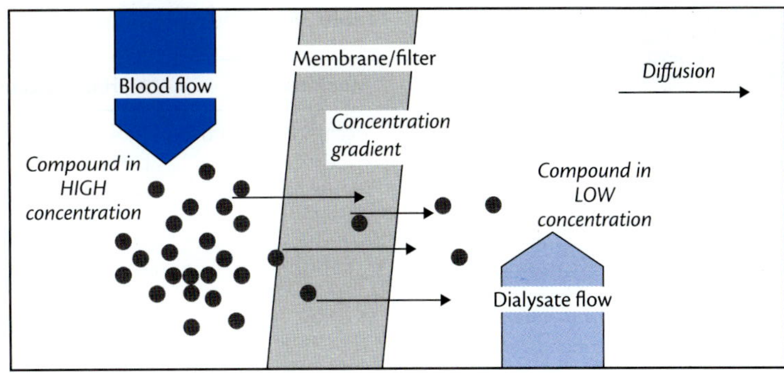


**Fig. 38.5** Diffusion (dialysis). (Courtesy of Patrick Neligan, Department of Intensive Care, University College Hospital, Galway, Ireland.)

specific CRRT modes, dialysate and replacement pumps may also be integrated. The safety features of the machines include pressure transducers, an air trap, and blood leak detectors that are all connected to alarms (see Table 38.4). In the operating room, long extension lines are needed to allow for additional space between the sterile field and the machine. As a consequence of long extension lines, hypothermia may result. Additional primed filters and consumables must also be readily available in the operating room.

There are many available commercial dialysate solutions. Customized solutions can also be made up by the hospital pharmacy. The concentration of the solutes will be ordered by the anaesthesiologist or nephrologist based on the needs of the patient. Sterility of the dialysate solution is essential. Contamination with bacteria or endotoxin can result in septic shock and cardiovascular collapse (Kraus, 2009). The dialysate solution requires buffering, with either lactate or bicarbonate. Patients with liver failure may be unable to adequately metabolize the extra lactate load. Bicarbonate-buffered solutions are an alternative. Bicarbonate solutions may confer improved haemodynamic stability with fewer cardiovascular events, particularly in patients with liver or cardiac dysfunction (Aucella et al., 2007). However, Agarwal et al. (2011) could demonstrate no difference in inotrope requirements or MAP in critically ill patients irrespective of whether bicarbonate or lactate was used. Further, lactate concentrations did not increase significantly during CRRT with lactate-buffered solutions in the liver failure group and control of acidosis was equivalent, whether lactate- or bicarbonate-based CRRT was used. Bicarbonate solutions are more expensive, have a higher risk of bacterial contamination, are unstable in the presence of calcium, and have a shorter shelf-life than lactate-based solutions.

**Table 38.2** Modes of continuous renal replacement therapy

| Mode | Solute removal | Molecule size | Dialysate | Replacement fluid |
|---|---|---|---|---|
| CVVH | Convection | Medium | No | Yes |
| CVVHD | Diffusion | Small | Yes | No |
| CVVHDF | Convection and diffusion | Small and medium | Yes | Yes |

CVVH, Continuous venovenous haemofiltration; CVVHD, continuous venovenous haemodialysis; CVVHDF, continuous venovenous haemodiafiltration.

## Circuit anticoagulation

Clotting within the dialysis circuit can lead to loss of blood, poor solute clearance, compromised electrolyte and acid-base balance, and inadequate volume management (O'Reilly and Tolwani, 2005). Anticoagulation is thus often necessary for the effective delivery of CRRT. Circuit anticoagulation is most commonly achieved with heparin, but this presents a challenge in patients with liver failure. CRRT without anticoagulation is feasible in patients with severe coagulopathies (Uchino et al., 2007). There are reports of intraoperative CRRT in OLT being undertaken successfully without anticoagulation (Townsend et al., 2009) and with regional citrate or prostacyclin. Prostacyclin causes vasodilation and hypotension, is expensive, and its routine use cannot be recommended at this time.

Citrate is infused into the blood at the beginning of the circuit. It exerts its anticoagulant activity by chelating ionized calcium. The majority of the citrate–calcium complex is filtered and the remainder returns to the patient and is metabolized to bicarbonate (and calcium) by the liver and other tissues (Tolwani and Wille,

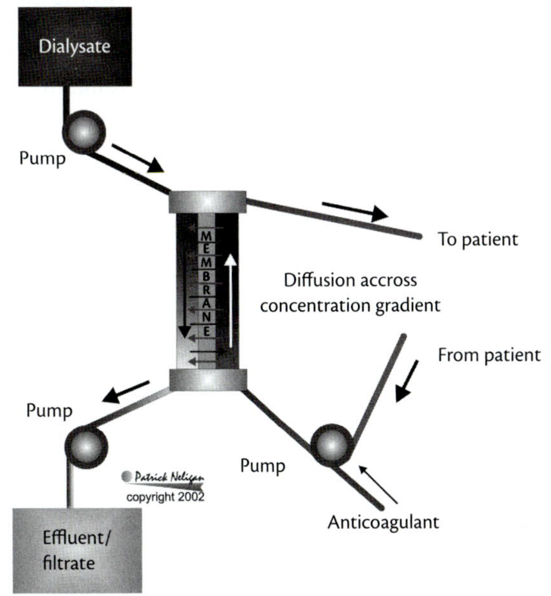


**Fig. 38.6** Continuous venovenous haemodialysis. (Courtesy of Patrick Neligan, Department of Intensive Care, University College Hospital, Galway, Ireland.)

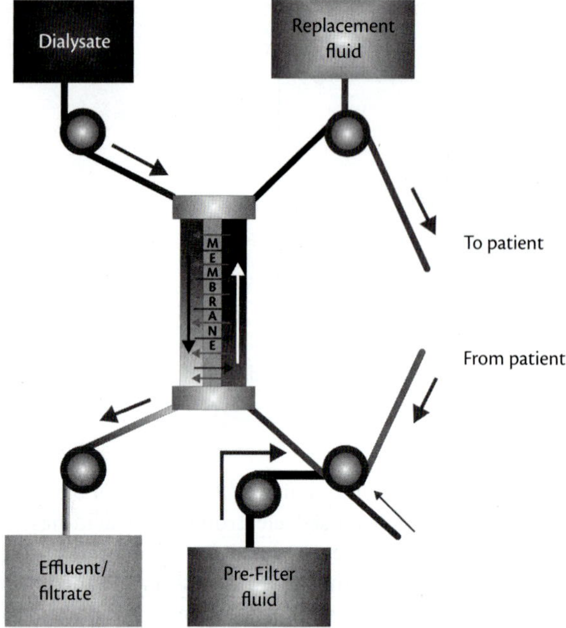


**Fig. 38.7** Continuous venovenous haemodialysis and filtration. (Courtesy of Patrick Neligan, Department of Intensive Care, University College Hospital, Galway, Ireland.)

2009). Most patients with liver disease adequately metabolize citrate, but it can accumulate and cause toxicity in patients with ALF and severe primary non-function (Agarwal and Davenport, 2009). Calcium must be infused into the patient whenever they are on citrate CRRT and careful monitoring of serum calcium levels is essential. This is of particular relevance in the intraoperative setting when large blood product transfusion may worsen the hypocalcaemia due to citrate exposure. Another option is regional anticoagulation of the dialysis circuit using heparin and protamine. The heparin in infused proximally prior to the filter and protamine is given either at the return lumen of the vascath or directly into the patient's other venous access. The dose of protamine is balanced to counter the heparin infused into the circuit and patient blood aPTT is performed to ensure the patient is not systemically anticoagulated.

## Operator

The equipment and the setup are the responsibility of the dialysis or ICU nurse, who is informed of the transplant start time. There are many challenges for the dialysis nurse, aside from working in an unfamiliar environment, often after-hours, and with limited clinical support. Communication with the transplant team is also essential and may be challenging due to a lack of familiarity. Therefore it is vitally important to maintain a core set of skilled and experienced nursing staff to perform CRRT intraoperatively. Nurses should be trained to independently assess and identify complications and be familiarized with the layout and functioning of the operating rooms. They need to be educated in the theoretical aspects of intraoperative dialysis and be provided with regular educational sessions (Henson and Carpenter, 2010). ICU nursing staff are an invaluable resource as they are already familiar with the running of CRRT in critically ill patients. The intraoperative dialysis prescription should be discussed regularly

**Table 38.3** Dialysis machines

| Machines | Modes |
|---|---|
| Prisma | CVVH, CVVHD, CVVHDF |
| Prisma Flex | CVVH, CVVHD, CVVHDF |
| Nx Stage | CVVH, CVVHD |
| Accura | CVVH, CVVHD, CVVHDF |
| B. Braun | CVVH, CVVHD, CVVHDF |
| Fresnius | CVVHD |

**Table 38.4** Troubleshooting

| Monitors | Alarms and cause | Troubleshooting |
|---|---|---|
| Access pressure from patient to machine (normally negative) | Excessive negative pressure due to occlusion | Check stop cocks, check for kinks<br>Check site for position or swelling<br>Position patient to decrease flexion at line insertion site<br>Flush port |
| Return pressure from machine to patient | Low pressure due to disconnection | Check all connections<br>Patient position change |
| | High pressure due to occlusion | Check stop cocks, check for kinks<br>Check site for position or swelling<br>Position patient to decrease flexion at line insertion site<br>Flush port |
| Filter pressure | Trend up or sudden increase due to clotting or clogged filter | Change filter |
| Blood leak detectors | Presence of blood, myoglobin, or bilirubin in effluent | Send sample of effluent to look for RBCs<br>Change filter |
| Bubble detector | Air in line—stops the blood pump | Large bubbles—reprime or change filter set<br>Undetectable bubbles—machine specific<br>Prevention—clear all air on priming, ensure connections are tight, use Luer-lock connectors |
| Fluid and effluent pump | Fluid—empty bag<br>Effluent—full bag | Ensure all clampsopen<br>Ensure bags properly spiked |

with the consultant anaesthesiologist and adjusted according to hourly blood gases and serum biochemistry. The anaesthesiologist must also have a thorough understanding of the procedure to be able to direct and adjust therapies. Transplant anaesthesiologists themselves may need to be trained in the basic operation and maintenance of the system.

### Intraoperative continuous renal replacement therapy

Throughout the procedure, the operator and the anaesthesiologist must be vigilant in monitoring the CRRT circuit to ensure disruptions do not occur. There are multiple alarms that monitor pressure and flow built into the dialysis machine that will signal both mechanical and functional problems (see Table 38.5) (Boyle and Baldwin, 2010). Blood loss can be caused by filter clotting, inadvertent disconnection, blood-filter leakage, or the vascular access site. Hypothermia can be prevented by in-line heating within the circuit either via the dialysis machine itself or through a Ranger pressure infusion system (maximum flow rate 500 mL/min) on the return line. The addition of space blankets around extension lines can further mitigate against heat loss. The effect of CRRT on intraoperative intravenous drug dosing should also be taken into consideration even though most drugs can be safely titrated to clinical effect. Drugs that are not eliminated by the kidney are unlikely to be removed during CRRT and thus will not require dose adjustment. The available literature on clearance of individual drugs with CRRT is limited and correct dosing is made more difficult due to the disturbed pharmacokinetics in critically ill patients. The dose of antibiotic prophylaxis need not be corrected for renal impairment.

### Special considerations for intraoperative continuous renal replacement therapy

#### *Metabolic acidosis*

Lactic acidosis is defined as an increased anion gap metabolic acidosis with pH < 7.35 and lactate > 5 mmol/L (Vitin et al., 2010). The liver is primarily responsible for lactate clearance. Lactic acidosis is common in ALF. Further, patients undergoing liver transplantation develop a lactic acidosis that commences during the dissection phase and worsens during the anhepatic phase (Sedra and Strum, 2011). The development of this acidosis is multifactorial. Vascular clamping, use of catecholamines and anaesthetic agent that result in reduction of hepatic blood flow, tissue hypoxia, and hypothermia may all contribute (Vitin et al., 2010). The fixed minute volume of mechanical ventilation makes the degree of acidosis worse and in the presence of renal failure more difficult to reverse or correct. CRRT can be used for management and correction of intraoperative metabolic acidosis during liver transplant surgery.

#### *Hyperkalaemia*

Hyperkalaemia is a major contributing factor to the haemodynamic instability following reperfusion of the transplanted liver. It can manifest as bradycardia, hypotension, and life-threatening dysrhythmias. The severity of the instability depends on several other factors including cross-clamp time, quality of the donor graft, and pre-existing recipient comorbidities. High potassium concentrations during liver transplant can be caused or exacerbated by pre-existing renal impairment or failure, high concentration of potassium in the preservation solution, acidosis, and high potassium load from blood and blood product transfusion (Sedra and Strum, 2011). Xia et al. (2007) identified factors associated with hyperkalaemia at three different time points during liver transplantation (see Table 38.6). Intraoperative CRRT facilitates control of potassium over time, but it should not be relied upon for the treatment of acute hyperkalaemia as potassium removal via haemodialysis is time dependent. Measurement of potassium is of great importance, especially just prior to reperfusion of the transplanted liver, and evidence of hyperkalaemia should be treated by the administration of calcium and then insulin-glucose or bicarbonate to drive intracellular uptake of potassium. Other methods such as washing of blood-banked products prior to infusion (using cell salvage equipment) may also be employed to curtail rises in potassium.

#### *Volume management*

During liver transplantation large volumes of blood products, colloids, and crystalloids may be administered. In the presence of renal impairment with oliguria or anuria, the management of a transplant candidate's volume status becomes a challenge. Invasive haemodynamic monitoring and TOE guide monitoring of intravascular volume help determine fluid replacement intraoperatively. CRRT may be used to facilitate volume removal in oliguric/anuric patients. High central pressures may translate to congestion of the transplanted liver and impair graft function. Most commonly, euvolaemia is achieved during intraoperative dialysis. The anaesthesiologist needs to have an accurate record of the total amount of fluids given to the patient and relate this to the dialysis nurse. Townsend et al. (2009) reviewed 41 patients who had intraoperative dialysis and found that 92.7% of them achieved an even or negative intraoperative balance with careful fluid management.

**Table 38.5** Problems with continuous renal replacement therapy

| Mechanical | Functional |
|---|---|
| Disconnection | Circuit/filter clotting |
| Air embolism | Haemorrhage |
| Catheter and circuit kinking | Citrate toxicity |
| Insufficient blood flow | Electrolyte imbalance |
| | Hypothermia |
| | Intraoperative drug dosing |

**Table 38.6** Factors associated with hyperkalaemia at three different time points

| Time point | Factors associated with increased potassium |
|---|---|
| 2 hours before reperfusion | Transfusion > 5 units of RBCs |
| 15 minutes after reperfusion | DCD donor |
| 1 hour after reperfusion | Intraoperative urine output < 500 mL |
| | Use of VVB |
| | Warm ischaemia time > 50 minutes |
| | Donor hospital stay > 5 days |

### Acute liver failure

Acute renal failure is common in patients with ALF. Acute renal failure also contributes to worsened prognosis and mortality in ALF patients (Polson and Lee, 2005). ALF may result in increased ICP secondary to cerebral oedema. Elevated ICP is the primary cause of morbidity and mortality in these patients (Stravitz et al., 2007). Intermittent haemodialysis is poorly tolerated in ALF and may exacerbate rises in ICP. CRRT is better tolerated in ALF due to slower changes in plasma osmolality and greater cardiovascular stability (Davenport, 2009b). CRRT initiated in the ICU should be continued in the intraoperative period to facilitate fluid volume, electrolyte, and acid-base management. Currently there are no specific criteria to start RRT in patients with ALF, but the decision should be based on the degree of renal dysfunction, fluid balance, and metabolic derangements.

## Conclusion

This chapter has covered specialized equipment used during transplantation and other major non-transplant surgery in patients exposed to major blood loss and in critically ill patients with renal failure and significant electrolyte and metabolic derangements. Intraoperative red blood cell salvage is used to reduce exposure to allogeneic blood products (with its attendant risks) and to reduce demands upon the limited resources of blood banks. Rapid infusion systems were developed during the advent of liver transplantation, and systems have been modified and improved to meet changing requirements. The section on renal replacement therapy describes a range of treatment modalities used to manage metabolic derangements, fluid overload, and electrolyte disturbances in critically ill patients, with a focus primarily on the care of patients presenting for liver transplantation.

## References


Adhikary GS, Massey SR (1998) Massive air embolism: a case report. *J Clin Anesth*, **10**(1):70–72.

Agarwal B, Davenport A (2009) Renal replacement therapy in patients undergoing liver transplantation. *US Nephrol*, **4**(2):64–68.

Agarwal B, Kovari F, Saha R, Shaw S, Davenport A (2011) Do bicarbonate-based solutions for continuous renal replacement therapy offer better control of metabolic acidosis than lactate-containing fluids? *Nephron Clin Prac*, **118**:392–398.

Antoun TA, Palevsky PM (2009) Selection of modality of renal replacement therapy. *Semin Dialysis*, **22**(2):108–113.

Ashworth A, Klein AA (2010) Cell salvage as part of a blood conservation strategy in anaesthesia, *Br J Anaesth*, **105**(4):401–416.

Aucella F, Di Paolo S, Gesualdo L (2007) Dialysate and replacement fluid composition for CRRT. *Contrib Nephrol*, **156**:287–296.

Barcelona SL, Vilich F, Coté CJ (2003) A comparison of flow rates and warming capabilities of the level 1 and rapid infusion system with various-size intravenous catheters. *Anesth Analg*, **97**(2):358–363.

Bellomo R (2009) Dialytic therapies. In: Bersten A, Soni N (eds) *Oh's Intensive Care Manual*, 7th edn, pp. 515–518. Elsevier, Amsterdam.

Blackwell MM, Chavin KD, Sistino JJ (2003) Perioperative perfusion strategies for optimal fluid management in liver transplant recipients with renal insufficiency. *Perfusion*, **18**:55–60.

Bowley DM, Barker P, Boffard KD (2006) Intraoperative blood salvage in penetrating abdominal trauma: a randomized, controlled trial. *World J Surg*, **30**(6):1074–1080.

Boyle M, Baldwin I (2010) Understanding the continuous renal replacement therapy circuit for acute renal failure support. *AACN Adv Crit Care*, **21**(4):367–375.

Burman JF, Westlake AS, Davidson SJ, et al. (2002) Study of five cell salvage machines in coronary artery surgery. *Transfusion Med*, **12**(3):173–179.

Catling S, Williams S, Freites O, Rees M, Davies C, Hopkins L (2008) Use of a leucocyte filter to remove tumor cells from intra-operative cell salvage blood. *Anaesthesia*, **63**(12):1332–1338.

Council of Scientific Affairs (1986) Autologous blood transfusions. *J Am Med Assoc*, **256**:2378–2380.

Davenport A (2009a) Continuous renal replacement therapies in patients with liver disease. *Semin Dialysis*, **22**(2):169–172.

Davenport A (2009b) Continuous renal replacement therapies in patients with acute neurological injury. *Semin Dialysis*, **22**(2):165–168.

De Boer, Christensen MC, Asmussen M, et al. (2008) The impact of intraoperative transfusion of platelets and red blood cells on survival after liver transplantation. *Anesth Analg*, **106**(1):32–44.

Duffy G, Tolley K (1997) Cost analysis of autologous blood transfusion, using cell salvage, compared with allogeneic blood transfusion. *Transfus Med*, **7**(3):189–196.

Dzik WH, Jenkins R (1985 ) Use of intraoperative blood salvage during orthotopic liver transplantation. *Arch Surg*, **120**(8):946–948.

Eaton MP, Dhillon AK (2003) Relative performance of the level 1 and Ranger pressure infusion devices. *Anesth Analg*, **97**(4):1074–1077.

Esper SA, Waters JH (2011) Intra-operative cell salvage: a fresh look at the indications and contraindications. *Blood Transfus*, **9**(2):139–147.

Ezzedine H, Baele P, Robert A (1991) Bacteriologic quality of intraoperative autotransfusion. *Surgery*, **109**:259.

Feltracco P, Michieletto E, Barbieri S, et al. (2007) Microbiologic contamination of intraoperative blood salvaged during liver transplantation. *Transplant Proc*, **39**(6):1889–91.

Fergusson D, Khanna MP, Tinmouth A, Hébert PC (2004) Transfusion of leukoreduced red blood cells may decrease postoperative infections: two meta-analyses of randomized controlled trials. *Can J Anaesth*, **51**(5):417–424.

Findlay JY, Retke SR (2000 ) Poor prediction of blood transfusion requirements in adult liver transplantations from preoperative variables. *J Clin Anesth*, **12**(4):319–323.

Foltys D, Linkermann A, Heumann A, et al. (2009) Organ recipients suffering from undifferentiated neuroendocrine small-cell carcinoma of donor origin: a case report. *Transplant Proc*, **41**(6):2639–2642.

Foltys DB, Zimmerman T, Heise M, et al. (2011) Liver transplantation for hepatocellular carcinoma—is there a risk of recurrence caused by intraoperative cell salvage autotransfusion? *Eur Surg Res*, **47**(3):182–187.

Fujimoto J, Okamoto E, Yamanaka N, et al. (1991) Autotransfusion in hepatectomy for hepatocellular carcinoma. *Nippon Geka Gakkai Zasshi*, **92**(7):825–830.

Ginés P, Schrier RW (2009) Renal failure in cirrhosis. *N Engl J Med*, **36**:1279–1290.

Gwak MS, Lee KW, Kim SY, et al. (2005) Can a leukocyte depletion filter (LDF) reduce the risk of reintroduction of hepatocellular carcinoma cells? *Liver Transplant*, **11**(3):331–335.

Henson A, Carpenter S (2010) Intra-operative hemodialysis during liver transplantation: an expanded role of the nephrology nurse. *Nephrol Nurs J*, **37**(4):351–354, 356

Jeng JC, Boyd TM, Jablonski KA, Harviel JD, Jordan MH (1998) Intraoperative blood salvage in excisional burn surgery: an analysis of yield, bacteriology and inflammatory mediators. *J Burn Care Rehab*, **19**:305–311

Jones CC, Stammers AH, Fristoe LW, et al. (1999) Removal of hepatocarcinoma cells from blood via cell washing and filtration techniques. *J Extra Corporeal Technol*, **31**(4):169–176.

Kang Y, Aggarwal S, Virji M, et al. (1991) Clinical evaluation of autotransfusion during liver transplantation. *Anesth Analg*, **72**(1):94–100.

Kar S, Carr BI (1995) Detection of liver cells in peripheral blood of patients with advanced-stage hepatocellular carcinoma. *Hepatology*, **21**(2):403–407.

Kempen PM, Hudson ME, Planinsic RM (2000) The rapid infusion system: user error in tubing connection mimicking severe hemorrhage. *Anesthesiology*, **93**(1):278–279.

Kemper RR, Menitove JE, Hanto DW (1997) Cost analysis of intraoperative blood salvage during orthotopic liver transplantation. *Liver Transplant Surg*, **3**(5):513–517.

Koch CG, Li L, Duncan AI, et al. (2006) Morbidity and mortality risk associated with red blood cell and blood-component transfusion in isolated coronary artery bypass grafting. *Crit Care Med*, **34**:1608–1616.

Kraus MA (2009) Selection of dialysate and replacement fluids and management of electrolyte and acid-base disturbances. *Semin Dialysis*, **22**(2):137–140.

Kudo H, Fujita H, Hanada Y, Hayami H, Kondoh T, Kohmura E (2004) Cytological and bacteriological studies of intraoperative autologous blood in neurosurgery. *Surg Neurol*, **62**(3):195–199.

Liang TB, Li DL, Liang L, et al. (2008) Intraoperative blood salvage during liver transplantation in patients with hepatocellular carcinoma: efficiency of leukocyte depletion filters in the removal of tumor cells. *Transplantation*, **85**(6):863–869.

Liang TB, Li JJ, Li DL, Liang L, Bai XL, Zheng SS (2010) Intraoperative blood salvage and leukocyte depletion during liver transplantation with bacterial contamination. *Clin Transplant*, **24**(2):265–272.

Linden JV, Kaplan HS, Murphy MT (1997) Fatal air embolism due to perioperative blood recovery. *Anesth Analg*, **84**(2):422–426.

Mangus RS, Kinsella SB, Nobari MM, et al. (2007) Predictors of blood products use in orthotopic liver transplantation using the piggyback hepatectomy technique. *Transplant Proc*, **39**(10):3207–3213.

Margarit C, Charco R, Hildago E, Allende H, Castell S, Bilbao I (2002) Liver transplantation for malignant disease: selection and pattern of recurrence. *World J Surg*, **26**:257.

Marsh JW, Dvorchik I, Subotin M, et al. (1997) The prediction of risk of recurrence and time to recurrence of hepatocellular carcinoma after orthotopic liver transplantation. *Hepatology*, **26**(2):444–450.

Massicotte L, Sassine MP, Lenis S, Seal RF, Roy A (2005) Survival rate changes with transfusion of blood products during liver transplantation. *Can J Anaesth*, **52**(2):148–155.

Massicotte L, Lenis S, Thibeault L, Sassine MP, Seal RF, Roy A (2006) Effect of low central venous pressure and phlebotomy on blood product transfusion requirements during liver transplantations. *Liver Transplant*, **12**(1):117–123.

Massicotte L, Thibeault L, Beaulieu D, Roy JD, Roy A (2007) Evaluation of cell salvage autotransfusion utility during liver transplantation. *HPB (Oxford)*, **9**(1):52–57.

Mazzaferro V, Llovet JM, Miceli R, et al. (2009) Predicting survival after liver transplantation in patients with hepatocellular carcinoma beyond the Milan criteria: a retrospective, exploratory analysis. *Lancet Oncol*, **10**(1):35–43.

Muscari F, Suc B, Vigouroux D, et al. (2005) Blood salvage autotransfusion during transplantation for hepatocarcinoma: does it increase the risk of neoplastic recurrence? *Transplant Int*, **18**(11):1236–1239.

Naumenko KS, Kim SF, Cherkanova MS, Naumenko SE (2008) The Haemonetics Cell Saver 5 washing properties: effect of different washing pump and centrifuge speeds. *Interact Cardiovasc Thorac Surg*, **7**(5):759–763.

NICE (2008) *Intraoperative Red Blood Cell Salvage During Radical Prostatectomy or Radical Cystectomy IPG 258 2008*. <http://publications.nice.org.uk/ipg258>.

Nieder AM, Carmack AJ, Sved PD, Kim SS, Manoharan M, Soloway MS (2005) Intraoperative cell salvage during radical prostatectomy is not associated with greater biochemical recurrence rate. *Urology*, **65**(4):730–734.

O'Reilly P, Tolwani A (2005) Renal replacement therapy III: IHD, CRRT, SLED. *Crit Care Clin*, **21**:367–378.

Ozmen V, McSwain NE, Nichols RL, Smith J, Flint LM (1992) Autotransfusion of potentially culture-positive blood in abdominal trauma: preliminary data from a prospective study. *J Trauma*, **32**:36–9.

Petroni KC, Cohen NH (2002) Continuous renal replacement therapy: anesthetic implications. *Anesth Analg*, **94**:1288–1297.

Phillips SD, Maguire D, Deshpande R, et al. (2006) A prospective study investigating the cost effectiveness of intraoperative blood salvage during liver transplantation, *Transplant*, **81**(4):536–540.

Polson J, Lee WM (2005) AASLD position paper: the management of acute liver failure. *Hepatology*, **41**:1179–1197.

Sedra AH, Strum S (2011) The role of intraoperative hemodialysis in liver transplant patients. *Curr Opin Organ Transplant*, **16**:323–325.

Shander A, Hofmann A, Gombotz H, Theusinger OM, Spahn DR (2007) Estimating the cost of blood: past, present, and future directions. *Best Practice Res Clin Anaesth*, **21**(2):271–289.

Steneker I, van Luyn MJ, van Wachem PB, Biewenga J (1992) Electron microscopic examination of white cell reduction by four white cell-reduction filters. *Transfusion*, **32**:450–457.

Stoffel JT, Topjian L, Libertino JA (2005) Analysis of peripheral blood for prostate cells after autologous transfusion given during radical prostatectomy. *Br J Urol Int*, **96**(3):313–315.

Stravitz RT, Kramer AH, Davern T, et al. (2007) Intensive care of patients with acute liver failure: recommendations of the US Acute Liver Failure Study Group. *Crit Care Med*, **35**(11):2498–2508.

Tolwani AJ, Wille KM (2009) Anticoagulation for continuous renal replacement therapy. *Semin Dialysis*, **22**(2):141–145.

Townsend DR, Bagshaw, SM, Jacka MJ, Bigam D, Cave D, Gibney RTN (2009) Intraoperative renal support during liver transplantation. *Liver Transplant*, **15**:73–78.

Uchino S, Bellomo R, Morimatsu H, et al. (2007) Continuous renal replacement therapy: a worldwide practice survey. *Intens Care Med*, **33**:1563–1570.

Van Voorst SJ, Peters TG, Williams JW, Vera SR, Britt LG (1985) Autotransfusion in hepatic transplantation. *Am J Surg*, **51**:623–626.

Vijayan A (2009) Vascular access for continuous renal replacement therapy. *Semin Dialysis*, **22**(2):133–136.

Vitin A, Muczynski K, Bakthavatsalam R, Martay K, Dembo G (2010) Treatment of severe lactic acidosis during the pre-anhepatic stage of liver transplant surgery with intraoperative hemodialysis. *J Clin Anesth*, **22**:466–472.

Waters JH, Tuohy MJ, Hobson DF, Procop G (2003) Bacterial reduction by cell salvage washing and leukocyte depletion filtration. *Anesthesiology*, **99**(3):652–655.

Williamson KR, Taswell HF, Rettke SR, Krom RA (1989) Intraoperative autologous transfusion: its role in orthotopic liver transplantation. *Mayo Clin Proc*, **64**(3):340–345.

Wong LP, Blackley MP, Andreoni KA, Chin H, Falk RJ, Klemmer PJ (2005) Survival of liver transplant candidates with acute renal failure receiving renal replacement therapy. *Kidney Int*, **68**:362–370.

Xia VW, Ghobrial RM, Du B, et al. (2007) Predictors of hyperkalemia in the prereperfusion, early postreperfusion and late postreperfusion periods during adult liver transplantation. *Anesth Analg*, **105**(3):780–785.

Yokoyama I, Carr B, Saitsu H, Iwatsuki S, Starzl TE (1991) Accelerated growth rates of recurrent hepatocellular carcinoma after liver transplantation. *Cancer*, **68**(10):2095–2100.

Zand MS, Orloff MS, Abt P, et al. (2011) High mortality in orthotopic liver transplant recipients who require hemodialysis. *Clin Transplant*, **25**:213–221.

Zoremba N, Gruenewald C, Zoremba M, Rossaint R, Schaelte G (2011) Air elimination capability in rapid infusion systems. *Anaesthesia*, **66**(11):1031–1034.

# CHAPTER 39

# Anaesthesia for non-transplant surgery in the organ transplant recipient

Luz Aguina and Ernesto A. Pretto, Jr.

## Introduction

According to the OPTN, in the US over 59,000 patients received a transplanted organ in 2014 alone (OPTN, 2015). Post-transplant survival ranges between 60 and 90% at 5 years, with good functional outcome. In general, 50% of organ transplant recipients enjoy good quality of life and return to work. However, restoration of pretransplant functionality is highly dependent on the organ transplanted. For example, 61.5% of kidney transplant recipients, 57% of liver recipients, and 37% of lung transplant recipients experience full recovery (Paris et al., 1998). Irrespective of functionality, all transplant recipients require some form of immunosuppression. Immunosuppressive agents may cause side effects. Patients may experience episodes of infection, which may lead to changes in health status. In fact, post-transplant status can be considered a new chronic illness that can affect physiological function, requiringa tailored anaesthetic management plan (Keegan and Plevak, 2004). Since the post-transplant period constitutes a new complex state, the transplant recipient deserves meticulous attention during preoperative preparation and during anaesthetic management for non-transplant surgery.

These patients may need re-operation for early or late complications of post-transplant surgery, or require elective diagnostic and surgical procedures, or suffer traumatic events or other emergencies (Karam et al., 2003). From the simplest procedures to the higher risk ones, the transplanted population can represent a challenge for the anaesthesia provider.

## Perioperative management

In general, preoperative evaluation and screening of the transplant recipient for non-transplant surgery should be guided by the medical and surgical history of the organ transplanted, as well as the risks of the planned surgical procedure. Transplant recipients in most cases experience a protracted state of end-stage organ disease prior to transplantation. Depending on the duration and severity of end-stage illness, secondary organ function may be compromised, particularly cardiovascular (CAD) and pulmonary (i.e. portopulmonary hypertension) complications. Therefore meticulous cardiopulmonary screening is mandatory. A few patients will receive a transplant in the early stages of the disease, such as in the case of malignancies (i.e. hepatocellular carcinoma), and will present in relatively good health. But the majority will be transplanted in the late stages of end-stage organ disease, with multiple systems affected, and, in some instances, poor nutritional status. However, many of the non-functional and systemic organ-related complications are corrected with successful transplantation (Gohn and Warren, 2006).

A complete blood count (CBC) should be performed in every transplanted patient, as well as establishment of baseline coagulation status (PT-INR, PTT, and platelet count) prior to surgery. *Anaemia* is a common denominator in solid organ transplant recipients and is multifactorial, commonly associated with a variety of related chronic conditions, such as poor nutrition, kidney dysfunction and failure, haemodilution, hypersplenism, and the side effects of immunosuppressive or anti-infective medications, among other non-specific causes. In a recent study, upwards of 30% of transplant recipients were found to have haemoglobin concentrations below 12 g/dL (Malyszko et al., 2012). *Thrombocytopaenia* secondary to hypersplenism is another common finding among patients with cirrhosis and ESLD in liver transplantation. It may also result from immunosuppressors (Gohn, 2006). It is important to note that transplanted patients as a group experience some degree of *renal insufficiency*. The incidence of renal insufficiency varies with the organ transplanted but is estimated at 18% of liver recipients, 32% of heart recipients, and 20% of lung recipients (Ojo et al., 2003). Approximately 29% of patients on long-term CNI therapy will eventually progress to ESRD and require RRT.

Metabolic assessment is important in the preoperative evaluation of the transplant recipient, especially electrolytes (serum $Na^{+}$, $Ca^{2+}$, $K^{+}$, and $Mg^{2+}$), acid-base status, and serum BUN and Cr levels. Patients receiving RRT should be dialysed as close to the day of surgery as possible, to correct these values. Intestinal transplant recipients with or without indwelling catheters for supplemental TPN can be suffering from *diarrhoea* or *dehydration* and *hypercoagulation* or *thrombosis*. Diarrhoea and dehydration can result in electrolyte imbalances, as well as acid-base disturbances (Kostopanagiotou et al., 2008). Thrombosis can create vascular access problems. Metabolic alterations may be chronic or reflect an acute underlying condition, such as infection with or without septicaemia or graft thrombosis. In the liver transplant recipient, standard LFTs should be evaluated (AST, ALT, bilirubin, and PT/PTT).

Transplanted patients receive routine immunosuppressive medications that may aggravate risk factors for CAD, such as *hypertension, hyperlipidaemia* and *diabetes.* As a result, CAD is highly prevalent and multifactorial in the transplant population and it is not reversible after transplantation. For this reason, careful cardiovascular evaluation and screening is paramount. Among kidney transplant recipients younger than 45 years of age, perioperative cardiovascular mortality is almost ten-fold higher than in older surgical patients (Foley et al., 1998). A review of cardiovascular indices within 30 days of surgery should be done. If more recent evaluation is warranted, this should be dictated by the patient's clinical status and the procedure to be undertaken. *Hyperglycaemia* requiring perioperative management for glycaemic control in any transplanted patient, including patients with a failed pancreatic graft, will be the same as in any diabetic patient. Hyperglycaemia in the setting of high-dose steroid immunosuppression is a common finding among transplanted patients. Tight glycaemic control in the perioperative period results in improved survival in surgical patients (Coursin et al., 2004).

## Immunosuppression

Immunosuppression is the common denominator in every transplanted patient. There is a delicate balance between organ acceptance, risk of rejection, and infection, on the one side, and risk of adverse effects and dose of immunosuppression, on the other. Immunosuppressive protocols (type and dose) will vary from centre to centre and depend on the graft, but usually consist of a cocktail of different agents (see Chapter 11). Plasma drug levels are monitored closely for prevention of side effects and fine-tuned to avoid rejection. 'Fine-tuning' of plasma levels is an art that determines the long-term success of organ transplantation. Other drugs that form part of the post-transplant drug regimen may include antibiotics, and antifungal and antiviral therapy, which will need to be verified and continued according to schedule by the anaesthesiologist in the perioperative period.

Immunosuppressive therapy should be continued during the perioperative period and the dose adjusted in the presence of hepatic or renal insufficiency. The stress of surgery may affect absorption and metabolism of these drugs, thereby altering plasma levels. It is extremely important for the surgical team to communicate to the anaesthesiologist the drug regimen and the doses of drug(s) utilized. It is also essential for the transplant anaesthesiologist to have an understanding of the actions, interactions, and potential side effects of immunosuppressive drugs.

There are insufficient data on anaesthesia and immunosuppressive drug interactions. Information on newer agents is limited and most available data deal with the use of cyclosporine A, which is no longer first-line therapy for immunosuppression. In the section 'Corticosteroids' we will present a brief synopsis of the most commonly used agents and implications for anaesthetic management.

### Corticosteroids

Corticosteroids are commonly used as adjuncts for induction and maintenance of immunosuppression and/or the management of acute or chronic rejection. These drugs cause immunosuppression mainly by sequestration of CD4+ T-lymphocytes of the reticuloendothelial system and by inhibiting the transcription of cytokines (Thomanson, 1999). Adverse effects of corticosteroids are well recognized as they impact virtually every organ system in the body, producing many dose-limiting side effects, such as hypertension, diabetes, obesity, and osteoporosis.

The decision to administer steroid stress-dose supplementation in the transplant recipient remains controversial. These patients will have a degree of hypothalamic–pituitary–adrenal suppression; hence the need for supplementation has not been well established. Several studies have suggested that there is no clear indication for stress doses of steroids in transplant recipients who present for minor risk procedures (Thomason et al., 1999). The recommendation is to continue maintenance doses up to the day of the surgery without supplementation (Mathis et al., 2004). In the case of a major surgical procedure, however, supplementation is advised. The usual stress dosage has been 100 mg of hydrocortisone every 8 hours. This dose, however, is far higher than the physiological cortisol response, which peaks at 150 mg/day after major surgery and returns quickly to baseline. A review of this topic recommends administration of the usual dose preoperatively, plus 50 mg of hydrocortisone every 8 hours for 48–72 hours, and then quickly return the dosage to baseline after surgery (Brown and Buie, 2001).This strategy is designed to mimic the physiological response of the normal adrenal gland to surgical stress (Axelrod, 2003).

### Calcineurin inhibitors

CNIs include cyclosporine and tacrolimus. They function by binding to calcineurin and preventing its translocation into the nucleus, thus affecting transcription and subsequent secretion of interleukin 2 (IL-2) by the T lymphocyte cell. Therapeutic drug monitoring is necessary to maintain adequate immunosuppression, but both drugs have a narrow therapeutic index, producing varying degrees of nephrotoxicity, neurotoxicity, and glucose intolerance. Their metabolism is dependent on cytochrome P450, and drugs that cause induction of P450 enzymes can affect plasma levels of these immunosuppressives. Examples of such drugs are amphotericin, non-steroidal anti-inflammatory drugs, ranitidine, cimetidine, co-trimoxazole, tobramycin, gentamicin, melphanan, and vancomycin. Cyclosporine may interfere with the metabolism of other medications (digoxin, lovastatin, and prednisolone), with resultant toxicity (Hirose and Vincenti, 2006).

To maintain therapeutic blood levels, it is important to administer oral cyclosporine or tacrolimus 4–7 hours before surgery (Brown et al., 1989). There have been reports of an increase in the MAC of isoflurane in rats pretreated with cyclosporine A, and delayed emergence when co-administered with barbiturates. This is most likely associated with metabolic CYP3 system interference. It is debatable whether this effect is relevant in clinical practice. Caution must be taken with the non-depolarizing neuromuscular blocking agents in patients receiving this class of immunosuppressives, since prolonged muscle relaxation and longer reversal times have been reported, and recommendations are to reduce neuromuscular relaxant dose (Gramstad et al., 1986).

### Antiproliferative agents

Azathioprine and mycophenolate are antimetabolites that inhibit the de-novo and salvage pathways of purine synthesis. This results in lymphocyte T and B suppression, but also toxicity to bone marrow, the gastrointestinal tract, and the liver. Previously, azathioprine was the drug of choice, but its use has been supplanted by mycophenolate, which is available in two forms: mycophenolate mofetil (CellCept, Roche) and enteric-coated mycophenolate sodium (Myfortic, Novartis). The enteric-coated form has better gastrointestinal tolerability and bioavailability, but both have similar haematological (anaemia, thrombocytopaenia, and leucopaenia) and neurological toxicity profiles. No major anaesthetic drug interactions have been described for these agents (Zolezzi, 2005).

### mTORinhibitors

Sirolimus (rapamycin) and everolimus inhibit large molecule kinase activity, termed the mTOR, thus causing arrest of the lymphocyte cell cycle. They are used concomitantly with CNIs in situations where there may be an increased risk for renal insufficiency (Murgia et al., 1996). Their use is associated with poor wound healing, and as such it is advisable not to initiate therapy until 6 weeks after transplantation or other surgical procedures. A complication described with these agents is pulmonary toxicity, presenting as interstitial pneumonitis, with fever, haemoptysis, and diffuse alveolar infiltrate in the absence of infection. This idiosyncratic toxicity frequently presents during the first 6 months of therapy, and usually patients respond well with drug discontinuation, with resolution of symptoms within 3 months (Augustine et al., 2007).

### Antibodies

This group of agents includes polyclonal and monoclonal antibodies. Even though some of these agents have been around for more than 30 years, the newest agents are the closest to the ideal immunosuppressant, exhibiting the lowest toxicity, specific activity, and prolonged effect.

#### OKT3

OKT3 is a murine monoclonal antibody directed against the CD3 component of the T-cell receptor, preventing T lymphocyte function (Berge et al., 1999). Acute administration of OKT3 causes cytokine release syndrome, which can include fevers, rigors, headache, dyspnoea, gastrointestinal side effects, and even life-threatening pulmonary oedema. Even though this syndrome has been described to occur within an hour of the first dose, close monitoring and premedication with tylenol, antihistaminic, and corticosteroid is required to prevent it. This syndrome improves with subsequent doses (Thillainathan et al., 2011).

#### Thymoglobulin

Thymoglobulin is a rabbit-derived polyclonal antithymocyte antibody. It is used as an induction agent and also as treatment of rejection in courses of up to 14 days. Thymoglobulin produces lymphocyte depletion, and can cause a milder form of cytokine release syndrome than OKT3 when administered. Therefore pretreatment with tylenol, antihistaminic, and steroid is recommended. Thrombocytopaenia and leucopaenia are common side effects and serum sickness has also been reported with its use (Lundquist et al., 2007).

#### Anti-interleukin-2 receptor monoclonal antibodies

Basiliximab and daclizumab block IL-2-mediated T-cell activation. The use of these antibodies is remarkable for its lack of toxicity when compared to monoclonal and polyclonal antibodies. Gastrointestinal upset and a case report of non-cardiogenic pulmonary oedema in young patients have been described (Bamgbola et al., 2003).

#### Alemtuzumab

Alemtuzumab (Campath-1H) is a humanized monoclonal antibody to the CD52 molecule that is expressed in lymphocytes (T greater than B cells) and results in its depletion both centrally and peripherally. It is widely used in haematological malignancies (Morgan et al., 2012).

## Common transplant-related complications

Transplant recipients, as a group, are at long-term risk of infection and rejection. It is important to be aware that these complications may arise at any time post-transplant.

### Rejection

Rejection is a worrisome condition in transplant recipients for obvious reasons, and expert evaluation is advised when detected. Transplanted organ function usually recovers almost fully after transplantation, and early organ dysfunction is an ominous sign. The signs and symptoms of chronic rejection and infection are similar and may be concurrent.

In heart transplant patients, a decrease of voltage on the ECG, presence of arrhythmias, especially of atrial origin, decreases in functional status, and dyspnoea can all be signs of rejection (Blasco et al., 2009). Lung transplant recipients may present acutely with fatigue, dyspnoea, oxygen desaturation on exertion or at rest,and abnormal pulmonary function tests. The presence of fever and signs of obliterative bronchiolitis are indicative of chronic rejection in this population (Feltracco et al., 2011).

Liver transplant recipients can present with a wide range of signs, including malaise, fever, and elevated serum bilirubin and/or other LFTs (Zeyneloglu et al., 2007). In the renal transplant recipient, increasing serum creatinine, hypertension, oliguria, and proteinuria should alert the anaesthesiologist to kidney graft dysfunction (Rao, 1998).

Graft dysfunction among recipients of intestinal transplant may present with enteritis and malabsorption syndrome. In these patients these findings are of special concern since this condition weakens the mucosal barrier of the intestinal allograft, allowing bacterial translocation and risk of septicaemia. Evaluation of the stoma and enteroscopy with biopsy are indicated if rejection is suspected, and any elective surgical procedure under these circumstances should be reconsidered (Ruiz et al., 2007).

The anaesthesiologist should be aware of graft organ dysfunction, since it may have a major impact on functional reserve. More importantly, anaesthetic drug pharmokinetics and pharmacodynamics may be altered. In general, patients with marginal graft function are best managed in a centre with experience in caring for patients with transplanted organs, particularly when major surgical procedures such as cardiovascular surgery are contemplated.

### Infections

Immunosuppression induces host tolerance of the new graft, but at the same time it makes the patient prone to infections. Over 80% of transplant recipients are expected to have at least one episode of infection after transplantation. Infection is associated with high mortality among transplant recipients. These patients are at risk of opportunistic infections related to viral, protozoan, or fungal pathogens. Among the most common infections are *Candida, Aspergillus*, and*Cytomegalovirus* (Loinaz et al., 2003).

Immunosuppressive medications such as steroids and azathioprine will render the white blood cell count unreliable. These patients may not present with the typical signs and symptoms of sepsis or may progress rapidly to severe sepsis. Early diagnosis and initiation of empiric treatment is mandatory.

### Neurological complications

Neurological complications should be of special concern to the anaesthesiologist. These may range from seizures and peripheral neuropathy, to brain infarcts and haemorrhages, and occur in up to 30–60% of transplant recipients (Patchell, 1994). The transplant recipient is more susceptible to neurological complications as a consequence of the combination of immunosuppressive regimens and shifts in electrolytes and fluids. Hypomagnesaemia causes aphasia and seizures. Central pontine myelinolysis (CPM) has an incidence of up to 17% after liver transplantation, based on autopsy results, and is associated with a high mortality rate of 50% or higher (Holmdahl et al., 2000). It has been associated with rapid correction of hyponatraemia, hypomagnesaemia, and other electrolytes, as well as the use of cyclosporine and tacrolimus (Fukazawa et al., 2011).

### Post-transplant malignancies

Malignancies have a higher incidence in transplanted recipients. Epithelial malignancies, including those affecting the colon, skin, vulva, bladder, lung, and testes, are not uncommon and behave more aggressively than those in the general population. PTLDcan present within 2 years after transplant and carries a high morbidity and mortality. This entity is associated with the EBV, causing proliferation in lymphoid tissue with progression to aggressive lymphoma. The treatment includes expert management of immunosuppression (Abu-Elmagd et al., 2004).

This population of patients is at risk for GVHD and cardiac allograft vasculopathy, among other complications.

## Perioperative management

### Preoperative evaluation

The type of surgical procedure to be undertaken dictates to a large degree the anaesthetic plan for intraoperative care, monitoring, and postoperative management. Early in the post-transplant period, anaesthetic management may encompass a continuation of perioperative transplant management. Early returns to the operating room for acute surgical complications such as bleeding require attention to resuscitation, haemodynamic stability, correction of coagulopathy, and correction of acid-base disturbances, as well as protection of transplanted organ function. Thrombosis of the graft may result in severe and rapid clinical deterioration with irreversible graft failure.

In the case of multivisceral transplantation a gastrointestinal anastomotic leak may require early reintervention. Months to years after transplant patients can present for elective procedures, diagnostic imaging, laparoscopy, abdominal incisional hernia, Nissen fundoplication for GORD, incision and drainage of abscesses, and caesarean section for childbirth, among others (Johnston and Katz, 1994). Orthopaedic procedures are common, since the transplanted patients may suffer from osteoporosis and bone fragility (Aaron and Ciombor, 2006).

Irrespective of the reason for surgery, if it involves areas of previous surgeries the anaesthesiologist should be prepared for a difficult surgical approach and the possibility of bleeding, requiring large volumes of blood. Trauma in a transplant recipient should be managed initially with the same resuscitation goals as in any other patient, but consideration and evaluation by a transplant team whenever possible is mandatory (Barone et al., 1997; Goffin and Devogelaer, 2005). Long hours of surgery with graft reconstructions may require postoperative critical care.

### Intraoperative management

#### General anaesthesia

General anaesthesia is administered in the majority of organ transplant recipients who are scheduled for non-transplant surgery. The type of surgical procedure planned, whether or not the operation is elective or emergent, and airway assessment will dictate airway management, as usual. The anaesthesiologist should be aware of special considerations. For example, rapid sequence induction should be considered in patients with ascites and in intestinal transplant recipients, since gastric emptying is delayed for a prolonged period after transplantation (Mousa et al., 1998). Large lymphomas obstructing the airway have been described in the transplanted patient with PTLD (Hammer et al., 1998). In these cases, awake fibreoptic intubation may be required. There are no data on specific agents or combinations of agents as the best choice in transplanted patients. All anaesthetic agents and techniques have been safely used in this patient population (Cheng and Ong, 1993). Etomidate is still the drug of choice in patients with cardiovascular instability. Propofol is the most popular induction agent and its use has been described in euvolaemic heart transplant patients without complication, as well as in patients with uraemic kidney failure (Kirvela et al., 1992).

The requirement for neuromuscular blockade may be altered as mentioned earlier by immunosuppressive medications. Succinyl choline can be used as usual in rapid sequence induction in the absence of hyperkalaemia and kidney dysfunction; rocuronium and mivacurium are other options. Atracurium and cisatracurium undergo plasma Hoffman elimination and they seem ideal for most procedures (Smith and Hunter, 1995). Vecuronium use is discouraged in liver-transplanted patients due to its reliance on hepatic metabolism and accumulation in patients with kidney dysfunction. In fact, studies have been done in the liver transplant recipient to predict quality of liver graft function based on the duration of vecuronium neuromuscular block (Lukin et al., 1995).

The inhalational agents sevoflurane, isoflurane, and desflurane have all been used in transplanted patients without complications. Isoflurane seems to be the preferred inhalational agent, especially in liver transplant patients, because it undergoes minimal biotransformation, with only 0.17% of the isoflurane taken up recovered in the form of urinary metabolites; it also has a safe haemodynamic profile, and organ-protective characteristics have been described.

The combination of intraoperative opioid analgesics is the practice of choice, and there are no major contraindications for their use. Caution is advised, however, in transplant recipients with renal dysfunction, since accumulation of active metabolites of morphine can cause prolonged sedation (Hanna et al., 1993).

The use of short-acting opioids like remifentanil that undergo Hoffman metabolism has been recommended in abdominal surgery and is accepted practice in some centres, allowing for easier titration and early extubation. However, short-acting opioids present the disadvantage of poor postoperative pain control, in which case multimodal analgesia may be considered (Park et al., 2000).

### Regional anaesthesia

Some transplant recipients will require long-term anticoagulation as a consequence of an underlying hypercoagulable state, and some others will be clinically hypocoagulopathic. Either way, careful assessment of coagulation is necessary prior to the use of regional blockade. Regional anaesthesia may be preferred when possible in the lung transplant recipient to avoid airway manipulation. Conversely, central neuraxial blockade in heart transplant patients (where the denervated heart is dependent upon preload for cardiac output) may cause haemodynamic instability due to sudden sympathetic blockade and loss of cardiac filling (Grimsehl and Levack, 2002). In this case, continuous epidural anaesthesia is preferred to spinal anaesthesia, and the safe use of bupivacaine or ropivacaine has been described (Riley, 1995). Lidocaine should be used with caution because of its negative inotropic actions, and adrenaline should be avoided in the heart transplant recipient.

### Monitoring

Standard monitoring is recommended in every case, to include ECG, pulse oximetry, non-invasive blood pressure, end-tidal $CO_2$, anaesthesia gas analysis, and temperature control. The type, duration, and potential for bleeding associated with the planned surgical procedure, together with an assessment of the patient's baseline preoperative cardiovascular stat, will determine the type of advanced monitoring modalities to be employed.

When large volume shifts or prolonged procedures are anticipated or the patient's underlying metabolic condition dictates frequent serum glucose, acid-base, and electrolyte monitoring, large-bore peripheral intravenous lines and/or invasive monitoring may be indicated. Whenever possible, ultrasound imaging for placement of central venous catheters and non-invasive haemodynamic monitors is recommended, for two main reasons: (1) the majority of these patients have had prior indwelling central venous catheters and this may create unexpected challenges to safe placement; and (2) these are immune-compromised patients with increased risk of catheter-related sepsis. TOE use in the transplant field has increased in recent years and is the routine monitor for high-risk procedures performed on kidney, liver, lung, and heart transplant recipients. The routine use of TOE is primarily governed by expertise and availability, as well as clinical indication. Other forms of non-invasive cardiac output monitoring, such as by pulse contour analysis, and indications for their use are discussed elsewhere in this book (Section 9). In our institution TOE is used instead of PA catheterization for haemodynamic monitoring (Cowie, 2011), when indicated. Needless to say, strict asepsis is essential when establishing venous and arterial access in these immune-compromised patients (Slota et al., 2001).

Antibiotic-impregnated catheters are routinely used in the transplant population in some centres; their use has proven to reduce colonization and associated infections in up to 60% of cases. Their use has been advocated when planning to use lines for a period in excess of 2 weeks (George et al., 1997).

### Haemodynamic control

Haemodynamic stability is the main objective in the transplanted patient during high-risk procedures. Adequate volume status and monitoring is the basis of good haemodynamic control, and the maintenance of preload results in better perfusion in most uncomplicated cases (Della Rocca et al., 2002, 2009).

### Electrolytes

Immunosuppressive therapy is associated with electrolyte imbalance. Therefore anaesthesia and surgery may aggravate electrolyte disequilibrium (Adu et al., 1983).

Careful intraoperative management of electrolytes is very important, especially potassium and magnesium; these are of special importance in the transplanted heart patient with conduction abnormalities. Since total body magnesium is difficult to measure and ionized magnesium is not always available, empiric magnesium supplementation may be necessary in the transplanted patient (June et al., 1985). It is important to remember that severe electrolyte shifts can worsen neurological complications for which some of these patients are already at higher risk.

### Glycaemic Control

There is controversy regarding intraoperative glycaemic targets and these apply to the transplant recipient as well. Pancreas transplant recipients should experience restoration of normal glucose metabolism unless there is graft dysfunction (Rickels, 2012).

Diabetic patients should be managed as any other diabetic patient. Post-transplant diabetes develops in 4–20% of patients. Careful glycaemic monitoring is recommended in all transplant recipients undergoing surgical procedures, since perioperative hyperglycaemia is associated with electrolyte imbalance, impaired wound healing, and a higher incidence of nosocomial infections.

Tight glycaemic control targets (80–110 mg/dL) are associated with hypoglycaemia; a recent review suggests a wider range of glucose maintenance below 150 and avoidance of hyperglycaemia (Russo, 2012).

## Special considerations in the kidney transplant recipient

The kidney transplant recipient is the most commonly encountered transplanted patient undergoing non-transplant surgery. It is important to note that it is a misconception to believe kidney function is completely restored after kidney transplantation. In fact, kidney transplant recipients have a lower GFR than normal individuals, and despite a near-normal Cr value, perioperative management should incorporate a renal-protective approach. These patients will present with multiple comorbidities, such as hyperlipidaemia, hypertension, diabetes, and CAD. CAD is the leading cause of death among kidney transplant recipients during the first year after transplantation. Therefore the preoperative evaluation should focus on blood pressure and glycaemic control, optimization of electrolytes and acid-base status, as well as careful screening of cardiovascular function, preferably with 2-D ECG and/or stress testing (Lindholm et al., 1995).

Kidney allograft function is assessed with urine analysis, and serum BUN and Cr levels. Elevated BUN or Cr may indicate dysfunction due to graft rejection. The type of surgical procedure and the patient's medical condition will dictate the selection of anaesthetic technique. Regional anaesthesia, including central neuraxial blocks, can be performed in patients with normal coagulation status.

The anaesthetic plan should be established with the understanding that drugs that rely heavily on renal excretion for clearance will result in prolonged effects. Most induction agents have been used successfully, but caution must be taken with the use of ketamine in the hypertensive patient. Succinylcholineis contraindicated when potassium levels are elevated. Inhaled agents such as isoflurane, desflurane, and sevoflurane have been used without complications.

The newly transplanted and functional kidney is able to clear neuromuscular blocking and anticholinesterase agents at the same rate as normal kidneys. However, whenever there is clinically detectable renal dysfunction the use of drugs not excreted by the kidney is advised (Kostopanagiotou et al., 1999).

Opiates for pain management area concern, since these patients will have the tendency to accumulate active metabolites, especially patients with graft dysfunction. Fentanyl is a good choice because it is well tolerated and lacks active metabolites (Sear, 1995). Non-steroidal anti-inflammatory medications should be avoided or used with caution.

The kidney graft may have suboptimal autoregulation of renal blood flow, making it susceptible to sudden blood pressure variations. Studies have demonstrated that adequate hydration during kidney transplantation results in less incidence of perioperative acute tubular necrosis (Carlier et al., 1982); this depends on the patient's underlying status. In general, volume should be optimized prior to the institution of diuretics to maintain urine output.

## Anaesthetic considerations in the liver and multivisceral transplant recipient

Liver transplantation is the definitive treatment for patients with cirrhosis/ESLD. The procedure has an average survival rate of 90% at 1 year. The number of liver transplant recipients requiring non-transplant surgery is on the rise, and perioperative outcome is in part dependent on time since transplant, as well as the adequacy of liver graft function at the time of surgery.

In the post-liver transplant period, any necessary follow-on surgery usually is aimed at the correction of early liver transplant-related complications, such as bleeding and bile duct anastomotic leaks. It is prudent for the transplant anaesthesiologist to manage these patients during these early surgical complications, since expert management of coagulopathy and haemodynamics is usually warranted. Moreover, extrahepatic complications of ESLD, such as severe portopulmonary hypertension, or hypoxaemia from pleural effusions, hydrothorax, HPS, or persistent ascites may not be completely resolved within the first two postoperative weeks. In patients with delayed graft function, continuation of mechanical ventilatory support with supplemental oxygen may be required to maintain adequate oxygenation. Invasive haemodynamic monitoring may also be necessary to monitor and treat pulmonary hypertension (Kato et al., 2006). Furthermore, the hyperdynamic circulation typical of the patient with ESLD reverses itself slowly after liver transplantation (Eriksson et al., 1990).

In the first few weeks after liver transplant a variety of late complications may require surgical re-exploration. These include hepatic artery thrombosis or stenosis, portal or hepatic vein thrombosis, biliary anastomotic leaks, and/or biliary tract reconstruction (Faenza et al., 2006). In these cases, general anaesthesia is indicated.

LFTs usually return to normal within 2 weeks after transplant, although some degree of elevation in AST can remain for years afterwards, as a result of immunosuppression. Persistently elevated LFTs, total bilirubin, or INR PT/PTT may be indicative of delayed function or acute rejection. Chronic rejection will also lead to a rise in liver function indices.

In the months and years after liver or multivisceral transplantation, indications for surgery will vary. Regional anaesthesia can be considered on a case-by-case manner in the absence of coagulopathy.

If the surgical plan includes an abdominal approach, difficult dissection is expected, and the anaesthesiologist should be prepared with available blood products and resuscitation fluids. Most general procedures will not require massive transfusion. There is debate regarding absolute haemoglobin or haematocrit value as a target for transfusion therapy. It is important to understand that overtransfusion and haemo-concentration can lead to graft thrombosis (Tisone et al., 1988). Because of the high prevalence of renal dysfunction in these patients, fluid status and electrolyte balance should be carefully monitored. Depending on fluid shifts and electrolyte disturbances and the severity of renal dysfunction, haemodialysis may be needed perioperatively (Gines et al., 2003). Increase in splanchnic vascular resistance, which may occur when there is such high airway pressure, hypoxia, hypercapnia, coughing and bucking, or volume overload, will decrease the perfusion of the graft and should be treated promptlyor avoided altogether (Kostopanagiotou, 1999).

Since hepatic metabolic capacity for drug metabolism is restored early after reperfusion of the graft, most induction agents have been used successfully, but the net effect and duration of action of any drug is unpredictable. It is advisable to titrate to effect and select drugs with extrahepatic metabolism, particularly muscle relaxants. Isoflurane is the inhaled agent of choice for this population. Pain management with opioids is still the best option, although even with a functional graft some patients still require low opioid doses for pain management; patient-controlled analgesia can be a good choice in this population (Eisenach, 1989).

## Anaesthetic considerations in the heart transplant recipient

The heart transplant recipient has a denervated heart. The donor graft has no parasympathetic, sympathetic, or sensory innervation. Therefore reflex sympathetic activity is absent. Beta-receptor density increases and myocyte sensitivity to circulating catecholamines is enhanced, with intrinsic myocardial contractility remaining unaffected (Blasco, 2009). Since heart-transplanted patients are preload dependent and lack reflex tachycardia, they are very sensitive to vasodilatation and changes in position (Cheng and Day, 2003). Crystalloid and colloids can be used for fluid management. However, the denervated heart will not respond to drugs that act on the autonomic nervous system, such as anticholinergic, anticholinesterase, phenylephrine, or nitroprusside. Additionally, neostigmine can cause severe bradycardia by activation of cholinergic receptors on cardiac ganglionic cells. Alpha- and beta-adrenergic receptors are present in the myocardium; hence endogenous or exogenous catecholamines will increase contractility in response to epinephrine, norepinephrine, isoproterenol, or dobutamine. Conversely, there can be a decrease in contractility in response to beta-blockers (Backman et al., 1997). The effect of beta-blockers, however, may result in severe hypotension, and their use should be avoided.

Left and right ventricular ejection fraction as well as stroke volume are normal in the transplant heart, and will remain so over at least the first 5 years after heart transplantation (Von Scheidt et al., 1991). Normally a higher resting heart rate of 90–100 is present, since the transplanted heart is dependent on preload for inotropy. This is extremely important in the anaesthetic management of these patients, since the normal physiological response to hypovolaemia is absent. On the ECG two P waves may be present: one of the recipient native atrium, which is non-conductive because of the suture lines, and the other from the donor atrium.

These patients frequently present with conduction abnormalities and 5% will require a pacemaker. The management of the pacemaker is similar to that of any other patient, requiring evaluation of proper function and change of pacing mode around the time of the surgical procedure when indicated (Von Scheidt, 1991).

Heart transplant patients will present for endocardial biopsies. Biopsies are usually performed through the right internal jugular vein, thus avoiding catheterization. However, communication with the transplant surgeon regarding the necessity for multiple biopsies during the course of surgery is important (Firestone, 1991).

## Anaesthetic considerations in the lung transplant recipient

Lung transplant recipients may require routine bronchoscopic evaluation in the days following transplantation. This is usually done with light sedation (Murthy et al., 2007). In addition, early complications include re-exploration for cardiac tamponade, pleural bleeding, thrombosis, and wound dehiscence. Pulmonary function tests and arterial gas analysis are of special importance in the management of these patients. Patients with lung transplantation require months to achieve total recovery of arterial oxygenation, but the outcomes have improved markedly in recent years, especially among bilateral lung transplant recipients (Pochettino et al., 2000). These patients will achieve normal arterial oxygenation almost at the time of hospital discharge. In contrast, outcome among single lung transplant recipients is highly dependent on the underlying disease and functionality of the remaining lung. The FEV1 in patients with single lung transplant can increase to 50–60% of the predicted value, but with persistence of a restrictive pattern (Pochettino et al., 2000). Hypercapnia in patients with emphysema and the ventilatory response to fluctuations in $PaCO_2$ is normalized within weeks of lung transplantation.

Careful clinical evaluation of symptoms such as progressive dyspnoea, cough with purulent tracheobronchial secretions, and deterioration of pulmonary function tests indicate bronchiolitis obliterans (BOB), a complication associated with chronic rejection. This condition affects 50–60% of patients who survive 5 years after lung transplantation. It carries a mortality rate of 40% (Feltracco et al., 2011). Any deterioration in oxygen saturation prior to surgery should prompt immediate arterial blood gas evaluation, with postponement of non-emergent surgical procedures.For this reason, arterial line placement is indicated in patients undergoing general endotracheal anaesthesia.

Furthermore, the lung transplant patient may present with tracheal stenosis or a stricture at the site of the tracheal anastomosis. In this case extreme care should be taken during placement of the endotracheal tube when general anaesthesia is warranted (Chacon et al., 1998). During airway manipulation, aseptic technique is recommended. It is important to note that the loss of the cough reflex may predispose these patients to silent aspiration and/or accumulation of secretions (Boscoe, 1995).

In general, the double lung transplanted patient will present with lower overall compliance when compared to normal (Haddow, 1997). In emphysematous patients with single lung transplants, over distention of bullae can produce pneumothorax. In patients with fibrous lung tissue, over inflation of the lung may cause barotrauma (Feltracco et al., 2011). Lung-protective ventilation entails limiting peak inspiratory pressure (PIP) to 30–35 cm/$H_2O$, plateau pressures to 20–25 cm/$H_2O$, and tidal volumes <7 mL/kg of predicted ideal body weight, and adjusting respiratory rate to desired $PaCO_2$ (40–45 mmHg).

Cardiopulmonary function will gradually normalize after transplantation, with reduction of pulmonary vascular resistance and pulmonary pressures, increases in cardiac index, and remodelling and improvement of right heart function (Mendelo et al., 2002). During surgery, ideal positioning is lateral decubitus with the transplanted lung in the non-dependent position. The lack of adequate lymphatic drainage of the transplanted lung requires conservative fluid management (Baker et al., 2005).

## Postoperative considerations and pain management

Previous organ transplant does not require a mandatory postoperative ICU stay (Mandell et al., 2002). On the contrary, exposure to patients with highly resistant nosocomial infections should be avoided wherever possible. The need for intensive care should be considered on a case-by-case basis, as in any other patient, and will ultimately depend on the patient's medical condition, comorbidities, haemodynamic and oxygenation status, and the complexity of the planned surgical procedure, or mandated by complications encountered during surgery (Haddow and Brock-Utne, 1999).

Extubation is a primary goal in these patients. It decreases the risk of ventilator-associated complications such as barotrauma or ventilator-associated pneumonia. The usual criteria for extubation will apply. However, some authors advocate extubation of lung transplant patients in the lateral decubitus position to prevent aspiration into the graft.

Postoperative analgesia with a multimodal approach to pain management is important to ensure extubation and early ambulation (Siniscalchi et al., 2000). Patient-controlled analgesia should be used where appropriate. However, morphine metabolites may accumulate in patients with impaired renal function. Some transplant patients may have tolerance to opioids due to enzyme induction from previous intravenous drug use or for chronic pain management. This may make perioperative management more complicated. In these patients, multimodal analgesia or the use of ketamine or regional analgesia may be of particular benefit. Epidural or regional analgesia can be used when appropriate, and depends upon institutional preferences as well as postoperative protocols by the acute pain service. Non-steroid anti-inflammatory drugs should be used sparingly, if at all, because of the added risk of nephrotoxicity among patients on immunosuppressive drugs (Harris et al., 1988).

## Conclusion

In this chapter we have addressed the perioperative care of the organ transplant patient undergoing non-transplant surgery. We have provided guidelines for each transplanted organ system, the preoperative evaluation and screening necessary to ensure the integrity of the patient with a transplanted organ, as well as the interactions presented by anaesthesia and immunosuppressive therapies. The population of organ transplant recipients among non-transplant surgical patients is increasing exponentially. One of the important points highlighted in this chapter is the fact that the vast majority of transplant recipients who are scheduled for elective non-transplant surgery are completely functional patients with good quality of life. We have emphasized the importance of a thorough assessment to include a careful review of the health status since transplantation, while taking into account pre-existing comorbidities and the risks associated with the type and scope of the planned surgical procedure. In particular, it is important to assess the type of immunosuppression regimen and their side effects, anaesthetic and drug interactions, as well as graft function.

## References


Aaron RK, Ciombor DM (2006) Orthopedic complications of solid-organ transplantation. *Surg Clin N Am*, **86**:1237–1255.

Abu-Elmagd KM, et al. (2004) De novo malignancies after intestinal and multivisceral transplantation. *Transplantation*, **77**:1719.

Adu D, et al. (1983) Hyperkalemia in cyclosporine treated renal allograft recipients. *Lancet*,**132**(8346):370–372.

Augustine JJ, Bodziak KA, Hricik DE (2007)The use of sirolimus in solid organ transplant. *Drugs*, **67**(3):360–391.

Axelrod L (2003) Perioperative management of patients treated with glucocorticoids. *Endocrinol Metabolism ClinN Am*, **32**:367–383.

Backman SB, Fox GS, Ralley FE (1997) Pharmacological properties of the denervated heart. *Can J Anaesth*, **44**:900–901.

Baker J, Yost CS, Niemann CU (2005) Organ transplantation.In: Miller RD (ed) *Miller's Anesthesia*, pp. 2271–2272.Elsevier, Philadelphia.

Bamgbola FO, Del Rio M, Kaskel FJ, et al. (2003) Non-cardiogenic pulmonary edema during induction in three adolescent renal transplant patients. *Pediatric Transplant*, **7**(4):315–320.

Barone GW, Sailors DM, Hudec WA, Ketel BL (1997) Trauma management in solid organ transplant recipients. *J Emerg Med*, **15**:169–176.

Berge JM, et al. (1999) Guidelines for the optimal use of muromonab CD3 in transplantation. *Bio Drugs*, **11**:277–284.

Blasco L,Parameshwar J, Vuylsteke A (2009) Anaesthesia for noncardiac surgery in the heart transplant recipient. *Curr Opin Anaesthesiol*, **22**:109–113.

Boscoe M (1995) Anesthesia for patients with transplanted lungs and heart and lungs. *Int Anesthesiol Clin*, **33**:21–44.

Boscoe M (1995) Anesthesia for patients with transplanted lungs and heart and lungs. *Int Anesthesiol Clin*, **33**:21–44.

Brown C, Buie D (2001) Perioperative stress dose steroids: do they make a difference? *J Am Coll Surg*, **193**(6):678–686.

Brown MR, et al. (1989) Efficacy of oral cyclosporine given prior to liver transplantation. *Anesth Analg*, **69**:773–775.

Carlier M. et al. (1982) Maximal hydration during anesthesia increases pulmonary arterial pressures and improves early function of human renal transplants. *Transplantation*,**34**:201–204.

Chacon RA, et al. (1998) Comparison of the functional results of single lung transplantation for pulmonary fibrosis and chronic airway obstruction. *Thorax*, **53**(1):43–49.

Cheng DC, Ong DD (1993) Anaesthesia for non-cardiac surgery in heart-transplanted patients. *Can J Anaesth*, **40**:981–986.

Cheng D, Day F (2003) Heart transplantation and subsequent non-cardiac surgery. In: Yao FSF (ed)*Anesthesiology: Problem Oriented Patient Management*, pp. 409–423. Lippincott Williams& Wilkins, Philadelphia.

Coursin DB, Connery LE, Ketzler JT (2004) Perioperative diabetic and hyperglycemic management issues. *Crit Care Med*, **32**:S116–125.

Cowie B (2011) Does the pulmonary artery catheter still have a role in the perioperative period? *Anaesth Intens Care*, **39**(3):345–355.

Della Roca G, Brondani A, Costa GM (2009) Intraoperative hemodynamic monitoring during organ transplantation: what's new? *Curr Opin Organ Transplant*, **14**:291–296.

Della Roca G, Costa GM, Coccia C, et al. (2002)Preload index: pulmonary artery occlusion pressure versus intrathoracic blood volume monitoring during lung transplantation. *Anesth Analg*, **95**:835–843.

Eisenach JC, et al. (1989) Comparison of analgesic requirements after liver transplantation and cholecystectomy. *MayoClin Proc*,; **64**:356–359.

Eriksson LS,Sodeman C, Bo Goran E, Eleborg L, Wahren J, Hedenstierna G (1990) Normalization of ventilation/perfusion relationships after liver transplantation in patients with decompensated cirrhosis: evidence for a hepatopulmonary syndrome. *Hepatology*, **12**:1350–1357.

Faenza S,Arpesella G, Bernardi E, et al. (2006) Combined liver transplants: main characteristics from the standpoint of anesthesia and support in intensive care. *Transplant Proc*, **38**:1114–1117.

Feltracco P, et al. (2011) Anesthetic considerations for nontransplant procedures in lung transplant patients. *J Clin Anesth*, **23**:508–516.

Firestone L (1991) Heart transplantation. *Int Anesth Clin*, **29**:41–58.

Foley RN, Parfrey PS, Sarnak MJ (1998) Clinical epidemiology of cardiovascular disease in chronic renal disease. *Am J Kidney Dis*, **32**:S112–S119.

Fukazawa K, et al. (2011) CPM associated with tacrolimus (FK506) after liver transplantation.*Annal Transplant*, **16**(3):139–142.

George SJ, Vuddamalay P, Boscoe MJ (2007) Antiseptic-impregnated central venous catheters reduce the incidence of bacterial colonization and associated infection in immunocompromised transplant patients. *Eur J Anaesth*, **14**:428–431.

Gines P, et al. (2003) Hepatorenal syndrome. *Lancet*, **362**:1819–1827.

Goffin E, Devogelaer JP (2005) Bone disorders after transplantation. *Transplant Proc*, **37**(6):2832–2833.

Gohn R, Warren G (2006) The preoperative evaluation of the transplanted patient for nontransplant surgery. *Surg Clin N Am*, **86**:1147–1166.

Gramstad L, et al. (1986) Interaction of cyclosporine and its solvent, cremophor, with atracurium and vecuronium: studies in the cat. *Br J Anaesth*, **58**:1149–1155.

Grimsehl K, Levack ID (2002) Combined epidural and general anaesthesia in a patient with a transplanted heart undergoing upper abdominal surgery. *Br J Anaesth*, **88**:612–613.

Haddow GR (1997) Anaesthesia for patients after lung transplantation. *Can J Anaesth*, **44**:182–197.

Haddow GR, Brock-Utne JG (1999) A non-thoracic operation for a patient with single lung transplantation. *Acta Anaesthesiol Scand*, **43**:960–963.

Hammer GB, et al. (1998) Post-transplant lymphoproliferative disease may present with severe airway obstruction. *Anesthesiology*, **89**:263–265.

Hanna MH, D'Costa F, Peat FJ, et al (1993)Morphine-6-glucuronide disposition in renal impairment. *Br J Anaesth*, **70**(5):511–514.

Harris KP, Jenkins D, Walls J (1988) Nonsteroidal anti-inflammatory drugs and cyclosporine. *Transplantation*, **46**:598–599.

Hirose R, Vincenti F (2006) Immunosuppression: today, tomorrow, and withdrawal. *Semin Liver Dis*, **26**(3):201–210.

Holmdahl MH, et al. (2000) The place of THAM in the management of acidemia in clinical practice. *Acta Anaesthesiol Scand*, **44**:524–527.

Johnston TD, Katz SM (1994) Special considerations in the transplant patient requiring other surgery. *Surg Clin N Am*, **74**(5):1211–1221.

June CH, et al. (1985) Profound hypomagnesemia and renal magnesium wasting associated with the use of cyclosporine for marrow transplantation. *Transplant*, **39**(6):620–624.

KaramV, et al. (2003) Longitudinal prospective evaluation of quality of life in adult patients before and one year after liver transplantation. *Liver Transplant*, **9**:703–711.

Kato T, et al. (2006) Intestinal transplantation in children: a summary of clinical outcomes and prognostic factors in 108 patients from a single center. *Annal Surg*, **243**(6):756–764.

Keegan MT, Plevak DJ (2004)The transplant recipient for nontransplant surgery. *Anesthesiol Clin N Am*, **22**(4):827–861.

Kirvela M, et al. (1992) Pharmacokinetics of propofol and haemodynamic changes during induction of anaesthesia in uraemic patients. *Br J Anaesth*, **68**:178–182.

Kostopanagiotou G, et al. (2008) Anesthetic and perioperative management of intestinal and multivisceral allograft recipient in nontransplant surgery. *Eur Soc Organ Transplant*, **21**:415–427.

Kostopanagiotou G, et al. (1999). Anesthetic and perioperative management of adult transplant recipients in nontransplant surgery. *Anesth Analg*, **89**:613–622.

Lindholm A, et al. (1995) Ischemic heart disease – major cause of death and graft loss after renal transplantation in Scandinavia. *Transplantation*, **60**:451–457.

LoinazC, et al. (2003) Bacterial infections after intestinal and multivisceral transplantation. *Transplant Proc*, **35**:1929–1930.

Lukin CL, et al. (1995) Duration of vecuronium-induced neuromuscular block as a predictor of liver allograft dysfunction. *Anesth Analg*, **80**:526–533.

Lundquist AL, et al. (2007) Serum sickness following rabbit antithymocyte-globulin induction in a liver transplant recipient: case report and literature review. *Liver Transplant*, **13**(5):647–650.

Małyszko J, et al. (2012) Anemia in solid organ transplantation.*Ann Transplant*, **17**(2):86–100.

Mandell MS, et al. (2002) Reduced use of intensive care after liver transplantation: influence of early extubation. *Liver Transplant*, **8**:676–681.

Mathis AS, Shah NK, Mulgaonkar S (2004) Stress dose steroids in renal transplant patients undergoing lymphocele surgery. *Transplant Proc*, **36**(10):3042–3045.

Mendelo EN, et al. (2002) Lung transplantation for pulmonary vascular disease. *Annal Thorac Surg*, **73**:209–217.

Morgan R, et al. (2012) Alemtuzumab induction therapy in kidney transplantation: a systematic review and meta-analysis. *Transplantation*, **93**:1179–1188.

Mousa H, et al. (1998) Intestinal motility after small bowel transplantation. *Transplant Proc*, **30**:25–35.

Murgia MG, Jordan S, Kahan BD (1996) The side effect profile of sirolimus: a phase I study in quiescent cyclosporine-prednisone-treated renal transplant patients. *Kidney Int*, **49**:209–216.

Murthy SC, et al. (2007) Members of Cleveland Clinic's Pulmonary Transplant Team. Impact of anastomotic airway complications after lung transplantation. *Annal Thorac Surg*, **84**:401–409.

Ojo AO, et al. (2003) Chronic renal failure after transplantation of a non-renal organ. *N Engl J Med*, **349**:931.

OPTN (2015) *Donation and Transplantation Data.*<http://optn.transplant.hrsa.gov/latestdata/rptdata.asp>.

Paris W, et al. (1998) Return to work after lung transplantation. *J Heart Lung Transplant*, **17**:430–436.

Park GR, et al. (2000) Reducing the demand for admission to intensive care after major abdominal surgery by a change in anaesthetic practice and the use of remifentanil. *Eur J Anaesthesiol*, **17**:111–119.

Patchell RA (1994) Neurological complications of organ transplantation. *Annal Neurol*, **36**:688–703.

Pochettino A,Kotloff RM, Rosengard BR, et al. (2000) Bilateral versus single lung transplantation for chronic obstructive pulmonary disease: intermediate-term results. *Annal Thorac Surg*, **70**:1813–1818.

Rao VK (1998) Post transplant medical complications. *Surg Clin N Am*, **78**:113–132.

Rickels MR (2012)Recovery of endocrine function after islet and pancreas transplantation.*Curr Diabetes Rep*, **12**(5):587–596.

Riley ET (1995) Obstetric management of patients with transplants. *Int Anesthesiol Clin*, **33**:125–140.

Ruiz P, Kato T, Tzakis A (2007) Current status of transplantation of the small intestine. *Transplantation*, **83**:1–6.

Russo N (2012) Perioperative glycemic control. *Anesthesiol Clin*, **30**(3):445–466.

Sear JW (1995) Kidney transplants: induction and analgesic agents. *Int Anesthesiol Clin*, **33**(2):45–68.

Siniscalchi A, et al. (2002) Pain management after small bowel/multivisceral transplantation. *Transplant Proc*, **34**:969–970.

Slota M, et al. (2001)The role of gown and glove isolation and strict hand washing in reduction of nosocomial infection in children with solid organ transplantation. *Crit Care Med*, **29**:405–412.

Smith CE, Hunter JM (1995) Anesthesia for renal transplantation: relaxants and volatiles. *Int Anesthesiol Clin*, **33**:69–92.

Thillainathan V, Loh-Trivedi M, Rajagopal A(2011) Pulmonary capillary leak syndrome as a result of OKT-3 therapy. *Int Anesthesiol Clin*, **49**(2):68–70.

Thomason JM, Girdler NM, Kendall-Taylor P (1999) An investigation into the need for supplementary steroids in organ transplant patients undergoing gingival surgery. A double blind, split-mouth, crossover study. *J Clin Periodontol*, **26**(9):577–582.

Tisone G,Gunson BK, Buckels JA, McMaster P (1988) Raised hematocrit: a contributing factor to hepatic artery thrombosis following liver transplantation. *Transplantation*, **46**: 162–163.

Von Scheidt W, et al. (1991) Heart transplantation: hemodynamics over a five-year period. *J Heart Lung Transplant*, **10**(3):342–350.

Zeyneloglu P, et al. (2007) Perioperative anesthetic management for recipients of OLT undergoing nontransplant surgery. *Exp Clin Transplant*, **2**:690–692.

Zolezzi M (2005) Mycophenolate sodium versus mycophenolate mofetil: a review of their comparative features. *Saudi J Kidney Dis Transplant*, **16**(2):140–145.

# CHAPTER 40

# The anaesthetic implications of pregnancy after organ transplantation

Katherine G. Hoctor and J. Sudharma Ranasinghe

## Introduction

As the medical world continues to evolve, more women of childbearing age are successfully undergoing organ transplantation, and many of those women are safely delivering babies. As anaesthesiologists we are faced with the challenge of caring for these high-risk obstetrical patients, in and out of the operating room. Since the first successful live birth to a woman with a kidney transplant in 1958 (Murray et al., 1963), more and more post-transplantation women are safely delivering babies. The US National Transplantation Pregnancy Registry (NTPR) in December 2012 reported a total of 2,270 live births to 1,281 female transplant recipients since 1991 (Armenti et al., 2012), and not all pregnancies to transplant patients are reported to the NTPR, so there are many more unreported cases.

Kidney and liver continue to be the most common organs transplanted in the US and they make up the majority of pregnant transplant patients. The 2011 annual data report from the OPTN and SRTR shows a total of 16,055 kidney transplants in 2011, with 6,286 of those being women. The OPTN and SRTR report for liver transplantations has 5,805 total adult liver transplants in 2011, with 1,935 female liver transplant recipients (SRTR, 2012). Thoracic organ transplantation is less common than liver or kidney transplantation, but the rate of heart transplantation in women has increased, according to the 2011 OPTN and SRTR report (SRTR, 2012). Of all the many women having solid organ transplants annually, only a handful of those go on to become pregnant. The findings from the 2012 NTPR annual report showed that from 1991–2012 there were 1,576 pregnancies in kidney transplant patients, 357 pregnancies in liver transplant patients, 116 pregnancies in heart transplant patients, 31 pregnancies in lung transplant patients, and 120 pregnancies in multiple organ transplant patients (Table 40.1) (Armenti et al., 2012). Pregnancy in transplant patients continues to become a growing field for high-risk obstetrical management; physicians must be aware of the many challenges involved in caring for these patients.

## Timing of pregnancy following transplantation

Although women are living better, healthier lives after transplantation, there are still many risks a transplanted woman who would like to become pregnant must face. Graft rejection, infection, and fetal-related issues are only some of the possible complications that must be discussed with transplant patients of childbearing age. Before women of childbearing age who have had a transplant decide to become pregnant, optimally they will have a discussion with their physician regarding the risks to mother and baby. Many factors are involved when determining the safety of pregnancy in a transplant recipient. Graft function plays a major role in the ability of a woman to manage the physiological changes of pregnancy. A well-functioning graft means a healthier mother and, hence, a healthier baby. Immunosuppressive agents must be evaluated and changed if necessary and women must be counselled regarding continuing immunosuppressive drugs throughout pregnancy in order to avoid graft rejection. Women must also be informed of the potential effects that immunosuppressive drugs may have on their fetus. Currently there are not enough data to determine the full risk to the fetus of a female transplant recipient on immunosuppressive agents, and long-term effects to a child are a potential risk. Although there is no definitive time scale that should be used when planning to become pregnant after an organ transplant, in 2005 the Women's Health Committee of the AST released a consensus statement that suggests pregnancy 1 year after transplant is safe as long as the patient has stable graft function (McKay et al., 2005).

Along with all the above risks and issues that need to be addressed prior to pregnancy, women with transplants must think about their own long-term health status and their future ability to parent. Pregnancy in the transplant population is not a benign condition and must be decided upon carefully and with the guidance of a knowledgeable physician.

## Evaluating graft function

Graft function and overall maternal health play a major role in determining pregnancy outcomes in transplant patients. From the 2011 OPTN and SRTR report we can ascertain the most current transplantation outcome data. Kidney, liver, heart, and lung recipients have shown increasing short- and long-term graft survival rates (SRTR, 2012). In regards to women of childbearing age, the better the graft organ functions and the longer transplant patients live a healthy life, the more chance for a woman to become pregnant.

**Table 40.1** NTPR participants as of 31 December 2012 (Reproduced from Armenti VT et al., 'Report from the National Transplantation Pregnancy Registry (NTPR): outcomes of pregnancy after transplantation', *Clinical Transplantation*, pp. 65–85, copyright 2012, with permission from Gift of Life Institute)

| Solid organ(s) transplanted | Recipients | Pregnancies | Outcomes [a] |
|---|---|---|---|
| **Kidney** | 904 | 1576 | 1625 |
| **Liver** | 198 | 357 | 364 |
| **Liver–kidney** | 6 | 8 | 9 |
| **Intestine** | 2 | 2 | 2 |
| **Pancreas–kidney** | 54 | 97 | 103 |
| **Pancreas** | 3 | 8 | 9 |
| **Heart** | 67 | 116 | 120 |
| **Heart–lung** | 5 | 5 | 5 |
| **Lung** | 22 | 31 | 33 |
| **Total** | 1261 | 2200 | 2270 |

[a] Includes multiple births.

A study from Spain evaluating kidney transplant graft function found that worsening GFR and increased proteinuria are good predictors of deteriorating renal graft function (Marcen et al., 2010). In a renal transplant patient, careful attention should be paid to the patient's current GFR, creatinine levels, and level of proteinuria, along with signs of kidney disease such as oliguria, peripheral oedema, and uraemia. Singh and Watt published a review article on management of liver transplant patients, and they consider good graft function to be liver enzymes (AST, ALT, and alkaline phosphatase) and liver function tests (bilirubin and INR) all less than 1.5 times the normal range (Singh and Watt, 2012). For lung transplant patients, data from a study by the Pulmonary Retransplant Registry showed that FEV1 changes and the presence or absence of bronchiolitis obliterans were the best predictors for lung transplant graft function (Novick et al., 1998).

The International Society of Heart and Lung Transplantation released guidelines for perioperative care of heart transplant recipients in which they suggest that measures of good cardiac graft function are CI > 2.0 L/min/m$^2$, right atrial pressure (RAP) < 15 mmHg, and PCWP > 15 mmHg (Costanzo et al., 2010). Endomyocardial biopsy is another way to evaluate and follow heart transplant patients for possible rejection (Cowan et al., 2012). Needless to say, the function of a transplant graft is extremely important in determining the overall health of the transplant recipient, and before becoming pregnant patients should be evaluated by their physician to evaluate graft function. As transplant medicine continues to improve, we will see more and more women delivering babies after transplantation, and the level of graft function will play a major role in medical management during pregnancy.

## Immunosuppression

The current mainstays of transplant patient maintenance immunosuppression are CNIs (calcenurin inhibitors, cyclosporine and tacrolimus), corticosteroids, and antiproliferative agents (azathioprine, sirolimus, and mycophenolate mofetil).

### Mycophenolate mofetil

Of all the immunosuppressive drugs used currently, mycophenolate mofetil has been the drug most consistently discussed in regard to fetal malformations. Multiple animal studies have shown a pattern of consistent fetal malformations with the use of mycophenolate mofetil (Tendron et al., 2002; Perez-Aytes et al., 2008). Through review of multiple studies using mycophenolate mofetil, Vento et al. (2008) found that there appears to be a specific phenotype of mutations seen in animal models as well as human fetuses. They recommend not taking mycophenolate mofetil during pregnancy to avoid possible fetal malformations and developmental issues. A case report by Le Ray et al. (2004) documents a case of a woman with a kidney transplant on mycophenolate mofetil who had an unplanned pregnancy and at 13 weeks gestation stopped the mycophenolate mofetil. The fetus describe by Le Ray et al. was aborted at 22 weeks gestation due to multiple malformations, including cleft lip and palate, external auditory duct atresia, microtia, ocular hypertelorism, micrognathia, and corpus callosum agenesis. Le Ray et al. note that the deformities seen in the fetus were similar to malformations seen in animal studies using mycophenolate mofetil (Le Ray et al., 2004) (Figures 40.1 and 40.2).

### Sirolimus

Sirolimus is another drug under contention regarding its safety profile in pregnancy due primarily to the fact that it is a newer drug with little clinical data to support or refute its safety. Multiple case reports have documented successful pregnancies with sirolimus therapy (Jankowska et al., 2004; Guardia et al., 2006; Framarino dei Malatesta et al., 2011).

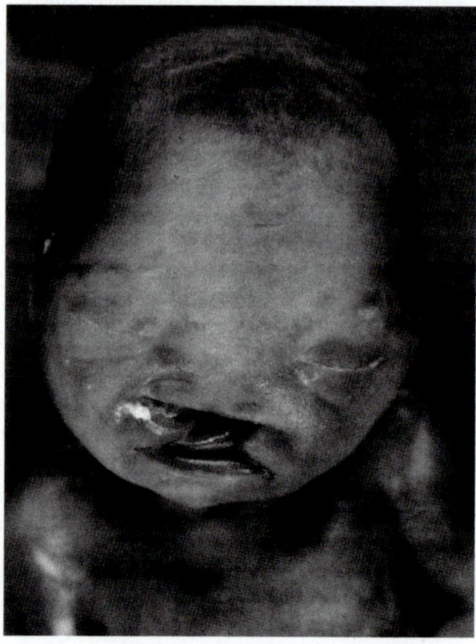

**Fig. 40.1** Fetus with mycophenolate mofetil exposure with cleft lip and palate, ocular hypertelorism, and micrognathia (Le Ray et al., 2004). (Reproduced with permission from Lippincott Williams and Wilkins/Wolters Kluwer Health: *Obstetrics & Gynecology*, Camille Le Ray et al., 'Mycophenolate Mofetil in Pregnancy After Renal Transplantation: A Case of Major Fetal Malformations', 103, 5, pp. 1091–1094, 2004.)

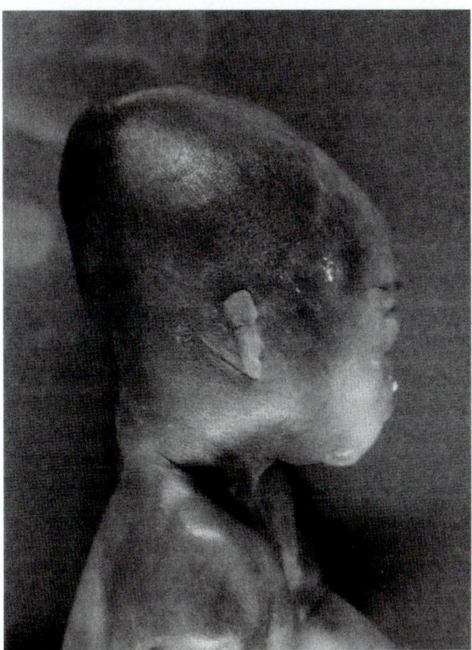

**Fig. 40.2** Fetus with mycophenolate exposure with external ear deformity, microtia, and external auditory duct atresia (Le Ray et al., 2004). (Reproduced with permission from Lippincott Williams and Wilkins/Wolters Kluwer Health: *Obstetrics & Gynecology*, Camille Le Ray et al., 'Mycophenolate Mofetil in Pregnancy After Renal Transplantation: A Case of Major Fetal Malformations', 103, 5, pp. 1091–1094, 2004.)

## Corticosteroids

Corticosteroids such as prednisone used for the maintenance of transplant grafts have shown to cross the placenta, but as much as 90% is metabolized before reaching the fetus (Blanford and Murphy, 1977). Placental metabolism of prednisone confers a fetal safety from adrenal suppression, but because some of the drug does reach the fetus, experts recommend using lower doses of prednisone throughout pregnancy (Bar et al., 1997).

## Azathioprine

In 2004 Matalon et al. (2004) reviewed the placental and embryonic effects of azathioprine. They discussed the high placental uptake (63–94% of maternal levels) of azathioprine and the very low levels of azathioprine found in fetal blood (1–5% of maternal levels). Antenatal exposure of azathioprine has been implicated in fetal complications such as spontaneous abortion, prematurity, low birth weight, and intrauterine growth retardation (Tendron et al., 2002; Langagergaard et al., 2007).

## Cyclosporine

Cyclosporine and tacrolimus are CNIs that have been used for many years in pregnant transplant patients. Cyclosporine became part of the transplant immunosuppression regime in the 1980s, and since that time transplant patient survival has greatly improved. The drug readily crosses the placenta and a study by Venkataramanan et al. (1988) found that the placenta is a reservoir for cyclosporine, housing 5–10 times the amount of cyclosporine found in maternal blood. The amount that gets to the fetus is still not fully known. We do know that it has been used for many years in pregnant transplant patients, and although it has a 2–3% risk of fetal anomalies (Bar Oz et al., 2001) and data suggest cyclosporine increases the incidence of prematurity and low birth weight (Bar Oz et al., 2001), many pregnant women on cyclosporine have had safe and healthy pregnancies. It is known to be nephrotoxic in humans and animals, but fetuses with cyclosporine exposure in utero have shown normal renal function (Shaheen et al., 1993).

## Tacrolimus

Tacrolimus has been gaining popularity as maintenance immunosuppression for pregnant transplant patients. The NTPR in 2012 collected data on 1,073 patients taking cyclosporine and 609 patients taking tacrolimus (Armenti et al., 2012). Data in one study suggest very low rates of congenital malformations (Garcia-Donaire et al., 2005) and another study shows a 4% rate of congenital malformations with tacrolimus (Kainz et al., 2000). Tacrolimus crosses the placenta and has been found to have a fetal blood level up to 71% of maternal blood levels (Zheng et al., 2012).

Pregnancy is a time where most women try to avoid medications, but in the transplant population, immunosuppressive medications are necessary to ensure the maternal graft function. All immunosuppressive medications have the potential to harm the fetus, whether by physical malformations, prematurity, growth restriction, electrolyte disturbances, or fetal organ dysfunction (Kainz et al., 2000; Tendron et al., 2002). It is important to inform patients that there are known, and potential unknown, risks to their fetus. Table 40.2 illustrates the current FDA classification of commonly used immunosuppressive drugs and their potential effect on the fetus.

The immune system in a pregnant woman goes through some changes to allow the safe growth of the fetus, which helps explain the decreased severity of autoimmune diseases and increased severity of viral infections during pregnancy (Pazos et al., 2012). These authors reported decreased B-cells and T-cells in pregnancy. Although pregnant patients are somewhat immune depressed, it is still very important for them to remain on immunosuppressive agents throughout pregnancy. Maternal graft rejection and even death have been reported in patients who have stopped their immunosuppressive drugs during pregnancy (Hebert et al., 2013).

**Table 40.2** FDA categories for common immunosuppressive drugs in transplant patients[a] (Data from the US Food and Drug Administration (FDA))

| Immunosuppressive drugs | FDA category |
|---|---|
| Cyclosporine (Gengraf, Neoral, Sandimmune) | C |
| Tacrolimus (Hecoria, Prograf) | C |
| Azathioprine (Azasan, Imuran) | D |
| Sirolimus (Rapamune) | C |
| Mycophenolate mofetil (CellCept) | D |
| Corticosteroids | C |

[a] Definitions of FDA categories: A, well-controlled human studies have shown no risk to the fetus; B, no risk to the fetus seen in animal reproductive studies, but there are no well-controlled studies in pregnant women; C, adverse fetal outcome seen in animal reproductive studies, but there are no well-controlled studies in pregnant women; D, evidence of adverse fetal outcome; X, evidence of fetal abnormalities and increased fetal risk.

## Liver transplant and pregnancy

Liver failure leads to decreased reproductive function secondary to hypothalamic–pituitary axis dysfunction causing decreased levels of some hormones such as follicle-stimulating hormone (FSH) and luteinizing hormone (LH), as well as increased levels of other hormones such as oestrogen and prolactin (Heneghan et al., 2008). Women of childbearing age with liver failure often find decreased reproductive capabilities that are frequently reversed after transplantation. Most women after transplant will regain menses within 1 month and have regular menstrual cycles within 1 year of transplant (Heneghan et al., 2008). Due to the reproductive changes after liver transplant, women who previously were unable to have children are finally able to become pregnant, and with the improving long-term survival of liver transplant patients (SRTR, 2012), pregnancy has become a relatively safe option for female transplant patients.

### Postliver transplant physiological changes

After liver transplantation there are many physiological changes due to metabolic- and medication-related changes. Immunosuppressive agents, although a necessary part of post-transplant care for graft function, can have many deleterious side effects. Hypertension (60–70% incidence) and chronic kidney disease (incidence of 8–25%) seen after liver transplantation may be related to immunosuppressive agents, specifically CNIs (Singh and Watt, 2012). Diabetes mellitus has an incidence of 30–40% after liver transplantation, with half of those patients having new-onset diabetes (Singh and Watt, 2012). Risks factors for diabetes postliver transplant are obesity, pretransplant diabetes, corticosteroids, CNIs, and hepatitis C infection (Singh and Watt, 2012). Patients with liver failure have low cholesterol levels due to decreased cholesterol synthesis by the liver, so after liver transplantation patients tend to have hyperlipidaemia (Singh and Watt, 2012). With the increased hypertension and hyperlipidaemia, as well as decreased renal function often seen in liver transplant patients, it is no surprise that these patients have an increased risk of cardiovascular events. Up to 25% of liver transplant patients will have a major cardiovascular event within 10 years post-transplant (Ciccarelli et al., 2005). Metabolic syndrome, which encompasses hypertension, obesity, diabetes, and cholesterol derangements, occurs in more than 50% of patients after transplant (Laish et al., 2011) and can lead to significant morbidity and mortality for transplant patients.

### Liver changes during pregnancy

As with most organ systems, the liver has some benign changes during pregnancy. Some of the tests used to determine liver function such as serum glutamic-oxaloacetic transaminase, lactic acid dehydrogenase, alkaline phosphatase, and cholesterol will increase during pregnancy (Suresh et al., 2013). Other liver-related parameters such as albumin, total protein, and antithrombin III will decrease during pregnancy (Wakim-Fleming and Zein, 2005). Liver aminotransferases, bilirubin, and PT should not change during pregnancy (Wakim-Fleming and Zein, 2005), so clinicians must be aware that changes in the above blood tests may be a sign of liver problems. Gall bladder contractility is decreased in pregnancy, so there is an increased rate of cholestasis in pregnant women that occurs at the end of the second trimester and beginning of the third trimester; this often resolves after delivery (Lorente and Montoro, 2007). Pseudocholinesterase is decreased in pregnant women by as much as 20%, but there is no clinically significant prolongation of succinylcholine duration (Blitt et al., 1977).

In light of all the normal changes to liver function during pregnancy, patients with liver transplantation can create a more complicated picture for peripartum management. Women with liver transplants should optimally meet with their primary care physician to evaluate their current liver function and other possible comorbidities prior to becoming pregnant, in order to have a safe and healthy pregnancy.

### Pregnancy-related complications with liver transplant patients

Liver transplant patients, as discussed in 'Liver changes during pregnancy', may possibly have chronic physiological comorbidities. Women who have had a liver transplant have a higher risk of some pregnancy-related conditions often due to the chronic physiological conditions related to liver transplantation. A systematic review and meta-analysis by Deshpande et al. with results from 450 pregnancies in 306 liver transplant patients reported that the rates of pre-eclampsia, preterm delivery, and caesarean delivery were all higher than the general population (Deshpande et al., 2012). They reported that pre-eclampsia rate in liver transplant patients is 21.9%, which is much higher than the 3.8% rate for the general pregnant population (Deshpande et al., 2012). The increased rate of pre-eclampsia in pregnant women with a liver transplant may be related to the hypertension and chronic renal failure seen in liver transplant patients.

Graft rejection and loss is a constant fear of most transplant recipients and many studies have reported graft function results after pregnancy (Jain et al., 2003; Nagy et al., 2003; Christopher et al., 2006), although there are no definitive answers as to whether pregnancy increases graft rejection and/or loss. The NTPR report liver transplant rejection during pregnancy to be 11% with cyclosporine and 3% with tacrolimus, and graft loss within 2 years of delivery to be 7% with cyclosporine and 4% with tacrolimus (Armenti et al., 2012). Coffin et al. (2010) did a case-control analysis to evaluate complications in 146 deliveries to pregnant liver transplant patients. They found that fetal complications such as prematurity, fetal distress, and growth restriction were more common in liver transplant patients, but congenital anomalies were the same in liver transplant and control groups. The 2012 NTPR report shows that babies born to liver transplant patients had newborn complications 26% of the time with cyclosporine and 36% of the time with tacrolimus (Armenti et al., 2012). Besides the known congenital anomalies seen with mycophenolate mofetil (Vento et al., 2008), no studies have proven that other immunosuppressive agents cause congenital malformations. There are many proven complications of pregnancy after liver transplantation; however, many women are delivering healthy babies. Women must be informed of the risks of pregnancy after liver transplant and physicians must be aware of the potential issues they face while caring for pregnant patients with liver transplants.

### Anaesthetic management of a parturient with a liver transplant

As anaesthesiologists we are constantly faced with challenging patients with varying degrees of medical conditions. Pregnancy itself has many challenges related to anaesthetic management and a pregnant woman with a liver transplant is a complicated patient to manage anaesthetically. Prior to determining an anaesthetic plan for a pregnant liver transplant patient, graft status and known complications of liver transplant should be assessed. Intravenous access may be difficult due to obesity or possible oedema related to pre-eclampsia or liver graft failure. Coagulopathies could exist secondary to pre-eclampsia, liver failure, or renal failure. Pregnant women with liver transplants have a higher rate of caesarean delivery (Deshpande et al., 2012), which could lead to airway management issues, surgical difficulties due to previous abdominal surgery, and post-partum haemorrhage if the parturient has coagulopathies. Neuraxial anaesthesia is a great choice for anaesthesia in liver transplant patients during labour, but particular attention must be paid to evaluation of possible coagulopathies prior to neuraxial placement.

Most liver transplant patients are taking long-term corticosteroids, which predisposes them to elevated blood glucose, hypertension, poor wound healing, oedema, obesity, adrenal suppression, and increased risk of infection. Adrenal suppression from corticosteroid can lead to perioperative hypotension, which can be dangerous and refractory to treatment. Historically patients on chronic corticosteroids have received stress-dose steroids intraoperatively. Many studies and review articles have been published on the subject (Brown and Buie, 2001; Jabbour, 2001; Rivers et al., 2001; Tasch, 2002,), but views on using stress-dose steroids have been conflicting. Jabbour reported that any patient with chronic use of corticosteroids (20 mg prednisone for more than 3 weeks) should receive stress-dose steroids perioperatively due to an inability to mount an appropriate cortisol stress response (Jabbour, 2001). Brown and Buie also reported on the use of stress-dose steroids and they suggest that there is no strong evidence for the use of such steroids perioperatively to prevent the hypotension related to adrenal insufficiency (Brown and Buie, 2001). In a review article published in 2002, Tasch discusses that although there are no studies to unequivocally prove the need for stress-dose steroids, the dangers of adrenal insufficiency-related hypotension and the historically safe use of stress-dose steroids give strong reasoning for their continued use perioperatively (Tasch, 2002).

## Kidney transplant and pregnancy

The kidney is the most frequently transplanted organ and has shown the best long-term survival rate of all transplanted organs (SRTR, 2012). After the first woman delivered a baby without immunosuppression with a kidney from her twin sister in 1958, hundreds of babies have been born annually to women with transplanted kidneys (Murray et al., 1963). As with liver disease (discussed in the section 'Liver transplant and pregnancy'), women with ESRD have impaired reproductive function due to lack of ovulation and amenorrhoea (Holley et al., 1997). After kidney transplantation most women return to normal menstrual function and hence experience improved reproductive capabilities to allow for pregnancy (Deshpande et al., 2011).

### Postkidney transplant physiological changes

After kidney transplantation the body adjusts to having a newly functioning kidney; this allows some physiological function to return to normal. As previously discussed in the section 'Liver transplant and pregnancy', reproductive capabilities frequently return to normal after renal transplant. Hyperlipidaemia is very common in renal transplant patients and considered to be due to immunosuppressive agents such as cyclosporine and corticosteroids (Silkensen, 2000). Diabetes, cardiovascular disease, and hypertension are also common comorbidities in renal transplant patients, most often due to pretransplant disease states, long-term uraemia, and immunosuppressive drugs (Silkensen, 2000). A study by Kasiske et al. found that renal transplant patients have four times higher incidence of ischaemic heart disease than the general population (Kasiske, 1988). Infection and malignancy are complications with any organ transplant, presumed to be due to immunosuppression. Most patients will have renal-related osteodystrophy prior to transplantation and, when combined with the osteoporotic effects of corticosteroids, this can lead to severe osteoporosis post-transplant (Kasiske, 1988). Prior to pregnancy women with kidney transplants should be evaluated for graft function and comorbidities.

### Kidney changes during pregnancy

During pregnancy blood volume increases as much as 40%, with an increase in plasma volume of up to 50% (Pritchard, 1965). GFR increases during pregnancy, from 100 to 150 mL/min, to accommodate the increased blood volume (Jeyabalan and Lain, 2007). The increased GFR subsequently leads to decrease in BUN and creatinine levels. Normal BUN and creatinine levels in pregnancy are 9 mg/dL and 0.5 mg/dl, respectively (Jeyabalan and Lain, 2007). Blood flow to the kidneys increases dramatically, as much as 80%, by the 26th week of gestation, and relaxin from the placenta causes renal vasodilation. Protein and glucose both have impaired renal reabsorption during pregnancy, which means that some proteinuria and glucosuria are both normal during pregnancy. Average 24-hour urine protein excretion during pregnancy is approximately 200 mg (Airoldi and Weinstein, 2007). Because often-times renal transplant graft function is measured by following creatinine and proteinuria, pregnancy changes in kidney function can confound or mask alterations in graft function. Women with a kidney transplant planning to become pregnant must have graft function evaluated prepregnancy in order to more efficiently follow graft function throughout pregnancy.

### Pregnancy-related complications with kidney transplant patients

Pregnancy itself is not a benign condition, and when compounded with pregnancy in a renal transplant patient there are increased risks to the mother and baby. In 2011 Deshpande et al. (2011) carried out a systematic review of pregnancy outcomes in kidney transplant patients, which included 4,706 pregnancies in 3,570 kidney transplant patients. They found increased maternal and fetal risk with pregnancy in the kidney transplant population, with high proportions of gestational diabetes, pre-eclampsia, caesarean delivery, preterm birth, and low birth weight (Deshpande et al., 2011).

Graft rejection in pregnant kidney transplant patients according to the NTPR's 2012 report is much lower than rejection seen with pregnant liver transplant patients. The 2012 NTPR report shows rejection episode occurrence is 1% in patients taking cyclosporine and 2% in patients taking tacrolimus, and graft loss occurrence is 8% in the cyclosporine group and 6% in the tacrolimus group (Armenti et al., 2012). Congenital malformations in relation to pregnancy after kidney transplant are equivalent to the incidence of malformations with other types of organ transplants, and congenital anomalies are likely related to genetic chance and immunosuppressive agents. There is an increased risk of fetal complications in babies born to mothers with kidney transplants, and this risk is due to the above-mentioned higher incidence of preterm delivery and low birth weight (see the section 'Pregnancy-related complications with kidney transplant patients'). The NTPR data report between 41 and 53% incidence of newborn complications in relation to pregnancy in kidney transplant females (Armenti et al., 2012). Female kidney transplant patients should be informed of the risks to themselves and their babies prior to conception, in order to allow for medical management of comorbidities so they can have the safest possible pregnancy.

### Anaesthetic management of the parturient with a kidney transplant

Graft function and comorbidities must be evaluated prior to and at the beginning of pregnancy. Women with kidney transplants can be anaesthetically challenging. Peripheral oedema and pre-eclampsia could make intravenous access difficult. Cardiovascular disease should be evaluated and managed appropriately. Renal graft failure could lead to decreased drug clearance, electrolyte abnormalities, oedema, and haemodynamic issues. Increased caesarean delivery rate could potentiate risks associated with airway, vascular access, and fluid dynamics. Previous abdominal surgery increases the risk of intraoperative bleeding and surgical complications if caesarean delivery is required. Chronic corticosteroid use is of concern because corticosteroids increase the risk of infection, oedema, haemodynamic changes, difficult wound healing, adrenal suppression, and elevated blood glucose. As long as the patient is amenable and has no contraindications, neuraxial anaesthesia can be a good choice for anaesthetic management of renal transplant patients in labour.

## Heart and lung transplant and pregnancy

Since the first successful delivery to a parturient with a heart transplant in 1986, hundreds of women have delivered babies after heart and/or lung transplantation (Lowenstein et al., 1988; Armenti et al., 2012). The 2012 data from the NTPR have 116 pregnancies in heart transplant patients, 31 pregnancies in lung transplant patients, and five pregnancies in heart–lung transplant patients (Armenti et al., 2012). Pregnancy for heart and lung transplant patients, just as with other solid organ transplants, is complicated by physiological changes of the graft organ and the physiological changes of pregnancy. Patients must be told of the risk to both mother and baby, as well as counselled on the long-term plans for childcare if the mother has morbidity and mortality related to the pregnancy and previous transplantation.

### Post-transplant physiological changes

#### Heart

The transplanted heart is denervated, which means that the heart rate is dependent on the intrinsic rate of the donated sinoatrial node. In a heart transplant patient the resting heart rate typically runs between 90 and 100 bpm and the vagal response is absent in the donor heart. The heart in a transplanted patient will not react normally to things such as carotid sinus massage, position changes, and valsalva manoeuvres (Dash, 1995). Due to the inability of the transplanted heart to adjust to stress with heart rate changes, the transplanted heart's primary response to stress or exercise is to increase the cardiac output via increased stroke volume. The donor heart is essentially preload dependent in order to maintain stroke volume increases in times of stress.

#### Lung

The transplanted lung, much like the transplanted heart, is considered a denervated organ due to the complete transection of pulmonary autonomic nerve supply during surgery (Studer et al., 2004). Bronchial hyperreactivity to methacholine, but not to exercise or dry air, is common in lung transplant patients and is postulated to be due to airway denervation leading to upregulation of muscarinic receptors and hence smooth muscle hypersensitivity (Liakakos et al., 1997). Resting minute ventilation, tidal volume, and ventilatory drive are unchanged in lung transplant patients, but such patients have decreased ventilatory responses to hypercapnia, specifically less respiratory rate changes (Sanders et al., 1989). Ventilation and perfusion of the transplanted lung is considered equivalent to that of the normal lung and gas exchange is thought to be normal within 8 weeks after transplantation (Studer et al., 2004).

### Cardiopulmonary physiological changes during pregnancy

#### Heart

Cardiac output begins increasing by the tenth week of gestation, reaches a 50% increase by 34 weeks, then stays stable until labour, when cardiac output continues to increase, eventually returning to baseline 2–5 days postpartum (Suresh, 2013). Blood volume, stroke volume, and heart rate all increase during pregnancy, while blood pressure and peripheral resistance decrease. Normal ECG changes in pregnancy are shortened PR, shortened QT interval, QRS axis deviation, and transient ST segment changes. Normal echocardiographic findings in pregnancy are regurgitation of the pulmonary and tricuspid valve in 94% of cases and regurgitation of the mitral valve in 27% (Campos et al., 1993). Accentuated first heart sound and later in pregnancy a third heart sound may be heard (Cutforth and MacDonald, 1966).

#### Lung

During pregnancy tidal volume increases almost 45% with increased inspiratory reserve and FRC decreases by up to 80%. The parturient is at risk for hypoxaemia while in the supine position due to possible decreased FRC below the closing capacity of the lungs. Progesterone, which is a direct respiratory stimulant, causes increased minute ventilation via increased tidal volume. Progesterone also sensitizes the central respiratory centre and increases the ventilatory response to $CO_2$ (Suresh, 2013). The $CO_2$ response curve is shifted to the left in pregnancy. Respiratory alkalosis is normal in pregnant women, with $PaCO_2$ values between 30 and 32 mmHg. A study by Jensen et al. (2008) showed that the hyperventilation during pregnancy is attributed to a complex interaction between changes in wakefulness, central chemoreceptors' drive to breath, acid-base balance, metabolic rate, and cerebral blood flow in the parturient. Pregnant women also have higher oxygen consumption due to delivery and use of oxygen by the fetus, uterus, and placenta. Oxygen consumption increases as much as 60% (Prowse and Gaensler, 1965). Due to high $O_2$ consumption and decreased FRC, pregnant women desaturate very quickly during apnoea. One study found that after 99% denitrogenation it only took 4 minutes for $SaO_2$ to drop below 90%, in comparison to non-pregnant patients who take more than 7 minutes to drop $SaO_2$ below 90% (McClelland et al., 2008).

### Pregnancy-related complications with heart and lung transplants

Data for pregnancy related to heart and/or lung transplants are limited in comparison to that available for liver and kidney transplants. Heart and/or lung transplant patients receive the same immunosuppressive agents discussed for other solid organ transplants, so the same complications apply, such as nephrotoxicity from cyclosporine, chronic corticosteroid side effects, and possible fetal complications. Data from the NTPR 2012 report show that maternal hypertension is common in heart and/or lung transplant patients during pregnancy, with as much as a 50% incidence of hypertension during pregnancy (Armenti et al., 2012). The risk of pre-eclampsia during pregnancy is equivalent to the amount of risk seen in liver and kidney transplant parturients (Armenti et al., 2012) and confounded by the chronic hypertension seen in transplant patients and the renal insufficiency likely from immunosuppression agents. Preterm delivery and low birth weight are common risks to the fetus in women with heart and/or lung transplants, as seen with other organ transplants (Armenti et al., 2012).

Immunosuppression in pregnant transplant patients leads to increased risk of infection (Cowan et al., 2012). Women should be followed for signs of infection, assessed for vaccine titres prior to pregnancy, and treated if infection does occur. Graft rejection is a concern with any transplant patient. NTPR data from 2012 show that 116 pregnancies in 67 women with heart transplants had 21% graft rejection with cyclosporine, 2% graft rejection with tacrolimus, no graft loss within 2 years of delivery with cyclosporine, and 2% graft loss within 2 years of delivery with tacrolimus (Armenti et al., 2012). NTPR 2012 data for lung transplant patients show that 31 pregnancies in 22 women had 16% graft rejection and 14% graft loss within 2 years of delivery (Armenti et al., 2012).

### Anaesthetic management of the parturient with heart and/or lung transplant

Patients with heart and/or lung transplant must have graft function evaluated prior to pregnancy and anaesthesia staff must be notified of graft function prior to administering anaesthesia. Besides the standard preoperative assessment, the anaesthesiologist must do a full review of the patient's surgical history, previous graft-related issues, current medications, ECG, echocardiograms, blood tests, myocardial biopsy results for heart transplant patients (Dash, 1995), and pulmonary function tests for lung transplant patients. Vaginal delivery is recommended and caesarean is reserved for patients who meet the obstetric requirements for caesarean delivery (McKay et al., 2005). There have been case reports of women with heart, lung, and heart–lung transplantation having successful neuraxial anaesthesia for labour and caesarean delivery (Camann et al., 1989; Rigg et al., 2000), although some sources feel that general anaesthesia is best for the heart transplant patient during caesarean deliveries in order to avoid exaggerated hypotension (Dash, 1995). Neuraxial anaesthesia seems to be a safe option for labour and caesarean delivery in heart and/or lung transplant patients, as long as the anaesthesiologist attempts to avoid high blockade levels to preclude decreased respiratory function and excessive sympathetic blockade. Immunosuppression side effects, graft function, comorbidities, and fetal complications must be assessed prior to managing heart and/or lung transplant patients.

#### Heart

Due to denervation of the transplanted heart, anaesthesiologists must be aware that the underlying heart rate will range between 90 and 100 bpm, the patient may have increased risk of arrhythmias, and cardiac output is dependent on stroke volume changes (Haddow, 1997). Circulating catecholamines may take up to 5 minutes to cause heart rate changes in the denervated heart. Many medications commonly used to change heart rate will be ineffective in the denervated heart, such as phenylephrine, anticholinergics, and anticholinesterases. The denervated heart requires direct-acting β-adrenergic agents to increase heart rate, such as epinephrine, ephedrine, and isoproterenol (Cheng and Ong, 1993; Stover and Siegel, 1995). Anaesthesiologists caring for pregnant women with heart transplants must be aware of the underlying mechanics of the heart graft and the effects of medications that are used.

#### Lung

Specifically for lung transplant patients, endotracheal intubation must be handled carefully with regards to the tracheal suture line, which is usually proximal to the carina (Haddow, 1997). The anaesthesiologist must be aware of autonomic denervation to the lung graft which may or may not have improved since transplantation, and also lymphatic circulation dysfunction that may also not yet be recovered (Haddow, 1997). Increased risk of pulmonary oedema, lack of cough reflex, decreased mucociliary clearance, and bronchial hyperreactivity may all be present in the pregnant patient with a lung transplant (Herve et al., 1993; Higenbottam et al., 1989; Haddow, 1997).

## Other solid organ transplants

Besides the liver, kidney, heart, and lung, other organs such as the intestine and pancreas and also combinations of multiple organs are frequently being transplanted. The NTPR 2012 database has the most documented information with regard to pregnancy after transplantation of some of the less frequently transplanted organs. In the 2012 report the NTPR had eight pregnancies in liver–kidney transplant patients, two pregnancies in intestine transplant patients, 97 pregnancies in pancreas–kidney transplant patients, and eight pregnancies in pancreas transplant patients (Armenti et al., 2012). There has also been one case report of a successful delivery in a pregnant woman with an intestine–liver–pancreas transplant (Srivastava et al., 2012). There are a few specific issues related to multiple organ transplant patients, such as more than one organ graft to evaluate, comorbidities related to each organ, and possible increased severity of the patient's underlying condition which may have led to the transplantation.

#### Intestine

Specific to intestinal transplant, clinicians should be aware of the increased risk of osteoporosis secondary to poor bone mineralization prior to transplant and corticosteroids postoperatively, as well as malnutrition from possible poor intestinal absorption

(Horslen, 2006). Many intestinal transplant patients have been on long-term TPN, which requires repeated intravenous access and has an increased risk of liver-related complications and poor nutrition status. The NTPR reports two successful pregnancies after intestinal transplant (Armenti et al., 2012); one of the two reported cases had an uncomplicated spontaneous vaginal delivery, with an acute rejection episode 3 months postpartum (Gomez-Lobo et al., 2012).

### Pancreas

Most frequently the pancreas is transplanted with a kidney, although solitary pancreas transplants do occur. SPK (simultaneous pancreas-kidney) transplants are commonly done for diabetic patients with nephropathy. Pancreatic transplant graft function is determined based on the patient's insulin dependence and blood levels of pancreatic enzymes, so patients with pancreatic transplants should be followed closely for changes in blood glucose, amylase, and lipase (Koehntop et al., 2000). During pregnancy a patient with a functioning pancreatic graft should be expected to maintain normoglycaemia. The rate of diabetes in pregnant women with SPK transplants, as per the NTPR 2012 report, is equivalent to that found in other solid organ transplants (Armenti et al., 2012). The anaesthesia for delivery in pancreas transplant patients is ideally neuraxial due to its maternal and fetal benefits. One case report showed a good outcome with epidural anaesthesia for caesarean delivery of a woman with an SPK transplant (Smyth et al., 2011).

## Conclusion

Pregnancy is a challenging time for the human body, with many transient organ changes to accommodate the growing fetus. Women who have had a solid organ transplant may have even more drastic changes during pregnancy and may risk the well-being of the fetus with physiological derangements and immunosuppressive therapy. Pregnancy in a woman with a transplanted organ should optimally be decided upon with the guidance of a knowledgeable physician and with prepregnancy evaluation of the woman's graft function and optimization of her possible other comorbidities. Due to the risks to the fetus, such as low birth weight, prematurity, and fetal malformations, the fetus must be regularly assessed throughout pregnancy by a qualified obstetrician. Both mother and baby require vigilant management during pregnancy to help decrease the risk of adverse events. The decision on when and how to deliver the baby should be made with a multidisciplinary team consisting of an obstetrician, anaesthesiologist, transplant physician, nursing staff, and any other specialists relating to the patient's comorbidities. Anaesthesiologists must consider the optimal anaesthetic approach on a patient-by-patient basis. Most women with solid organ transplants will be good candidates for neuraxial anaesthesia, with the main concern being possible coagulopathies. Of note, anaesthesiologists should be aware that chronic corticosteroid and immunosuppressive use in the transplant population can increase infection, specifically worrisome with neuraxial anaesthesia but also a concern with possible airway oedema, difficult intravenous access, and osteoporotic bone changes. Overall, the pregnant patient with a solid organ transplant can be challenging to manage; it is important for physicians to understand the underlying physiology and medication-related complications and to work as a team to protect the safety of both mother and baby.

## References


Airoldi J, Weinstein L (2007) Clinical significance of proteinuria in pregnancy. *Obstet Gynecol Surv*, **62**:117–124.

Armenti VT, Moritz MJ, Coscia LA, McGrory CH, Carlin FR, Armenti D (2012) Report from the National Transplantation Pregnancy Registry (NTPR): outcomes of pregnancy after transplantation. *Clin Transpl*, **2000**:65–85.

Bar J, Fisch B, Wittenberg C, Gelerenter I, Boner G, Hod M (1997) Prednisone dosage and pregnancy outcome in renal allograft recipients. *Nephrol Dial Transplant*, **12**:760–763.

Bar Oz B, Hackman R, Einarson T, Koren G (2001) Pregnancy outcome after cyclosporine therapy during pregnancy: a meta-analysis. *Transplantation*, **71**:1051–1055.

Blanford AT, Murphy BE (1977) In vitro metabolism of prednisolone, dexamethasone, betamethasone, and cortisol by the human placenta. *Am J Obstet Gynecol*, **127**:264–267.

Blitt CD, Petty WC, Alberternst EE, Wright BJ (1977) Correlation of plasma cholinesterase activity and duration of action of succinylcholine during pregnancy. *Anesth Analg*, **56**:78–83.

Brown CJ, Buie WD (2001) Perioperative stress dose steroids: do they make a difference? *J Am Coll Surg*, **193**:678–686.

Camann WR, Goldman GA, Johnson MD, Moore J, Greene M (1989) Cesarean delivery in a patient with a transplanted heart. *Anesthesiology*, **71**:618–620.

Campos O, Andrade JL, Bocanegra J, et al. (1993) Physiologic multivalvular regurgitation during pregnancy: a longitudinal Doppler echocardiographic study. *Int J Cardiol*, **40**:265–272.

Cheng DC, Ong DD (1993) Anaesthesia for non-cardiac surgery in heart-transplanted patients. *Can J Anaesth*, **40**:981–986.

Christopher V, al-Chalabi T, Richardson PD, et al. (2006) Pregnancy outcome after liver transplantation: a single-center experience of 71 pregnancies in 45 recipients. *Liver Transpl*, **12**:1138–1143.

Ciccarelli O, Kaczmarek B, Roggen F, et al. (2005) Long-term medical complications and quality of life in adult recipients surviving 10 years or more after liver transplantation. *Acta Gastroenterol Belg*, **68**:323–330.

Coffin CS, Shaheen AA, Burak KW, Myers RP (2010) Pregnancy outcomes among liver transplant recipients in the United States: a nationwide case-control analysis. *Liver Transpl*, **16**:56–63.

Costanzo MR, Dipchard A, Starling R, et al. (2010) Task force 1: peri-operative care of the heart transplant recipient. In: The International Society of Heart and Lung Transplantation Guidelines for the Care of Heart Transplant Recipients. *J Heart Lung Transplant*, **29**(8):915–926.

Cowan SW, Davison JM, Doria C, Moritz MJ, Armenti VT (2012) Pregnancy after cardiac transplantation. *Cardiol Clin*, **30**:441–452.

Cutforth R, MacDonald CB (1966) Heart sounds and murmurs in pregnancy. *Am Heart J*, **71**:741–747.

Dash A (1995) Anesthesia for patients with a previous heart transplant. *Int Anesthesiol Clin*, **33**:1–9.

Deshpande NA, James NT, Kucirka LM, et al. (2011) Pregnancy outcomes in kidney transplant recipients: a systematic review and meta-analysis. *Am J Transplant*, **11**:2388–2404.

Deshpande NA, James NT, Kucirka LM, et al. (2012) Pregnancy outcomes of liver transplant recipients: a systematic review and meta-analysis. *Liver Transpl*, **18**:621–629.

Framarino dei Malatesta M, Corona LE, De Luca L, et al. (2011) Successful pregnancy in a living-related kidney transplant recipient who received sirolimus throughout the whole gestation. *Transplantation*, **91**:e69–e71.

Garcia-Donaire JA, Acevedo M, Gutierrez MJ, et al. (2005) Tacrolimus as basic immunosuppression in pregnancy after renal transplantation. A single-center experience. *Transplant Proc*, **37**:3754–3755.

Gomez-Lobo V, Landy HJ, Matsumoto C,Fishbein TM (2012) Pregnancy in an intestinal transplant recipient. *Obstet Gynecol*, **120**:497–500.

Guardia O, Rial Mdel C, Casadei D (2006) Pregnancy under sirolimus-based immunosuppression. *Transplantation*, **81**:636.

Haddow GR (1997) Anaesthesia for patients after lung transplantation. *Can J Anaesth*, **44**:182–197.

Hebert MF, Zheng S, Hays K, et al. (2013) Interpreting tacrolimus concentrations during pregnancy and postpartum. *Transplantation*, **95**:908–915.

Heneghan MA, Selzner M, Yoshida EM, Mullhaupt B (2008) Pregnancy and sexual function in liver transplantation. *J Hepatol*, **49**:507–519.

Herve P, Silbert D, Cerrina J, Simonneau G, Dartevelle P (1993) Impairment of bronchial mucociliary clearance in long-term survivors of heart/lung and double-lung transplantation. The Paris-Sud Lung Transplant Group. *Chest*, **103**:59–63.

Higenbottam T, Jackson M, Woolman P, Lowry R, Wallwork J (1989) The cough response to ultrasonically nebulized distilled water in heart–lung transplantation patients. *Am Rev Respir Dis*, **140**:58–61.

Holley JL, Schmidt RJ, Bender FH, Dumler F, Schiff M (1997) Gynecologic and reproductive issues in women on dialysis. *Am J Kidney Dis*, **29**:685–690.

Horslen SP (2006) Optimal management of the post-intestinal transplant patient. *Gastroenterology*, **130**:S163–S169.

Jabbour SA (2001) Steroids and the surgical patient. *Med Clin N Am*, **85**:1311–1317.

Jain AB, Reyes J, Marcos A, et al. (2003) Pregnancy after liver transplantation with tacrolimus immunosuppression: a single center's experience update at 13 years. *Transplantation*, **76**:827–832.

Jankowska I, Oldakowska-Jedynak U, Jabiry-Zieniewicz Z, et al. (2004) Absence of teratogenicity of sirolimus used during early pregnancy in a liver transplant recipient. *Transplant Proc*, **36**:3232–3233.

Jensen D, Duffin J, Lam YM, et al. (2008) Physiological mechanisms of hyperventilation during human pregnancy. *Respir Physiol Neurobiol*, **161**:76–86.

Jeyabalan A, Lain KY (2007) Anatomic and functional changes of the upper urinary tract during pregnancy. *Urol Clin N Am*, **34**:1–6.

Kainz A, Harabacz I, Cowlrick IS, Gadgil SD, Hagiwara D (2000) Review of the course and outcome of 100 pregnancies in 84 women treated with tacrolimus. *Transplantation*, **70**:1718–1721.

Kasiske BL (1988) Risk factors for accelerated atherosclerosis in renal transplant recipients. *Am J Med*, **84**:985–992.

Koehntop DE, Beebe DS, Belani KG (2000) Perioperative anesthetic management of the kidney–pancreas transplant recipient. *Curr Opin Anaesthesiol*, **13**:341–347.

Laish I, Braun M, Mor E, Sulkes J, Harif Y, Ben Ari Z (2011) Metabolic syndrome in liver transplant recipients: prevalence, risk factors, and association with cardiovascular events. *Liver Transpl*, **17**:15–22.

Langagergaard V, Pedersen L, Gislum M, Norgard B, Sorensen HT (2007) Birth outcome in women treated with azathioprine or mercaptopurine during pregnancy: a Danish nationwide cohort study. *Aliment Pharmacol Ther*, **25**:73–81.

Le Ray C, Coulomb A, Elefant E, Frydman R, Audibert F (2004) Mycophenolate mofetil in pregnancy after renal transplantation: a case of major fetal malformations. *Obstet Gynecol*, **103**:1091–1094.

Liakakos P, Snell GI, Ward C, et al. (1997) Bronchial hyperresponsiveness in lung transplant recipients: lack of correlation with airway inflammation. *Thorax*, **52**:551–556.

Lorente S, Montoro MA (2007) Cholestasis of pregnancy. *Gastroenterol Hepatol*, **30**:541–547.

Lowenstein BR, Vain NW, Perrone SV, Wright DR, Boullon FJ, Favaloro RG (1988) Successful pregnancy and vaginal delivery after heart transplantation. *Am J Obstet Gynecol*, **158**:589–590.

Marcen R, Morales JM, Fernandez-Rodriguez A, et al. (2010) Long-term graft function changes in kidney transplant recipients. *NDT Plus*, **3**:ii2–ii8.

Matalon ST, Ornoy A, Lishner M (2004) Review of the potential effects of three commonly used antineoplastic and immunosuppressive drugs (cyclophosphamide, azathioprine, doxorubicin on the embryo and placenta). *Reprod Toxicol*, **18**:219–230.

McClelland SH, Bogod DG, Hardman JG (2008) Apnoea in pregnancy: an investigation using physiological modelling. *Anaesthesia*, **63**:264–269.

McKay DB, Josephson MA, Armenti VT, et al. (2005) Reproduction and transplantation: report on the AST Consensus Conference on Reproductive Issues and Transplantation. *Am J Transplant*, **5**:1592–1599.

Murray JE, Reid DE, Harrison JH, Merrill JP (1963) Successful pregnancies after human renal transplantation. *N Engl J Med*, **269**:341–343.

Nagy S, Bush MC, Berkowitz R, Fishbein TM, Gomez-Lobo V (2003) Pregnancy outcome in liver transplant recipients. *Obstet Gynecol*, **102**:121–128.

Novick RJ, Stitt LW, al-Kattan K, et al. (1998) Pulmonary retransplantation: predictors of graft function and survival in 230 patients. Pulmonary Retransplant Registry. *Ann Thorac Surg*, **65**:227–234.

Pazos M, Sperling RS, Moran TM, Kraus TA (2012) The influence of pregnancy on systemic immunity. *Immunol Res*, **54**:254–261.

Perez-Aytes A, Ledo A, Boso V, et al. (2008) In utero exposure to mycophenolate mofetil: a characteristic phenotype? *Am J Med Genet*, **146A**:1–7.

Pritchard JA (1965) Changes in the blood volume during pregnancy and delivery. *Anesthesiology*, **26**:393–399.

Prowse CM, Gaensler EA (1965) Respiratory and acid-base changes during pregnancy. *Anesthesiology*, **26**:381–392.

Rigg CD, Bythell VE, Bryson MR, Halshaw J, Davidson JM (2000) Caesarean section in patients with heart–lung transplants: a report of three cases and review. *Int J Obstet Anesth*, **9**:125–132.

Rivers EP, Gaspari M, Saad GA, et al. (2001) Adrenal insufficiency in high-risk surgical ICU patients. *Chest*, **119**:889–896.

Sanders MH, Owens GR, Sciurba FC, et al. (1989) Ventilation and breathing pattern during progressive hypercapnia and hypoxia after human heart–lung transplantation. *Am Rev Respir Dis*, **140**:38–44.

Shaheen FA, al-Sulaiman MH, al-Khader AA (1993) Long-term nephrotoxicity after exposure to cyclosporine in utero. *Transplantation*, **56**:224–225.

Silkensen JR (2000) Long-term complications in renal transplantation. *J Am Soc Nephrol*, **11**:582–588.

Singh S, Watt KD (2012) Long-term medical management of the liver transplant recipient: what the primary care physician needs to know. *Mayo Clin Proc*, **87**:779–790.

Smyth A, Gaffney G, Hickey D, Lappin D, Reddan D, Dunne F (2011) Successful pregnancy after simultaneous pancreas–kidney transplantation. *Case Rep Obstet Gynecol*, **2011** :983592.

Srivastava R, Clarke S, Gupte GL, Cartmill JL (2012) Successful pregnancy outcome following triple organ transplantation (small intestine, liver and pancreas). *Eur J Obstet Gynecol Reprod Biol*, **163**:238–239.

SRTR (2012) OPTN and SRTR Annual Data Report 2011. United States Organ Transplantation. US Department of Health and Human Services Health Resources and Services Administration. SRTR, Minneapolis.

Stover EP, Siegel LC (1995) Physiology of the transplanted heart. *Int Anesthesiol Clin*, **33**:11–20.

Studer SM, Levy RD, McNeil K, Orens JB (2004) Lung transplant outcomes: a review of survival, graft function, physiology, health-related quality of life and cost-effectiveness. *Eur Respir J*, **24**:674–685.

Suresh MS, Segal BS, Preston RL, Fernando R, Mason CL (2013) *Shnider and Levinson's Anesthesia for Obstetrics*. Lippincott Williams & Wilkins, Baltimore, Maryland.

Tasch MD (2002) Corticosteroids and anesthesia. *Curr Opin Anaesthesiol*, **15**:377–381.

Tendron A, Gouyon JB, Decramer S (2002) In utero exposure to immunosuppressive drugs: experimental and clinical studies. *Pediatr Nephrol*, **17**:121–130.

Venkataramanan R, Koneru B, Wang CC, Burckart GJ, Caritis SN, Starzl TE (1988) Cyclosporine and its metabolites in mother and baby. *Transplantation*, **46**:468–469.

Vento M, Perez Aytes A, Ledo A, Boso V, Carey JC (2008) Mycophenolate mofetil during pregnancy: some words of caution. *Pediatrics*, **122**:184–185.

Wakim-Fleming J, Zein NN (2005) The liver in pregnancy: disease vs benign changes. *Cleve Clin J Med*, **72**:713–721.

Zheng S, Easterling TR, Umans JG, et al. (2012) Pharmacokinetics of tacrolimus during pregnancy. *Ther Drug Monit*, **34**:660–670.

# CHAPTER 41

# Starting a new organ transplant programme

Karina Rando and Gebhard Wagener

## Introduction

The ability to provide organ transplant services to patients with terminal organ diseases has been one of the greatest advances of medicine in the last decades (Medlin et al., 2006; Rando et al., 2011). Organ transplantation has become the treatment of choice for eligible patients with end-stage organ disease. Yet, despite the unprecedented success of organ transplantation, the type, scope, and quality of transplantation programmes vary widely between countries. Setting up a transplant programme is exceedingly complex and involves many different stakeholders and participants. Aside from the need for an advanced healthcare infrastructure, societal (i.e. cultural, religious, legal, and economic) factors often shape and dictate the structure of the transplant programme. For example, certain approaches to the development of transplant programmes such as living organ donation may not be acceptable in some societies (Rios et al., 2006; Caplan, 2011; Cronin, 2011; Glannon, 2011; Hofmann, 2011; McGill and Ko, 2011). Furthermore, if patients travel to other countries for transplantation, unique challenges to the continued care of transplant patients may occur (Kapoor et al., 2011).

A major obstacle to building a new transplant programme is the associated high capital investment and labour intensity. A transplantation programme cannot function in isolation as it depends on the existence of a sophisticated hospital infrastructure to support transplant services. Services such as critical care medicine, advanced interventional radiology, and transplant-oriented infectious disease, pharmacy and laboratory support need to be available a priori (Gasper et al., 2008; Lampela et al., 2011; Pavlakis and Hanto, 2011). This type of integrated service is essential to minimize wait-list mortality and assure excellent transplant outcomes with patient follow-up care (Rando et al., 2010; Grattagliano et al., 2011; Trainor et al., 2011). Additionally, a network of community primary care physicians and specialists (i.e. nephrologists/hepatologists) is essential in order to secure the long-term sustainability of a transplant programme. Timely recognition of eligible transplant patients and their referral to transplant centres is of paramount importance. Likewise, close cooperation between community healthcare providers and the transplant centres during patient follow-up is essential for excellent long-term outcomes after transplantation (Jafferbhoy et al., 2011).

## When is it time to set up a new transplant centre?

In high-income countries the number of transplantation centres is regulated by either the government (the UK, France) or independent government-mandated and -financed agencies such as UNOS in the US. In either case the driving force is the need in each country to serve its citizens with end-stage organ disease in order to improve life expectancy and quality of life. To serve this demand, a national infrastructure needs to be in place and fully developed to supply the needed organs within a legal and ethical framework. This is achieved with the establishment of legislation to mandate brain death certification and organ sharing and procurement organizations (OPOs) for deceased donor and living donor programmes (Medlin et al., 2006). This infrastructure can be expensive to build and maintain, and consequently countries with limited resources may be reluctant to start transplant programmes that divert financial resources away from preventive healthcare. When geographically feasible, sending patients to experienced centres in foreign countries may be more cost-effective and beneficial for the patient but may entail complex logistic and legal challenges. For example, prior to starting its own liver transplant programme in 2010, Uruguay had an agreement with Argentina that allowed patients from Uruguay who required a liver transplant to be referred to transplant centres in Argentina. This may be a viable option for many countries that remain unable to offer transplantation services to their citizens with end-stage organ disease.

Among Latin American countries, organ donation and transplantation rates vary significantly. While most have kidney transplant programmes, liver, heart, and lung transplantation programmes remain in their infancy in many Latin American countries. To further complicate matters, access to transplant services in much of Latin America is limited to a small part of the population who can afford to pay for costly transplant procedures, since in many cases these services are usually available only at private clinics or hospitals. For example, 70% of the population in Perú and 75% in Ecuador have no access to advanced healthcare (Duro, 2001) and many other developing and emergent countries face similar situations. These countries need to expand access to advanced healthcare to the entire population and to include transplantation services for all patients with end-stage organ disease (Depine, 2009).

**Table 41.1** Donation and transplantation activities in Latin America, Portugal, and Spain during 2007 and/or 2008. (Data from Punta Cana web site: www.grupopuntacana.org/ (http://www.grupopuntacana.org/ 2012))

| COUNTRY | YEAR | POTENTIAL DONORS | DD | FAMILY DENIES | DD KIDNEY | LR KIDNEY | CARDIAC TRANSPLANTS | KIDNEY–PANCREAS | LIVER |
|---|---|---|---|---|---|---|---|---|---|
| | | (PMP) | | (%) | (TRANSPLANTS PMP) | | | | |
| ARGENTINA | 2008 | 29.1 | 13.1 | 47.8 | 19.3 | 4.6 | 2.7 | 1.9 | 7.3 |
| BOLIVIA | 2008 | n/d | 2.2 | n/d | 4.2 | 4.2 | n/d | n/d | n/d |
| BRAZIL | 2008 | n/d | 7.2 | n/d | 11 | 9.5 | 1.1 | 0.2 | 5.7 |
| CHILE | 2008 | n/d | 7.1 | 33 | 12.3 | n/d | 1.1 | n/d | 4.4 |
| COLOMBIA | 2008 | n/d | 9.6 | 40.1 | 13.3 | 1.33 | 1.72 | 0.1 | 4.12 |
| COSTA RICA | 2007 | n/d | 4.2 | n/d | 4 | 4.4 | 0.2 | n/d | n/d |
| CUBA | 2008 | n/d | 16.6 | 27 | 12.1 | 0.7 | 0.26 | 0.08 | 2.5 |
| DOMINICAN REPUBLIC | 2008 | 10.7 | 4.32 | 43.8 | 0.74 | 10 | n/d | n/d | 0.11 |
| ECUADOR | 2007 | n/d | 1.8 | n/d | 0.8 | 3.15 | n/d | n/d | n/d |
| EL SALVADOR | 2007 | n/d | 0 | n/d | n/d | 5.4 | n/d | n/d | n/d |
| HONDURAS | 2007 | n/d | 0.1 | n/d | 0.5 | n/d | n/d | n/d | n/d |
| MEXICO | 2008 | n/d | 3.11 | n/d | 5.26 | 15.91 | 0.13 | 0.009 | 0.89 |
| PANAMA | 2008 | n/d | 1.2 | n/d | 2.4 | 2.5 | n/d | n/d | n/d |
| PARAGUAY | 2007 | n/d | 2.7 | 30 | 0.5 | 3.4 | 0.38 | n/d | n/d |
| PERU | 2008 | n/d | 0.8 | n/d | n/d | n/d | n/d | n/d | n/d |
| URUGUAY | 2008 | n/d | 19.1 | 32 | 34.5 | 2.12 | 3.3 | 1.81 | n/d |
| VENEZUELA | 2008 | 7.09 | 3.329 | 28.28 | 6.372 | 3.58 | n/d | n/d | 0.36 |
| PORTUGAL | 2007 | n/d | 23.9 | n/d | 42 | 3.5 | 4.8 | 1.8 | 25.1 |
| SPAIN | 2008 | 41.6 | 34.2 | 17.9 | 44.95 | 154 | 6.3 | n/d | 1108 |

n/d, No data; pmp, per million people; DD, diseased donor(s); LR, .

Data from the Punta Cana Group (Iberoamerican Group of Transplant Coordinators—<www.grupopuntacana.org/>[1]) illustrate the paucity of transplantation in Latin America (Duro, 2001; Depine, 2009) (Table 41.1).

## The foundations of a successful transplant programme

A successful transplant programme has to operate within the cultural context of its country. Societal endorsement of the transplant process including its infrastructure for organ supply is of paramount importance and will require the inclusion of many stakeholders from different parts of society. Each country must have oversight mechanisms in place to ensure patient safety, ethics, and patient outcomes.

Some countries have dedicated organizations that monitor transplantation and transplantation outcomes, such as United Network for Organ Sharing (UNOS) in the US, Organización Nacional de Trasplantes (ONT) in Spain, and the Directorate of Organ Donation and Transplantation (formerly UK Transplant) in the UK. Eurotransplant International Foundation (formerly Eurotransplant (<http://www.eurotransplant.org/>)) is a similar but supranational organization that coordinates organ donation in European countries[2]. The general objective is to evaluate the results of organ transplantation in Europe. That allows a comprehensive overview of the quality and safety in solid organ transplantation and identification of best practices and safety standards. Special project objectives include the preparation of a registry of outcome data of cadaveric solid organ transplantation.

[1] The Latin-American transplant coordinators met in the Dominican Republic (Punta Cana) in 2001 during the XVI Latin American Congress of Transplantation and formed this group with the support of Spanish transplant coordinators. The objective of this group is to use the experience of the 'Spanish model' to develop donation and transplantation activity in Latin America and the Caribbean. The first activities of the Punta Cana Group were the elaboration of a document, the Declaration of Punta Cana, related to organ donation and to make a study on the reality of each country in terms of funding and legal and organizational aspects of transplantation.

[2] Eurotransplant members: Stichting Eurotransplant International Foundation (ETI); L'Agence de la Biomedécine (ABM)—France; European Society for Organ Transplantation (ESOT); Centro Nazionale Trapianti (ISS-CNT)—Italy; NHS Blood and Transplant (NHSBT)—UK; Organización Nacional de Transplantes (ONT)—Spain; Scandiatransplant (SKT).

Eurotransplant also promotes the promulgation of uniform guidelines, common definitions of terms, and methodologies to evaluate the results of transplantation.

While there is no supranational organization in Latin America that organizes organ donation, the 'Proyecto Siembra' (Grupo Punta Cana) provides a framework for Caribbean and Latin American countries to seek assistance with the establishment of national OPOs. Examples of national OPOs that started to work in Latin America using the Spanish ONT as a model were the National Council of Transplantation (CNT) and the National Institute of Transplant Coordination (INCORT) in the Dominican Republic (Morales, 2001). Argentina, Uruguay, and many other Latin American countries now also have OPOs with well-established bylaws and regulations.

During the planning phase on an institutional (hospital) level, early identification and involvement of essential medical staff across allied specialties and auxiliary staff (i.e. ultrasound, blood bank, radiology, pharmacy, and laboratory technicians) is critical. Consensus should be established on the required perioperative equipment and technologies for each transplant procedure. Equipment needs may range from minimal (i.e. kidney transplantation) to extensive (liver and thoracic transplantation) and decisions should be based on the best evidence available and cost-effectiveness for each centre (Fleisher et al., 1998; Schumann, 2003; Craig et al., 2008; Rando et al., 2011).

Twenty-four-hour availability of critical services such as blood bank, laboratory, radiology, and anaesthesiology and immediate access to the operating room are prerequisites for any type of major surgery but in particular for transplantation surgery. Similarly, reliable transportation systems for patients and organs are needed to minimize cold ischaemic time, as delays may adversely affect graft quality and graft and patient outcomes (Rauchfuss et al., 2011).

## Multidisciplinary teams

A multidisciplinary team approach is essential to provide excellent perioperative care and achieve good patient outcome. The identification of a dedicated anaesthesiology team (especially for lung, heart, and liver transplantation) is desirable. A study demonstrated that a designated anaesthesia team significantly reduces blood transfusion requirements, the need for mechanical ventilation, and intensive care length of stay (Hevesi et al., 2009). Similar benefits were observed when specialized transplant nurses were integrated into the multidisciplinary team (Russell and Van Gelder, 2008).

Intense patient and family education is also essential in order to guarantee good patient outcomes. Realistic patient expectations and the need for 100% compliance with immunosuppressive drug regimens and the importance of follow-up visits are critical to avoid postoperative complications such as episodes of rejections (Franco et al., 1996; Korus, Stinson et al., 2011).

## Use of standardized protocols and quality control

Standardized protocols should be implemented for the entire transplant pathway, ranging from management of patients on the transplant waiting list to long-term follow-up after transplantation. During the perioperative phase, protocols based on multidisciplinary consensus should be developed for preoperative evaluation and preparation for surgery as well as intraoperative and postoperative management. Standardized protocols serve multiple purposes: they facilitate patient throughput by identifying decision points, reduce risk by guiding less-experienced practitioners and providing clear instruction at decision points, and reduce the risk and cost of unnecessary procedures.

Standardized protocols should also include provisions for monitoring (Jarrett, 2009) quality of the services, safety, efficacy, and cost-effectiveness of the transplant programme (Devitt et al., 2008).

Quality and process indicators must be well defined and established prior to starting a programme. Review of nationally or regionally accepted outcomes should be used as initial guidelines. For example, post-transplant mortality is common to all types of transplants (Taioli et al., 2005). Other universally accepted quality or process indicators include time on the waiting list, wait-list mortality, improvement of quality of life (Neipp et al., 2006; Laba et al., 2008; Griva et al., 2011; Smith, Trauer et al., 2011), rate of complications, and frequency of retransplantation. Indicators may be more specific and need to be defined within the context of the transplant surgery. These may include transfusion requirements, frequency of early extubation, length of stay in the ICU, and incidence of postoperative infections (Sabate et al. 1996).

## Medical competency

Assuring medical competency of all participating healthcare providers is part of quality control and ideally a standardized accreditation process should be implemented. Accreditation is the process by which a programme or an individual healthcare provider is credentialed by a regulatory body or institution to participate in certain aspects of patient care. This process may vary between institutions and certainly between countries. The accreditation process should be uniform and needs to consider local factors. Minimum requirements need to be established and clearly communicated to all stakeholders.

In the US new transplant programmes are not fully certified by the Centers for Medicare & Medicaid Services (CMS) for at least 2 years (Benjey et al., 2007). Specialized fellowship training is now common for surgeons and some of the transplant-related medical specialties in the US. However, transplant fellowships for anaesthesiology and critical care medicine have not been well defined and are rarely required. Most recently, the American Board of Anesthesiologists (ASA) and UNOS have promulgated minimum credentialing criteria for the position of Director of Liver Transplant Anesthesiology.

In Europe the Division of Transplantation was formed in 2007 as part of the Section of Surgery of the Union Européenne des Médecins Spécialistes (UEMS) and the European Board of Surgery (EBS). The Division operates in close collaboration with European Society for Organ Transplantation (ESOT) and its main objective is to guarantee the best standard of care in organ transplantation in Europe by ensuring that training in transplantation surgery is maintained at the highest level. Certification can be obtained for the following (separate) areas: multi-organ retrieval, kidney transplantation, pancreas transplantation, and liver transplantation (Casanova, 2009). The Joint Accreditation Committee of the International Society for Cellular Therapy (ISCT) and the

European Group for Blood and Marrow Transplantation (EBMT) launched its first official inspection programme in January 2004. Most centres require at least 18 months to prepare for accreditation and 85% employed a quality manager and/or data manager on an ongoing basis (Samson et al., 2007).

Most Latin American and African programmes currently do not have specific certification requirements; however, even non-medical certification agencies can be useful in establishing standards of quality control. The International Organization for Standardization (ISO) (<http://www.iso.org/>), for example, has developed standards that define quality management and control systems for any kind of organizational structure (ISO 9001), and these standards can be adapted to certify transplant programmes. In Uruguay a new programme that started in 2009 has obtained International ISO 9001 certification for its Liver Center (Rando et al., 2010).

Moreover, to assure quality of care and patient outcomes, transparency and high ethical standards are a prerequisite. For new programmes in particular, all decisions related to organ donation and patient care should be based on consensus and involve all stakeholders. Initially, decisions have to consider not only patient factors such as severity of disease but also programme experience and institutional resources. It is not advisable to transplant a medically very challenging patient that will strain resources and may pose challenges that are beyond the expertise of a newly started transplant programme. Once experience is acquired and a higher point on the learning curve has been achieved, these criteria can be gradually relaxed and more complex patients considered for transplantation.

## Training and mentorship

Training and mentorship by experts in well-established programmes is key to the success of new transplant programmes (Sabate et al., 1996; Cohen et al., 2007; Michinov et al., 2008). A strong relationship and good communication (in person, by telephone, or email) with personnel from experienced programmes will help to overcome initial obstacles and may accelerate learning curves in new programmes (Broumand, 2005; Walia and Schumann, 2008; Peele et al., 2011). Overall, there is no consensus regarding adequate training or mentorship for anaesthesiologists participating in transplantation. A thorough understanding of the pathophysiology of end-stage organ disease as well as previous participation in complex surgical procedures is highly desirable. On an individual level, the benefits of mentorship for the mentee are well established; however, the advantages for the mentor are generally underreported in the medical literature. Frequently, mentors are very self-motivated and derive satisfaction from developing junior colleagues to enable them to improve the quality of programmes in their institutions (Cohen et al., 2007). Institutional or individual collaboration may foster research productivity and improve accountability by providing formalized progress reports with individualized feedback (Cohen et al., 2012).

Further, participation in national and international educational conferences is essential to enhance learning and exchange experiences. The first step in Latin America towards international cooperation was the creation of the Punta Cana Group in 2001 (Duro, 2001).

Training is essential for the achievement of good outcomes among anaesthesia staff (Wojcicki et al., 2003; Broumand, 2005; Rando et al., 2010; Rando et al., 2011); intraoperative management affects blood product utilization (Massicotte et al., 2005a, 2006), postoperative outcomes (Massicotte et al., 2005b), and resource utilization such as duration of ventilation and ICU and hospital stays. Therefore specialized training of anaesthesiologists could be considered as one of the most cost-effective actions that can be taken in liver transplantation (Rando et al., 2011) and possibly in all other transplants (Hevesi et al., 2009; Rando et al., 2010).

## Data management

Several studies have demonstrated that the use of information systems is conducive to more complete and accurate documentation of data by healthcare professionals (Simini et al., 2001; Mehrabi et al., 2008). Assuring high-quality data collection is particularly important in patient care but also provides important information for secondary purposes, such as quality assurance and health policy planning, evaluation, and research.

The complexity of clinical information collected on transplant patients makes paper records less useful and reliable. When establishing a new transplant programme, reliance on established data acquisition systems facilitates the evaluation of the programme (Hayrinen et al., 2008) and the systematic collection of health data using a comprehensive electronic health record (EHR) facilitates data access, from individual files compiled in single departments to the longitudinal collection of complex patient data across specialties. The Latter-day Saints Hospital in Salt Lake City, for example, developed a perioperative information system for transplant patients that includes forms to enter external laboratory results and transplant-related information. This system improved data availability and data flow processes following liver transplantation, with capability to easily transfer data to outside institutions (Staes et al., 2007).

A member of the transplant team trained in data management will ensure data integrity and completeness. The multitude of different EHRs and their interoperability, as well as varying requirements for different practitioners and semantic and terminology differences, however, frequently impede the implementation of national health record projects (Hayrinen et al., 2008).

## Patient-centred outcomes

With improvements in surgical technique and immunosuppressant therapy, survival after solid organ transplantation has increased dramatically. Survival can no longer be the sole outcome parameter measured after transplantation, and other sensitive measures should be included such as objective functional outcomes and subjective Quality of life (QOL) and health-related quality of life (HRQOL). A meta-analysis of patients with ESLD found an improvement of 32% in the Karnofsky score[3] (measuring general performance), an 11% improvement in the Sickness Impact Profile[4] score (Bergner et al., 1981), and a 20–50% increase in domains of the Nottingham Health

[3] The Karnofsky score runs from 100 to 0, where 100 is 'perfect' health and 0 is death. This scoring system is named after Dr David A. Karnofsky, who described the scale with Dr Joseph H. Burchenal in 1949.

[4] M. Bergner, R.A. Bobbitt, W.B. Carter, and B.S. Gilson developed this instrument, a 136-item behaviourally based, health status questionnaire. Every-day activities in 12 categories (sleep and rest, emotional behaviour, body care and movement, home management, mobility, social interaction, ambulation, alertness behaviour, communication, work, recreation and pastimes, and eating) are measured.

**Table 41.2** The cost of haemodialysis, peritoneal dialysis, and kidney transplantation in different countries (the latter includes the cost of surgery and immunosuppressant treatment in the first year) (Data from Punta Cana web site: www.grupopuntacana.org/ (http://www.grupopuntacana.org/2012)).

| Country | ANNUAL COST OF HAEMODIALYSIS | ANNUAL COST OF PERITONEAL DIALYSIS | ANNUAL COST OF KIDNEY TRANSPLANTATION |
|---|---|---|---|
| Chile (Pecoits-Filho et al., 2009) | US $20,810 | US $20,750 | US $106,000 |
| Sudan (Elsharif et al., 2010) | US $684,700 | — | US $148,2504 |
| Canada (Arredondo et al., 1998) | US $9,631.60 | US $5,643.07 | US $3,021.63 |
| Spain (Villa et al., 2011) | 8.929 Euros | 7.429 Euros | 5.487 Euros |

Profile (assessing the individual perception of health)[5] after liver transplantation. There were further significant improvements of post-transplantation physical health, sexual function, daily activities, and social functioning (but surprisingly not psychological health). The general HRQOL of the 3,576 patients studied was impaired pre-transplantation and significantly improved post-transplantation. Transplant recipients reported large gains in those areas of HRQOL that affected physical health and smaller improvements in areas affected by psychological functioning (Bravata et al., 1999). Other studies further confirmed long-lasting improvement of QOL. At 10–20 years after liver transplantation the QOL of transplant recipients was comparable to the general population (Aberg et al., 2011; Duffy et al., 2011). Pinson et al. (2000) studied QOL in 371 patients that underwent solid organ transplantation (100 livers, 94 hearts, 112 kidneys, and 65 lungs) and found that different types of transplant patients have different HRQOL before transplantation and performance improvements after surgery (Pinson et al., 2000).

Improvements in QOL after kidney transplantation are so impressive that some have suggested pre-emptive kidney transplant (PKT) as a new initiative ('Transplant First'), with the aim of transplanting patients prior to dialysis. PKT significantly improves long-term graft and recipient survival but also QOL, particularly for adolescents. Essential for this initiative is education to increase the rate of living donation and life-long availability of immunosuppression (Davis, 2011).

Elderly patients undergoing heart transplantation frequently suffer depression after surgery, so psychological support is mandatory (Ruzyczka et al., 2011). After liver transplantation depression can significantly reduce the ability to return to work and increase unemployment after transplantation (Gorevski et al., 2011).

[5] The Nottingham Health Profile is a generic QOL survey used to measure subjective physical, emotional, and social aspects of health.

## Financial implications and benefits

Transplantation is a highly effective but often extremely costly treatment option. For publicly funded health systems in countries with low to medium average incomes, transplant programmes must be well justified to obtain governmental support (Rando et al., 2011). However, with economic growth and improving results, more low- and medium-income countries will be reconsidering transplantation.

The cost of transplantation is not only limited to the procedure itself; lifelong requirement for immunosuppression poses an additional substantial financial burden on society and the patient. India has attempted to minimize these costs by developing a pharmaceutical industry that supplies the country with generic immunosuppressant drugs (tacrolimus and mycophenolate mofetil) for a fractional cost of the price in the developed world (Saigal and Shah, 2012). Bioequivalence and bioavailability studies are essential if generic drugs are to be used.

The costs of dialysis and kidney transplantation in different countries vary widely (Table 41.2). Frequently the cost of one year of dialysis is higher than the cost of medical care for the first year after kidney transplantation. Therefore kidney transplantation often does not only result in better quality of life but also makes economic sense (Neipp, Karavul et al., 2006, Davis, 2011).

## Conclusion

Setting up a new transplant programme is complicated by medical, organizational, and logistical challenges. The process involves many different stakeholders and participants as well as major social, political, ethical, and economic considerations. Multidisciplinary teamwork is essential for the successful planning and implementation of the legal national framework, the establishment of quality organ donation and procurement programmes, and the development of transplant education and training and continuing medical education programmes. In addition, team-training, informatics, evaluation and research, continuing quality assurance, and resource optimization are essential for long-term sustainability.

## References


Aberg F, Isoniemi H, Hockerstedt K (2011) Long-term results of liver transplantation. *Scand J Surg*, **100**(1):14–21.

Arredondo A, Ricardo R, Icaza E (1998) Cost-effectiveness of interventions for end-stage renal disease. *Rev Saúde Pública*, **32**(6):556–565.

Benjey J, Cunanan M, Thomson A (2007) Regulatory compliance in solid-organ transplantation: what you don't know can hurt your program. *Prog Transplant*, **17**(2):129–135.

Bergner M, Bobbitt RA, Carter WB, Gilson BS (1981) The Sickness Impact Profile: development and final revision of a health status measure. *Med Care*, **19**(8):787–805.

Bravata DM, Olkin I, Barnato AE, Keeffe EB, Owens DK (1999) Health-related quality of life after liver transplantation: a meta-analysis. *Liver Transpl Surg*, **5**(4):318–331.

Broumand B (2005) Transplantation activities in Iran. *Exp Clin Transplant*, **3**(1):333–337.

Caplan A (2011) The use of prisoners as sources of organs—an ethically dubious practice. *Am J Bioeth*, **11**(10):1–5.

Casanova D (2009) Surgical accreditation in liver transplantation. *Transplant Proc*, **41**(3):998–1000.

Cohen JG, Sherman AE, Kiet T, et al. (2012) Characteristics of success in mentoring and research productivity—a case-control study of academic centers. *Gynecol Oncol*, **125**(1):8–13.

Cohen MS, Jacobs JP, Quintessenza JA, et al. (2007) Mentorship, learning curves, and balance. *Cardiol Young*, **17**(Suppl 2):164–174.

Craig J, Aguiar-Ibanez R, Bhattacharya S, et al. (2008) *The Clinical and Cost Effectiveness of Thromboelastography/Thromboelastometry*. NHS Quality Improvement Scotland 2007; Health Technology Assessment, Issue Report 11. <http//www.nhshealthquality.org>.

Cronin AJ (2011) Is it unethical for doctors to encourage healthy adults to donate a kidney to a stranger? No. *BMJ*, **343**:d7140.

Davis CL (2011) Preemptive transplantation and the transplant first initiative. *Curr Opin Nephrol Hypertens*, **19**(6):592–597.

Depine S (2009) The role of government and competing priorities in minority populations and developing nations. *Ethn Dis*, **19**(Suppl 1):S73–S79.

Devitt J, Cass A, Cunningham J, Preece C, Anderson K, Snelling P (2008) Study Protocol—Improving Access to Kidney Transplants (IMPAKT): a detailed account of a qualitative study investigating barriers to transplant for Australian indigenous people with end-stage kidney disease. *BMC Health Serv Res*, **8**:31.

Duffy JP, Kao K, Ko CY (2011) Long-term patient outcome and quality of life after liver transplantation: analysis of 20-year survivors. *Ann Surg*, **252**(4):652–661.

Duro V (2001) The 'Punta Cana' Group. A proposal in Latin America. *Nefrologia*, **21**(Suppl 4):141–143.

Elsharif ME, Elsharif EG, Gadour WH (2010) Costs of hemodialysis and kidney transplantation in Sudan: a single center experience. *Iran J Kidney Dis*, **4**(4):282–284.

Fleisher LA, Metzger SE, Lam J, Harris A (1998) Perioperative cost-finding analysis of the routine use of intraoperative forced-air warming during general anesthesia. *Anesthesiology*, **88**(5):1357–1364.

Franco T, Warren JJ, Menke KL, et al. (1996) Developing patient and family education programs for a transplant center. *Patient Educ Couns*, **27**(1):113–120.

Gasper WJ, Sweet MP, Hoopes C, et al. (2008) Antireflux surgery for patients with end-stage lung disease before and after lung transplantation. *Surg Endosc*, **22**(2):495–500.

Glannon W (2011) Is it unethical for doctors to encourage healthy adults to donate a kidney to a stranger? Yes. *BMJ* **343**:d7179.

Gorevski E, Succop P, Sachdeva J, et al. (2011) Factors influencing post-transplantation employment: does depression have an impact? *Transplant Proc*, **43**(10):3835–3839.

Grattagliano I, Ubaldi E, Bonfrate L, Portincasa P (2011) Management of liver cirrhosis between primary care and specialists. *World J Gastroenterol*, **17**(18):2273–2282.

Griva K, Stygall J, Ng JH, Davenport A, Harrison MJ, Newman S (2011) Prospective changes in health-related quality of life and emotional outcomes in kidney transplantation over 6 years. *J Transplant*, **2011**:671571.

Grupo Punta Cana (2012) Actividad de trasplante en Latinoamérica y el Caribe. <http://www.grupopuntacana.org/>.

Hayrinen K, Saranto K, Nykanen P (2008) Definition, structure, content, use and impacts of electronic health records: a review of the research literature. *Int J Med Inform*, **77**(5):291–304.

Hevesi ZG, Lopukhin SY, Mezrich JD, Andrei AC, Lee M (2009) Designated liver transplant anesthesia team reduces blood transfusion, need for mechanical ventilation, and duration of intensive care. *Liver Transpl*, **15**(5):460–465.

Hofmann BM (2011) Commercialization of organs. *Tidsskr Nor Laegeforen*, **131**(22):2230–2231.

Jafferbhoy H, Gashau W, Dillon J (2011) Cost effectiveness and quality of life considerations in the treatment of hepatitis C infection. *Clinicoecon Outcome Res*, **2**:87–96.

Jarrett M (2009) Use of clinical practice guidelines to promote best practice when managing clinical interventions for liver transplant candidates. *Prog Transplant*, **19**(2):132–140; quiz 141.

Kapoor A, Kwan KG, Whelan JP (2011) Commercial renal transplantation: A risky venture? A single Canadian centre experience. *Can Urol Assoc J*, **5**(5):335–340.

Korus M, Stinson JN, Pool R, Williams A, Kagan S (2011) Exploring the information needs of adolescents and their parents throughout the kidney transplant continuum. *Prog Transplant*, **21**(1):53–60.

Laba M, Pszenny A, Gutowska D, et al. (2008) Quality of life after liver transplantation—preliminary report. *Ann Transplant*, **13**(4):67–71.

Lampela H, Ritvanen A, Kosola S, et al. (2011) National centralization of biliary atresia care to an assigned multidisciplinary team provides high-quality outcomes. *Scand J Gastroenterol*, **47**(1):99–107.

Massicotte L, Lenis S, Thibeault L, Sassine MP, Seal RF, Roy A (2005a) Reduction of blood product transfusions during liver transplantation. *Can J Anaesth*, **52**(5):545–546.

Massicotte L, Sassine MP, Lenis S, Seal RF, Roy A (2005b) Survival rate changes with transfusion of blood products during liver transplantation. *Can J Anaesth*, **52**(2):148–155.

Massicotte L, Lenis S, Thibeault L, Sassine MP, Seal RF, Roy A (2006) Effect of low central venous pressure and phlebotomy on blood product transfusion requirements during liver transplantations. *Liver Transpl*, **12**(1):117–123.

McGill RL, Ko TY (2011) Transplantation and the primary care physician. *Adv Chronic Kidney Dis*, **18**(6):433–438.

Medlin CA, Chowdhury M, Jamison DT, Measham A (2006) Improving the health of populations: lessons of experience. In: Jamison DT, Breman JG, Measham AR (eds) *Disease Control Priorities in Developing Countries*, Chapter 8. World Bank, Washington, DC.

Mehrabi A, Fonouni H, Muller SA, Schmidt J (2008) Current concepts in transplant surgery: liver transplantation today. *Langenbeck Arch Surg*, **393**(3):245–260.

Michinov E, Olivier-Chiron E, Rusch E, Chiron B (2008) Influence of transactive memory on perceived performance, job satisfaction and identification in anaesthesia teams. *Br J Anaesth*, **100**(3):327–332.

Morales F (2001) Influencia del modelo Español en República Dominicana. *Nefrología*, **20**(4):144–147.

Neipp M, Karavul B, Jackobs S (2006) Quality of life in adult transplant recipients more than 15 years after kidney transplantation. *Transplantation*, **81**(12):1640–1644.

Pavlakis M, Hanto DW (2011) Clinical pathways in transplantation: a review and examples from Beth Israel Deaconess Medical Center. *Clin Transplant*, **26**(3):382–386.

Pecoits-Filho R, Campos C, Cerdas-Calderon M, et al. (2009) Policies and health care financing issues for dialysis in Latin America: extracts from the roundtable discussion on the economics of dialysis and chronic kidney disease. *Perit Dial Int*, **29**(Suppl 2):S222–S226.

Peele AS, Goldberg S, Trompeta JA (2011) Collaborative use of the peer assist model in large transplant programs in the United States. *Prog Transplant*, **21**(2):124–130.

Pinson CW, Feurer ID, Payne JL, Wise PE, Shockley S, Speroff T (2000) Health-related quality of life after different types of solid organ transplantation. *Ann Surg*, **232**(4):597–607.

Rando K, Harguindeguy M, Leites A, et al. (2010) Quality standards in liver surgery: influence of multidiscilpinary team work and patient centralization. *Acta Gastroenterol Latinoam*, **40**(1):10–21.

Rando K, Niemann CU, Taura P, Klinck J (2011) Optimizing cost-effectiveness in perioperative care for liver transplantation: a model for low- to medium-income countries. *Liver Transpl*, **17**(11):1247–1278.

Rauchfuss F, Breuer M, Dittmar Y, et al. (2011) Implantation of the liver during reperfusion of the heart in combined heart–liver transplantation: own experience and review of the literature. *Transplant Proc*, **43**(7):2707–2713.

Rios A, Conesa C, Ramirez P, et al. (2006) Attitudes of resident doctors toward different types of organ donation in a Spanish transplant hospital. *Transplant Proc*, **38**(3):869–874.

Russell CL, Van Gelder F (2008) An international perspective: job satisfaction among transplant nurses. *Prog Transplant*, **18**(1):32–40.

Ruzyczka EW, Milaniak I, Przybylowski P, et al. (2011) Depression and quality of life in terms of personal resources in heart transplant recipients. *Transplant Proc*, **43**(8):3076–3081.

Sabate A, Sanzol R, Sopena R (1996) Quality in anesthetic management during hepatic transplant. Hepatic Transplant Anesthesia Group. *Rev Esp Anestesiol Reanim*, **43**(10):354–359.

Saigal S, Shah SR (2012) Liver transplantation—economics in the less developed world. *Indian J Gastroenterol*, **31**(1):13–14.

Samson D, Slaper-Cortenbach I, Pamphilon D, et al. (2007) Current status of JACIE accreditation in Europe: a special report from the Joint Accreditation Committee of the ISCT and the EBMT (JACIE). *Bone Marrow Transplant*, **39**(3):133–141.

Schumann R (2003) Intraoperative resource utilization in anesthesia for liver transplantation in the United States: a survey. *Anesth Analg*, **97**(1):21–28, table of contents.

Simini F, Fernandez A, Sosa C, Diaz Rossello JL (2001) Perinatal information system. Incorporation latency and impact on perinatal clinical registry. *Ginecol Obstet Mex*, **69**:386–389.

Smith GC, Trauer T, Kerr PG, Chadban SJ (2011) Prospective quality-of-life monitoring of simultaneous pancreas and kidney transplant recipients using the 36-item short form health survey. *Am J Kidney Dis*, **55**(4):698–707.

Staes CJ, Evans RS, Narus SP, Huff SM, Sorensen JB (2007) System analysis and improvement in the process of transplant patient care. *Stud Health Technol Inform*, **129**(Pt 2):915–919.

Taioli E, Venettoni S, Pretagostini R, et al. (2005) Quality evaluation of solid organ transplant in Italy for the period 2000 to 2002 data from the national transplant center. *Transplant Proc*, **37**(10):4163–4169.

Trainor D, Borthwick E, Ferguson A (2011) Perioperative management of the hemodialysis patient. *Semin Dial*, **24**(3):314–326.

Villa G, Rodríguez-Carmona A, Fernández-Ortiz L, et al. (2011) Cost analysis of the Spanish renal replacement therapy programme. *Nephrol Dial Transplant*, **26**(11):3709–3714.

Walia A, Schumann R (2008) The evolution of liver transplantation practices. *Curr Opin Organ Transplant*, **13**(3):275–279.

Wojcicki M, Lubikowski J, Czuprynska M, et al. (2003) Early results of a new liver transplant program in Szczecin, Poland. *Ann Transplant*, **8**(4):50–56.

# CHAPTER 42

# Quality improvement and data analysis in transplantation

Ryutaro Hirose and Justin Parekh

## Introduction

In the demanding and highly competitive environment of organ transplantation it is critical to determine and confirm that transplant centres are providing adequate, high-quality care to potential and actual transplant recipients and donors. In the US multiple efforts by interested parties have resulted in mandatory data collection, administrative databases, incentives, and regulations regarding performance. The systems in the US will be discussed as an example of the evolution of data analysis and quality improvement in transplantation.

## The regulatory environment of transplantation

In an effort to assure quality and to monitor the activity of transplant centres, the US Department of Health and Human Services has established regulations concerning the survey and certification of transplant programmes. The CMS has been given the authority and responsibility for monitoring the transplant centres' compliance with the Conditions of Participation. CMS conducts site visits to help determine compliance. Based on findings from on-site surveys and other documentation, CMS certifies transplant centres and covers solid organ transplants. CMS certification remains a critical element of maintaining viable transplant centres, as not only reimbursement from CMS depends on CMS certification, but also other third-party payers are sensitive to the certification status of a transplant centre. CMS, third-party payers, patients, and the general public's interests are served by assuring that all transplant centres meet standards and have acceptable outcomes.

## Mandated data submission

The US Congress by enacting the NOTA in 1984 established the OPTN. NOTA established that a unified transplant network should be operated by a private non-profit organization under federal contract. In 1986 UNOS was awarded the OPTN contract and has maintained it since then. In addition, the HRSA Division of Transplantation contracts the SRTR, currently held by the Minneapolis Medical Research Foundation. The SRTR provides statistical analysis and evaluates scientific and clinical data pertaining to solid organ transplantation.

Each US transplant centre is subject to Conditions of Participation from CMS, as well as the policies, procedures, and regulations established by UNOS to remain a member in good standing. UNOS collects, analyses, and publishes data with the assistance of the SRTR in an effort to characterize the status of solid organ transplantation in the US.

The source of data concerning wait-listed patients and transplanted patients is partially derived from mandatory data forms submitted by the transplant centres to UNOS. In order to place a patient on a transplant waiting list, UNOS requires that a transplant centre submit extensive data as captured by electronic forms that are submitted online. Transplant programmes are mandated to report data that encompasses patients on the waiting list, the conditions around the time of transplant, and both graft and recipient outcomes after transplant. Transplant programmes are also required to follow-up on living donors. Data are submitted via standard forms through Unet, the electronic transplant information application. These standard forms are largely conserved across different organs and consist of the Transplant Candidate Registration Form (TCR), the Transplant Recipient Registration Form (TRR), and the Transplant Recipient Follow-up Form (TRF).

Detailed information on potential recipient characteristics, the number of potential recipients on the wait-list, the number of potential recipients entering and exiting the wait-list, and the reasons why patients were removed from the wait-list are data elements that are mandated to be collected and submitted. Most importantly there is emphasis on the rate of transplantation, time to transplantation, and the death rate while on the wait-list. Based on the demographic and medical characteristics of the patients on a transplant centre's wait-list, an expected wait-list mortality is calculated and compared with the observed wait-list mortality.

For patients undergoing transplant, greater detail about the transplant itself is also reported to the SRTR. The data include recipient and donor characteristics, cold ischaemia time, HLA mismatch, and need for dialysis within the first week of transplant for kidney transplants. Details regarding post-transplant malignancy and other outcomes are reported on specific data forms. Finally, each programme is expected to report both short- and long-term patient and graft survival as long as the organ recipient is alive. Each programme is required to submit an updated data form on the anniversary of recipients' transplant for the remainder of their lives.

There are obvious advantages of collecting as much and as granular a dataset to examine outcomes, predictive variables, and modifiable practices in order to improve quality in transplantation. However, the collection of such data comes at a cost.

The burden of data submission on transplant centres is a significant one, and the AST and ASTS have expressed concerns to the OPTN about the increasing burden of adding data fields and the existing unfunded mandates of data submission. While all transplant professionals recognize the necessity of monitoring outcomes, the societies have argued that many of the data elements and variables currently being collected have not been scientifically proven to affect overall outcomes. In an open letter to UNOS, the AST and ASTS argued that new data elements should only be approved if the data elements were necessary to (1) develop policy and regulations to allocate organs for transplant, (2) determine if transplant centres were complying with OPTN policy, (3) determine programme-specific compliance, or (4) assure patient safety where no alternative data exist (Merion and Madsen, 2010). The controversy regarding the set of data that should be required of all transplant centres to submit to the national database registry continues. The debate is not a transplant specific one, as it is recognized by others that in the current environment of increasing requirements for reporting metrics of quality and performance, particularly those that result in differential reimbursement (pay-for-performance), the burden of data collection is significant and is increasing. One advantage of scientific analysis of risk factors and relevant variables is the potential elimination of redundant or irrelevant factors, the intelligent and rational prioritization of data collection for the purposes of measuring quality, and adequate and desirable risk adjustment.

## Data analysis and results of specific transplant programmes

With mandatory data reporting and close evaluation of recipient outcomes, UNOS and CMS have moved to objective measures in order to evaluate an individual centre's performance. The SRTR publishes programme reports on a biannual basis that summarize data regarding transplant centre characteristics and outcomes. The Program-Specific Reports (PSRs) are programme reports that are generated at regular intervals by the SRTR to aid in evaluating the performance of an individual programme. Acknowledging that each centre is faced with a unique population, transplant centres are currently evaluated based on the ratio of their observed to expected events, or O:E ratios. These events include the incidence of death and transplantation for potential recipients on the wait-list and recipient and graft survival.

To give a specific example, a given renal transplant centre will be assigned an O:E ratio for 1-year patient survival after renal transplant. The observed number of events is simply the incidence of deaths during the study period. The expected number of deaths is derived from a national database composed of data from all US transplant centres. These data are used to identify risk factors for death after transplantation. Recent risk adjustment models for kidney transplantation include 22 risk factors that include donor (age, race, cause of death, diabetes status, serum creatinine), recipient (age, race, gender, HCV status, diabetes status, cause of renal disease, body mass index, peak panel reactive antibody), and transplant factors (cold ischaemia time, HLA mismatch). The risk adjustment models are then employed to calculate an expected number of deaths for an individual transplant centre given their population's characteristics. The final O:E ratio is then calculated.

Designed with the goal of ensuring performance within a specified set of standards, these reports evaluate each programme based on the ratio of observed to expected events for a number of adverse events and monitor 3-month-, 1-year, and 3-year patient and graft survival. The observed outcomes are then characterized as being significantly poorer, significantly better, or not significantly different from the expected outcomes. The PSRs have been used to help CMS and the OPTN Membership and Professional Standards Committee (MPSC) identify programmes that are in need of review. Therefore one use of the PSRs has been to identify programmes that vary from expected performance in regards to the care of wait-listed patients and organ recipients.

Should a programme perform below expectations the CMS has the power to investigate and even suspend a transplant programme. Currently a centre that meets any of the following three criteria is subject to review:

- Outcome failures that exceed predetermined thresholds (currently O:E ratio >1.5)
- Total number of excess deaths > 3
- Discrepancy between observed and expected outcomes, which is statistically significant ($P$ value < 0.05) for more than two consecutive reporting periods

This level of regulation demands that transplant centres must perform a constant, data-driven evaluation of their performance and adverse events.

## CMS conditions of participation and QAPI requirements

In order to comply with CMS standards and to be certified as a transplant centre the conditions of participation require that transplant centres develop and maintain a data-driven QAPI programme that includes all transplant services. Each QAPI programme must constitute a dynamic process designed to identify adverse events and their root causes and evaluate methods to reduce adverse events in the future. The standard components of such a programme include:

- Objective measurement of the transplant centre's performance, including but not limited to donor management, accuracy of donor and recipient matching, selection criteria, rates of death and transplantation of patients on the waiting list, and recipient outcomes
- A process to identify and report adverse outcomes
- Systems to analyse adverse events and prevent future events

A major component of CMS surveys of transplant centres includes an assessment of the QAPI process that is in place at the transplant centre and documentation of the QAPI programme activities.

## Quality improvement in transplantation

In the US the National Veterans Administration Surgical Risk Study (NVASRS) was started within the Veterans Administration (VA) system to attempt to prospectively collect outcome data and to provide a risk-adjusted analysis of hospital performance.

Based on these data, the National Surgical Quality Improvement Program (NSQIP) was developed at the VA and in hospitals in the private sector. This effort was continued in the ACS and has provided benchmarks to participating hospitals to aid in quality improvement (Ingraham et al., 2010). The outcomes are documented by Surgical Clinical Reviewers and require a commitment of resources by the participating hospitals. Depending on the specific procedure under study and the volume at a specific hospital, a sample of the cases of appropriate size is analysed and a risk-adjusted expected rate of events is calculated. The O:E ratio and confidence intervals are reported. If the O:E ratio and confidence intervals are exclusive of 1.0, the ratio is considered an outlier. The NSQIP allows comparisons between a participating hospital and other hospitals in a blinded, risk-adjusted manner. Of 118 participating hospitals in the initial stages of NSQIP, risk-adjusted mortality improved in 66% of these hospitals in a 2-year time period (Ingraham et al., 2010). Other subsequent studies have confirmed quality improvement in participating medical centres (Hall et al., 2009).

Some authors have called for an NSQIP-type surgical quality improvement programme for transplantation (Englesbe et al., 2006). As the ACS NSQIP diversifies and includes other procedure-specific measures, and as collaboration of the ACS with other professional surgical societies increases, the development of a NSQIP-type programme for transplantation seems realistic and desirable.

## Improving quality improvement

More recently, statistical process control techniques such as the Shewhart chart (Shewhart, 1931), the sequential probability ratio test (SPRT) (Spiegelhalter et al., 2003), and the cumulative summation (CUSUM) have been taken from industry and applied to transplant outcomes (Axelrod et al., 2006, 2009). Originally designed to detect deviation from production standards, CUSUMs provide a very sensitive, real-time way to identify changes in outcomes. In transplantation, CUSUMs were initially adapted to monitor binary outcomes that could be rapidly ascertained, such as the number of patients that convert from waiting-list status to undergoing transplant. More recently, risk-adjusted CUSUM charts that can analyse survival, using time as a continuous variable, and incorporate events as they occur have been used in transplantation. For example, the number of observed deaths can be updated on a daily basis and repeatedly compared to the expected number of deaths, thereby allowing individual centres to detect deviation from expected outcomes. This technique has been shown to detect changes in performance more rapidly than current data reporting. Such techniques can therefore be incorporated into QAPI programmes with the goal of monitoring and improving overall care within a centre in a near real-time fashion or, at the very least, within a shorter timespan to monitor for outlying signals and also effects of interventions.

## Beyond data analysis

The reporting of data is only an initial step in the process necessary to improve performance and must be followed by careful analysis of outcome data as well as identification of processes to improve. This analysis must then lead to the planning and implementation of strategies to improve outcomes. Ultimately, a system that monitors the effects of the implemented plans and allows for modifications in a circular and iterative process, such as the one described as plan, do, study, act (PDSA), is necessary to sustain success and the continued process of improvement (Speroff and O'Connor, 2004). As the medical field and specifically transplantation seeks to improve outcomes, there is increased interest in borrowing methods from industry.

Originally designed to improve manufacturing process, Six Sigma has been adapted throughout industry to identify and improve any outcome that does not meet expectations. The term comes from the concept that if a specification limit is set six standard deviations beyond the mean, very few negative outcomes will occur. Overall, Six Sigma follows two methodologies: DMAIC (define, measure, analyse, improve, control), intended to control existing processes, and DMADV (define, measure, analyse, design, verify). It then incorporates other process tools and statistical methods such as cost:benefit analysis, regression, and root cause analysis to identify and measure outcomes. Key to the implementation of the Six Sigma system is the assignment of various roles at different levels of expertise. While there continues to be debate about the utility of Six Sigma in healthcare and other service-oriented industries, there are already examples of its use in medicine (Feng and Manuel, 2008). One of the first examples of Six Sigma strategies in medicine is its use at the Commonwealth Health Corporation to improve efficiency within the Corporation's system, eventually claiming large financial benefits in its radiology department by increasing throughput while decreasing average costs per procedure.

## Patient satisfaction as a quality measure

Patient satisfaction has been surveyed, using various tools such as those developed by Press-Ganey and others, and has been used as a quality measure in surgery (Farber, 2010) and medicine. CMS has approved Hospital Consumer Assessment of Healthcare Providers and Systems (HCAHPS) as a quality measure and will adjust reimbursement accordingly. Patients and others will be able to compare hospitals in patient satisfaction outcomes. Most recently, the ACS-sponsored Consumer Assessment of Healthcare Providers and Systems (CAHPS) Surgical Care Survey (Hoy, 2010) was endorsed as a quality measure by the National Quality Forum (NQF) (ACS, 2012). The current version of the surgical survey assesses patients' perioperative surgical experience. Transplant professionals will need to examine such surveys closely and help design modifications to reflect the differences and unique characteristics of the practice of transplantation medicine in the current environment so that the surveys accurately reflect quality in the delivery of healthcare in transplantation.

## Conclusion

Solid organ transplantation represents a zenith in the success of modern medicine and technology. Biomedical and technological advances have improved outcomes of solid organ transplantation to extraordinary levels. All transplant clinicians, no matter what the environment, are conscious of cost containment and cost-effectiveness. However, in transplantation, clinicians are also acutely aware that providing one patient with a transplant, e.g. a deceased donor organ, by definition will mean denying someone else a transplant because of the simple fact that the supply of organs does not meet the demand. Transplantation has in essence become a victim of its success. As success rates improve and as contraindications fade there has been an impressive rise in the number of potential candidates for solid organ transplant, without a concomitant rise in the number of donor organs, even with the expansion of the donor pool by reducing or eliminating historical contraindications to organ donation.

The expansion of living donation in many countries has ameliorated some of the need, but in all countries the supply is in general outstripped by the demand for transplants. As such, transplantation as a field has attempted to provide the best stewardship for the limited organs that are available for transplantation. This goal, by definition, mandates that we attempt to attain the most favourable post-transplant outcomes and maintain high quality, while at the same time serving those patients most in need of a transplant to maximize the utility and efficacy and overall benefit of transplantation and maximize the number of lives saved. In many transplant centres, multidisciplinary selection committees help determine which patients are appropriate candidates for transplantation and which patients are not. If there was a limitless source of organs, these decisions may not be as critical (inappropriate resource utilization notwithstanding) or as difficult. Therefore transplantation is a field that by definition involves rationing of healthcare, and always has been. If and when transplantation of artificial or bioengineered organs becomes a reality, then the resources may only be limited by financial and other access limitations, but, at present, transplant physicians ration transplantation in order to maximize utility of the precious resource of human organs.

As transplant centres take on riskier patients it behooves them to risk adjust as much as possible to report accurate reflection of the risk of the patient population. As much as low or no risk adjustment fosters risk-averse behaviour, more risk adjustment favours risk-taking behaviour. If sufficient risk adjustment results in exceedingly low expected rates of success, one may question whether this incentivizes and encourages a desired effect. Achieving the right balance between these competing forces and the degree to which risk adjustment should be performed are yet to be determined by society as well as the field of transplantation, where an absolute minimum rate of success may also be desired. In a field such as transplantation where the limited resource should be used in the most utilitarian and effective manner while balancing the sense of fairness, justice and equal access, it is a difficult task, but one that must involve the accurate collection, analysis, reporting, and use of robust outcome data.

## References

ACS (2012) *National Quality Forum Endorses Surgical Quality Alliance's Patient Focused Surgical Survey.* <http://www.facs.org/news/2012/surgical-survey0612.html>.

Axelrod DA, Guidinger MK, Metzger RA, Wiesner RH, Webb RL, Merion RM (2006) Transplant center quality assessment using a continuously updatable, risk-adjusted technique (CUSUM). *Am J Transplant*, **6**:313–323.

Axelrod DA, Kalbfleisch JD, Sun RJ, et al. (2009) Innovations in the assessment of transplant center performance: implications for quality improvement. *Am J Transplant*, **9**:959–969.

Englesbe MJ, Pelletier SJ, Kheterpal S, O'Reilly M, Campbell DA Jr (2006) A call for a national transplant surgical quality improvement program. *Am J Transplant*, **6**:666–670.

Farber J (2010) Measuring and improving ambulatory surgery patients' satisfaction. *AORN J*, **92**:313–321.

Feng Q, Manuel CM (2008) Under the knife: a national survey of six sigma programs in US healthcare organizations. *Int J Health Care Qual Assur*, **21**:535–547.

Hall BL, Hamilton BH, Richards K, Bilimoria KY, Cohen ME, Ko CY (2009) Does surgical quality improve in the American College of Surgeons National Surgical Quality Improvement Program: an evaluation of all participating hospitals. *Ann Surg*, **250**:363–376.

Hoy EW (2010) ACS-SQA surgical patient experience of care survey desgin project: a progress report. *Bull Am Coll Surg*, **94**:14–17.

Ingraham AM, Richards KE, Hall BL, Ko CY (2010) Quality improvement in surgery: the American College of Surgeons National Surgical Quality Improvement Program approach. *Adv Surg*, **44**:251–267.

Merion RM, Madsen JC (2010) *Public Comment Concerning Proposed Modifications to Data Elements on Tiedi Forms.* <http://asts.org/docs/default-source/optn-unos/proposal---modifications-to-data-elements---comments-to-optn-unos-april-15-2010.pdf?sfvrsn=6>.

Shewhart WA (1931) *Economic Control of Quality of Manufactured Product.* Van Nostrand, New York.

Speroff T, O'Connor GT (2004) Study designs for PDSA quality improvement research. *Qual Manag Health Care*, **13**:17–32.

Spiegelhalter D, Grigg O, Kinsman R, Treasure T (2003) Risk-adjusted sequential probability ratio tests: applications to Bristol, Shipman and adult cardiac surgery. *Int J Qual Health Care*, **15**:7–13.

## Further reading

SRTR: <http://www.srtr.org/ />.

UNOS: <http://www.unos.org/donation>.

# Index

## D

## M

## Q



## R